Using Medical Terminology

SECOND EDITION

Using Medical Terminology

SECOND EDITION

Judi L. Nath Ph.D.

Professor of Biology, Lourdes University, Sylvania, Ohio

Wolters Kluwer | Lippincott Williams & Wilkins
Health

Philadelphia • Baltimore • New York • London
Buenos Aires • Hong Kong • Sydney • Tokyo

Acquisitions Editor: David Troy
Senior Product Manager: Amy Millholen
Developmental Editor: Anne Reid
Design Coordinator: Doug Smock
Marketing Manager: Sarah Schuessler
Compositor: S4Carlisle Publishing Services
Printer: C&C Offset

351 West Camden Street
Baltimore, MD 21201

530 Walnut Street
Philadelphia, PA 19106

Printed in the People's Republic of China

DISCLAIMER
Care has been taken to confirm the accuracy of the information present and to describe generally accepted practices. However, the authors, editors, and publisher are not responsible for errors or omissions or for any consequences from application of the information in this book and make no warranty, expressed or implied, with respect to the currency, completeness, or accuracy of the contents of the publication. Application of this information in a particular situation remains the professional responsibility of the practitioner; the clinical treatments described and recommended may not be considered absolute and universal recommendations.

Library of Congress Cataloging-in-Publication Data

Nath, Judi Lindsley.
Using medical terminology / Judi L. Nath.—2nd ed.
p. ; cm.
Includes index.
ISBN 978-1-4511-1583-3 (pbk.)
I. Title.
[DNLM: 1. Terminology as Topic-Problems and Exercises. W 18.2]

610.1′4—dc23
2012026124

The publishers have made every effort to trace the copyright holders for borrowed material. If they have inadvertently overlooked any, they will be pleased to make the necessary arrangements at the first opportunity.

To purchase additional copies of this book, call our customer service department at **(800) 638-3030** or fax orders to **(301) 223-2320**. International customers should call **(301) 223-2300**.

Visit Lippincott Williams & Wilkins on the Internet:
http://www.lww.com. Lippincott Williams & Wilkins customer service representatives are available from 8:30 am to 5:00 pm, EST.

13

1 2 3 4 5 6 7 8 9 10

To my husband Mike—I could not have done it without you.

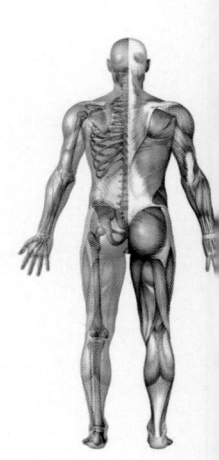

About the Author

*J*udi Nath, Ph.D., is a professor at Lourdes University, where she holds joint appointments in the Department of Biology & Health Science and the Nurse Anesthesia Program. Every semester, she teaches both undergraduate and graduate anatomy and physiology (A&P). Other courses she instructs include medical terminology and the occasional basic pharmacology class. She received her bachelor's and master's degrees from Bowling Green State University with majors in biology and German and her Ph.D. from the University of Toledo. As part of her undergraduate eduction, she also studied at the University of Salzburg in Austria. Dr. Nath is devoted to her students and strives to convey the intricacies of science in a captivating way that students find meaningful, interactive, and exciting. She is a multiple recipient of the Lourdes University Faculty Excellence Award, granted by the college to recognize her effective teaching, scholarship, and community service. Dr. Nath has also served as Biology Department Chair. She is active in many professional organizations, including the Human Anatomy & Physiology Society, where she has served several terms on the board of directors. Dr. Nath also holds professional memberships in the American Association of Anatomists, the Society for College Science Teaching, and the National Science Teachers Association. She is the sole author of *Using Medical Terminology: A Practical Approach* (published by Lippincott Williams & Wilkins), the first book to use a "foreign language and total immersion" approach to teaching medical terminology within the context of applied anatomy and physiology. Dr. Nath has reviewed several textbooks and written ancillary materials, including lecture outlines, PowerPoint presentations, and test banks for A&P textbooks. She is also the coauthor of *Fundamentals of Anatomy & Physiology, 8th* and *9th editions; Anatomy & Physiology, 2nd edition; Visual Anatomy & Physiology, first edition;* and *Visual Essentials of Anatomy & Physiology, first edition* (published by Pearson Benjamin Cummings), which are leading undergraduate A&P textbooks.

On a personal note, Dr. Nath thoroughly enjoys family life with her husband Mike and their three dogs, Bear, Quincy, and Gabbi. Piano playing and bicycling are welcome diversions from authoring and her favorite charities include the local Humane Society, the Cystic Fibrosis Foundation, and Real Partners Uganda.

Preface

$\mathcal{W}$elcome to the exciting and expanding field of medical terminology. This textbook is written to teach you the language of your medical career in an engaging and meaningful way. Textbooks often fail to adequately represent the real world, and expect students to leap from the confines of a classroom to actual practice without being acquainted with real application. By using medical terminology in context, you will be prepared to enter the workforce. This book's concept and practice exercises give you lifelong tools to use, regardless of your chosen medical profession. Your training in medical terminology is quick, yet covers a wide area of mainstream and allied health fields. You will be amazed by how much you learn!

NEW TO THE SECOND EDITION

Based on reviewer comments, student communications, and instructor usage (including my personal experiences using the book in the classroom), I've made several changes to improve this edition. Here is a sampling of what to expect in the second edition:

- **More** The number of exercises has expanded greatly. The opportunities to practice and review have doubled.
- **Exercises** Labeling exercises and word search puzzles have been added to enhance the learning experience.
- **Writing Style** The overall writing has been made more student friendly to help you comprehend medical terms without getting lost in scientific writing.
- **A&P Content** The content related to anatomy and physiology has been reduced, without compromising key terms or practical applications.
- **Figures and Photographs** The art program has been improved so that figure labels are less cluttered and include only those medical terms introduced in the chapter. The number of photographs has increased significantly.
- **Chapters** Former Chapter 5, *Skeletal System,* and Chapter 6, *Articulations*, have been combined into one cohesive unit, Chapter 5, *Skeletal System: Bones and Joints.* Former Chapter 8, *Nervous System and Special Senses,* has been divided into Chapter 7, *Nervous System*, and Chapter 8, *Special Senses.* Moreover, Chapter 20, *Oncology*, is new! Although oncology is still presented in the appropriate systems chapters, this new chapter focuses solely on cancer in its various forms. And, Chapter 21, *Gerontology*, is new! As geriatric medicine becomes increasingly important, so does its lexicon.
- **Design** The design for the second edition has been improved to make the text more appealing and much easier to use.

INNOVATIVE APPROACH

This workbook–textbook hybrid (called a "worktext") teaches medical terminology using a two-pronged approach: immersion and chunking. Within this framework you will learn whole terms in context (immersion) while the information is presented in manageable units (chunking). Understanding whole terms within context allows you to better understand and remember the terms. Because exercises are given at frequent intervals, you'll have ample opportunity to practice using the terms. This approach improves retention of information, enables written and verbal expression, and motivates learners. Basically, you learn by doing.

You will learn medical terminology while also learning very basic anatomy, physiology, and pathology. Because medical terms describe the human body in health and in disease, attaining a working knowledge of anatomy, physiology, and pathology will do much to ensure long-term memory of the language. At the end of the course, you will be astounded at the body of knowledge (or knowledge of the body) you possess.

Using the medical terms in context, rather than fully deconstructing the language, facilitates learning because you will be using the language from the very beginning, much like you might in a foreign-language class. In fact, grasping medical terminology is like learning a foreign language. The words sound odd and many are probably not part of your everyday vocabulary. However, just as you can learn to speak another language, you can learn another aspect of the English language. That is, medical terminology is just a variation of the language you already know!

This textbook provides a number of methods not only to encourage you but also to permit you to walk away with a thorough understanding of the words and with the ability to use them correctly in your new career. Throughout every chapter, you will be totally immersed in the language of medicine while practicing terms throughout each chapter. The sections are long enough to hold your interest, but not so difficult that you become frustrated. Right at the point where you've "had enough," there is a chance to pause and practice. Research has shown time and again that practice makes a skill perfect, permanent, automatic, and transferable to new situations. This book follows the proven methods of natural language acquisition that many instructors use in foreign-language courses while implementing a "chunking" approach that both teachers and students have used for centuries.

In addition, I designed each chapter to work independently of the others. Although you may read the chapters in any order, Chapter 1, *Introduction to Medical Terminology*, provides the blueprint for subsequent chapters and gives the foundation on which all other chapters are built.

You will not be bogged down with memorizing lists. Rather, the medical terms will appear in context to reinforce learning. Each chapter follows the same format, beginning with an introduction to the relevant word parts, accompanied by several exercises to boost retention. After the introductory content, the bulk of the chapter follows a predictable pattern: read, review, and practice. Terms appear in digestible chunks of discussions, followed by a review of the key terms and a practice of those terms. Each chapter then ends with a variety of exercises, including a spelling test using audio files. Profiles of healthcare professionals, case studies, and real medical reports will spark your interest while presenting medical terms as you would encounter them in life. Concepts are best learned through experience, and this book provides you with those experiential tools for successful learning.

LEARNING AND TEACHING RESOURCES

Using Medical Terminology is more than a textbook. It is a package of learning resources. A suite of ancillary material is available for both students and instructors. These supplemental materials were created specifically to enhance and strengthen both student learning and instructor teaching.

Student Site

The online student resources that accompany this textbook include numerous opportunities for enhancing your learning experience. Student resources include an all-new suite of games and activities, in addition to an audio pronunciation glossary and flash cards, animations and videos of selected concepts and materials presented in the textbook, chapter quizzes, a final exam, and student PowerPoint slides.

Teaching Resources

In addition to the ancillary material available for students, this text also comes with extensive instructor resources. The free Instructor Resource site contains the following:

- Comprehensive lesson plans
- Test generator
- Image bank
- *PowerPoint* slides, instructor version

Using Medical Terminology utilizes an innovative method to learning medical terminology by chunking information into manageable blocks of text and immersing learners into the language of medicine. Throughout the pages, the student is exposed to the use of medical terms in a variety of contexts, while consistency among the chapters creates a predictable pattern to ensure achievement. As the healthcare system and medical fields continue to expand, this textbook will provide an invaluable resource for practitioners in all health professions.

Judi L. Nath, Ph.D.
Professor of Biology
Lourdes University
Sylvania, Ohio

User's Guide

This User's Guide shows you how to the put the features of *Using Medical Terminology, Second Edition,* to work for you.

Objectives

Each chapter begins with a list of learning objectives, which are goals to guide you toward success in the course. After completing the chapter, you can assess whether you have achieved these learning goals.

Professional Profile

This profile introduces you to a person working in a healthcare field related to the chapter's content. That person then serves as a tour guide, leading you through the chapter by demonstrating the significance of medical terminology to his or her particular field. You will encounter this person again at the end of the chapter when he or she presents an actual patient case study and medical report.

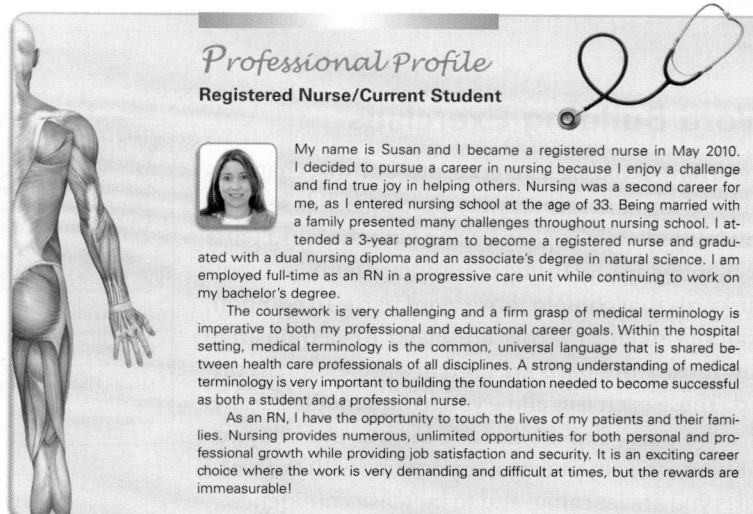

Professional Profile
Registered Nurse/Current Student

My name is Susan and I became a registered nurse in May 2010. I decided to pursue a career in nursing because I enjoy a challenge and find true joy in helping others. Nursing was a second career for me, as I entered nursing school at the age of 33. Being married with a family presented many challenges throughout nursing school. I attended a 3-year program to become a registered nurse and graduated with a dual nursing diploma and an associate's degree in natural science. I am employed full-time as an RN in a progressive care unit while continuing to work on my bachelor's degree.

The coursework is very challenging and a firm grasp of medical terminology is imperative to both my professional and educational career goals. Within the hospital setting, medical terminology is the common, universal language that is shared between health care professionals of all disciplines. A strong understanding of medical terminology is very important to building the foundation needed to become successful as both a student and a professional nurse.

As an RN, I have the opportunity to touch the lives of my patients and their families. Nursing provides numerous, unlimited opportunities for both personal and professional growth while providing job satisfaction and security. It is an exciting career choice where the work is very demanding and difficult at times, but the rewards are immeasurable!

INTRODUCTION

Radiology is the branch of science dealing with the medical use of imaging techniques to diagnose and treat disease. Examination of body structures is made using ionizing radiation, radionuclides, other forms of penetrating radiation, nuclear magnetic resonance, and ultrasound. This is an area of health care with broadening applicability.

As technology increases and noninvasive procedures replace exploratory surgery, this field will continue to expand. Interventional radiology uses fluoroscopy (x-ray examination using a fluoroscope), computed tomography (CT), and ultrasound to guide other medical

Introduction

The first section introduces the chapter and emphasizes the importance of the body system or topic to the comprehension of medical terms. Common medical problems associated with the particular system may also be presented here.

Medical Term Parts

This table consists of word parts that are relevant to the content of each chapter.

MEDICAL TERM PARTS

Word Parts

Medical term prefixes, suffixes, and combining forms related to the integumentary system are introduced in this section.

Word Part	Meaning
adip-, adipo-	fat
aut-, auto-	self
cero-	wax
chrom-, chromat-, chromato-, -chrome, chromo-	color
cry-, cryo-	cold
cyan-, cyano-	blue
cyt-, -cyte, cyto-	cell
derm-, derma-, dermat-, dermato-, dermo-	skin
erythr-, erythro-	red or red blood cell
hidr-, hidro-	sweat

Word Grouping Exercises: Bones

Using the *Medical Term Parts* table, identify the prefix, suffix, or combining form for each of the following definitions. The first one has been done as an example.

Definition	Word Part
tibia, shin bone	*tibio-*
bone	A.
	B.
bone marrow	
calcaneus	
calcium	
carpus (wrist), carpal	
cartilage	
cranium	
ethmoid bone	
ilium	
immature precursor cell	
passage	
pelvis	
pubic	
rib	

Word Grouping Exercises

To reinforce retention of the *Medical Term Parts* table, these exercises require you to identify the word part for each definition. This section helps you group the chapter's word parts by common meanings. For example, you will learn that there are two word parts that refer to the kidney: *neph-* and *ren-*. So, when you encounter the word *kidney*, you will be able to provide two word parts that refer to it. In essence, if you know that $3 + 2 = 5$, you also know that $5 - 3 = 2$. This analogy may seem elementary, but it actually begins the process of learning the language of medical terminology. You, as the student, must provide the links, and this reinforces learning.

Word Building Exercises

The *Word Building Exercises* present the chapter's medical terms in an everyday context. In this section, you immediately begin working with the word parts by identifying and listing common or familiar medical words that contain those word parts. In addition, example medical terms are given to demonstrate how those word parts are used in a professional context. These exercises allow you to find medical terms or word parts that are already in your everyday vocabulary, to gain practical experience with the word parts you are learning, and to increase confidence.

Word Building Exercises

Word parts introduced in the *Medical Term Parts* section are listed in the following table. For this exercise, first supply the meaning of each word part, then use the word part to build a word you already know. The word you list under *Common or Known Word* does not have to be a medical term; a commonly used word is fine. Be sure, however, that the word correctly reflects the intended meaning. The first one has been done as an example. Check your answers in a dictionary.

Word Part	Meaning	Common or Known Word	Example Medical Term
cardi-, cardio-	*heart*	*cardiac*	cardiomyopathy
fibr-, fibro-			fibromyalgia
kinesi-, kinesio-, kineso-			kinesiology
tendo-, teno-			tendinitis

ANATOMY AND PHYSIOLOGY

Nervous System Preview

The nervous system has two main divisions, the **central nervous system (CNS)** and the **peripheral nervous system (PNS)**. The CNS consists of the brain and spinal cord, and the PNS consists of the supporting cranial and spinal nerves that connect the CNS to other body parts.

The brain and spinal cord are the only components of the central nervous system. The peripheral nervous system has two divisions: the **somatic nervous system (SNS)** and **autonomic nervous system (ANS)**. The SNS is under voluntary control, but the ANS is entirely automatic and cannot be consciously controlled. There are two divisions of the ANS:

Anatomy and Physiology

This short narrative section provides an overview of the body system and serves as a backdrop for the anatomy and physiology content of the chapter.

Key Terms Table and Practice

Each section of narrative contains boldface medical terms that are introduced in context. These key terms, their pronunciations, and their definitions appear in a table following the narrative.

Practice questions reinforce your understanding of the newly introduced terms.

KEY TERM	Definition
serum (SEER-um)	blood plasma without the clotting protein fibrinogen

KEY TERM PRACTICE: *Blood Preview*

1. Plasma without the clotting protein fibrinogen is called _____.

The Clinical Dimension

This section is divided into blocks of narrative on different disorders, which integrate terms and definitions for signs and symptoms, clinical tests and diagnostic procedures, and treatments. These terms commonly appear in medical reports or in health-related courses.

THE CLINICAL DIMENSION

This section identifies signs and symptoms, pathological conditions, and treatments rela to the endocrine system. Endocrine disorders can be assessed through a variety of clin tests and diagnostic procedures. Laboratory analyses used to evaluate endocrine function clude plasma, serum, blood, urine, glucose tolerance, and glycosylated hemoglobin (A_{1c}) te Common disorders and treatments of the endocrine system are described.

Disorders of the endocrine system are generally the result of tumors or the hyperfunct (hypersecretion) or hypofunction (hyposecretion) of specific glands. They can also be seco ary to some other primary condition. The pathological disorders discussed in this section

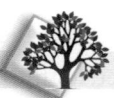

LIFE SPAN

Blood cells develop from the mesoderm germ layer, one of the primary layers formed early in embryonic life. While in utero, the mesoderm gives rise to other tissues and blood, which then forms from several sites, including the liver and spleen. By the seventh gestational month, the bone marrow takes over the role of hemopoiesis.

Fetal hemoglobin (HbF) is the form found in the body while still in the womb. It is different from infant and adult hemoglobin (HbA). HbF has a greater affinity for oxygen than does HbA, the form produced after birth and throughout life. After birth, HbF is destroyed by the infant's liver and replaced by newly formed HbA.

In the News

This feature takes a story from the popular media and offers another opportunity to put the chapter's medical terminology in context. It provides interesting, real-life scenarios related to the topic studied. This feature links mainstream science with medical terminology and provides additional application of the terms.

Common Abbreviations Table and Exercises

This table lists the common, accepted abbreviations and acronyms introduced in the chapter. Practice exercises also accompany these sections.

Life Span

This section contains information on developmental anatomy and physiology and significant alterations seen throughout human life. While focusing on the chapter's topic, the discussion covers lifespan issues from the "womb to the tomb," paying special attention to key changes that occur in utero, childhood, adolescence, adulthood, and older adulthood.

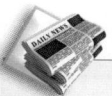

IN THE NEWS: Aspirin

The phrase is familiar: "Aspirin, the wonder drug." Is it really? Or is this marketing hype? The pharmaceutical name for aspirin is acetylsalicylic acid (ASA), and it is a common nonsteroidal anti-inflammatory drug (NSAID). Its properties are numerous, ranging from anti-inflammatory effects to acting as an analgesic, antipyretic (fever reducer), and thrombolytic.

Studies indicate that prophylactic aspirin therapy is beneficial for secondary prevention of vascular events in individuals with a history of CV disease. The U.S. Food and Drug Administration (FDA) has approved aspirin use at 325 mg/day for primary myocardial infarction prevention. Aspirin used clinically at a dosage level of 81 mg/day (baby aspirin) demonstrated antiplatelet effects that last 8 to 10 days, the life span of a platelet.

Other research demonstrated that aspirin administration of 325 mg/day decreased the incidence of transient ischemic attacks (TIAs; also known as mini-strokes, which

COMMON *Abbreviations*

Abbreviation	Term
ABG	arterial blood gas
AFB	acid-fast bacilli
ARDS	adult respiratory distress syndrome
CF	cystic fibrosis
CO	carbon monoxide
CO_2	carbon dioxide

COMMON ABBREVIATIONS EXERCISES

1. CO is the abbreviation for _____

Case Study

In this section, we follow the healthcare professional introduced in the beginning of the chapter as he or she treats a patient. Each case emphasizes the relevance of medical terminology to professional practice. Each *Case Study* is followed by questions that allow you to test your understanding of the chapter's terms. This method gives you opportunities to interact with the chapter's topic in a medical context.

Case Study

Mrs. Eleanor Chime is 67 years old and has a history of melanoma (cancer derived from skin melanocytes) on her back. The melanoma metastasized to regional lymph nodes with concomitant splenomegaly and hepatomegaly. Her lungs and brain are not affected.

She is not very ambulatory because of arthritis and suffers from lymphedema, notably in her legs. Analgesics and nonsteroidal anti-inflammatory drugs (NSAIDs) provide some relief. Mrs. Chime's oncologist recommended massage therapy for lymphedema relief.

Case Study Questions

Select the best answer to each of the following questions.

1. **Splenomegaly is best described as**
   _____
   a. enlargement of the spleen
   b. a papule on the epidermis
   c. cancer of the spleen
   d. non-Hodgkin lymphoma

2. **Lymphedema is best described as**
   _____
   a. enlargement of the lymph nodes
   b. swelling of lymphatic tissue
   c. an autoimmune disease
   d. all of these

3. **Lymphedema could result from**
   _____
   a. obstructed lymphatics
   b. immobility
   c. decreased fluid intake
   d. a and b

4. **Why might Mrs. Chime experience relief after having massage therapy?** _____
   a. The oils used increase lymph flow.
   b. Manual manipulation and compression enhance lymph flow.
   c. Reclining while receiving a massage increases lymph flow.
   d. Massage therapy is counterintuitive, and the benefit she proclaims is merely perceived and not actual.

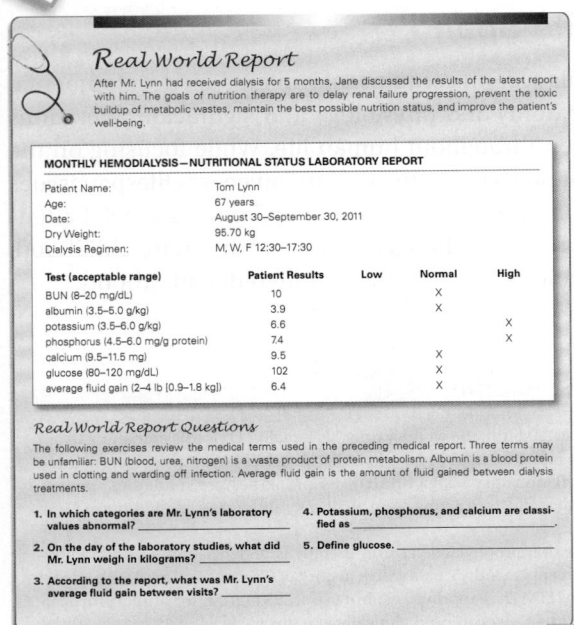

Real World Report

After Mr. Lynn had received dialysis for 5 months, Jane discussed the results of the latest report with him. The goals of nutrition therapy are to delay renal failure progression, prevent the toxic buildup of metabolic wastes, maintain the best possible nutrition status, and improve the patient's well-being.

MONTHLY HEMODIALYSIS—NUTRITIONAL STATUS LABORATORY REPORT

Patient Name:	Tom Lynn
Age:	67 years
Date:	August 30–September 30, 2011
Dry Weight:	95.70 kg
Dialysis Regimen:	M, W, F 12:30–17:30

Test (acceptable range)	Patient Results	Low	Normal	High
BUN (8–20 mg/dL)	10		X	
albumin (3.5–5.0 g/kg)	3.9		X	
potassium (3.5–6.0 g/kg)	6.6			X
phosphorus (4.5–6.0 mg/g protein)	7.4			X
calcium (9.5–11.5 mg)	9.5		X	
glucose (80–120 mg/dL)	102		X	
average fluid gain (2–4 lb [0.9–1.8 kg])	6.4		X	

Real World Report Questions

The following exercises review the medical terms used in the preceding medical report. Three terms may be unfamiliar: BUN (blood, urea, nitrogen) is a waste product of protein metabolism. Albumin is a blood protein used in clotting and warding off infection. Average fluid gain is the amount of fluid gained between dialysis treatments.

1. In which categories are Mr. Lynn's laboratory values abnormal? _____

2. On the day of the laboratory studies, what did Mr. Lynn weigh in kilograms? _____

3. According to the report, what was Mr. Lynn's average fluid gain between visits? _____

4. Potassium, phosphorus, and calcium are classified as _____.

5. Define glucose. _____

Real Word Report

This feature uses a medical report compiled for the patient introduced in the *Case Study* to demonstrate how medical terms are used in clinical practice. The questions for this section highlight the terms that appear in the report. Because the report is linked to both the *Case Study* and the chapter's *Professional Profile,* it caps a unifying theme:

- A professional working in the field sees a patient with a particular medical history.
- Diagnostic testing or treatment on that patient results in a medical report.
- This report must then be understood by the healthcare professionals who interact with that patient. The report must also be understood by people who deal with that patient's medical records.

All forms included in this section are factual reports, although all identifying information has been removed and every name is fictitious.

Review and Application

Each chapter ends with a variety of *Review and Application* exercises for recall, concept analysis, application, and critical thinking. The questions, designed to enhance learning and reinforce term usage, consist of a variety of exercises, such as multiple choice, matching, defining, giving alternate terms, spelling, unscrambling, abbreviating, providing analogies, labeling, and word searching.

Review and Application

Multiple–Choice Questions

Select the best answer to each of the following questions.

1. The hollow chambers within the kidneys are called _____.
   a. vestibules   b. sinuses   c. hila   d. capsules

2. The word part *nephr-* means _____, and the word part *-osis* means _____.
   a. kidney; condition of   b. renin; pathology of   c. urine; inflammation of   d. nephron; condition

3. Surgical removal of a kidney is termed _____.
   a. lithotomy   b. lithotripsy   c. nephrectomy   d. pyelotomy

4. The _____ delivers urine to the outside.
   a. urinary tubule   b. papillary duct   c. ureter   d. urethra

5. The structure connecting the kidney to the bladder is the _____.
   a. renal tubule   b. papillary duct   c. ureter   d. urethra

Vocabulary Review

Vocabulary Review

Review the key terms from this chapter, study the spelling and pronunciation of each term, and write its definition in the space provided. Listen to the audio available for most terms at http://thepoint.lww.com/nath2e and pronounce each term for yourself. Then check the box when you feel confident that you know the definition and can pronounce the term correctly.

Key Term	Pronunciation	Definition
☐ abstinence		_____
☐ acquired immunodeficiency syndrome (AIDS)	(im-yoo-noh-dee-FISH-un-see)	_____
☐ acrosome	(ACK-roh-sohm)	_____
☐ adnexa	(ad-NECK-suh)	_____

Vocabulary Review

This section links the text to audio pronunciations provided on the online student resource site. You listen to the audio pronunciation and write the definition of the term in the space provided.

Answers

Each chapter concludes with answers to all the exercises, allowing you to check your responses easily and quickly. Also, justifications for correct answers and rationales for incorrect answers are given for the *Case Study* questions.

Answers

Word Grouping Exercises

Definition	Word Part	Definition	Word Part
food, nutrition	troph-, tropho-	appearance	phen-, pheno-
allantois (a fetal membrane), allantoid, sausage-shaped	allant-, allanto-	brain	encephal-, encephalo-
amnion (innermost embryonic membrane)	amnio-	child	ped-, pedi-, pedo-

Additional Learning Resources

- **Companion site for students** includes student PowerPoints, animations, videos, audio glossary, flash cards, chapter quizzes, final exam, and a variety of new games and activities. The companion site can be accessed at http://thepoint.lww.com/Nath2e
- **Instructor Resource site** includes lesson plans, image bank, test generator, and PowerPoint lecture slides.

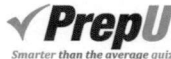

PrepU: a personalized learning solution proven to improve your students' success.

PrepU for Nath's Using Medical Terminology, Second Edition is designed with thousands of questions that remediate back to this text. The questions not only provide an explanation for the correct answer, but also reference the text page for the student to review the source material. *PrepU for Nath's Using Medical Terminology* challenges students with questions and activities that coincide with the material they've learned in this text and gives students a proven tool to learn Medical Terminology more effectively. PrepU gives instructors a tool to assess students learning while benefiting from data that is useful for accreditation.

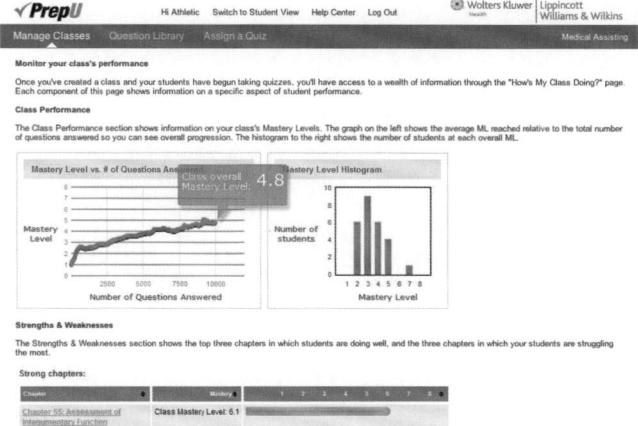

PrepU offers an INDIVIDUALIZED LEARNING EXPERIENCE for each student.

An adaptive learning engine, PrepU offers questions customized for each student's level of understanding, challenging them at an appropriate pace and difficulty level, while dispelling common misconceptions. PrepU not only helps students to improve their knowledge, but also helps foster their test-taking confidence.

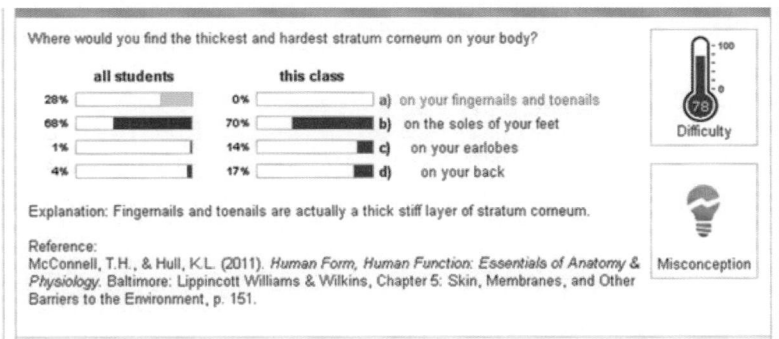

PrepU WORKS—and not just because we say so. PrepU efficacy is backed by data:

1. In an introductory nursing course at Central Carolina Technical College, student course outcomes were positively associated with PrepU usage. The students who answered the most PrepU questions in the class also had the best overall course grades.
2. In a randomized, controlled study at UCLA, students using PrepU (for biology) achieved 62% higher learning gains than those who did not.

Reviewers

Tammie Bolling, EdD
Master Instructor
Department of Business Systems
  Technology
Tennessee Technology Center at
  Jacksboro
Jacksboro, Tennessee

Marianne Bovee, CCMA, CET, CHI
Department Head
Department of Medical Assisting/
  Phlebotomy
Duluth Business University
Duluth, Minnesota

Cyndi Caviness, AAS
Director/Senior Instructor
Department of Medical Assisting
Montgomery Community College
Troy, North Carolina

**Anna Hilton, BS Management,
AAS Medical Assisting**
Faculty CMA (AAMA)
Department of Medical Assisting
Forsyth Technical Community College
Winston-Salem, North Carolina

**Jacqueline M. Johnson,
CCMA, BS**
Instructor
Department of Allied Health
Lincoln College of Technology–
  Tri-County Campus
Cincinnati, Ohio

**Tamara E. Mottler, BA, CMA
(AAMA)**
Program Manager
Department of Medical Assisting
Daytona State College
Daytona Beach, Florida

Yvette Pawlowski, BA, RHIT, CMT
Professor
Department of Office Technology
Central Texas College
Killeen, Texas

**Karen Scott, MA Adult
Education/Distance Learning**
Division Chair
Department of Business and
  Social Science
Pierce College at Puyallop
Tacoma, Washington

**Claire Maday Travis, MA, MBA,
CPHQ**
Surgical Residency Coordinator
Department of Surgery
University of Colorado
Aurora, Colorado

Jackie Waite, MA
Business/Medical Office Instructor
Department of Business Technology
Hinds Community College
Jackson, Mississippi

Acknowledgments

Writing a textbook requires more than putting ink to the page or fingers to the keyboard. The endeavor needs an orchestra of key people to bring the product to its finished form. Individuals from diverse areas gave of their time and talent to bring this book to you. It is those key people that I am thankful worked with me on this project. To begin, kudos are extended to my LWW editorial team. Senior Product Manager Amy Millholen kept all the iterations organized and made sure that every component of every chapter was in order. Her keen attention to detail and assistance on this edition were both warmly welcomed and greatly appreciated. Developmental Editor Annie Reid edited and read several versions of each chapter, providing expert analysis. Her skill was invaluable. Artist Susan Caldwell reworked all the figures and photos to enhance this edition—all with great talent and patience. Freelance Developmental Editor Molly Ward did a stellar job preparing the ancillaries for the textbook. Additionally, she caught a few items before they slipped through the process. Thanks to Editorial Assistant Courtney Shell who was continuously available. Thank you to Senior Publisher Julie Stegman who certified that a second edition was essential. And, a special note of acknowledgment goes to Acquisitions Editor David Troy. This second edition was possible because he not only endorsed the concept, he also believed in the approach.

Many thanks to the professionals profiled in each chapter, who provided biographies and real world reports to make medical terminology come alive and attach realism to the pages. My own students were quite helpful, provided constructive feedback, and were quick to let me know "what worked" and what didn't. Student Kelsey Lindsley read pages of manuscript and eagerly assisted with narrative development. Thanks are also due my colleagues at Lourdes University, who have been supporting this project for nearly a decade.

I am indebted to instructors and students from across the United States, who sent me feedback over the years. Your suggestions and comments should be evident in the following pages. Thanks, Team!

Figure Credits

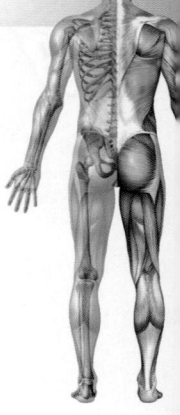

Figure 1-3 From Willis MC, CMA-AC. *Medical Terminology: A Programmed Learning Approach to the Language of Health Care.* Baltimore: Lippincott Williams & Wilkins, 2002.

Figure 1-4 From Willis MC, CMA-AC. *Medical Terminology: A Programmed Learning Approach to the Language of Health Care.* Baltimore: Lippincott Williams & Wilkins, 2002.

Figure 1-6 Image provided by LifeART, © 2013 Lippincott Williams & Wilkins. All rights reserved.

Figure 1-8 Courtesy of G. Avery.

Figure 2-1 Reprinted with permission from Pillitteri A. *Maternal and Child Health Nursing*, 4th ed. Philadelphia: Lippincott Williams & Wilkins, 2003.

Figure 2-3 Asset provided by Anatomical Chart Co.

Figure 2-14 Courtesy of Lindsey Lemons.

Figure 3-1 Image provided by LifeART, © 2013 Lippincott Williams & Wilkins. All rights reserved.

Figure 3-2 Reprinted with permission from Becker KL, Bilezikian JP, Brenner WJ, et al. *Principles and Practice of Endocrinology and Metabolism*, 3rd ed. Philadelphia: Lippincott Williams & Wilkins, 2001.

Figure 3-4 Reprinted with permission from Bucholz RW, Heckman JD. *Rockwood & Green's Fractures in Adults*, 5th ed. Baltimore: Lippincott Williams & Wilkins, 2001.

Figure 3-5 From Snell, MD, PhD, *Clinical Anatomy*, 7th ed. Lippincott, Williams & Wilkins, 2003.

Figure 3-6 From Snell, MD, PhD, *Clinical Anatomy*, 7th ed. Lippincott, Williams & Wilkins, 2003.

Figure 3-7 Donald S. Baim, *Grossman's Cardiac Catheterization, Angiography, and Intervention*, 7th ed. Philadelphia: Lippincott Williams & Wilkins, 2006.

Figure 3-8 Image provided by LifeART, © 2013 Lippincott Williams & Wilkins. All rights reserved.

Figure 3-9 Image provided by LifeART, © 2013 Lippincott Williams & Wilkins. All rights reserved.

Figure 3-10 From Snell, MD, PhD, *Clinical Anatomy*, 7th ed. Philadelphia: Lippincott, Williams & Wilkins, 2003.

Figure 3-13 Terry R. Yochum, Lindsay J. Rowe, *Yochum and Rowe's Essentials of Skeletal Radiology*, 3rd ed.. Philadelphia: Lippincott Williams & Wilkins, 2004.

Figure 3-15 From Smeltzer SC, Bare BG. *Textbook of Medical-Surgical Nursing*, 9th ed. Philadelphia: Lippincott Williams & Wilkins, 2000.

Figure 3-16 Michael W. Mulholland, Ronald V. Maier, et al. *Greenfield's Surgery Scientific Principles and Practice*, 4th ed. Philadelphia: Lippincott Williams & Wilkins, 2006.

Figure 3-19 William J. Koopman, Larry W. Moreland, *Arthritis and Allied Conditions: A Textbook of Rheumatology*, 15th ed. Philadelphia: Lippincott Williams & Wilkins, 2005.

Figure 3-20 From Moore KL, PhD, FRSM, FIAC & Dalley AF II, PhD. *Clinical Oriented Anatomy*, 4th ed. Baltimore: Lippincott Williams & Wilkins, 1999.

Figure 3-21 Courtesy of TSA.

Figure 4-1 Asset provided by Anatomical Chart Co.

Figure 4-3 From Weber JW, Kelley J. *Health Assessment in Nursing*. Philadelphia: Lippincott-Raven, 1998.

Figure 4-4 Image provided by Stedman's.

Figure 4-5 Fletcher M. *Physical Diagnosis in Neonatology*. Philadelphia: Lippincott-Raven, 1998.

Figure 4-6 From Weber J, RN, EdD, and Kelley J, RN, PhD. *Health Assessment in Nursing*, 2nd ed. Philadelphia: Lippincott Williams & Wilkins, 2003.

Figure 4-8 Image provided by Anatomical Chart Co.

Figure 4-9 Goodheart H. *A Photoguide of Common Skin Disorders*. Baltimore: Williams & Wilkins, 1999.

Figure 4-11 From Goodheart HP, MD. *Goodheart's Photoguide of Common Skin Disorders*, 2nd ed. Philadelphia: Lippincott Williams & Wilkins, 2003.

Figure 4-12 From *Stedman's Medical Dictionary*, 27th ed. Baltimore: Lippincott Williams & Wilkins 2000.

Figure 4-14 From Goodheart HP, MD. *Goodheart's Photoguide of Common Skin Disorders*, 2nd ed. Philadelphia: Lippincott Williams & Wilkins, 2003.

Figure 4-15 From Goodheart HP, MD. *Goodheart's Photoguide of Common Skin Disorders*, 2nd ed. Philadelphia: Lippincott Williams & Wilkins, 2003.

Figure 4-16 From Goodheart HP, MD. *Goodheart's Photoguide of Common Skin Disorders*, 2nd ed. Philadelphia: Lippincott Williams & Wilkins, 2003.

Figure 4-17 From Goodheart HP, MD. *Goodheart's Photoguide of Common Skin Disorders*, 2nd ed. Philadelphia: Lippincott Williams & Wilkins, 2003.

Figure 4-18 From Goodheart HP, MD. *Goodheart's Photoguide of Common Skin Disorders*, 2nd ed. Philadelphia: Lippincott Williams & Wilkins, 2003.

Figure 4-19 From Goodheart HP, MD. *Goodheart's Photoguide of Common Skin Disorders*, 2nd ed. Philadelphia: Lippincott Williams & Wilkins, 2003.

Figure 4-20 From Goodheart HP, MD. *Goodheart's Photoguide of Common Skin Disorders*, 2nd ed. Philadelphia: Lippincott Williams & Wilkins, 2003.

Figure 4-21 Dale Berg and Katherine Worzala, *Atlas of Adult Physical Diagnosis*. Philadelphia: Lippincott Williams & Wilkins, 2006.

Figure 4-22 From Weber J, RN, EdD, and Kelley J, RN, PhD. Health Assessment in Nursing, 2nd ed. Philadelphia: Lippincott Williams & Wilkins, 2003.

Figure 4-23 From Goodheart HP, MD. *Goodheart's Photoguide of Common Skin Disorders*, 2nd ed. Philadelphia: Lippincott Williams & Wilkins, 2003.

Figure 4-24 From Smeltzer SC, Bare BG. *Textbook of Medical-Surgical Nursing*, 9th ed. Philadelphia: Lippincott Williams & Wilkins, 2000.

Figure 4-25 From Goodheart HP, MD. *Goodheart's Photoguide of Common Skin Disorders*, 2nd ed. Philadelphia: Lippincott Williams & Wilkins, 2003.

Figure 4-26 From Goodheart HP, MD. *Goodheart's Photoguide of Common Skin Disorders*, 2nd ed. Philadelphia: Lippincott Williams & Wilkins, 2003.

Figure 4-27 From Goodheart HP, MD. *Goodheart's Photoguide of Common Skin Disorders*, 2nd ed. Philadelphia: Lippincott Williams & Wilkins, 2003.

Figure 4-28 Image provided by Stedman's.

Figure 4-29 From Goodheart HP, MD. *Goodheart's Photoguide of Common Skin Disorders*, 2nd ed. Philadelphia: Lippincott Williams & Wilkins, 2003.

Figure 4-30 From Sweet RL, Gibbs RS. *Atlas of Infectious Diseases of the Female Genital Tract*. Philadelphia: Lippincott Williams & Wilkins, 2005.

Figure 4-32 From Goodheart HP, MD. *Goodheart's Photoguide of Common Skin Disorders*, 2nd ed. Philadelphia: Lippincott Williams & Wilkins, 2003.

Figure 5-4 Image from Rubin E MD and Farber JL MD. *Pathology*, 3rd ed. Philadelphia: Lippincott Williams & Wilkins, 1999.

Figure 5-9 Asset provided by Anatomical Chart Co.

Figure 5-14 From Oatis CA. *Kinesiology. The Mechanics and Pathomechanics of Human Movement*. Baltimore: Lippincott Williams & Wilkins 2003.

Figure 5-15 From Moore KL, PhD, FRSM, FIAC, and Dalley AF II, PhD. *Clinical Oriented Anatomy*, 4th ed. Baltimore, Lippincott Williams & Wilkins 1999.

Figure 5-19 Moore KL, PhD, FRSM, FIAC, and Dalley AF II, PhD. *Clinical Oriented Anatomy*, 4th ed. Baltimore, Lippincott Williams & Wilkins 1999.

Figure 5-21A Courtesy of Martin Herman, MD.

Figure 5-21C Dale Berg and Katherine Worzala, *Atlas of Adult Physical Diagnosis*. Philadelphia: Lippincott Williams & Wilkins, 2006.

Figure 5-23 Image from Rubin E MD and Farber JL MD. *Pathology*, 3rd ed. Philadelphia: Lippincott Williams & Wilkins, 1999.

Figure 5-27 From Becker KL, Bilezikian JP, Brenner WJ, et al. *Principles and Practice of Endocrinology and Metabolism*, 3rd ed. Philadelphia: Lippincott Williams & Wilkins, 2001.

Figure 5-28 Raphael Rubin, David S. Strayer, Rubin's Pathology: Clinicopathologic Foundations of Medicine, Fifth ed. Philadelphia: Lippincott Williams & Wilkins, 2008.

Figure 5-34 Image provided by Stedman's.

Figure 5-36 Asset provided by Anatomical Chart Co.

Figure 5-37 From Strickland JW, Graham TJ. *Master Techniques in Orthopeadic Surgery: The Hand*, 2nd ed. Philadelphia: Lippincott Williams & Wilkins, 2005.

Figure 5-38 Dale Berg and Katherine Worzala, *Atlas of Adult Physical Diagnosis*. Philadelphia: Lippincott Williams & Wilkins, 2006.

Figure 5-41 From Bickley, LS, and Szilagyi, P. *Bates' Guide to Physical Examination and History Taking*, 8th ed. Philadelphia: Lippincott Williams & Wilkins 2003.

Figure 5-42 From Weber J, RN, EdD, and Kelley J, RN, PhD. *Health Assessment in Nursing*, 2nd ed. Philadelphia: Lippincott Williams & Wilkins, 2003.

Figure 5-44 From Goodheart HP, MD. *Goodheart's Photoguide of Common Skin Disorders*, 2nd ed. Philadelphia: Lippincott Williams & Wilkins, 2003.

Figure 6-2 From Moore KL and Agur A. *Essential Clinical Anatomy*, 2nd ed. Philadelphia: Lippincott Williams & Wilkins, 2002.

Figure 6-4 From Strickland JW, Graham TJ. *Master Techniques in Orthopeadic Surgery: The Hand*, 2nd ed. Philadelphia: Lippincott Williams & Wilkins, 2005.

Figure 6-8 From Premkumar K. *The Massage Connection Anatomy and Physiology*. Baltimore: Lippincott Williams & Wilkins 2004.

Figure 6-9 Image provided by Stedman's.

Figure 6-10 From Strickland JW, Graham TJ. *Master Techniques in Orthopeadic Surgery: The Hand*, 2nd ed. Philadelphia: Lippincott Williams & Wilkins, 2005.

Figure 7-3 From Bear M, Conner B, Paradiso M. *Neuroscience, Exploring the Brain*, 2nd ed. Baltimore: Lippincott Williams and Wilkins, 2000.

Figure 7-4 Cohen BJ, Taylor JJ. *Memmler's The Human Body in Health and Disease*, 11th ed. Baltimore: Wolters Kluwer Health, 2009.

Figure 7-6 From Weber J, RN, EdD and Kelley J, RN, PhD. *Health Assessment in Nursing*, 2nd ed. Philadelphia: Lippincott Williams & Wilkins, 2003.

Figure 7-7 From Bear M, Conner B, Paradiso M. *Neuroscience, Exploring the Brain*, 2nd ed. Baltimore: Lippincott Williams and Wilkins, 2000.

Figure 7-8 Asset provided by Anatomical Chart Co.

Figure 7-9 Asset provided by Anatomical Chart Co.

Figure 7-10A Asset provided by Anatomical Chart Co.

Figure 7-10B From Bear MF, Connors BW, and Parasido, MA. *Neuroscience, Exploring the Brain*, 2nd ed. Philadelphia: Lippincott Williams & Wilkins. 2001.

Figure 7-12 From Fleisher GR, MD, Ludwig W, MD, Baskin MN, MD. *Atlas of Pediatric Emergency Medicine*. Philadelphia: Lippincott Williams & Wilkins, 2004.

Figure 7-13 Rubin E., Farber J.L. (1999). *Pathology*, 3rd ed., p. 1511. Philadelphia: Lippincott-Raven.

Figure 7-16 Reprinted with permission from Pillitteri A. *Maternal and Child Health Nursing*, 4th ed. Philadelphia: Lippincott Williams & Wilkins, 2003.

Figure 8-2 Photo reprinted by permission of the *New England Journal of Medicine*, 328: 186, 1993.

Figure 8-3 From Weber J, RN, EdD and Kelley J, RN, PhD. *Health Assessment in Nursing*, 2nd ed. Philadelphia: Lippincott Williams & Wilkins, 2003.

Figure 8-6 Image from Rubin E MD and Farber JL MD. *Pathology*, 3rd ed. Philadelphia: Lippincott Williams & Wilkins, 1999.

Figure 8-7 Dale Berg and Katherine Worzala, *Atlas of Adult Physical Diagnosis*. Philadelphia: Lippincott Williams & Wilkins, 2006.

Figure 8-8 From Tasman W, Jaeger E. *The Wills Eye Hospital Atlas of Clinical Ophthalmology*, 2e. Lippincott Williams & Wilkins, 2001.

Figure 8-10 From Tasman W, Jaeger E. *The Wills Eye Hospital Atlas of Clinical Ophthalmology*, 2e. Lippincott Williams & Wilkins, 2001.

Figure 8-11 Thomas H. McConnell. *The Nature of Disease Pathology for the Health Professions*, Philadelphia: Lippincott Williams & Wilkins, 2007.

Figure 8-12 From Tasman W, Jaeger E. *The Wills Eye Hospital Atlas of Clinical Ophthalmology*, 2e. Lippincott Williams & Wilkins, 2001.

Figure 8-13 From Fuller J and Schaller-Ayers J. *Health Assessment: A Nursing Approach.* 2nd ed. Philadelphia: JP Lippincott 1994.

Figure 8-15 From Tasman W, Jaeger E. *The Wills Eye Hospital Atlas of Clinical Ophthalmology*, 2e. Lippincott Williams & Wilkins, 2001.

Figure 8-16 From Weber J, RN, EdD, and Kelley J RN, PhD. *Health Assessment in Nursing,* 2nd ed. Philadelphia: Lippincott Williams & Wilkins, 2003.

Figure 8-17 From Fleisher GR, MD, Ludwig W, MD, Baskin MN, MD. *Atlas of Pediatric Emergency Medicine.* Philadelphia: Lippincott Williams & Wilkins, 2004.

Figure 8-18 From Tasman W, Jaeger E. *The Wills Eye Hospital Atlas of Clinical Ophthalmology*, 2e. Lippincott Williams & Wilkins, 2001.

Figure 9-2 Thomas H. McConnell. *The Nature of Disease Pathology for the Health Professions.* Philadelphia: Lippincott Williams & Wilkins, 2007.

Figure 9-3 Asset provided by Anatomical Chart Co.

Figure 9-4 From Smeltzer SC, Bare BG. *Textbook of Medical–Surgical Nursing*, 9th ed. Philadelphia: Lippincott Williams & Wilkins, 2000.

Figure 9-7 Adapted from Coleman RM. 1986. *Wide Awake at 3:00 A.M. by Choice or by Chance?* New York: W.H. Freeman. Fig. 2.1.

Figure 9-9 Thomas H. McConnell. *The Nature of Disease Pathology for the Health Professions.* Philadelphia: Lippincott Williams & Wilkins, 2007.

Figure 9-11 Image from Rubin E MD and Farber JL MD. *Pathology*, 3rd ed. Philadelphia: Lippincott Williams & Wilkins, 1999.

Figure 9-12 Image provided by Stedman's.

Figure 9-15 Gagel R.F., McCutcheon I.E. (1999). Images in Clinical Medicine. *New England Journal of Medicine 340*, 524. Copyright © 2003. Massachusetts Medical Society.

Figure 9-19 From Rubin E. *Essential Pathology*, 3rd ed. Philadelphia: Lippincott Williams & Wilkins, 2000.

Figure 9-20 Rubin E., Farber J.L. (1999). *Pathology*, 3rd ed., p. 1167. Philadelphia: Lippincott-Raven.

Figure 10-1 Asset provided by Anatomical Chart Co.

Figure 10-2 Asset provided by Anatomical Chart Co.

Figure 10-4 LifeART image copyright © 2013 Lippincott Williams & Wilkins. All rights reserved.

Figure 10-5 From Smeltzer SCO, Bare BG. *Brunner and Suddarth's Textbook of Medical–Surgical Nursing*, 9e, Lippincott Williams & Wilkins 2002.

Figure 10-6 Asset provided by Anatomical Chart Co.

Figure 10-7 Asset provided by Anatomical Chart Co.

Figure 10-9 Asset provided by Anatomical Chart Co.

Figure 10-11 From Smeltzer SC, Bare BG. *Textbook of Medical–Surgical Nursing*, 9th ed. Philadelphia: Lippincott Williams & Wilkins, 2000.

Figure 10-12 Courtesy of Sidney Sussman, MD.

Figure 10-13 From Gold DH, MD, and Weingeist TA, MD, PhD. *Color Atlas of the Eye in Systemic Disease.* Baltimore: Lippincott Williams & Wilkins, 2001.

Figure 10-15 LifeART image copyright © 2013 Lippincott Williams & Wilkins. All rights reserved.

Figure 10-16 From Gold DH, MD, and Weingeist TA, MD, PhD. *Color Atlas of the Eye in Systemic Disease.* Baltimore: Lippincott Williams & Wilkins, 2001.

Figure 10-17 Image from Rubin E MD and Farber JL MD. *Pathology*, 3rd ed. Philadelphia: Lippincott Williams & Wilkins, 1999.

Figure 10-18 Image from Rubin E MD and Farber JL MD. *Pathology*, 3rd ed. Philadelphia: Lippincott Williams & Wilkins, 1999.

Figure 11-1 From Smeltzer SCO, Bare BG. *Brunner and Suddarth's Textbook of Medical-Surgical Nursing*, 9th ed. Philadelphia: Lippincott Williams & Wilkins 2002.

Figure 11-2 Asset provided by Anatomical Chart Co.

Figure 11-5 Asset provided by Anatomical Chart Co.

Figure 11-6 Cohen BJ, Taylor JJ. *Memmler's The Human Body in Health and Disease*, 10th ed. Baltimore: Lippincott Williams & Wilkins, 2005.

Figure 11-9 Carol Mattson Porth, *Pathophysiology Concepts of Altered Health States*, 7th ed. Philadelphia: Lippincott Williams & Wilkins, 2005.

Figure 11-10 From Bickley, LS and Szilagyi, P. *Bates' Guide to Physical Examination and History Taking*, 8th ed. Philadelphia: Lippincott Williams & Wilkins 2003.

Figure 11-11A From *Stedman's Medical Dictionary*, 27th ed. Baltimore: Lippincott Williams & Wilkins 2000.

Figure 11-11B Asset provided by Anatomical Chart Co.

Figure 11-13 Springhouse. *Lippincott's Visual Encyclopedia of Clinical Skills*. Philadelphia: Wolters Kluwer Health, 2009.

Figure 11-14 Image provided by LifeART, © 2013, Lippincott Williams & Wilkins. All rights reserved.

Figure 11-15 From Pillitteri, A. (2003). *Maternal and Child Nursing*, 4th ed., Philadelphia: Lippincott, Williams & Wilkins.

Figure 11-16 From Pillitteri, A.(2003), *Maternal and Child Nursing*, 4th ed., Philadelphia: Lippincott, Williams & Wilkins.

Figure 11-17 Neil O. Hardy, Westport, CT.

Figure 11-19 From Pillitteri, A.(2003), *Maternal and Child Nursing*, 4th ed., Philadelphia: Lippincott, Williams & Wilkins.

Figure 11-21 Asset provided by Anatomical Chart Co.

Figure 11-22 Neil O. Hardy. Westport, CT. From *Stedman's Medical Dictionary*, 27th ed. Baltimore: Lippincott Williams & Wilkins, 2000. pg. 84.

Figure 11-23 Cohen BJ. *Medical Terminology*, 4th ed. Philadelphia: Lippincott Williams & Wilkins, 2004.

Figure 11-24 From Cohen BJ. *Medical Terminology*, 4th ed. Philadelphia. Lippincott Williams & Wilkins, 2003.

Figure 11-25 Raphael Rubin, David S. Strayer, *Rubin's Pathology: Clinicopathologic Foundations of Medicine*, 5th ed. Philadelphia: Lippincott Williams & Wilkins, 2008.

Figure 11-29 Asset provided by Anatomical Chart Co.

Figure 11-31 Neil O. Hardy. Westport, CT. From *Stedman's Medical Dictionary*, 27th ed. Baltimore: Lippincott Williams & Wilkins, 2000. pg. 79.

Figure 11-32 Bickley LS. Bates. *Guide to Physical Examination and History Taking*, 8th ed. Philadelphia: Lippincott Williams & Wilkins, 2003.

Figure 11-33 Effeney, D J & Stoney, RJ. *Wylie's Atlas of Vascular Surgery: Disorders of the Extremities*. Philadelphia: Lippincott Williams & Wilkins, 1993.

Figure 12-2 From *Stedman's Medical Dictionary*, 27th ed. Baltimore: Lippincott Williams & Wilkins 2000.

Figure 12-4 Asset provided by Anatomical Chart Co.

Figure 12-5 From Cohen BJ, Taylor JJ. *Memmler's The Human Body in Health and Disease*, 10th ed. Baltimore: Lippincott Williams & Wilkins, 2005.

Figure 12-6 Image provided by LifeART, © 2013 Lippincott Williams & Wilkins. All rights reserved.

Figure 12-7 Richard S. Snell, *Clinical Anatomy by Regions*, 8th ed. Philadelphia: Lippincott Williams & Wilkins, 2008.

Figure 12-9 Springhouse. *Lippincott's Visual Encyclopedia of Clinical Skills*. Philadelphia: Wolters Kluwer Health, 2009.

Figure 16-14 Courtesy of T. Ernesto Figueroa, MD.

Figure 16-15 Courtesy of T. Ernesto Figueroa, MD

Figure 16-18 From Cohen BJ. *Medical Terminology*, 4th ed. Philadelphia. Lippincott Williams & Wilkins 2003.

Figure 16-19 From Beckmann CRB M.D., M.H.P.E., Ling FW M.D., Laube DW M.D., M.ED., Smith RP M.D., Barzansky BM PH.D., M.H.P.E., and Herbert WNM.D. *Obstetrics and Gynecology*, 4th ed. Baltimore: Lippincott Williams & Wilkins, 2002.

Figure 16-20 Thomas H. McConnell. *The Nature of Disease Pathology for the Health Professions*. Philadelphia: Lippincott Williams & Wilkins, 2007.

Figure 16-22 American Society of Plastic and Reconstructive Surgeons, Arlington Heights, Illinois.

Figure 16-23 From Cohen BJ. *Medical Terminology*, 4th ed. Philadelphia. Lippincott Williams & Wilkins 2003.

Figure 16-26 From Pillitteri, A.(2003), *Maternal and Child Nursing*, 4th ed., Philadelphia: Lippincott, Williams & Wilkins.

Figure 16-27 From Pillitteri, A.(2003), *Maternal and Child Nursing*, 4th ed., Philadelphia: Lippincott, Williams & Wilkins.

Figure 16-28 From Goodheart HP, MD. *Goodheart's Photoguide of Common Skin Disorders*, 2nd ed. Philadelphia: Lippincott Williams & Wilkins, 2003.

Figure 16-29 From Goodheart HP, MD. *Goodheart's Photoguide of Common Skin Disorders*, 2nd ed. Philadelphia: Lippincott Williams & Wilkins, 2003.

Figure 16-31 From Sweet RL, Gibbs RS. *Atlas of Infectious Diseases of the Female Genital Tract*. Philadelphia: Lippincott Williams & Wilkins, 2005.

Figure 16-32 From Sanders CV and Nesbitt LT. *The Skin and Infection*. Baltimore: Williams & Wilkins, 1995.

Figure 16-33 From Goodheart HP, MD. *Goodheart's Photoguide of Common Skin Disorders*, 2nd ed. Philadelphia: Lippincott Williams & Wilkins, 2003.

Figure 16-34 Courtesy of Ansell Health Care, Inc., Personal Products Group and Carter-Wallace, Inc. From Westheimer R, Lopater S. 2002. *Human Sexuality—A Psychosocial Perspective*. Baltimore: Lippincott Williams & Wilkins.

Figure 16-35 From Smeltzer SC, Bare BG. *Textbook of Medical–Surgical Nursing*, 9th ed. Philadelphia: Lippincott Williams & Wilkins, 2000.

Figure 16-36 Courtesy of Ortho-McNeil. From Westheimer R, Lopater S. 2002. Human *Sexuality—A Psychosocial Perspective*. Baltimore: Lippincott Williams & Wilkins.

Figure 17-1 Image provided by LifeART, © 2013 Lippincott Williams & Wilkins. All rights reserved.

Figure 17-3 Reprinted with permission from Blechmidt E. *The Stages of Human Development Before Birth*. Philadelphia: WB Saunders, 1961.

Figure 17-4 Copyright Petit Format/Nestle/Science Source/Photo Researchers.

Figure 17-5 From Goodheart HP, MD. *Goodheart's Photoguide of Common Skin Disorders*, 2nd ed. Philadelphia: Lippincott Williams & Wilkins, 2003.

Figure 17-7 From Bickley, LS and Szilagyi, P. *Bates' Guide to Physical Examination and History Taking*, 8th ed. Philadelphia: Lippincott Williams & Wilkins 2003.

Figure 17-10 From Pillitteri, A.(2003). *Maternal and Child Nursing*, 4th ed., Philadelphia: Lippincott, Williams & Wilkins.

Figure 17-11 Neil O. Hardy, Westport, CT.

Figure 17-12 Laura and Michael Wahl.

Figure 17-14 From Pillitteri, A.(2003), *Maternal and Child Nursing*, 4th ed., Philadelphia: Lippincott, Williams & Wilkins.

Figure 17-15 Reprinted with permission from Cohen BJ, Wood DL. *Memmler's The Human Body in Health and Disease*, 9th ed. Philadelphia: Lippincott Williams & Wilkins, 2000.

Figure 17-16 Klossner NJ. *Introductory Maternity and Pediatric Nursing*. Philadelphia: Lippincott Williams & Wilkins, 2006.

Figure 17-17 Thomas H. McConnell. *The Nature of Disease Pathology for the Health Professions*. Philadelphia: Lippincott Williams & Wilkins, 2007.

Figure 17-18 Michael S. Baggish, Rafael F. Valle, Hubert Guedj. *Hysteroscopy: Visual Perspectives of Uterine Anatomy, Physiology and Pathology*. Philadelphia: Lippincott Williams & Wilkins, 2007.

Figure 17-19A Richard S. Snell, *Clinical Anatomy by Regions*, 8th ed. Philadelphia: Lippincott Williams & Wilkins, 2008.

Figure 17-19B Image from Rubin E MD and Farber JL MD. *Pathology*, 3rd ed. Philadelphia: Lippincott Williams & Wilkins, 1999.

Figure 17-24 From Gold DH, MD, and Weingeist TA, MD, PhD. *Color Atlas of the Eye in Systemic Disease*. Baltimore: Lippincott Williams & Wilkins, 2001.

Figure 17-25 Image from Rubin E MD and Farber JL MD. *Pathology*, 3rd ed. Philadelphia: Lippincott Williams & Wilkins, 1999.

Figure 17-26 From Bickley, LS and Szilagyi, P. *Bates' Guide to Physical Examination and History Taking*, 8th ed. Philadelphia: Lippincott Williams & Wilkins 2003.

Figure 17-27 Courtesy of J. Adams.

Figure 17-28 From McConnell TH. *The Nature of Disease Pathology for the Health Professions*. Philadelphia: Lippincott Williams & Wilkins, 2007.

Figure 17-29 From Weber J, RN, EdD, and Kelley J, RN, PhD. *Health Assessment in Nursing*, 2nd ed. Philadelphia: Lippincott Williams & Wilkins, 2003.

Figure 17-31 Tim, Julie, and Brianna Cheek.

Figure 17-32 Image provided by Stedman's.

Figure 17-33 Courtesy of Kathleen Cronan, MD.

Figure 17-34 Photo courtesy of Centers for Disease Control and Prevention.

Figure 17-35 Centers for Disease Control Public Health Image Library.

Figure 17-36 From Gold DH, MD, and Weingeist TA, MD, PhD. *Color Atlas of the Eye in Systemic Disease*. Baltimore: Lippincott Williams & Wilkins, 2001.

Figure 18-1 From Bear M, Conner B, Paradiso M. *Neuroscience, Exploring the Brain*, 2nd ed. Baltimore: Lippincott Williams and Wilkins, 2000.

Figure 18-4 From Pillitteri, A.(2003), *Maternal and Child Nursing*, 4th ed., Philadelphia: Lippincott, Williams & Wilkins.

Figure 18-5 Thomas H. McConnell. *The Nature of Disease Pathology for the Health Professions*. Philadelphia: Lippincott Williams & Wilkins, 2007.

Figure 18-7 Image courtesy of Medical & Scientific Illustration.

Figure 18-8 From Bickley, LS and Szilagyi, P. *Bates' Guide to Physical Examination and History Taking*, 8th ed. Philadelphia: Lippincott Williams & Wilkins 2003.

Figure 18-9 From Westheimer R, Lopater S. 2002. *Human Sexuality—A Psychosocial Perspective*. Baltimore: Lippincott Williams & Wilkins.

Figure 18-10 Courtesy of Carl Allen, D.D.S., M.S.D.

Figure 19-1 From Willis MC, CMA-AC. *Medical Terminology: A Programmed Learning Approach to the Language of Health Care*. Baltimore: Lippincott Williams & Wilkins, 2002.

Figure 19-2 Thomas N. Tozer, Malcolm Rowland, *Introduction to Pharmacokinetics and Pharmacodynamics: The Quantitative Basis of Drug Therapy*, Philadelphia: Lippincott Williams & Wilkins, 2006.

Figure 19-4 Engleberg NC, Dermody T, DiRita V. *Schaecter's Mechanisms of Microbial Disease*, 4th ed. Baltimore: Lippincott Williams & Wilkins, 2007.

Figure 19-5 From Weber J, RN, EdD, and Kelley J, RN, PhD. *Health Assessment in Nursing*, 2nd ed. Philadelphia: Lippincott Williams & Wilkins, 2003.

Figure 19-8 Image provided by LifeART, © 2013 Lippincott Williams & Wilkins. All rights reserved.

Figure 19-10 Courtesy of Jason Dietz. From Westheimer R, Lopater S. 2002. *Human Sexuality—A Psychosocial Perspective*. Baltimore: Lippincott Williams & Wilkins.

Figure 19-11 Courtesy of Noven Pharmaceuticals, Inc. From Westheimer R, Lopater S. 2002. *Human Sexuality—A Psychosocial Perspective*. Baltimore: Lippincott Williams & Wilkins.

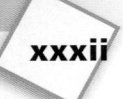

Contents

About the Author   vii

Preface   ix

Reviewers   xix

Acknowledgments   xxi

Figure Credits   xxiii

CHAPTER 1	**Introduction to Medical Terminology** 1
	Professional Profile 2
	Introduction 3
	The Medical Record 4
	A Brief Lesson in Language 9
	Pronunciation Key 11
	Rules for Plurals 13
	Medical Term Parts 14
	Common Abbreviations 27
	Review and Application 29
	Vocabulary Review 32
	Answers 33

CHAPTER 2	**Anatomical and Physiological Terminology** 41
	Professional Profile 42
	Introduction 42
	Medical Term Parts 43
	Anatomy and Physiology Defined 46
	The Clinical Dimension 65
	Life Span 70
	In the News: Wrong-Site Surgery 71
	Common Abbreviations 72
	Case Study 73
	Real World Report 74
	Review and Application 76
	Vocabulary Review 80
	Answers 84

CHAPTER 3	**Radiology and Nuclear Medicine** 93
	Professional Profile 94
	Introduction 94
	Medical Term Parts 95
	Radiology 97
	The Clinical Dimension 100
	Life Span 124
	In the News: Airport Screening 124
	Common Abbreviations 125

Case Study   126
Real World Report   127
Review and Application   128
Vocabulary Review   134
Answers   137

CHAPTER 4   **Integumentary System**   145

Professional Profile   146
Introduction   146
Medical Term Parts   147
Anatomy and Physiology   149
The Clinical Dimension   160
In the News: Necrotizing Fasciitis   173
Life Span   183
Common Abbreviations   184
Case Study   185
Real World Report   186
Review and Application   188
Vocabulary Review   193
Answers   198

CHAPTER 5   **Skeletal System: Bones and Joints**   207

Professional Profile   208
Introduction to the Skeletal System   208
Medical Term Parts: Bones   209
Anatomy and Physiology: Bones   211
The Clinical Dimension: Bones   229
Introduction to Joints   238
Medical Term Parts: Joints   239
Anatomy and Physiology: Joints   240
The Clinical Dimension: Joints   246
Life Span   257
In the News: Lyme Arthritis   258
Common Abbreviations   259
Case Study   260
Real World Report   261
Review and Application   263
Vocabulary Review   269
Answers   274

CHAPTER 6   **Muscular System**   285

Professional Profile   286
Introduction   286
Medical Term Parts   287
Anatomy and Physiology   289
In the News: Botox   292
The Clinical Dimension   299
Life Span   304
Common Abbreviations   304
Case Study   305

Real World Report   307
Review and Application   309
Vocabulary Review   313
Answers   314

CHAPTER 7   **Nervous System**   319

Professional Profile   320
Introduction   320
Medical Term Parts   321
Anatomy and Physiology   322
The Clinical Dimension   332
In The News: Bicycling Alleviates the Symptoms
   of Parkinson Disease   338
Life Span   348
Common Abbreviations   349
Case Study   350
Real World Report   351
Review and Application   352
Vocabulary Review   355
Answers   358

CHAPTER 8   **Special Senses**   365

Professional Profile   366
Introduction   366
Medical Term Parts   366
Anatomy and Physiology   369
The Clinical Dimension   376
In the News: Bionic Eyes   379
Life Span   391
Common Abbreviations   392
Case Study   393
Real World Report   394
Review and Application   396
Vocabulary Review   400
Answers   403

CHAPTER 9   **Endocrine System**   411

Professional Profile   412
Introduction   412
Medical Term Parts   413
Anatomy and Physiology   415
In the News: DHEA   422
The Clinical Dimension   425
Life Span   437
Common Abbreviations   437
Case Study   439
Real World Report   440
Review and Application   441
Vocabulary Review   446
Answers   448

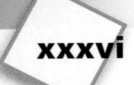

CHAPTER 10   **Blood**   455

Professional Profile   456
Introduction   456
Medical Term Parts   457
Anatomy and Physiology   459
The Clinical Dimension   472
In the News: Blood Doping   480
Life Span   486
Common Abbreviations   487
Case Study   488
Real World Report   489
Review and Application   491
Vocabulary Review   495
Answers   499

CHAPTER 11   **Cardiovascular System**   507

Professional Profile   508
Introduction   508
Medical Term Parts   509
Anatomy and Physiology   511
The Clinical Dimension   525
In the News: Aspirin   537
Life Span   547
Common Abbreviations   548
Case Study   550
Real World Report   551
Review and Application   553
Vocabulary Review   558
Answers   562

CHAPTER 12   **Respiratory System**   571

Professional Profile   572
Introduction   572
Medical Term Parts   573
Anatomy and Physiology   576
In the News: Hypothermia and the Diving Reflex   586
The Clinical Dimension   588
Life Span   612
Common Abbreviations   612
Case Study   614
Real World Report   615
Review and Application   617
Vocabulary Review   623
Answers   628

CHAPTER 13   **Lymphatic System and Immunity**   637

Professional Profile   638
Introduction   638
Medical Term Parts   639
Anatomy and Physiology   641
The Clinical Dimension   652

In the News: Antimicrobial Resistance   660
Life Span   665
Common Abbreviations   666
Case Study   667
Real World Report   668
Review and Application   669
Vocabulary Review   674
Answers   677

CHAPTER 14   **Digestive System**   685

Professional Profile   686
Introduction   686
Medical Term Parts   687
Anatomy and Physiology   690
The Clinical Dimension   707
In the News: Obesity in America   716
Life Span   734
Common Abbreviations   735
Case Study   736
Real World Report   738
Review and Application   739
Vocabulary Review   745
Answers   751

CHAPTER 15   **Urinary System**   761

Professional Profile   762
Introduction   762
Medical Term Parts   763
Anatomy and Physiology   766
The Clinical Dimension   772
In the News: Hemolytic Uremic Syndrome   781
Life Span   790
Common Abbreviations   791
Case Study   792
Real World Report   794
Review and Application   796
Vocabulary Review   803
Answers   806

CHAPTER 16   **Reproductive Systems**   815

Professional Profile   816
Introduction   816
Medical Term Parts   817
Anatomy and Physiology   820
The Clinical Dimension   839
In the News: Male Birth Control from
   an Indonesian Plant   865
Life Span   870
Common Abbreviations   871
Case Study   873
Real World Report   874

Review and Application   875
Vocabulary Review   881
Answers   886

CHAPTER 17   **Pregnancy, Human Development, and Child Health**   897

Professional Profile   898
Introduction   898
Medical Term Parts   899
Anatomy and Physiology   901
In the News: A Twin Inside a Twin   915
The Clinical Dimension   919
Life Span   947
Common Abbreviations   948
Case Study   950
Real World Report   951
Review and Application   952
Vocabulary Review   957
Answers   961

CHAPTER 18   **Mental Health**   971

Professional Profile   972
Introduction   972
Medical Term Parts   973
Anatomy and Physiology   975
The Clinical Dimension   979
In the News: Alzheimer Disease Present Physically
    but Not Psychologically   989
Life Span   1014
Common Abbreviations   1015
Case Study   1016
Real World Report   1017
Review and Application   1019
Vocabulary Review   1023
Answers   1028

CHAPTER 19   **Pharmacology**   1037

Professional Profile   1038
Introduction   1038
Medical Term Parts   1039
Fundamentals   1040
In the News: Color Does Matter   1048
The Clinical Dimension   1048
Life Span   1070
Common Abbreviations   1070
Case Study   1072
Real World Report   1073
Review and Application   1074
Vocabulary Review   1078
Answers   1083

CHAPTER 20   **Oncology**   1091

Professional Profile   1092
Introduction   1092
Medical Term Parts   1093
Anatomy and Physiology   1095
The Clinical Dimension   1102
In the News: Cancer-Sniffing Canines   1122
Life Span   1126
Common Abbreviations   1127
Case Study   1128
Real World Report   1129
Review and Application   1130
Vocabulary Review   1134
Answers   1139

CHAPTER 21   **Gerontology**   1149

Professional Profile   1150
Introduction   1150
Medical Term Parts   1151
Fundamentals   1153
The Clinical Dimension   1155
In the News: Long-Lived Okinawans   1188
Common Abbreviations   1189
Case Study   1190
Real World Report   1191
Review and Application   1193
Vocabulary Review   1197
Answers   1202

Index   1211

CHAPTER 1

Introduction to Medical Terminology

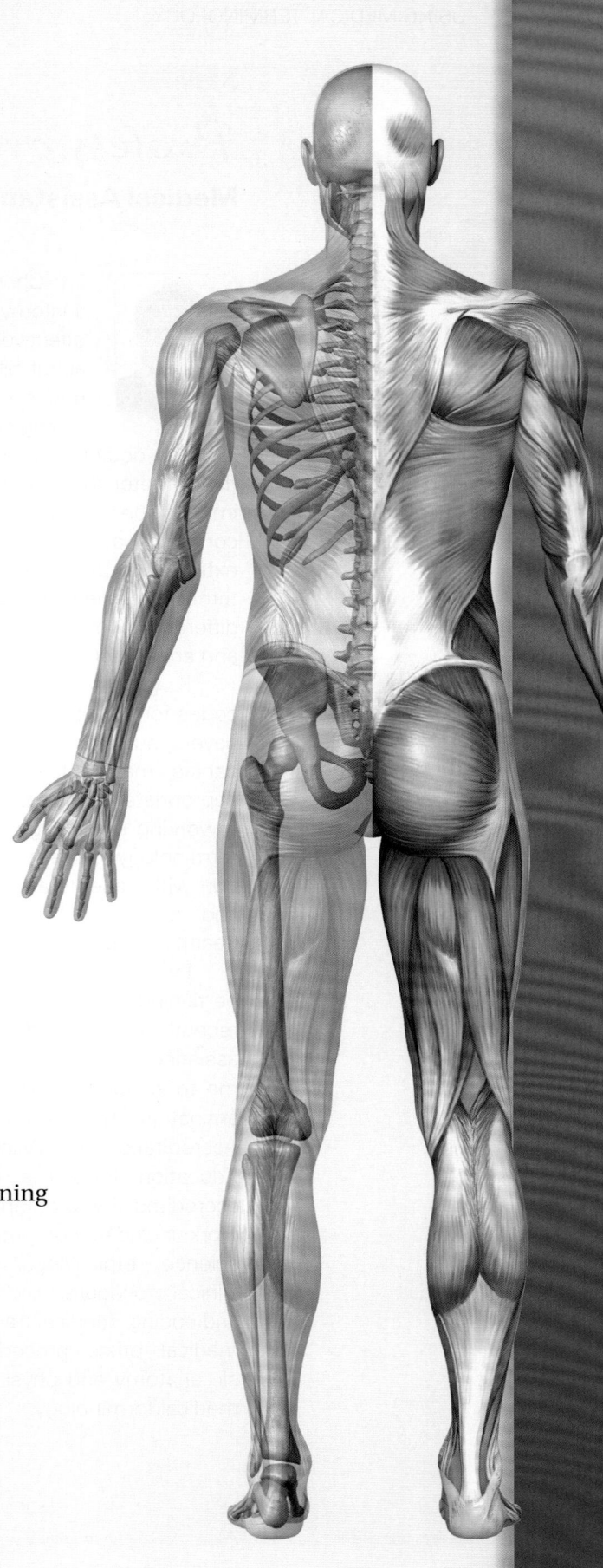

OBJECTIVES

After completing this chapter, you should be able to:

1. Summarize how medical terms are derived.

2. State the importance of coding guidelines as outlined in *Current Procedural Terminology* and *International Classification of Diseases.*

3. Define the terms *prefix, suffix, root,* and *combining form.*

4. Write scientific names correctly.

5. State the general rules for pronouncing medical terms.

6. State the rules for making plural forms of singular words.

7. Define the meanings of common medical prefixes, combining forms, and suffixes.

8. Pronounce medical terms correctly.

9. Define abbreviations of common medical terms.

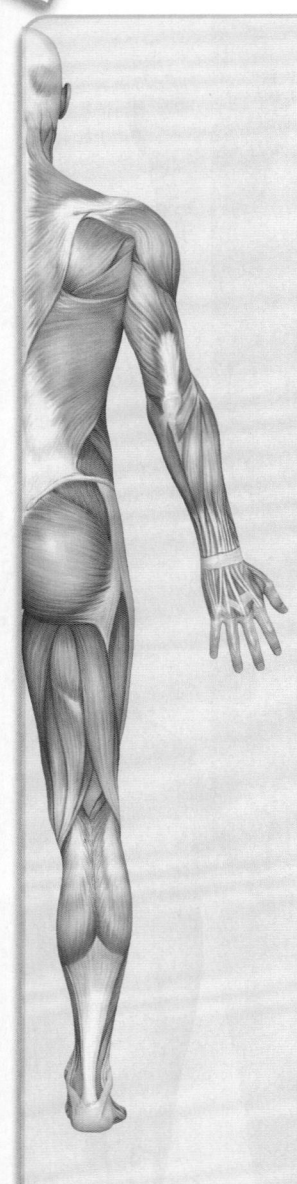

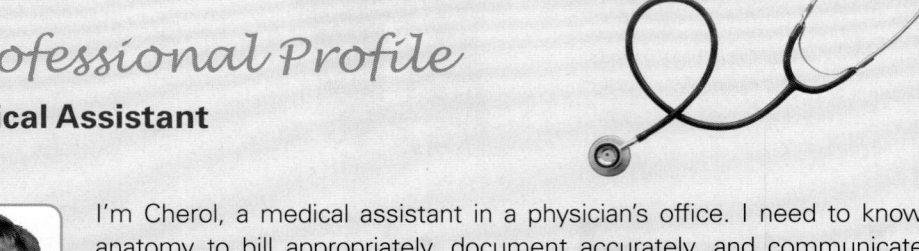

Professional Profile

Medical Assistant

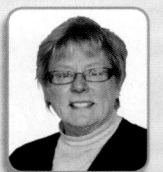

I'm Cherol, a medical assistant in a physician's office. I need to know anatomy to bill appropriately, document accurately, and communicate effectively within the medical field. In our office we recently had an issue about billing codes. (The code is a system of numbers that stands for medical procedures and is used for reimbursement purposes.) The following situation shows the importance of anatomy in the work that I do.

The doctor had accessed the left femoral artery (upper leg artery), maneuvered the catheter to the right common iliac artery (extension of femoral artery), and then imaged the renal artery (kidney artery), which was anastomosed (connected) to the common iliac. A coder in our office questioned whether this should be coded as an extremity angio (vessel in the leg) or a selective renal (kidney vessel) procedure. As it turned out, the procedure could be coded as a selective renal into the iliac with two different codes. You can see how important it is to understand medical terminology and anatomy (**Figure 1-1**)!

If we assign inappropriate codes for a procedure, third-party payers such as insurance companies may not reimburse us appropriately. In addition, I need a working knowledge of medical terminology for clear communication with patients and physicians and for understanding written health records.

I've taken an array of courses pertaining to health careers. Most recently, I completed the medical assisting program, which enabled me to sit for the certification examination. The Commission on Accreditation of Allied Health Education Programs (CAAHEP) accredited this program. Coursework included computers, basic science, ethical/legal concerns, clinical procedures, medical billing and coding, medical transcription, medical office procedures, basic anatomy and physiology, and medical terminology.

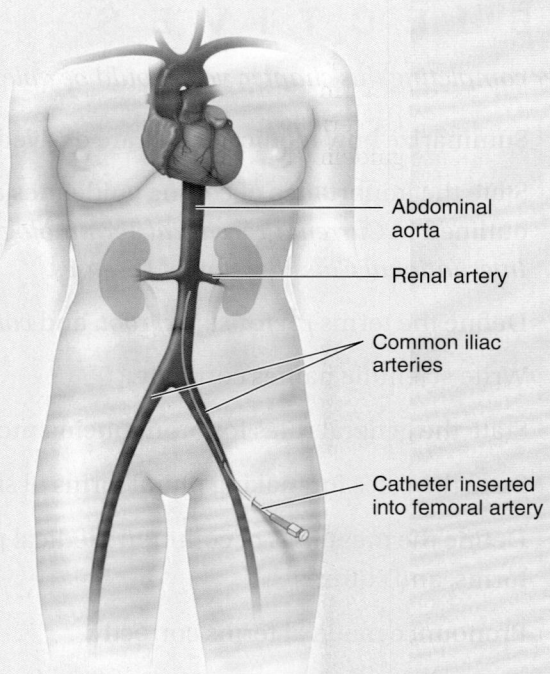

Abdominal aorta

Renal artery

Common iliac arteries

Catheter inserted into femoral artery

Figure 1-1 Is this procedure an "extremity angio" or a "selective renal"? It is important to understand anatomy even for a simple billing procedure in a medical office.

INTRODUCTION

*A*natomical and physiological language is the foundation of medical terminology. The book that serves as the authority on correct anatomical naming, called **nomenclature**, is *Terminologia Anatomica*. It is also referred to by its English title, *International Anatomical Terminology*. Its purpose is to ensure that scientists and doctors worldwide use the same name for each body structure. To achieve this goal, *Terminologia Anatomica* provides standardized terms for all body parts. Despite valiant attempts, the language of medicine is not yet uniform, as you can see by reading medical reports and textbooks, which often refer to the same structure by two different terms.

Medical terms derived from a person's name are called **eponyms**. Body parts, diseases, syndromes, tests, and procedures are often named after their discoverer, or the person who first described it, or a scientist who perfected or invented a particular test or procedure. Eponyms are still used, but there is a general trend toward eliminating them. It is simpler to use the correct anatomical name for a body part or disease description because that eliminates confusion and creates standardization. For example, Cowper glands are more correctly identified as bulbourethral glands. The word *Cowper* does not assist in locating these glands, whereas the word *bulbourethral* indicates that the structures are bulbs found around a portion of the urethra (**Figure 1-2**).

Eponyms can be written in either a possessive or nonpossessive form. Adding an apostrophe s (*'s*) to the nonpossessive form changes it to the possessive form. For example, *Alzheimer disease* becomes *Alzheimer's disease* and *Huntington disease* becomes *Huntington's disease*. A person's medical training or geographic location often determines which form is used. As a result, eponyms—with or without the *'s*—and their alternate medical terms may be cited in general medical writing. This book will use eponyms without the *'s*.

Many medical terms are derived from the Greek and Latin languages. For this reason, when learning these terms it may seem as if you are taking a foreign language course. Fortunately, there are guidelines and rules to assist you. Once you conquer the terms, a world of opportunity exists. The number of careers for which a knowledge of medical terminology is

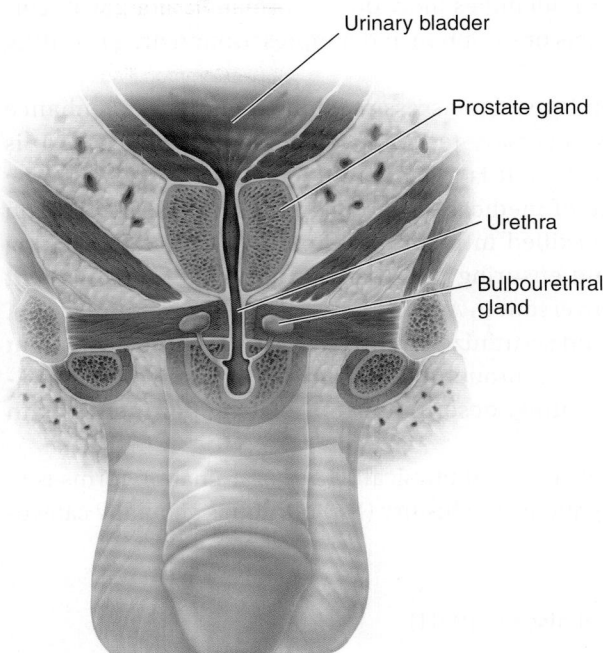

Urinary bladder

Prostate gland

Urethra

Bulbourethral gland

Figure 1-2 Bulbourethral (Cowper) glands. The glands are more correctly identified as bulbourethral glands, which indicates that the structures are bulbs surrounding a portion of the urethra.

BOX 1-1

PROFESSIONAL FIELDS THAT
REQUIRE KNOWLEDGE OF MEDICAL TERMINOLOGY

- Allied health
- Biology
- Chemistry
- Cytotechnology
- Dentistry
- Dietetics
- Engineering
- Epidemiology
- General technology
- Genetics/genetic counseling
- Health education
- Health services
- Law
- Massage therapy
- Medical assisting
- Medical billing
- Medical coding

- Medical editing
- Medical illustration
- Medical transcription
- Medicine
- Microbiology
- Nursing
- Occupational therapy
- Optometry
- Pharmacy
- Phlebotomy
- Physical therapy
- Psychiatry
- Psychology
- Radiology technology
- Respiratory therapy
- Stenography
- Technical writing

beneficial is growing. Medical billing and related occupations are among the fastest growing careers in the United States. As the allied health fields expand, so will the job market. Some occupations and fields of study that require a solid foundation in medical terminology are given in **Box 1-1**.

THE MEDICAL RECORD

A patient's **medical record** provides the person's physical, emotional, nutritional, and social history. The personal medical history form identifies individual information along with current and past medical conditions. It also lists prescription and nonprescription drug use, drug sensitivities, and allergies.

Patient medical record information is used to assess previous treatment, to enhance the continuity of care, and to avoid unnecessary tests and/or procedures. Because it is an invaluable tool for health care providers, it is a working document that needs to be as complete as possible. So, knowledge of medical terminology is essential. The person documenting the information must be skilled in recording the data accurately, making sure the terms are spelled correctly, and ensuring that the facts supplied by the patient make sense within the context of the conversation. As a primary means of communication, this collection of facts and data is read and scrutinized by all clinicians treating the patient or office personnel servicing the person. A thorough understanding of medical terminology is necessary for adequately documenting, describing, and relaying pertinent health information.

The aim of the questions on typical history and physical (H&P) examination forms is to obtain a complete representation of the patient. The history (Hx) portion is generally categorized into the following headings:

- Chief complaint (CC)
- Medical/surgical history or past medical history (PMH)
- History of present illness (HPI)

- Family history (FH)
- Social history (SH)
- Occupational history (OH)
- Diet/exercise history
- Review of systems (ROS).

Females also answer questions pertaining to menstrual, gynecologic, pregnancy, contraceptive, and sexual history. Males answer questions of contraception, sexual history, and performance status.

Once the personal medical history has been obtained, practitioners typically evaluate the patient through a physical examination (PE or Px). The physical examination includes assessment of the following:

- General appearance
- Vital signs
- Head, eyes, ears, nose, and throat (HEENT)
- Neck, lungs, heart, rectopelvis, extremities, and neurological condition
- Laboratory data.

The report ends with the general impression (IMP), or general view, of the patient's condition and a plan (P). An example history and physical form is shown in **Figure 1-3**.

Through conversation, written documentation, and a quick examination, more information is obtained for the H&P form. Commonly used terms and phrases (with their abbreviations) to document findings include:

- Complains of (c/o)
- Diagnosis (Dx)
- Family members living and well (L&W)
- No acute distress (NAD)
- No known allergies (NKA)
- No known drug allergies (NKDA)
- Pupils equal, round, and reactive to light and accommodation (PERRLA)
- Rule out (R/O)
- Symptom (Sx)
- Usual childhood diseases (UCHD)
- Within normal limits (WNL).

Progress notes, also called **SOAP notes**, are made in a patient's medical record after the H&P has been finished. These notes are used in patient records for organizing follow-up data, evaluating, and planning. SOAP is an acronym for **s**ubjective, **o**bjective, **a**ssessment, and **p**lan. The subjective portion identifies the patient's symptoms, and the objective section lists the signs. **Symptoms** are experienced by the patient and may include such things as pain and dizziness. **Signs** include functions that can be measured, such as blood pressure, respiration rate, temperature, height, and weight. The assessment is the professional judgment made of the patient's progress. Finally, the plan is the outline for treatment. **Figure 1-4** shows a typical progress note using the SOAP method.

Federal law mandates that patient health information be treated with respect and confidentiality. Public Law 104–191—the **Health Insurance Portability & Accountability Act (HIPAA)** of 1996—is a set of national standards that protects the privacy and personal health information of Americans. It applies to all medical information that is conveyed orally, in written form, or by electronic means. The law provides standards for security, transactions, and coding. It further serves as a guide for privacy, research, and public health.

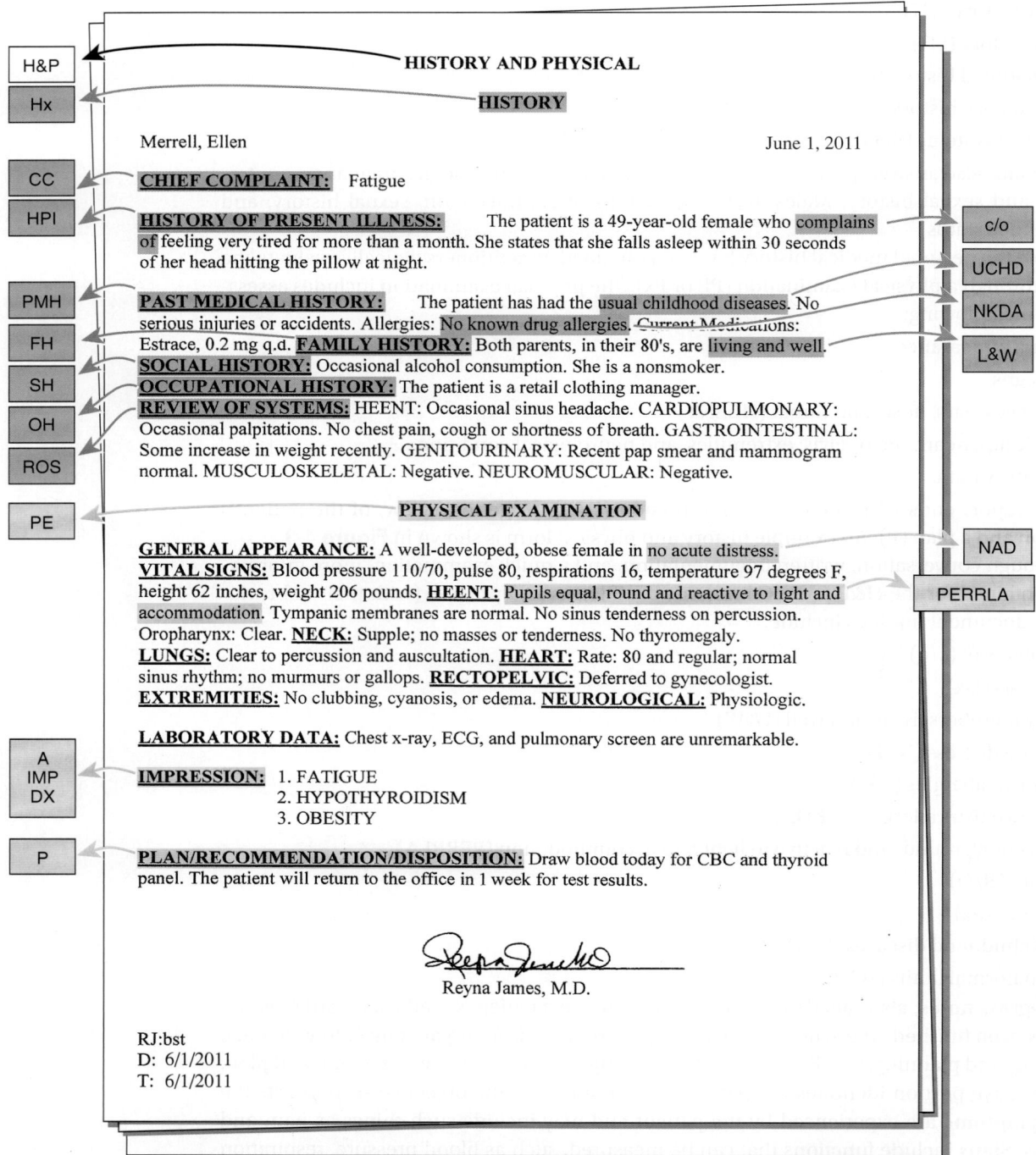

HISTORY AND PHYSICAL

H&P

HISTORY

Hx

Merrell, Ellen   June 1, 2011

CC   **CHIEF COMPLAINT:**   Fatigue

HPI   **HISTORY OF PRESENT ILLNESS:**   The patient is a 49-year-old female who complains   c/o
            of feeling very tired for more than a month. She states that she falls asleep within 30 seconds
            of her head hitting the pillow at night.   UCHD

PMH   **PAST MEDICAL HISTORY:**   The patient has had the usual childhood diseases. No   NKDA
            serious injuries or accidents. Allergies: No known drug allergies. Current Medications:
FH   Estrace, 0.2 mg q.d. **FAMILY HISTORY:** Both parents, in their 80's, are living and well.   L&W
            SOCIAL HISTORY: Occasional alcohol consumption. She is a nonsmoker.
SH   **OCCUPATIONAL HISTORY:** The patient is a retail clothing manager.
            REVIEW OF SYSTEMS: HEENT: Occasional sinus headache. CARDIOPULMONARY:
OH   Occasional palpitations. No chest pain, cough or shortness of breath. GASTROINTESTINAL:
            Some increase in weight recently. GENITOURINARY: Recent pap smear and mammogram
ROS   normal. MUSCULOSKELETAL: Negative. NEUROMUSCULAR: Negative.

PE   **PHYSICAL EXAMINATION**

            GENERAL APPEARANCE: A well-developed, obese female in no acute distress.   NAD
            VITAL SIGNS: Blood pressure 110/70, pulse 80, respirations 16, temperature 97 degrees F,
            height 62 inches, weight 206 pounds. **HEENT:** Pupils equal, round and reactive to light and   PERRLA
            accommodation. Tympanic membranes are normal. No sinus tenderness on percussion.
            Oropharynx: Clear. **NECK:** Supple; no masses or tenderness. No thyromegaly.
            LUNGS: Clear to percussion and auscultation. **HEART:** Rate: 80 and regular; normal
            sinus rhythm; no murmurs or gallops. **RECTOPELVIC:** Deferred to gynecologist.
            EXTREMITIES: No clubbing, cyanosis, or edema. **NEUROLOGICAL:** Physiologic.

            LABORATORY DATA: Chest x-ray, ECG, and pulmonary screen are unremarkable.

A   **IMPRESSION:**   1. FATIGUE
IMP   2. HYPOTHYROIDISM
DX   3. OBESITY

P   **PLAN/RECOMMENDATION/DISPOSITION:** Draw blood today for CBC and thyroid
            panel. The patient will return to the office in 1 week for test results.

                                            Reyna James, M.D.

            RJ:bst
            D: 6/1/2011
            T: 6/1/2011

Figure 1-3 A typical history and physical form.

In addition to the history and physical reports and progress notes of individual patients, many health care professionals must be acquainted with two important general references: *Current Procedural Terminology* (*CPT*) and *International Classification of Diseases* (*ICD*). The *CPT* lists codes for working clinical nomenclature. The codes describe procedures and services performed in health care settings that are used for reporting medical services. These HIPAA-mandated procedure codes are used in all medical billing. The *CPT* provides a means of communication among physicians, patients, and third parties

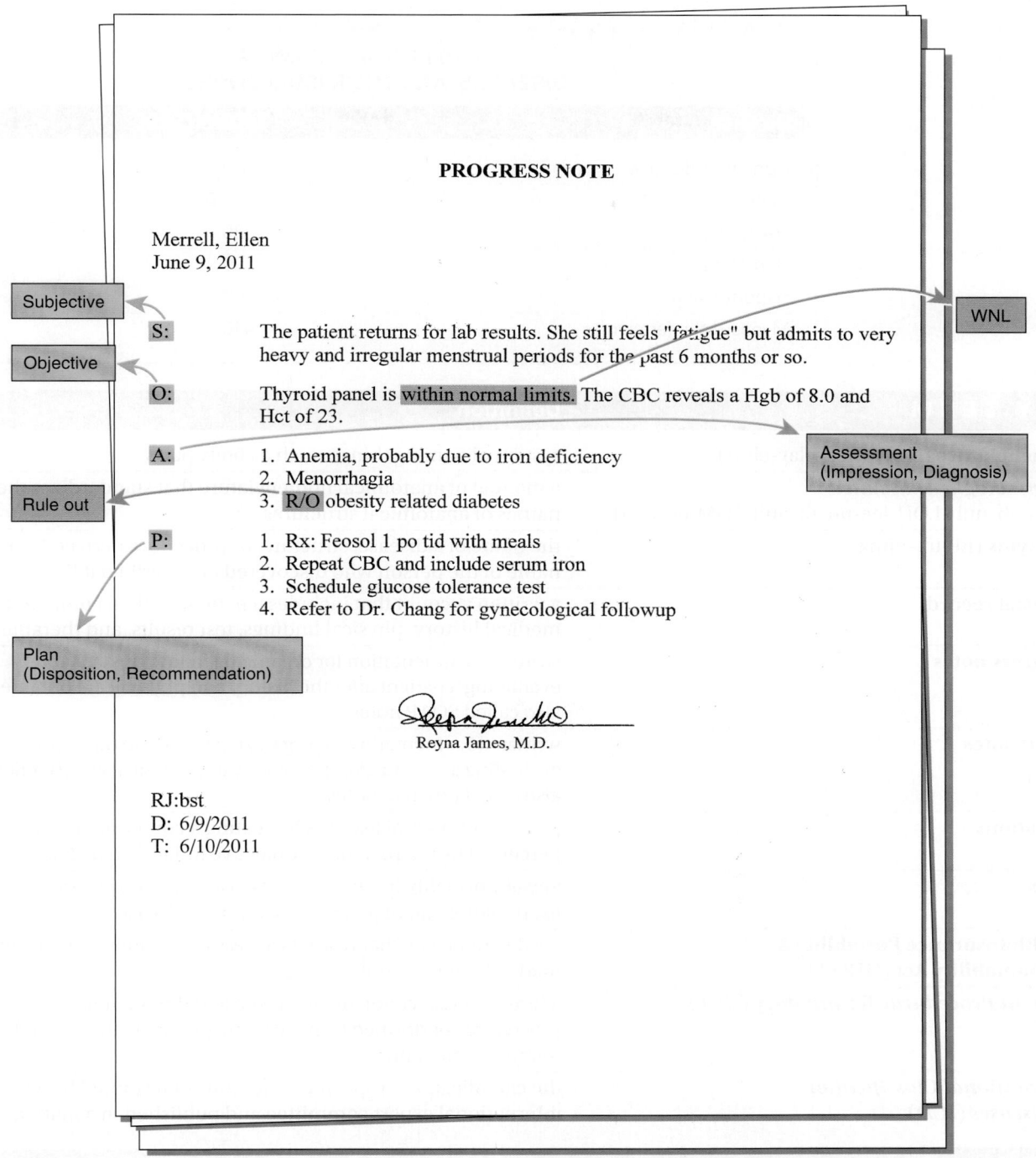

Figure 1-4 A progress note utilizing the SOAP method of charting.

(insurance companies, Medicare, and Medicaid). The *ICD* is similar to the *CPT,* but its focus is on coding related to human disease. The code sets are necessary for statistical purposes, medical documentation, and reimbursement. Accurate coding is essential to the reimbursement process. At the writing of this text, the 2010 *ICD-10, Standard Edition Draft,* was available, but the 2009 ICD-9 was still readily used. Regardless of edition, these manuals will be referred to as *CPT* and *ICD* in this textbook. Examples of ICD codes are given in **Table 1-1**.

T A B L E **1-1**

EXAMPLES OF COMMON DISEASES AND THEIR ICD-9 CODES

Disease	ICD-9 Code
Alzheimer disease	331.0
Asthma	493.90
Fracture	829.0
Hematuria	599.7
Hypertension	401.9
Myocardial infarction	410.9

KEY TERM	Definition
nomenclature (NOH-men-clay-chur)	system of naming things, such as body parts
Terminologia Anatomica (tur-mih-nuh-LOH-jee-uh ah-nuh-TOM-eh-kuh)	a manual of anatomical nomenclature that standardizes the names of anatomical structures
eponyms (EP-uh-nimz)	the name of a disease, structure, or procedure derived from the name of the person who discovered or described it first
medical record	a written account that includes a patient's initial complaints, medical history, physical findings, test results, and therapies
progress notes	written documentation for organizing follow-up data and evaluating a patient after the history and physical are obtained; also called SOAP notes
SOAP notes	written documentation for organizing follow-up data and evaluating a patient after the history and physical are obtained; also called progress notes
symptoms	physical or mental features indicating a condition that are perceived by the patient; a subjective indication of disease
signs	any abnormality indicative of disease that is discovered on examination; an objective indication of disease
Health Insurance Portability & Accountability Act (HIPAA)	1996 Federal law that restricts access to an individual's private medical information
Current Procedural Terminology (CPT)	a formal classification of diagnostic and therapeutic procedures performed by health care providers that is used for reimbursement purposes
International Classification of Diseases (ICD)	the classification of specific conditions determined by an international expert committee and published in a manual

KEY TERM PRACTICE: *Introduction and The Medical Record*

1. A _____ is an objective indication of disease.

2. A _____ is a subjective indication or feeling about a disease.

3. The federal law that restricts access to an individual's private medical information is known as the _____, which is abbreviated as _____.

4. _____ are medical names derived from the name of a person.

5. The manual that classifies specific conditions by codes is called the _____.

A BRIEF LESSON IN LANGUAGE

The purpose of language is to communicate effectively and accurately, so spelling counts! This is particularly true for medical terms. For example, an incision in the *ilium* or the *ileum* could be the difference between cutting a hip bone (ilium) or a segment of the small intestine (ileum) (**Figure 1-5**)!

We will concern ourselves primarily with vocabulary and secondarily with pronunciation, also called phonetics. Vocabulary is governed by rules for word formation. However, written and spoken languages are dynamic—for example, our language is constantly changing as terms are created for new technology and new knowledge. These changes are occurring rapidly in the field of medicine, and keeping pace can be challenging.

Word Parts

Word parts is the general phrase used in this text to identify **prefixes** (beginnings of words), **suffixes** (word endings), and **combining forms** (a word element used in combination with another element to form a word). For example, *bio-*, which means "life," forms *biology*. A **word root** is the main part of a medical term and conveys its main meaning. Memorizing the definition of a word root and its combining form will help you figure out the meaning of new medical terms.

In the word part tables, hyphens are used to signify prefixes, suffixes, and combining forms. The hyphen indicates that a particular word element forms part of a compound word and indicates the placement of the word part when used to form a medical term. For example, a hyphen placed after the word part, as in *hypo-*, means the part is a prefix or a combining form. A hyphen placed before the word part, as in *-ology*, means the part is a suffix.

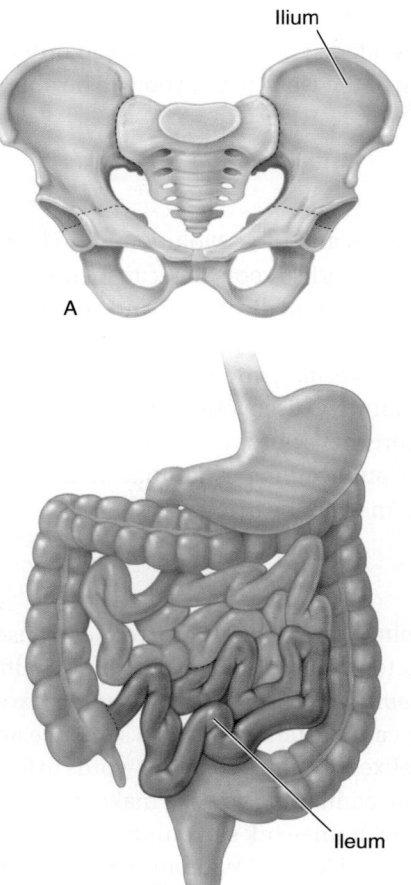

Ilium

A

Ileum

B

Figure 1-5 Correct spelling is important for medical terms, when an incision in the ilium **(A)** or the ileum **(B)** could mean the difference between surgery on the hipbone or a segment of the small intestine.

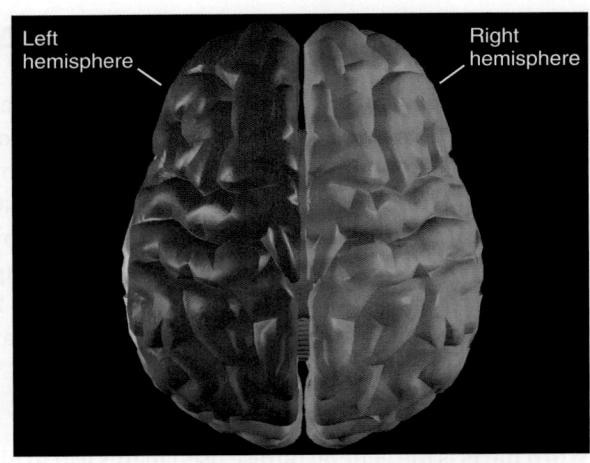

Figure 1-6 The brain is made up of two hemispheres, or two halves. This figure shows areas of the brain, which have been colorized.

Many medical terms are made by combining word parts. To illustrate, the word *cardiology,* which means "the study of the heart and its functions," is made by joining the word part *cardio-,* which means "heart," with *-logy,* which means "study of."

Prefixes and suffixes are not independent words but word parts that modify the word root's meaning. As mentioned, prefixes are word parts that appear at the beginning of the medical word or base. Not all medical terms have prefixes; but when present, prefixes make the meaning more specific. For example, the word *sphere* means "round." Adding the prefix *hemi-,* which means "half," creates the word *hemisphere,* meaning "half of a sphere," as in the sentence "The brain has two hemispheres" (**Figure 1-6**).

Suffixes are word parts that appear at the end of the word or base. In medical words, a suffix may describe a body condition. For example, *-itis* means "inflammation," so *prostatitis* refers to an "inflamed prostate." You do not need to be skilled at dissecting words in order to learn medical terminology, but if you learn the meaning of the word parts, you will be able to figure out many of the new medical terms you read.

Word Etymology and Word Roots

Etymology is the study of the origins of words or word parts and their evolution to their current form and meaning. Medical terms in particular have historical roots that can be traced to Greek and Latin origins. Recall that a *word root* is the basis of a medical term and conveys its main meaning. Think of the root as the word form without a prefix or a suffix. Other terms that mean the same thing as "root" are *base, stem, theme,* and *radical.* Remember that language is always evolving and changing as new terms are coined for new discoveries, inventions, techniques, procedures, processes, and therapies. Furthermore, new words often develop through everyday spoken or written use before they appear in publications. Note that dictionaries include words that have a history of use, so newer words may not be listed yet.

Combining Vowels

To make medical terms easier to pronounce, the combining vowels *o* and *i* are frequently used between word parts. These combining vowels are added to word roots when attaching a suffix that begins with a consonant or another root. The term *combining form* describes the word root with its associated combining vowel. A combining form cannot stand alone in a sentence and makes sense only when it occurs in combination with prefixes or suffixes or other words to form compound words. For example, *viscer* means "organ." The combining vowel *o* makes the word part *viscero-.* An example term is *visceroskeleton,* "the bony framework surrounding an organ." Another example is *hepatorenal,* which refers to the liver and kidney. Without the combining vowel, it would be *hepatrenal,* which is more difficult to pronounce. Again, if you know the meaning of a medical term's prefix, suffix, and root, you can figure out what the term means.

Biological Naming System

Medical reports may cite names of various types of organisms, ranging from plants and worms to viruses and bacteria. Technical notation of such names follows an accepted standard for naming organisms. Organisms have two words in their name, a genus name and a species name. The names of organisms are set in italics (or when written by hand, underlined). The genus name appears first and is capitalized, and the species name appears next and begins with a lowercase letter. This is the accepted international classification system, or taxonomy. For example, the common bacterium found in yogurt is *Lactobacillus acidophilus* (or Lactobacillus acidophilus). The genus name is *Lactobacillus,* and the species name is *acidophilus*. After it has been spelled out once, the genus name is often abbreviated; for example, the yogurt bacterium is abbreviated *L. acidophilus*. Names of microbes often appear on laboratory reports and are mentioned in everyday life, such as when a contaminated food is recalled.

PRONUNCIATION KEY

Correct pronunciation of medical terms is necessary for good communication. For example, in spoken language, *renin* (REE-nin), an enzyme released by the kidneys, is often mispronounced as *rennin* (REN-in), an enzyme found in the stomach of calves. The difference in meaning is profound because renin is an enzyme in the kidney that converts one compound to another and plays a role in blood pressure, but rennin is an enzyme found in calf stomach juice. Note, however, that complete uniformity in pronunciation of medical terms, like other words in any language, is not possible. Geography, training, and common practice all influence pronunciation, so medical dictionaries commonly give variant pronunciations. For that reason, any pronunciation key should be used only as a guide.

Table 1-2 is the pronunciation guide for the terms in this book. In parentheses, after most terms in the key term tables, the words are spelled just as they sound, or phonetically. The syllables are separated by a hyphen, and individual words are separated by a double space within the parentheses. Stressed, or accented, syllables are in capital letters. Alternate spelling and singular/plural forms are given when appropriate. Audio is available for most terms at www.thepoint.lww.com/nath2e.

TABLE 1-2

PRONUNCIATION KEY

Letters	Phonetics	Examples	Pronunciation
Long vowel sounds			
a	ay	bay	BAY
		fatal	FAY-tul
e	ee	bee	BEE
		fetal	FEE-tul
i	eye	eye	EYE
		island	EYE-lund
i	igh	arthritis	ahr-THRIGH-tis
o	oh	post	POHST
		low	LOH
u	yoo	union	YOON-yun
u	soo	supine	SOO-pine
		superficial	soo-per-FISH-ul
u	ew	mute	mewt

continued

continued from page 11

Letters	Phonetics	Examples	Pronunciation
In-between vowel sounds[a]			
a, e, i, o, u, y	uh	anatomy	uh-NAT-uh-mee
Short vowel sounds			
a	a	fat	FAT
e	e	get	GET
i	i	bit	BIT
o	o	not	NOT
u	u	but	BUT
Combination vowels			
ae	ee	bursae	BER-see
oe	e	roentgen	RENT-gen
oi	oi	void	VOID
eu at the beginning of a word	yoo	eupnea	yoop-NEE-uh.
Hard and Soft Sounds			
c before e, i, and y	soft s	cerebrum	se-REE-brum
		cicatrix	SIK-uh-triks
		cystic	SIS-tick
c before a, o, and u	hard k	cava	KAY-vuh
		colon	KOH-lun
		culture	KUL-chur
g before e, i, and y	soft j	gene	JEEN
		gingivitis	jin-ji-VYE-tis
		gyrus	JYE-rus
g before a, o, and u	hard g	galactometer	gal-ack-TOM-eh-tur
		goiter	GOY-tur
		gustation	gus-TAY-shun
Other consonant/vowel sounds			
ch at the beginning of a word	sometimes k	cholesterol	koh-LES-tur-ol
		chronic	KRON-ick
dys at the beginning of a word	dis	dystrophy	DIS-truh-fee
i at the end of a word	eye	nuclei	NEW-klee-eye
gn at the beginning of a word	n	gnathic	NATH-ick
ph at the beginning of a word	f	pharmacology	fahr-muh-KOL-uh-jee
pn at the beginning of a word	n	pneumonia	new-MOH-nyuh
pn in the middle of a word	hard p, hard n	apnea	AP-nee-uh
ps at the beginning of a word	s	psychosis	sigh-KOH-sis
pt at the beginning of a word	t	pterygoid	TERR-i-goid
rh at the beginning of a word	r	rheumatoid	ROO-muh-toid
x at the beginning of a word	z	xiphoid	ZYE-foid

[a]*Note:* This sound is referred to as a *schwa,* which is a neutral or unstressed vowel sound. It is the most common sound in the American English language and can be found in words such as *about* (uh-BOWT), *synthesis* (SIN-thuh-sis), *harmony* (HAR-muh-nee), *medium* (MEE-dee-um), and *syringe* (suh-RINJ).

RULES FOR PLURALS

It is important to follow the general rules for making plural forms of singular words. **Table 1-3** lists the rules for common endings.

TABLE 1-3

RULES FOR PLURALS

Singular Ending	Rule	Plural Ending	Example
-a	keep the -a and add -e	-ae	vertebra → vertebrae
-ax	drop -ax and add -aces	-aces	thorax → thoraces
-en	drop -en and add -ina	-ina	foramen → foramina
-ex	drop -ex and add -ices	-ices	pollex → polices
-ion	drop -ion and add -ia	-ia	ganglion → ganglia
-is	drop -is and add -es	-es	axis → axes
-itis	drop -itis and add -itides	-itides	dermatitis → dermatitides
-ium	drop -ium and add -ia	-ia	epithelium → epithelia
-ix	drop -ix and add -ices	-ices	appendix → appendices
-oma	keep -oma and add -ta	-omata	hematoma → hematomata
	keep -ma and add -s	-omas	hematoma → hematomas
-sis	drop -sis and add -ses	-ses	diagnosis → diagnoses
-um	drop -um and add -a	-a	ovum → ova
-us	drop -us and add -i	-i	embolus → emboli
-x	drop -x and add -ges	-ges	phalanx → phalanges
-y	drop -y and add -ies	-ies	biopsy → biopsies

KEY TERM	Definition
word parts	prefixes, suffixes, or combining forms
prefixes	word elements that are attached to the beginning of a word
suffixes	word elements that are added to the end of a word
combining forms	elements used in combination with another element to form a word
word root	the basic, meaningful part of a word that is left when any prefixes or suffixes are removed
etymology (et-uh-MOL-uh-jee)	the study of the origins of words or word parts and how they have arrived at their current form and meaning

KEY TERM PRACTICE: *A Brief Lesson in Language*

1. A _____ is a word element that is attached to the beginning of a word.

2. _____ is the study of the origins of words or word parts and how they have arrived at their current form and meaning.

3. Write the plural form of septum. _____

4. Write the singular form of pharynges. _____

5. The _____ is the basic, meaningful part of a word that is left when any prefixes or suffixes are removed.

MEDICAL TERM PARTS

Common Prefixes

Commonly used medical term prefixes, suffixes, and combining forms are introduced in this section. Note that some combining forms are also used as prefixes.

Word Part	Meaning	Example with Definition
a-	without	*arrhythmia*; without a regular heart rhythm
ab-	away from	*abduct*; to move a limb away from the midline of the body
ad-	toward	*adduct*; to move a limb toward the midline of the body
ambi-	both sides	*ambidextrous*; able to use both the right and the left hand with equal skill
an-	without	*anaerobic*; living without oxygen
ana-	up	*anacrotic*; referring to the upstroke of the arterial pulse tracing
ante-	before, in front of	*antecubital*; referring to the front of the elbow
anti-	against	*antibacterial*; an agent that works against bacteria growth
auto-	self	*autoimmunity*; condition in which the immune response is directed against the body's own (self) tissues
brady-	slow	*bradycardia*; slow heart rate
caud-, caudo-	tail	*caudal ligament*; fibrous bands that extend from the skin to the coccyx (tail region)
cephal-, cephalo-	head	*cephalgia*; headache
chrom-, chromo-	color, colored	*chromotherapy*; treatment of disease with colored light
circum-	around	*circumcision*; to cut around an anatomical part
contra-	against	*contraindicant*; method of treatment that is against the advised treatment; favoring the reverse
cry-, cryo-	cold, freezing	*cryotherapy*; the use of cold in the treatment of disease
cyst-, cysti-, cysto-	bladder	*cystogram*; x-ray of the bladder
de-	from, away	*deaminase*; any enzyme that removes (takes away) an amino group from a compound
dextr-, dextro-	right, toward the right	*dextral*; right-handed
dys-	painful, difficult	*dysuria*; pain or difficult in urinating
ec-	out of, away from	*eccentric amputation*; limb removal with the scar of the stump off-center
encephal-, encephalo-	brain	*encephalitis*; inflammation of the brain
end-, endo-	within, inner	*endocardium*; the innermost layer of the heart
epi-	upon, following	*epicondyle*; a projection on a bone above or upon the condyle
equi-	equal, equally	*equilibrium*; a state of balance
eu-	good, well, normal	*eupnea*; normal breathing
ex-, exo-	out, outside	*exoenzyme*; an enzyme that performs its function outside the cell
extra-	without, outside of	*extracellular*; outside of the cell
heter-, hetero-	other, different	*heterozygous*; used to describe a cell that has two or more different versions of at least one of its genes

continued

continued from page 14

Word Part	Meaning	Example with Definition
homo-	same	*homozygous*; having two identical genes at the corresponding loci of homologous chromosomes
hydro-	water	*hydrocephalus*; a condition marked by an excessive amount of cerebrospinal fluid within the spaces of the brain; also called "water on the brain"
hyper-	above, beyond, over	*hyperthyroidism*; the overproduction of thyroid hormones
hypo-	below, under, beneath	*hypothyroidism*; the underproduction of thyroid hormones
im-	not, in, within	*impotence*; not able to perform sexual intercourse
in-	not, in, within; appears as im- before b, p, or m	*in utero*; within the womb
infra-	below, under	*infraorbital*; below the orbit
inter-	among, between	*interatrial*; between the atria of the heart
intra-	within, inside	*intraarticular*; within the cavity of a joint
juxta-	near	*juxtaglomerular*; close to a renal glomerulus
mal-	abnormal, bad, ill	*malady*; a disease or illness
mes-, meso-	middle	*mesoderm*; the middle of the three primary germ layers
meta-	between, behind, after, beyond	*metacarpus*; group of five bones of the hand between the wrist (carpus) and the fingers
mid-	middle	*midtarsal*; referring to the middle of the tarsus (ankle)
neo-	new, recent	*neonate* ; newborn
pan-	all, entire	*panacea*; a cure-all
par-, para-	adjacent to, near	*parathyroid*; in the area near the thyroid
per-	through	*percutaneous*; the passage of substances through the skin
peri-	around	*periodontal*; around a tooth
post-	after, behind	*postpartum*; immediately after childbirth
pre-	before	*preanesthetic*; before anesthesia
pro-	supporting, in front of, before	*procephalic*; relating to the front part of the head
pseudo-	false	*pseudoparaplegia*; false paralysis
re-	backward, again	*reactivate*; to render active again, as in an infection
retro-	behind, backward	*retrocecal*; behind the cecum
sinistro-	left, toward the left	*sinistrocardia*; displacement of the heart beyond the normal position toward the left side
sub-	below, under, beneath	*subcutaneous*; beneath the skin
super-	above, beyond	*superinfection*; a new infection beyond one already present
supra-	above, upon	*suprarenal*; above the kidney
sym-	together, with	*symphysis*; growing together
syn-	together, with	*synchondrosis*; a joint in which two bones are united
tachy-	rapid	*tachycardia*; rapid heart rate
trans-	through, across	*transection*; a cross-section or cutting across
ultra-	beyond, excess	*ultraligation*; tying a blood vessel beyond the point where a branch is given off

Word Grouping Exercises

Using the *Common Prefixes* table, identify the prefix for each of the following definitions. The first one has been done as an example.

Definition	Word Part
away from	ab-
abnormal, bad, ill	
above, beyond	
above, beyond, over	
above, upon	
adjacent to, near	
after, behind	
against	A. B.
all, entire	
among, between	
around	A. B.
backward, again	
before	
before, in front of	
behind, backward	
below, under	
below, under, beneath	A. B.
between, behind, after, beyond	
beyond, excess	
bladder	
both sides	
brain	
cold, freezing	
color, colored	
equal, equally	
false	
from, away	
good, well, normal	
head	
left, toward the left	
middle	A. B.
near	

continued

continued from page 16

Definition	Word Part
new, recent	
not	
not, into	
other, different	
out, outside	
out of, away from	
painful, difficult	
rapid	
right, toward the right	
same	
self	
slow	
supporting, in front of, before	
tail	
through	
through, across	
together, with	A. B.
toward	
up	
upon, following	
water	
within, inner	
within, inside	
without	A. B.
without, outside of	

Word Building Exercises

Word parts introduced in the *Common Prefixes* section are listed in the following table. For this exercise, first supply the meaning of each word part, then use the word part to build a word you already know. The word you list under *Common or Known Word* does not have to be a medical term; a commonly used word is fine. Be sure, however, that the word correctly reflects the intended meaning. The first one has been done as an example. Check your answers in a dictionary.

Word Part	Meaning	Common or Known Word	Example Medical Term
ab-	*away from*	*abduct*	abduction
ad-			adduction
ante-			anterior
anti-			antibody
auto-			autoimmune
circum-			circumcision
contra-			contraceptive
dys-			dysuria
ex-, exo-			exhale
heter-, hetero-			heterozygous
homo-			homozygous
hyper-			hypertension
hypo-			hypotonic
inter-			interosseous
intra-			intramuscular
juxta-			juxtaglomerular
meta-			metaphysis
neo-			neoplasm
post-			postpartum
retro-			retroperitoneal
sub-			subdural

Prefixes Related to Number and Size

Commonly used medical prefixes and combining forms pertaining to number or size are introduced in this section. An example showing two prefixes relating to numbers is shown in **Figure 1-7**.

Word Part	Meaning
bi-	two
di-	two
diplo-	double
hemi-	half
hex-, hexa-	six
macr-, macro-	large
maxi-	extra large
mega-	big, large, great
micro-	small
mini-	small, miniature
mono-	one
multi-	many
noni-	nine
oct-, octa-, octo-	eight
pent-, penta-	five
poly-	many, much
quadri-, quadru-	four
semi-	half, partial
sept-, septi-	seven
sex-, sexi-	six
tetra-	four
tri-	three
uni-	one

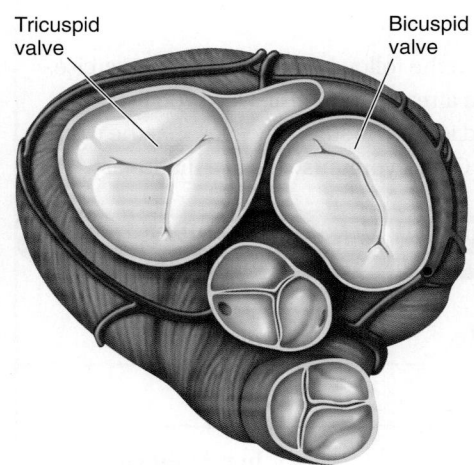

Tricuspid valve

Bicuspid valve

Figure 1-7 The heart has a bicuspid valve and a tricuspid valve. The prefixes *bi-* and *tri-* indicate number. In this case, they refer to the number of cusps, or flaps, in the heart valves.

Word Grouping Exercises

Using the *Prefixes Related to Number and Size* table, identify the prefix or combining form for each of the following definitions. The first one has been done as an example.

Definition	Word Part
two	A. bi- B. di-
big, large, great	
double	
eight	
extra large	
five	
four	A. B.
half	
half, partial	
large	
many	
many, much	
nine	
one	A. B.
seven	
six	A. B.
small	
small, miniature	
three	

Word Building Exercises

Word parts introduced in the *Prefixes Related to Number and Size* section are listed in the following table. For this exercise, first supply the meaning of each word part, then use the word part to build a word you already know. The word you list under *Common or Known Word* does not have to be a medical term; a commonly used word is fine. Be sure, however, that the word correctly reflects the intended meaning. The first one has been done as an example. Check your answers in a dictionary.

Word Part	Meaning	Common or Known Word	Example Medical Term
bi-	two	bicycle	bicuspid
di-			diotic
hemi-			hemisphere

continued

continued from page 20

Word Part	Meaning	Common or Known Word	Example Medical Term
macr-, macro-			macromastia
micro-			microorganism
mono-			monozygous
multi-			multicellular
poly-			polyuria
quadri-, quadru-			quadrigemina
semi-			semicomatose
tri-			tricuspid

Prefixes Related to Measurement

Commonly used medical term prefixes relating to measurement are introduced in this section. Laboratory reports often include measurements, which may be reported in terms that use the following prefixes.

Word Part	Meaning
dec-, deca-	ten (10)
deci-	one-tenth (0.1 or 10^{-1})
hecto-	one hundred (100 or 10^2)
centi-	one-hundredth (0.01 or 10^{-2})
kilo-	one thousand (1000 or 10^3)
milli-	one-thousandth (0.001 or 10^{-3})
mega-	one million (1,000,000 or 10^6)
micro-	one-millionth (0.000001 or 10^{-6})
giga-	one billion (1,000,000,000 or 10^9)
nano-	one-billionth (0.000000001 or 10^{-9})

Word Grouping Exercises

Using the *Prefixes Related to Measurement* table, identify the prefix or combining form for each of the following definitions. The first one has been done as an example.

Definition	Word Part
ten	*dec-, deca-*
one billion	
one million	

continued

continued from page 21

Definition	Word Part
one-billionth	
one hundred	
one-hundredth	
one-millionth	
one-tenth	
one-thousandth	
one thousand	

Word Building Exercises

Word parts introduced in the *Prefixes Relating to Measurement* section are listed in the following table. For this exercise, first supply the meaning of each word part, then use the word part to build a word you already know. The word you list under *Common or Known Word* does not have to be a medical term; a commonly used word is fine. Be sure, however, that the word correctly reflects the intended meaning. The first one has been done as an example. Check your answers in a dictionary.

Word Part	Meaning	Common or Known Word	Example Medical Term
centi-	*one-hundredth*	*centiliter*	centimeter
dec-, deca-			decagram
deci-			deciliter
kilo-			kilogram
micro-			micrometer
milli-			milliliter

Medical Term Parts Used as Suffixes

Commonly used medical term suffixes are introduced in this section. **Table 1-4** lists several subcategories of these word parts.

Word Part	Meaning
-ac	pertaining or relating to
-ad	toward
-al	pertaining or relating to
-algia	pain
-ase	enzyme
-blast	immature precursor cell

continued

continued from page 22

Word Part	Meaning
-cele	swelling, hernia
-centesis	surgical puncture to remove fluid
-cide	kill
-cise	cut
-clast	something that breaks; to break
-cyte	cell
-desia	surgical fixation, fusion
-eal	pertaining to
-ectasis	expansion, dilation
-ectomy	surgical removal
-emia	condition of the blood
-esis	condition, action, process
-genesis	origination
-genic	produced by
-gram	written record or picture
-graph	record or picture
-graphy	writing, description
-ia, -iac	condition of, pertaining to
-iasis	presence of
-ic	pertaining to
-id	condition of
-ior	pertaining to
-ism	process
-itis	inflammation
-lith	stone
-logia, -logy	study of
-lysis	breakdown, destruction
-malacia	abnormal softening
-megaly	large, enlargement
-oid	resembling
-ology	study of
-oma	tumor or neoplasm
-osis	condition
-parous	giving birth
-pathy	disease
-penia	few, deficiency
-pexy	fixation
-phasia	speech
-phil-, -phile, -philia	attraction for
-phobia	abnormal fear
-plasia	growth

continued

continued from page 23

Word Part	Meaning
-plasty	surgical repair
-plegia	paralysis
-pnea	breathing
-poiesis	production, formation
-praxia	movement
-rrhage, -rrhagia	excessive, abnormal flow
-rrhaphy	surgical suturing
-rrhea	fluid discharge or flow
-rrhexis	rupture
-scope	instrument for viewing
-scopy	viewing
-sis	state of
-spasm	twitch, involuntary muscle contraction
-stalsis	constriction, contraction
-stenosis	abnormal narrowing, stricture
-stomy	artificial or surgical opening
-taxis	movement toward a stimulus
-tome	part or section; instrument or cutting
-tomy	incision, cutting
-tripsy	crushing
-trophy	growth, nourishment
-uria	pertaining to the urine

TABLE 1-4 — SUBCATEGORIES OF SUFFIXES

Category	Suffix	Example Medical Term
Condition of	-ia	myalgia
	-iac	cardiac
	-id	invalid
	-osis	cirrhosis
Pertaining to	-ac	iliac
	-al	brachial
	-eal	peroneal
	-ia	insomnia
	-iac	cardiac
	-ic	cephalic
Medical specialty	-logy	physiology
	-ist	dentist
	-ian	pediatrician
	-iatrics	geriatrics
	-iatry	podiatry

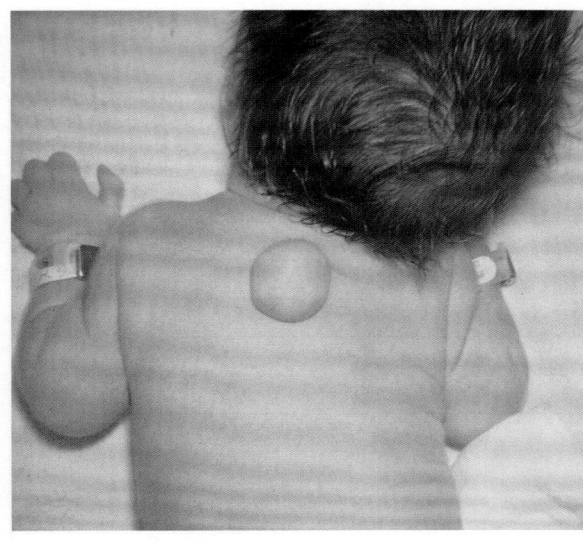

Figure 1-8 The suffix *-cele* means swelling. This is a meningomyelocele, or a swelling of the spinal cord.

Word Grouping Exercises

Using the table of *Medical Term Parts Used as Suffixes*, identify the suffix form for each of the following definitions. The first one has been done as an example, and a photo showing a swelling on the spinal cord is given in **Figure** 1-8.

Definition	Word Part
swelling, hernia	-cele
abnormal fear	
abnormal narrowing, stricture	
abnormal softening	
artificial or surgical opening	
attraction for	
breakdown, destruction	
breathing	
cell	
condition	
condition, action, process	
condition of	
condition of, pertaining to	
condition of the blood	
constriction, contraction	
crushing	
cut	
disease	
enzyme	
excessive, abnormal flow	
expansion, dilation	

continued

continued from page 25

Definition	Word Part
few, deficiency	
fixation	
fluid discharge or flow	
giving birth	
growth	
growth, nourishment	
immature precursor cell	
incision, cutting	
inflammation	
instrument for viewing	
kill	
large, enlargement	
movement	
movement toward a stimulus	
origination	
pain	
paralysis	
part or section; instrument for cutting	
pertaining to	A. B. C.
pertaining to or relating to	A. B.
pertaining to the urine	
presence of	
process	
produced by	
production, formation	
record or picture	
resembling	
rupture	
something that breaks; to break	
speech	
state of	
stone	
study of	A. B.
surgical fixation, fusion	
surgical puncture to remove fluid	
surgical removal	

continued

continued from page 26

Definition	Word Part
surgical repair	
surgical suturing	
toward	
tumor or neoplasm	
twitch, involuntary muscle contraction	
visualize, to	
writing, description	
written record or picture	

Word Building Exercises

Word parts introduced in the *Medical Term Parts Used as Suffixes* section are listed in the following table. For this exercise, first supply the meaning of each word part, then use the word part to build a word you already know. The word you list under *Common or Known Word* does not have to be a medical term; a commonly used word is fine. Be sure, however, that the word choice correctly reflects the intended meaning. The first one has been done as an example. Check your answers in a dictionary.

Word Part	Meaning	Common or Known Word	Example Medical Term
-ac	*pertaining or relating to*	*cardiac*	cardiac
-ad			cephalad
-gram			angiogram
-graph			radiograph
-ic			pelvic
-ology			histology
-phobia			claustrophobia
-scope			otoscope

COMMON Abbreviations

Abbreviation	Term
A	assessment
CAAHEP	Commission on Accreditation of Allied Health Education Programs
CC	chief complaint
c/o	complains of

continued

continued from page 27

Abbreviation	Term
CPT	Current Procedural Terminology
Dx or DX	diagnosis
FH	family history
HEENT	head, eyes, ears, nose, and throat
H&P	history and physical
HIPAA	Health Insurance Portability & Accountability Act
HPI	history of present illness
Hx	history
ICD	International Classification of Diseases
IMP	impression
L&W	living and well
NAD	no acute distress
NKA	no known allergies
NKDA	no known drug allergies
O	objective
OH	occupational history
P	plan
PE	physical examination
PERRLA	pupils equal, round, and reactive to light and accommodation
PMH	past medical history
Px	physical examination
R/O	rule out
ROS	review of systems
S	subjective
SH	social history
SOAP	subjective, objective, assessment, plan
Sx	symptom
UCHD	usual childhood diseases
WNL	within normal limits

COMMON ABBREVIATIONS EXERCISES

1. The abbreviation for *symptom* is _____.

2. SOAP is an abbreviation for _____.

3. NKA refers to _____.

4. The abbreviation for diagnosis is _____.

5. HEENT is the abbreviation for _____.

Review and Application

Multiple-Choice Questions

Select the best response to each of the following questions.

1. An eponym is a medical term derived from _____.
    a. a person's name   b. Latin roots   c. Greek roots   d. its anatomical location

2. Standardized anatomical naming is determined by _____.
    a. your instructor   b. the text book industry   c. *Terminologia Anatomica*   d. *Index Medicus*

3. Commonly used combining vowels are _____.
    a. *a* and *e*   b. *o* and *i*   c. *i* and *u*   d. *i* and *y*

4. A combining form is defined as a _____.
    a. word root plus a prefix   b. prefix plus a suffix   c. word root plus a vowel   d. word root plus a suffix

5. A word root _____.
    a. is another term for *affix*   b. is the main part of a word   c. conveys the primary meaning of the word   d. b and c

6. A suffix _____.
    a. occurs at the beginning of the term   b. occurs in the middle of the term   c. occurs at the end of the term   d. conveys the main meaning of the term

7. Medical term suffixes _____.
    a. can describe a body condition   b. can serve as verbs   c. usually do not affect the root meaning   d. usually end in *s*

8. If a word is spelled phonetically, it is written _____.
    a. in consonants only   b. just as it sounds   c. in vowels only   d. using the Greek alphabet

9. If a suffix begins with a consonant, a combining _____ is needed.
    a. vowel   b. consonant   c. affix   d. prefix

10. Which of the following terms is an eponym? _____
    a. calcaneal tendon   b. Achilles tendon   c. phalanx   d. biceps

Plurals

Write the plural form for each term.

11. phalanx _____   14. cervix _____

12. nucleolus _____   15. sclerosis _____

13. mitochondrion _____   16. epithelium _____

Singulars

Write the singular form for each term.

17. fungi _____

18. ganglia _____

19. fractures _____

20. atria _____

21. sarcomata _____

Matching Exercises

Match the prefix with its correct meaning.

_____ 22. hyper-

_____ 23. endo-

_____ 24. mal-

_____ 25. hypo-

_____ 26. par-, para-

a. within
b. above, beyond
c. below, under
d. abnormal, bad
e. adjacent to

Match the meaning with its correct prefix.

_____ 27. four

_____ 28. seven

_____ 29. six

_____ 30. nine

a. sex-, sexi-
b. sept-, septi-
c. noni-
d. quadri-, quadru-

Match the suffix with its correct meaning.

_____ 31. -al

_____ 32. -emia

_____ 33. -poiesis

_____ 34. -taxis

_____ 35. -pnea

a. condition of the blood
b. breathing
c. pertaining to
d. formation, production
e. movement toward a stimulus

Definitions

Write the prefix for each of the following terms.

36. one hundred _____

37. ten _____

38. one-tenth _____

39. one-hundredth _____

40. million _____

Define the following word parts.

41. -itis _____

42. -cyte _____

43. -osis _____

44. -pathy _____

45. hypo- _____

Define the following terms.

46. hemiplegia _____

47. polyuria _____

48. lithotripsy _____

49. hypertrophy _____

50. apraxia _____

Spelling

Identify the correctly spelled term in each set.

51. _____
   a. epponym
   b. aponym
   c. eponym
   d. eponim

52. _____
   a. diarrea
   b. diarrhea
   c. diarhea
   d. diarrhia

53. _____
   a. myalgia
   b. myoalgia
   c. myialgia
   d. mylgia

Identify the correctly styled scientific name in each set.

54. _____
   a. mycobacterium tuberculosis
   b. Mycobacterium Tuberculosis
   c. *Mycobacterium Tuberculosis*
   d. *Mycobacterium tuberculosis*

55. _____
   a. escherichia coli
   b. escherichia Coli
   c. <u>Escherichia coli</u>
   d. <u>Escherichia Coli</u>

56. _____
   a. *Clostridium* botulinum
   b. *clostridium Botulinum*
   c. *C. botulinum*
   d. *clostridium botulinum*

Unscramble

Unscramble the letters to form a medical term.

57. ginss _____

58. drow toro _____

59. iiomgnnbc rofms _____

60. xfsseuif _____

Abbreviations

Provide the term for the abbreviations and then define the terms.

61. CC = _____

62. Px = _____

63. ROS = _____

Short Answer

Answer the following question.

64. Tina works in a medical office, where she files medical records and answers the telephone. One afternoon, she received a phone call from an irate parent requesting sensitive medical information about her 20-year-old daughter. Tina told the mother she was unable to divulge any information contained in any patient's medical record. Did Tina act appropriately under these circumstances? Why?

_____

_____

_____

Word Search

....

Find the medical terms hidden in the puzzle.

```
E  N  L  M  L  S  E  X  I  F  E  R  P  C
P  R  O  C  E  D  U  R  A  L  N  S  L  A
A  S  U  T  E  B  T  P  C  Y  O  A  Y  I
N  M  D  T  E  T  R  K  S  A  S  G  E  G
A  O  R  W  A  S  Y  S  P  S  O  A  P  O
T  T  O  O  I  L  E  M  I  L  D  Q  O  L
O  P  C  R  D  R  C  F  O  I  G  A  N  O
M  M  E  D  G  C  I  N  S  L  A  D  Y  N
I  Y  R  O  C  C  I  E  E  P  O  J  M  I
C  S  R  J  A  M  A  L  I  M  O  G  S  M
A  P  E  T  R  S  M  H  K  U  O  F  Y  R
N  G  I  E  E  W  C  U  R  R  E  N  T  E
N  O  T  S  L  A  C  I  D  E  M  G  H  T
N  L  A  N  O  I  T  A  N  R  E  T  N  I
H  W  O  U  U  N  O  P  A  R  T  S  C  C
L  L  P  H  T  A  Q  G  F  A  W  F  G  F
```

CPT
ICD
current
international
procedural
classification
diseases
terminology
eponyms
etymology
hipaa
medical record
nomenclature
symptoms
progress notes
prefixes
soap
terminologia
anatomica
word parts

Vocabulary Review

Review the key terms from this chapter, study the spelling and pronunciation of each term, and write its definition in the space provided. Listen to the audio available for most terms at http://thepoint.lww.com/nath2e and pronounce each term for yourself. Then check the box when you feel confident that you know the definition and can pronounce the term correctly.

Key Term	Pronunciation	Definition
❑ combining forms		_____
❑ Current Procedural Terminology (CPT)		_____
❑ eponyms	(EP-uh-nimz)	_____
❑ etymology	(et-uh-MOL-uh-jee)	_____
❑ Health Insurance Portability & Accountability Act (HIPAA)		_____
❑ International Classification of Diseases (ICD)		_____
❑ medical record		_____
❑ nomenclature	(NOH-men-clay-chur)	_____

Key Term	Pronunciation	Definition
❏ prefixes		_____
❏ progress notes		_____
❏ signs		_____
❏ SOAP notes		_____
❏ suffixes		_____
❏ symptoms		_____
❏ *Terminologia Anatomica*	(tur-mih-nuh-LOH-jee-uh ah-nuh-TOM-eh-kuh)	_____
❏ word parts		_____
❏ word root		_____

Answers

Key Term Practice

Introduction and The Medical Record

1. sign
2. symptom
3. Health Insurance Portability & Accountability Act; HIPAA
4. Eponyms
5. International Classification of Diseases (ICD)

A Brief Lesson in Language

1. prefix
2. Etymology
3. septa
4. pharynx
5. word root

Word Grouping Exercises: Common Prefixes

Definition	Word Part	Definition	Word Part
away from	ab-	backward, again	re-
abnormal, bad, ill	mal-	before	pre-
above, beyond	super-	before, in front of	ante-
above, beyond, over	hyper-	behind, backward	retro-
above, upon	supra-	below, under	infra-
adjacent to, near	par-, para-	below, under, beneath	A. hypo- B. sub-
after, behind	post-	between, behind, after, beyond	meta-
against	A. anti- B. contra-	beyond, excess	ultra-
all, entire	pan-	bladder	cyst-, cysti-, cysto-
among, between	inter-	both sides	ambi-
around	A. circum- B. peri-	brain	encephal-, encephalo-

Definition	Word Part	Definition	Word Part
cold, freezing	cry-, cryo-	right, toward the right	dextr-, dextro-
color, colored	chrom-, chromo-	same	homo-
equal, equally	equi-	self	auto-
false	pseudo-	slow	brady-
from, away	de-	supporting, in front of, before	pro-
good, well, normal	eu-	tail	caud-, caudo-
head	cephal-, cephalo-	through	per-
left, toward the left	sinistro-	through, across	trans-
middle	A. mes-, meso- B. mid-	together, with	A. sym- B. syn-
near	juxta-	toward	ad-
new, recent	neo-	up	ana-
not	im-	upon, following	epi-
not, into	in-	water	hydro-
other, different	heter-, hetero-	within, inner	end-, endo-
out, outside	ex-, exo-	within, inside	intra-
out of, away from	ec-	without	A. a- B. an-
painful, difficult	dys-	without, outside of	extra-
rapid	tachy-		

Word Building Exercises: Common Prefixes

Word Part	Meaning	Common or Known Word	Example Medical Term
ab-	away from	abduct	abduction
ad-	toward	adduct	adduction
ante-	before, in front of	anteroom	anterior
anti-	against	antibacterial	antibody
auto-	self	automobile	autoimmune
circum-	around	circumvent	circumcision
contra-	against	contraband	contraceptive
dys-	painful, difficult	dysfunction	dysuria
ex-, exo-	out, outside	exit	exhale
heter-, hetero-	other, different	heterogenous	heterozygous
homo-	same	homosexual	homozygous
hyper-	above, beyond, over	hyperextend	hypertension
hypo-	below, under, beneath	hypodermic	hypotonic
inter-	among, between	interstate	interosseous
intra-	within, inside	intramural	intramuscular
juxta-	near	juxtaposition	juxtaglomerular
meta-	between, behind, after, beyond	metabolism	metaphysis
neo-	new, newly formed	neoimpressionism	neoplasm

Word Part	Meaning	Common or Known Word	Example Medical Term
post-	after, behind	postgraduate	postpartum
retro-	behind, backward	retrofit	retroperitoneal
sub-	below, under	submarine	subdural

Word Grouping Exercises: Prefixes Related to Number and Size

Definition	Word Part	Definition	Word Part
two	A. bi- B. di-	large	macr-, macro-
big, large, great	mega-	many, much	A. multi- B. poly-
double	diplo-	nine	noni-
eight	oct-, octa-, octo-	one	A. mono- B. uni-
extra large	maxi-	seven	sept-, septi-
five	pent-, penta-	six	A. hex-, hexa- B. sex-, sexi-
four	A. quadri-, quadru- B. tetra-	small	micro-
half	hemi-	small, miniature	mini-
half, partial	semi-	three	tri-

Word Building Exercises: Prefixes Related to Number and Size

Word Part	Meaning	Common or Known Word	Example Medical Term
bi-	two	bicycle	bicuspid
di-	two	diameter	diotic
hemi-	half	hemisphere	hemisphere
macr-, macro-	large	macrobiotic	macromastia
micro-	small	microbiology	microorganism
mono-	one	monogram	monozygous
multi-	many	multicolor	multicellular
poly-	many, much	polyester	polyuria
quadri-, quadru-	four	quadruple	quadrigemina
semi-	half, partial	semicircle	semicomatose
tri-	three	triathlete	tricuspid

Word Grouping Exercises: Prefixes Related to Measurement

Definition	Word Part	Definition	Word Part
ten	dec-, deca-	one-hundredth	centi-
one billion	giga-	one-millionth	micro-
one million	mega-	one-tenth	deci-
one-billionth	nano-	one-thousandth	milli-
one hundred	hecto-	one thousand	kilo-

Word Building Exercises: Prefixes Related to Measurement

Word Part	Meaning	Common or Known Word	Example Medical Term
centi-	one-hundredth	centiliter	centimeter
dec-, deca-	ten	decagram	decagram
deci-	one-tenth	deciliter	deciliter
kilo-	thousand	kilogram	kilogram
micro-	one-millionth	microbiology	micrometer
milli-	one-thousandth	millipede	milliliter

Word Grouping Exercises: Medical Term Parts Used as Suffixes

Definition	Word Part	Definition	Word Part
swelling, hernia	-cele	excessive, abnormal flow	-rrhage, -rrhagia
abnormal fear	-phobia	expansion, dilation	-ectasis
abnormal narrowing, stricture	-stenosis	few, deficiency	-penia
abnormal softening	-malacia	fixation	-pexy
artificial or surgical opening	-stomy	fluid discharge or flow	-rrhea
attraction for	-phil, -phile, -philia	giving birth	-parous
breakdown, destruction	-lysis	growth	-plasia
breathing	-pnea	growth, nourishment	-trophy
cell	-cyte	immature precursor cell	-blast
condition	-osis	incision, cutting	-tomy
condition, action, process	-esis	inflammation	-itis
condition of	-id	instrument for viewing	-scope
condition of, pertaining to	-ia, iac	kill	-cide
condition of the blood	-emia	large, enlargement	-megaly
constriction, contraction	-stalsis	movement	-praxia
crushing	-tripsy	movement toward a stimulus	-taxis
cut	-cise	origination	-genesis
disease	-pathy	pain	-algia
enzyme	-ase	paralysis	-plegia

Definition	Word Part	Definition	Word Part
part or section; instrument for cutting	-tome	stone	-lith
pertaining to	A. -eal B. -ic C. -ior	study of	A. -logia, -logy B. -ology
pertaining to or relating to	A. -ac B. -al	surgical fixation, fusion	-desia
pertaining to the urine	-uria	surgical puncture to remove fluid	-centesis
presence of	-iasis	surgical removal	-ectomy
process	-ism	surgical repair	-plasty
produced by	-genic	surgical suturing	-rrhaphy
production, formation	-poiesis	toward	-ad
record or picture	-graph	tumor or neoplasm	-oma
resembling	-oid	twitch, involuntary muscle contraction	-spasm
rupture	-rrhexis	visualize, to	-scopy
something that breaks; to break	-clast	writing, description	-graphy
speech	-phasia	written record or picture	-gram
state of	-sis		

Word Building Exercises: Medical Term Parts Used as Suffixes

Word Part	Meaning	Common or Known Word	Example Medical Term
-ac	pertaining or relating to	cardiac	cardiac
-ad	toward	caudad	cephalad
-gram	written record or picture	telegram	angiogram
-graph	record or picture	telegraph	radiograph
-ic	pertaining to	psychic	pelvic
-ology	study of	biology	histology
-phobia	abnormal fear	arachnophobia	claustrophobia
-scope	an instrument for viewing	telescope	otoscope

Common Abbreviations Exercises

1. Symptom = Sx
2. SOAP = subjective, objective, assessment, plan
3. NKA = no known allergies
4. diagnosis = Dx
5. HEENT = head, eyes, ears, nose, and throat

Review and Application

1. a
2. c
3. b
4. c
5. d
6. c
7. a
8. b
9. a
10. b
11. phalanges
12. nucleoli
13. mitochondria
14. cervices
15. scleroses
16. epithelia
17. fungus
18. ganglion
19. fracture
20. atrium
21. sarcoma
22. b
23. a
24. d
25. c
26. e
27. d
28. b
29. a
30. c
31. c
32. a
33. d
34. e
35. b
36. hect-, hecto-
37. dec-, deca-
38. deci-
39. centi-
40. meg-, mega-
41. inflammation
42. cell
43. condition
44. disease
45. below
46. paralysis on half of the body
47. excessive urination
48. stone crushing
49. excessive growth
50. without movement
51. c
52. b
53. a
54. d
55. c
56. c
57. signs
58. word root
59. combining forms
60. suffixes
61. CC = chief complaint; the main point that is bringing the patient to the health care provider
62. Px = physical examination; evaluation of the patient by means such as visual inspection, percussion (tapping), and auscultation (listening with a stethoscope) to collect information or form a diagnosis
63. ROS = review of systems; analysis of the body's organ systems
64. Yes, Tina acted appropriately. Medical information is private information and cannot be divulged without patient consent.

Word Search

E	N	+	+	+	S	E	X	I	F	E	R	P	C
P	R	O	C	E	D	U	R	A	L	+	+	L	A
A	S	U	T	E	+	T	P	C	+	+	A	Y	I
N	M	D	T	E	T	+	+	S	+	S	G	E	G
A	O	R	W	A	S	Y	S	+	S	O	A	P	O
T	T	O	O	+	L	E	M	I	L	D	+	O	L
O	P	C	R	D	R	C	F	O	I	+	A	N	O
M	M	E	D	G	C	I	N	S	L	A	+	Y	N
I	Y	R	O	+	C	I	E	E	P	O	+	M	I
C	S	R	+	A	M	A	+	I	M	+	G	S	M
A	P	+	T	R	S	+	H	+	+	O	+	Y	R
+	+	I	E	E	+	C	U	R	R	E	N	T	E
+	O	T	S	L	A	C	I	D	E	M	+	+	T
N	L	A	N	O	I	T	A	N	R	E	T	N	I
+	+	+	+	+	+	P	A	R	T	S	+	+	+
+	+	+	+	+	+	+	+	+	+	+	+	+	+

CPT
ICD
current
international
procedural
classification
diseases
terminology
eponyms
etymology
hipaa
medical
nomenclature
record
symptoms
progress notes
prefixes
soap
terminologia anatomica
word
parts

Vocabulary Review

Key Term	Definition	Key Term	Definition
combining forms	elements used in combination with another element to form a word	**prefixes**	word elements that are attached to the beginning of a word
Current Procedural Terminology (CPT)	a formal classification of diagnostic and therapeutic procedures performed by health care providers that is used for reimbursement purposes	**progress notes**	written documentation for organizing follow-up data and evaluating a patient after the history and physical are obtained; also called SOAP notes
eponyms	the name of a disease, structure, or procedure derived from the name of the person who discovered or described it first	**signs**	any abnormality indicative of disease that is discovered on examination; an objective indication of disease
etymology	the study of the origins of words or word parts and how they have arrived at their current form and meaning	**SOAP notes**	written documentation for organizing follow-up data and evaluating a patient after the history and physical are obtained; also called progress notes
Health Insurance Portability & Accountability Act (HIPAA)	1996 Federal law that restricts access to an individual's private medical information	**suffixes**	word elements that are added to the end of a word
International Classification of Diseases (ICD)	the classification of specific conditions determined by an international expert committee and published in a manual	**symptoms**	physical or mental features indicating a condition that are perceived by the patient; a subjective indication of disease
medical record	a written account that includes a patient's initial complaints, medical history, physical findings, test results, and therapies	***Terminologia Anatomica***	a manual of anatomical nomenclature that standardizes the names of anatomical structures
nomenclature	system of naming things, such as body parts	**word parts**	prefixes, suffixes, or combining forms
		word root	the basic, meaningful part of a word that is left when any prefixes or suffixes are removed

CHAPTER 2

Anatomical and Physiological Terminology

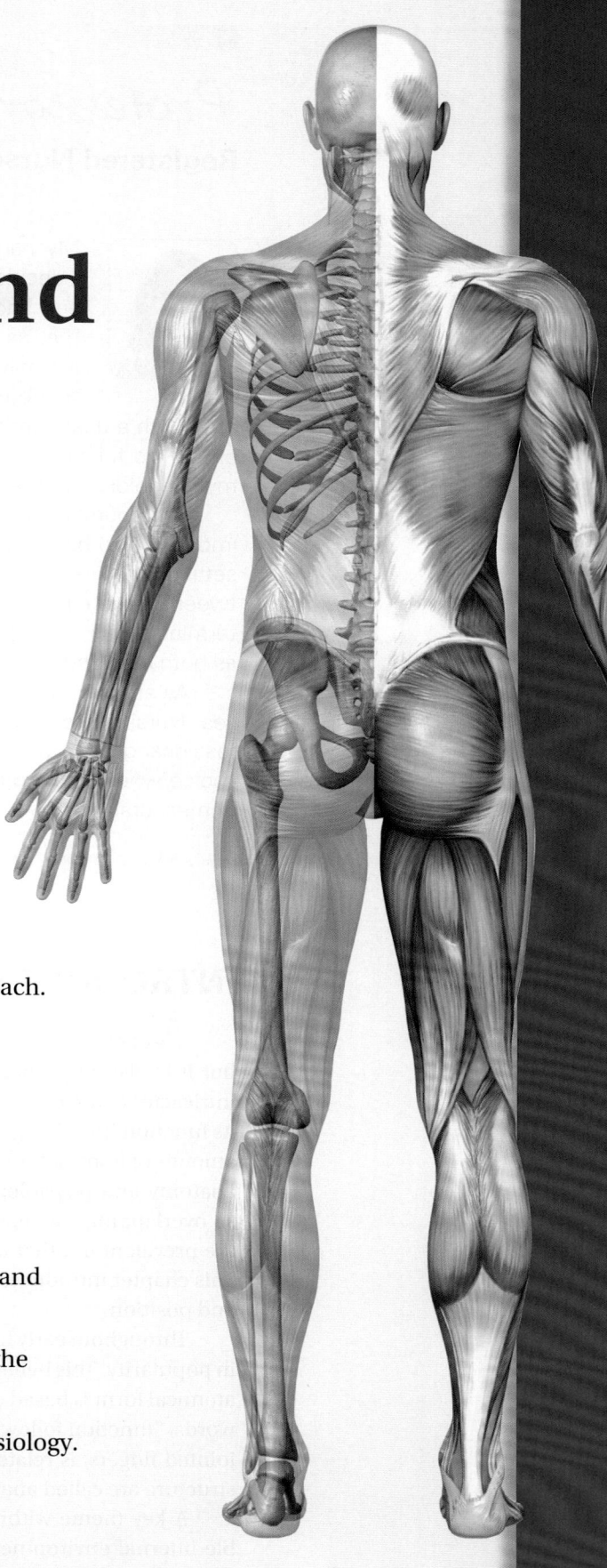

OBJECTIVES

After completing this chapter, you should be able to:

1. Explain the difference between anatomy and physiology.

2. List the levels of organization within the human body.

3. Identify key cellular organelles and give a key function of each.

4. Describe the anatomic position.

5. Identify the body cavities, quadrants, and regions.

6. Use directional terms to describe body planes.

7. Define word parts used for describing the human body.

8. Provide definitions for key terms.

9. Define various signs, symptoms, treatments, clinical tests, and procedures.

10. Cite anatomical and physiological alterations throughout the lifespan.

11. Define common abbreviations related to anatomy and physiology.

12. Define, spell, and pronounce the chapter's medical terms correctly.

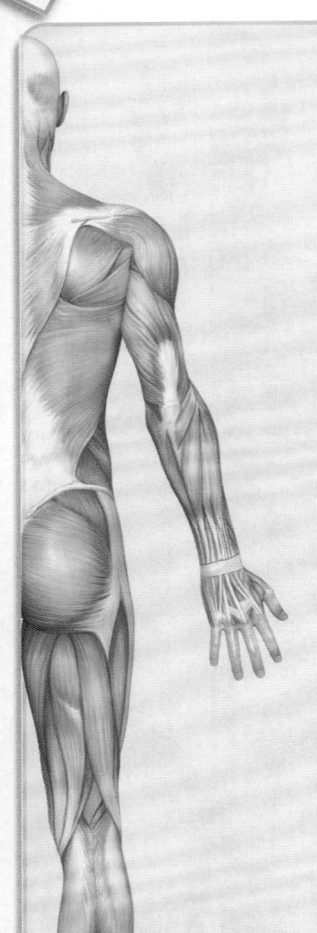

Professional Profile

Registered Nurse/Current Student

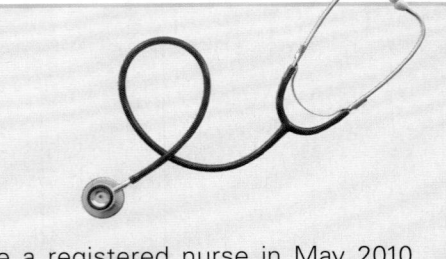

My name is Susan and I became a registered nurse in May 2010. I decided to pursue a career in nursing because I enjoy a challenge and find true joy in helping others. Nursing was a second career for me, as I entered nursing school at the age of 33. Being married with a family presented many challenges throughout nursing school. I attended a 3-year program to become a registered nurse and graduated with a dual nursing diploma and an associate's degree in natural science. I am employed full-time as an RN in a progressive care unit while continuing to work on my bachelor's degree.

The coursework is very challenging and a firm grasp of medical terminology is imperative to both my professional and educational career goals. Within the hospital setting, medical terminology is the common, universal language that is shared between health care professionals of all disciplines. A strong understanding of medical terminology is very important to building the foundation needed to become successful as both a student and a professional nurse.

As an RN, I have the opportunity to touch the lives of my patients and their families. Nursing provides numerous, unlimited opportunities for both personal and professional growth while providing job satisfaction and security. It is an exciting career choice where the work is very demanding and difficult at times, but the rewards are immeasurable!

INTRODUCTION

Not only is knowledge of anatomy and physiology critical in any health care profession, but it is also important for understanding our own bodies. No book can do justice to the intricacies of the human body. Yet we can learn a great deal about its structure (anatomy) and its function (physiology) by studying medical terminology. Furthermore, we can absorb a vast amount of information about medical terminology and the language of medicine by studying anatomy and physiology. There are no clearly defined borders among the health sciences, so overlapping concepts are commonplace. Terms associated with anatomy and physiology are prevalent in other aspects of human biology, disease, medicine, and allied health fields. This chapter introduces you to general terms associated with the body, its structure, function, and position.

Throughout early history, the belief that humans could understand natural processes grew in popularity. This belief in turn stimulated people to think about physiology and anatomy. Anatomical form is based on its function; and the purpose depends on the construction. In other words, "function follows form." For example, the arrangement of parts in the hand, with long, jointed fingers, is related to the hand's function of grasping objects. People who study body structure are called anatomists, and physiologists are people who focus on body function.

A key theme within physiology is that of homeostasis, the tendency to maintain a stable internal environment in relationship to the external surroundings. When the body is in homeostatic balance, it remains fairly constant in terms of chemical composition, temperature, and pressure. This enables optimum function. All body systems attempt to maintain homeostasis. For this reason, homeostasis is a fundamental concept in physiology. The nervous and endocrine systems play key roles in preserving homeostasis. Common examples of homeostasis include maintaining blood glucose levels, regulating temperature, and controlling blood gas concentrations.

Body parts function most efficiently when the concentration of water, food substances, oxygen, heat, and pressure remains within specific narrow limits. This delicate balance is accomplished partly by a process called metabolism. Metabolism refers to the physical and chemical changes occurring in the body that are necessary for life.

This chapter focuses on the body as a whole. It provides an overview of anatomical and physiological disciplines, outlines the different body systems, and describes the various terms used for anatomical orientation.

MEDICAL TERM PARTS

Word Parts

Medical term prefixes, suffixes, and combining forms related to anatomical and physiological terminology are introduced in this section.

Word Part	Meaning
abdomin-, abdomino-	abdomen, abdominal
acro-	extremity, end, tip
ante-	before, in front of
antero-	anterior, front
brachio-	arm
bucco-	cheek
calcaneo-	heel, calcaneus
cardi-, cardio-	heart
cephal-, cephalo-	head
cervic-, cervico-	neck, cervix
chem-, chemo-	chemistry
costo-	rib
crani-, cranio-	skull, cranium
cyt-, cyto-	cell
embry-, embryo-	embryo
etio-	cause
facio-	face
-genesis	origin, beginning process
histio-, histo-	tissue
homeo-	same, steady
ili-, ilio-	ilium, hip bone
latero-	lateral, to one side
mamm-, mammo-	breasts

continued

continued from page 43

Word Part	Meaning
morph-, morpho-	form, shape
naso-	nose
nucl-, nucleo-	nucleus
occipito-	occiput, back part of head
oro-	mouth
ot-, oto-	ear
parieto-	body wall or parietal bone
path-, patho-, -pathy	disease
ped-, pedi-, pedo-	foot or child
pelvi-, pelvio-, pelvo-	pelvis
peritoneo-	peritoneum
physi-, physio-	physiological
pleur-, pleura-, pleuro-	lung membrane, side
postero-	posterior, at the back
prox-, proxi-, proximo-	proximal
pubo-	pubic
retro-	back, backward, behind
sacr-, sacro-	sacrum
somat-, somatico-, somato-	body
spin-, spino-	spine
stern-, sterno-	sternum
tars-, tarso-	tarsus (root of foot)
thorac-, thoracico-, thoraco-	chest (thorax)
vertebro-	vertebra (backbone)
viscero-	viscera (internal organs)

Word Grouping Exercises

Using the *Medical Term Parts* table, identify the prefix, suffix, or combining form for each of the following definitions. The first one has been done as an example.

Definition	Word Part
body wall or parietal bone	*parieto-*
abdomen, abdominal	
anterior, front	
arm	
back, backward, behind	
before, in front of	
body	
breasts	

continued

continued from page 44

Definition	Word Part
cause	
cell	
cheek	
chemistry	
chest (thorax)	
disease	
ear	
embryo	
extremity, end, tip	
face	
foot or child	
form, shape	
head	
heart	
heel, calcaneus	
ilium, hip bone	
lateral, to one side	
lung membrane, side	
mouth	
neck, cervix	
nose	
nucleus	
occiput, back part of head	
origin, beginning process	
pelvis	
peritoneum	
physiological	
posterior, at the back	
proximal	
pubic	
rib	
sacrum	
same, steady	
skull, cranium	
spine	
sternum	
tarsus (root of foot)	
tissue	
vertebra (backbone)	
viscera (internal organs)	

Word Building Exercises

Word parts, introduced in the *Medical Term Parts* section, are listed in the following table. For this exercise, first supply the meaning of each word part, then use the word part to build a word you already know. The word you list under *Common or Known Word* does not have to be a medical term; a commonly used word is fine. Be sure, however, that the word correctly reflects the intended meaning. The first one has been done as an example. Check your answers in a dictionary.

Word Part	Meaning	Common or Known Word	Example Medical Term
antero-	*anterior, front*	*anterior*	anterior
cardi-, cardio-			pericardium
chem-, chemo-			chemotherapy
embry-, embryo-			embryo
-genesis			osteogenesis
homeo-			homeostasis
latero-			lateral
mamm-, mammo-			mammary gland
naso-			nasopharynx
nucl-, nucleo-			nucleus
retro-			retroperitoneal
vertebro-			vertebral column

ANATOMY AND PHYSIOLOGY DEFINED

Anatomy is the study of the physical structure of the human body. The shape of a specific structure is referred to as its **morphology**. For instance, the patella (kneecap) is an anatomical structure whose morphology is round. The study of the form and structure of something is also called morphology. A few examples of fields of anatomical study—cytology, embryology, gross anatomy, histology, and pathology—are described here.

The word part *cyto-* refers to "cell" and *-ology* means "study of." Hence, **cytology** is the study of cells. It is microscopic anatomy and requires special slide preparation and staining techniques so that the cells can be seen under the microscope. Much study of the human body is done using a microscope. It is interesting that the tiny human egg cell, or oocyte, is the only cell in the body that can be seen without a microscope.

Embryology is the study of development from the fertilized egg through the eighth week in utero, meaning in the mother's womb, or uterus. While in the uterus, the developing human is termed an embryo until the end of the eighth gestational week (**Figure 2-1A**). After the eighth week, the embryo is called a fetus (**Figure 2-1B**).

Gross anatomy is the study of anatomy that can be seen without a microscope. Courses in gross anatomy generally involve cadaver dissection. **Histology** is a form of microscopic anatomy that studies the cells, tissues, and organs in relation to their function.

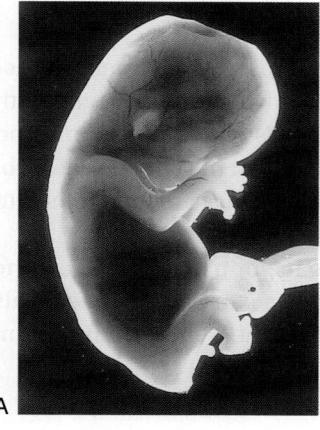 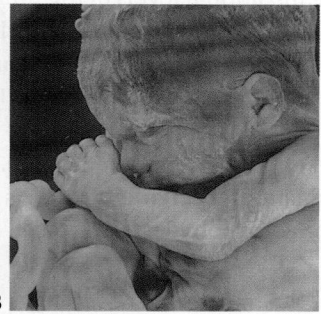

A   B

Figure 2-1 (A) Embryo at 41 days. The developing human is termed an embryo until the end of the eighth gestational week. **(B)** Fetus between 12 and 15 weeks.

The study of diseased body structures is referred to as **pathology** because the prefix *path-* indicates disease. A **pathologist** is a physician with special training who studies the causes of disease and death .

Physiology is the study of the function of body structures. Think of it in terms of "what the body parts do and how they do it." It is difficult to separate anatomy from physiology because the structures of body parts are so closely related to their functions. As with anatomy, there are several disciplines within the broader field of physiology that focus on different aspects of how an organism functions. An **organism** is any living individual, whether plant or animal, considered as a whole, with all body parts functioning together. Hence, a human organism is a collection of structurally and functionally integrated systems.

KEY TERM	Definition
anatomy (uh-NAT-uh-mee)	the study of structure
morphology (mor-FOL-uh-jee)	shape of a specific structure
cytology (si-TOL-uh-jee)	branch of biology that studies cells
embryology (em-bree-OL-uh-jee)	study of the embryo (from fertilization through week eight) and its development
gross anatomy (GROCE uh-NAT-uh-mee)	study of the body that does not require magnification
histology (his-TOL-uh-jee)	study of cells, tissues, and organs in relation to their function
pathology (pa-THOL-uh-jee)	scientific study of disease
pathologist (pa-THOL-uh-jist)	a physician trained in pathology who studies the causes of disease and death
physiology (fiz-ee-OL-uh-jee)	study of body function
organism (OR-guh-NIZ-um)	any living individual, whether plant or animal, considered as a whole

KEY TERM PRACTICE: *Anatomy and Physiology Defined*

1. If *-ology* refers to the *study of*, and *hist-* refers to *tissue*, what is the medical term that means *the study of body tissues*? _____

2. The study of diseases of the body is known as _____.

3. Anatomy is the study of human structure. What is the word that describes *the study of human function*? _____

4. The study of the human embryo and its development is termed _____.

5. _____ is the study of body structures.

Cells and Organizational Structure

Larger body structures are made up of smaller parts, which are composed of yet smaller structures. **Figure 2-2** presents the organizational levels of the human body. The figure begins with the smallest structures and builds up to include the following levels: chemical (atoms and molecules), organelle, cell, tissue, organ, organ system, and organism. At the chemical level of organization, atoms are bound together to form molecules. The molecules are then joined to form organelles inside cells.

Cells are the basic structural and functional units of life. The major parts of a cell are the membrane, organelles, and cytoplasm. The **cell membrane** is a barrier composed of chemicals known as lipids, proteins, and some carbohydrates. The cell membrane is an extremely thin,

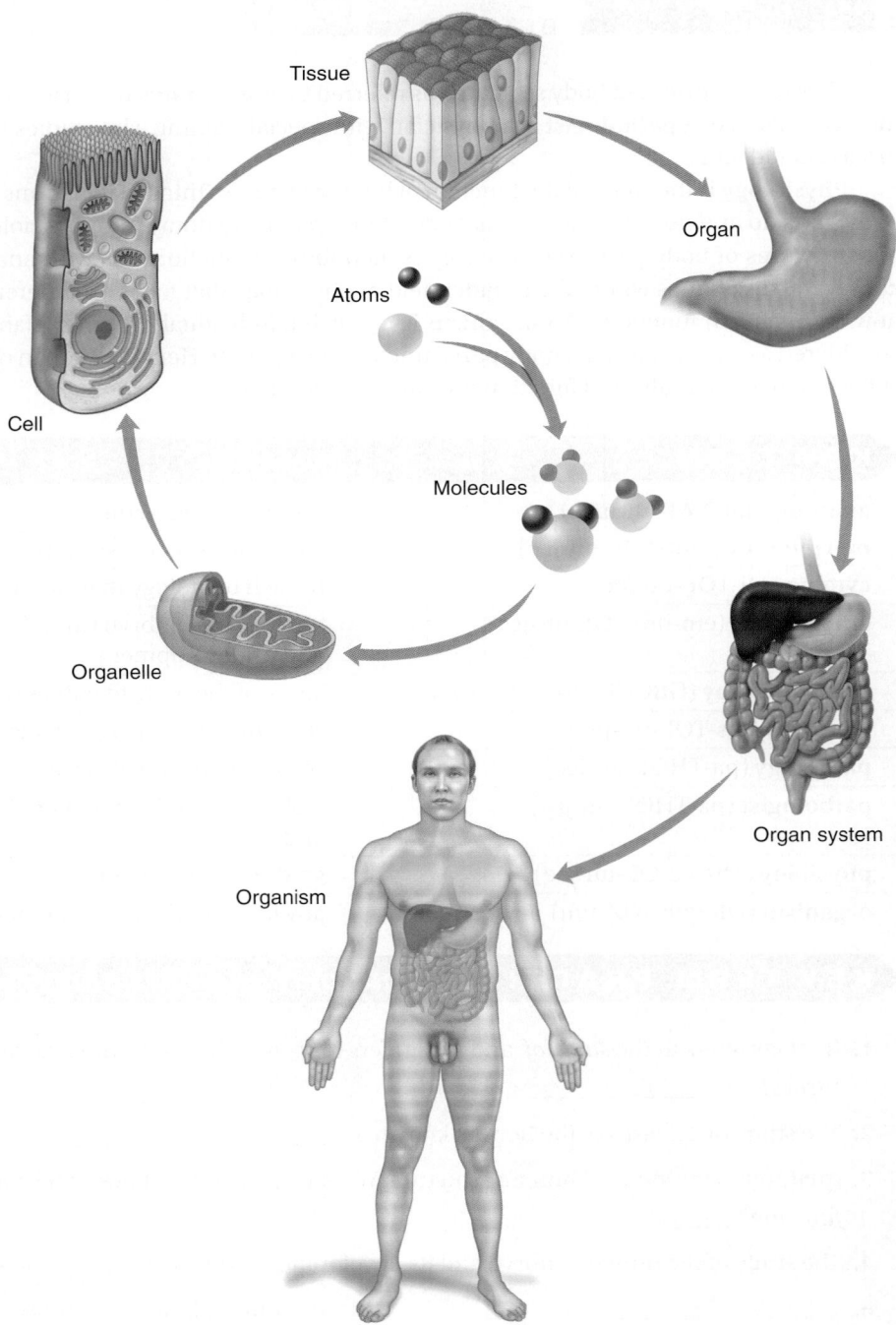

Figure 2-2 The structural organizational levels of the human body, beginning with the smallest (the atom).

yet flexible double layer that controls the movement of particles into and out of the cell. The fluid contained by a cellular membrane is the cytoplasm. Within the cytoplasm are structures called **organelles**, which are living parts of the cells that perform specialized functions. Approximately two dozen human cellular organelles have been identified. Examples of organelles filling the cytoplasm are the ribosomes, mitochondria, and nucleus. **Ribosomes** are clusters of proteins and RNA (ribonucleic acid) that manufacture proteins. **Mitochondria** are membranous sacs with inner partitions that release energy from food and use it to make molecules of ATP (adenosine triphosphate). ATP then transfers this energy to where it is needed. For this reason, mitochondria are commonly referred to as the cell's "power house." The **nucleus** is a fairly large, spherical structure that directs activities of the cell. It contains the cell's DNA (deoxyribonucleic acid). A typical human cell is shown in **Figure 2-3**.

Chromosomes are rod-shaped structures within the nucleus that carry genetic information in the form of genes. **Genes** are specific sequences of DNA on a chromosome that determine our heredity. Each chromosome consists of DNA, and humans have 22 pairs of somatic chromosomes plus two sex chromosomes. The sex chromosomes are designated X and Y, and females have two X chromosomes (designated XX), while males have one X chromosome and one Y chromosome (designated XY). To survive, cells must undergo a series of chemical and physical changes in a process called metabolism. On the cellular level, specialization is necessary for an organism to function well, thus cells differentiate (change) into various types that perform specific jobs. For example, nerve cells have long, thread-like extensions that transmit nerve impulses; epithelial cells are thin, flattened, tightly packed cells that protect underlying cells; and muscle cells, which pull parts closer together, are slender and rod-like.

Tissues are the next level of organization. A **tissue** is a grouping of comparable cells that performs a specific function. Thus tissues consist of groups of similarly specialized cells. Humans have four basic types of tissues: epithelial, connective, muscular, and nervous. Each of these tissue types has various divisions. **Epithelial tissue** is the type of tissue that covers body surfaces and lines internal organs. Epithelial tissue is also called **epithelium**. The *-al* ending in *epithelial* indicates the adjective form, whereas the *-um* ending is the noun form. **Connective tissue**, such as adipose (fat) tissue, bones, and cartilage, supports and protects. **Muscle tissue** produces movement. There are three types of muscle tissue: skeletal (attached to bones), cardiac (found in the heart), and smooth (found lining organs). The fourth type of tissue is **nervous tissue**, which conducts nerve impulses.

A grouping of two or more tissues that is integrated to perform a particular function is an **organ**. Organs vary greatly in size and have definite forms and functions. Lungs, kidneys, and hearts are examples of organs.

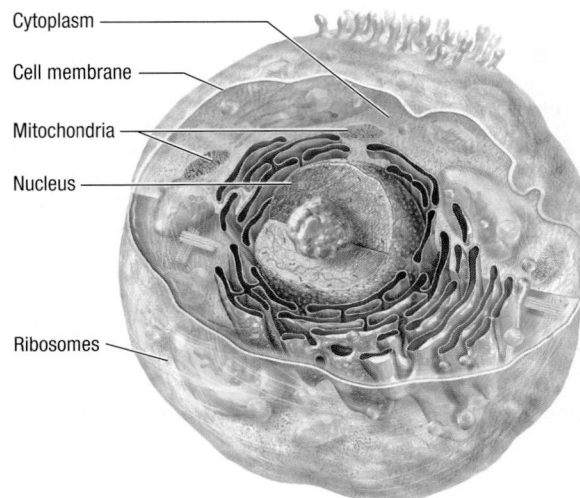

Cytoplasm

Cell membrane

Mitochondria

Nucleus

Ribosomes

Figure 2-3 A typical human cell with various organelles.

The next level of organization is the systemic level. An **organ system** consists of various organs that have similar or related functions. The 11 major human organ systems are the integumentary, skeletal, muscular, nervous, endocrine, cardiovascular, respiratory, lymphatic, digestive, urinary, and reproductive. This final level of organization involves the interplay of these systems to form a complete organism.

KEY TERM	Definition
cells	basic structural and functional units of life
cell membrane (MEM-brane)	barrier that surrounds the cytoplasm
organelles (OR-guh-nelz)	specialized cellular structures with specific functions
ribosomes (RYE-boh-sohmz)	sites of protein synthesis within the cytoplasm
mitochondria (migh-toh-KON-dree-uh)	organelles that make ATP
nucleus (NEW-klee-us)	cellular center that contains DNA
chromosomes (KROH-muh-somes)	structures in the nucleus that carry genetic information in the form of genes
genes	sequences of DNA on a chromosome that determine our heredity
tissue	grouping of similar cells that perform a specific function
epithelial (ep-i-THEE-lee-ul) **tissue**	type of tissue that covers body surfaces and lines internal organs; also called epithelium
epithelium (ep-i-THEE-lee-um)	type of tissue that covers body surfaces and lines internal organs; also called epithelial tissue
connective tissue	supporting and connecting tissue in the body
muscular tissue	tissue that has the ability to contract
nervous tissue	tissue that has the ability to conduct nerve impulses
organ	grouping of two or more tissues that are integrated to perform a particular function
organ system	combination of organs with similar or related functions

KEY TERM PRACTICE: *Cells and Organizational Structure*

1. A _____ is basic structural and functional unit of life.

2. The definition for a _____ is a grouping of similar cells specialized for a particular function.

3. Name the structures found within a cell's cytoplasm that perform specific functions. _____.

4. _____ are sequences of DNA on chromosomes that determine our heredity.

5. Name the four types of tissues. _____

Human Body Systems

The human is complex, with 11 different body systems (**Figure 2-4**). These systems and their key functions are as follows:

- The **integumentary system**, which includes the skin, serves a protective function and helps regulate body temperature.

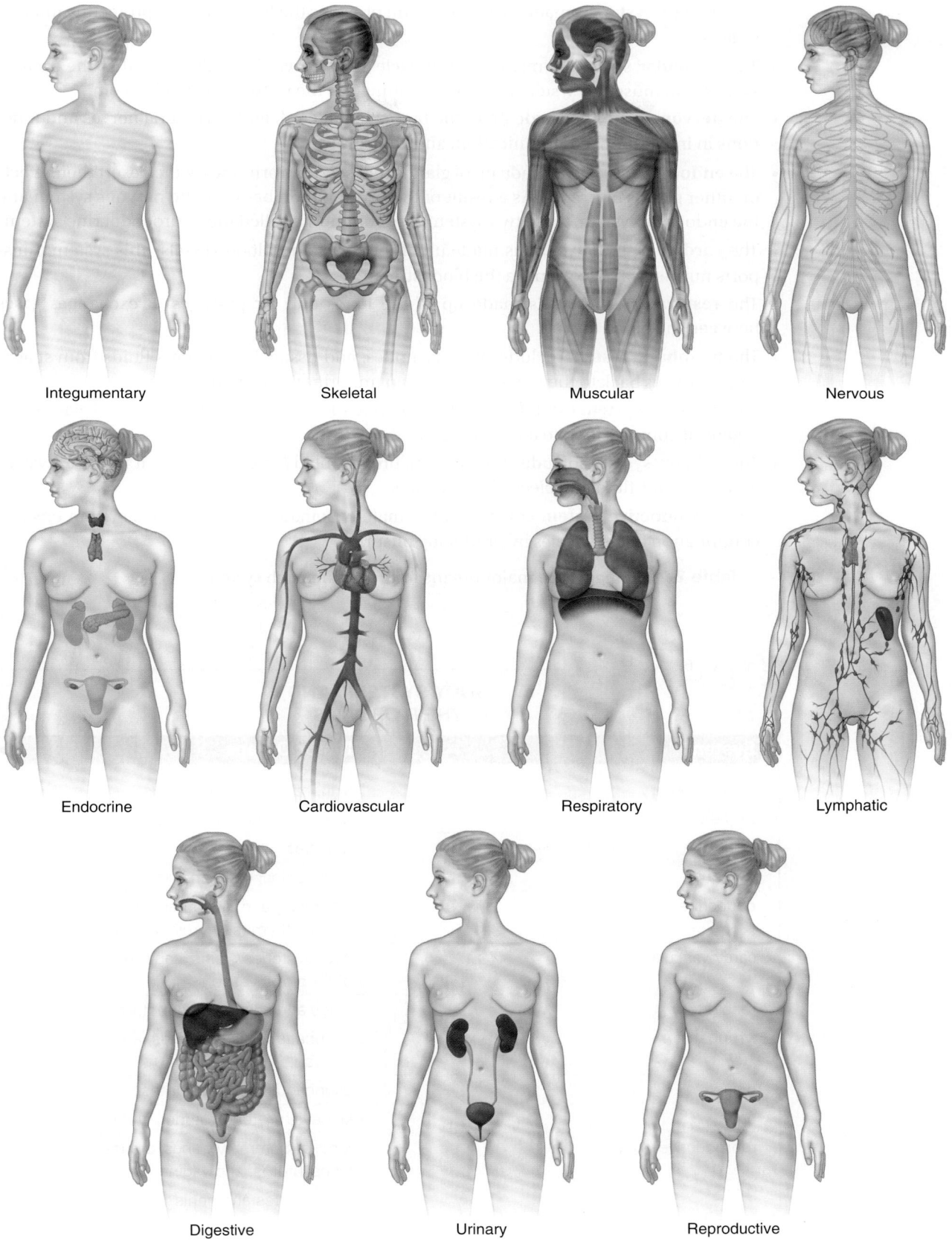

Integumentary   Skeletal   Muscular   Nervous

Endocrine   Cardiovascular   Respiratory   Lymphatic

Digestive   Urinary   Reproductive

Figure 2-4 The 11 body systems of the human.

- The **skeletal system** is made up of bones and provides the framework for protecting internal organs.
- The **muscular system** is made up of muscles that move the body. Note that the skeletal system and muscular system are often combined as the musculoskeletal system.
- The **nervous system** is made up of the brain, spinal cord, and peripheral nerves and functions in integration, communication, and control.
- The **endocrine system** is made up of glands that secrete hormones, which exert their effects on other glands or tissues. As a result of the coordination between the nervous system and the endocrine system, these two systems are commonly called the neuroendocrine system.
- The **cardiovascular system** is made up of the heart and blood vessels. This system transports nutrients and oxygen via the bloodstream.
- The **respiratory system** is made up of the lungs and air passages. It exchanges gases between the blood and air.
- The **lymphatic system** includes vessels, nodes, and tissue. It transports fluids from spaces within tissues back to the blood and plays an important role in immunity.
- The **digestive system** extends from the mouth to the anus with all its associated glands and organs. It converts food to a usable form.
- The **urinary system** includes the kidneys, ureters, bladder, and urethra. It removes wastes and maintains fluid and electrolyte balance.
- The **reproductive system** consists of the male or female sex organs. This system ensures continuation of the species by producing offspring.

Table 2-1 highlights the major organs found within each system.

TABLE 2-1

BODY SYSTEMS AND THEIR ORGANS

System	Major Organs
integumentary	skin, hair, nails, and glands
skeletal	bones, ligaments, and cartilage
muscular	muscles
nervous	brain, spinal cord, and nerves
endocrine	pituitary gland, hypothalamus, adrenal glands, thymus, thyroid, and pancreas
cardiovascular	heart, arteries, veins, capillaries, and other blood vessels
respiratory	lungs and accessory structures
lymphatic	lymphatic vessels, glands, and lymph nodes
digestive	esophagus, stomach, intestines, and liver
urinary	kidneys, ureters, bladder, and urethra
reproductive	*female:* mammary glands, ovaries, uterine tubes, uterus, and vagina *male:* testes and penis

KEY TERM	Definition
integumentary (in-teg-yoo-MEN-tuh-ree) **system**	system that includes the skin and serves a protective function
skeletal (SKEL-e-tul) **system**	system that is made up of bones and provides the framework for protecting internal organs
muscular (MUS-kew-lur) **system**	system made up of muscles that move the body
nervous system	system made up of the brain, spinal cord, and peripheral nerves that function in communication, integration, and control
endocrine (EN-doh-krin) **system**	system made up of glands that secrete hormones and it interacts with the nervous system
cardiovascular (karr-dee-oh-VAS-kew-lur) **system**	system made up of the heart and blood vessels and transports nutrients and oxygen via the bloodstream
respiratory (RES-pi-ruh-toh-ree) **system**	system made up of the lungs and air passages that exchange gases between the blood and air
lymphatic (lim-FAT-ik) **system**	system that includes vessels, nodes, and tissues that transport fluids from spaces within tissues back to the blood and plays an important role in immunity
digestive (di-JES-tiv) **system**	system that extends from the mouth to the anus with all its associated glands and organs and converts food to a usable form
urinary (YOOR-i-nerr-ee) **system**	system made up of the kidneys, ureters, bladder, and urethra that is involved with waste removal and fluid and electrolyte balance
reproductive (ree-pruh-DUCK-tiv) **system**	system consisting of male or female sex organs that is involved with producing offspring

KEY TERM PRACTICE: *Human Body Systems*

1. Identify the 11 human body systems._____
   _____
   _____
   _____

2. The systems making up the neuroendocrine system are the _____ system and the _____ system.

3. Name the systems making up the musculoskeletal system. _____

Body Membranes

A **membrane** is a thin tissue layer that surrounds a body part, separates cavities, lines cavities, or connects adjacent body structures. The human body has four primary membranes: the serous, pleural, pericardial, and peritoneal.

   Serous membranes, also called the **serosa**, line the thoracic (chest) and abdominal (lower trunk) cavities. Serous membranes cover organs and secrete a watery fluid called serous fluid. Composed of connective tissue and a single layer of flattened cells (called simple squamous epithelium), serous membranes compartmentalize, protect, and lubricate organs.

   Two main body linings are the parietal and visceral. **Parietal** means pertaining to the wall of a body cavity. **Visceral** means pertaining to an internal organ. Parietal membranes line body cavities and visceral membranes cover organs. For example, the parietal pleura is the inside lining of the thoracic cavity, and the visceral pleurae cover the lungs. Viscera refers to internal organs and the term can be used in place of the word *organ*. **Mesentery** is a double layer of peritoneum that attaches abdominal organs, such as the intestines, to the abdominal wall.

Pleural membranes are associated with the lungs or pleural cavity (**Figure 2-5A**). The word part *pleur-* means "lung." **Pericardial membranes** are associated with the heart and pericardial cavity (**Figure 2-5B**). The **peritoneal membranes**, or **peritoneum**, are associated with the abdominopelvic cavity and cover the organs contained there (**Figure 2-5C**).

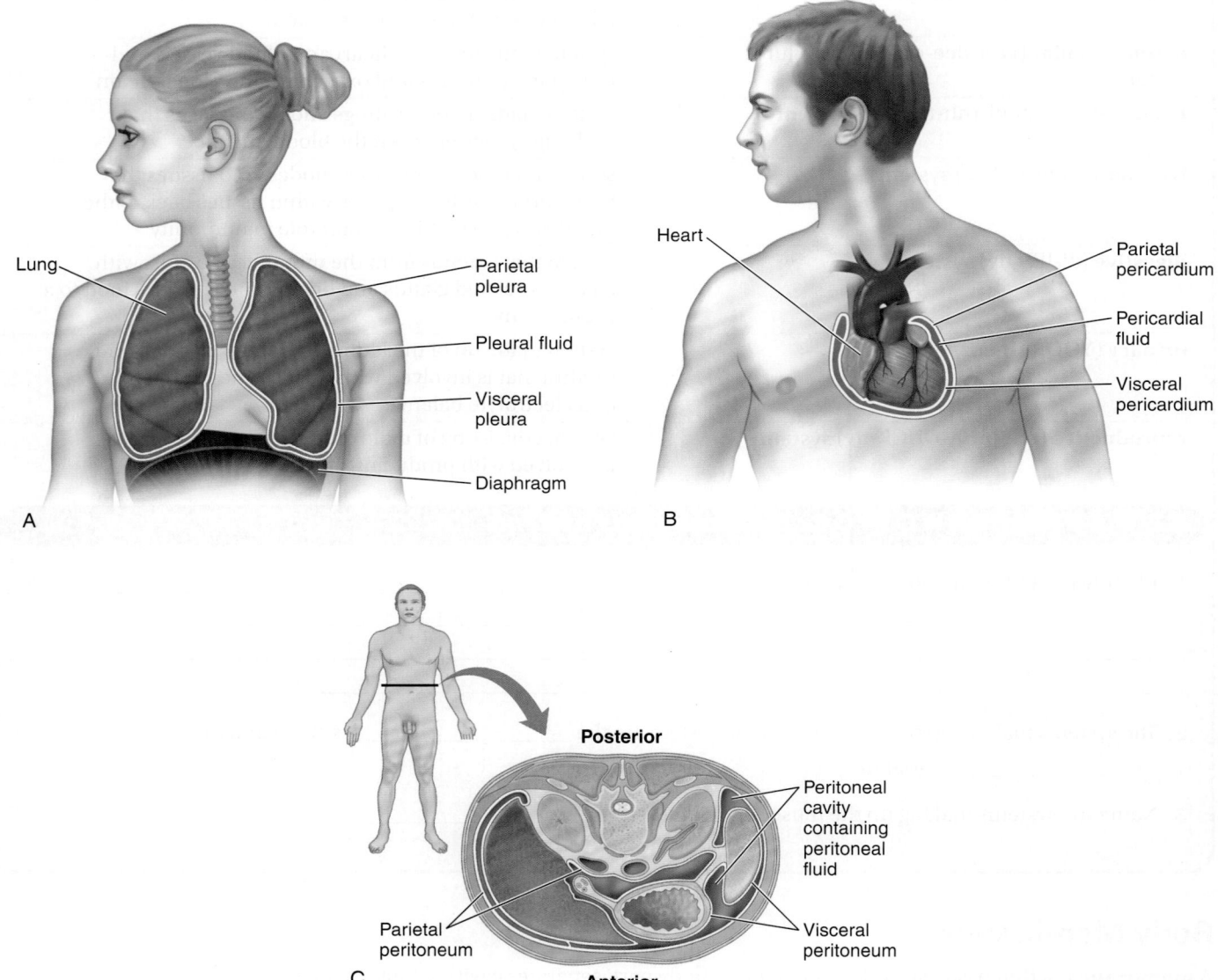

Figure 2-5 (A) The pleural membranes associated with the lungs. **(B)** The pericardial membranes associated with the heart. **(C)** The peritoneal membranes associated with the abdominopelvic cavity.

KEY TERM	Definition
membrane (MEM-brane)	thin tissue layer surrounding, separating, lining, or connecting a body part
serous (SEER-us) **membranes**	membranes lining the thoracic and abdominal cavities that secrete a watery fluid; also called the serosa
serosa (se-ROH-suh)	membranes lining the thoracic and abdominal cavities that secrete a watery fluid; also called serous membranes
parietal (puh-RYE-e-tul)	pertaining to a body wall
visceral (VIS-ur-al)	pertaining to internal organs
mesentery (MES-un-terr-ee;-MEZ-un-terr-ee)	double layer of peritoneum that attaches abdominal organs to the abdominal wall
pleural (PLOOR-ul) **membranes**	membranes associated with the lungs
pericardial (perr-i-KAHR-dee-ul) **membranes**	membranes associated with the heart
peritoneal (perr-i-toh-NEE-ul) **membranes**	membranes associated with the abdominopelvic cavity that cover the organs contained therein; also called the peritoneum
peritoneum (PER-i-toh-NEE-um)	membranes associated with the abdominopelvic cavity that cover the organs contained therein; also called peritoneal membranes

KEY TERM PRACTICE: *Body Membranes*

1. If a membrane is associated with an organ, it is termed _____.

2. If a membrane is associated with a body wall or cavity, it is termed _____.

3. Give the two names for the membranes that are associated with the abdominopelvic cavity and cover abdominopelvic organs. _____

4. Give the two names for the membranes that line the thoracic and abdominal cavities that secrete a watery fluid. _____

5. The _____ is a double layer of peritoneum that attaches abdominal organs to the abdominal wall.

Anatomic Position and Body Cavities

Anatomical terms are used to identify direction and position. To avoid confusion, all bodily references are made in accordance with the anatomic position, illustrated in **Figure 2-6**. The **anatomic position** refers to a person standing erect, facing an observer, with the arms placed at the sides and the palms of the hands turned forward (anteriorly). When using anatomical terminology, **anterior** refers to the front, and **posterior** refers to the back. In medical charts, **anteroposterior** (**AP**) is often used to describe the anterior–posterior perspective of x-ray images.

For reference purposes, the human body is divided into two major divisions: axial and appendicular. Bones, muscles, and nerves of the head, neck, shoulders, and torso make up the **axial** division, while structures of the appendages (arms and legs) make up the **appendicular** division. For general orientation, specific terms describe the body while lying. The positional term **supine** refers to lying on the back, face upward, and **prone** refers to lying face downward. The word *up* is found in *sup*ine, thus the face is *up* while in a supine position.

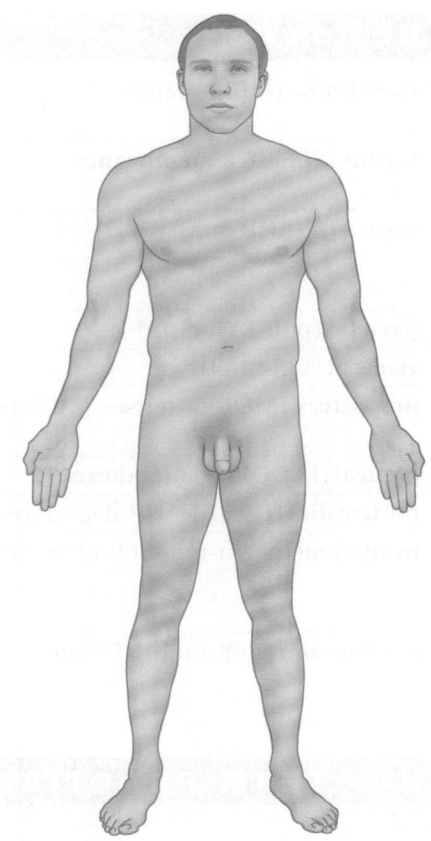

Figure 2-6 The anatomic position. The person is standing erect, facing the observer, with the arms placed at the sides and the palms of the hands turned forward.

The body is also made up of several cavities, which are hollow spaces (**Figure 2-7**). The main body cavities are the thoracic, abdominal, and pelvic. The abdominopelvic cavity is the combination of the abdominal and pelvic cavities.

The **thoracic cavity** is the space within the thoracic walls bordered by the base of the neck above and the diaphragm below. The **diaphragm** is the dome-shaped muscle of breathing that

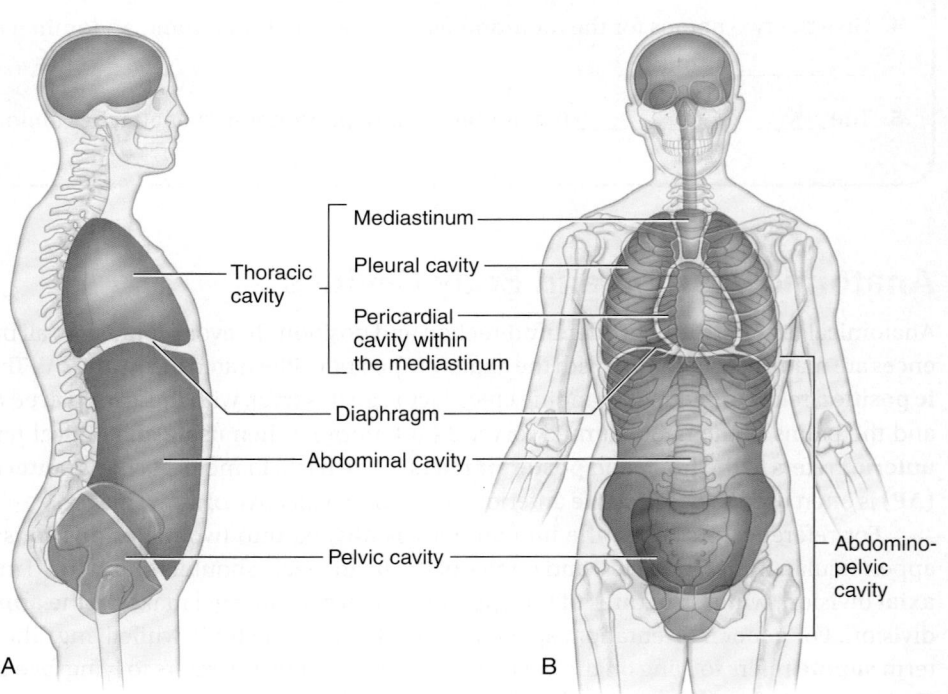

Figure 2-7 The body cavities:
(A) lateral view; **(B)** anterior view.

A

B

Thoracic cavity

Diaphragm

Abdominal cavity

Pelvic cavity

Mediastinum

Pleural cavity

Pericardial cavity within the mediastinum

Abdomino-pelvic cavity

divides the anterior cavity into an upper thoracic region and a lower abdominopelvic region. The middle region of the thoracic cavity between the lungs is known as the **mediastinum**. The mediastinum contains the heart, trachea (windpipe), and other organs.

The **abdominopelvic cavity** is divided into the superior (upper) **abdominal cavity** and the inferior (lower) **pelvic cavity** by an imaginary line that extends from the symphysis pubis (where the pubic bones meet) to a specific point on the sacrum known as the sacral promontory. Be careful of the tricky spelling of *abdominopelvic*, as you might be tempted to incorrectly call it the "abdomin*al*pelvic" cavity. Organs of the abdominal cavity include the stomach, spleen, pancreas, liver, gallbladder, small intestine, and most of the large intestine. Organs of the pelvic cavity include the urinary bladder, sigmoid colon, rectum, and internal male and female reproductive structures. The visceral peritoneum covers all abdominal organs. Some other body cavities, including the oral cavity with the teeth and tongue, and the nasal cavity within the nose, will be discussed in other chapters.

KEY TERM	Definition
anatomic (an-uh-TOM-ick) **position**	pose in which a person is facing forward, standing erect, with the arms at the side and palms turned forward
anterior (an-TEER-ee-ur)	toward the human front side
posterior (pos TEER ee ur)	toward the human back side
anteroposterior (an-TEER-oh-pos-TEER-ee-or) **(AP)**	in x-ray imaging, describes the direction of the beam through a patient from anterior to posterior
axial (ACK-see-ul)	body portion consisting of head, neck, and torso
appendicular (ap-en-DICK-yoo-lur)	body portion consisting of the arms and legs
supine (suh-PINE;-SOO-pine)	lying face up
prone	lying face down
thoracic (thoh-RAS-ick) **cavity**	space occupied by the lungs, heart, and trachea
diaphragm (DYE-uh-fram)	the dome-shaped muscle of breathing that separates the thoracic cavity from the abdominal cavity
mediastinum (mee-dee-uh-STYE-num)	region in the middle of the chest between the lungs that contains the heart, trachea, and other organs
abdominopelvic (ab-dom-i-noh-PEL-vick) **cavity**	combination of the abdominal and pelvic cavities
abdominal (ab-DOM-i-nul) **cavity**	space between the diaphragm and the pelvic floor
pelvic (PEL-vick) **cavity**	space within the bones of the pelvis

KEY TERM PRACTICE: *Anatomic Position and Body Cavities*

1. Explain what is meant by *anatomic position*. _____

   _____

   _____

2. The combination of the abdominal cavity and pelvic cavity is commonly known as the _____ cavity.

3. The body portion consisting of the arms and legs is called the _____ division, whereas the portion consisting of the head, neck, and chest is referred to as the _____ division.

4. Lying face down is termed _____.

5. The term that means *toward the front* is _____.

Directional Terms

Directional terms are used to indicate the relationship of one body part to another (**Figure 2-8**). Common terms are described in pairs with opposite meanings. For instance, the word *anterior* means near or at the front of the body, and the term *posterior* refers to a structure near or at the back of the body: The nipple is on the anterior surface, and the kidneys are posterior to the intestines. **Ventral** and **dorsal** are alternate terms for anterior and posterior, respectively. Although the terms are often used within human anatomy, ventral and dorsal are usually reserved for describing nonhuman animals.

Medical terms used to indicate directions that can be described using the common words *up* and *down* include cephalic, caudal, superior, and inferior:

- **Cephalic** means toward the head, and the opposite of cephalic is caudal.
- **Caudal** refers to the lower portion of the spine, and the word *cauda* means "tail." *Caudal* is a term used in human anatomy but is more appropriate for describing animals that actually have a tail, such as dogs and cats.
- **Superior** means toward the head or upper part of a structure. The opposite of superior is inferior.
- **Inferior** means away from the head.
- **Cranial** is another term that means toward the head or top.

To illustrate the correct use of these terms, the feet are inferior to the hips, whereas the thoracic region is superior to the abdominal region.

Words specifying location include *deep* and *superficial*. **Deep** means internal or away from the body surface. *Deep* is used in reference to an internal structure, as in "the brain is deep to the skull." **Superficial** means external, toward the surface, or on the body. This term can be used to describe a structure located on the body's exterior or to describe muscles that

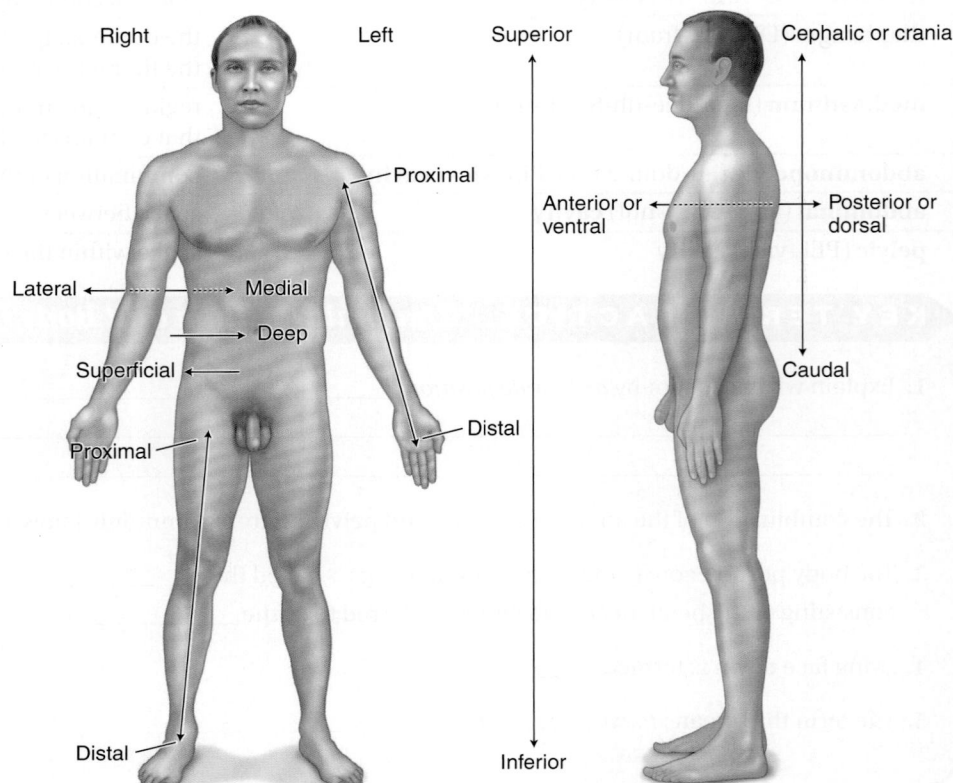

Figure 2-8 Directional terms are used to indicate the relationship of one body part to another.

overlay other muscles. For example, the skin is superficial to the bones, and the pectoralis major muscle is superficial to the pectoralis minor muscle.

Proximal is used to describe a structure that is toward the point of attachment or toward the center of the body. For example, the knee is proximal to the foot. **Distal** means that a structure is away from the point of attachment. Think of it as being toward the end. For example, the hand is distal to the elbow.

Lateral (lat.) means toward the side of the body. The ears are lateral to the head. **Medial** means closer to the midline of the body or nearest to the middle of a body structure. For example, the heart is medial to the lungs. The term **peripheral** is used to describe the position of anything around an organ or extending outward from the body trunk. For example, peripheral nerves form networks extending from the spinal cord.

KEY TERM	Definition
ventral (VEN-trul)	anterior, belly side
dorsal (DOR-sul)	back side
cephalic (se-FAL-ick)	toward the head or pertaining to the head
caudal (KAW-dul)	toward the tail
superior (soo-PEER-ee-ur)	toward the head or upper part of a structure
inferior (in-FEER-ee-ur)	away from the head
cranial (KRAY-nee-ul)	toward the head or top
deep	away from the surface
superficial (soo-pur-FISH-ul)	pertaining to the surface
proximal (PROCK-si-mul)	toward the attachment of an extremity to the trunk
distal (DIS-tul)	farther from the attachment of an extremity to the trunk
lateral (LAT-ur-ul)	pertaining to the side
medial (MEE-dee-ul)	toward the midline
peripheral (puh-RIF-uh-rul)	around an organ or extending outward from the body trunk

KEY TERM PRACTICE: *Directional Terms*

1. The hand is _____ to the shoulder.

2. The head is _____ to the feet.

3. The opposite of anterior is _____.

4. The opposite of deep is _____.

5. The eyes are _____ to the nose.

Abdominopelvic Quadrants and Regions

To describe the location of body structures and provide points of reference, the abdominopelvic cavity is divided into quadrants. These are important because they enable medical professionals to work from the same point of reference. **Quadrants** are four descriptive regions of the abdominopelvic cavity that are used in physical examinations. Imaginary horizontal and vertical lines passing through the umbilicus (belly button) create the following four sections (**Figure 2-9**): **left upper quadrant (LUQ)**, **right upper quadrant (RUQ)**, **left lower quadrant (LLQ)**, and **right lower quadrant (RLQ)**.

A different approach divides the lower trunk into nine separate regions. **Regions** are abdominopelvic body divisions. The regions are arranged like a tic-tac-toe game, divided by two vertical lines and two horizontal lines that run through the body to create nine squares (**Figure 2-10**): the **epigastric**, **left** and **right hypochondriac**, **umbilical**, **left** and **right lumbar**,

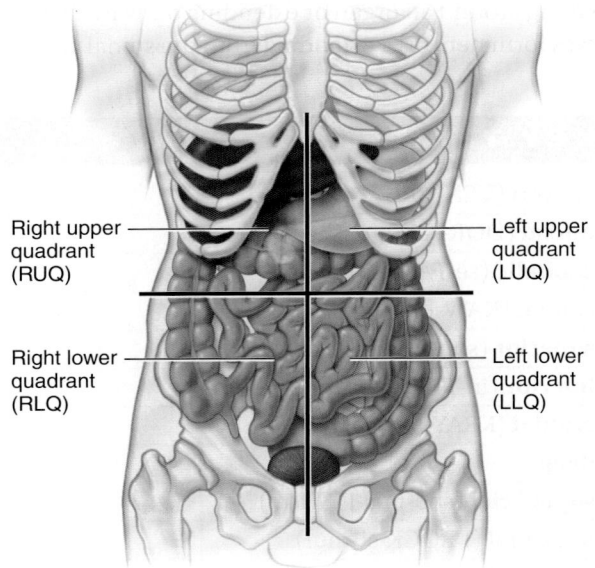

Right upper quadrant (RUQ)

Left upper quadrant (LUQ)

Right lower quadrant (RLQ)

Left lower quadrant (LLQ)

Figure 2-9 Abdominopelvic quadrants are four regions of the abdominopelvic cavity that are used in physical examinations.

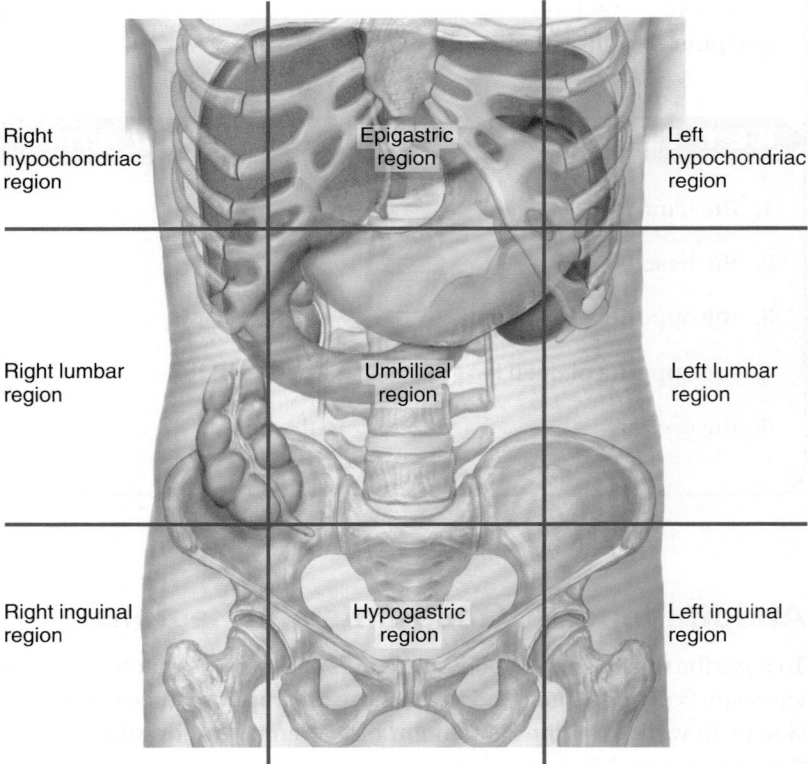

Right hypochondriac region

Epigastric region

Left hypochondriac region

Right lumbar region

Umbilical region

Left lumbar region

Right inguinal region

Hypogastric region

Left inguinal region

Figure 2-10 The nine abdominopelvic regions.

hypogastric, and **left** and **right inguinal**. Knowing the location of specific organs in these regions is necessary because it helps clinicians isolate sources of aches and pains. For example, pain in the right hypochondriac region may indicate a gallbladder problem.

KEY TERM	Definition
quadrants (KWAH-drunts)	four areas of the abdominopelvic cavity
left upper quadrant (KWAH-drunt) **(LUQ)**	one area of the abdominopelvic cavity on the superior left side
right upper quadrant (KWAH-drunt) **(RUQ)**	one area of the abdominopelvic cavity on the superior right side
left lower quadrant (KWAH-drunt) **(LLQ)**	one area of the abdominopelvic cavity on the inferior left side
right lower quadrant (KWAH-drunt) **(RLQ)**	one area of the abdominopelvic cavity on the inferior right side
regions	nine divisions of the abdominopelvic cavity
epigastric (ep-i-GAS-trick) **region**	upper middle region between the two hypochondriac regions
left hypochondriac (high-poh-KON-dree-ack) **region**	left upper lateral region below the lower ribs
right hypochondriac (high-poh-KON-dree-ack) **region**	right upper lateral region below the lower ribs
umbilical (um-BIL-i-kul) **region**	middle region below the epigastric region and above the pubic region
left lumbar (LUM-bahr) **region**	region to the left side of the umbilical region
right lumbar (LUM-bahr) **region**	region to the right side of the umbilical region
hypogastric (high-poh-GAS-trick) **region**	pubic region
left inguinal (ING-gwi-nul) **region**	left lower region beside the pubic region
right inguinal (ING-gwi-nul) **region**	right lower region beside the pubic region

KEY TERM PRACTICE: *Abdominopelvic Quadrants and Regions*

1. The abdominopelvic cavity can be divided into nine _____.

2. The four areas of the abdominopelvic cavity are termed _____.

3. Name the four quadrants. _____

4. Name the nine abdominopelvic regions. _____

Anatomical Planes

The body can be diagrammed according to planes of reference. This enables medical personnel to study and visualize the structural arrangement of various organs. **Planes** are imaginary flat surfaces used to divide the body or organs into definite areas. **Figure 2-11** shows the three fundamental planes of reference: sagittal, frontal, and horizontal.

A **sagittal plane** divides the body into left and right sides. A specific type of sagittal plane is a **midsagittal**, which is a vertical surface through the midline of the body that divides it into *equal* left and right sides. The key is *equal* because it passes through the midplane of the body.

A **frontal plane**, also called a **coronal plane**, is a plane passing lengthwise to divide the body or organs into anterior and posterior portions. In essence, the body or part is sectioned into front and back segments.

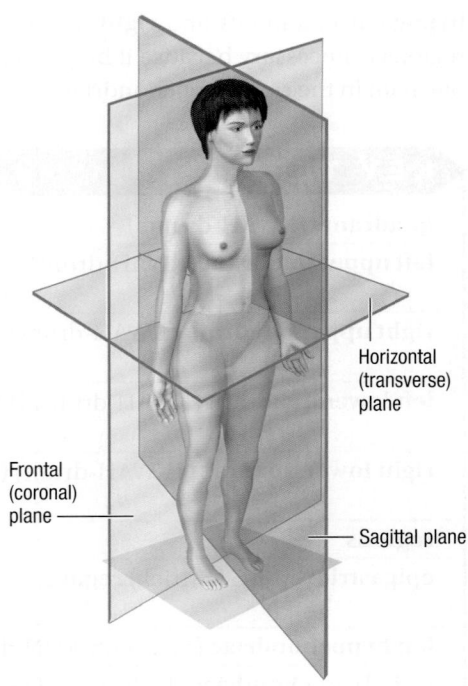

Horizontal (transverse) plane

Frontal (coronal) plane

Sagittal plane

Figure 2-11 The body can be sectioned and diagrammed according to planes of reference.

A **horizontal plane**, or **transverse plane**, is a line drawn parallel to the ground at a right angle to the sagittal and frontal planes. It divides the body or organ into superior (upper) and inferior (lower) portions.

KEY TERM	Definition
planes	imaginary lines representing flat surfaces used to divide the body
sagittal (SAJ-i-tul) **plane**	line dividing the body into left and right sides
midsagittal (mid-SAJ-i-tul) **plane**	line dividing the body at the middle creating equal left and right halves
frontal plane	line dividing the body into front and back parts; also called a coronal plane
coronal (KOR-oh-nul) **plane**	line dividing the body into front and back parts; also called a frontal plane
horizontal plane	line parallel to the ground or the body's axis creating superior and inferior portions; also called a transverse plane
transverse (trans-VURCE) **plane**	line parallel to the ground or the body's axis creating superior and inferior portions; also called a horizontal plane

KEY TERM PRACTICE: *Anatomical Planes*

1. Two terms that describe a plane that divides the body into inferior and superior portions are _____ and _____.

2. Which planes divide the body into anterior and posterior parts? _____

3. A plane that divides the body or structure into equal right and left sides is called a _____ plane.

4. _____ are imaginary lines representing flat surfaces that are used to divide the body.

5. The plane that divides the body into left and right sides is termed a _____.

Anatomical Terms

Anatomical terms are words describing superficial landmarks used for body orientation. All references are based on the person being in the anatomic position. **Figure 2-12** demonstrates these landmarks in (A) anterior view and (B) posterior view. **Tables 2-2** and **2-3** list anatomical terms in their adjective form along with their common name for the anterior and posterior views, respectively. For example, the area around the nose is known as the *nasal* region. Many of these terms provide the foundation for the names of other anatomical structures. For this reason, learning the terms now will make the later chapters more understandable.

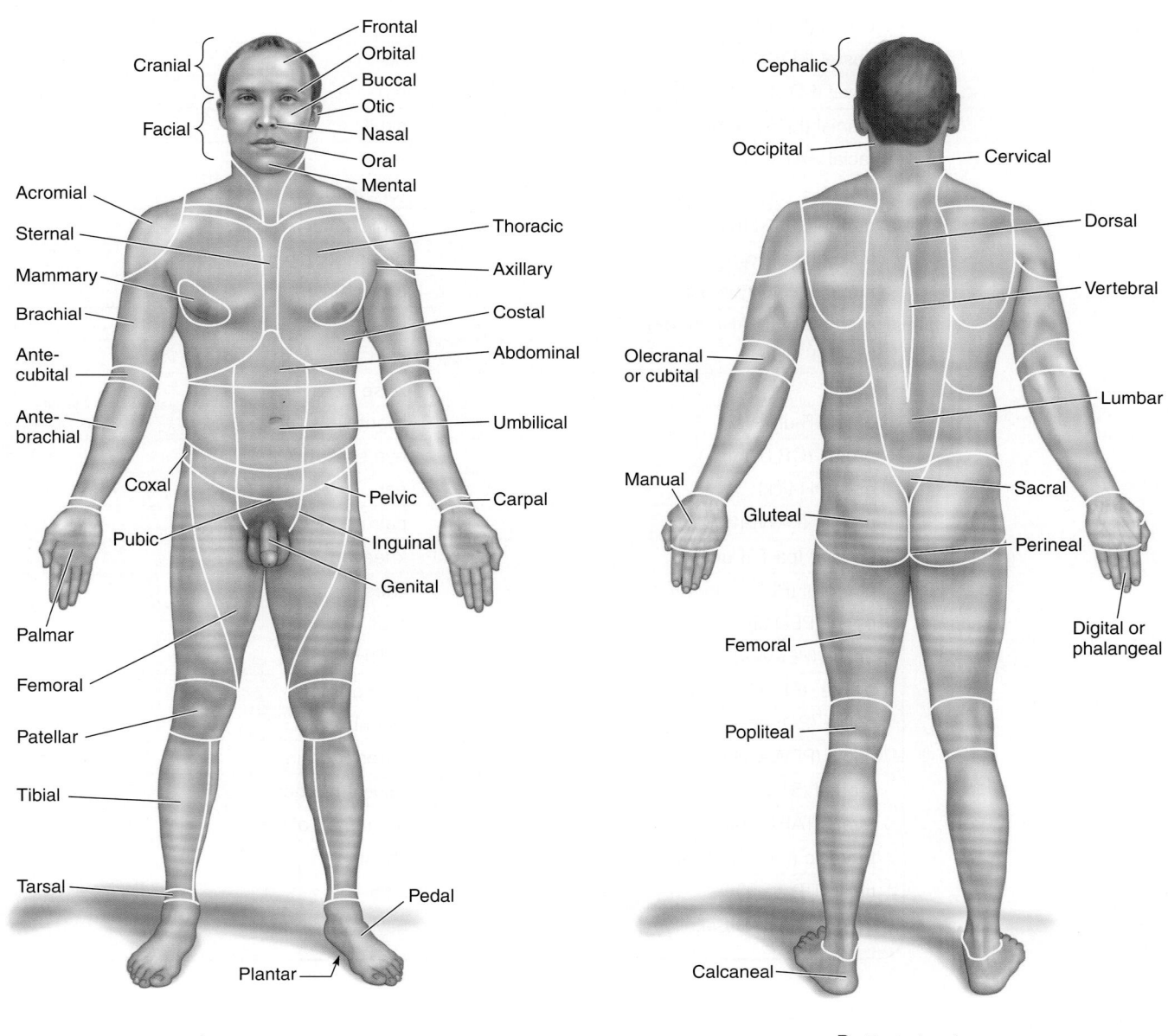

A   Anterior view

B   Posterior view

Figure 2-12 Anatomical terms describing superficial landmarks used for body orientation: **(A)** anterior view; **(B)** posterior view.

T A B L E **2-2**

ANATOMICAL TERMS
(ANTERIOR VIEW)

Adjective Form for Describing Region	Common Name
abdominal (ab-DOM-i-nul)	abdomen; inferior cavity of the trunk
acromial (uh-KROH-mee-ul)	point of shoulder
antebrachial (an-te-BRAY-kee-ul)	forearm
antecubital (an-te-KEW-bi-tul)	front of elbow; inner elbow
axillary (ACK-si-lerr-ee)	armpit
brachial (BRAY-kee-ul)	arm
buccal (BUCK-ul)	cheek
carpal (KAHR-pul)	wrist
costal (KOS-tul)	rib
coxal (KOCK-sul)	hip
cranial (KRAY-nee-ul)	skull
facial (FAY-shul)	face
frontal	forehead
genital (JEN-i-tul)	reproductive organs
hallux (HAL-ucks)	great toe; big toe
inguinal (ING-gwi-nul)	groin
mammary (MAM-uh-ree)	breast
mental	chin
nasal	nose
oral (OR-ul)	mouth
orbital (OR-bi-tul)	eye socket
otic (OH-tick)	ear
palmar (PAWL-mur)	palm
patellar (pa-TEL-ur)	kneecap
pectoral (PECK-tuh-rul)	chest or breast
pedal (PED-ul)	foot
pelvic (PEL-vick)	pelvis
plantar (PLAN-tur)	sole of foot
pollex (POL-ecks)	thumb
pubic (PEW-bick)	anterior groin
sternal (STUR-nul)	middle of chest
tarsal (TAHR-sul)	top instep of foot
thoracic (thoh-RAS-ick)	chest
tibial (TIB-ee-ul)	shin
umbilical (um-BIL-i-kul)	navel; bellybutton

TABLE 2-3

ANATOMICAL TERMS
(POSTERIOR VIEW)

Adjective Form for Describing Region	Common Name
calcaneal (kal-KAY-nee-ul)	heel of foot
cephalic (se-FAL-ick)	head
cervical (SUR-vi-kul)	neck
cubital (KEW-bi-tul)	elbow
digital (DIJ-i-tul)	finger or toe
dorsal (DOR-sul)	back
femoral (FEM-uh-rul)	thigh
gluteal (GLOO-tee-ul)	buttocks
lumbar (LUM-bahr)	lower back
manual	hand
occipital (ock-SIP-i-tul)	lower back of head
olecranal (oh-LECK-ruh-nul)	back of elbow
perineal (perr-i-NEE-ul)	*females:* between the vulva and anus
	males: between the scrotum and anus
phalangeal (fa-LAN-jee-ul)	finger or toe
popliteal (pop-LIT-ee-ul)	back of knee
sacral (SAY-krul)	lowest area of back
vertebral (VER-te-brul)	spinal column

KEY TERM PRACTICE: *Anatomical Terms*

1. What is the anatomical term used to describe the anterior lower leg? _____

2. The _____ region is found at the inner elbow.

3. The _____ region is located on the back of the knee.

4. The anatomical terms for the elbow are the _____ region or _____ region.

5. The term used to describe the bottom of the foot is _____ .

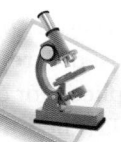

THE CLINICAL DIMENSION

Generalized terms identifying signs and symptoms, clinical tests and diagnostic procedures, pathology, and treatments are defined in this section. Disorders affecting various body systems and chapter-specific medical terms related to those conditions will be given in the appropriate chapters that follow.

Signs and Symptoms

Disease is an indication that the body's homeostatic balance has been disrupted. Signs and symptoms indicate abnormal states. **Signs** are objective evidence of disease—that is, they can be determined by physical examination and clinical tests. Irregular pulse and respiratory rates, fever, and abnormal blood pressure are examples of signs. **Symptoms** are less obvious because they are subjective—that is, symptoms are something that the person experiences, such as dizziness, pain, and itching. Signs and symptoms (S&S) pertaining to diseases that affect particular body systems are presented in subsequent chapters.

KEY TERM	Definition
signs	objective evidence of disease
symptoms	subjective state of disease

KEY TERM PRACTICE: *Signs and Symptoms*

1. Dizziness and headache are examples of _____.

2. Fever and high blood pressure are examples of _____.

Clinical Tests and Diagnostic Procedures

Disease diagnosis is based on information gathered from professional experience, physical examination, visual inspection, and the results of clinical tests and investigative procedures. Despite the clinician's great knowledge of physiology and the advances in technology, medicine remains an art as well as a science.

Using their fingers, clinicians often detect landmarks or attempt to isolate tender spots and sore lumps by applying firm pressure to the body surface. This procedure is termed **palpation**. When a clinician taps sharply on various body locations, this is called **percussion** (**Figure 2-13A**). To determine fluid accumulation and organ densities, the thoracic and abdominal regions are percussed to detect resonating vibrations. Tapping over the chest determines the presence of normal air content in the lungs, and tapping over the abdomen evaluates air in the intestines and the sizes of the solid organs.

Another common procedure, **auscultation**, refers to using a medical instrument called a **stethoscope** to listen to various organs as they perform their functions (**Figure 2-13B**). The stethoscope usually has a small disk-shaped resonator that is placed against the body and two tubes connected to earpieces. For example, clinicians can listen to breathing sounds, heartbeats, and digestive noises.

To determine the state of certain parts of the nervous system and specific organs of innervation, reflex responses are used. A **reflex response** is the involuntary movement that occurs after a stimulus has been applied. For example, a clinician uses a rubber hammer to strike the knee directly below the patella (kneecap); in response to this, the lower leg kicks out (knee-jerk response).

Various anatomy scanning instruments and equipment used to visualize the internal body are available. Some of these include conventional radiography (x-ray imaging), computed tomography (CT), positron emission tomography (PET), and magnetic resonance imaging (MRI).

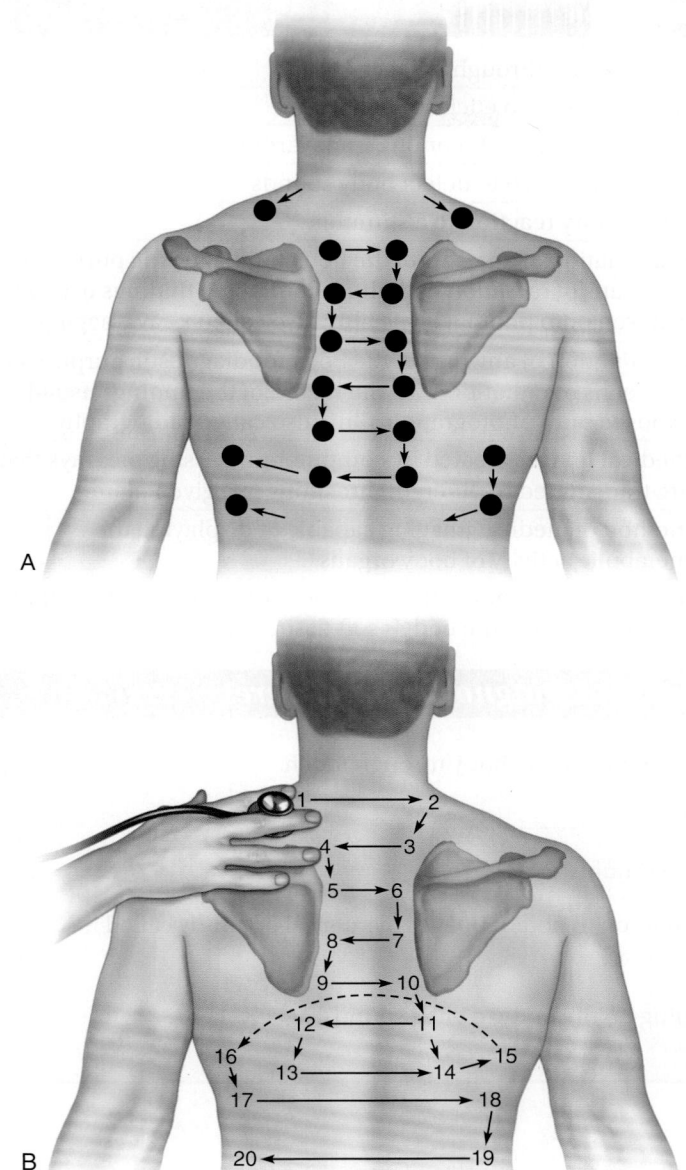

A

B

Figure 2-13 (A) Sites of percussion. Percussion can determine fluid accumulation and organ densities. **(B)** Sites of auscultation. During auscultation, a clinician can listen through a stethoscope to various organs as they perform their functions.

Radiography or **x-ray imaging** is used in medical examinations to produce images of internal structures by x-rays, gamma rays, or similar radiation. With **computed tomography (CT)**, images of anatomical structures are generated by a computer synthesis of x-ray transmission data obtained in many different directions in a given plane. **Positron emission tomography (PET)** is a medical imaging technique that utilizes gamma rays to produce a three-dimensional image or picture of body processes. PET scans create images of the metabolic activity in the body and are useful in diagnosing cancer, locating brain tumors, and assessing other brain disorders. An imaging technique that uses electromagnetic radiation to obtain images of the body's soft tissues, such as the brain and spinal cord, is called **magnetic resonance imaging (MRI)**. These diagnostic tools are discussed in greater detail in other chapters, beginning with Chapter 3.

KEY TERM	Definition
palpation (pal-PAY-shun)	examination through touch
percussion (pur-KUSH-un)	firmly tapping to elicit sounds
auscultation (aws-kul-TAY-shun)	listening for sounds coming from various organs
stethoscope (STETH-uh-skope)	instrument used to detect body sounds
reflex response	involuntary reaction to a stimulus
radiography (ray-dee-OG-ruh-fee)	examination of any part of the body for diagnostic purposes by means of radiation with the record of the findings usually exposed onto photographic film; also called x-ray imaging
x-ray imaging	examination of any part of the body for diagnostic purposes by means of radiation with the record of the findings usually exposed onto photographic film; also called radiography
computed tomography (CT) (tuh-MOG-ruh-fee)	medical images created by computer processing of x-rays that are transmitted in different directions in a given plane
positron emission tomography (PET) (POZ-ih-tron eh-MISH-un tuh-MOG-ruh-fee)	method of medical imaging capable of displaying the metabolic activity of body organs
magnetic resonance imaging (MRI) (mag-NET-ick REZ-uh-nants)	an imaging technique that uses electromagnetic radiation to obtain images of the body's soft tissues

KEY TERM PRACTICE: *Clinical Tests and Diagnostic Procedures*

1. The term _____ refers to physical examination of the body through touch.

2. Listening to heart sounds through a stethoscope is called _____.

3. A _____ is an involuntary reaction to a stimulus.

4. An imaging technique that utilizes electromagnetic radiation to obtain images of internal organs is called _____.

5. _____ describes the technique of tapping on the body to elicit sounds.

Disorders

The mechanisms of disease are varied and numerous. Common causes of disease are related to pathogens (disease-causing microorganisms such as bacteria and viruses), autoimmunity (triggered by the body's own antibodies), inflammation, malnutrition, and chemicals. The following chapters describe how many of these agents promote the onset of disease. Other disease risk factors include genetics, age, lifestyle, stress, environment, and preexisting conditions that lead to ill health.

Pathology is the scientific study of the nature, origin, progress, characteristics, and effects of disease. Some frequently used terms in the field of pathology are pathogenesis, pathophysiology, and epidemiology. **Pathogenesis** refers to the origin and course of disease development. It attempts to provide the **etiology**, factors that contribute to the occurrence of the disease. If the cause cannot be determined, it is termed **idiopathic**. The study of body function or physiological processes modified by disease is termed **pathophysiology**. The study of disease occurrence, distribution, and transmission is called **epidemiology**. For example, when there is an outbreak of a particular disease, such as Ebola fever, specialists called epidemiologists track the course and development of the disease. They also try to locate the very first person, or **index case**, who exhibited signs and symptoms of the illness they are studying.

KEY TERM	Definition
pathogenesis (path-oh-JEN-i-sis)	origin and course of disease development
etiology (ee-tee-OL-uh-jee)	study of the cause and course of disease development
idiopathic (id-ee-oh-PATH-ick)	disease or condition that arises for which there is no known cause
pathophysiology (path-oh-fiz-ee-OL-uh-jee)	study of body function modified by disease
epidemiology (ep-i-dee-mee-OL-uh-jee)	study of disease occurrence and distribution
index case	first documented person identified with a particular disease

KEY TERM PRACTICE: *Disorders*

1. The first person identified with an outbreak of chickenpox is called the _____.

2. If the suffix *-gist* refers to a person who works in a particular field, then a person who studies pathology would be called a _____.

3. The suffix *-gist* refers to a person who works in a particular field, so a person who studies the distribution and occurrence of disease is called an _____.

4. The term _____ is used to describe a disease or disorder that has no known cause.

5. The study of the factors that contribute to the cause and occurrence of a disease is _____.

Treatments

Pathological conditions may be resolved or altered through treatment. Treatment is often synonymous with therapy and involves therapeutic measures to alleviate signs and symptoms or to cure the disease. Treatment can include medication, physical rehabilitation, exercise, nutrition strategies, surgery, radiation therapy, or psychological therapy.

The prevention or treatment of disease by chemicals and medicines is termed **chemotherapy**. **Physical rehabilitation** is a type of therapy that helps the individual regain functional use of a particular body part or the body as a whole. The goal of physical rehabilitation is to restore the ability to function in a normal or near-normal manner after disease, illness, or injury. It may involve the professional services of physical therapists. Moreover, exercise is often a treatment option to preserve or restore health.

Nutrition strategies are used to maintain and/or repair the body. Nutrition involves the ingestion of the appropriate vitamins, minerals, and nutrients (carbohydrates, fats, and proteins). There is growing evidence that good nutrition plays a large role in preventing and treating disease.

Surgery is an operative procedure used to treat various conditions. In many cases, surgery is a last resort when other treatment options fail, or it is used because research has demonstrated its superiority over the alternatives.

Radiation therapy treats disease with ionizing radiation such as x-rays, β-rays (beta rays), and γ-rays (gamma rays). It is commonly used for cancer treatment. **Psychological therapy** is used for treating the mind. It involves counseling with a psychiatrist, psychologist, or counselor.

KEY TERM	Definition
chemotherapy	use of medications or chemicals to treat disease
physical rehabilitation	physical therapy to regain function
nutrition strategies	eating well for health
surgery	an operation or operative procedure
radiation therapy	treatment using ionizing radiation
psychological therapy	treatment for the mind

KEY TERM PRACTICE: *Treatments*

1. What sort of treatment is likely to be prescribed for a patient who has just had a cast removed from her arm?
_____

2. The umbrella term describing the use of chemical agents to treat disease is _____.

3. Another term for an operation or operative procedure is _____.

4. Treatment using ionizing radiation is called _____.

5. _____ is a treatment for the mind and uses the services of a psychologist.

LIFE SPAN

Lifespan is the maximum number of years a human is able to live. Despite available products aimed at increasing our years on earth, the human lifespan appears to be fixed at approximately 120 years. Many have approached her record, but the world's longest-lived person at 122 years was Jeanne Calment of France, who was born February 21, 1875, and died August 4, 1997.

The lifespan varies by species, ranging from 1 day for mayflies to about 13 years for medium-size dogs to 5,000 years for a bristle-cone pine tree. Lifespan should not be confused with life expectancy, which is the number of years a person can look forward to living under particular circumstances. For example, cigarette smoking greatly increases the risks of cardiovascular disease, which decreases a person's chances of living a very long life. According to 2005–2010 statistics compiled by the World Health Organization (WHO), the life expectancy for the world is 67.2 years (65.0 years for males and 69.5 years for females). Those figures are markedly different across the globe. For example, the life expectancy in Japan is 82.6 years (78.0 years for males and 86.1 years for females), while the life expectancy in Swaziland is 39.6 years (39.8 years for males and 39.4 years for females.) In the United States, the average life expectancy is 79.4 years (75.5 years for males and 83.3 years for females).

Throughout the human lifespan, from conception to death, many changes take place within the various levels of body organization. A critical period in human development is the first few weeks when embryonic membranes form and then transform into three primary germ layers: endoderm, ectoderm, and mesoderm. These germ layers then differentiate into all body cells, tissues, organs, and systems.

Human life phases are marked by embryonic development, fetal stage, neonatal period (the first 4 weeks of infant life), infancy, childhood, puberty and adolescence, and adulthood. Aging occurs at all levels of organization, but the manifestations may not necessarily be experienced until advanced old age. In subsequent chapters, the lifespan section will focus on key system-specific physiological, anatomical, and pathological changes that occur throughout the aging process.

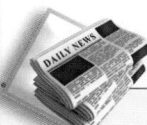

IN THE NEWS: Wrong-Site Surgery

Imagine the horror of waking up from anesthesia to discover that the wrong limb had been amputated. On February 20, 1995, that is exactly what happened to Willie King of Tampa, Florida. Due to complications of diabetes, Mr. King was scheduled for a below-the-knee right-leg amputation. Surgeons had mistakenly removed his *left* leg. Two weeks later, his diseased right leg was removed, greatly affecting his quality of life.

There is limited research on wrong-site surgeries, but all are preventable medical errors. According to a study supported by the Agency for Healthcare Research and Quality (AHRQ), the rate of wrong-site surgeries was 1 in 112,994 cases between 1985 and 2004. Wrong-site surgical procedures fall into four broad categories: (1) wrong-side surgery, (2) wrong-level/wrong-part surgery, (3) correct-site/wrong-procedure surgery, and (4) wrong-patient surgery. Wrong-side surgeries are described as those procedures performed on the opposite anatomical extremity or body structure. Wrong-level and wrong-part surgeries are done in proximity to the correct spot. Correct-site/wrong-procedure surgeries occur when the correct anatomical structure is treated but the incorrect procedure is performed. Last, the wrong-patient category includes procedures performed on the wrong person and the wrong surgery performed on the right person.

The Joint Commission, formerly called the Joint Commission on Accreditation of Healthcare Organizations (JCAHO) lists wrong-site surgery as the fourth most commonly reported event. The most commonly occurring anatomic location of wrong-site orthopedic surgery was the knee, followed by the ankle/foot, hip, leg, hand/fingers, and wrist.

It is estimated that the Joint Commission's Universal Protocol might have prevented only 62% of the cases of wrong-site surgery. The American College of Surgeons and individual hospitals each have site-verification protocols. The practice with the greatest potential seems to be the "sign your site" program. Patients undergoing a surgical procedure involving a limb sign their initials at the surgical site; physicians also sign the site. Use of an anatomical marking, such as "wrong," "cut here," "no," or "correct" on limbs is recommended to prevent wrong-site surgeries (**Figure 2-14**). This initial double-check system is used in conjunction with a verification checklist to ensure procedures are performed on the proper body part. Knowing correct anatomical terminology and position is crucial for preventing wrong-site amputations.

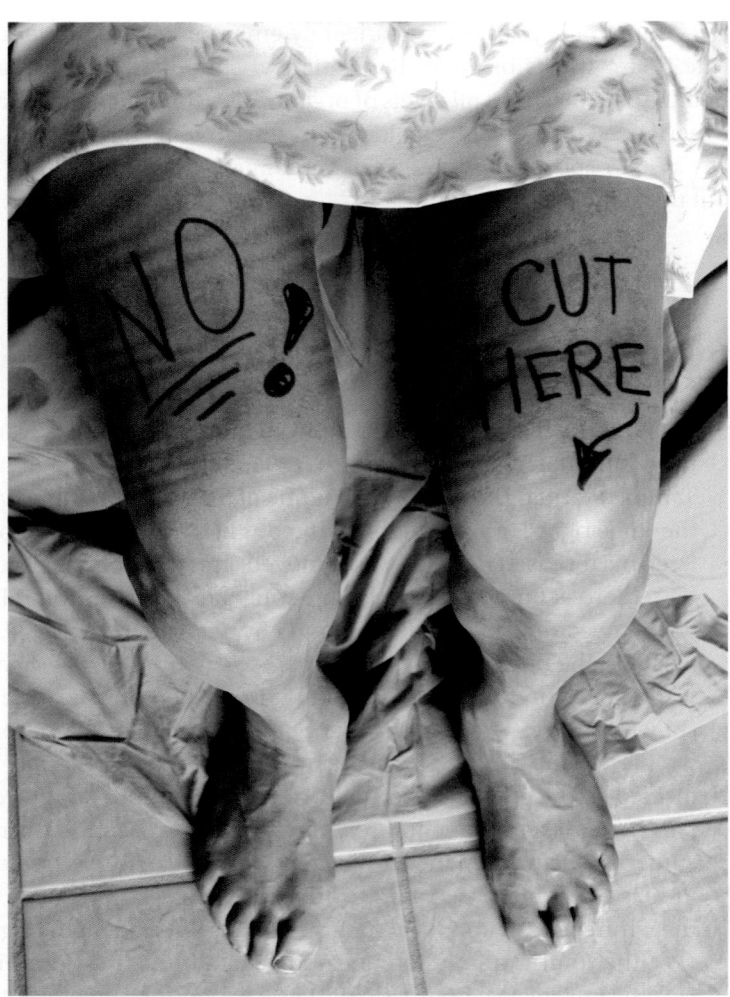

Figure 2-14 An example of marking a limb to prevent wrong-site surgery.

COMMON Abbreviations

Abbreviation	Term
AHRQ	Agency for Healthcare Research and Quality
AP	anteroposterior
ATP	adenosine triphosphate
CT	computed tomography
DNA	deoxyribonucleic acid
JCAHO	Joint Commission on Accreditation of Healthcare Organizations
lat.	lateral
LLQ	left lower quadrant
LUQ	left upper quadrant
MRI	magnetic resonance imaging
PET	positron emission tomography
RLQ	right lower quadrant

continued

continued from page 72

Abbreviation	Term
RNA	ribonucleic acid
RUQ	right upper quadrant
S&S	signs and symptoms
WHO	World Health Organization

COMMON ABBREVIATIONS EXERCISES

1. Write the abbreviation for right lower quadrant. _____

2. Computed tomography is abbreviated _____.

3. Write the abbreviation for adenosine triphosphate. _____

4. S&S is the abbreviation for _____.

5. Write the abbreviation for lateral. _____

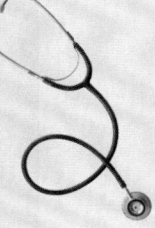

Case Study

Mr. Smythe, a 67-year-old male with diabetes, arrived in the hospital with pain in his right back. His history indicates that he has had diabetes for 30 years, takes regular insulin injections, gets no exercise, and that he had a right nephrectomy 1 month ago. He also had a right hip replacement several years ago. He is 6 feet 3 inches tall and weighs 200 lbs. The physical examination revealed nothing remarkable other than pain when palpating the right lumbar region. Chemical analysis of the urine was negative. He was admitted and his nurse, Susan, is taking him to the radiology department, where CT scans of the abdomen and pelvis will be performed.

Case Study Questions

Select the best answer to each of the following questions.

1. Mr. Smythe had a right nephrectomy 1 month ago. This means that he had _____.

a. both kidneys removed
b. his right kidney removed
c. tests performed on his kidney
d. an artificial kidney operation

2. What does the phrase "palpating the right lumbar region" mean? _____

a. listening to sounds through a stethoscope
b. during the physical examination, the clinician is examining the right, lower back by touching and pressing on specific areas
c. tapping in the upper back
d. trying to elicit an involuntary reaction to a stimulus

3. Why might right lumbar pain be expected after a right nephrectomy? _____

a. That is the location of the right kidney.
b. That is the location of the bladder.
c. That is the location of the right lung.
d. That is the location of the heart.

4. CT scans of the abdomen and pelvis were ordered. CT images are created from which type of technology? _____

a. magnetic resonance
b. sound waves
c. x-rays
d. fluoroscopy

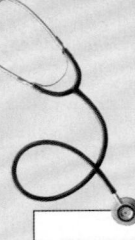

Real World Report

Susan transported Mr. Smythe by wheelchair to the hospital's radiology department. He underwent CT scanning of his abdominal and pelvic areas. The radiologist's report follows.

IMAGING DEPARTMENT: CT SCAN

NAME: Matt Smythe
DATEORD: August 10, 2011
ORDPHYS: Dr. Flagg
TEST: Abdomen CT
ATTENDING: N/A
REFERRING: N/A
CLINIC: Hospital
ADDORD: N/A
PT: Smythe
EXAM: N/A
ROOM: CT
ACCT: 0010213
TYPE: N/A
DATE: August 10, 2011

CLINICAL INFORMATION:

Status post previous right nephrectomy; follow-up.

CT ABDOMEN

CT scans of the abdomen were obtained before and after intravenous contrast administration. The enteric contrast was given before the examination. The previous examination of July 20, 2009, was compared.

The liver is of unremarkable size without focal mass or biliary dilation. The spleen and the adrenal glands are unremarkable. There is moderate atrophy of the pancreas, which is probably an unremarkable finding.

Previous right nephrectomy is evident. There is no evidence of recurrent retroperitoneal mass or lymphadenopathy. The left kidney shows clustered perinephric cysts, which are of no clinical significance. No focal mass or hydronephrosis is demonstrated at the left kidney. No paranephric fluid collection is noted. There is no ascites.

There is a small ventral hernia in the midline of the midabdomen. A small, nondilated small-bowel loop is present within the hernia without evidence of obstructive phenomenon.

There is a metallic device at the lower anterior abdominal wall to reinforce the previous anterior abdominal incision in the midline. There is also a small hernia present along the left side of the metallic device within the lower abdomen. A small nondilated small-bowel loop is present within this second ventral hernia.

CT PELVIS

CT scans of the pelvis were obtained before and after intravenous contrast administration. The enteric contrast was given before the examination.

continued

continued from page 74

There is no pelvic mass or lymph nodal enlargement. The anatomical details of the soft tissue structures are somewhat limited at the right lower pelvis resulting from the metallic right hip prosthesis.

IMPRESSION

- Status post previous right nephrectomy; no evidence of recurrent retroperitoneal mass or lymphadenopathy.
- Peripelvic cysts at the left kidney; otherwise the left kidney is unremarkable.
- Normal appearing liver.
- Two ventral hernias within the mid and the lower abdomen.

DICTATED BY: Dr. Amy Weissen

Real World Report Questions

The following exercises review the medical terms used in the preceding medical report.

1. The first section of the report describes a CT scan of the abdomen.

   a. CT is the medical abbreviation for _____.

   b. Using directional terminology, describe the location of the abdomen.

   _____

   _____

   _____

2. What organs were found in the abdominal scan?

   _____

   _____

   _____

3. The report indicated a "small ventral hernia in the midline of the midabdomen."

   a. Is this hernia located toward the front or toward the back of the abdomen?

   _____.

   b. Is this hernia located in the middle of, left of center of, or right of center of the abdomen?

   _____.

4. The report cited an "anterior abdominal incision in the midline." In nonmedical terms, describe the location of the incision.

   _____

   _____

   _____

5. Describe the location of the pelvis.

   _____

   _____

   _____

6. The report states that "tissue structures are somewhat limited at the right lower pelvis." Using the medical terminology for the abdominopelvic regions and quadrants, give alternate terms for this specific area.

   a. _____

   b. _____

7. *Retroperitoneal* is a common word used in medical reports to describe structures in the abdominopelvic region.

   a. Word part *retro-* means _____.

   b. Word part *peritoneo-* means _____.

   c. What does *retroperitoneal* mean?

   _____.

8. If the prefix *nephr-* means "kidney" and the suffix *-ectomy* means "surgical removal," what word from the report means removal of a kidney?

   _____

Review and Application

Multiple-Choice Questions

Select the best answer to each of the following questions.

1. The study of body structure is termed _____.
   a. anatomy   b. physiology   c. biology   d. pathophysiology

2. The study of body function is termed _____.
   a. anatomy   b. physiology   c. systemic anatomy   d. homeostasis

3. _____ is the term used to describe an anatomical shape.
   a. Somatotype   b. Anatomy   c. Axial   d. Morphology

4. Embryology is the study of _____.
   a. disease processes
   c. human development in utero until the end of the eighth week
   b. human development after birth
   d. body structures

5. The membrane covering the lung is the _____.
   a. parietal pleura   b. visceral pleura   c. pericardial pleura   d. serous pleura

6. The _____ peritoneum adheres to the abdominal wall.
   a. parietal   b. visceral   c. pericardial   d. pleural

7. Identify the word part that means "head." _____
   a. cyt-, cyto-   b. etio-   c. cephal-, cephalo-   d. bucco-

8. Identify the correct sequence, from *smallest* to *largest*, of the levels of organization. _____
   a. cell → organ → tissue → system → organism
   c. cell → molecule → organ → system → tissue
   b. tissue → cell → organ → system → organism
   d. cell → tissue → organ → system → organism

9. This type of plane divides the body into left and right halves. _____
   a. sagittal   b. frontal   c. coronal   d. midsagittal

10. This type of plane divides the body into anterior and posterior portions. _____
    a. coronal or frontal   b. coronal or sagittal   c. transverse or horizontal   d. frontal or median

11. In which region is the bladder located? _____
    a. lumbar region   b. hypogastric region   c. inguinal region   d. epigastric region

12. The lungs are located in the _____ cavity.
    a. abdominal   b. pelvic   c. thoracic   d. vertebral

13. Signs of an infection may include _____.
    a. fever   b. tiredness   c. sweating   d. a and c

14. Nursing notes indicate that sutures were placed superior to the right tarsal region, inferior to the patellar region. Identify the location in common terms. _____
    a. right shin   b. right thigh   c. right forearm   d. right shoulder

15. Dr. Cutter is about to amputate a patient's left leg inferior to the patella. Standing at the foot of the patient's bed, facing the patient, the leg that is to be removed should be closest to _____.
    a. Dr. Cutter's left arm   b. Dr. Cutter's right arm

Word Parts Exercises

Define the following word parts.

16. acro- = _____

17. homeo- = _____

18. parieto- = _____

19. pelvi-, pelvio-, pelvo- = _____

20. brachio- = _____

Matching Exercises

Match the system with its primary function.

21. _____ nervous

22. _____ endocrine

23. _____ cardiovascular

24. _____ muscular

25. _____ urinary

26. _____ skeletal

a. movement
b. integration
c. hormone secretion
d. nutrient transport
e. protection
f. waste removal

Match the body system with organs found in that system.

27. _____ urinary

28. _____ endocrine

29. _____ digestive

30. _____ respiratory

a. esophagus and stomach
b. kidneys and bladder
c. trachea and lungs
d. thyroid and thymus

Match the cellular organelle with its description.

31. _____ ribosome

32. _____ nucleus

33. _____ mitochondrion

a. power house of cell
b. protein synthesis
c. contains DNA

Supply a directional term to make each statement correct.

34. The right knee is _____ to the right hip.

35. The feet are _____ to the head.

36. The elbow is _____ to the hand.

Supply a regional name to make each statement correct.

37. The neck is called the _____ region.

38. The _____ region refers to the posterior knee.

39. The upper arm is the _____ region.

For each of the following terms, write the term that has the opposite meaning.

40. distal / _____

41. deep / _____

42. anterior / _____

43. inferior / _____

Spelling

Identify the correctly spelled term in each set.

44. _____   45. _____   46. _____   47. _____   48. _____

a. adominopelvic	a. iliac	a. saggital	a. popliteal	a. hypochondriak
b. abdamenopelvic	b. illiac	b. sagattal	b. poplliteal	b. hypochondriack
c. abdominopelvic	c. ileaic	c. saggittal	c. poplitial	c. hypochondriac
d. abdomialpelvic	d. illeac	d. sagittal	d. popplitial	d. hypocondriac

Write the plural form for each given term.

49. coxa _____

50. phalanx _____

51. umbilicus _____

Write the singular form for each given term.

52. crura _____   54. pelves _____

53. buccae _____   55. mitochondria _____

Unscramble

Unscramble the letters to form a medical term.

56. aeildm _____   59. rbosimoes _____

57. nipsue _____   60. rhirt erupp aadrtnqu _____

58. albidmona ycvtia _____

Abbreviations

Provide the term for the abbreviations and then define the terms.

61. AP = _____

62. PET = _____

63. LLQ = _____

Analogies

Provide a medical term to complete a meaningful analogy.

64. Atoms are to molecules as cells are to _____.
    a. organelles   b. tissues   c. organs   d. systems

65. Cranial is to skull as gluteal is to _____.
    a. head   b. chest   c. buttocks   d. knee

66. Calcaneal is to calcaneus as sternal is to _____.
    a. sternum   b. stern   c. sternus   d. sternial

Short Answer

Answer the following questions.

67. Mikey has had abdominal aches all evening. He thought it was just gas pains from eating too many beans. Since the pain was so severe, he went to the emergency clinic. After palpating the hypogastric region, the physician concluded it was appendicitis. What probably led to this diagnosis?

_____

_____

_____

68. Jim and John were riding bicycles when John stopped suddenly, causing Jim to crash into him. This minor accident caused Jim to have a pulled muscle in his femoral region and a pain in his cervical region. John's only complaint was in his axillary region. Where were Jim's and John's injuries?

_____

_____

Labeling

Using anatomical terms, label the regions in the following figures.

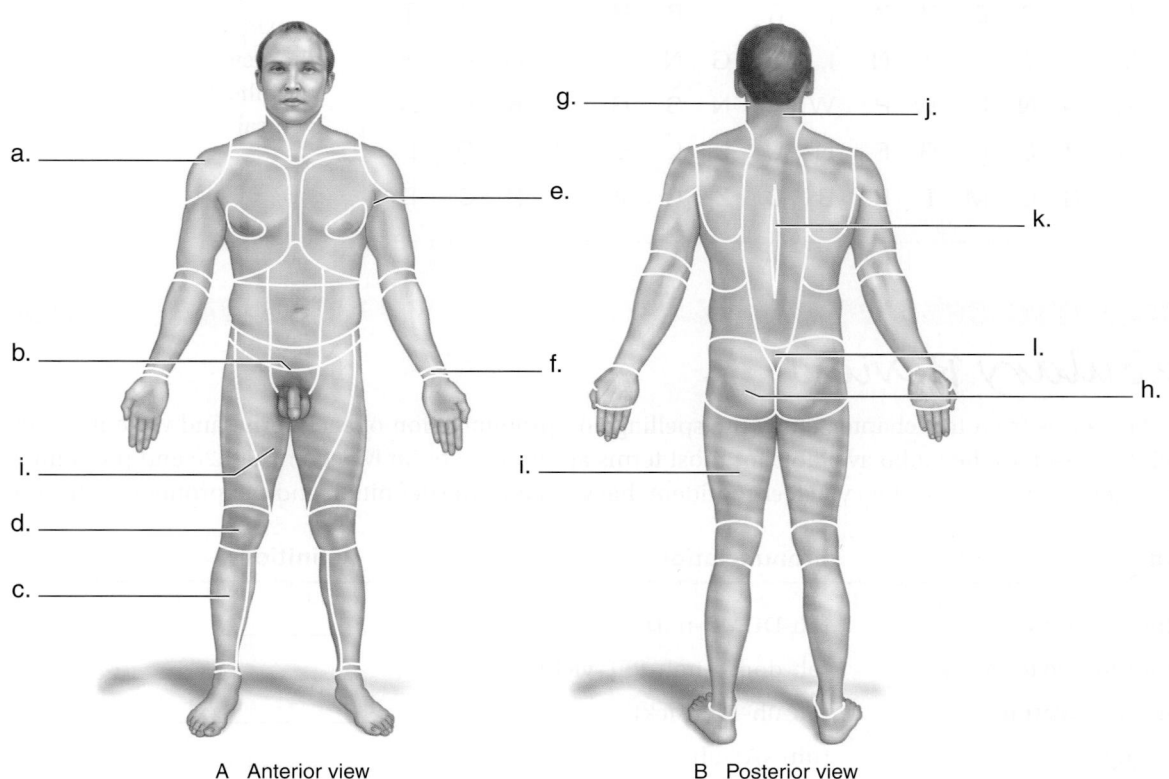

A   Anterior view   B   Posterior view

Word Search

Find the medical terms hidden in the puzzle.

```
C  Y  T  O  L  O  G  Y  V  E  T  S  A  P  N  I  X
L  A  R  R  E  A  L  U  P  L  E  F  I  E  H  N  C
M  N  I  J  G  A  M  I  T  M  P  W  R  R  T  F  I
L  G  B  R  I  M  G  I  O  F  C  Z  D  I  N  E  C
P  W  A  N  D  A  E  S  X  I  S  C  N  C  L  R  A
W  L  A  R  S  N  O  D  L  O  A  V  O  A  A  I  R
F  R  E  T  H  M  O  A  I  U  R  F  H  R  C  O  O
C  C  R  U  O  P  H  H  D  A  G  P  C  D  I  R  H
W  I  P  R  R  P  A  A  C  Z  S  Q  O  I  L  Z  T
C  U  H  W  E  A  L  I  Q  O  A  T  T  A  I  V  V
U  C  E  C  W  F  L  C  D  V  P  J  I  L  B  S  E
H  Y  P  O  G  A  S  T  R  I  C  Y  M  N  M  U  N
O  B  L  A  R  E  H  P  I  R  E  P  H  B  U  P  T
W  C  T  A  J  L  A  N  I  U  G  N  I  S  Q  M  R
K  B  H  D  N  I  W  P  W  F  N  S  G  Y  B  H  A
L  A  S  R  O  D  G  F  N  U  C  L  E  U  S  O  L
C  C  B  G  O  M  T  R  B  C  Z  C  V  Y  H  C  D
```

caudal
cephalic
chromosomes
cranial
cytology
diaphragm
dorsal
epigastric
hypochondriac
hypogastric
inferior
inguinal
mediastinum
mitochondria
nucleus
pericardial
peripheral
pleural
proximal
thoracic
umbilical
ventral

Vocabulary Review

Review the key terms from this chapter, study the spelling and pronunciation of each term, and write its definition in the space provided. Listen to the audio available for most terms at http://thepoint.lww.com/nath2e and pronounce each term for yourself. Then check the box when you feel confident that you know the definition and can pronounce the term correctly.

Key Term	Pronunciation	Definition
❏ **abdominal cavity**	(ab-DOM-i-nul)	
❏ **abdominopelvic cavity**	(ab-dom-i-noh-PEL-vick)	
❏ **anatomic position**	(an-uh-TOM-ick)	
❏ **anatomy**	(uh-NAT-uh-mee)	
❏ **anterior**	(an-TEER-ee-ur)	
❏ **anteroposterior (AP)**	(an-TEER-oh-pos-TEER-ee-or)	
❏ **appendicular**	(ap-en-DICK-yoo-lur)	
❏ **auscultation**	(aws-kul-TAY-shun)	
❏ **axial**	(ACK-see-ul)	
❏ **cardiovascular system**	(karr-dee-oh-VAS-kew-lur)	

Key Term	Pronunciation	Definition
❏ caudal	(KAW-dul)	
❏ cell membrane	(MEM-brane)	
❏ cells		
❏ cephalic	(se-FAL-ick)	
❏ chemotherapy		
❏ chromosomes	(KROH-muh-somes)	
❏ computed tomography (CT)	(tuh-MOG-ruh-fee)	
❏ connective tissue		
❏ coronal plane	(KOR-oh-nul)	
❏ cranial	(KRAY-nee-ul)	
❏ cytology	(si-TOL-uh-jee)	
❏ deep		
❏ diaphragm	(DYE-uh-fram)	
❏ digestive system	(di-JES-tiv)	
❏ distal	(DIS-tul)	
❏ dorsal	(DOR-sul)	
❏ embryology	(em-bree-OL-uh-jee)	
❏ endocrine system	(EN-doh-krin)	
❏ epidemiology	(ep-i-dee-mee-OL-uh-jee)	
❏ epigastric region	(ep-i-GAS-trick)	
❏ epithelial tissue	(ep-ih-THEE-lee-ul)	
❏ epithelium	(ep-ih-THEE-lee-um)	
❏ etiology	(ee-tee-OL-uh-jee)	
❏ frontal plane		
❏ genes		
❏ gross anatomy	(GROCE uh-NAT-uh-mee)	
❏ histology	(his-TOL-uh-jee)	
❏ horizontal plane		
❏ hypogastric region	(high-poh-GAS-trick)	
❏ idiopathic	(id-ee-oh-PATH-ick)	
❏ index case		
❏ inferior	(in-FEER-ee-ur)	
❏ integumentary system	(in-teg-yoo-MEN-tuh-ree)	
❏ lateral	(LAT-ur-ul)	
❏ left hypochondriac region	(high-poh-KON-dree-ack)	
❏ left inguinal region	(ING-gwi-nul)	
❏ left lower quadrant (LLQ)	(KWAH-drunt)	
❏ left lumbar region	(LUM-bahr)	
❏ left upper quadrant (LUQ)	(KWAH-drunt)	

Key Term	Pronunciation	Definition
❏ lymphatic system	(lim-FAT-ik)	_____
❏ magnetic resonance imaging (MRI)	(mag-NET-ick REZ-uh-nants)	_____
❏ medial	(MEE-dee-ul)	_____
❏ mediastinum	(mee-dee-uh-STYE-num)	_____
❏ membrane	(MEM-brane)	_____
❏ mesentery	(MES-un-terr-ee;-MEZ-un-terr-ee)	_____
❏ midsagittal plane	(mid-SAJ-i-tul)	_____
❏ mitochondria	(migh-toh-KON-dree-uh)	_____
❏ morphology	(mor-FOL-uh-jee)	_____
❏ muscular system	(MUS-kew-lur)	_____
❏ muscular tissue		_____
❏ nervous system		_____
❏ nervous tissue		_____
❏ nucleus	(NEW-klee-us)	_____
❏ nutrition strategies		_____
❏ organ		_____
❏ organ system		_____
❏ organelle	(OR-guh-nel)	_____
❏ organism	(OR-guh-NIZ-um)	_____
❏ palpation	(pal-PAY-shun)	_____
❏ parietal	(puh-RYE-e-tul)	_____
❏ pathogenesis	(path-oh-JEN-i-sis)	_____
❏ pathologist	(pa-THOL-uh-jist)	_____
❏ pathology	(pa-THOL-uh-jee)	_____
❏ pathophysiology	(path-oh-fiz-ee-OL-uh-jee)	_____
❏ pelvic cavity	(PEL-vick)	_____
❏ percussion	(pur-KUSH-un)	_____
❏ pericardial membranes	(perr-i-KAHR-dee-ul)	_____
❏ peripheral	(puh-RIF-uh-rul)	_____
❏ peritoneal membranes	(perr-i-toh-NEE-ul)	_____
❏ peritoneum	(PER-i-toh-NEE-um)	_____
❏ physical rehabilitation		_____
❏ physiology	(fiz-ee-OL-uh-jee)	_____
❏ planes		_____
❏ pleural membranes	(PLOOR-ul)	_____
❏ positron emission tomography (PET)	(POZ-ih-tron eh-MISH-un tuh-MOG-ruh-fee)	_____
❏ posterior	(pos-TEER-ee-ur)	_____

Key Term	Pronunciation	Definition
❏ prone		
❏ proximal	(PROCK-si-mul)	
❏ psychological therapy		
❏ quadrants	(KWAH-drunts)	
❏ radiation therapy		
❏ radiography	(ray-dee-OG-ruh-fee)	
❏ reflex response		
❏ regions		
❏ reproductive system	(ree-pruh-DUCK-tiv)	
❏ respiratory system	(RES-pi-ruh-toh-ree)	
❏ ribosomes	(RYE-boh-sohmz)	
❏ right hypochondriac region	(high-poh-KON-dree-ack)	
❏ right inguinal region	(ING-gwi-nul)	
❏ right lower quadrant (RLQ)	(KWAH-drunt)	
❏ right lumbar region	(LUM-bahr)	
❏ right upper quadrant (RUQ)	(KWAH-drunt)	
❏ sagittal plane	(SAJ-i-tul)	
❏ serosa	(se-ROH-suh)	
❏ serous membranes	(SEER-us)	
❏ signs		
❏ skeletal system	(SKEL-e-tul)	
❏ stethoscope	(STETH-uh-skope)	
❏ superficial	(soo-pur-FISH-ul)	
❏ superior	(soo-PEER-ee-ur)	
❏ supine	(suh-PINE;-SOO-pine)	
❏ surgery		
❏ symptoms		
❏ thoracic cavity	(thoh-RAS-ick)	
❏ tissue		
❏ transverse plane	(trans-VURCE)	
❏ umbilical region	(um-BIL-i-kul)	
❏ urinary system	(YOOR-i-nerr-ee)	
❏ ventral	(VEN-trul)	
❏ visceral	(VIS-ur-al)	
❏ x-ray imaging		

Answers

Word Grouping Exercises

Definition	Word Part	Definition	Word Part
body wall or parietal bone	parieto-	lateral, to one side	latero-
abdomen, abdominal	abdomin-, abdomino-	lung membrane, side	pleur-, pleura-, pleuro-
anterior, front	antero-	mouth	oro-
arm	brachio-	neck, cervix	cervico-
back, backward, behind	retro-	nose	naso-
before, in front of	ante-	nucleus	nucl-, nucleo-
body	somat-, somatico-, somato-	occiput, back part of head	occipito-
breasts	mamm-, mammo-	origin, beginning process	-genesis
cause	etio-	pelvis	pelvi-, pelvio-, pelvo-
cell	cyt-, cyto-	peritoneum	peritoneo-
cheek	bucco-	physiological	physi-, physio-
chemistry	chem-, chemo-	posterior, at the back	postero-
chest (thorax)	thorac-, thoracico-, thoraco-	proximal	prox-, proxi-, proximo-
disease	path-, patho-, -pathy	pubic	pubo-
ear	ot-, oto-	rib	costo-
embryo	embry-, embryo-	sacrum	sacro-
extremity, end, tip	acro-	same, steady	homeo-
face	facio-	skull, cranium	crani-, cranio-
foot or child	ped-, pedi-, pedo-	spine	spin-, spino-
form, shape	morph-, morpho-	sternum	stern-, sterno-
head	cephal-, cephalo-	tarsus (root of foot)	tars-, tarso-
heart	cardi-, cardio-	tissue	histio-, histo-
heel, calcaneus	calcaneo-	vertebra (backbone)	vertebro-
ilium, hip bone	ili-, ilio-	viscera (internal organs)	viscero-

Word Building Exercises

Word Part	Meaning	Common or Known Word	Example Medical Term
antero-	anterior, front	anterior	anterior
cardi-, cardio-	heart	cardiac arrest	pericardium
chem-, chemo-	chemistry	chemistry	chemotherapy
embry-, embryo-	embryo	embryo	embryo
-genesis	origin, beginning process	genesis	osteogenesis
homeo-	same, steady	homeopathy	homeostasis

Word Part	Meaning	Common or Known Word	Example Medical Term
latero-	lateral, to one side	lateral	lateral
mamm-, mammo-	breasts	mammary	mammary gland
naso-	nose	nasal	nasopharynx
nucl-, nucleo-	nucleus	nucleus	nucleus
retro-	back, backward, behind	retrofit	retroperitoneal
vertebro-	vertebra (backbone)	vertebrate	vertebral column

Key Term Practice

Anatomy and Physiology Defined

1. histology
2. pathology
3. physiology
4. embryology
5. anatomy

Cells and Organizational Structure

1. cell
2. tissue
3. organelles
4. Genes
5. epithelial tissue (epithelium), connective tissue, muscular tissue, and nervous tissue

Human Body Systems

1. integumentary, skeletal, nervous, muscular, endocrine, digestive, urinary, reproductive, respiratory, lymphatic, and cardiovascular
2. nervous; endocrine
3. muscular system and skeletal system

Body Membranes

1. visceral
2. parietal
3. peritoneal membranes or peritoneum
4. serous membranes or serosa
5. mesentery

Anatomic Position and Body Cavities

1. The person is standing erect, facing forward, with the arms at the sides and the palms facing forward.
2. abdominopelvic
3. appendicular; axial
4. prone
5. anterior

Directional Terms

1. distal
2. superior
3. posterior
4. superficial
5. lateral

Abdominopelvic Quadrants and Regions

1. regions
2. quadrants
3. left upper quadrant (LUQ), right upper quadrant (RUQ), left lower quadrant (LLQ), and right lower quadrant (RLQ)
4. left hypochondriac region, epigastric region, right hypochondriac region, left lumbar region, umbilical region, right lumbar region, left inguinal region, hypogastric region, and right inguinal region

Anatomical Planes

1. horizontal and transverse
2. frontal plane or coronal plane
3. midsagittal
4. Planes
5. sagittal plane

Anatomical Terms

1. tibial
2. antecubital
3. popliteal
4. olecranal region or cubital region
5. plantar

Signs and Symptoms

1. symptoms
2. signs

Clinical Tests and Diagnostic Procedures

1. palpation
2. auscultation
3. reflex response
4. magnetic resonance imaging (MRI)
5. Percussion

Disorders

1. index case
2. pathologist
3. epidemiologist
4. idiopathic
5. etiology

Treatments

1. physical rehabilitation
2. chemotherapy
3. surgery
4. radiation therapy
5. Psychological therapy

Common Abbreviations Exercises

1. right lower quadrant = RLQ
2. computed tomography = CT
3. adenosine triphosphate = ATP
4. S&S = signs and symptoms
5. lateral = lat.

Case Study

1. b is the correct answer.
   - a is incorrect because there are two kidneys (one on the left, and one on the right), he had his right one removed.
   - c and d are incorrect because *nephrectomy* refers to a kidney removal.
2. b is the correct answer.
   - a is incorrect because auscultating is the term used for listening, not palpating, which means examining by touch.
   - c is incorrect because percussing is the term for tapping, and the right lumbar region is located in the lower back, not the upper back.
   - d is incorrect because reflex response is the involuntary reaction to a stimulus; palpating refers to examining by touch.
3. a is the correct answer.
   - b is incorrect because the bladder is found in the hypogastric region.
   - c is incorrect because the lungs are found in the thoracic region.
   - d is incorrect because the heart is found in the mediastinum of the chest.
4. c is the correct answer.
   - a, b, and d are all incorrect; these technologies refer to other techniques for body visualization.

Real World Report

1. a. computed tomography
   b. The abdomen is located in the inferior cavity of the body trunk. It is bordered superiorly by the diaphragm.
2. Organs found in this CT abdominal scan were the spleen, adrenal glands, pancreas, liver, kidneys, and small bowel.
3. a. toward the front; b. middle of the abdomen
4. An incision had been made on the front of the body, along the center of the belly.
5. The pelvis is located inferiorly to the abdominal region and is bordered by the pelvic bones.
6. a. right inguinal (iliac) region; b. right lower quadrant (RLQ)
7. a. behind; b. peritoneum; c. behind the peritoneum
8. nephrectomy

Review and Application

1. a
2. b
3. d
4. c
5. b
6. a
7. c
8. d
9. d
10. a
11. b
12. c
13. d
14. a
15. b
16. extremity, end
17. same, steady
18. wall, parietal
19. pelvis
20. arm
21. b
22. c
23. d
24. a
25. f
26. e
27. b
28. d
29. a
30. c
31. b
32. c
33. a
34. distal
35. inferior
36. proximal
37. cervical
38. popliteal
39. brachial
40. proximal
41. superficial
42. posterior
43. superior
44. c
45. a
46. d
47. a
48. c
49. coxae
50. phalanges
51. umbilici
52. crus
53. bucca
54. pelvis
55. mitochondrion
56. medial
57. supine
58. abdominal cavity
59. ribosomes
60. right upper quadrant
61. AP = anteroposterior; relating to or directed toward both front and back
62. PET = positron emission tomography; nuclear medicine imaging technique capable of displaying the metabolic activity of body organs
63. LLQ = left lower quadrant; area of the abdominopelvic cavity on the inferior left side
64. b
65. c
66. a
67. The appendix is found in this specific region.
68. Jim's injuries were in his thigh (femoral region) and neck (cervical region). John's injury was in his armpit (axillary region).

Labeling

a. acromial
b. pubic
c. tibial
d. patellar
e. axillary
f. carpal
g. occipital
h. gluteal
i. femoral
j. cervical
k. vertebral
l. sacral

Word Search

```
C  Y  T  O  L  O  G  Y  +  E  +  S  A  P  N  I  +
+  A  +  +  +  A  L  +  P  +  E  +  I  E  +  N  C
M  +  I  +  +  A  M  I  +  M  +  +  R  R  +  F  I
+  G  +  R  I  M  G  I  O  +  C  +  D  I  +  E  C
P  +  A  N  D  A  E  S  X  I  +  C  N  C  L  R  A
+  L  A  R  S  N  O  D  L  O  A  +  O  A  A  I  R
+  R  E  T  H  M  O  A  I  U  R  +  H  R  C  O  O
C  +  R  U  O  P  H  H  D  A  +  P  C  D  I  R  H
+  I  +  R  R  P  A  A  C  +  S  +  O  I  L  +  T
C  +  H  +  E  A  L  I  +  O  +  T  T  A  I  +  V
+  C  +  C  +  +  L  +  D  +  P  +  I  L  B  +  E
H  Y  P  O  G  A  S  T  R  I  C  Y  M  N  M  +  N
+  +  L  A  R  E  H  P  I  R  E  P  H  +  U  +  T
+  +  +  +  L  A  N  I  U  G  N  I  +  +  M  R
+  +  +  +  +  +  +  +  +  +  +  +  +  +  +  A
L  A  S  R  O  D  +  +  N  U  C  L  E  U  S  +  L
+  +  +  +  +  +  +  +  +  +  +  +  +  +  +  +  +
```

caudal
cephalic
chromosomes
cranial
cytology
diaphragm
dorsal
epigastric
hypochondriac
hypogastric
inferior
inguinal
mediastinum
mitochondria
nucleus
pericardial
peripheral
pleural
proximal
thoracic
umbilical
ventral

Vocabulary Review

Key Term	Definition	Key Term	Definition
abdominal cavity	space between the diaphragm and the pelvic floor	**cardiovascular system**	system made up of the heart and blood vessels and transports nutrients and oxygen via the bloodstream
abdominopelvic cavity	combination of the abdominal and pelvic cavities		
anatomic position	pose in which a person is facing forward, standing erect, with the arms at the side and palms turned forward	**caudal**	toward the tail
		cell membrane	barrier that surrounds the cytoplasm
anatomy	the study of structure	**cells**	basic structural and functional units of life
anterior	toward the human front side		
anteroposterior (AP)	in x-ray imaging, describes the direction of the beam through a patient from anterior to posterior	**cephalic**	toward the head or pertaining to the head
		chemotherapy	use of medications or chemicals to treat disease
appendicular	body portion consisting of the arms and legs	**chromosomes**	structures in the nucleus that carry genetic information in the form of genes
auscultation	listening for sounds coming from various organs	**computed tomography (CT)**	medical images created by computer processing of x-rays that are transmitted in different directions in a given plane
axial	body portion consisting of head, neck, and torso		

Key Term	Definition	Key Term	Definition
connective tissue	supporting and connecting tissue in the body	horizontal plane	line parallel to the ground or the body's axis creating superior and inferior portions; also called a transverse plane
coronal plane	line dividing the body into front and back parts; also called a frontal plane	hypogastric region	pubic region
cranial	toward the head or top	idiopathic	disease or condition that arises for which there is no known cause
cytology	branch of biology that studies cells		
deep	away from the surface	index case	first documented person identified with a particular disease
diaphragm	the dome-shaped muscle of breathing that separates the thoracic cavity from the abdominal cavity	inferior	away from the head
		integumentary system	system that includes the skin and serves a protective function
digestive system	system that extends from the mouth to the anus with all its associated glands and organs and converts food to a usable form	lateral	pertaining to the side
		left hypochondriac region	left upper lateral region below the lower ribs
		left inguinal region	left lower region beside the pubic region
distal	farther from the attachment of an extremity to the trunk	left lower quadrant (LLQ)	one area of the abdominopelvic cavity on the inferior left side
dorsal	back side	left lumbar region	region to the left side of the umbilical region
embryology	study of the embryo (from fertilization through week eight) and its development	left upper quadrant (LUQ)	one area of the abdominopelvic cavity on the superior left side
endocrine system	system made up of glands that secrete hormones and it interacts with the nervous system	lymphatic system	system that includes vessels, nodes, and tissues that transport fluids from spaces within tissues back to the blood and plays an important role in immunity
epidemiology	study of disease occurrence and distribution		
epigastric region	upper middle region between the two hypochondriac regions	magnetic resonance imaging (MRI)	an imaging technique that uses electromagnetic radiation to obtain images of the body's soft tissues
epithelial tissue	type of tissue that covers body surfaces and lines internal organs; also called epithelium		
epithelium	type of tissue that covers body surfaces and lines internal organs; also called epithelial tissue	medial	toward the midline
		mediastinum	region in the middle of the chest between the lungs that contains the heart, trachea, and other organs
etiology	study of the cause and course of disease development	membrane	thin tissue layer surrounding, separating, lining, or connecting a body part
frontal plane	line dividing the body into front and back parts; also called a coronal plane	mesentery	double layer of peritoneum that attaches abdominal organs to the abdominal wall
genes	sequences of DNA on a chromosome that determine our heredity	midsagittal plane	line dividing the body at the middle creating equal left and right halves
gross anatomy	study of the body that does not require magnification		
histology	study of cells, tissues, and organs in relation to their function	mitochondria	organelles that make ATP
		morphology	shape of a specific structure

Key Term	Definition	Key Term	Definition
muscular system	system made up of muscles that move the body	physical rehabilitation	physical therapy to regain function
muscular tissue	tissue that has the ability to contract	physiology	study of body function
nervous system	system made up of the brain, spinal cord, and peripheral nerves that function in communication, integration, and control	planes	imaginary lines representing flat surfaces used to divide the body
		pleural membranes	membranes associated with the lungs
nervous tissue	tissue that has the ability to conduct nerve impulses	positron emission tomography (PET)	method of medical imaging capable of displaying the metabolic activity of body organs
nucleus	cellular center that contains DNA	posterior	toward the human back side
nutrition strategies	eating well for health	prone	lying face down
organ	grouping of two or more tissues that are integrated to perform a particular function	proximal	toward the attachment of an extremity to the trunk
		psychological therapy	treatment for the mind
organelles	specialized cellular structures with specific functions	quadrants	four areas of the abdominopelvic cavity
organism	any living individual, whether plant or animal, considered as a whole	radiation therapy	treatment using ionizing radiation
organ system	combination of organs with similar or related functions	radiography	examination of any part of the body for diagnostic purposes by means of radiation with the record of the findings usually exposed onto photographic film; also called x-ray imaging
palpation	examination through touch		
parietal	pertaining to a body wall		
pathogenesis	origin and course of disease development		
pathology	scientific study of disease	reflex response	involuntary reaction to a stimulus
pathologist	a physician trained in pathology who studies the causes of disease and death	regions	nine divisions of the abdominopelvic cavity
pathophysiology	study of body function modified by disease	reproductive system	system consisting of male or female sex organs that is involved with producing offspring
pelvic cavity	space within the bones of the pelvis	respiratory system	system made up of the lungs and air passages that exchanges gases between the blood and air
percussion	firmly tapping to elicit sounds		
pericardial membranes	membranes associated with the heart	ribosomes	sites of protein synthesis within the cytoplasm
peripheral	around an organ or extending outward from the body trunk	right hypochondriac region	right upper lateral region below the lower ribs
peritoneal membranes	membranes associated with the abdominopelvic cavity that cover the organs contained therein; also called the peritoneum	right inguinal region	right lower region beside the pubic region
		right lower quadrant (RLQ)	one area of the abdominopelvic cavity on the inferior right side
peritoneum	membranes associated with the abdominopelvic cavity that cover the organs contained therein; also called peritoneal membranes	right lumbar region	region to the right side of the umbilical region
		right upper quadrant (RUQ)	one area of the abdominopelvic cavity on the superior right side

Key Term	Definition	Key Term	Definition
sagittal plane	line dividing the body into left and right sides	thoracic cavity	space occupied by the lungs, heart, and trachea
serosa	membranes lining the thoracic and abdominal cavities that secrete a watery fluid; also called serous membranes	tissue	grouping of similar cells that perform a specific function
		transverse plane	line parallel to the ground or the body's axis creating superior and inferior portions; also called a horizontal plane
serous membranes	membranes lining the thoracic and abdominal cavities that secrete a watery fluid; also called the serosa	umbilical region	middle region below the epigastric region and above the pubic region
signs	objective evidence of disease		
skeletal system	system that is made up of bones and provides the framework for protecting internal organs	urinary system	system made up of the kidneys, ureters, bladder, and urethra that is involved with waste removal and fluid and electrolyte balance
stethoscope	instrument used to detect body sounds		
superficial	pertaining to the surface	ventral	anterior, belly side
superior	toward the head or upper part of a structure	visceral	pertaining to internal organs
		x-ray imaging	examination of any part of the body for diagnostic purposes by means of radiation with the record of the findings usually exposed onto photographic film; also called radiography
supine	lying face up		
surgery	an operation or operative procedure		
symptoms	subjective state of disease		

CHAPTER 3

Radiology and Nuclear Medicine

OBJECTIVES

After completing this chapter, you should be able to:

1. Define the meaning of word parts related to radiology.

2. Explain basic radiology terms.

3. Describe components of diagnostic radiology, ultrasound, radiation oncology, and nuclear medicine.

4. Recognize clinical tests and diagnostic procedures related to diagnostic radiology, ultrasound, radiation oncology, and nuclear medicine.

5. Explain variations in diagnostic procedures throughout the lifespan.

6. Define abbreviations related to radiology and nuclear medicine.

7. Define terms used in medical reports.

8. Define, spell, and pronounce the chapter's medical terms correctly.

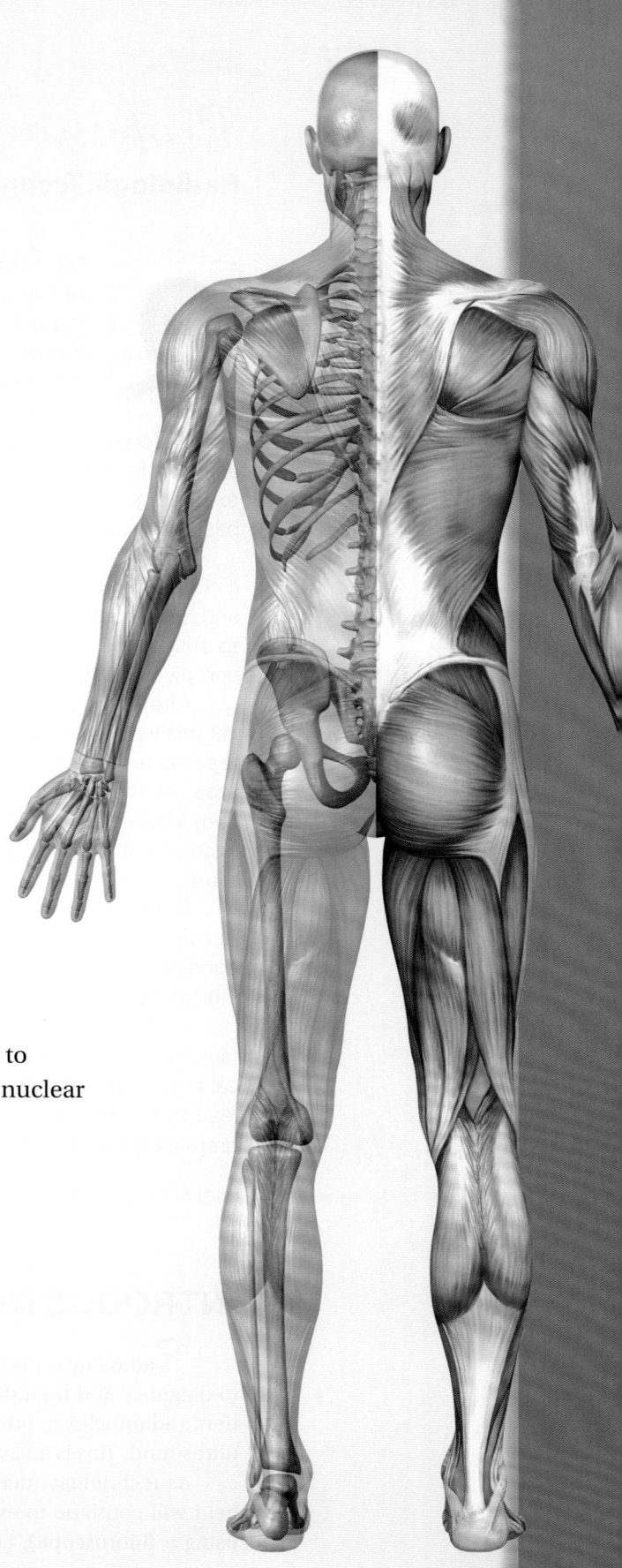

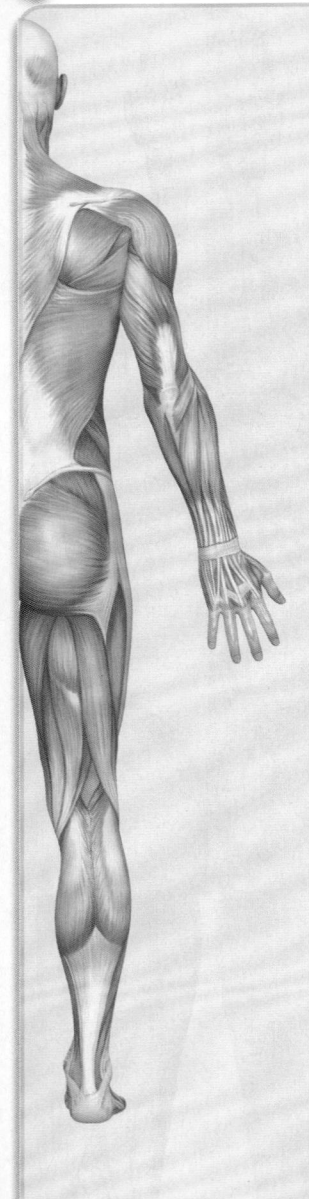

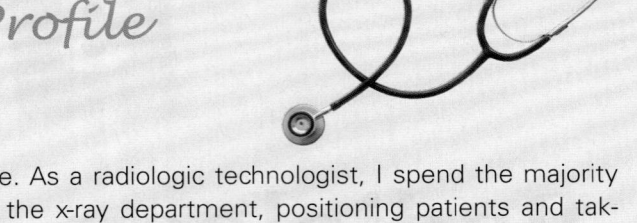

Professional Profile

Radiologic Technologist

My name is Lynne. As a radiologic technologist, I spend the majority of my day within the x-ray department, positioning patients and taking radiographs. I work in a hospital equipped with x-ray machines, a computed tomography (CT) scanner, and magnetic resonance imaging (MRI) equipment.

One aspect of my job that is particularly appealing is patient interaction. Before performing any imaging procedure, I explain it thoroughly to the person in an effort to alleviate fears and anxieties. This is especially important for a patient about to undergo an MRI study, because he or she may feel claustrophobic while being passed through a close-fitting cylindrical tube.

In addition to situating the patient, I oversee the operation of the machinery. This includes keying commands into the computer, setting exposure time and distance, and documenting scan sequences. Working with radiation requires health precautions to ensure the safety of all those in the area. Furthermore, measures must be taken to comply with government regulations.

After the CT scan, x-ray, or MRI pictures have been taken, I review them for technical quality. If the image is substandard, the procedure must be repeated. Experience teaches technologists how best to position a given individual, based on his or her body type, on the examination table to achieve the highest quality images. However, less-than-ideal conditions may make it difficult to obtain usable images on the first try—for example, if I must use a mobile unit in the emergency department or the patient's room.

Once I obtain good-quality images, I forward them to the radiology division, where radiologists interpret the images and provide detailed reports. These reports are of diagnostic value for identifying pathology, confirming the presence of an abnormality, or indicating if follow-up tests are necessary.

To become a certified radiologic technologist, I completed a 2-year radiology technician program and passed a qualification test. The only entrance requirement for typical programs is a high school diploma. Programs range in length from 1 to 4 years and lead to a certificate plus an associate's degree or a bachelor's degree. The 2-year programs are the most popular and currently exist in 35 states and Puerto Rico.

INTRODUCTION

*R*adiology is the branch of science dealing with the medical use of imaging techniques to diagnose and treat disease. Examination of body structures is made using ionizing radiation, radionuclides, other forms of penetrating radiation, nuclear magnetic resonance, and ultrasound. This is an area of health care with broadening applicability.

As technology increases and noninvasive procedures replace exploratory surgery, this field will continue to expand. Interventional radiology uses fluoroscopy (x-ray examination using a fluoroscope), computed tomography (CT), and ultrasound to guide other medical procedures. For example, biopsies, fluid drainage, catheter insertion, and vessel stenting and dilation are all performed using interventional radiology. Interventional radiology is becoming a leading therapeutic measure for treatment of disease.

Furthermore, demand for skilled professionals in every aspect of this area from billing and coding to technicians and physicians is currently greater than the supply. Radiologic technologists have the highest vacancy rate of any hospital profession. In 2009, the Joint Review Committee on Education in Radiologic Technology accredited 213 certificate programs, 397 associate degree programs, and 35 bachelor's degree programs.

This chapter focuses on the relationship between anatomy and physiology, medical terminology, and the numerous clinical tests and diagnostic procedures related to radiology, including diagnostic radiology, nuclear medicine, radiation oncology, and ultrasound.

MEDICAL TERM PARTS

Word Parts

Medical term prefixes, suffixes, and combining forms related to radiology, nuclear medicine, and diagnostic ultrasound are introduced in this section.

Word Part	Meaning
brachy-	short
cine-	movement, relating to motion pictures
electro-	electricity
end-, endo-	within, inner
fluo-	flow
-gram	recording, usually by an instrument
-graph	something written, instrument for making a recording
grapho-, -graphy	a writing, description
nucl-, nucleo-	nuclear, nucleus
onco-, oncho-	tumor
phon-, phono-	sound, speech
porto-	portal
ptyal-, ptyalo-	salivary glands, saliva
pyr-, pyro-	fever, fire, heat
radio-	radiation
sial-, sialo-	saliva, salivary glands
spectro-	spectrum
tel-, tele-, telo-	distant
-tome	section
ultra-	excess, beyond
xero-	dry

Word Grouping Exercises

Using the *Medical Term Parts* table, identify the prefix, suffix, or combining form for each of the following definitions. The first one has been done as an example.

Definition	Word Part
movement, relating to motion pictures	*cine-*
distant	
dry	
electricity	
excess, beyond	
fever, fire, heat	
flow	
nuclear, nucleus	
portal	
radiation	
recording, usually by an instrument	
saliva, salivary glands	
salivary glands, saliva	
section	
short	
something written, instrument for making a recording	
sound, speech	
spectrum	
tumor	
within, inner	
a writing, description	

Word Building Exercises

Word parts, introduced in the *Medical Term Parts* section, are listed in the following table. For this exercise, first supply the meaning of each word part, then use the word part to build a word you already know. The word you list under *Common or Known Word* does not have to be a medical term; a commonly used word is fine. Be sure, however, that the word correctly reflects the intended meaning. The first one has been done as an example. Check your answers in a dictionary.

Word Part	Meaning	Common or Known Word	Example Medical Term
brachy-	*short*	*brachycephalic*	brachytherapy
cine-			cineradiography
electro-			electromyography

continued

continued from page 96

Word Part	Meaning	Common or Known Word	Example Medical Term
end-, endo-			endoscopic catheterization
fluo-			fluoroscopy
-gram			sonogram
-graph			angiograph
grapho-, -graphy			arteriography
nucleo-			nuclear medicine
onco-, oncho-			oncology
phon-, phono-			phonocardiography
pyr-, pyro-			hyperpyrexia
radio-			radiology
tel-, tele-, telo-			teletherapy
-tome			tomography
ultra-			ultrasound
xero-			xeromammography

RADIOLOGY

Radiology is the science of radiation and radioactive substances and their application to medicine. It deals with radioactive substances, x-rays, and ionizing radiation for treating and diagnosing disease. The field has expanded to include various forms of imaging techniques, such as **ultrasound** (imaging technique that uses high-frequency sound waves) and magnetic resonance imaging, that may not necessarily use radiation yet are used to view internal body structures.

As a diagnostic tool, radiology has been in use since the early 1900s. Diagnostic imaging encompasses all imaging modalities used in radiology, such as ultrasound, magnetic resonance imaging, computed tomography, mammography, positron emission tomography, and traditional x-rays (radiographs). A **radiologist** is a physician specializing in the diagnostic and/or therapeutic use of x-rays, radionuclides, and other imaging techniques. It takes 10 to 12 years of training to become a radiologist. Diagnostic radiologists assist in treatments by inserting thin, flexible tubes called catheters and delivering therapy through interventional methods. Radiologists are the professionals who interpret images, regardless of the modality used.

An imaging technique that uses high-frequency sound waves reflecting off internal body parts to create pictures for identifying the nature or cause of a disorder or for recognition and treatment purposes is termed **diagnostic ultrasound**.

Radiation oncology (radiotherapy) is the treatment of cancer using radioactive substances. **Nuclear medicine** is the branch of clinical medicine in which radioactive materials are used to diagnose and treat diseases. Nuclear medicine is a more recent addition to the medical arsenal. Interventional radiology, which uses guided procedures, is advancing the treatment of disease and enhancing health by providing less invasive procedures. Various forms of radiology, nuclear medicine, diagnostic ultrasound, and radiation oncology are described in this chapter.

KEY TERM	Definition
radiology (ray-dee-OL-uh-jee)	branch of medicine that deals with radioactive substances, x-rays, and ionizing radiation for treating and diagnosing disease
ultrasound	imaging technique that uses high-frequency sound waves
radiologist (ray-dee-OL-uh-jist)	physician specializing in radiology
diagnostic (dye-ug-NOS-tik) **ultrasound**	use of high-frequency sound waves in diagnosing and treating conditions
radiation oncology (ray-dee-AY-shun ong-KOL-uh-jee)	use of radioactive materials for cancer; also called radiotherapy
nuclear (NEW-klee-ur) **medicine**	clinical branch of medicine that deals with the use of radioactive materials in diagnosis and therapy

KEY TERM PRACTICE: *Radiology*

1. The use of high-frequency sound waves for diagnosing and treating disorders is termed _____.

2. _____ is the clinical branch of health care that uses radioactive materials for treating and diagnosing disease.

3. The use of radioactive materials for treating cancer is called _____.

4. _____ is the branch of medicine dealing with the use of x-rays.

5. A physician who specializes in radiology is known as a _____.

Radiology Basic Terms

In 1901, German physicist Wilhelm K. Roentgen won the Nobel Prize in Physics for his discovery of x-rays in November 1895. Thus, the eponym *Roentgen rays* is another term for x-rays. An x-ray is electromagnetic radiation that penetrates various thickness of solids, ionizes tissues, and causes some substances to fluoresce (glow). A photograph taken with Roentgen rays (x-rays) is known as a radiograph or x-ray (also spelled X-ray, but always with a hyphen).

Radiographs (x-rays) are photographs made by projecting x-rays or gamma-rays through the body and onto sensitive film (**Figure 3-1**). They are often used to diagnose musculoskeletal and lung disorders. To highlight organs and tissues during these diagnostic procedures, various media are used. Because it absorbs radiation to a different degree than body tissues, a dye or other substance called a **contrast medium** highlights radiographic images of structures or spaces. This type of medium is **radiopaque**, meaning that light or radiation does not pass through it, making the outline of the body part easier to visualize on x-ray images. Commonly used contrast media are barium for the gastrointestinal tract; water-soluble compounds

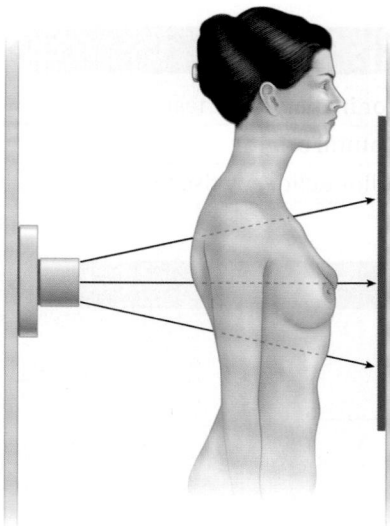

Figure 3-1 Radiography technique showing an x-ray procedure.

containing iodine for blood vessels, glands, and genitourinary imaging; air for a variety of images; and weakly magnetized substances for magnetic resonance imaging.

Knowing a few basic radiology terms is essential to understand fundamental procedures while providing the foundation for their application in medicine. Atomic nuclei that emit alpha-, beta-, or gamma-rays are termed **radioactive**. Radioactive substances give off energy in the form of streams of particles, due to the decay of their unstable atoms. The half-life ($T_{1/2}$) refers to the time a radioactive substance takes to lose half of its radioactivity through decay. The half-life of a particular radioactive material determines the substance's use as a radiotracer and is used to calculate appropriate dosages. A **radiotracer** is a radioactive substance introduced into the body as a detector or tag to locate diseased cells or tissue. This substance is generally a **radionuclide**, also called a radioisotope, which is a radioactive substance of artificial or natural origin. The absorption of the radiotracer by a tissue is known as **uptake**.

Finally, the side effects of radiation exposure require consideration. Patients undergoing oncology radiation commonly experience adverse reactions. Some are described here. Alopecia is hair loss, especially from the head, and mucositis refers to inflammation of the mucous membranes. Dry mouth, **xerostomia**, often accompanies mucositis. Nausea is the unsettling feeling in the stomach that accompanies the urge to vomit. Emesis is vomiting, or expelling the contents of the stomach through the mouth. Reduced development of white blood cells and platelets from the bone marrow is called myelosuppression.

KEY TERM	Definition
radiographs (RAY-dee-oh-grafs)	images produced on film by x-rays passing through a body part; another term for x-rays
x-rays	images produced on film by x-rays passing through a body part; another term for radiographs
contrast medium	dye or other substance introduced into the body that is opaque to x-rays, thereby allowing a structure's image to appear on film
radiopaque (ray-dee-oh-PAKE)	impenetrable by light or x-rays
radioactive	atomic nuclei emitting ionizing radiation or particles

continued

continued from page 99

KEY TERM	Definition
radiotracer	radioactive chemical used as a detector in diagnostic tests
radionuclide (RAY-dee-oh-NEW-klide)	radioactive substance of artificial or natural origin
uptake	absorption of something, such as a radionuclide, by tissue
xerostomia (zeer-oh-STOH-mee-uh)	dry mouth

KEY TERM PRACTICE: *Radiology Basic Terms*

1. Absorption of an introduced substance in the body is termed _____.

2. A dye or substance that cannot be penetrated by x-rays is known as a _____.

3. The alternate term for an x-ray is a _____.

4. _____ refers to the emission of ionizing radiation.

5. If a body structure cannot be penetrated by x-rays, it is said to be _____.

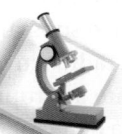

THE CLINICAL DIMENSION

This section focuses on pathology related to radiology and is organized according to the area of radiology. Diagnostic radiology, along with its subspecialties, is described first. Diagnostic ultrasound, including its diverse applications, is discussed next. Finally, elements of radiation oncology and nuclear medicine are introduced. When appropriate, a procedure is explained in context with the specific body system for which it is used. This organization reflects real-world radiologic practice.

Diagnostic Radiology

Diagnostic radiology, also called diagnostic imaging, is the branch of medicine that determines the nature of a patient's disease through x-rays, radioactive substances, nuclear magnetic resonance, ultrasound, and other forms of ionizing radiation. In some cases, it also provides treatment for pathology. **Interventional radiology** is a subspecialty that uses fluoroscopy, computed tomography, and ultrasound to guide other procedures, such as performing biopsies, draining fluids, inserting catheters, and dilating or stenting narrowed ducts or vessels. The following text describes a number of diagnostic and interventional techniques. **Box 3-1** provides a list of diagnostic radiology procedures.

B O X 3-1

DIAGNOSTIC RADIOLOGY PROCEDURES

Angiocardiography
Angiography
Antegrade pyelography
Aortography
Arteriography
Arthrography
Barium enema, lower gastrointestinal (GI)
Barium swallow, upper gastrointestinal (GI)
Bronchography
Cardiac catheterization
Cholangiography
Cholecystography
Cinefluoroscopy
Cineradiography
Computed tomography (CT)
Corpora cavernosography
Cystography
Cystourethrography
Densitometry/photodensitometry
Digital subtraction angiography
Diskography
Duodenography
Electromyography
Hysterosalpingography
Intravenous pyelography (IVP)

Lymphangiography
Magnetic resonance angiography (MRA)
Magnetic resonance imaging (MRI)
Magnetic resonance spectroscopy
Mammography
Pelvimetry
Percutaneous needle biopsy
Percutaneous transhepatic cholangiography
   (PCT; PTHC)
Percutaneous transhepatic portography
Percutaneous transluminal angioplasty (PTA)
Phonocardiography
Ptyalography
Pyelography
Radiography
Retrograde pyelography (RP)
Shuntogram
Sialography
Transcatheter biopsy
Transluminal atherectomy
Urethrocystography
Urography
Vasography
X-ray

KEY TERM	Definition
diagnostic radiology (dye-ug-NOS-tik ray-dee-OL-uh-jee)	use of x-rays and other ionizing radiation for the diagnosis and treatment of disease; also called diagnostic imaging
interventional radiology (in-ter-VEN-shun-ul ray-dee-OL-uh-jee)	specialty area of radiology that uses catheters, scopes, and various procedures to guide instruments for the diagnosis and treatment of pathology

KEY TERM PRACTICE: *Diagnostic Radiology*

1. A specialty area of radiology that uses catheters and scopes for the diagnosis and treatment of diseased states is called _____.

2. Give the alternate term for *diagnostic imaging*. _____

Radiography

The examination of any part of the body using x-rays is termed **radiography**. A **shunt** is a surgically created bypass or diversion. A radiographic study to determine shunt placement is referred to as a **shuntogram**.

Joints can be imaged via arthrography or diskography. The word part *arthro-* means joint, so **arthrography** is an x-ray of the joint space taken after a contrast dye has been injected into the joint. Arthrography is used to diagnose knee and shoulder injuries. X-ray examination of intervertebral discs (pads of fibrocartilage between the bones of the spine called vertebrae) after the injection of a contrast dye into the structures is termed **diskography**.

KEY TERM	Definition
radiography (ray-dee-OG-ruh-fee)	making and using radiographs (x-rays) for medical purposes
shunt	a surgically created bypass
shuntogram (SHUNT-oh-gram)	x-ray examination to determine shunt placement
arthrography (ahr-THROG-ruh-fee)	examination of a joint's interior after the injection of a contrast dye
diskography (disk-OG-ruh-fee)	examination of the intervertebral discs after the direct injection of a contrast dye

KEY TERM PRACTICE: *Radiography*

1. The word part *arthro-* means joint; the word part _____ means "a writing, description"; therefore, the term _____ means "radiographic assessment of a joint."

2. Radiographic evaluation of intervertebral discs is termed _____.

3. A _____ is a surgically created bypass.

4. X-ray examination to determine shunt placement is called a _____.

5. Making and using x-rays for medical purposes is termed _____.

Radiography in Motion

Organs in motion can be viewed using specialized imaging techniques. Radiography of an organ while it is moving is called **cineradiography** or **cinefluoroscopy**. The term cineradiography is derived from the word part *cine-,* which means *motion picture*. A fluorescent screen of crystals excited by x-rays produces an image. This technique is commonly used to obtain views of the heart and gastrointestinal tract and to assist in catheter placement.

KEY TERM	Definition
cineradiography (sin-e-ray-dee-OG-ruh-fee)	radiography of an organ in motion; another term for cinefluoroscopy
cinefluoroscopy (sin-e-floor-OS-kuh-pee)	radiography of an organ in motion; another term for cineradiography

continued

continued from page 102

KEY TERM PRACTICE: *Radiography in Motion*

1. The word part *cine-* means _____; the word part *radio-* means _____; and the word part _____ means *description*. So, the term _____ describes the procedure of viewing an organ in motion.

2. In the term *cinefluoroscopy*, the word part *fluo-* means _____.

Tomography

The term **tomography** refers to radiography that highlights structures in one selected plane at a time as the x-ray tube moves, leaving structures in other planes unfocused. **Computed tomography (CT)** uses a moving scanner and detector that encircle the patient while a computer creates cross-sectional x-ray images. This procedure is useful for diagnosing conditions of the brain, abdomen, and chest. It is known by several terms, including computer-assisted tomography (CAT), computed axial tomography (CAT), and computerized axial tomography (CAT) (**Figure 3-2**). A technique combining CT with angiography to view blood or lymphatic vessels is termed **computed tomographic angiography**.

CT pelvimetry is the procedure for measuring the bony pelvis and fetal head through the use of CT images. Pelvimetry is performed to assess whether there will be any difficulty during vaginal childbirth.

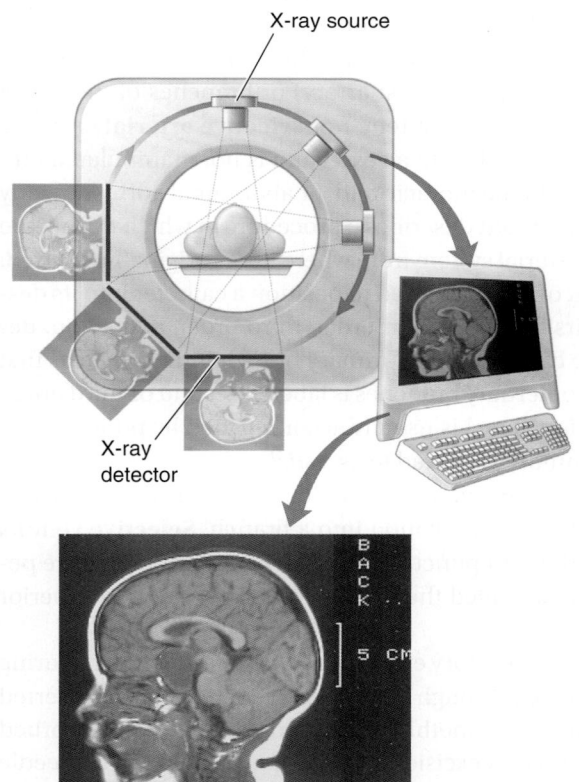

X-ray source

X-ray detector

Figure 3-2 A CT scan of the head. The scanner takes a series of cross-sectional images one slice at a time in a full-circle rotation. A computer calculates and converts each image into a picture on a screen.

KEY TERM	Definition
tomography (toh-MOG-ruh-fee)	radiography in which images in certain planes are focused while images in other planes are blurred
computed tomography (toh-MOG-ruh-fee) **(CT)**	technique for producing x-ray images of body cross-sections
computed tomographic angiography (toh-moh-GRAF-ik an-jee-OG-ruh-fee)	combination CT and angiography for visualizing blood vessels or lymphatic vessels
CT pelvimetry (pel-VIM-uh-tree)	measurement of the dimensions of the bony pelvis and fetal head using CT scans

KEY TERM PRACTICE: *Tomography*

1. A procedure that combines CT imaging with angiography is termed _____.

2. A technique for producing cross-sectional images of the body is known as _____.

3. _____ is a technique for displaying cross-sections through the human body using x-rays.

4. The measurement of the dimensions of the pelvis and fetal head to help determine whether a woman can give birth normally is termed _____.

Catheterization, Biopsy, and Percutaneous Radiographic Procedures

Placement of the thin, flexible tubes known as catheters requires knowledge of anatomy. The clinician must understand the anatomy related to the puncture site and final catheter position as well as the pathways of the blood vessels. Arteries are blood vessels that carry blood away from the heart, and veins carry blood toward the heart. The **vascular family** refers to a group of vessels fed by a primary branch of the aorta (the largest artery) or branches of the vessel that are being punctured. With respect to the arterial system, **nonselective arterial catheter placement** means that the needle is placed directly into a vessel and is not manipulated into a branch, or that the catheter is negotiated into the thoracic and/or abdominal aorta from any approach. A **selective arterial catheter placement** describes a procedure in which the needle is manipulated into another portion of the arterial system from where it was originally inserted.

Vessel ordering describes the amount of work required to position a catheter into its destination. Vessel ordering is identified as first order, second order, third order, and so on, depending on the pathway taken. Placing the catheter into a primary branch is described as first order; passing the catheter into secondary or tertiary branches is labeled second or third order, respectively. The approach to the destination vessel is usually accomplished by puncturing a readily accessible vessel. A *puncture* is commonly referred to as a *stick*.

In regard to the venous system, **nonselective venous** describes the procedure in which a needle is placed directly into a vein with no manipulation into a branch. **Selective venous** procedures require manipulation beyond the vein puncture site. Direct puncture sites are peripheral veins and large veins. The large veins, called the inferior vena cava and the superior vena cava, are used most often.

The removal of a living tissue sample for laboratory examination is called a biopsy. During a **transcatheter biopsy**, a tissue sample is taken through a thin, flexible tube which is inserted into the body. The term *percutaneous* refers to something being administered or absorbed through the skin. **Percutaneous needle biopsy** is excision of tissue performed with a needle through a skin incision.

A generalized procedure that uses an instrument called an endoscope, which transmits light and carries images of the internal body back to the observer, is termed **endoscopic catheterization**. The long tube is usually inserted through a small incision. Endoscopic catheterization is used for diagnostic examination and surgical procedures.

Another type of tissue removal is transluminal atherectomy. *Transluminal* means across or through a lumen, which is the space inside a blood vessel. A lipid (fat) deposit or atherosclerotic plaque is known as an **atheroma**. The surgical removal or catheterization of an atheroma is called an atherectomy. So, a **transluminal atherectomy** is the removal of plaque or lipid deposits from the inner lining of an artery.

An operation that enlarges narrowed vascular lumen via a balloon on the tip of a catheter is known as **percutaneous transluminal angioplasty (PTA)**. Once the catheter tip reaches the blockage, the balloon is enlarged to crush the obstruction, thereby restoring circulation. **Figure 3-3** demonstrates this procedure.

During a **cardiac catheterization**, a tubular instrument is passed through an artery or vein to the heart for visualization. Blood samples can be withdrawn, pressures within the heart and vessels can be measured, and contrast media can be injected for angiography. Images obtained by the procedure enable the physician to identify cardiac structures and possible obstructions. Cardiac catheterization is used to diagnose heart disorders, anomalies, and stenosed (narrowed, occluded) vessels.

Radiography of the bile ducts with a contrast medium is known as **cholangiography**. It is used to diagnose tumors or stones. **Percutaneous transhepatic cholangiography (PTC, PTHC)** is radiography of bile ducts via needle puncture. For this procedure, radiopaque dye is delivered through a needle that is inserted into a hepatic (liver) bile duct.

The process of taking radiographic views of the hepatic portal venous system after the injection of contrast medium into the spleen or portal vein is termed **percutaneous transhepatic portography**. The portal system refers to the hepatic portal vein and its branches found in the liver. Blood passes from gastrointestinal (GI) capillaries and the spleen to the liver via the portal circulation. Several routes provide portal access.

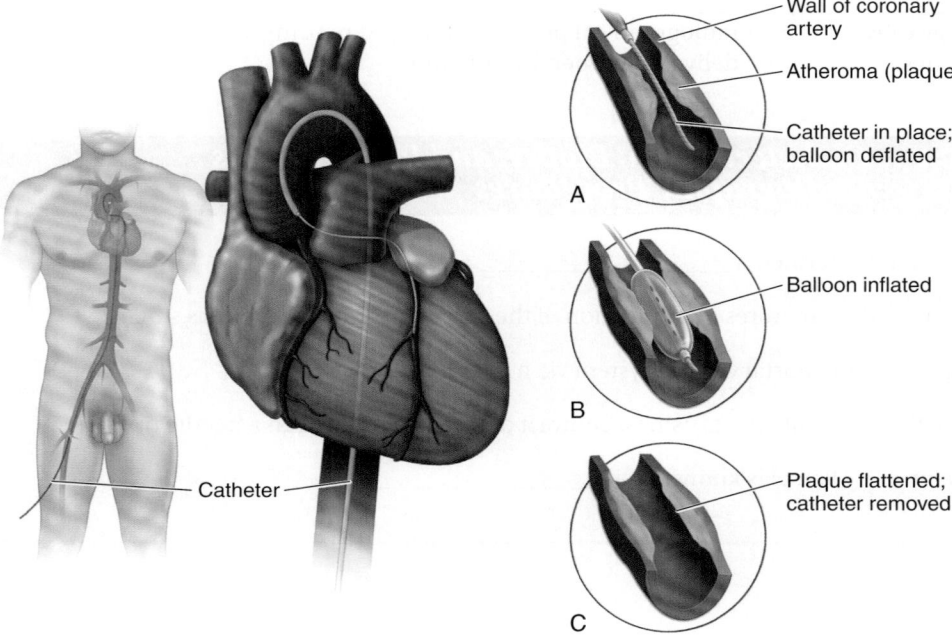

Wall of coronary artery

Atheroma (plaque)

Catheter in place; balloon deflated

A

Balloon inflated

B

Plaque flattened; catheter removed

C

Catheter

Figure 3-3 Percutaneous transluminal angioplasty. **(A)** A guide catheter is threaded into the coronary artery. **(B)** A balloon catheter is then inserted through the occluded (blocked) artery, and the balloon is inflated and deflated until **(C)** the atheroma (plaque) is flattened and the vessel is open.

KEY TERM	Definition
vascular family	group of blood vessels fed by a primary vessel
nonselective arterial catheter placement	catheter placed into an arterial vessel and not manipulated to another arterial site
selective arterial catheter placement	catheter placed into another portion of the arterial system from where it was originally inserted
vessel ordering	term describing the amount of work required to place a catheter at its destination
nonselective venous	catheter placed into a vein and not manipulated to another venous site
selective venous	catheter placed into a vein and manipulated into another venous site
transcatheter biopsy (trans-KATH-e-tur BYE-op-see)	tissue sample taken via a catheter
percutaneous (pur-kew-TAY-nee-us) **needle biopsy** (BYE-op-see)	excision of tissue by a guided needle through the skin
endoscopic catheterization (en-duh-SKOP-ick kath-e-tur-i-ZAY-shun)	procedure that uses an endoscope to view internal body structures
atheroma (ath-er-OH-muh)	fat deposit in an artery
transluminal atherectomy (trans-LEW-mi-nul ath-e-RECK-toh-me)	removal of fatty deposits on the inner lining of an artery
percutaneous transluminal angioplasty (pur-kew-TAY-nee-us trans-LEW-mi-nul AN-jee-oh-plas-tee) **(PTA)**	use of a balloon catheter to widen a narrowed artery
cardiac catheterization (kath-e-tur-i-ZAY-shun)	examination of the heart after threading a catheter through a vessel into the heart for diagnostic, therapeutic, or visualization purposes
cholangiography (koh-lan-jee-OG-ruh-fee)	examination of the bile ducts using a contrast medium
percutaneous transhepatic cholangiography (pur-kew-TAY-nee-us trans-he-PAT-ick koh-lan-jee-OG-ruh-fee) **(PCT, PTHC)**	radiography of the bile ducts using contrast medium delivered via needle puncture
percutaneous transhepatic portography (pur-kew-TAY-nee-us trans-he-PAT-ick por-TOG-ruh-fee)	radiography of portal venous system using a contrast medium delivered via needle puncture

KEY TERM PRACTICE: *Catheterization, Biopsy, and Percutaneous Radiographic Procedures*

1. A tissue sample obtained via a catheter is termed a _____.

2. A _____ venous procedure requires manipulation of the catheter to another venous site.

3. _____ is radiography of the portal venous system via a needlestick.

4. _____ is radiography of the bile ducts using a contrast dye delivered through a needle puncture.

5. A group of blood vessels fed by a primary vessel is known as a _____.

Magnetic Resonance Imaging (MRI)

Magnetic resonance imaging (MRI) is a radiology tool that does not use ionizing radiation. Instead, it uses magnetic fields. Magnetic resonance imaging is used to determine blood flow and identify tumors of bone and fluid-filled soft tissues.

During magnetic resonance imaging, the patient is placed within a tube and is surrounded by electromagnetic coils that excite hydrogen atoms in the body. Radiofrequency waves are aimed at the body, which cause internal hydrogen nuclei to change their alignment. This, in turn, causes the body to emit signals that a computer translates into images of body organs. Another term for MRI is nuclear magnetic resonance (NMR) imaging. Open and stand-up MRI machines have been developed to make the experience less claustrophobic for patients. **Figure 3-4** illustrates the MRI technique.

Imaging of blood vessels using magnetic resonance sequences that enhance the signal of flowing blood and suppress signals from other tissues is called **magnetic resonance angiography (MRA)**.

Another MRI variation is **magnetic resonance spectroscopy**, which is the detection and measurement of the absorbed light energy of molecules in a tissue sample. Spectroscopy involves measuring absorbed light energy (spectrum) in a body structure.

KEY TERM	Definition
magnetic resonance imaging (MRI)	imaging technique that uses electromagnetic radiation to obtain pictures of the body's soft tissues
magnetic resonance angiography (an-jee-OG-ruh-fee) **(MRA)**	imaging blood vessels using MRI
magnetic resonance spectroscopy (speck-TROS-kuh-pee)	imaging structures using lightwaves

KEY TERM PRACTICE: *Magnetic Resonance Imaging (MRI)*

1. Imaging blood vessels using MRI is termed _____, which is derived from the word part *angio-*, which means *vessels*, and the word part _____, which means *a description*.

2. A noninvasive technique that uses lightwaves to create images is called _____.

3. An imaging technique that uses electromagnetic radiation to obtain pictures of the body's soft tissues is known as _____.

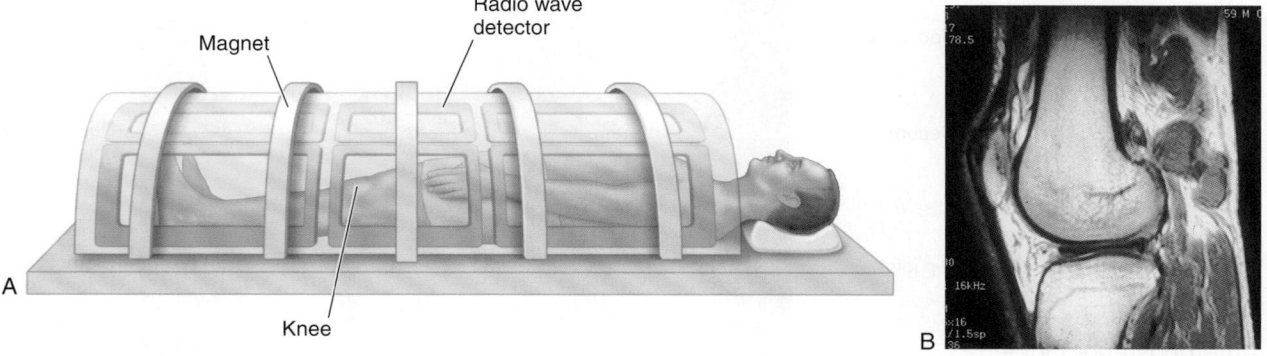

Figure 3-4 An MRI study of the knee. **(A)** MRI uses magnetic fields and radiofrequency waves to visualize anatomical structures. **(B)** Image of the knee obtained from an MRI.

Contrast Studies and Digestive System Radiography

Contrast studies are used for comparative purposes to highlight marked differences in the appearance of organs or tissues. Structures are made more visible when radiographs are taken after a contrast medium has been introduced. Types of gastrointestinal (GI) contrast studies include the barium enema for lower GI evaluation and the barium swallow for upper GI study. **Barium sulfate (BaSO₄)** is a water-insoluble salt used as an opaque radiographic contrast medium. A **barium enema** study involves infusing the rectum with barium sulfate for radiographic study of the lower GI tract to identify obstructions and tumors (**Figure 3-5**). The oral administration of barium sulfate for radiographic study of the upper GI tract is termed a **barium swallow**. The barium swallow is used to diagnose disorders of the esophagus, stomach, and duodenum (first segment of the small intestine). A radiographic depiction of only the duodenum using a contrast medium is **duodenography**.

The salivary glands can be viewed via a unique procedure. Radiographic examination of the salivary glands and ducts after they have been injected with an opaque dye is termed **sialography** or **ptyalography**. Both terms are derived from the word parts meaning "saliva": *sialo-* and *ptyalo-*.

Examination of the bile ducts and gallbladder is accomplished through cholangiography and cholecystography, which come from the word part *chol-*, which means "bile." Recall that radiography of the bile ducts with a contrast medium is known as **cholangiography** and is used to diagnose tumors or stones. If no obstruction exists, the biliary structures readily empty into the intestinal tract. **Cholecystography** is radiography of the gallbladder after ingestion or intravenous (IV) injection of a radiopaque dye that is then excreted in bile. Usually, the patient swallows a tablet containing the dye the night before the x-ray examination. **Splenoportography** is radiographic examination of the splenic and portal vein system after a contrast medium has been injected into the spleen.

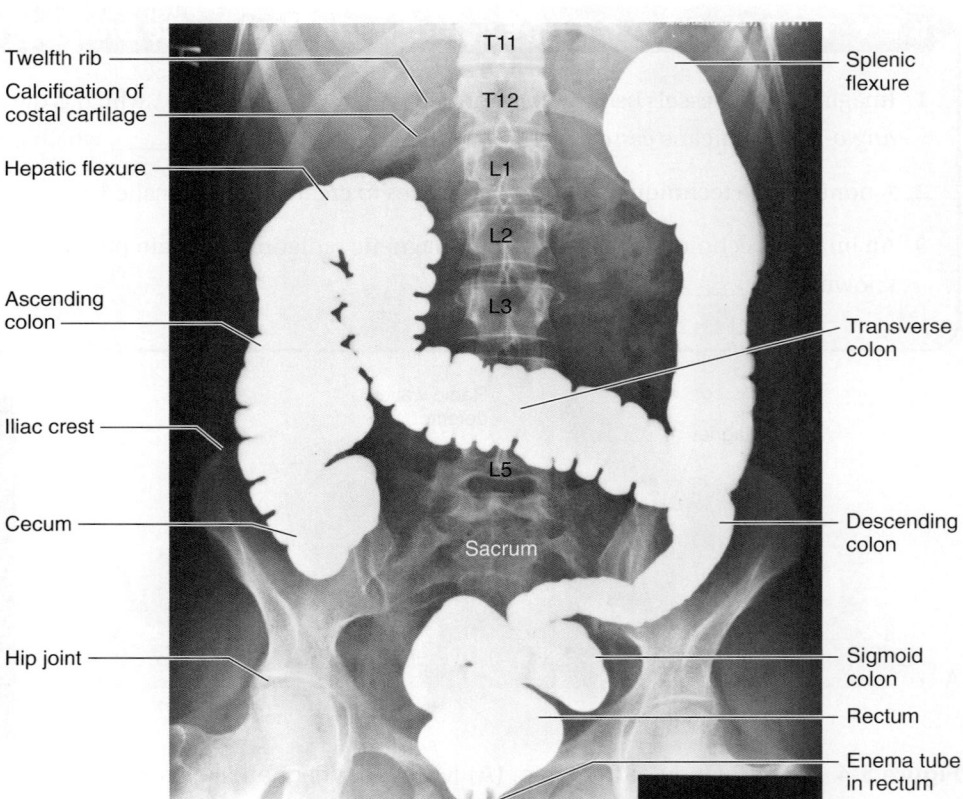

Figure 3-5 Anteroposterior radiograph of the large intestine after a barium enema.

KEY TERM	Definition
barium (BAIR-ee-um) **sulfate (BaSO$_4$)**	compound used as a contrast medium because it is not penetrated by x-rays
barium enema (BAIR-ee-um EN-e-muh)	introduction of a contrast medium containing barium sulfate into the rectum and colon for x-ray examination
barium (BAIR-ee-um) **swallow**	ingestion of barium sulfate for x-ray examination of the upper GI tract
duodenography (dew-oh-de-NOG-ruh-fee)	x-ray examination of the duodenum after introduction of a contrast medium
sialography (sigh-uh-LOG-ruh-fee)	x-ray examination of the salivary glands after administration of a contrast medium; also called ptyalography
ptyalography (tigh-uh-LOG-ruh-fee)	x-ray examination of the salivary glands after administration of a contrast medium; also called sialography
cholangiography (koh-lan-jee-OG-ruh-fee)	examination of the bile ducts using a contrast medium
cholecystography (koh-lee-sis-TOG-ruh-fee)	examination of the gallbladder after injection or ingestion of a contrast medium
splenoportography (splee-noh-por-TOG-ruh-fee)	x-ray examination of the splenic and portal vein system after injection of a contrast medium

KEY TERM PRACTICE: *Contrast Studies and Digestive System Radiology*

1. The procedure in which digestive structures are viewed after the ingestion of barium sulfate (BaSO$_4$) is known as a
   _____.

2. The radiographic examination of the duodenum using a contrast medium is termed a _____.

3. List the two terms that describe an examination of the salivary glands after introduction of a contrast dye.
   _____

4. Introduction of barium sulfate into the rectum and colon for x-ray examination describes the procedure known as a
   _____.

5. Examination of the gallbladder after injection or ingestion of a contrast medium is termed a _____.

Nervous System Radiography

Several areas of the brain and spinal cord can be visualized with x-rays. **Myelography** is radiographic demonstration of the spinal cord, nerve roots, and subarachnoid space after introduction of a contrast medium or air into the space (**Figure 3-6**). Myelography is used to detect lesions, herniated discs, tumors, and cysts.

KEY TERM	Definition
myelography (migh-e-LOG-ruh-fee)	radiographic examination of the spinal cord after injection of radiopaque dye

KEY TERM PRACTICE: *Nervous System Radiography*

1. _____ is the x-ray examination of the spinal cord after injection of a radiopaque dye.

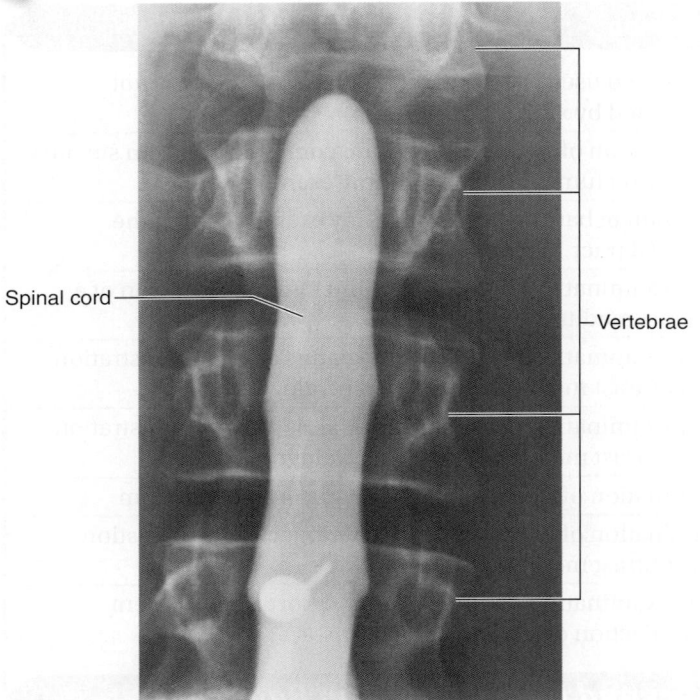

Figure 3-6 Posteroanterior myelogram of the lumbar region.

Spinal cord

Vertebrae

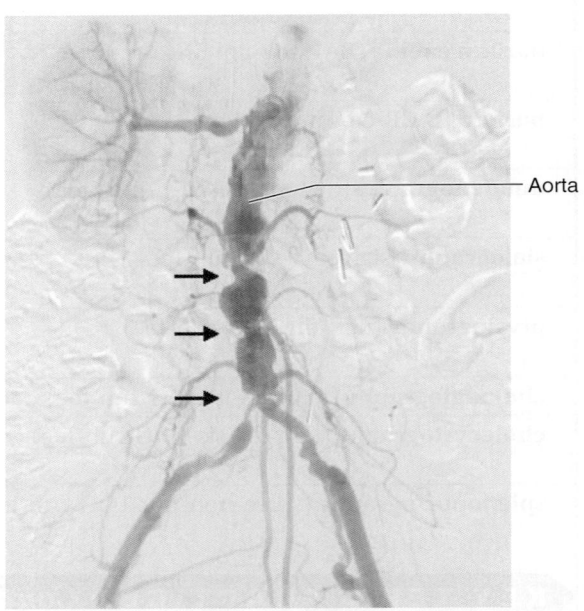

Figure 3-7 Digital subtraction angiography (DSA) showing narrowing of the aorta as shown at the arrows.

Aorta

Heart and Vessel Radiography

Several radiology techniques are used on the heart and vessels. **Angiography** is the x-ray examination of blood vessels after injection of a radiopaque (contrast) dye. Common types of angiography are cardiac, cerebral, peripheral, and pulmonary. Presurgical vessel mapping accomplished by angiography is used for vascular surgery procedures such as creating fistulas (passages connecting structures) and grafting.

Computer-assisted radiography that permits imaging of blood vessels separate from images of bone or soft tissue is termed **digital subtraction angiography (DSA)**. Structures not enhanced by the contrast medium are removed from the picture to improve the visualization of the vessels (**Figure 3-7**). Radiographic examination of veins after the administration of a contrast dye is termed **venography** or *phlebography*. Incomplete vein filling indicates an obstruction.

Radiographic examination of thoracic vessels and the heart chambers after intravascular injection of radiopaque dye is called **angiocardiography**. An x-ray of the aorta after intravascular injection of a contrast dye is termed **aortography**, and x-ray examination of arteries after the intravascular injection of a dye is known as **arteriography**.

Radiographic visualization of lymph channels and nodes after the injection of a radiopaque dye into lymphatic vessels is termed **lymphography**. In cases of cancer, lymph node mapping by lymphography enables the clinician to locate the sentinel node, which is the first lymph node into which a tumor drains. This knowledge allows the surgeon to remove only those nodes likely to be cancerous rather than all nodes in an area.

KEY TERM	Definition
angiography (an-jee-OG-ruh-fee)	examination of blood vessels after introduction of a radiopaque (contrast) dye
digital subtraction angiography (an-jee-OG-ruh-fee) (DSA)	computer-assisted radiography of vascular structures without superimposed bone or soft tissue
venography (vee-NOG-ruh-fee)	x-ray examination of veins after injection of a contrast dye; also called phlebography
angiocardiography (an-jee-oh-kahr-dee-OG-ruh-fee)	x-ray examination of heart and blood vessels after injection of a radiopaque dye
aortography (ay-or-TOG-ruh-fee)	x-ray examination of the aorta after injection of a contrast dye
arteriography (ahr-teer-ee-OG-ruh-fee)	x-ray examination of arteries after injection of a contrast dye
lymphography (limf-OG-ruh-fee)	x-ray examination of lymphatic vessels after introduction of a radiopaque dye

KEY TERM PRACTICE: *Heart and Vessel Radiography*

1. _____ is the examination of blood vessels after intravenous administration of a radiopaque (contrast) dye.

2. X-ray examination of arteries after injection of a contrast dye is termed _____.

3. _____ is the x-ray examination of veins after injection of a contrast dye.

4. The word part _____ means *a writing or description*, and the term used to describe the x-ray examination of lymphatic vessels is known as _____.

5. Computer-assisted radiography of vascular structures without superimposed bone or soft tissue is called _____.

Reproductive System Radiography

Studies of the male and female reproductive systems are possible through several diagnostic radiology procedures.

The vas deferens is one of a pair of ducts that carries sperm from structures in the testicles to the urethra, which opens to the outside. Radiography of the vas deferens, known as **vasography**, is done to determine patency (state of being freely open) of the structures. This test might be performed on a male to rule out infertility issues and to determine if the sperm are obstructed

Mammography is radiographic examination of breast tissue, occasionally performed with a contrast medium (**Figure 3-8**). It is used to detect breast tumors and cysts. Mammography screening does not prevent or cure breast cancer, but it may detect disease before signs and symptoms become apparent. One out of nine women in the United States will develop breast cancer. Tumors can exist for 6 to 10 years before they are large enough to be detected by mammography. Mammary **galactography**, also known as **ductography**, is an x-ray examination that uses mammography and a contrast medium that is injected into the milk ducts. It is used to evaluate a woman who has a discharge from her breast nipple and an otherwise normal mammogram.

Radiographic examination of the uterus and uterine tubes after injection of a contrast medium into the cavities is called **hysterosalpingography** (*hystero-* means "uterus"; *salpingo-* means "tube"). Hysterosalpingography is used to diagnose uterine pathology and identify possible causes of infertility.

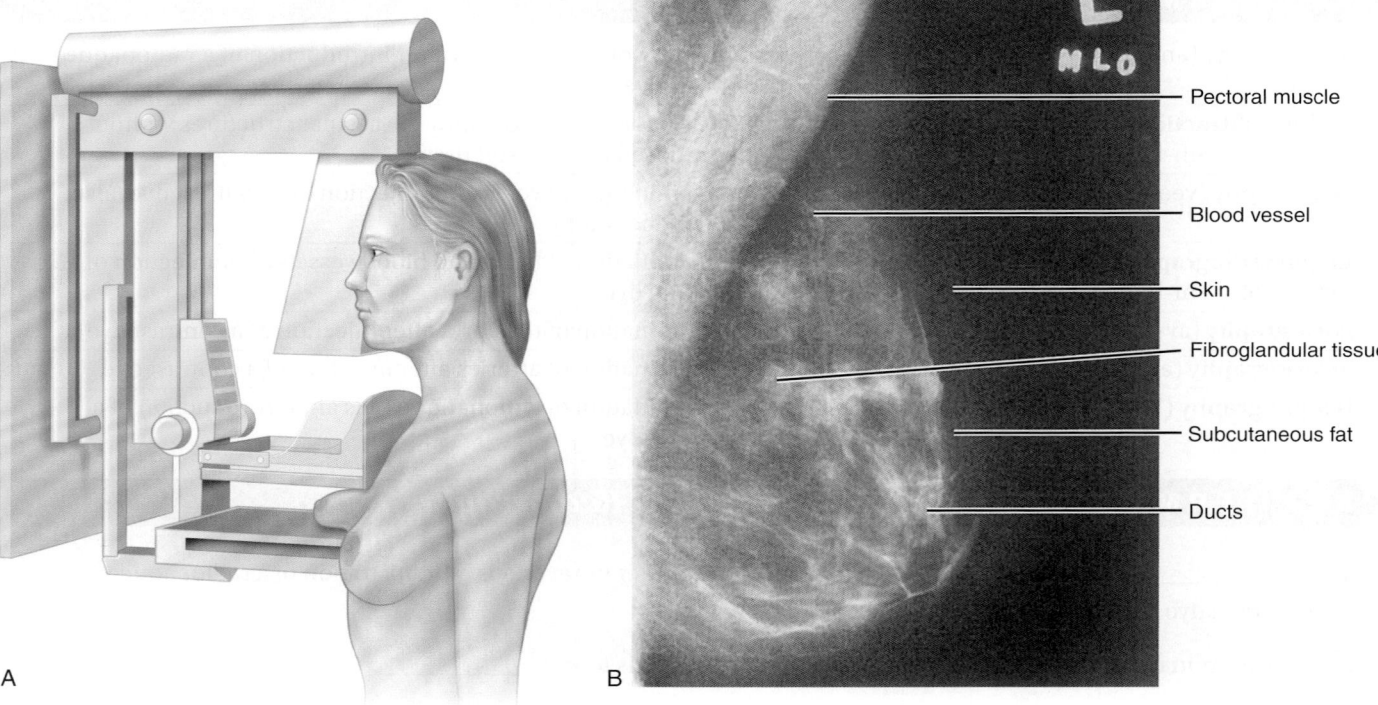

A   B

Figure 3-8 Mammography. **(A)** Mammography is the radiologic examination of the breast by means of x-ray, ultrasound, or nuclear magnetic resonance imaging. **(B)** Image displayed from a mammogram.

KEY TERM	Definition
vasography (vay-SOG-ruh-fee)	x-ray examination of the vas deferens using a contrast medium to determine if blockages are present
mammography (ma-MOG-ruh-fee)	x-ray examination of the breast
galactography (gal-ak-TOG-ruh-fee)	mammographic imaging of the milk ducts using a contrast medium; also called ductography
ductography (duk-TOG-ruh-fee)	mammographic imaging of the milk ducts using a contrast medium; also called galactography
hysterosalpingography (his-tur-oh-sal-ping-OG-ruh-fee)	x-ray examination of the uterus and uterine tubes using a contrast dye

KEY TERM PRACTICE: *Reproductive System Radiography*

1. The word part *mammo-* refers to "breast"; *-graphy* means "a description"; so _____ is the x-ray evaluation of breast tissue.

2. Cite two terms that describe a radiologic examination of the milk ducts of the breast. _____

3. X-ray examination of the vas deferens using a contrast medium to determine if blockages are present is termed a _____.

4. A _____ is an x-ray examination of the uterus and uterine tubes after introduction of a contrast dye.

Respiratory System Radiography

The **chest x-ray** is a noninvasive medical test to evaluate the lungs, heart, and bones of the thoracic area. It is useful for diagnosing lung obstructions and pneumonia. Both an anterior (A) and a posterior (P) view are normally taken (**Figure 3-9**). Not only is it the oldest form of medical imaging, it is the most commonly performed diagnostic x-ray examination.

   Laryngography is the radiographic examination of the larynx (voice box) after the mucosal surfaces have been coated with a contrast dye. The test is performed to evaluate vocal cord function.

KEY TERM	Definition
chest x-ray	imaging technique that uses a small dose of ionizing radiation to produce pictures of body structures in the thoracic cavity
laryngography (luh-rin-GOG-ruh-fee)	radiography of the larynx (voice box) after coating the surface with a contrast dye

KEY TERM PRACTICE: *Respiratory System Radiography*

1. X-ray examination of the larynx is termed _____.

2. Examination of the thoracic region utilizing a small dose of ionizing radiation is known as a _____.

Urinary System Radiography

Pyelography is the branch of radiography dealing with the kidneys and surrounding tissue. An x-ray of the kidneys, ureters (tubes connecting the kidneys to the bladder), and the urinary bladder after filling with an opaque solution is termed a **pyelogram**. **Intravenous pyelography (IVP)** is the x-ray examination of the renal pelvis (where urine collects in the kidney), ureters, and urinary bladder after a contrast dye is administered into a vein (**Figure 3-10**).

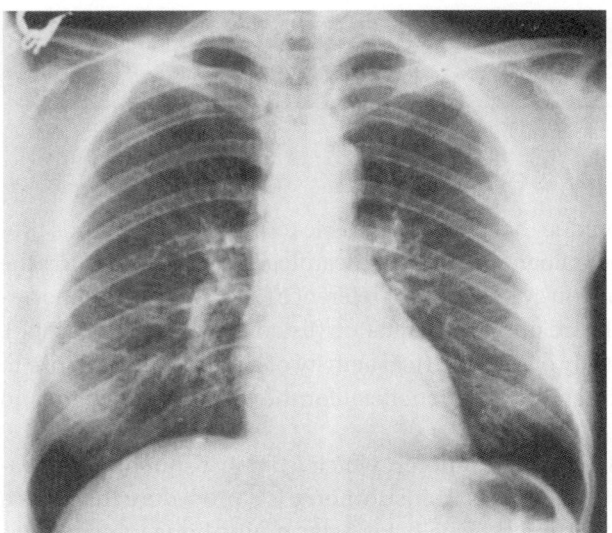

Figure 3-9 Plain chest x-ray.

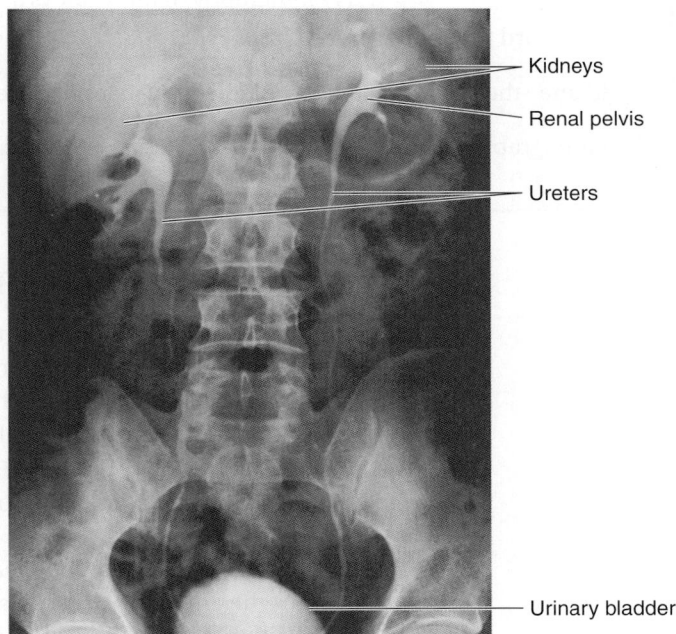

Kidneys
Renal pelvis
Ureters
Urinary bladder

Figure 3-10 Intravenous pyelogram of the kidneys, ureters, and urinary bladder.

During a **retrograde pyelography (RP)** procedure, a contrast medium is injected into the ureters from an endoscope placed in the bladder. It is called *retrograde* because the fluid is moving in the opposite direction of the normal flow.

Radiography of any part of the urinary tract is termed **urography**. Radiography of only the urinary bladder after introduction of a contrast medium is termed **cystography** (*cyst-* = bladder). A procedure that simultaneously measures pressure in the urinary bladder and urethra is called **urethrocystometry**. This procedure provides images during urination. Radiography of the urinary system helps clinicians identify tumors, defects, reflux (backflow), and stones.

KEY TERM	Definition
pyelography (pye e-LOG-ruh-fee)	radiography of the kidneys, ureters, and urinary bladder using a contrast dye
pyelogram (pye-e-loh-gram)	x-ray of the kidneys, ureters, and urinary bladder obtained after introducing a contrast dye
intravenous pyelogram (pye-e-loh-gram) **(IVP)**	x-ray of the urine-collecting part of the kidneys, ureters, and bladder using a contrast dye
retrograde pyelography (RP) (RET-roh-grade pye-e-LOG-ruh-fee)	radiography of the kidneys after a contrast dye is injected into the ureters, resulting in backward fluid movement
urography (yoo-ROG-ruh-fee)	radiography of any part of the urinary tract
cystography (sis-TOG-ruh-fee)	x-ray examination of the bladder using a contrast dye
urethrocystometry (yoo-re-throh-sis-TOM-e-tree)	procedure that simultaneously measures pressures in the urinary bladder and urethra

KEY TERM PRACTICE: *Urinary System Radiography*

1. Radiography of the kidneys, ureters, and bladder after introduction of a contrast dye is called _____.

2. _____ is an x-ray examination of the bladder using a contrast dye.

3. _____ is radiography of the kidneys after a contrast dye is injected into the ureters, resulting in backward fluid movement.

4. Identify the procedure that simultaneously measures pressures in the urinary bladder and urethra. _____

5. Radiography of any part of the urinary tract is referred to as _____.

Other Diagnostic Radiology Services

Phonocardiography is a diagnostic technique that creates a graphic record of heart sounds produced during contraction. During phonocardiography, an electrocardiogram (ECG) measures the heart's electrical activity, which is simultaneously recorded for reference (**Figure 3-11**). Phonocardiography supplements the information heard during auscultation (listening with a stethoscope).

Electromyography (EMG) is the study of the electrical activity of a muscle in response to electrical stimulation. Electromyography studies are beneficial for the diagnosis of nerve and muscle disorders.

Bone density can be measured using a **densitometer**, which is an instrument that measures the amount of light a tissue absorbs or reflects. **Densitometry** is a procedure that uses a densitometer in a clinical setting, and it is used especially for determining bone mineral density (**Figure 3-12**). For this reason, it is a valuable diagnostic tool for detecting osteoporosis, a disease marked by bone loss.

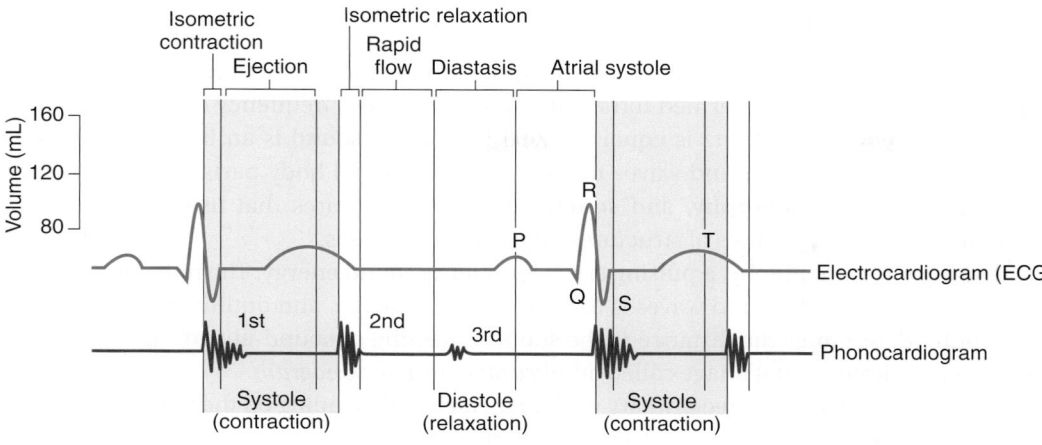

Figure 3-11 Phonocardiography. This technique provides a graphic recording of heart sounds and murmurs and is recorded along with an ECG.

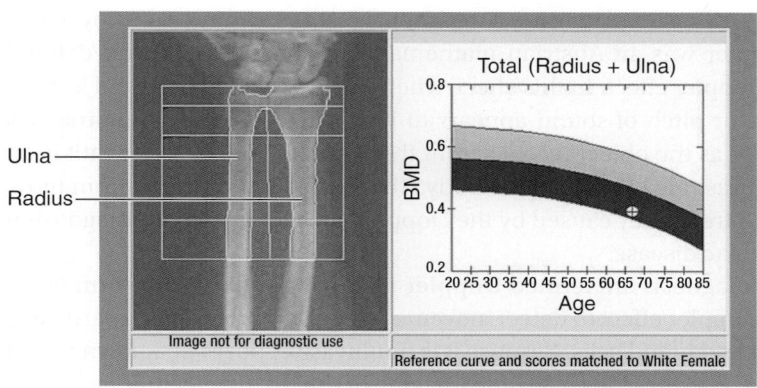

Figure 3-12 This bone density scan shows the bone mineral density (BMD) for the radius and ulna (forearm bones).

KEY TERM	Definition
phonocardiography (foh-noh-kahr-dee-OG-ruh-fee)	procedure for obtaining a graph of heart sounds using a phonocardiograph and an electrocardiogram
electromyography (EMG) (ee-leck-troh-migh-OG-ruh-fee)	procedure used to diagnose nerve and muscle disorders by measuring electrical activity of muscle tissue
densitometer (den-si-TOM-e-ter)	instrument used to measure the amount of light a tissue absorbs or reflects
densitometry (den-si-TOM-uh-tree)	examination of bone density using a densitometer

KEY TERM PRACTICE: *Other Diagnostic Radiology Services*

1. The procedure used to diagnose nerve and muscle disorders by measuring the electrical activity of muscles is known as _____.

2. _____ is examination of bone density using a densitometer.

3. The procedure for obtaining a graph of heart sounds using a phonocardiograph and an electrocardiogram is termed _____.

4. Name the instrument used to measure the amount of light that a tissue absorbs or reflects. _____

Diagnostic Ultrasound

Sound waves that have frequencies above the upper limit of the normal range of human hearing, about 20 kilohertz, are termed ultrasonic. A hertz (Hz) is a frequency equal to one cycle per second; hence, a kilohertz is equal to 1,000 hertz. Ultrasound is an imaging technique that uses high-frequency sound waves that bounce off internal body parts to create images. **Ultrasonography**, **echography**, and **sonography** are procedures that use high-frequency sound waves to make pictures of structures for medical purposes.

During ultrasonography, a pulsing crystal produces sound energy. The reflection of high-frequency (ultrasound) sound waves is used to locate, measure, and outline deep structures. A computer determines the distance to the sound-reflecting or sound-absorbing surface and creates a two-dimensional image called an *ultrasonogram* or *sonogram*.

Ultrasound is used in three primary ways in medicine, depending on the power level: diagnostic, therapeutic, and treatment. Diagnostic ultrasound uses sound waves below 0.1 watt per square centimeter (W/cm^2). For example, obstetric ultrasound is used during pregnancy to assess embryonic and fetal status (**Figure 3-13**). Ultrasound at 1 to 3 W/cm^2 is used for physiotherapy in joint and muscle disorders. Ultrasound for cancer treatment is set at 5 W/cm^2 to destroy tissue.

Johann Christian Doppler was an Austrian mathematician and physicist who defined what is now known as the Doppler effect. In this effect, when a source of light or sound is moving rapidly, the wavelength or pitch of sound appears to increase as the object approaches the observer and to decrease as the object recedes from the observer. The Doppler unit is an instrument that emits an ultrasonic beam into the body. The ultrasound reflected from moving structures has a changed frequency caused by the Doppler effect. It is used for diagnosing peripheral vascular and cardiac disease.

Pulse echoes used for diagnosis are termed **Doppler ultrasonography**. This form of ultrasonography applies the Doppler effect to detect movements of scatters (beams of particles), which are usually caused by red blood cells. Because it is noninvasive, poses no known risk to patients, is of moderate cost, and provides real-time imaging of organs, this technique has replaced radiography in many instances. It is particularly useful for viewing tissues, blood flow, heart structures, embryos, and fetuses. **Figure 3-14** illustrates Doppler ultrasonography via an image of normal blood flow in the internal carotid artery.

Echocardiography is also known as *ultrasonic cardiography* or *ultrasound cardiography*. **Doppler echocardiography** uses Doppler ultrasonographic techniques to enhance two-dimensional echocardiography by registering velocity of blood flow within the image on a strip chart. It is used to diagnose valve and structural abnormalities in the heart and blood vessels (**Figure 3-15**).

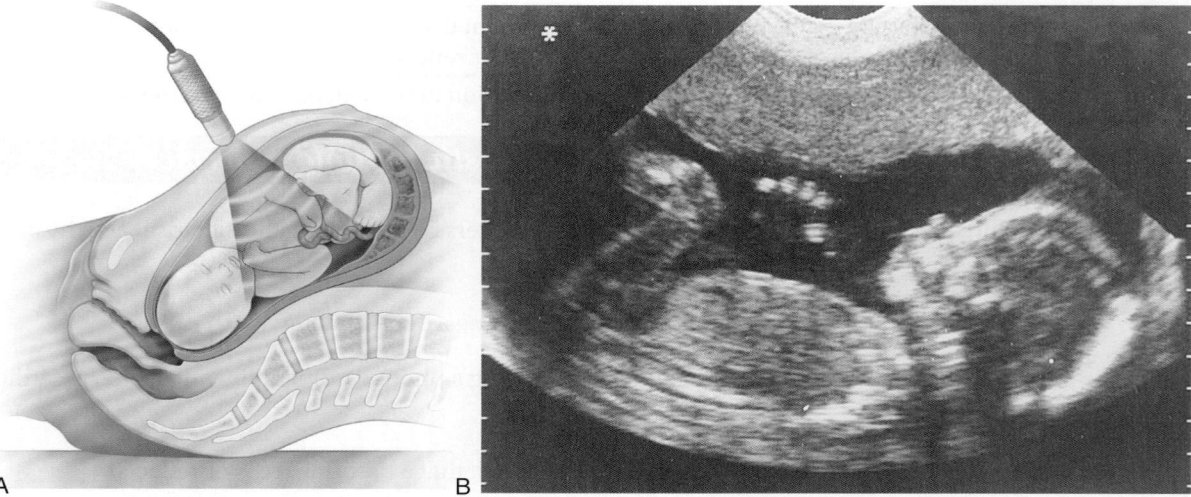

Figure 3-13 (A) Sonography technique. **(B)** A sonogram showing a fully formed normal fetus.

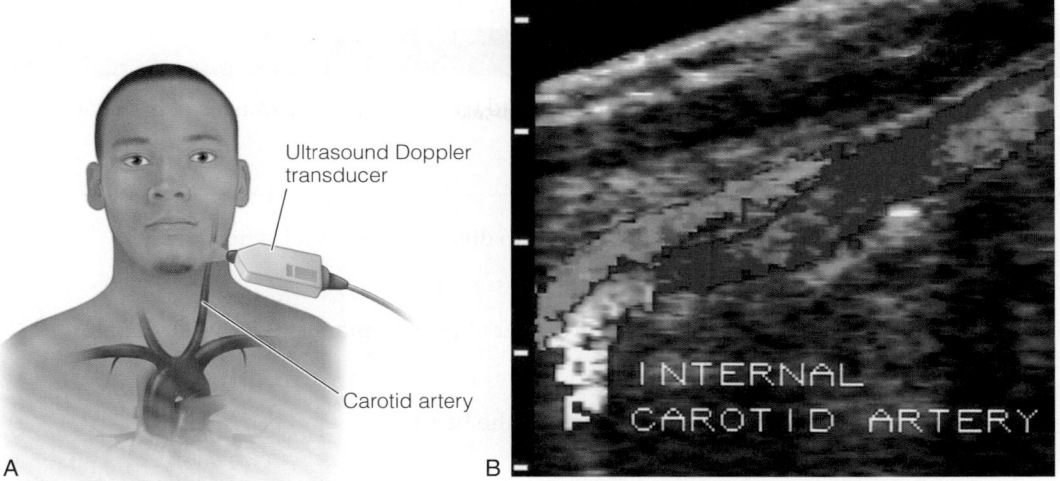

Figure 3-14 (A) Doppler ultrasonography. **(B)** Normal Doppler of internal carotid artery.

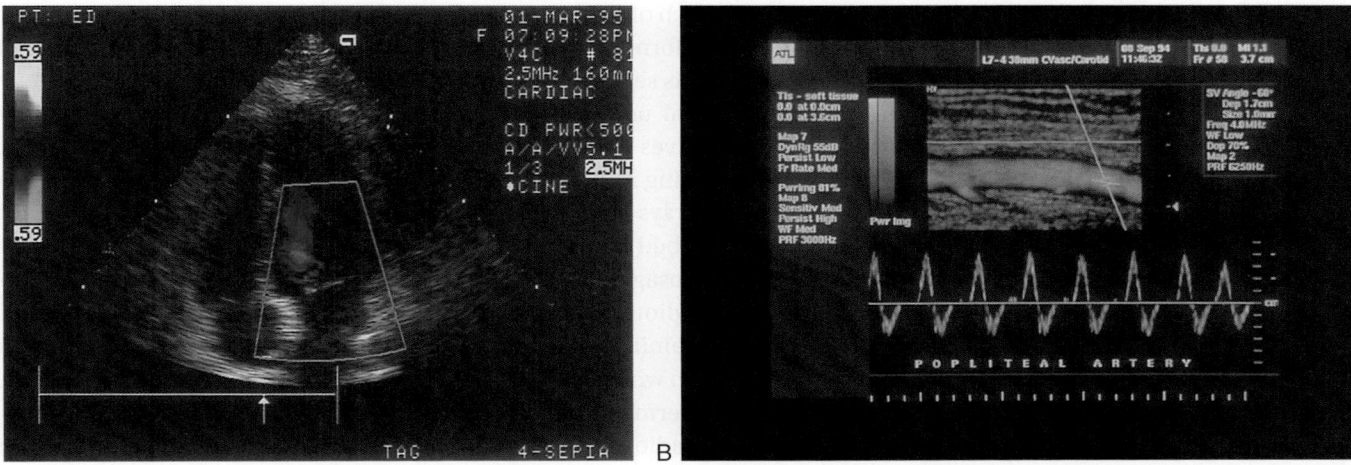

Figure 3-15 (A) Two-dimensional echocardiogram, four-chamber view in a normal patient. The heart's ventricles (lower chambers) and atria (upper chambers) are the dark areas outlined by the lighter coppery tones. **(B)** Echocardiogram of popliteal artery.

KEY TERM	Definition
ultrasonography (ul-truh-suh-NOG-ruh-fee)	imaging technique that uses high-frequency sound waves; another term for echography or sonography
echography (ECK-oh-graf-ee)	imaging technique that uses high-frequency sound waves; another term for ultrasonography or sonography
sonography (so-NOG-ruh-fee)	imaging technique that uses high-frequency sound waves; another term for echography or ultrasonography
Doppler ultrasonography (DOP-ler ul-truh-suh-NOG-ruh-fee)	application of the Doppler effect in ultrasound to detect movement
echocardiography (eck-oh-kahr-dee-OG-ruh-fee)	ultrasound technique for observing and examining the heart
Doppler echocardiography (DOP-ler eck-oh-kahr-dee-OG-ruh-fee)	ultrasound technique that uses the Doppler effect to enhance two-dimensional echocardiography

continued

continued from page 117

KEY TERM PRACTICE: *Diagnostic Ultrasound*

1. List the three terms that describe the imaging technique that uses sound waves to produce images of internal structures.

   _____

2. The ultrasound technique that applies the Doppler effect and is used to detect movement is known as

   _____.

3. _____ is an ultrasound technique that uses the Doppler effect to enhance two-dimensional echocardiography.

4. _____ is the ultrasound technique used for observing the heart.

Radiation Oncology

Radiation oncology is the branch of medicine that deals with the study and treatment of cancer using ionizing radiation. This form of radiation therapy is also called **radiotherapy**. Several procedures are described in this section.

Irradiation is the medical use of x-rays, gamma-rays, and other radioactive sources. Irradiation of body tissue involves bombarding the site with ionizing radiation to destroy unwanted cells and tissues or giving radionuclides in pill form. Measuring the amount of exposure or dosage of delivered x-rays is known as **dosimetry**. The instrument used to measure the amount of radiation absorbed by the body is called a *dosimeter*. Calculations are necessary to determine medicinal dosages. **Total body irradiation** exposes the whole body to ionizing radiation. This form of radiotherapy is often given in several doses before bone marrow transplantation to kill any remaining cancerous cells in the patient. If is often used along with chemotherapy. Radiotherapy in which the source of irradiation is placed close to the body surface or within a body cavity is termed **brachytherapy**. **Interstitial brachytherapy** is a form of radiation treatment in which radioactive needles or other sources are implanted directly into and around tissue to be irradiated (**Figure 3-16**).

Intraoperative cone irradiation involves aiming a beam of x-rays directly at the target through a cylinder during a surgical procedure. The goal is to eradicate cancerous growth.

A palliative cancer therapy (designed to relieve symptoms) involving radiation to half of the body is termed **hemibody radiation**. Hemibody radiation can treat multiple disease sites simultaneously and is effective in treating cancer that has spread throughout the body. Some pain and symptoms are alleviated, but the cause is not eliminated.

Prostate cancer is often treated with **radionuclide seeds**. Treatment with radionuclide seeds involves the planting of radioactive particles directly in the cancerous tissue. Treatment

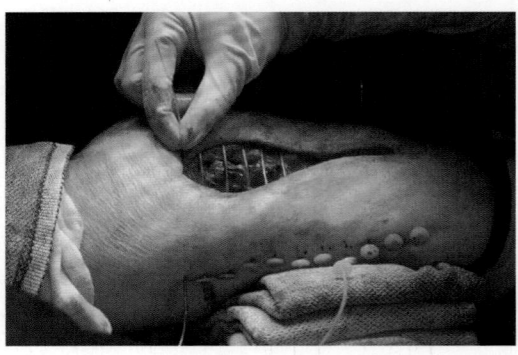

Figure 3-16 Brachytherapy catheters placed after resection of a soft tissue cancer.

with radiation from a source that is far from the body is known as **teletherapy** or external radiation therapy. Teletherapy uses a beam of radiation positioned above the patient that is aimed directly at the tumor. After the initial treatment, a small ink tattoo is fixed to the skin so that during future treatments the exact location can be identified and the radiation beam can be focused on the same site. Teletherapy is usually performed once a day, 5 to 6 days per week, for several weeks.

Treatment of disease by inducing a fever through inoculation with an infection or by physical means is known as **hyperthermia** or **hyperpyrexia**. Cancer cells are more sensitive to heat than are normal body cells, and raising the body temperature by either internal or external methods has therapeutic merit in selectively destroying malignant cells. External methods include using thermal blankets, radiofrequencies, and ultrasound. Internal methods involve administering pyrogens (fever-inducing agents). Some research suggests that hyperthermia combined with radiation therapy provides greater benefit than radiation treatment alone for treating cancer.

KEY TERM	Definition
radiotherapy (ray-dee-oh-THERR-uh-pee)	treating cancer by radiation; another term for radiation oncology
irradiation (i-ray-dee-A-Y-shun)	medical use of radiation—such as x-rays, gamma-rays, or other radioactive sources—to treat cancer
dosimetry (doh-SIM-e-tree)	measurement of exposure to radiation
total body irradiation (i-ray-dee-A-Y-shun)	exposing the entire body to ionizing radiation
brachytherapy (brack-ee-THERR-uh-pee)	radiotherapy in which the source is placed directly on or in close proximity to the body
interstitial brachytherapy (in-tur-STISH-ul brack-ee-THERR-uh-pee)	radiation treatment via implanted sources
intraoperative cone irradiation (in-truh-OP-ur-uh-tiv KONE i-ray-dee-A-Y-shun)	using x-rays aimed at a target to destroy cancerous cells during surgery
hemibody (HEM-i-bod-ee) **radiation**	radiotherapy of one half of the body
radionuclide (ray-dee-oh-NEW-klide) **seeds**	radioactive particles that are implanted in the body for treating cancer
teletherapy (tel-e-THERR-uh-pee)	radiation treatment administered with the source at a distance from the body
hyperthermia (high-pur-THUR-mee-uh)	therapeutically induced fever; another term for hyperpyrexia
hyperpyrexia (high-pur-PYE-rex-ee-uh)	therapeutically induced fever; another term for hyperthermia

KEY TERM PRACTICE: *Radiation Oncology*

1. Give the term that means treatment of cancer with radiation. _____

2. _____ is medical exposure to ionizing radiation.

3. Radiation treatment that is administered with the source at a distance from the body is called _____.

4. Radiotherapy in which the source is placed directly on or in close proximity to the body is termed _____, which is derived from the word part _____, which means "short."

5. Measuring the amount of exposure to radiation is termed _____.

Nuclear Medicine

Nuclear medicine is the branch of medicine that uses radioactive substances in diagnosis and therapy. Radionuclides or radioisotopes are used for diagnostic or therapeutic measures or as tracers to be detected in the body. They are observed in contained compartments of the body such as the vascular, urinary, or lymphatic systems.

Nuclear scan studies use radionuclides and radiation detectors with imaging instruments and computers to view internal structures. The radionuclide is administered either orally or intravenously (IV) and can then be measured by a camera that detects the amount of radiation emitted. The data are then converted into a two-dimensional image.

Radionuclide ejection fraction is a nuclear medicine study that determines the amount of blood ejected out of either ventricle in the heart. It assesses the motion of the heart wall.

Another variation of tomography has an application in nuclear medicine. **Positron emission tomography (PET)** creates images by computer analysis when low-dose radioactively tagged substances are incorporated into tissue. PET scans assess metabolic activity and physiologic function rather than anatomical structure. They are a useful tool for performing experimental living brain investigations. Diagnostic information can be obtained for central nervous system and cardiac function and for cancer evaluation. These scans can recognize some dementias like Alzheimer disease, Parkinson disease, Huntington disease, and epilepsy (**Figure 3-17**). Blood flow and viable heart tissue can also be identified. This technique is useful in the noninvasive assessment of tumor behavior in cancer patients.

Radioisotopes of iodine are used as radiopharmaceuticals for nuclear medicine studies. A **radiopharmaceutical** is a radioactive chemical or pharmaceutical preparation labeled with a tracer used as a diagnostic or therapeutic agent. Radioisotopes of iodine are used for studies of thyroid disease and renal function and as a treatment for some thyroid disorders.

Radioimmunoassay is a method for determining and quantifying antigens (substances that cause the body's immune system to react) or antibodies (substances produced by the body's immune system to fight foreign substances or organisms) in the blood using radiolabeled reactants. The tracer-tagged antigen will bind with an antibody, if one exists. If the antigen–antibody complex forms, the attached tracer allows the clinician to readily identify it (**Figure 3-18**).

Scintigraphy determines the distribution of a radioactive tracer in intact tissue via an external scintillation camera placed over the area. A photo obtained by scintigraphy is also called a *scintophotogram* or *scintiphotograph* (**Figure 3-19**).

A radioisotope of thallium (Tl), thallium-201 (^{201}Tl), is used for nuclear imaging of the heart. This test is called a **thallium scan**. Thallium is also taken up by some tumors so it can be easily detected.

The **urea breath test** is used to detect the presence of *Helicobacter pylori,* the bacterium that causes stomach ulcers. Patients swallow a capsule containing a radioisotope of carbon. If the radioactive substance is detected in the breath, it indicates the presence of the bacterium.

The **Schilling test** is a method of assessing vitamin B_{12} absorption. It determines the amount excreted in the urine using a substance tagged with a radioisotope of cobalt.

Bone scans use technetium-99 (^{99}Tc), a synthetic radioactive metallic element. A **bone scan** is a radiograph of the entire body that is used to evaluate the skeletal system. A high dose of a radioactive substance is injected into the body and the scan reads the distribution of radioactivity. The test identifies connective tissue disease, bone fractures, and bone infections (**Figure 3-20**). In the **gallium scan**, gallium-67 (^{67}Ga) is used as a tracer to identify tumors and inflammation.

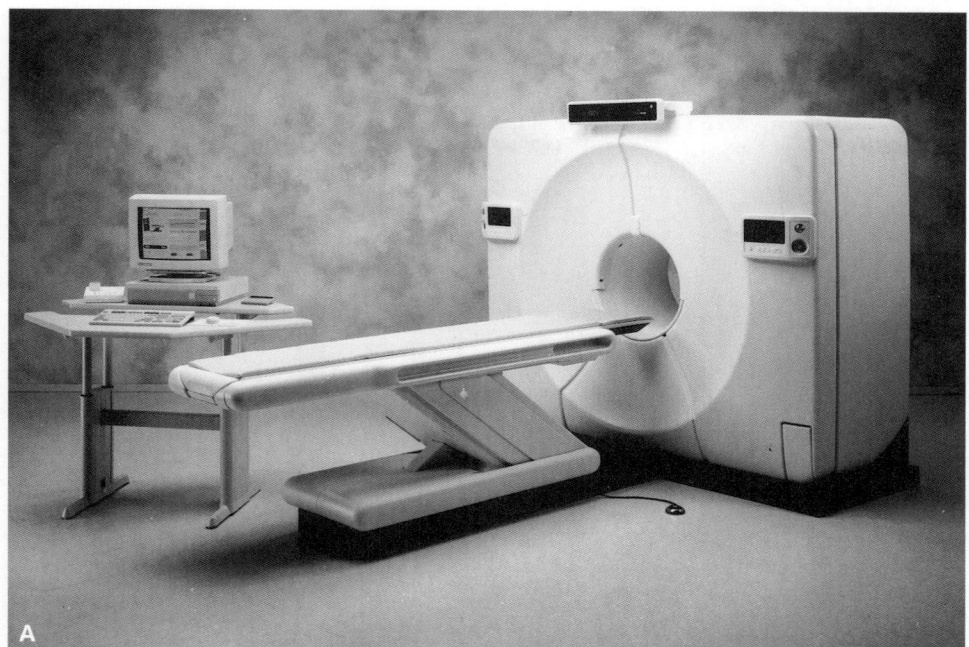

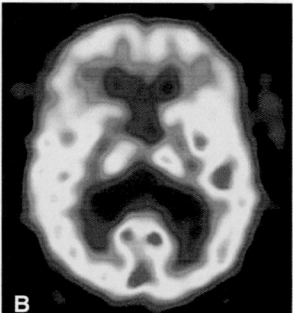 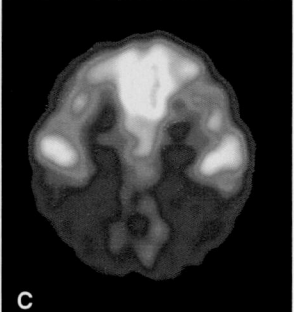

Figure 3-17 (A) Positron emission tomography. This technique combines nuclear medicine and computed tomography to create images of body parts. **(B)** PET scan of the brain of a healthy person. The red and yellow areas indicate areas of high metabolic activity. **(C)** PET scan of the brain of a person with Alzheimer disease. The blue areas indicate reduced brain activity.

Other organs visualized with nuclear scans are the spleen and thyroid. **Spleen imaging** is accomplished by administering a radionuclide intravenously. The spleen then absorbs the radionuclide and an image can be made. Spleen scans are used to diagnose cysts, abscesses, tumors, ruptures, or splenomegaly (enlarged spleen). **Thyroid imaging** is a picture of the thyroid gland after it takes up (absorbs) radioactive iodine. Radioactive iodine is either given orally or intravenously in the **radioactive iodine uptake** test. A normal function of the thyroid gland is to absorb iodine to make hormones. So, during this test, the thyroid traps and retains the radioactive iodine. The ability to capture the iodine then indicates how well the thyroid functions.

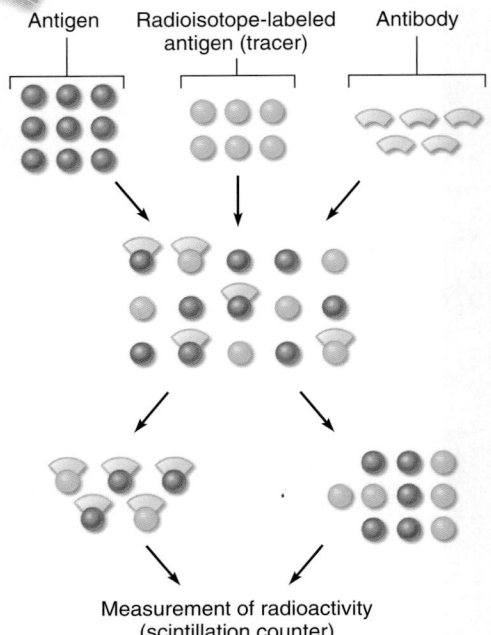

Figure 3-18 Radioimmunoassay.

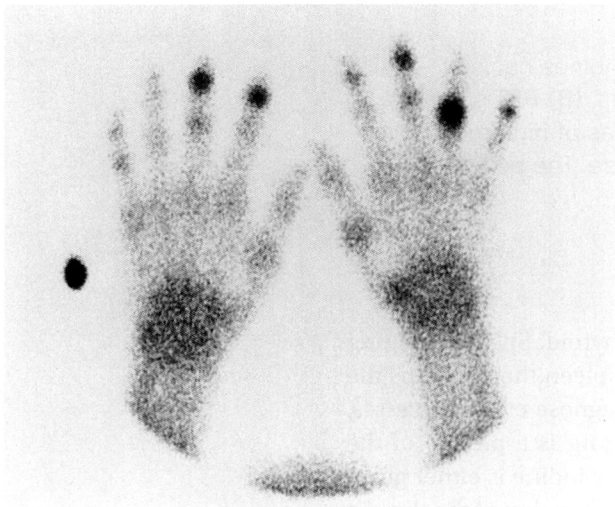

Figure 3-19 Scintigraphy. This scintophotogram shows radiotracer uptake in the joints of both hands, indicating arthritis.

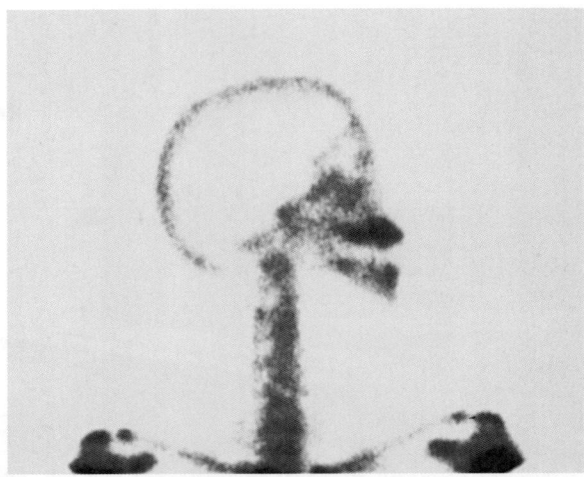

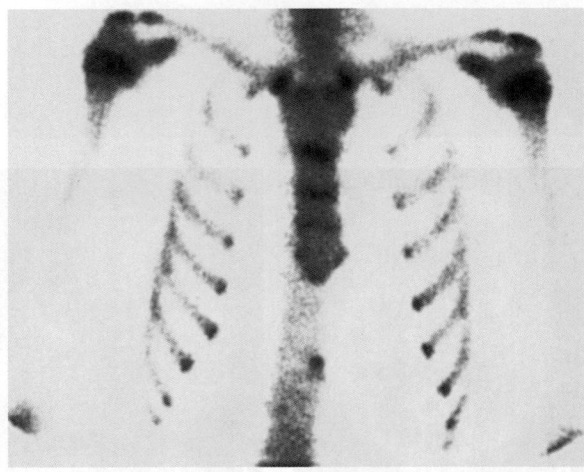

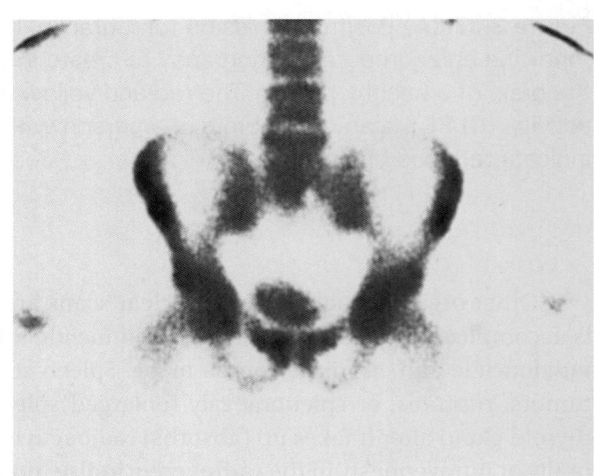

Figure 3-20 Bone scans of the head and neck, thoracic region, and pelvis. The images can be viewed as a whole or in cross-section.

KEY TERM	Definition
nuclear (NEW-klee-ur) **scan studies**	procedures that use radioactive substances in the body for diagnostic purposes
radionuclide ejection fraction (RAY-dee-oh-NEW-klide ee-JECK-shun FRACK-shun)	a nuclear medicine study to determine the amount of blood ejected out of either ventricle in the heart
positron (POZ-i-tron) **emission tomography** (toh-MOG-ruh-fee) **(PET)**	nuclear medicine technique for assessing metabolic activity of organs, diagnosing cancer, locating brain tumors, and investigating brain function
radiopharmaceutical (ray-dee-oh-far-muh-SOO-ti-kul)	radioactive substance used in nuclear medicine
radioimmunoassay (ray-dee-oh-im-yoo-noh-as-SAY)	technique for identifying antibodies using a radioactive tracer
scintigraphy (sin-TIG-ruh-fee)	two-dimensional imaging technique that uses a radioactive tracer
thallium (THAL-ee-um) **scan**	nuclear imaging technique that uses a radioisotope of thallium
urea (yoo-REE-uh) **breath test**	test that uses a radioisotope of carbon to determine the presence of *Helicobacter pylori*
Schilling (SHIL-ing) **test**	technique for determining vitamin B$_{12}$ absorption
bone scan	radiograph of the entire skeletal system using technetium-99 as a tracer
gallium (GAL-ee-um) **scan**	imaging technique that uses gallium-67 for the identification of tumors and inflammation
spleen imaging	radiograph of the spleen after administering a radionuclide
thyroid imaging	radiograph of the thyroid after administering a radionuclide such as radioactive iodine
radioactive iodine uptake	test used to determine thyroid function by assessing the amount of radioactive iodine absorbed by the thyroid gland

KEY TERM PRACTICE: *Nuclear Medicine*

1. A radiograph of the entire skeletal system using ^{99}Tc is termed a _____.

2. _____ is an imaging technique that uses radioactively tagged substances to assess the metabolic activity in organs instead of organ structure.

3. _____ are procedures that use radioactive substances in the body for diagnostic purposes.

4. The test that uses a radioisotope of carbon to determine the presence of *Helicobacter pylori* is called the _____.

5. Identify the test that is used for determining the absorption of vitamin B$_{12}$. _____

LIFE SPAN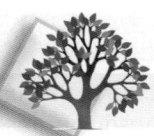

Many procedures identified in this chapter can be used at any point in life. Diagnostic ultrasound can detect the presence of embryonic life and can be performed as early as the fourth week of pregnancy. Although some procedures carry considerable risk, others such as magnetic resonance imaging have very little, because they do not use radioactive substances. Hence, ultrasound and MRI are deemed safe throughout the lifespan.

IN THE NEWS: Airport Screening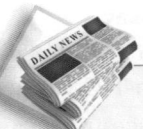

Probably the area of radiology that receives the most attention is airport screening. The Transportation Security Administration (TSA) uses two types of imaging technology to screen passengers: millimeter wave and backscatter. With millimeter wave technology, electromagnetic waves are bounced off the body to create black-and-white three-dimensional images. With backscatter technology, low-level x-ray beams are projected over the person to create a reflection of the body that is displayed on the monitor (**Figure 3-21**). Both techniques are safe and have met national health and safety standards.

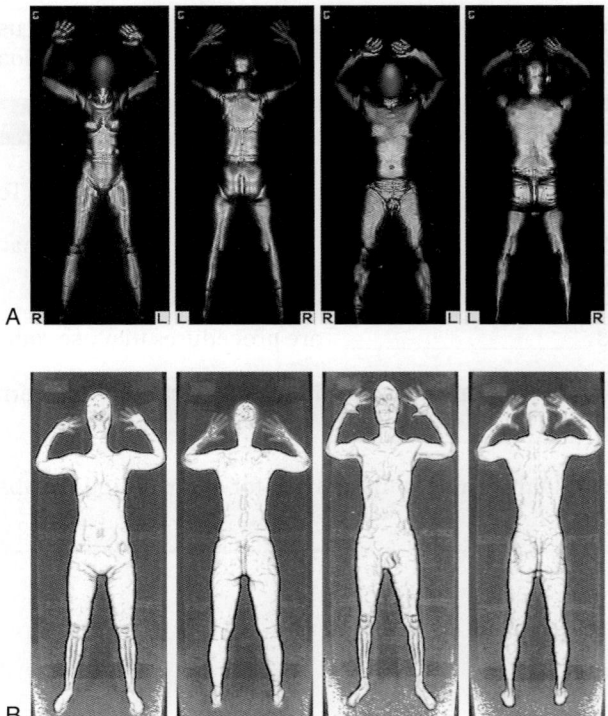

Figure 3-21 (A) Millimeter wave technology. **(B)** Backscatter technology.

COMMON Abbreviations

Abbreviation	Term
A	anterior
$BaSO_4$	barium sulfate
CAT	computed axial tomography computer-assisted tomography computerized axial tomography
CT	computed tomography
DSA	digital subtraction angiography
ECG	electrocardiogram
EMG	electromyography
Ga	gallium
^{67}Ga	gallium-67
GI	gastrointestinal
Gy	gray (unit of absorbed dose of ionizing radiation)
Hz	hertz
IV	intravenous
IVP	intravenous pyelogram
μCi	microcurie
MRA	magnetic resonance angiography
MRI	magnetic resonance imaging
NMR	nuclear magnetic resonance
P	posterior
PCT	percutaneous transhepatic cholangiography
PET	positron emission tomography
PTA	percutaneous transluminal angioplasty
PTHC	percutaneous transhepatic cholangiography
RP	retrograde pyelography
$T_{1/2}$	half-life
^{99}Tc	technetium-99
Tl	thallium
^{201}Tl	thallium-201

COMMON ABBREVIATIONS EXERCISES

1. DSA is the abbreviation for which procedure? _____

2. PET is the abbreviation for _____

3. Give the abbreviation for half-life. _____

4. MRA is the abbreviation for which procedure? _____

5. Write the abbreviation for barium sulfate. _____

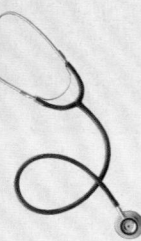

Case Study

Max Korinna's case is typical of the type seen in Lynne's radiology office. The medical report indicated that a chest x-ray was performed to determine intravenous catheter placement. Clinical information stated the patient was a 67-year-old male. The test performed was a chest radiography and was marked "chest, 1 view AP."

Report Information

AP view obtained of the chest with the patient erect shows cardiac monitoring electrodes overlying the anterior chest wall. A radiopaque catheter is identified extending from the left side, the tip of which is localized to the superior vena cava. The heart is prominent in regard to size. The lungs demonstrate no evidence of acute pulmonary pathology. There is no evidence of pneumothorax.

Impression

1. Cardiomegaly exists with underlying chronic pulmonary changes.

2. The tip of the indwelling catheter is thought to reside within the superior vena cava.

Case Study Questions

Select the best answer to each of the following questions.

1. **AP view refers to** _____.
   a. anatomy and physiology
   b. axial and proximal
   c. anterior and posterior
   d. appendicular and physical

2. **The word part *cardio-* refers to** _____,
   and the word part *-megaly* means
   _____; **so *cardiomegaly* refers**
   to _____.
   a. vessel; large; large vessel
   b. heart; small; an atrophied (small, wasting) heart
   c. chest; large; enlarged chest cavity
   d. heart; large; enlarged heart

3. **Which is the correct definition for catheter?**
   _____
   a. a thin flexible tube inserted into a body part
   b. an artificially created passage to redirect circulation

   c. a unit of measurement for the absorbed dose of ionizing radiation
   d. a substance opaque to x-rays that is used to make the outline of a body part easier to see on radiographs

4. **The term *radiopaque* means that the catheter** _____.
   a. could be visualized on radiographic examination because it blocked the passage of x-rays
   b. could not be visualized on radiographic examination because it blocked the passage of x-rays
   c. contained radioactive material
   d. was colored

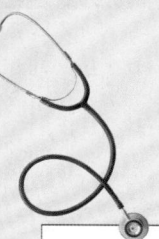

Real World Report

Lynne's office received Max Korinna's medical report from the imaging department for coding and billing purposes.

CENTRAL IMAGING DEPARTMENT

NAME:	Max Korinna		
DATE ORDERED:	January 20, 2011	AGE: 67Y	
ORDPHYS:	M. R. Tambo, M.D.	EXAM DATE: 01/20/2011	
DOB:	02/02/1944	TEST: ANGIO, CAR/CRBRL, BIL, RS&I	
ATTENDING:	M. R. Tambo, M.D.	REFERRING: P. J. Miter, M.D.	

CLINICAL INFORMATION:

Follow-up for possible lesion at distal cervical segment of the right internal carotid.

NONSELECTIVE RIGHT CAROTID ANGIOGRAM

Following right brachial arterial puncture at the antecubital region, a 4 French straight catheter was placed at the innominate artery for nonselective right carotid angiogram. Frontal and oblique projections were made. The patient tolerated the procedure well and left the department in stable condition.

Comparison was made to previous cerebral and carotid angiogram of January 18, 2009. The previously noted segmental narrowing at the distal portion of the cervical segment of the right internal carotid is no longer demonstrated on this examination; therefore, the previous finding is from spasm. There is no significant plaque formation or narrowing of the right internal or external carotid arteries. Incidentally noted is plaque formation at the origin of the left internal carotid without significant stenosis. Bilateral vertebral arteries appear unremarkable.

Refer to the previous cerebral and carotid angiogram for anatomical details of the intracranial circulation. DICTATED BY: M. J. Manju, M.D.

Real World Report Questions

The following exercises review the medical terms used in the preceding medical report.

1. The term *nonselective* means _____.

2. Provide a brief description of an angiogram.

_____

3. Was this procedure performed to evaluate arteries or veins?

_____

4. The regions of the body through which the catheter passed include _____.

a. arm, neck, and head

b. leg, neck, and arm

c. head, chest, and leg

d. leg, neck, and head

Review and Application

Multiple-Choice Questions

Select the best response to each of the following questions.

1. The branch of medicine that deals with radioactive substances in the diagnosis and treatment of disease is known as _____.

   a. urology   b. radiology   c. oncology   d. hematology

2. A physician specializing in the diagnostic and/or therapeutic use of x-rays and radionuclides is a/an _____.

   a. radiologist   b. urologist   c. professional coder   d. radiographer

3. _____ is the branch of medicine that uses radioisotopes in diagnosis and therapy.

   a. Nuclear medicine   b. Diagnostic medicine   c. Therapeutic medicine   d. Mammography

4. The branch of radiology that uses guided procedures for diagnosing and treating pathology is _____ radiology.

   a. oncology   b. nuclear   c. interventional   d. diagnostic

5. An x-ray of the joint interior after introduction of a contrast dye is termed _____.

   a. shuntogram   b. CT pelvimetry   c. cineradiography   d. arthrography

6. _____ is an imaging technique in which certain planes of the body are focused while other planes are blurred.

   a. Scintigraphy   b. Ultrasound   c. Radiology   d. Tomography

7. Which of the following is a therapy in which half of the body is radiated to treat multiple cancer sites simultaneously? _____

   a. hemibody radiation   b. teletherapy   c. brachytherapy   d. interstitial brachytherapy

8. Examination of blood vessels after introduction of a contrast dye is called _____.

   a. angiography   b. atheroma   c. irradiation   d. interstitial brachytherapy

9. The branch of medicine that uses radioactive substances specifically for cancer treatment is called _____.

   a. nuclear medicine   b. ultrasonography   c. diagnostic ultrasound   d. radiation oncology

10. Examination of the intervertebral discs after direct injection of a contrast medium is known as _____.

    a. vessel ordering   b. cineradiography   c. diskography   d. cinefluoroscope

11. A procedure in which a tubular instrument is passed through a blood vessel to the heart for imaging purposes is termed _____.

    a. cardiac catheterization   b. percutaneous transluminal angioplasty
    c. percutaneous balloon angioplasty   d. percutaneous needle biopsy

12. Imaging blood vessels using MRI is termed _____.

    a. vessel ordering   b. CT scanning   c. magnetic resonance angiography   d. all of these

13. A group of vessels fed by a primary vessel is called a _____.

    a. vessel ordering   b. vascular family   c. millicurie   d. rad

14. A catheter placed into an arterial vessel and not manipulated is _____, whereas a catheter placed into a vein and not manipulated to another site is _____.

    a. nonselective venous; nonselective arterial catheter placement
    b. nonselective arterial catheter placement; nonselective venous
    c. selective venous; selective arterial catheter placement
    d. selective arterial catheter placement; selective venous

15. A _____ is a radiolabeled chemical used as a detector in diagnostic tests.

    a. gray   b. radionuclide   c. radiotracer   d. rad

16. A dye or other substance introduced into the body that is opaque to x-rays is termed a _____.

    a. chest x-ray   b. contrast medium   c. myelography   d. shunt

17. A _____ is an imaging technique that uses a small dose of ionizing radiation to produce pictures of body structures in the thoracic cavity.

    a. CT pelvimetry   b. computed tomographic angiography   c. chest x-ray   d. percutaneous trans-hepatic portography

18. A radiograph of the entire skeletal system is a _____.

    a. gallium scan   b. biopsy   c. bone scan   d. scintigraphy

19. _____ is an imaging technique that uses electromagnetic radiation.

    a. X-ray   b. MRI   c. CAT   d. Ultrasound

20. Excision of tissue by a guided needle through the skin is called _____.

    a. subcutaneous needle incision   b. percutaneous needle incision
    c. percutaneous needle biopsy   d. percutaneous subcutaneous needle biopsy

21. Use of a balloon catheter to widen a narrowed artery is _____.

    a. percutaneous transluminal angioplasty   b. subcutaneous transluminal angioplasty
    c. percutaneous subcutaneous angioplasty   d. none of these

22. Examination of bone density using light absorption and reflection is termed _____.

    a. ultrasonography   b. densitometry   c. angioplasty   d. electromyography

23. An x-ray of the urine-collecting part of the kidneys after IV administration of a dye is termed _____.

    a. antegrade pyelography   b. retrograde pyelography   c. anterograde pyelography   d. intravenous pyelogram

24. An imaging technique that uses radionuclides to assess metabolic function is _____.

    a. positron emission tomography   b. radioimmunoassay   c. computed axial tomography   d. ultrasound

25. _____ studies use isotopes in the body for diagnostic purposes.

    a. Ultrasound   b. Nuclear scan   c. Densitometry   d. Teletherapy

26. During a _____ catheter placement, the catheter is threaded into another artery from the original puncture site.

    a. selective arterial   b. nonselective arterial   c. selective venous   d. nonselective venous

27. _____ pyelography shows backward flow.

    a. Retrograde   b. Antegrade   c. Uptake   d. Radioactive

Word Parts Exercises

Using the following word parts, form a medical term for each definition. Each word part is used only once.

aorto-	-graphy	hystero-
angio-	-graphy	mammo-
arterio-	-graphy	phono-
cardio-	-graphy	sono-
cardio-	-graphy	vaso-
epididymo-	-graphy	veno-
-graphy-	-graphy	vesiculo-
-graphy	-graphy	

28. ultrasound of the uterus = _____

29. x-ray examination of the aorta after injection of a contrast medium = _____

30. x-ray examination of veins after injection of an opaque dye = _____

31. x-ray examination of the heart and blood vessels after administration of a contrast dye = _____

32. x-ray examination of arteries after injection of a contrast dye = _____

33. procedure for obtaining a visual record of heart sounds = _____

34. x-ray examination of the seminal vesicles after administration of a contrast medium = _____

35. x-ray examination of the vas deferens after introducing a contrast medium = _____

36. x-ray examination of the epididymis after introducing a contrast medium = _____

37. radiographic examination of the breast tissue = _____

Matching Exercises

Match the term or procedure with its description.

_____ 38. barium swallow

_____ 39. x-ray

_____ 40. endoscopic catheterization

_____ 41. shuntogram

_____ 42. barium enema

a. x-ray examination to determine shunt placement
b. procedure that uses an endoscope to view internal structures
c. rectal infusion with barium sulfate for x-ray examination of the lower GI tract
d. ingestion of barium sulfate for x-ray examination of the upper GI tract
e. image produced on film by passing x-rays through a body part

Match the term or procedure with its description.

_____ 43. cholangiography

_____ 44. cholecystography

_____ 45. cisternography

_____ 46. sialography

_____ 47. splenoportography

a. x-ray examination of the salivary glands
b. x-ray examination of bile ducts after administration of a contrast dye
c. x-ray examination of the gallbladder after administration of a contrast dye
d. x-ray examination of the spleen and portal vein after administration of a contrast dye
e. x-ray examination of the subarachnoid space after administration of a contrast dye

Match the term or procedure with its description.

_____ 48. digital subtraction angiography
_____ 49. cardiac catheterization
_____ 50. lymphography
_____ 51. cinefluoroscopy
_____ 52. electromyography

a. x-ray examination of the heart after threading a catheter through a vessel into the heart
b. radiography of an organ in motion
c. computer-assisted radiography of vascular structures without superimposed bone or soft tissue
d. procedure used to diagnose nerve and muscle disorders
e. x-ray examination of lymphatic vessels after introduction of a contrast dye

Match the term or procedure with its description.

_____ 53. corpora cavernosography
_____ 54. hysterosalpingography
_____ 55. CT pelvimetry
_____ 56. cystography
_____ 57. urography

a. x-ray examination of the urinary tract
b. x-ray examination of the bladder after administration of a contrast medium
c. x-ray examination of the penile erectile tissue
d. measurements of pelvic dimensions and fetal head
e. x-ray examination of the uterus and uterine tubes using a contrast dye

Match the term or procedure with its description.

_____ 58. echocardiography
_____ 59. echoencephalography
_____ 60. Doppler echocardiography
_____ 61. Doppler ultrasonography
_____ 62. ultrasonography

a. imaging technique that uses high-frequency sound waves
b. imaging technique that applies the Doppler effect to detect movement
c. ultrasound technique for observing the heart
d. ultrasound technique that uses the Doppler effect to enhance two-dimensional echocardiography
e. ultrasound technique for studying intracranial structures

Match the term or procedure with its description.

_____ 63. brachytherapy
_____ 64. hemibody radiation
_____ 65. hyperthermia
_____ 66. scintigraphy
_____ 67. urea breath test

a. therapeutically induced fever
b. radiotherapy in which the source is placed close to or directly on the body
c. radiotherapy of half of the body
d. two-dimensional imaging technique that uses a radioactive tracer
e. test that uses a radioisotope of carbon to determine the presence of *Helicobacter pylori*

Match the term or procedure with its description.

_____ 68. gallium scan
_____ 69. Schilling test
_____ 70. thallium scan
_____ 71. radioimmunoassay
_____ 72. ductography

a. nuclear imaging technique that uses a radioisotope of thallium
b. mammographic imaging of the milk ducts using a contrast medium
c. technique used to determine absorption of vitamin B_{12}
d. imaging technique that uses ^{67}Ga
e. technique for identifying antibodies using a radioactive tracer

Definitions

Define the following terms.

73. radionuclide _____
74. spleen imaging _____
75. barium sulfate ($BaSO_4$) _____
76. transluminal atherectomy _____

What is the term described by each of the following definitions?

77. term describing the amount of work required to position a catheter at its destination _____

78. absorption of radionuclide by tissue _____

79. radiology of bile ducts via needle puncture through the skin _____

80. introduction of a barium salt suspension into the rectum and colon for x-ray examination _____

81. aiming a beam of x-rays directly at the target tissue through a cylinder _____

82. tissue sample taken via a catheter _____

Spelling

Identify the correctly spelled term in each set.

83. _____
   a. veinography
   b. venography
   c. venegraphy
   d. venogrephy

84. _____
   a. galacktogram
   b. glactiogram
   c. galactogram
   d. gelactogram

85. _____
   a. yoorography
   b. uregraphy
   c. urrography
   d. urography

86. _____
   a. radiopaque
   b. radioopaque
   c. radipaque
   d. radiopake

87. _____
   a. telatherapy
   b. teletherapy
   c. telotherapy
   d. telletherpy

88. _____
   a. radinuclide
   b. radionucleide
   c. radionuclide
   d. radionuklide

89. _____
   a. radiofarmaceutical
   b. radiopharmacutical
   c. radiopharmeceutical
   d. radiopharmaceutical

Unscramble

Unscramble the letters to form a medical term.

90. lluimaht acns _____

91. diveaaoritc _____

92. mitesdryo _____

93. aaadiioommnussyr _____

94. tatol odyb idinoirraat _____

95. ridthoy ginmiag _____

Abbreviations

Provide the terms for the abbreviations and then define the terms.

96. μCi = _____

97. PTA = _____

98. PET = _____

99. CT = _____

100. MRI = _____

101. EMG = _____

Analogies

Provide a medical term to complete a meaningful analogy.

102. Ultrasonic cardiography and ultrasound cardiography are to _____ as _____ is to echography or sonography.

103. Urethrocystography is to _____ as _____ is to ptyalography.

104. Radiograms are to shadowgraphs as _____ are to roentgenograms.

Short Answer

Answer the following question.

105. A physician orders a procedure that involves catheter placement through the aorta to the left common carotid artery, ending in the left external carotid artery.

    a. The primary branch is the _____.

    b. The secondary branch is the _____.

Word Search

Find the medical terms hidden in the puzzle.

```
T  G  L  R  K  B  D  N  N  D  W  W  E  Y  M  H
G  A  A  T  H  E  R  O  M  A  Z  R  D  H  R  M
S  Q  O  P  Y  M  A  R  G  O  L  E  Y  P  U  K
U  X  Y  H  P  A  R  G  O  G  N  Y  R  A  L  P
J  W  H  U  E  P  A  P  V  S  O  D  G  R  T  B
Q  M  P  X  R  B  D  F  I  Q  I  K  U  G  R  X
B  T  A  E  P  S  I  T  A  M  T  T  P  O  A  B
B  G  R  R  Y  X  O  D  B  X  A  Z  R  N  S  E
R  W  G  O  R  M  G  N  B  G  I  O  V  E  O  N
X  V  O  S  E  R  R  E  O  T  D  H  R  D  U  T
L  M  L  T  X  R  A  C  U  G  A  W  M  O  N  Y
N  B  E  O  I  A  P  X  X  H  R  R  O  U  D  Q
L  R  Y  M  A  H  H  R  M  K  R  A  H  D  D  F
C  G  M  I  S  Z  Y  E  X  H  I  S  P  B  Y  W
C  D  Q  A  H  V  A  S  O  G  R  A  P  H  Y  I
E  P  L  B  N  E  E  O  Y  I  V  U  E  C  Y  D
```

atheroma
densitometer
duodenography
hyperpyrexia
irradiation
laryngography
myelography
pyelogram
radiography
shunt
sonography
ultrasound
vasography
xerostomia

Vocabulary Review

Review the key terms from this chapter, study the spelling and pronunciation of each term, and write its definition in the space provided. Listen to the audio available for most terms at http://thepoint.lww.com/nath2e and pronounce each term for yourself. Then check the box when you feel confident that you know the definition and can pronounce the term correctly.

Key Term	Pronunciation	Definition
☐ angiocardiography	(an-jee-oh-kahr-dee-OG-ruh-fee)	_____
☐ angiography	(an-jee-OG-ruh-fee)	_____
☐ aortography	(ay-or-TOG-ruh-fee)	_____
☐ arteriography	(ahr-teer-ee-OG-ruh-fee)	_____
☐ arthrography	(ahr-THROG-ruh-fee)	_____
☐ atheroma	(ath-er-OH-muh)	_____
☐ barium enema	(BAIR-ee-um-EN-e-muh)	_____
☐ barium sulfate (BaSO$_4$)	(BAIR-ee-um)	_____
☐ barium swallow	(BAIR-ee-um)	_____
☐ bone scan		_____
☐ brachytherapy	(brack-ee-THERR-uh-pee)	_____
☐ cardiac catheterization	(kath-e-tur-i-ZAY-shun)	_____
☐ chest x-ray		_____
☐ cholangiography	(koh-lan-jee-OG-ruh-fee)	_____
☐ cholecystography	(koh-lee-sis-TOG-ruh-fee)	_____
☐ computed tomographic angiography	(toh-moh-GRAF-ik an-jee-OG-ruh-fee)	_____
☐ computed tomography (CT)	(toh-MOG-ruh-fee)	_____
☐ contrast medium		_____
☐ CT pelvimetry	(pel-VIM-uh-tree)	_____
☐ cystography	(sis-TOG-ruh-fee)	_____
☐ densitometer	(den-si-TOM-e-ter)	_____
☐ densitometry	(den-si-TOM-uh-tree)	_____
☐ diagnostic radiology	(dye-ug-NOS-tik ray-dee-OL-uh-jee)	_____
☐ diagnostic ultrasound	(dye-ug-NOS-tik)	_____
☐ digital subtraction angiography (DSA)	(an-jee-OG-ruh-fee)	_____
☐ diskography	(disk-OG-ruh-fee)	_____
☐ dosimetry	(doh-SIM-e-tree)	_____
☐ Doppler echocardiography	(DOP-ler eck-oh-kahr-dee-OG-ruh-fee)	_____
☐ Doppler ultrasonography	(DOP-ler ul-truh-suh-NOG-ruh-fee)	_____
☐ ductography	(duk-TOG-ruh-fee)	_____
☐ duodenography	(dew-oh-de-NOG-ruh-fee)	_____

Key Term	Pronunciation	Definition
❑ echocardiography	(eck-oh-kahr-dee-OG-ruh-fee)	_____
❑ echography	(ECK-oh-graf-ee)	_____
❑ electromyography (EMG)	(ee-leck-troh-migh-OG-ruh-fee)	_____
❑ endoscopic catheterization	(en-duh-SKOP-ick kath-e-tur-i-ZAY-shun)	_____
❑ galactography	(gal-ak-TOG-ruh-fee)	_____
❑ gallium scan	(GAL-ee-um)	_____
❑ hemibody radiation	(HEM-i-bod-ee)	_____
❑ hyperpyrexia	(high-pur-PYE-rex-ee-uh)	_____
❑ hyperthermia	(high-pur-THUR-mee-uh)	_____
❑ hysterosalpingography	(his-tur-oh-sal-ping-OG-ruh-fee)	_____
❑ interstitial brachytherapy	(in-tur-STISH-ul brack-ee-THERR-uh-pee)	_____
❑ interventional radiology	(in-ter-VEN-shun-ul ray-dee-OL-uh-jee)	_____
❑ intraoperative cone irradiation	(in-truh-OP-ur-uh-tiv KONE i-ray-dee AY-shun)	_____
❑ intravenous pyelogram (IVP)	(pye-e-loh-gram)	_____
❑ irradiation	(i-ray-dee-AY-shun)	_____
❑ laryngography	(luh-rin-GOG-ruh-fee)	_____
❑ lymphography	(limf-OG-ruh-fee)	_____
❑ magnetic resonance angiography	(an-jee-OG-ruh-fee)	_____
❑ magnetic resonance imaging (MRI)		_____
❑ magnetic resonance spectroscopy	(speck-TROS-kuh-pee)	_____
❑ mammography	(ma-MOG-ruh-fee)	_____
❑ myelography	(migh-e-LOG-ruh-fee)	_____
❑ nonselective arterial catheter placement		_____
❑ nonselective venous		_____
❑ nuclear medicine	(NEW-klee-ur)	_____
❑ nuclear scan studies	(NEW-klee-ur)	_____
❑ percutaneous needle biopsy	(pur-kew-TAY-nee-us) (BYE-op-see)	_____
❑ percutaneous transhepatic cholangiography (PCT, PTHC)	(pur-kew-TAY-nee-us trans-he-PAT-ick koh-lan-jee-OG-ruh-fee)	_____
❑ percutaneous transhepatic portography	(pur-kew-TAY-nee-us trans-he PAT-ick por-TOG-ruh-fee)	_____
❑ percutaneous transluminal angioplasty (PTA)	(pur-kew-TAY-nee-us trans-LEW-mi-nul AN-jee-oh-plas-tee)	_____

Key Term	Pronunciation	Definition
❏ phonocardiography	(foh-noh-kahr-dee-OG-ruh-fee)	_____
❏ positron emission tomography (PET)	(POZ-i-tron toh-MOG-ruh-fee)	_____
❏ ptyalography	(tigh-uh-LOG-ruh-fee)	_____
❏ pyelogram	(pye-e-loh-gram)	_____
❏ pyelography	(pye-e-LOG-ruh-fee)	_____
❏ radiation oncology	(ray-dee-AY-shun ong-KOL-uh-jee)	_____
❏ radioactive		_____
❏ radioactive iodine uptake		_____
❏ radiograph	(RAY-dee-oh-graf)	_____
❏ radiography	(ray-dee-OG-ruh-fee)	_____
❏ radioimmunoassay	(ray-dee-oh-im-yoo-noh-as-SAY)	_____
❏ radiologist	(ray-dee-OL-uh-jist)	_____
❏ radiology	(ray-dee-OL-uh-jee)	_____
❏ radionuclide	(RAY-dee-oh-NEW-klide)	_____
❏ radionuclide ejection fraction	(RAY-dee-oh-NEW-klide ee-JECK-shun FRACK-shun)	_____
❏ radionuclide seeds	(ray-dee-oh-NEW-klide)	_____
❏ radiopaque	(ray-dee-oh-PAKE)	_____
❏ radiopharmaceutical	(ray-dee-oh-far-muh-SOO-ti-kul)	_____
❏ radiotherapy	(ray-dee-oh-THERR-uh-pee)	_____
❏ radiotracer		_____
❏ retrograde pyelography (RP)	(RET-roh-grade pye-e-LOG-ruh-fee)	_____
❏ Schilling test	(SHIL-ing)	_____
❏ scintigraphy	(sin-TIG-ruh-fee)	_____
❏ selective arterial catheter placement		_____
❏ selective venous		_____
❏ shunt		_____
❏ shuntogram	(SHUNT-oh-gram)	_____
❏ sialography	(sigh-uh-LOG-ruh-fee)	_____
❏ sonography	(so-NOG-ruh-fee)	_____
❏ spleen imaging		_____
❏ splenoportography	(splee-noh-por-TOG-ruh-fee)	_____
❏ teletherapy	(tel-e-THERR-uh-pee)	_____
❏ thallium scan	(THAL-ee-um)	_____
❏ thyroid imaging		_____
❏ tomography	(toh-MOG-ruh-fee)	_____

Key Term	Pronunciation	Definition
❏ **total body irradiation**	(i-ray-dee-AY-shun)	
❏ **transcatheter biopsy**	(trans-KATH-e-tur BYE-op-see)	
❏ **transluminal atherectomy**	(trans-LEW-mi-nul ath-e-RECK-toh-me)	
❏ **ultrasonography**	(ul-truh-suh-NOG-ruh-fee)	
❏ **ultrasound**		
❏ **uptake**		
❏ **urea breath test**	(yoo-REE-uh)	
❏ **urethrocystometry**	(yoo-re-throh-sis-TOM-e-tree)	
❏ **urography**	(yoo-ROG-ruh-fee)	
❏ **vascular family**		
❏ **vasography**	(vay-SOG-ruh-fee)	
❏ **venography**	(vee-NOG-ruh-fee)	
❏ **vessel ordering**		
❏ **xerostomia**	(zeer-oh-STOH-mee-uh)	
❏ **x-rays**		

Answers

Word Grouping Exercises

Definition	Word Part	Definition	Word Part
movement, relating to motion pictures	cine-	saliva, salivary glands	sial-, sialo-
distant	tel-, tele-, telo-	salivary glands, saliva	ptyal-, ptyalo-
dry	xero-	section	-tome
electricity	electro-	short	brachy-
excess, beyond	ultra-	something written, instrument for making a recording	-graph
fever, fire, heat	pyr-, pyro-	sound, speech	phon-, phono-
flow	fluo-	spectrum	spectro-
nuclear, nucleus	nucleo-	tumor	onco-, oncho-
portal	porto-	within, inner	end-, endo-
radiation	radio-	a writing, description	grapho-, -graphy
recording, usually by an instrument	-gram		

Word Building Exercises

Word Part	Meaning	Common or Known Word	Example Medical Term
brachy-	short	brachycephalic	brachytherapy
cine-	motion picture	cinema	cineradiography
electro-	electricity	electronics	electromyography
end-, endo-	within, inner	endothermic	endoscopic catheterization
fluo-	flow	fluorescent	fluoroscopy
-gram	recording, usually by an instrument	sonogram	sonogram
-graph	something written, instrument for making a recording	photograph	angiograph
grapho-, -graphy	a writing, description	photography	arteriography
nucleo-	nuclear, nucleus	nuclear reaction	nuclear medicine
onco-, oncho-	tumor	oncogene	oncology
phon-, phono-	sound, speech	phonics	phonocardiography
pyr-, pyro-	fever, fire, heat	pyrotechnics	hyperpyrexia
radio-	radiation	radioactive	radiology
tel-, tele-, telo-	distant	telephone	teletherapy
-tome	section	dermatome	tomography
ultra-	beyond, excess	ultraviolet	ultrasound
xero-	dry	Xerox	xeromammography

Key Term Practice

Radiology

1. diagnostic ultrasound
2. Nuclear medicine
3. radiation oncology
4. Radiology
5. radiologist

Radiology Basic Terms

1. uptake
2. contrast medium
3. radiograph
4. Radioactive
5. radiopaque

Diagnostic Radiology

1. interventional radiology
2. diagnostic radiology

Radiography

1. -graphy; arthrography
2. diskography
3. shunt
4. shuntogram
5. radiography

Radiography in Motion

1. motion picture; radiation; -graphy; cineradiography
2. flow

Tomography

1. computed tomography angiography
2. computed tomography (CT); the following are also correct: computerized axial tomography (CAT), computer-assisted tomography (CAT), and computed axial tomography (CAT)
3. Tomography
4. CT pelvimetry

Catheterization, Biopsy, and Percutaneous Radiographic Procedures

1. transcatheter biopsy
2. selective
3. Percutaneous transhepatic portography
4. Percutaneous transhepatic cholangiography (PCT, PTHC)
5. vascular family

Magnetic Resonance Imaging (MRI)

1. magnetic resonance angiography (MRA); -graphy
2. magnetic resonance spectroscopy
3. magnetic resonance imaging (MRI)

Contrast Studies and Digestive System Radiology

1. barium swallow
2. duodenography
3. sialography and ptyalography
4. barium enema
5. cholangiography

Nervous System Radiography

1. Myelography

Heart and Vessel Radiography

1. Angiography
2. arteriography
3. Venography
4. -graphy; lymphography
5. digital substraction angiography

Reproductive System Radiography

1. mammography
2. galactography and ductography
3. vasography
4. hysterosalpingography

Respiratory System Radiography

1. laryngography
2. chest x-ray

Urinary System Radiography

1. pyelography
2. Cystography
3. Retrograde pyelography (RP)
4. urethrocystometry
5. urography

Other Diagnostic Radiology Services

1. electromyography
2. Densitometry
3. phonocardiography
4. densitometer

Diagnostic Ultrasound

1. ultrasonography, sonography, and echography
2. Doppler ultrasonography
3. Doppler echocardiography
4. Echocardiography

Radiation Oncology

1. radiotherapy
2. Irradiation
3. teletherapy
4. brachytherapy; brachy-
5. dosimetry

Nuclear Medicine

1. bone scan
2. Positron emission tomography (PET)
3. Nuclear scan studies
4. urea breath test
5. Schilling test

Common Abbreviations Exercises

1. DSA = digital subtraction angiography
2. PET = positron emission tomography
3. half life = $T_{1/2}$
4. MRA = magnetic resonance angiography
5. barium sulfate = $BaSO_4$

Case Study

1. c is the correct answer.
   - a, b, and d are incorrect because in reference to radiology, AP means anterior and posterior, or anteroposterior.
2. d is the correct answer.
   - a, b, and c are incorrect because the term *cardiomegaly* is formed from the word parts meaning "heart" and "large."
3. a is the correct answer.
   - b is incorrect because an artificially created passage to redirect circulation is a shunt.
   - c is incorrect because a unit of measurement for the absorbed dose of ionizing radiation is a gray (Gy).
   - d is incorrect because a substance opaque to x-rays that is used to make the outline of a body part easier to see on radiographs is a contrast medium.
4. a is the correct answer.
   - b is incorrect because it could be visualized on radiographic examination.
   - c is incorrect because the term *radioactive* indicates that an object emits energy in the form of particle streams.
   - d is incorrect because the color of the catheter would not be evident on an x-ray.

Real World Report

1. The term *nonselective* means that the needle is placed directly into a vessel and is not manipulated into a branch.
2. An angiogram is an x-ray of a blood vessel after introducing a contrast dye.
3. This procedure was done to evaluate arteries.
4. a is the correct answer.

Review and Application

1. b	19. b	37. mammography	55. d
2. a	20. c	38. d	56. b
3. a	21. a	39. e	57. a
4. c	22. b	40. b	58. c
5. d	23. d	41. a	59. e
6. d	24. a	42. c	60. d
7. a	25. b	43. c	61. b
8. a	26. a	44. a	62. a
9. d	27. a	45. e	63. b
10. c	28. hysterosonography	46. b	64. c
11. a	29. aortography	47. d	65. a
12. c	30. venography	48. c	66. d
13. b	31. angiocardiography	49. a	67. e
14. b	32. arteriography	50. e	68. d
15. c	33. phonocardiography	51. b	69. c
16. b	34. vesiculography	52. d	70. a
17. c	35. vasography	53. c	71. e
18. c	36. epididymography	54. e	72. b

73. radioactive substance of artificial or natural origin
74. radiograph of the spleen after administering a radionuclide
75. compound used as a contrast medium because it is not penetrated by x-rays
76. removal of fatty deposits on the inner lining of an artery
77. vessel ordering
78. uptake
79. percutaneous transhepatic cholangiography
80. barium enema
81. intraoperative cone irradiation
82. transcatheter biopsy
83. b
84. c
85. d
86. a
87. b
88. c
89. d
90. thallium scan
91. radioactive
92. dosimetry
93. radioimmunoassay
94. total body irradiation
95. thyroid imaging
96. μCi = microcurie; unit of radioactivity
97. PTA = percutaneous transluminal angioplasty; use of a balloon catheter to widen a narrowed artery
98. PET = positron emission tomography; nuclear medicine technique for assessing metabolic activity of organs, diagnosing cancer, locating brain tumors, and investigating brain function
99. CT = computed tomography; technique for producing x-ray images of body cross-sections
100. MRI = magnetic resonance imaging; imaging technique that uses electromagnetic radiation to obtain pictures of the body's soft tissues
101. EMG = electromyography; procedure used to diagnose nerve and muscle disorders by measuring electrical activity of muscle tissue
102. echocardiography; ultrasonography
103. cystourethrography; sialography
104. radiographs or x-rays
105. a. left common carotid; b. left external carotid artery

Word Search

```
+  +  +  +  +  +  +  +  +  +  +  +  +  Y  +  +
+  +  A  T  H  E  R  O  M  A  +  +  D  H  +  +
+  +  +  +  Y  M  A  R  G  O  L  E  Y  P  U  +
+  +  Y  H  P  A  R  G  O  G  N  Y  R  A  L  +
+  +  H  +  E  +  A  +  +  S  O  +  +  R  T  +
+  +  P  X  R  +  D  +  I  +  I  +  +  G  R  +
+  +  A  E  P  S  I  T  +  +  T  +  +  O  A  +
+  +  R  R  Y  +  O  +  +  +  A  +  +  N  S  +
+  +  G  O  R  M  G  N  +  +  I  +  +  E  O  +
+  +  O  S  E  +  R  +  O  +  D  +  +  D  U  T
+  +  L  T  X  +  A  +  +  G  A  +  +  O  N  +
+  +  E  O  I  +  P  +  +  +  R  +  +  U  D  +
+  R  Y  M  A  +  H  +  +  +  R  A  H  D  +  +
+  +  M  I  +  +  Y  +  +  +  I  S  P  +  +  +
+  +  +  A  +  V  A  S  O  G  R  A  P  H  Y  +
+  +  +  +  +  +  +  +  +  +  +  +  +  +  Y  +
```

atheroma
densitometer
duodenography
hyperpyrexia
irradiation
laryngography
myelography
pyelogram
radiography
shunt
sonography
ultrasound
vasography
xerostomia

Vocabulary Review

Key Term	Definition	Key Term	Definition
angiocardiography	x-ray examination of heart and blood vessels after injection of a radiopaque dye	contrast medium	dye or other substance introduced into the body that is opaque to x-rays, thereby allowing a structure's image to appear on film
angiography	examination of blood vessels after introduction of a radiopaque (contrast) dye	CT pelvimetry	measurement of the dimensions of the bony pelvis and fetal head using CT scans
aortography	x-ray examination of the aorta after injection of a contrast dye	cystography	x-ray examination of the bladder using a contrast dye
arteriography	x-ray examination of arteries after injection of a contrast dye	densitometer	instrument used to measure the amount of light a tissue absorbs or reflects
arthrography	examination of a joint's interior after the injection of a contrast dye	densitometry	examination of bone density using a densitometer
atheroma	fat deposit in an artery	diagnostic radiology	use of x-rays and other ionizing radiation for the diagnosis and treatment of disease; also called diagnostic imaging
barium enema	introduction of a contrast medium containing barium sulfate into the rectum and colon for x-ray examination	diagnostic ultrasound	use of high-frequency sound waves in diagnosing and treating conditions
barium sulfate (BaSO$_4$)	compound used as a contrast medium because it is not penetrated by x-rays	digital subtraction angiography (DSA)	computer-assisted radiography of vascular structures without superimposed bone or soft tissue
barium swallow (BAIR ee um)	ingestion of barium sulfate for x-ray examination of the upper GI tract	diskography	examination of the intervertebral discs after the direct injection of a contrast dye
bone scan	radiograph of the entire skeletal system using technetium-99 as a tracer	dosimetry	measurement of exposure to radiation
brachytherapy	radiotherapy in which the source is placed directly on or in close proximity to the body	Doppler echocardiography	ultrasound technique that uses the Doppler effect to enhance two-dimensional echocardiography
cardiac catheterization	examination of the heart after threading a catheter through a vessel into the heart for diagnostic, therapeutic, or visualization purposes	Doppler ultrasonography	application of the Doppler effect in ultrasound to detect movement
chest x-ray	imaging technique that uses a small dose of ionizing radiation to produce pictures of body structures in the thoracic cavity	ductography	mammographic imaging of the milk ducts using a contrast medium; also called galactography
		duodenography	x-ray examination of the duodenum after introduction of a contrast medium
cholangiography	examination of the bile ducts using a contrast medium	echocardiography	ultrasound technique for observing and examining the heart
cholecystography	examination of the gallbladder after injection or ingestion of a contrast medium	echography	imaging technique that uses high-frequency sound waves; another term for ultrasonography or sonography
computed tomographic angiography	combination CT and angiography for visualizing blood vessels or lymphatic vessels	electromyography (EMG)	procedure used to diagnose nerve and muscle disorders by measuring electrical activity of muscle tissue
computed tomography (CT)	technique for producing x-ray images of body cross-sections		

Key Term	Definition	Key Term	Definition
endoscopic catheterization	procedure that uses an endoscope to view internal body structures	nonselective arterial catheter placement	catheter placed into an arterial vessel and not manipulated to another arterial site
galactography	mammographic imaging of the milk ducts using a contrast medium; also called ductography	nonselective venous	catheter placed into a vein and not manipulated to another venous site
gallium scan	imaging technique that uses gallium-67 for the identification of tumors and inflammation	nuclear medicine	clinical branch of medicine that deals with the use of radioactive materials in diagnosis and therapy
hemibody radiation	radiotherapy of one half of the body	nuclear scan studies	procedures that use radioactive substances in the body for diagnostic purposes
hyperpyrexia	therapeutically induced fever; another term for hyperthermia	percutaneous needle biopsy	excision of tissue by a guided needle through the skin
hyperthermia	therapeutically induced fever; another term for hyperpyrexia	percutaneous transhepatic cholangiography (PCT, PTHC)	radiography of the bile ducts using contrast medium delivered via needle puncture
hysterosalpingography	x-ray examination of the uterus and uterine tubes using a contrast dye	percutaneous transhepatic portography	radiography of portal venous system using a contrast medium delivered via needle puncture
interstitial brachytherapy	radiation treatment via implanted sources	percutaneous transluminal angioplasty (PTA)	use of a balloon catheter to widen a narrowed artery
interventional radiology	specialty area of radiology that uses catheters, scopes, and various procedures to guide instruments for the diagnosis and treatment of pathology	phonocardiography	procedure for obtaining a graph of heart sounds using a phonocardiograph and an electrocardiogram
intraoperative cone irradiation	using x-rays aimed at a target to destroy cancerous cells during surgery	positron emission tomography (PET)	nuclear medicine technique for assessing metabolic activity of organs, diagnosing cancer, locating brain tumors, and investigating brain function
intravenous pyelogram (IVP)	x-ray of the urine-collecting part of the kidneys, ureters, and bladder using a contrast dye	ptyalography	x-ray examination of the salivary glands after administration of a contrast medium; also called sialography
irradiation	medical use of radiation—such as x-rays, gamma-rays, or other radioactive sources—to treat cancer	pyelogram	x-ray of the kidneys, ureters, and urinary bladder obtained after introducing a contrast dye
laryngography	radiography of the larynx (voice box) after coating the surface with a contrast dye	pyelography	radiography of the kidneys, ureters, and urinary bladder using a contrast dye
lymphography	x-ray examination of lymphatic vessels after introduction of radiopaque dye	radiation oncology	use of radioactive materials for treating cancer; also called radiotherapy
magnetic resonance angiography	imaging blood vessels using MRI	radioactive	atomic nuclei emitting ionizing radiation or particles
magnetic resonance imaging (MRI)	imaging technique that uses electromagnetic radiation to obtain pictures of the body's soft tissues	radioactive iodine uptake	test used to determine thyroid function by assessing the amount of radioactive iodine absorbed by the thyroid gland
magnetic resonance spectroscopy	imaging structures using lightwaves		
mammography	x-ray examination of the breast		
myelography	radiographic examination of the spinal cord after injection of radiopaque dye		

Key Term	Definition	Key Term	Definition
radiographs	images produced on film by x-rays passing through a body part; another term for x-rays	spleen imaging	radiograph of the spleen after administering a radionuclide
radiography	making and using radiographs (x-rays) for medical purposes	splenoportography	x-ray examination of the splenic and portal vein system after injection of a contrast medium
radioimmunoassay	technique for identifying antibodies using a radioactive tracer	teletherapy	radiation treatment administered with the source at a distance from the body
radiologist	physician specializing in radiology	thallium scan	nuclear imaging technique that uses a radioisotope of thallium
radiology	branch of medicine that deals with radioactive substances, x-rays, and ionizing radiation for treating and diagnosing disease	thyroid imaging	radiograph of the thyroid after administering a radionuclide such as radioactive iodine
radionuclide	radioactive substance of artificial or natural origin	tomography	radiography in which images in certain planes are focused while images in other planes are blurred
radionuclide ejection fraction radionuclide seeds	a nuclear medicine study to determine the amount of blood ejected out of either ventricle in the heart	total body irradiation	exposing the entire body to ionizing radiation
radiopaque	impenetrable by light or x-rays	transcatheter biopsy	tissue sample taken via a catheter
radiopharmaceutical	radioactive substance used in nuclear medicine	transluminal atherectomy	removal of fatty deposits on the inner lining of an artery
radiotherapy	treating cancer by radiation; another term for radiation oncology	ultrasonography	imaging technique that uses high-frequency sound waves; another term for echography or sonography
radiotracer	radioactive chemical used as a detector in diagnostic tests	ultrasound	imaging technique that uses high-frequency sound waves
retrograde pyelography (RP)	radiography of the kidneys after a contrast dye is injected into the ureters, resulting in backward fluid movement	uptake	absorption of something, such as a radionuclide, by tissue
Schilling test	technique for determining vitamin B_{12} absorption	urea breath test	test that uses a radioisotope of carbon to determine the presence of *Helicobacter pylori*
scintigraphy	two-dimensional imaging technique that uses a radioactive tracer	urethrocystometry	procedure that simultaneously measures pressures in the urinary bladder and urethra
selective arterial catheter placement	catheter placed into another portion of the arterial system from where it was originally inserted	urography	radiography of any part of the urinary tract
selective venous	catheter placed into a vein and manipulated into another venous site	vascular family	group of blood vessels fed by a primary vessel
shunt	a surgically created bypass	vasography	x-ray examination of the vas deferens using a contrast medium to determine if blockages are present
shuntogram	x-ray examination to determine shunt placement	venography	x-ray examination of veins after injection of a radiopaque dye
sialography	x-ray examination of the salivary glands after administration of a contrast medium; also called ptyalography	vessel ordering	term describing the amount of work required to place a catheter at its destination
sonography	imaging technique that uses high-frequency sound waves; another term for echography or ultrasonography	xerostomia	dry mouth
		x-rays	images produced on film by x-rays passing through a body part; another term for radiographs

CHAPTER 4

Integumentary System

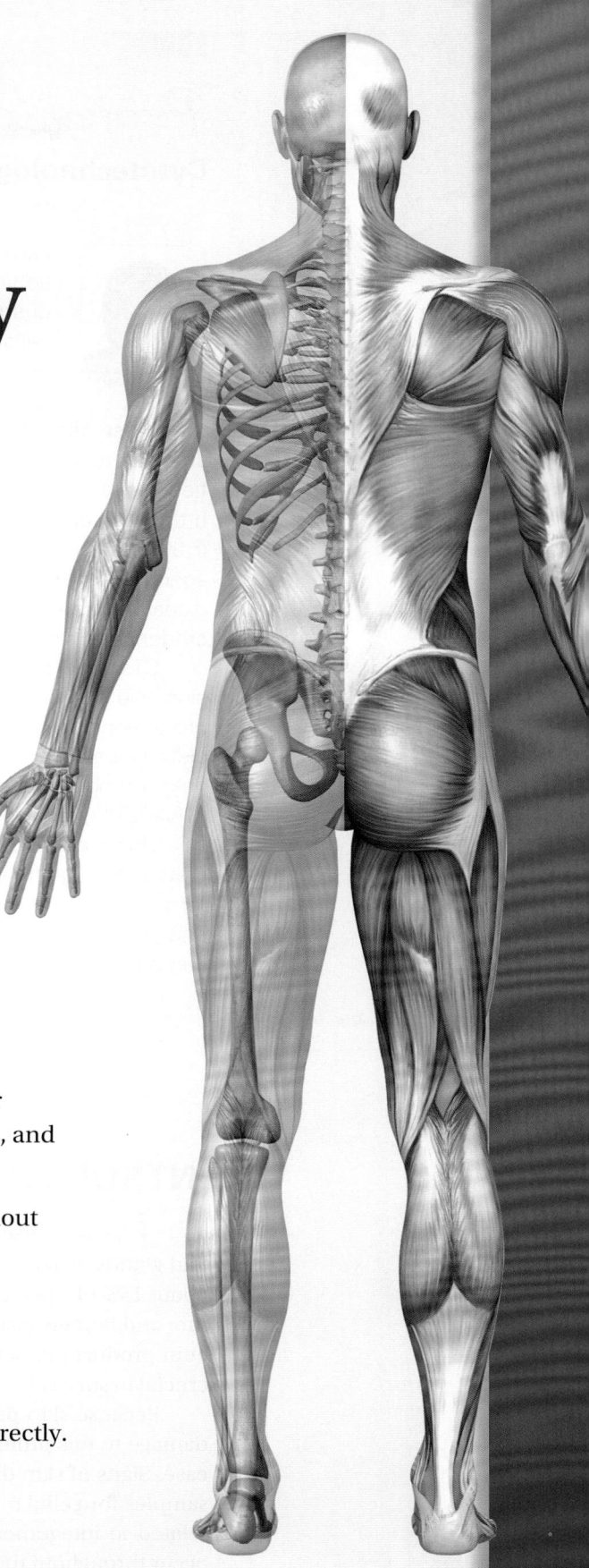

OBJECTIVES

After completing this chapter, you should be able to:

1. Identify structures of the skin, hair, and nails.

2. Describe the primary function of each component of the skin and the integumentary system.

3. Label anatomical structures of the integumentary system.

4. Define word parts used for the integumentary system.

5. Recognize common integumentary system diseases and their various signs, symptoms, clinical tests, diagnostic procedures, and treatments.

6. Summarize anatomical and physiological alterations throughout the life span.

7. Define common abbreviations related to the integumentary system.

8. Define terms used in medical reports.

9. Define, spell, and pronounce the chapter's medical terms correctly.

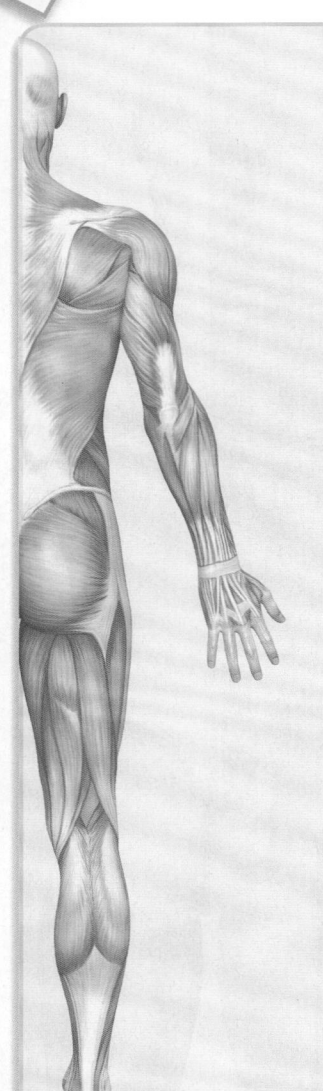

Professional Profile

Cytotechnologist

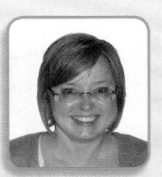

I am Lindsey, a cytotechnologist (CT) at a private laboratory in an urban setting. Hospitals, for-profit labs, clinics, public health facilities, and industry employ many CTs. CTs view specially prepared slides of human cells under the microscope, looking for early signs of disease. Findings obtained by the CT directly affect a patient because treatments are generally designed around the test results.

Most often the cultures and tissue samples come from physicians' offices or small area hospitals and clinics. When viewing the slide, I look for cellular abnormalities in color, size, and morphology (shape) that could be clues to pathology (disease). If the slide appears normal, a final report is issued to the ordering physician. However, if there are indications of irregularity, I work with the pathologist to reach a final diagnosis. A pathologist is a physician who identifies the nature, origin, and cause of disease. I view dermatology slides daily, and much of my work is subjective. This lends credence to the phrase "as much of an art as a science."

CTs are proficient in problem solving, and we work independently with little supervision. We need excellent verbal and written communication skills, because many other professionals read the reports and are involved with patient care. To become a CT, I completed a bachelor's degree plus one year of clinical education in an accredited cytotechnology program. The Commission on Accreditation of Allied Health Education Programs (CAAHEP) grants accreditation of cytotechnology programs.

This is a growing field. Students are qualified for a job immediately after they complete the program and pass the boards. The Board of Registry of the American Society for Clinical Pathology (ASCP) is responsible for the national certification examination. The job outlook for CTs is bright because there are more positions available than qualified people to fill them.

INTRODUCTION

*T*he skin, also called the integument, and its associated structures such as hair, nails, and glands, make up the integumentary system. Skin is the body's largest organ. It makes up about 15% of a person's weight. Its primary functions include maintenance of body temperature and homeostasis, protection, stimuli reception, excretion, vitamin D synthesis, and melanin production. Serving as a covering for the body's internal structures, the integument is crucial to survival.

Because skin provides the first line of defense against a host of environmental insults, damage to this protective covering allows the entry of microorganisms, which can cause disease. Signs of skin disorders are usually obvious, yet at times it is necessary to obtain tissue samples for cellular analysis. Symptoms, signs, tests, diagnostic procedures, and treatments related to integumentary disorders are discussed in this chapter. Age-related changes that occur throughout the life span are also given.

MEDICAL TERM PARTS

Word Parts

Medical term prefixes, suffixes, and combining forms related to the integumentary system are introduced in this section.

Word Part	Meaning
adip-, adipo-	fat
aut-, auto-	self
cero-	wax
chrom-, chromat-, chromato-, -chrome, chromo-	color
cry-, cryo-	cold
cyan-, cyano-	blue
cyt-, -cyte, cyto-	cell
derm-, derma-, dermat-, dermato-, dermo-	skin
erythr-, erythro-	red or red blood cell
hidr-, hidro-ₐ	sweat
histio-, histo-	tissue
ichthyo-	fish
kerat-, kerato-	horny tissue or cornea
leuc-, leuco-, leuk-, leuko-	white or white blood cell
lip-, lipo-	fatty
melan-, melano-	black
myco-	fungus
necr-, necro-	death
-oma	tumor
onych-, onycho-	fingernail or toenail
papulo-	pimple, circumscribed solid elevation
path-, patho-, -pathy	disease
phyt-, phyto-	plants
pilo-	hair
-plasia	formation
pyo-	pus accumulation
-rrhea	flowing
scler-, sclero-	hardness
squamo-	epidermal scale
seb-, sebi-, sebo-	sebum (oil)
sub-	beneath
sudor-	sweat
trich-, trichi-, tricho-	hair
vesic-, vesico-, vesiculo-	vesicle, blister
xanth-, xantho-	yellow
xero-	dry

ᵃ*Note:* The word parts *hidr-* and *hidro-* mean *sweat*. Do not confuse them with *hydr-* and *hydro-*, which mean *water*. Notice the difference in spelling.

Word Grouping Exercises

Using the *Medical Term Parts* table, identify the prefix, suffix, or combining form for each of the following definitions. The first one has been done as an example.

Definition	Word Part
beneath	*sub-*
black	
blue	
cell	
cold	
color	
death	
disease	
dry	
epidermal scale	
fat	A. B.
fatty	
fingernail or toenail	
fish	
flowing	
formation	
fungus	
hair	A. B.
hardness	
horny tissue or cornea	
pimple, circumscribed solid elevation	
plants	
pus accumulation	
red or red blood cell	
sebum (oil)	
self	
skin	
sweat	A. B.
tissue	
tumor	
vesicle, blister	
wax	
white or white blood cell	
yellow	

Word Building Exercises

Word parts introduced in the *Medical Term Parts* section are listed in the following table. For this exercise, first supply the meaning of each word part, then use the word part to build a word you already know. The word you list under *Common or Known Word* does not have to be a medical term; a commonly used word is fine. Be sure, however, that the word correctly reflects the intended meaning. The first one has been done as an example. Check your answers in a dictionary.

Word Part	Meaning	Common or Known Word	Example Medical Term
adip-, adipo-	*fat*	*adipose*	adipocytes
aut-, auto-			autoimmune
cyt-, -cyte, cyto-			erythrocyte
derm-, derma-, dermat-, dermato-, dermo-			epidermis
erythr-, erythro-			erythrocyte
histio-, histo-			histology
lip-, lipo-			liposuction
melan-, melano-			melanocyte
path-, patho-, -pathy			pathophysiology
-rrhea			seborrhea
scler-, sclero-			scleroderma
sub-			subcutaneous
vesic-, vesico-, vesiculo-			vesicle

ANATOMY AND PHYSIOLOGY

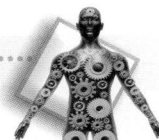

Integumentary System Preview

Skin is considered an organ because two or more kinds of tissues are grouped together to perform its specialized functions. It is also considered a membrane and is composed of epithelial and connective tissues. The skin is sometimes called the **cutaneous** (relating to the skin) membrane. The **integumentary system** consists of associated structures such as **hair** (keratinized filaments covering the body), **nails** (protective coverings on the fingers and toes), **sudoriferous glands** or **sweat glands** (glands that secrete sweat), and **sebaceous glands**

(glands that secrete oil). The skin and its epidermal structures such as hair, fingernails, toenails, and glands make up the integumentary system. The study of the skin and the integumentary system is termed **dermatology**. A physician who specializes in this field is called a **dermatologist**.

The skin is responsible for maintaining body temperature, thus keeping homeostatic balance. When the body becomes too warm, heat is carried away from the body in sweat, which is a mixture of water, salt, and organic wastes.

Hair and nails are skin derivatives. Hair is made of **keratin**, a tough, waterproof protein that develops in the membranes. Every hair has an associated sebaceous gland that secretes **sebum**, an oil, to keep the skin soft and pliable. Nails are made of epithelial cells that cover the distal portion of each finger and toe.

The integumentary system serves a protective function by creating a physical barrier that prevents microbes from entering. Broken skin increases the risk of infection. Additional protective features include the production of melanin and keratin. **Melanin** is a dark brown to black pigment that gives the skin its color. It is produced by **melanocytes**, cells in the epidermal layer of the skin (**Figure 4-1**). The primary purpose of melanin is to filter ultraviolet (UV) radiation, which can disrupt underlying cellular activity. The interaction of UV radiation with melanocytes gives you suntanned skin. Cells called keratinocytes produce keratin, which is a protein that acts as a water repellent. About 90% of skin cells are of this type because keratin is the main element of the outer skin.

Furthermore, the epidermal cells of the skin synthesize vitamin D. Vitamin D is important for normal bone development throughout life. Recent research also suggests a variety of other roles for vitamin D—so stay tuned!

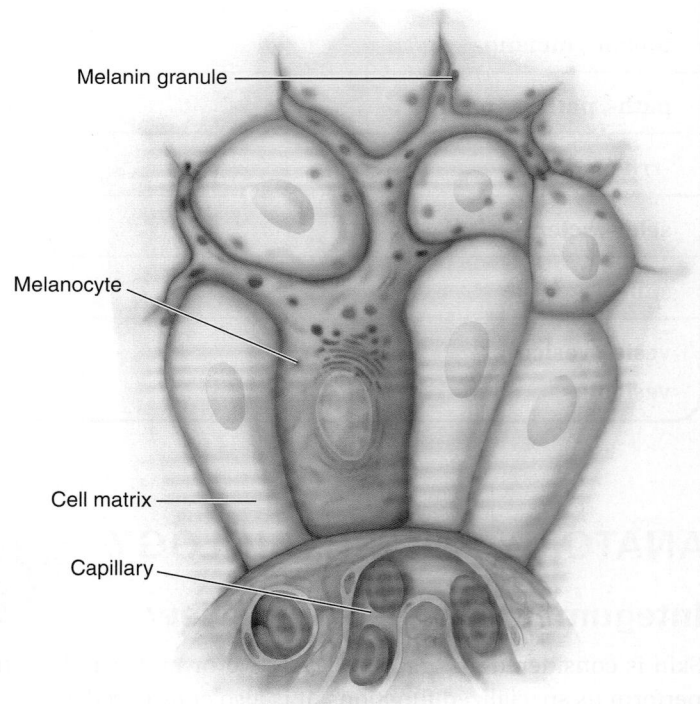

Melanin granule

Melanocyte

Cell matrix

Capillary

Figure 4-1 Melanocytes are cells that release the brown pigment melanin.

KEY TERM	Definition
cutaneous (kew-TAY-nee-us)	relating to the skin
integumentary system (in-teg-yoo-MEN-tuh-ree SIS-tem)	skin and its associated hair, nails, and glands
hair	keratinized filaments covering the body
nails	protective coverings on the fingers and toes
sudoriferous (sue-dur-IF-ur-us) **glands**	glands that secrete sweat; also called sweat glands
sweat glands	glands that secrete sweat; also called sudoriferous glands
sebaceous (se-BAY-shus) **glands**	glands that secrete oil
dermatology (dur-muh-TOL-uh-jee)	the study of skin
dermatologist (dur-muh-TOL-uh-jist)	physician specializing in skin and the integumentary system
keratin (KERR-uh-tin)	tough protein associated with hair and nails
sebum (SEE-bum)	oil
melanin (MEL-uh-nin)	dark brown to black pigment produced by cells called melanocytes
melanocytes (me-LAN-oh-sites)	cells that produce the pigment melanin

KEY TERM PRACTICE: *Integumentary System Preview*

1. _____ is a tough protein associated with the hair and nails.

2. The term that means relating to the skin is _____.

3. Name the gland that secretes sebum. _____

4. The word part *dermato-* means "skin." The suffix *-ology* means "study of. What word means "the study of skin"?
_____

5. Cells that secrete melanin are termed _____, which is derived from the word part _____, meaning "black," and the word part _____, which means "cell."

Skin Layers

The main layers of the skin are the epidermis, dermis, and subcutaneous layer. These layers and other structures associated with the skin are shown in **Figure 4-2**. The **epidermis** is the outermost layer. The epidermis itself contains several layers, called **strata** (*stratum* = singular). Its deepest layer is the stratum basale, or basal cell layer. Its most superficial layer is the stratum corneum, or horny layer. It is commonly called the horny layer because under a microscope the layer appears to have horns.

The deeper layers of the epidermis contain melanin-secreting melanocytes. Cells of the stratum basale divide to create new skin cells. As specialized cells called keratinocytes age, they harden through a process called **keratinization**, which forms the horny layer of the epidermis. Newer cells composed of tough keratin push the older cells toward the skin surface. Keratin is a waterproof protein that makes up the dead outer layer of the epidermis, creating the stratum corneum. This layer is extremely thick on the soles of the feet.

The stratum lucidum is a clear layer found in the epidermis of the skin covering the palms of the hands and the soles of the feet. This layer is called *thick skin*. The stratum lucidum is absent in all other body locations.

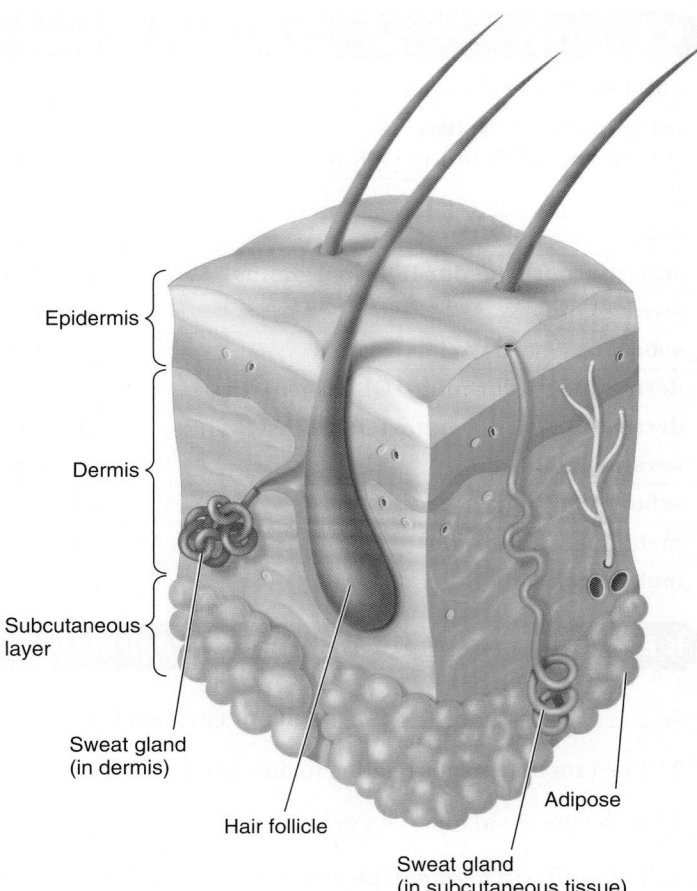

Epidermis {

Dermis {

Subcutaneous {
layer

Sweat gland
(in dermis)

Hair follicle

Adipose

Sweat gland
(in subcutaneous tissue)

Figure 4-2 Anatomy of
the skin.

The **dermis** is the middle inner layer of the skin. It is composed of a variety of tissues, including fibrous connective, epithelial, smooth muscle, nerve, and blood. The dermis is thicker than the epidermis and binds the epidermis to underlying tissues. Hair, sebaceous (oil) glands, sudoriferous (sweat) glands, and blood vessels are derived from this layer. The sebum that is secreted by the sebaceous glands makes the skin soft and pliable. The sudoriferous glands allow excess body heat to escape in sweat that evaporates from the skin surface (**Figure 4-3**). **Collagen**, a fibrous protein, is a major component of the connective tissue; *colla* means "glue." Collagen and elastic fibers make skin tough, yet stretchable.

Turgor refers to normal skin tension as a result of its elasticity. It is often used to assess signs of dehydration or connective tissue disorders. After a fold of skin is gently grasped and pulled, it should return to its normal state in about 3 seconds after release. Stretch marks, or **striae** (*stria* = singular), are linear tears in the dermal layer. They occur when there is rapid skin growth and stretching, such as in pregnancy or weight gain.

The **subcutaneous layer**, or **hypodermis**, is the innermost layer of skin. It connects the dermis to underlying tissues. In medical records, subcutaneous should either be written in its entirety or should be abbreviated as *subcut*. Because many medical abbreviations are ambiguous, the Institute for Safe Medication Practices (ISMP) maintains a list of error-prone abbreviations, symbols, and dose designations that should be avoided. Masses of loose connective and adipose tissue are found in the subcutaneous layer. **Adipose** (fat) tissue is formed by **lipocytes** (fat cells) within this layer. Adipose tissue insulates the body and protects organs.

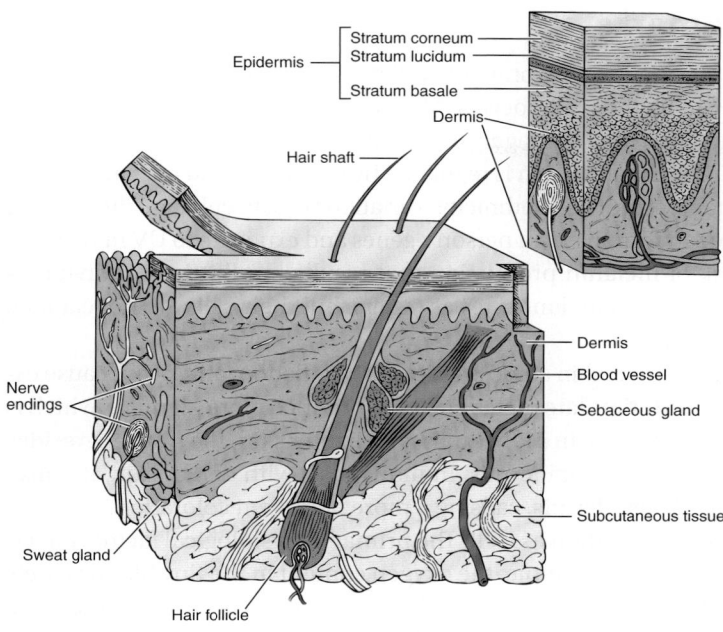

Figure 4-3 The skin in cross-section with the layers of the epidermis exposed.

KEY TERM	Definition
epidermis (ep-i-DER-mis)	superficial skin layer
strata (STRA-tuh)	layers
keratinization (kerr-uh-tin-i-ZAY-shun)	formation of keratin and the horny layer
dermis (DUR-mis)	middle layer of skin, below the epidermis
collagen (KOL-uh-jin)	fibrous protein
turgor (TUR-gur)	normal skin tension
striae (STRYE-ee)	stretch marks
subcutaneous (sub-kew-TAY-nee-us) **layer**	innermost skin layer; also called the hypodermis
hypodermis (high-poh-DER-mis)	innermost skin layer; also called the subcutaneous layer
adipose (AD-i-poce)	fat
lipocytes (LIP-oh-sights)	fat cells

KEY TERM PRACTICE: *Skin Layers*

1. The outer layer of the skin is called the _____.

2. The _____ is the innermost layer of the skin.

3. The middle layer of the skin is termed the _____.

4. What are the singular and plural forms of the term that means *layer*?

   A. Singular = _____

   B. Plural = _____

5. Fat cells are called _____, which is formed by combining the word part _____, meaning "fat," and the word part _____, meaning "cell."

Skin Color and Birthmarks

Human skin color is the result of genetics, environment, and physiology. In all cases, it is due to the quantity of melanin produced by the melanocytes. Melanin is a dark pigment that absorbs light energy and prevents UV radiation from damaging deeper skin cells. Individuals inherit genes from both parents for melanin production, which is regulated by hormones and enzymes. Melanocyte numbers are fairly constant regardless of ethnicity. Variations in skin color are the result of the amount of melanin produced in response to a person's genes and exposure to UV radiation.

Mutant genes cause a lack of melanin production that results in **albinism**. Individuals with albinism have the same number of melanocytes as others, but their cells are not capable of producing melanin (**Figure 4-4**).

Several environmental factors affect skin color. Sunlight, UV radiation, and x-rays cause existing melanin to darken quickly and stimulate melanocytes to produce more pigment, which is then transferred to nearby epidermal cells. In individuals with lighter skin, the pigment resides primarily in more superficial layers of the epidermis. In individuals with darker skin, it is also transferred into a deeper layer of the epidermis, causing a more persistent coloration.

Physiology plays a role in skin coloration as well. The primary physiological factors affecting skin color are blood and disease. For example, the oxygen content in the tiny blood vessels in the dermis of people with light skin affects skin color. When the blood is rich in oxygen, the skin has a characteristic red-pink color. If blood oxygen levels are low, hemoglobin is dark, and the skin may appear bluish, a condition called **cyanosis** (**Figure 4-5**). Various skin diseases may affect skin color as well. When a person suffers from liver disease, the skin may appear yellow from an accumulation of the bile pigment bilirubin. This is referred to as **jaundice**.

Birthmarks are congenital skin **lesions** (structural or functional alterations of the anatomy). **Nevi** (*nevus* = singular), or moles, are masses of pigmented tissue. A **port wine stain** is a large, reddish birthmark that may be removed by laser surgery. The colored skin patch can occur singly or in

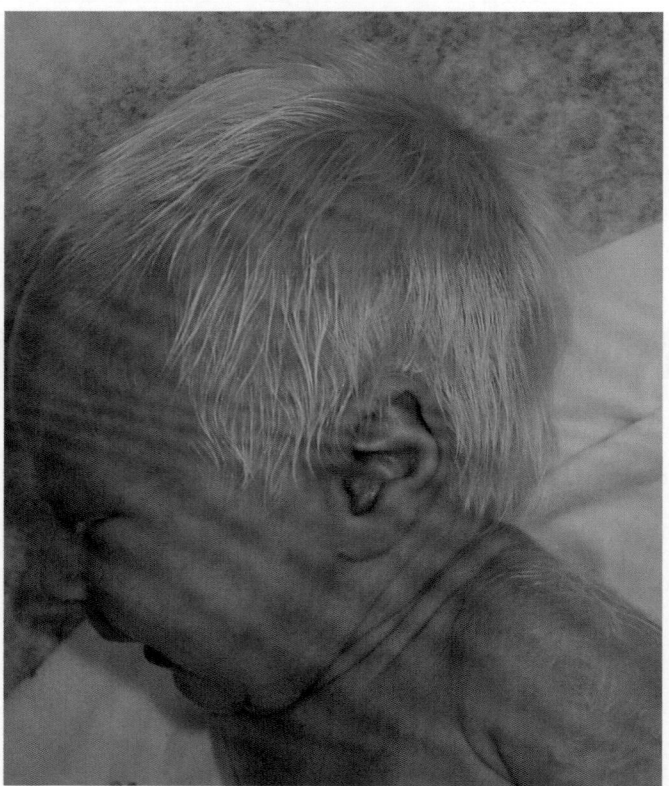

Figure 4-4 An infant with albinism.

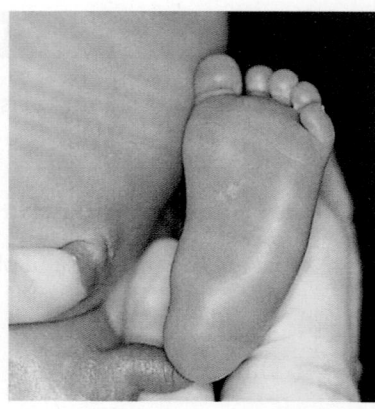

Figure 4-5 Cyanosis in the first half hour of life in a 32-week infant.

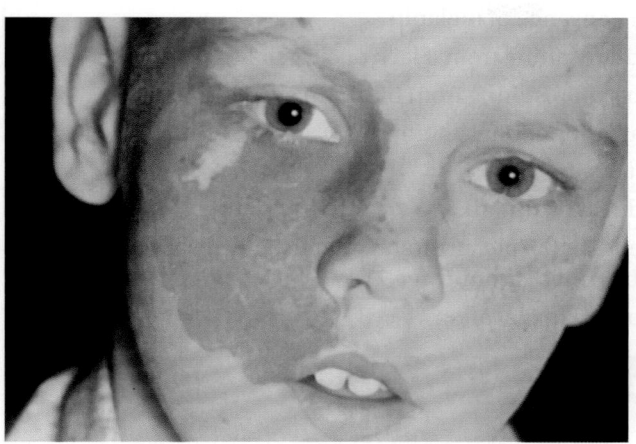

Figure 4-6 Port wine stain birthmark. The birthmark is dark red and will not fade with time.

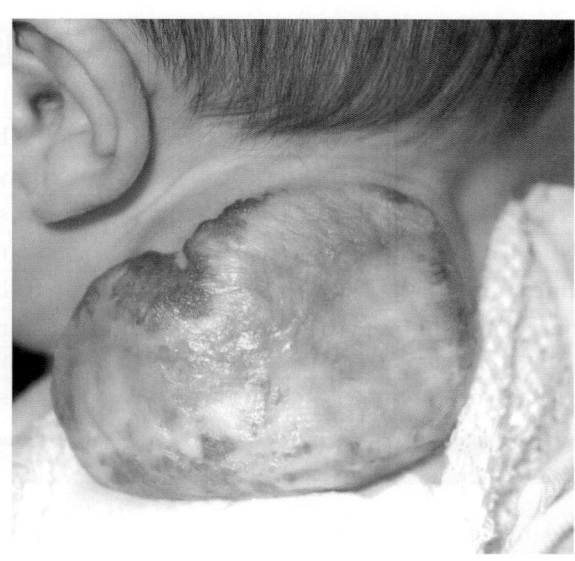

Figure 4-7 Strawberry hemangioma.

multiples, can be raised or flat, and typically occurs on the face (**Figure 4-6**). A raised, reddish purple birthmark that usually disappears without treatment around age 7 years is termed a **strawberry hemangioma**. Strawberry hemangiomas often have a lumpy, lobed appearance (**Figure 4-7**).

A solid, round skin elevation is called a **papule**. Mosquito bite bumps are examples of papules.

Conditions of the skin and the integumentary system are frequently described in medical terms denoting color. **Table 4-1** provides common word parts and terms used to describe a variety of colors associated with the skin. Examples are also given in the table.

T A B L E 4-1	WORD PARTS PERTAINING TO THE COLOR OF SKIN	
Word Part and Term Origin	**Color**	**Example**
albus	white	albinism
anthraco-	black	anthracosis
chlor-, chloro-	green	chlorophyll
cyan-, cyano-	blue	cyanosis
eryth-, erytho-	red	erythematous
jaune	yellow	jaundice
kirrkos	yellow	cirrhosis
leuk-, leuko-	white	leukoderma
luteus	yellow	corpus luteum
melan-, melano-	black	melanin
polio-	gray	poliomyelitis
porphyra	purple	allergic purpura
rosaceus, roseus	rosy	roseola
ruber	red	rubeola
xanth-, xantho-	yellow	xanthoderma

KEY TERM	Definition
albinism (AL-bi-niz-um)	hereditary absence of melanin
cyanosis (sigh-uh-NOH-sis)	bluish skin resulting from a lack of oxygen in the blood
jaundice (JAWN-dis)	yellowish skin resulting from bilirubin accumulation
lesions (LEE-zhunz)	structural or functional alterations
nevi (NE-VIGH)	medical term for moles
port wine stain	large, reddish birthmark
strawberry hemangioma (he-man-jee-OH-muh)	raised, reddish purple birthmark that usually disappears without treatment around age 7
papule (PAP yool)	solid, round skin elevation

KEY TERM PRACTICE: *Skin Color and Birthmarks*

1. Name the hereditary condition in which melanin is not produced. _____

2. A condition in which the skin appears bluish is termed _____.

3. The condition in which the skin appears yellow as a result of bilirubin accumulation is called _____.

4. A _____ is a solid, round skin elevation.

5. The medical term for moles is _____.

Hair

Hair, nails, and skin glands develop from the embryonic epidermis. Hair covers all body surfaces except the palms of the hands, the soles of the feet, portions of the external genitalia, and the lips. Our genes determine hair color by directing the amount of pigment produced by melanocytes.

Hair is composed of a root and a shaft. Hair is found within a hair **follicle**, which is the tube-like depression extending from the surface into the dermis that contains the hair root. The **shaft** is the visible part that extends beyond the surface. The **root** penetrates the dermis and is embedded in the hair follicle. The root anchors the hair in the skin. New hair develops at the base of the hair follicle when epidermal cells divide, forcing older cells to move outward. As new cells are pushed toward the surface, they undergo keratinization. Hair goes through periods of growth, rest, and replacement. On average, head hair grows about 12.5 cm (5 inches) per year.

Bundles of smooth muscle cells, referred to as the **arrector pili muscles**, are attached to each hair follicle (**Figure 4-8**). When nerve impulses stimulate these muscles to contract, they create "goose bumps."

KEY TERM	Definition
follicle (FOL-i-kul)	tube-like depression containing the hair root
shaft	visible portion of the hair
root (hair)	hair portion embedded in the hair follicle that attaches the hair to the skin
arrector pili (a-RECK-tur PYE-lye) **muscles**	bundles of smooth muscle cells attached to hair follicles that cause goose bumps when contracted

continued

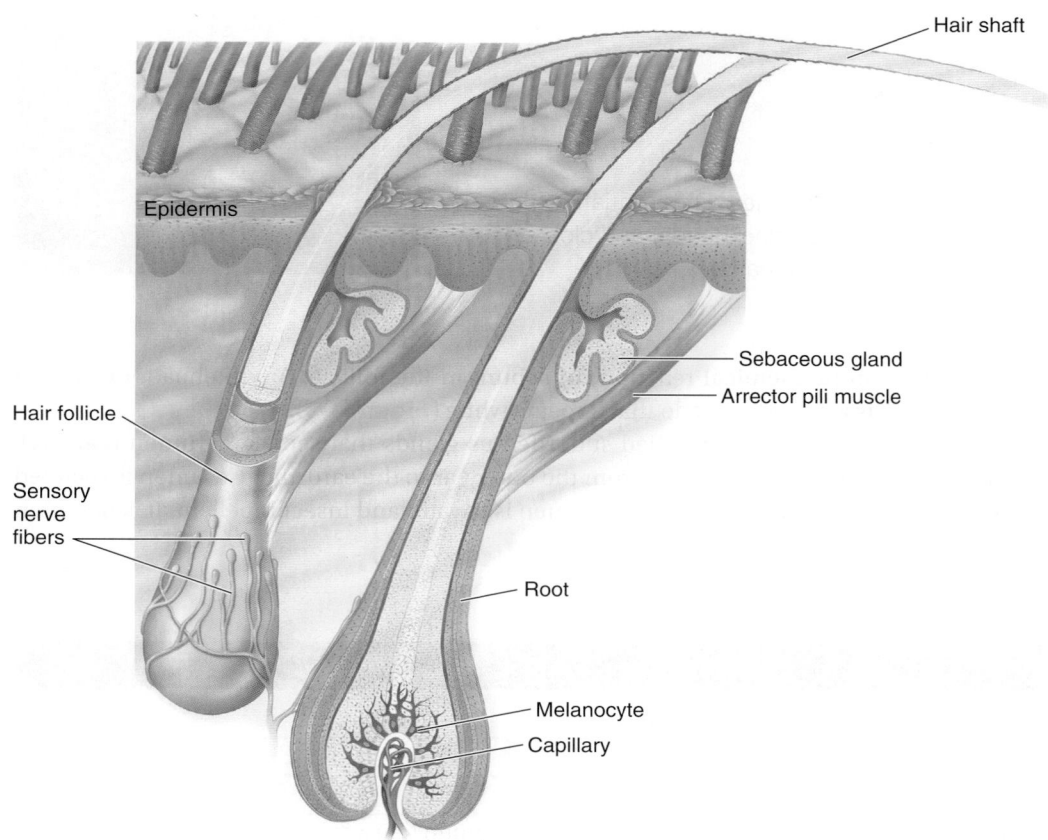

Hair shaft

Epidermis

Sebaceous gland

Arrector pili muscle

Hair follicle

Sensory nerve fibers

Root

Melanocyte

Capillary

Figure 4-8 Cross section of hair and accessory structures.

continued from page 156

KEY TERM PRACTICE: *Hair*

1. The principal parts of hair are _____, _____, and _____.

2. These muscles contract to create goose bumps on the flesh. _____

Glands

Basic skin glands secrete oil, sweat, or wax. As noted earlier, those secreting oil are termed sebaceous, and those secreting sweat are called sudoriferous. Glands secreting wax are called ceruminous. Sebaceous glands are usually connected to hair follicles and secrete an oily substance called sebum. Sebum keeps skin soft, pliable, and relatively waterproof. Sebaceous glands are not found on the palms and soles.

Sudoriferous glands produce sweat, which carries water, waste products, and heat to the skin surface to assist in maintaining body temperature and homeostasis. **Hidrosis** is the medical term for sweating. Sweat glands are most numerous on the palms, soles, forehead, armpits, neck, and back. Ducts that end at **pores** (openings) on the epidermal surface allow the secretions to escape.

Enlarged sebaceous or sudoriferous glands may produce blackheads, pimples, and boils. **Comedo** is the medical term for a blackhead, resulting from an enlarged pore that becomes clogged with sebum, bacteria, and pigment. The black dot at the skin surface results

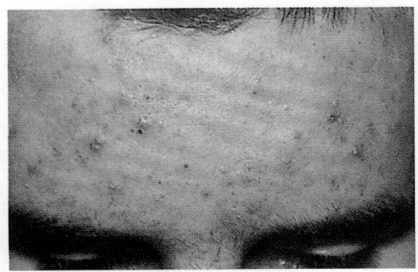

Figure 4-9 Comedones. Differentiate between open comedones (blackheads) and closed comedones (whiteheads).

from the oxidation (a chemical reaction) of sebum in the follicle. A whitehead, or milium (*milia* = plural), is a closed comedo that appears white (**Figure 4-9**).

Ceruminous glands are modified sudoriferous glands that secrete cerumen (earwax). They are found in the canal that leads from the outer ear to the eardrum. Cerumen is secreted to keep the eardrum pliable. Moreover, cerumen is a water and insect repellent. It is not often that a bug flies into your ear!

KEY TERM	Definition
hidrosis (high-DROH-sis)	sweating
pores	openings
comedo (KOM-ee-doh)	blackhead
ceruminous (se-ROO-mi-nus) **glands**	glands that secrete cerumen (earwax)

KEY TERM PRACTICE: *Glands*

1. _____ is the medical term for a blackhead.

2. The medical term for sweating is _____, which is derived from the word part _____, which means "sweat."

3. Glands that secrete cerumen are termed _____.

4. _____ are openings onto the skin surface.

Nails

Nails are hard, keratinized epidermal cells located over the posterior surfaces of the ends of fingers and toes. The principal parts of nails are shown in **Figure 4-10**. The last term is derived from the word part *onych-*, which means "nail." The medical term for nail biting is **onychophagia**.

The **nail body** is the visible part of the nail that rests on the **nail bed**, which is a layer of epithelium. The **nail root** is the part of the nail hidden by a fold of skin called the **eponychium** or **cuticle**. The white moon-shaped growth area nearest the root is called the **lunula**. The distal **free edge** (the part you clip with nail scissors) extends beyond the nail bed. The matrix is the growth layer. Cell division of this matrix produces new nails through the keratinization process. The average fingernail turnover is 3 to 5 months, but it may take 12 to 18 months for total toenail replacement.

CHAPTER 4 Integumentary System

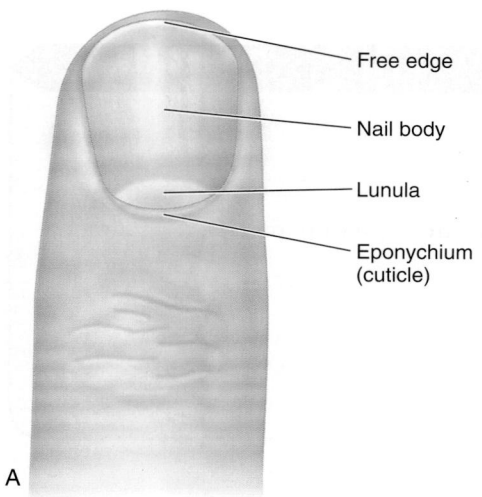

Free edge

Nail body

Lunula

Eponychium
(cuticle)

A

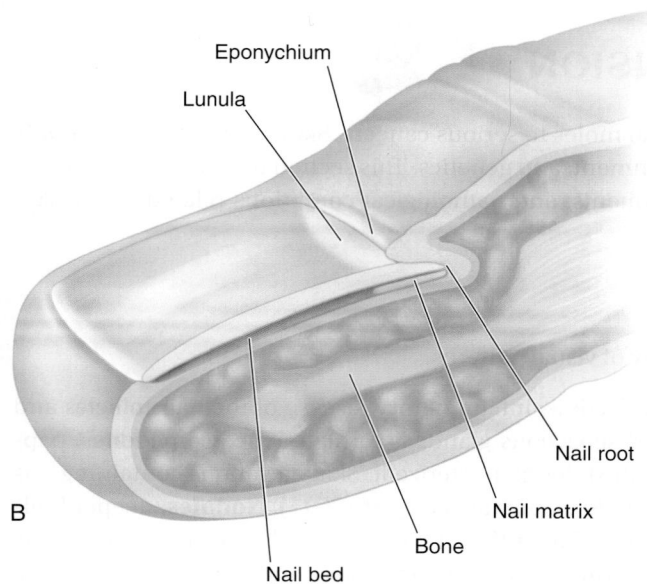

Eponychium

Lunula

Nail root

Nail matrix

Bone

Nail bed

B

Figure 4-10 (A) Surface structures of the fingernail.
(B) Cross section of fingertip.

KEY TERM	Definition
onychophagia (on-i-koh-FAY-jee-uh)	nail biting
nail body	main part of the nail
nail bed	epithelial tissue on which the nail rests
nail root	nail part beneath the cuticle
eponychium (ep-oh-NICK-ee-um)	fold of skin near the nail root; also called the cuticle
cuticle (KEW-ti-kul)	fold of skin near the nail root; also called the eponychium
lunula (LOO-new-luh)	white, moon-shaped growth area of nail near the root
free edge	portion of the nail growing beyond the tips of fingers or toes

continued

continued from page 159

KEY TERM PRACTICE: *Nails*

1. The part of the nail you clip is called the _____.

2. The white, moon-shaped area of the nail is termed the _____.

3. *Eponychium* is the medical term for the _____, and is derived from the word part _____, meaning "nail."

4. _____ is the medical term for nail biting.

5. The nail part beneath the cuticle is called the _____.

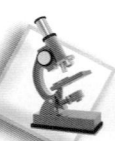

THE CLINICAL DIMENSION

Disorders of the skin range from trivial moles to serious cancers. Skin pathologies commonly result from sun exposure, diet, environment, and genetics. This section describes signs, symptoms, clinical tests, procedures, treatments, and pathological conditions related to the skin and the integumentary system.

Skin Conditions

Skin conditions are evident in a variety of visual patterns.

acne

The noninfectious inflammatory disease of the hair follicles and associated sebaceous glands is termed **acne**. Comedones, papules, and pustules characterize it. Skin elevations containing pus are referred to as **pustules** (**Figure 4-11**). **Nodules**, deeper boil-like structures larger than a papule, can also occur. Acne vulgaris is located primarily on the face, neck, and back and has a peak onset during adolescence.

Although the cause of acne is unknown, it is suspected that hormonal changes, stress, and endocrine disorders lead to its development. Treatment involves the use of topical or oral antibiotics and the topical application of keratolytic agents. Keratolytic agents cause increased **exfoliation** (shedding of the skin layer) of the epidermis.

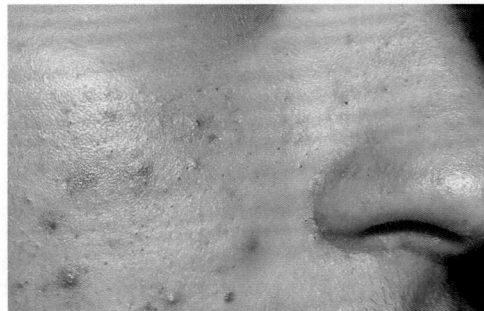

Figure 4-11 Adolescent acne showing comedones, papules, and pustules.

contusion	Commonly referred to as a bruise, a **contusion** is an injury to subcutaneous tissue in which the skin is not broken.
abrasion	An **abrasion** is damaged skin caused by scraping or rubbing.
causalgia	**Causalgia** is a persistent burning sensation that develops after injury to a nerve.
ichthyosis	A hereditary skin condition that gives the outward appearance of fish scales is **ichthyosis**.
pemphigus	**Pemphigus** is a nonspecific term for blistering skin diseases. Burning sensations and itching are also commonly associated with it.
bullae (*bulla* = singular)	**Bullae** (bulla = singular) are large fluid-filled blisters.
xeroderma	**Xeroderma** is extremely dry skin. The skin appears hard and scaly.
pachyderma and elephantiasis	Abnormally thick skin is called **pachyderma**, derived from the word part pachy- meaning "thick." **Elephantiasis**, a condition characterized by pachyderma, is the result of years of infection by filarial worms such as Wuchereria bancrofti. The worm causes obstruction in the lymphatic system leading to **edema** (swelling) (**Figure 4-12**).
purpura	**Purpura** is a condition in which purple hemorrhages (bleeding) occur in the skin. Signs include **petechiae** (small, rounded spots of bleeding on the skin surface).

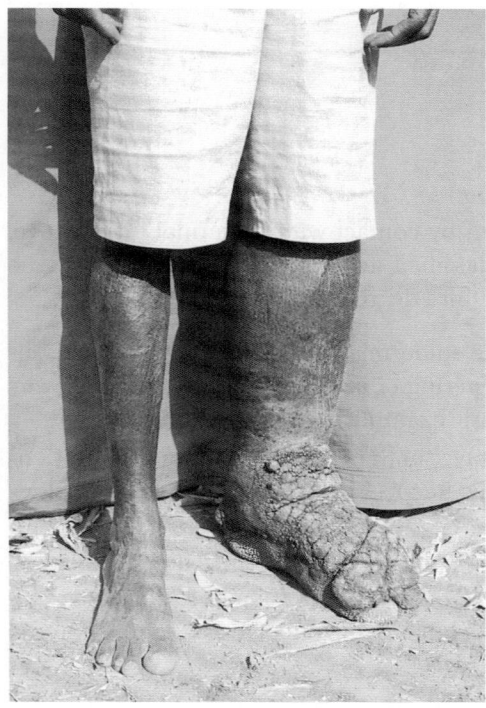

Figure 4-12 Elephantiasis of the left leg.

KEY TERM	Definition
acne (ACK-nee)	inflammation of the hair follicle and associated sebaceous glands
pustules (PUS-tyoolz)	skin elevations containing pus
nodules (NOD-yoolz)	deep, boil-like structures
exfoliation (ecks-foh-lee-AY-shun)	peeling and shedding of the epidermis
contusion (con-TEW-zhun)	bruise
abrasion (uh-BRAY-zhun)	damaged skin caused by scraping or rubbing
causalgia (kaw-SAL-jee-uh)	persistent burning sensation caused by nerve damage
ichthyosis (ick-thee-OH-sis)	hereditary skin condition giving the appearance of scales
pemphigus (PEM-fi-gus)	nonspecific term for blistering skin diseases
bullae (BULL-ee)	blisters
xeroderma (zeer-oh-DUR-muh)	extremely dry skin
pachyderma (pack-i-DUR-muh)	abnormally thick skin
elephantiasis (el-e-fan-TYE-uh-sis)	abnormally thick skin and edema caused by a filarial worm infection
edema (e-DEE-muh)	swelling
purpura (PUR-pew-ruh)	condition with purple skin hemorrhages
petechiae (pee-TEE-kee-uh)	spots on skin that result from bleeding

KEY TERM PRACTICE: *Skin Conditions*

1. _____ is a condition characterized by burning sensations as a result of nerve damage.

2. The shedding of the epidermal layer of skin tissue is termed _____.

3. _____ are spots on the skin caused by bleeding.

4. The medical term for swelling is _____.

5. _____ is the medical term for a bruise.

Burns

burn A **burn** is defined as a tissue injury caused by contact with a thermal, radioactive, chemical, or electrical agent. Burns are classified according to the depth of tissue damage as first degree, second degree, and third degree (**Figure 4-13**).

- With a **first-degree** (or superficial) **burn**, only the epidermis is affected. Characteristics include redness, pain, and edema. There is no blistering or scarring, and the surface layers shed within a few days. A minor sunburn is a classic example.

- A **second-degree** (or partial-thickness) **burn** involves both the epidermis and dermis. Generally, there is severe pain, blistering, and edema. Recovery is usually complete but slow, and scarring is common.

- A **third-degree** (full-thickness) **burn** destroys the epidermis and dermis along with some underlying muscle and nerves. There is no *immediate* pain because nerve endings are affected. Ulcerating wounds characterize this type of burn. Skin grafts are frequently required and a **scar** (permanent mark) often results.

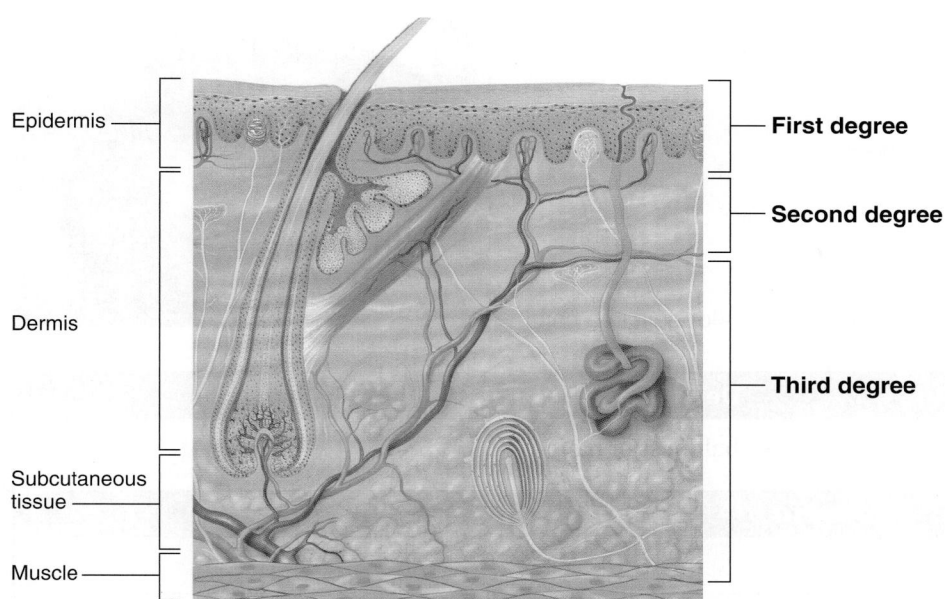

Epidermis

Dermis

Subcutaneous tissue

Muscle

First degree

Second degree

Third degree

Figure 4-13 Classification of burns according to the depth of damage to tissue.

KEY TERM	Definition
burn	tissue injury as a result of contact with a thermal, radioactive, chemical, or electrical agent
first-degree burn	superficial burn with damage to the epidermis
second-degree burn	partial-thickness burn with damage to the epidermis and dermis
third-degree burn	full-thickness burn, with damage to epidermis and dermis and some underlying muscle and nerves
scar	a permanent mark that forms where a wound heals

KEY TERM PRACTICE: *Burns*

1. Give a brief definition of the term *burn.* _____

2. Burns are categorized according to the extent of damage to the underlying tissue. List the three categories of burns.

_____

3. A _____ is a permanent mark that forms on the skin as a result of wound healing.

Alopecia

alopecia   **Alopecia**, commonly known as baldness, is loss of hair. The loss is typically from the scalp and may be partial, total, or complete (**Figure 4-14**).

Diagnosis is made by physical and visual examination and is accompanied by blood and thyroid studies. If an underlying pathology exists, correcting it generally causes hair growth to resume. Drug therapies (minoxidil [Rogaine] and finasteride [Propecia]) and hair transplants are often successful.

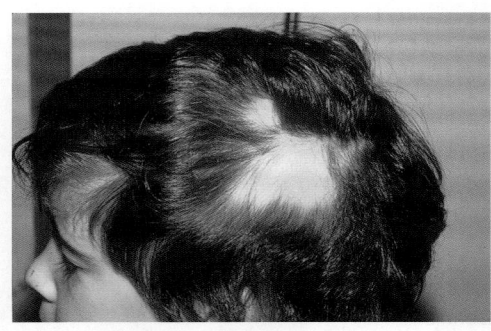

Figure 4-14 Alopecia in a child.

KEY TERM	Definition
alopecia (al-oh-PEE-shee-uh)	baldness or hair loss

KEY TERM PRACTICE: *Alopecia*

1. The medical term for hair loss or baldness is _____.

Autoimmune Disorders

Several autoimmune disorders affect the skin. An **autoimmune disorder** is one in which immune cells are directed against the body. In essence, the system that is supposed to protect the body from harm instead causes the damage. The common autoimmune disorders that affect the skin are dermatomyositis, scleroderma, systemic lupus erythematosus, and psoriasis.

dermatomyositis	As its name suggests, **dermatomyositis** is an inflammation of the dermal and muscular layers of tissue. It is often accompanied by muscle weakness and extremely taut skin.
scleroderma	**Scleroderma** is an autoimmune disease characterized by increased collagen formation in connective tissues. It causes the skin to become very thick and tight (**Figure 4-15**).
systemic lupus erythematosus (SLE)	**Systemic lupus erythematosus (SLE)**, frequently shortened to lupus, is another autoimmune disease of connective tissue (**Figure 4-16**). Lupus is characterized by **erythema** (redness) and a typical "butterfly" rash on the cheeks. Diagnosis is usually made by blood test, tissue biopsy, patient history, and physical examination. A **biopsy (bx)** involves the excision of living tissue for diagnostic study. General treatment consists of physical exercise, sun avoidance, and immunosuppressive drugs.

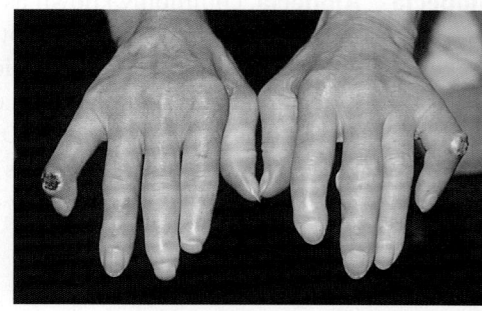

Figure 4-15 This patient with scleroderma has tapered shiny, stiff, waxy fingers with lesions on the fingertips.

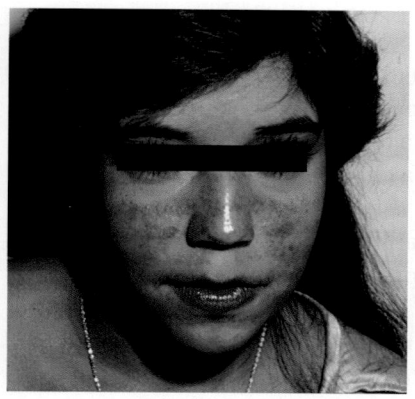

Figure 4-16 This young girl has the characteristic butterfly rash of lupus.

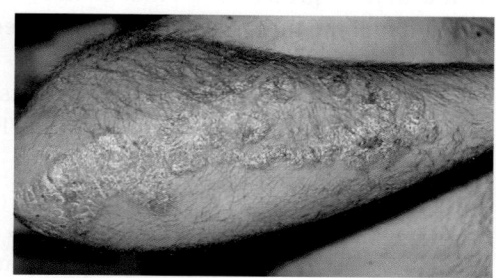

Figure 4-17 Psoriasis. Thick lesions are on the forearms of this patient.

psoriasis

Psoriasis is a chronic, inflammatory autoimmune skin disorder characterized by red, itchy, scaly patches (**Figure 4-17**). In plaque psoriasis, hardened patches on the skin give the skin a silvery-white appearance. Although psoriasis can occur at any age, disease onset is typically between the ages of 10 and 30 years. It is diagnosed by the presence of white, silvery skin scales. Remissions and exacerbations (flare-ups) commonly occur. Treatment options include UV light therapy to retard cellular division and the application of topical steroid ointments.

KEY TERM	Definition
autoimmune (aw-toh-i-MEWN) **disorder**	condition in which the immune response is directed against the body
dermatomyositis (dur-muh-toh-migh-oh-SIGH-tis)	autoimmune disease characterized by inflammation of skin and muscles
scleroderma (skleer-oh-DUR-muh)	autoimmune disease characterized by increased collagen formation in connective tissues
systemic lupus erythematosus (SLE) (LOO-pus er-ih-thee-mah-TOH-sus)	autoimmune disease of connective tissue; also called lupus
erythema (er-ih-THEE-mah)	redness on the skin
biopsy (BYE-op-see)	excision of live tissue for diagnostic study
psoriasis (soh-RYE-uh-sis)	chronic, inflammatory autoimmune skin disease characterized by red, itchy, scaly patches

KEY TERM PRACTICE: *Autoimmune Disorders*

1. Increased collagen formation in connective tissues is seen in this autoimmune disease. _____

2. _____ is the medical term for the autoimmune disease that is characterized by inflammation of the skin and underlying muscles.

3. A _____ is the excision of live tissue for diagnostic purposes.

4. _____ is a skin disease marked by red, itchy, scaly patches.

5. An _____ is caused by a reaction of the body against its own tissues.

Noncancerous Tumors

Noncancerous skin growths and tumors are classified as either benign or premalignant. A tumor that is **malignant** spreads to other body sites to hinder health or cause death. **Benign** means that the growth is not malignant. **Premalignant** is a term meaning precancerous, indicating that if the tumor is not treated immediately, it has a chance of developing into **cancer**, malignant tumors that may result in death.

Benign tumors include sebaceous cysts, cutaneous papillomas (skin tags), hemangiomas, keloids, lipomas, and seborrheic keratosis. Two common premalignant skin tumors are actinic keratoses and nevi (moles).

sebaceous cysts	**Sebaceous cysts** are palpable (capable of being felt), movable, fluid-filled cysts that develop in sebaceous glands. They may take several years to build up, are usually painless, and generally require no treatment, although they may be surgically removed.
cutaneous papillomas	Also called skin tags, **cutaneous papillomas** are flaps of skin held to the body by a thin stalk. They are frequently found in the axillary and cervical regions (armpits and neck). Skin tags tend to be a nuisance, because they get caught on clothing, so they are often removed in the dermatologist's office by freezing or snipping.
hemangioma	A benign, reddish purple tumor composed of a mass of blood vessels is a **hemangioma**. It looks like a red birth mark.
keloid	A **keloid** is an area of irregular fibrous tissue that develops at the site of a scar (**Figure 4-18**). The condition is observed more commonly in female adults and in dark-skinned people than in others. Laser treatment, corticosteroid injections, and surgery are options for removing or diminishing unsightly keloids.
lipoma	A benign tumor composed of adipocytes (fat cells) is a **lipoma**. Lipomas generally do not require treatment but are often removed because they are unsightly.
seborrheic keratosis	**Seborrheic keratosis** is a benign tumor composed of cells arranged in various patterns that produce a purple-brown papule. Yellow flecks may give the papule a greasy appearance. The cause is unknown, but their sudden appearance or an increase in their numbers could indicate an internal malignancy, notably a stomach cancer. Diagnosis is made by visual examination.

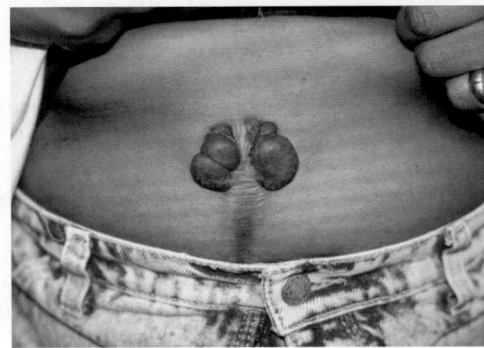

Figure 4-18 This keloid is growing well beyond the border of the cesarean section scar.

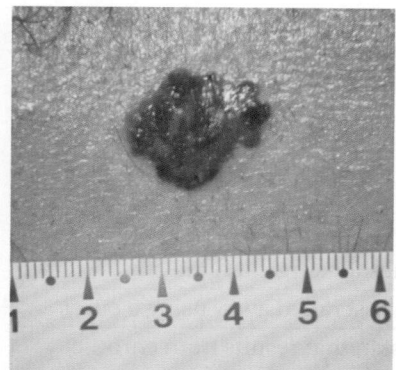

Figure 4-19 Note the ABCD features: asymmetry, notched border, varied colors, and diameter of more than 6 mm.

If treatment is necessary, the options include cryosurgery and curettage. **Cryosurgery** involves the localized freezing of tissue for removal. Once the tissue has been frozen, special instruments aid in removing the diseased area. Another surgical method for removing tissue is called **curettage**. With this procedure, a specially designed spoon-shaped instrument called a curet is used to scrape away tissue.

actinic keratosis

Chronic exposure to sunlight may cause a premalignant warty lesion called **actinic keratosis**. The term actinic means "pertaining to radiant energy." Actinic keratosis can be treated with topical ointments, curettage, and desiccation (drying).

melanoma

Moles typically appear as round, darkened spots on the skin surface and generally remain benign but can be precancerous. When in doubt about a mole, follow the ABCDs of **melanoma** (cancer of melanocytes) to assess the situation. Under this scheme, each letter represents a specific characteristic of the mole's physical appearance:

- A = asymmetry
- B = border
- C = color
- D = diameter

Moles that are asymmetrical, have irregular borders, uneven color, and diameters larger than 6 mm (0.24 inch) should be clinically tested (**Figure 4-19**).

KEY TERM	Definition
malignant (muh-LIG-nunt)	having a tendency to spread, endangering health or life
benign (be-NINE)	not malignant; noncancerous
premalignant (PREE-muh-LIG-nunt)	precancerous
cancer	malignant tumor that can lead to death
sebaceous cysts (se-BAY-shus SISTS)	fluid-filled sebaceous glands
cutaneous papillomas (kew-TAY-nee-us pap-i-LOH-muhz)	skin tags
hemangioma (hee-man-jee-OH-muh)	benign tumor made up of a blood vessel mass

continued

continued from page 167

KEY TERM	Definition
keloid (KEE-loid)	an area of irregular fibrous tissue that develops at the site of a scar
lipoma (li-POH-muh)	benign, fatty tumor
seborrheic keratosis (seb-oh-REE-ick kerr-uh-TOH-sis)	benign purple-brown skin tumor
cryosurgery (krye-oh-SUR-juh-ree)	localized freezing of diseased tissues for surgical removal
curettage (kewr-e-TAHZH)	surgical procedure in which tissue is scraped away using a curet
actinic keratosis (ack-TIN-ick ker-uh-TOH-sis)	premalignant warty lesion on the skin that results from chronic exposure to sunlight
melanoma (mel-uh-NOH-muh)	cancer of melanocytes

KEY TERM PRACTICE: *Noncancerous Tumors*

1. A noncancerous tumor is termed a _____ tumor.

2. Give the term that refers to a fatty tumor. _____

3. _____ is a skin condition characterized by a premalignant warty lesion that results from chronic exposure to sunlight.

4. A _____ is an area of irregular fibrous tissue that develops at the site of a scar.

5. A benign tumor made up of blood vessels is termed a _____, and is derived from the word part _____, meaning "blood."

Cancerous Tumors

Common skin cancers, called **carcinomas**, are malignant tumors arising from the epithelial layer of the skin (or other organs) and include basal cell carcinoma, squamous cell carcinoma, and malignant melanoma. Sun exposure is the primary cause of all skin carcinomas, and this is the most commonly occurring type of cancer.

Treatment options of the various skin carcinomas are numerous and are case specific. These include, but are not limited to, surgical excision, electrodesiccation, cryosurgery, Mohs surgery, laser surgery, and chemotherapy. **Mohs surgery** is performed under the microscope using zinc oxide paste to remove skin layers. As each cell layer is removed, it is examined under the microscope. The procedure ends when all cancerous cells have been removed.

basal cell carcinoma	**Basal cell carcinoma** is a cancer caused by malignant stem cells in the basal layer. Stem cells are early cells that give rise to other types of cells. Locally invasive and rarely metastasizing (spreading), it is common in individuals with a history of chronic sun exposure.

squamous cell carcinoma	**Squamous cell carcinoma**, the most common type of skin cancer, develops in the skin's epidermis. Both basal cell carcinoma and squamous cell carcinoma form hard coverings resulting from dried skin exudates (fluid) called **crusts** on the skin surface. Squamous cell carcinoma is more serious than basal cell carcinoma as it may spread to other body parts.
malignant melanoma	**Malignant melanoma**, the most serious type of skin cancer, is a rapidly spreading cancer of melanocytes. This type of cancer is generally detected by observing mole changes. Malignant melanoma has particular risk factors, such as family history, prior case of melanoma, and history of blistering sunburns, that may make an individual more susceptible.
Kaposi sarcoma	**Kaposi sarcoma**, occurring often in patients with AIDS (acquired immunodeficiency syndrome), is a tumor characterized by multiple bluish-red or brown nodules and plaques (**Figure 4-20**). It is typically seen on the extremities. Diagnosis is made by physical and visual examination and biopsy.

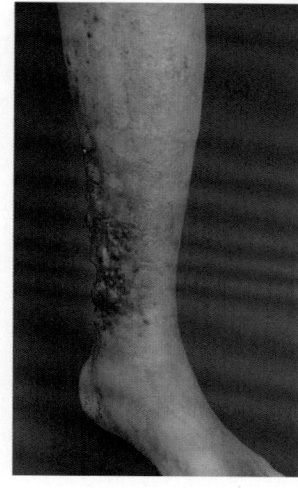

Figure 4-20 Kaposi sarcoma. Multiple papules and nodules are present on this patient's leg.

KEY TERM	Definition
carcinomas (kahr-si-NOH-muhs)	malignant tumors arising from the epithelial layer of the skin (or other organs)
Mohs (MOHZ) **surgery**	microscopically controlled surgery using zinc oxide paste to remove skin layers
basal cell carcinoma (BAY-sul SELL kahr-si-NOH-muh)	cancer of the basal cell layer
squamous cell carcinoma (SKWAY-mus SELL kahr-si-NOH-muh)	cancer that develops in the epidermis
crusts	hard coverings that result when exudate dries on the skin
malignant melanoma (muh-LIG-nunt mel-uh-NOH-muh)	cancer of the melanocytes, typically rapidly spreading
Kaposi sarcoma (KAH-poh-zee sahr-KOH-muh)	bluish-red, brown tumor occurring often in patients with AIDS

KEY TERM PRACTICE: *Cancerous Tumors*

1. _____ is cancer of the melanocytes.

2. Malignant tumors (cancer) of epithelial cells are termed _____.

3. _____ are hard coverings on the skin that result when exudate dries.

4. Skin cancer that originates in the basal cell layer is termed _____.

5. _____ is skin cancer that develops in the epidermis.

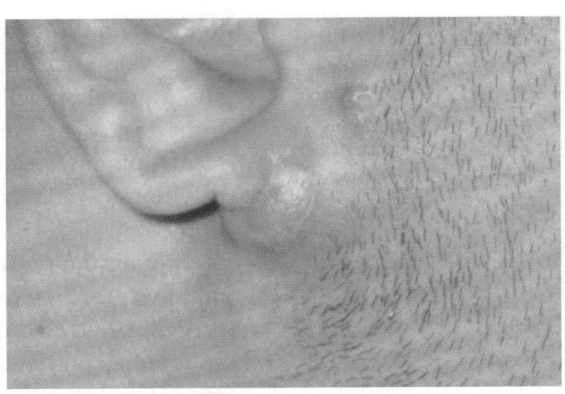

Figure 4-21 Carbuncle.

Carbuncles and Furuncles

furuncle or **boil**   A **furuncle**, or boil, is a localized infection originating in or near a hair follicle that develops into an abscess. It is caused by staphylococcal infection.

abscess   An **abscess** is a furuncle involving entire hair follicles and adjoining subcutaneous tissues.

carbuncle   A **carbuncle** is a large furuncle or multiple furuncles that form an interconnected mass. Symptoms include erythema, edema, and pain. It is caused by staphylococcal infection (**Figure 4-21**).

Treatment consists of the application of warm, moist heat to aid fluid drainage. In several cases, **incision and drainage (I&D)**, in which a surgical cut is made to release tissue fluid, and antibiotic therapy may be necessary.

KEY TERM	Definition
furuncle (FEW-rung-kul)	a boil
abscess (ab-SES)	furuncle involving hair follicles and adjacent tissue
carbuncle (KAHR-bunk-ul)	large furuncle
incision and drainage (I&D)	surgical cut to drain fluid from tissue

KEY TERM PRACTICE: *Carbuncles and Furuncles*

1. I&D is the abbreviation for what procedure? _____

2. Give the medical term for a boil. _____

3. A very large furuncle is termed a _____.

4. A furuncle that involves hair follicles and adjacent tissues is known as an _____.

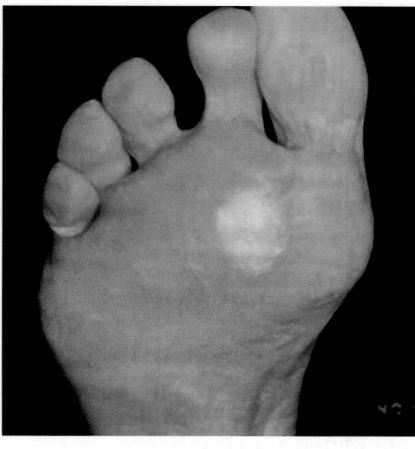

Figure 4-22 Calluses are thickened skin that occur at pressure points.

Corn (Clavus) and Callus

corn or **clavus**   A **corn** or **clavus** is a small, painful area of thickened skin, usually on a toe. Clavi usually result from pressure or friction.

callus   A **callus** is a thickening of epithelial tissue. Calluses are larger than corns and typically develop on the palms of the hands and the balls of the feet (**Figure 4-22**). Pain and tenderness are common symptoms. Repeated trauma or overuse, such as from playing stringed musical instruments, engaging in manual labor, or having impaired circulation, may also cause calluses. Treatments include avoiding or removing the causative agent, using creams, and undergoing exfoliation.

KEY TERM	Definition
corn	small, painful area of thickened skin, usually on the toe; also called a clavus
clavus (KLAY-vus)	small, painful area of thickened skin, usually on the toe; also called a corn
callus (KAL-us)	thickening of epithelial tissue resulting from overuse

KEY TERM PRACTICE: *Corn (Clavus) and Callus*

1. Give the two terms for a small, painful area of thickened skin, usually on the toe. _____

2. A _____ is a thickening of epithelial tissue that typically results from repeated hand trauma, such as playing a guitar.

Decubitus Ulcers

ulcers   **Ulcers** are sores that result from epithelial tissue destruction.

decubitus ulcers   **Decubitus ulcers**, also known as pressure sores or bedsores, are caused by a chronic deficiency of blood to tissues subjected to prolonged pressure. Decubitus ulcers are so named because they frequently occur in individuals who have been immobile in the decubitus (lying down) position. These ulcers generally occur over a bony prominence or joint (**Figure 4-23**).

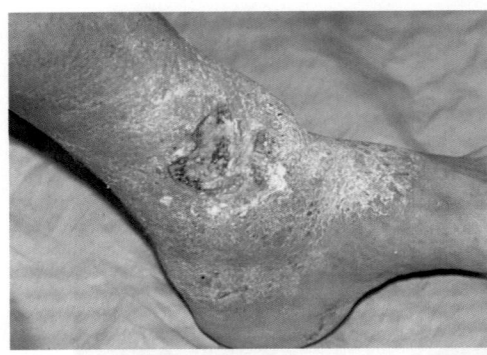

Figure 4-23 Ulcer on the ankle of a patient.

Thus, it is extremely important that bedridden or paralyzed individuals be moved on a regular basis to increase blood flow into tissues.

Decubitus ulcers can affect all layers of the skin, and the more severe cases penetrate to the bone. Signs include shiny, red skin in the early stages, and blisters, open wounds, and exudates in later stages. Pungent odors are common, because the flesh creates a nice environment for germs. Necrosis and gangrene are two terms that describe tissue death. **Necrosis** is death of one or more cells, or of a portion of tissue or organ, resulting from irreversible damage. **Gangrene** (or mortification) is necrosis due to obstruction or diminished blood supply.

A tissue culture may be necessary to choose the appropriate antibiotic therapy. Treatment must be vigorous and rapid to delay further damage to underlying tissue. Options include topical agents, gelatin sponges to absorb excess fluid drainage, antibiotics, antiseptic irrigations to flush the area, and débridement. **Débridement** involves removal of the necrotized (dead) tissue in order to expose healthy tissue and allow the wound to heal. Ulcers can be prevented or alleviated by changing position frequently, doing range-of-motion exercises, and using specially designed air mattresses that ease pressure on the tissues.

KEY TERM	Definition
ulcers (UL-surz)	sores that result from destruction of epithelial tissue
decubitus ulcers (dee-KEW-bi-tus UL-surs)	pressure sores or bedsores
necrosis (ne-KROH-sis)	death of one or more cells, or of a portion of tissue or organ, resulting from irreversible damage
gangrene (GANG-green)	necrosis due to obstruction or diminished blood supply; also called mortification
débridement (dih-BREED-ment)	removal of dead tissue to expose healthy tissue and allow the wound to heal

KEY TERM PRACTICE: *Decubitus Ulcers*

1. What is another term for a pressure sore? _____

2. _____ refers to the removal of dead tissue.

3. _____ are sores that result from destruction of epithelial tissues, usually resulting from immobility.

4. Give two terms that mean death of tissue as a result of interrupted blood flow. _____

IN THE NEWS: Necrotizing Fasciitis

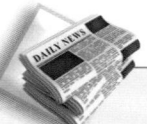

Do you remember cases of necrotizing fasciitis, the flesh-eating infection? If not, then here is the news. It sounded like something out of a horror film. Reports from England in 1994, San Francisco in 1996, and Texas in 1998 focused on this disease, when people died as their flesh was literally eaten away at the rate of several inches per hour. The culprit was the very common bacterium *Streptococcus pyogenes*. The *Streptococcus* bacteria killed the infected tissue, thrived in the remaining dead flesh, and produced toxins that diffused into the surrounding healthy tissue to continue the process. The disease was named necrotizing fasciitis because, as the term suggests, it flourished in the *fascia* (tissue layers under the skin), *necrotizing* (killing) tissue in its path.

Symptoms of necrotizing fasciitis were described as early as the fifth century B.C.E. by Hippocrates, the Greek physician regarded as the father of medicine. More than 2,000 cases were reported among soldiers during the Civil War. Signs and symptoms include fever, severe pain and swelling, large fluid-filled purple bullae, and rapid invasive infection of tissue. The release of foul-smelling pus from the vesicles is a telltale sign. Dermal gangrene is often apparent. It often originates from a minor trauma or skin injury that allows the bacteria to gain entry into the body. There are no preventive measures and its onset cannot be predicted. However, for unknown reasons, the flesh-eating strain recurs every 10 years.

Treatment must be swift to prevent its rampant spread and increase the chances of survival. Urgent tissue excision is usually necessary to remove infected areas and relieve edema. Amputation of limbs is frequently necessary. Antibiotics are useless for the initial infection because they cannot reach the target site due to inadequate circulatory function in the dead tissue layers. Antibiotic agents also have no effect on the toxins produced by the bacteria. Thus, surgery is the therapy of choice, and broad-spectrum antibiotics are given intravenously afterward. Further management involves aggressive antimicrobial therapy, fluid replacement, and the use of a hyperbaric oxygen chamber to promote wound healing.

Flesh-eating bacteria affect between 500 and 1,500 people annually in the United States. The mortality rate is 40% to 60%.

Dermatitis

dermatitis	The general term for inflammation of the skin is **dermatitis**. Several types of dermatitis exist, and each has distinguishing skin characteristics. Treatment of all forms of dermatitis is aimed at controlling inflammation and itching (pruritus). It usually involves application of topical steroid creams that contain cortisone or hydrocortisone and possibly administration of an oral steroid.
contact dermatitis	Skin inflammation caused by an irritant coming in contact with the skin is **contact dermatitis**. Causes of contact dermatitis are varied, ranging from a minor skin irritant resulting from brushing up against a surface to an allergic reaction to food ingested. Symptoms include erythema, edema, and **vesicles**, which are small blisters that leak fluid. **Pruritus** (itching), burning at the site, and stinging sensations are frequent.

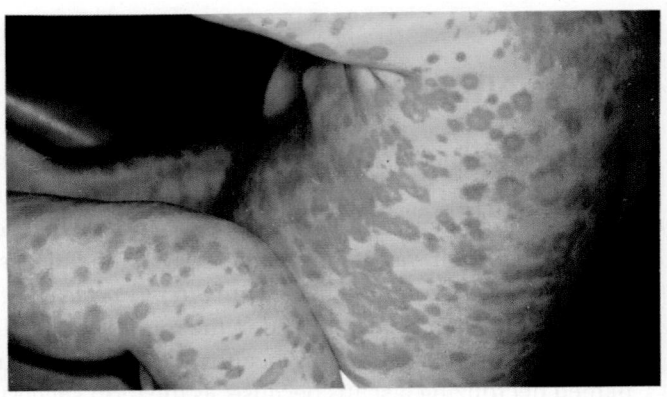

Figure 4-24 Urticaria in an infant as a result of a drug reaction.

seborrheic dermatitis Inflammation of the skin at the sebaceous glands is **seborrheic dermatitis**. It is characterized by inflammation of the skin at the sebaceous glands. The irritation is greatest in areas of high sebaceous gland concentration, notably the scalp, eyebrows, eyelids, lateral margins of the nose, behind the ears, and on the chest. In infants, it is referred to as **cradle cap**.

Seborrheic dermatitis is not a secondary condition to any other illness, and its cause is not known, thus its onset is said to be **idiopathic**. Seborrheic dermatitis affecting the scalp can be treated using medicated shampoos.

atopic dermatitis (atopic eczema) **Atopic dermatitis**, also known as **atopic eczema**, is a genetically determined inflammatory allergic skin disorder characterized by itching. **Atopy** means that the condition is genetically determined. A rash with vesicles and **exudative** (leaky) eruptions may also be seen. There is no known cure for atopic eczema.

urticaria **Urticaria** (hives) is a rash of round, red welts on the skin that itch. The medical term for these welts is **wheals**. The condition is generally acute, lasting a few hours, but chronic cases have been reported. Urticaria is generally caused by allergic reactions to food, drugs, insect bites or stings, or sunlight (**Figure 4-24**). Treatment consists of removing the allergen (substance that caused the allergy) if known, administering antihistamines, or injecting epinephrine in serious cases.

KEY TERM	Definition
dermatitis (dur-muh-TYE-tis)	skin inflammation
contact dermatitis (dur-muh-TYE-tis)	skin inflammation caused by an irritant coming in contact with the skin
vesicles (VES-i-kuls)	blisters that leak fluid
pruritus (proo-RYE-tus)	itching
seborrheic dermatitis (seb-oh-REE-ick dur-muh-TYE-tis)	inflammation of the skin at the sebaceous glands
cradle cap	seborrheic dermatitis in infants
idiopathic (id-ee-OH-path-ick)	of unknown cause
atopic dermatitis (ay-TOP-ick dur-muh-TYE-tis)	a genetically determined inflammatory allergic skin disorder characterized by itching; also called atopic eczema

continued

continued from page 174

KEY TERM	Definition
atopic eczema (ay-TOP-ick ECK-zuh-muh)	a genetically determined inflammatory allergic skin disorder characterized by itching; also called atopic dermatitis
atopy (ah-TUH-pee)	genetically determined
exudative (ig-zoo-DAY-tiv)	leaking out of tissues
urticaria (ur-tih-KAHR-ee-ah)	rash of round, red welts on the skin that itch; also called hives
wheals (WHEELZ)	rash of round, red welts

KEY TERM PRACTICE: *Dermatitis*

1. Skin inflammation is termed _____.

2. If a disease occurs with no known cause, it is said to be _____.

3. Inflammation of sebaceous glands in infants is commonly called _____.

4. The other medical term for atopic eczema is _____.

5. Another term for hives is _____.

6. The raised bump on the arm after an insect bite could be described as a _____.

Dermatophytosis

A pathogenic fungus called a **dermatophyte** is responsible for skin infections called **dermatophytoses** (*dermatophytosis* = singular). The fungi (*fungus* = singular) invade the superficial keratinized areas such as the skin, hair, and nails.

Fungal infections invade the skin through cuts, scrapes, or wounds. They are transmitted via direct contact with the fungus or its spores. Identification of specific fungi is made through culturing affected tissue. Treatment options are available, but persistence is key when attempting to eradicate this type of infection. Along with oral and topical antifungal medications, it is critical that the affected site be kept clean and dry.

tinea   A fungal infection of the hair, skin, or nails is called **tinea** or ringworm. The affected body part gives rise to the medical term describing the infection.
- **Tinea capitis** affects the scalp (**Figure 4-25**).
- **Tinea corporis** is found anywhere on the body (**Figure 4-26**).
- **Tinea pedis**, or athlete's foot, is on the foot.
- **Tinea unguium** involves the nails.

The lesions are generally round, ringed, scaled vesicles that resemble targets. Signs and symptoms can include burning sensations; stinging pruritus; and dry, peeling **fissures** (skin cracks). Characteristics of tinea unguium include thickened, brittle, and dull nails without pain or itching.

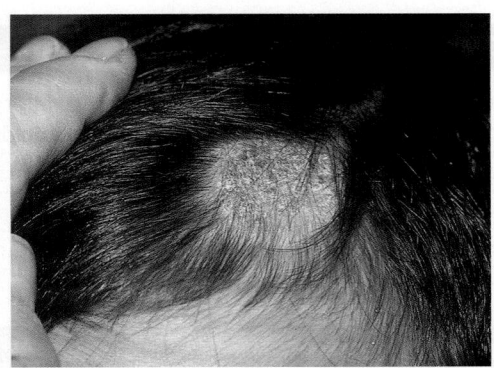

Figure 4-25 Tinea capitis, a dermatophytosis affecting the scalp.

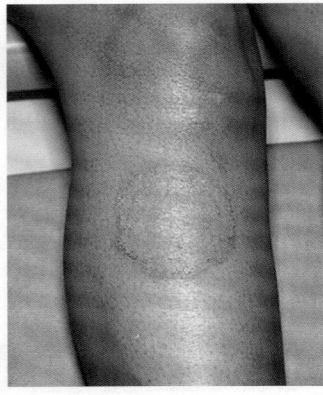

Figure 4-26 Tinea corporis on the leg.

KEY TERM	Definition
dermatophyte (der-MAT-oh-fite)	pathogenic fungus
dermatophytoses (dur-muh-toh-figh-TOH-seez)	skin infections caused by fungi
tinea (TIN-ee-uh)	fungal infection; commonly called ringworm
tinea capitis (TIN-ee-uh KAP-i-tis)	ringworm of the scalp
tinea corporis (TIN-ee-uh KOR-po-ris)	ringworm anywhere on the body
tinea pedis (TIN-ee-uh PED-is)	ringworm of the foot; commonly called athlete's foot
tinea unguium (TIN-ee-uh UNG-gwee-um)	ringworm of the nails
fissures (FISH-urz)	cracks in the skin

KEY TERM PRACTICE: *Dermatophytosis*

1. Infections caused by fungi are termed _____.

2. The medical term for ringworm is _____.

3. _____ is ringworm of the scalp.

4. _____ is ringworm of the foot, and is commonly called athlete's foot.

5. Cracks in the skin are known as _____.

Cellulitis

cellulitis   **Cellulitis** is an inflammation of the skin and subcutaneous tissue (**Figure 4-27**). It results from a streptococcal or staphylococcal bacterial infection. It typically occurs on the legs, but any part of the body can be affected.

     Signs and symptoms include erythema, edema, and skin that is hot and tender to touch. Bacteria enter through an abrasion. Definitive diagnosis may include a blood culture to identify the microorganism. Treatment aims include mobilization and elevation of the affected limb, cool magnesium sulfate application, system antibiotics, and **analgesics** (drugs that relieve pain).

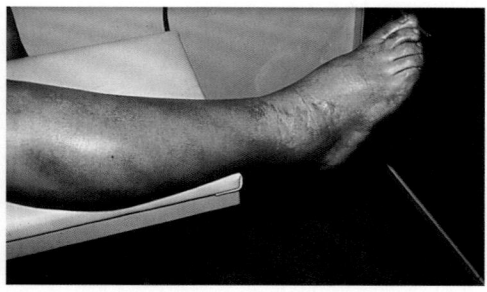

Figure 4-27 This patient with cellulitis has a painful, tender lower leg.

KEY TERM	Definition
cellulitis (sell-yoo-LYE-tis)	inflammation of the skin and subcutaneous tissue caused by a bacterial infection
analgesics (an-al-JEE-zicks)	drugs that relieve pain

KEY TERM PRACTICE: *Cellulitis*

1. Inflammation of the skin and subcutaneous tissue that is caused by a bacterial infection is termed _____.

2. Drugs that relieve pain are termed _____.

Hair, Follicle, and Gland Disorders

folliculitis **Folliculitis** is an inflammation of hair follicles that produces small boils. Shaving is a precipitating factor. Treatment involves cleansing the affected area daily and applying antiseptics.

hirsutism **Hirsutism** is a condition of excessive body hair, particularly in women. In females, the condition causes hair growth in patterns that are typically male. For example, facial hair is very noticeable. It results from a physiological hormone imbalance or anabolic steroid use.

hypertrichosis Excessive growth of normal hair is referred to as **hypertrichosis** (**Figure 4-28**). This condition is responsible for the werewolf syndrome.

rosacea **Rosacea** is a recurring inflammatory disorder characterized by redness on the cheeks, forehead, nose, and chin that results from dilation of capillaries and follicles. It is often mistaken for a sunburn or acne. Rosacea has an unknown cause. Treatment consists of avoiding sunlight, cold weather, and wind. Routine use of facial creams is also suggested.

rhinophyma **Rhinophyma** is a form of rosacea that affects the nose. The condition results from **hyperplasia** (excessive cell growth) of the sebaceous glands and connective tissue causing the nose to appear red and knobby (**Figure 4-29**).

seborrhea A disease of the sebaceous glands characterized by excessive sebum secretion and excessively oily skin is called **seborrhea**. The oily sebum collects on the skin, forming a greasy coating that eventually becomes crusty. It occurs in areas where sebaceous glands are most numerous. Treatment for rhinophyma and seborrhea includes antiseptic cleansers and medicated facial creams.

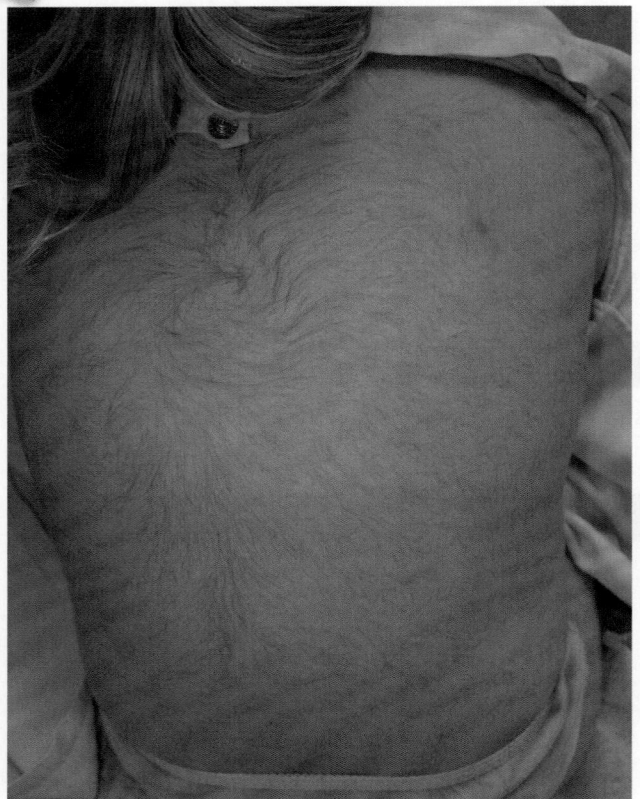

Figure 4-28 Girl with hypertrichosis on her back.

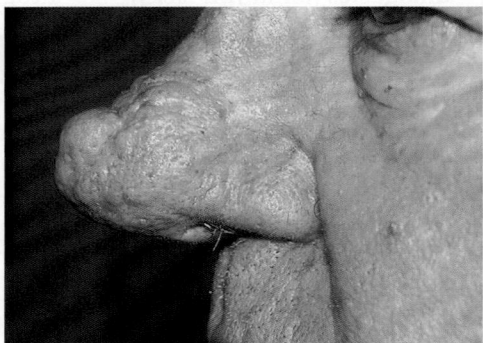

Figure 4-29 Rhinophyma.

KEY TERM	Definition
folliculitis (fol-ick-yoo-LYE-tis)	inflammation of the hair follicles that produces small boils
hirsutism (HER-soot-izm)	excessive body hair, especially in women
hypertrichosis (high-pur-tri-KOH-sis)	excessive growth of normal hair
rosacea (roh-ZAY-shee-uh)	recurring inflammatory disorder characterized by redness on the cheeks, forehead, nose, and chin that results from dilation of capillaries and follicles
rhinophyma (rye-noh-FIH-muh)	form of rosacea affecting the nose
hyperplasia (high-pur-PLAY-zhuh)	excessive cell growth
seborrhea (seb-oh-REE-uh)	disease of the sebaceous glands involving excessive sebum secretion

KEY TERM PRACTICE: *Hair, Follicle, and Gland Disorders*

1. _____ is the term used to describe inflammation of the hair follicles.

2. Excessive growth of normal hair is called _____.

3. Anabolic steroid use can result in unusual hairiness in women. This condition is called _____.

4. _____ is characterized by excessive sebum secretion that results in extremely oily skin.

5. A recurring inflammatory disorder characterized by redness on the cheeks, forehead, nose, and chin that results from dilation of capillaries and follicles is termed _____.

Infectious Diseases

Infectious disorders result from bacterial, viral, or other pathogens. Several forms are described.

varicella (chickenpox)

The causative agent for both varicella (chickenpox) and herpes zoster (shingles) is the varicella-zoster virus (VZV). Affecting children and young adults, **varicella** (chickenpox) is a highly contagious, acute, viral infection. **Figure 4-30** illustrates the characteristic skin lesions, macules, vesicles, and crusts. A small, discolored spot on the skin is termed a **macule**. The macules progress to papules, which eventually form vesicles, which in turn form crusts in the end stage of the disease. Pruritus is intense. A person is contagious 1 to 2 days before the rash appears and until all the lesions have crusted (about 4 to 5 days). It takes about 14–17 days after contact with an infected person for you to develop chickenpox. **Palliative** (relieving or soothing without eliminating the cause) measures are the primary treatment options and include anti-itch creams and baths as well as administration of acetaminophen. A varicella vaccine is currently available.

herpes zoster (shingles)

Herpes zoster, also known as **shingles**, is reactivation of the varicella-zoster virus (VZV). Signs and symptoms include acute inflammation, redness and banding along a dermatome, and pain. A **dermatome** is a specific area of skin supplied by a particular peripheral nerve. The characteristic rash develops along a dermatome. The rash eventually forms vesicles, which may become pustulant and finally crust (**Figure 4-31**). The typical period of duration ranges from 10 days to 5 weeks, but the disease persists in some elderly individuals. Although the cause of reactivation of this virus is not clear, stress appears to play a role. Treatment is palliative and antiviral medication may be administered. There is no cure, but a vaccine, Zostavax, is currently available.

rubella

A contagious infection in children caused by the rubella virus, **rubella** (German measles) is characterized by fever, pale pink rash, and lymph node swelling. Children are routinely immunized against rubella.

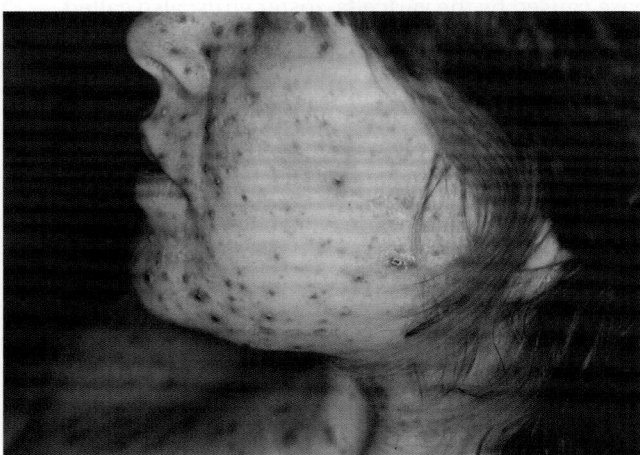

Figure 4-30 Rash of varicella (chickenpox).

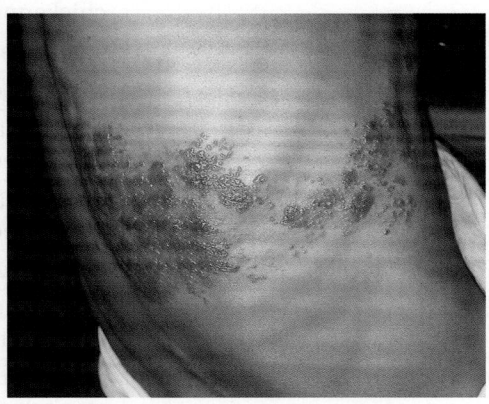

Figure 4-31 Rash of herpes zoster (shingles).

impetigo	**Impetigo** is an acute, contagious inflammatory skin rash caused by streptococcal or staphylococcal bacteria. Characteristically, vesicles develop and then burst, forming yellow-brown crusts. The lesions are typically located on the face, arms, legs, and trunk. Diagnosis is made through visual inspection of the characteristic lesions and a skin test. Impetigo is treated with systemic antibiotic therapy and thorough cleansing.
scabies	**Scabies** is a contagious skin disorder caused by the *Sarcoptes scabiei* mite. Intense pruritus and lesions characterize it. The itching occurs primarily at night when the female insect burrows beneath the skin to lay eggs. Scabies treatment involves the use of special shampoos, sulfur creams, and topical steroids.
pediculosis	**Pediculosis** is a highly contagious skin disease caused by lice infestation. Signs and symptoms include intense pruritus, cutaneous lesions, and nits (eggs) on the hair shafts. Several forms affect humans, each caused by a specific species of louse. *Pediculus humanus capitis* infests the head and scalp, causing **pediculosis capitis**. Lice infestation is treated by using special shampoos, meticulously combing the hair, and cleaning affected personal items. Mites and lice are transmitted via physical contact with other infected individuals or through contact with their personal belongings, clothes, or bed sheets.
verrucae (warts)	**Verrucae** (*verruca* = singular) are warts caused by the human papillomavirus (HPV). **Verruca vulgaris**, better known as the common wart, often occurs on the fingers. The most common type of wart is found on the foot; hence the name **plantar wart**. Plantar warts are small, hard lumps speckled with black dots. The dots are actually clotted blood vessels. Pruritus may be present. Most warts disappear naturally without any treatment. However, treatment in the form of creams, surgical excision, cryosurgery, and electrodesiccation is available.

KEY TERM	Definition
varicella (vair-i-SELL-uh)	contagious disease caused by the varicella-zoster virus; also called chickenpox
macule (MACK-yool)	small, discolored skin spot
palliative (PAL-ee-uh-tiv)	relieving or soothing without eliminating the cause
herpes zoster (HUR-peez ZOS-tur)	disease caused by reactivation of the varicella-zoster virus (VZV); also called shingles
shingles	disease caused by reactivation of the varicella-zoster virus (VZV); also called herpes zoster
dermatome (DUR-muh-tome)	area of skin supplied by a peripheral nerve
rubella (roo-BEL-uh)	a contagious infection caused by the rubella virus; also called German measles
impetigo (im-pe-TYE-goh)	contagious skin condition caused by streptococcal or staphylococcal bacteria

continued

continued from page 180

KEY TERM	Definition
scabies (SKAY-beez)	skin disease with itching caused by mites
pediculosis (pe-dick-yoo-LOH-sis)	skin disease caused by lice
pediculosis capitis (pe-dick-yoo-LOH-sis KAP-i-tis)	lice infestation on the head
verrucae (ve-ROO-kee)	warts caused by the human papillomavirus (HPV)
verruca vulgaris (ve-ROO-kuh vul-GAIR-us)	common wart that occurs on the fingers
plantar wart	wart on the foot

KEY TERM PRACTICE: *Infectious Diseases*

1. An area of skin supplied by a peripheral nerve is termed a _____.

2. Itch mites are also referred to as _____.

3. Pediculosis _____ is the term used to describe lice infestation on the scalp.

4. The medical term for warts caused by the human papillomavirus (HPV) is _____.

5. _____, also known as _____, is caused by the reactivation of the varicella-zoster virus (VZV).

Nail Disorders

The fingernails and toenails provide an excellent source for quickly assessing health status because their appearance can often suggest underlying conditions. Many diseases cause nail discoloration, and white patches on the nail beds indicate vitamin and/or mineral deficiency. Diagnosis of nails disorders is usually through physical examination. Correcting underlying pathologies typically corrects nail discoloration.

onychia and onychomycosis   A basic inflammation of the nail matrix (growth layer) is **onychia**. **Onychomycosis** is a fungal nail infection.

Edema, erythema, and pain are classic signs and symptoms of nail disorders. Antibiotics and antifungal creams and medications are used to treat these various conditions.

KEY TERM	Definition
onychia (oh-NICK-ee-uh)	inflammation of the nail matrix
onychomycosis (on-i-koh-migh-KOH-sis)	fungal infection of the nail

KEY TERM PRACTICE: *Nail Disorders*

1. _____ is the medical term used to describe a fungal infection of the nails.

2. _____ is the medical term for inflammation of the nail matrix.

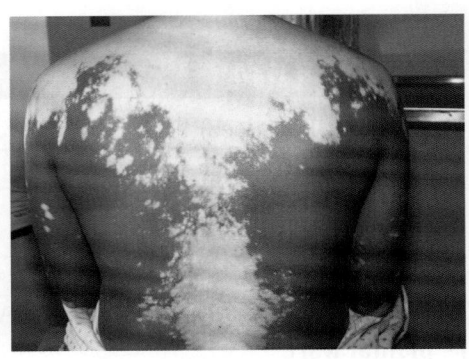

Figure 4-32 A case of vitiligo with extensive depigmentation.

Pigment Disorders

Recall that skin color variation is a result of genetic, physical, and environmental influences. Alterations in pigmentation are named according to the specific skin abnormality. Diagnosis of pigmentation disorders is made through physical and visual examination.

leukoderma	An absence of pigment is termed **leukoderma**.
ecchymosis	Skin discoloration as a result of a ruptured blood vessel or bleeding into the subcutaneous space is known as **ecchymosis**. A bruise is an example of an ecchymosis.
chloasma	**Chloasma** describes hyperpigmentation occurring on the forehead, temples, cheeks, and nipples. It results from hormonal factors during pregnancy, menstruation, or with oral contraceptive use. Chloasma is made worse by sunlight.
vitiligo	**Vitiligo** is a skin disorder characterized by areas of white patches on otherwise normal pigmented skin (**Figure 4-32**). Note that the borders of these achromic regions are hyperpigmented.

KEY TERM	Definition
leukoderma (lew-koh-DUR-muh)	absence of pigment
ecchymosis (eck-i-MOH-sis)	discoloration because of a ruptured blood vessel
chloasma (kloh-AZ-muh)	hyperpigmentation caused by hormonal factors
vitiligo (vit-i-LYE-go)	skin disease characterized by white patches on otherwise normal pigmented skin

KEY TERM PRACTICE: *Pigment Disorders*

1. Which skin disease is characterized by regions of white patches on otherwise normal pigmented skin? _____

2. The absence of pigment is termed _____, which is derived from the word part _____, meaning "white," and the word part _____, meaning "skin."

3. _____ is dark coloration caused by hormonal changes related to pregnancy, menstruation, or oral contraceptive use.

4. Discoloration that results from a ruptured blood vessel is termed _____.

LIFE SPAN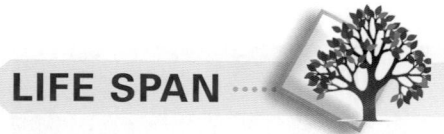

All human tissues develop from three primary germ layers. Skin develops from two of these layers. During embryological development, the epidermis is derived from the ectoderm, whereas the dermis and hypodermis (subcutaneous layer) are derived from the mesoderm. The skin is nearly developed by the fourth gestational month. Lanugo—soft, downy, peach-fuzz-like hair—covers the fetus beginning around the fifth month.

At birth, the body's skin is covered with vernix caseosa, which literally means "varnish of cheese." It is produced by the sebaceous glands. Newborn skin is thin, and small white spots called milia on the face are common. Milia are caused by particles clogging the sebaceous glands. These white dots gradually disappear within several weeks.

As children develop, the skin thickens, the subcutaneous fat layer increases, and sweat glands become increasingly functional. During adolescence, there is a marked increase in sebaceous gland activity, often resulting in acne. Skin function and appearance are optimum between the ages of 20 and 40 years. However, many age-associated skin changes are not evident until age 45 years and beyond.

As the integumentary system ages, there are noticeable changes, such as wrinkling, thinner and drier skin, loss of subcutaneous fat, atrophy of sebaceous glands, pigmentation alterations, and a decrease in the number of melanocytes. As a result of having fewer melanocytes, there is less filtering of UV radiation, increasing the risk of skin cancers. Graying hair is another result of the decrease in melanocytes. Moreover, an increase in the size of some melanocytes causes patches of increased pigmentation known as age spots.

The decrease in dermal thickness gives aging skin a thin, translucent appearance. Wrinkling occurs as a result of decreased numbers of fibroblasts, which produce collagen and elastic fibers. For this reason, the skin is less flexible, resulting in wrinkling.

Hair and nail growth also diminish with the aging process. Beginning around the age of 50 years, only about one-third of the hair follicles are active. It is also common for hair to become thinner.

Dry skin in the elderly population is attributed to atrophy of sweat and sebaceous glands. Wound healing is delayed in response to decreased blood supply, reduced cell proliferation, and diminished immune response. The immune response is weakened because there are fewer Langerhans cells, which are responsible for resisting disease. Temperature regulation is compromised in aging people as a result of diminished fat reserves, decreased vascular function, and reduced sweat production.

The skin is the organ that shows the most obvious signs of aging. Proper fluid intake and nutrition, good hygiene, and avoidance of too much UV radiation are essential to maintaining healthy skin throughout the life span.

COMMON Abbreviations

Abbreviation	Term
ABCD	asymmetry, border, color, diameter
AIDS	acquired immunodeficiency syndrome
ANA	antinuclear antibody
ASCP	American Society for Clinical Pathology
bx	biopsy
CAAHEP	Commission on Accreditation of Allied Health Education Programs
CT	cytotechnologist
HPV	human papillomavirus
I&D	incision and drainage
ISMP	Institute for Safe Medication Practices
SLE	systemic lupus erythematosus
subcut.	subcutaneous
UV	ultraviolet
VZV	varicella-zoster virus

COMMON ABBREVIATIONS EXERCISES

1. When referring to a mole, to what does ABCD refer? _____

2. VZV is the abbreviation for _____.

3. Write the abbreviation for ultraviolet. _____

4. AIDS is the abbreviation for _____.

5. SLE is the abbreviation for what condition? _____

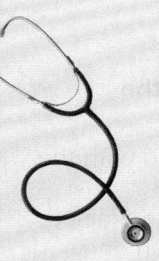

Case Study

Mrs. Walford, a 55-year-old, arrived in her dermatologist's office with a yearlong history of a skin lesion on her right temple. History of the present illness indicated that this spot has occasionally bled in response to minor trauma. Surgical, social, and psychosocial histories were unremarkable. Family history was noncontributory.

Mrs. Walford's physical examination revealed that she appeared healthy and was in no acute distress. Because her chief complaint was a neoplasm (new growth) on the right temple, she was questioned about outdoor activities, sunscreen use, and history of blistering sunburns. It was discovered that in her youth, Mrs. Walford remembered having at least one blistering sunburn. She also stated that she rarely uses any type of sunscreen while she gardens, which she does on a regular basis.

Physical examination of the integumentary system revealed the following regarding the lesion:

LOCATION: right temple at temporal hair line
SIZE: 1.7 cm × 1.3 cm
SHAPE: irregular
COLOR: erythematous
ELEVATION: slightly elevated
IRRITATION: slightly irritated

Dr. Byron, her dermatologist, diagnosed probable basal cell carcinoma of right temple and suggested that the most reasonable treatment would be excision of the lesion with pathological examination of the tissue by a CT.

Case Study Questions

Select the best answer to each of the following questions.

1. **Mrs. Walford made an appointment with her dermatologist for her lesion. Why is this the most appropriate medical specialty for her condition?**
   _____.
   a. Dermatologists specialize in diseases of the skin and integumentary system; thus Dr. Byron would be a wise choice.
   b. A better choice would have been a family physician because these doctors see a lot of different cases.
   c. She should have gone directly to a pathologist because that specialty area deals with the study of disease.
   d. A dermatologist is okay, but a cytotechnologist is better trained to deal with skin conditions.

2. **What sign or symptom suggested to the doctor that this might be basal cell carcinoma?** _____
   a. There was nothing in particular to suggest this.
   b. The doctor believed a "better safe than sorry" approach was best.

   c. The lesion had irregular borders, was elevated, and was irritated.
   d. The lesion had been there a long time.

3. **The lesion was described as erythematous. This means the lesion**
   _____.
   a. has a redness
   b. has a bluish hue
   c. is fluid filled
   d. is hard

4. **What is the significance of the skin being exposed to the sun without using sunscreen?**
   _____
   a. There is no significance because sun-exposed skin can hold up to UV radiation.
   b. There is no significance because there is no evidence that sunscreen protects against harmful sun rays.
   c. Continuous sun exposure without sunscreen increases the risk of developing skin cancer.
   d. Sunscreen use has been linked to an increased risk of skin cancer.

continued

continued from page 185

5. Basal cell carcinoma is

_____.

a. locally invasive, rarely metastasizes, and is common in individuals with a history of chronic sun exposure
b. the most serious type of skin cancer and is generally associated with changes in a mole
c. a tumor characterized by multiple bluish-red or brown nodules and plaques
d. a minor lesion that does not require medical treatment

6. Excision of the lesion with pathological examination means that the

_____.

a. growth will be frozen and viewed with the naked eye
b. lesion will be lanced and the fluid drained
c. lesion will be removed and grown on a Petri plate
d. lesion will be removed and evaluated by trained professionals to arrive at a conclusive diagnosis

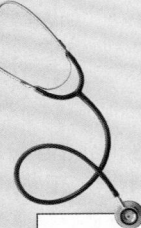

Real World Report

COMMUNITY HOSPITAL: DEPARTMENT OF PATHOLOGY

NAME: Charon Walford
DATE ORDERED:COLLECTION DATE: 05/30/2011
SURGEON: Richard Kelley
ADMITTER: Mary Anne Edinburgh
DOB: 02/21/1956
AGE: 55
SEX: F
CONSULTOR: Lindsey Limpson
PATH NO.: F002434
HOSPITAL NO.: 01478
ACCOUNT NO.: 47891s
LOCATION: Clinic

PATHOLOGICAL DIAGNOSIS

Right temple, excisional biopsy: Basal cell carcinoma

COMMENT

- *All* margins of resection are free of neoplasm
- Sources: *Skin,* Rt temple neoplasm

continued

continued from page 186

CLINICAL INFORMATION

Excision neoplasm right temple

GROSS DESCRIPTION

In fixative is a solitary elliptical segment of light tan skin measuring 4 × 1.6 × 0.5 cm. A poorly defined gray-tan macular lesion measuring 1.2 × 0.8 cm is present in the center of the specimen, approximately 1 to 2 mm from the short axis margin of resection. All margins are inked in blue. Serial sections across the short axis to include the lesion are submitted in cassette no. 1. The opposite pointed margins are submitted in cassette no. 2.

MICROSCOPIC DESCRIPTION

Sections of skin and subcutaneous tissue demonstrate mild hyperkeratosis. The epidermis is focally atrophic. There is mild basophilic degeneration of the reticular collagen. Arising at the dermal–epidermal junction and involving the reticular dermis is a neoplasm consisting of broad-based islands and ribbons of basaloid cells having a hyperchromatic, spindled nucleus with finely stippled chromatin. The peripheral cell layer of these tumor lobules shows prominent palisading. Focal central necrosis is at times identified as well as scattered mitotic figures within the tumor nests. A slightly basophilic fibromyxoid stroma containing chronic inflammation surrounds the tumor nests. All margins of resection are free of neoplasm.
SIGNATURE: Pathologist (signed out 06/01/2011)

Real World Report Questions

The following exercises review the medical terms used in the preceding medical report. A term that may be unfamiliar is *palisading,* which is used in microbiology to describe cells that are lined up next to each other much like a white picket fence.

1. What is a neoplasm?

_____

2. Hyperkeratosis

    a. Word part *hyper-* = _____

    b. Word part *kerat-* = _____

    c. Word part *-osis* = _____

    d. What does *hyperkeratosis* mean?

_____

3. What word literally means "a reduction in tissue size"?

_____

4. The dermal–epidermal junction was mentioned. Refer to the diagram in the text and describe this area.

_____

5. The margins of the section were free of neoplasm, thus _____.

    a. cancerous tissue remains

    b. all cancerous tissue was removed

Review and Application

Multiple-Choice Questions

Select the best answer to each of the following questions.

1. These types of burns are characterized by severe pain; blisters; edema; and slow, complete recovery. _____
   - a. first-degree burn
   - b. second-degree burn
   - c. third-degree burn
   - d. a and c

2. Skin functions include _____.
   - a. maintaining body temperature and serving
   - b. serving and synthesizing blood as a protective barrier
   - c. maintaining body temperature and synthesizing nerve cells
   - d. all of the above

3. The correct order of epidermal layers from deep to superficial is _____.
   - a. stratum corneum, stratum basale, and stratum granulosum
   - b. stratum granulosum, stratum corneum, and stratum basale
   - c. stratum basale, stratum corneum, and stratum granulosum
   - d. stratum basale, stratum granulosum, and stratum corneum

4. The primary purpose of _____ is to absorb UV radiation to prevent damage to underlying cells.
   - a. carotene
   - b. melanin
   - c. lipocytes
   - d. follicles

5. Factors influencing skin color include all of the following *except* _____.
   - a. genetics
   - b. environment
   - c. gender
   - d. physiology

6. The correct meaning of the word part *derm-* is _____.
   - a. horn
   - b. black
   - c. skin
   - d. carotene

7. The word part _____ means "hair."
   - a. trich-
   - b. unguo-
   - c. onych-
   - d. scler-

8. The word part *hidr-* refers to _____.
   - a. water
   - b. sweat
   - c. tissue
   - d. a and b

9. The stratum lucidum is _____.
   - a. an extra layer found covering the eyes
   - b. another skin layer that occurs only in some people
   - c. a very thick layer of skin that develops during puberty
   - d. a clear layer located on palms and soles of feet

10. _____ occur as a result of weight gain.
    - a. Turgor
    - b. Tinea
    - c. Bullae
    - d. Striae

11. _____ is an inflammation of the hair follicle and associated sebaceous glands.
    - a. Acne
    - b. Pruritus
    - c. Stratum
    - d. Vitiligo

12. Excessive cell growth is termed _____.
    - a. hirsutism
    - b. seborrhea
    - c. hyperplasia
    - d. atopy

13. The term that means "genetically determined" is _____.
    - a. bullae
    - b. atopy
    - c. abscess
    - d. root

14. The skin is an organ because _____.
    a. there are so many different types
    b. it is composed of two or more kinds of tissue
    c. it is very large
    d. it covers the entire body surface

15. Melanin is important because it _____.
    a. filters UV radiation, thereby preventing damage to underlying tissue
    b. darkens the skin, thereby deterring microbial activity
    c. aids in absorbing nutrients, thus keeping the skin healthy
    d. screens the body of toxins that would otherwise penetrate its surface

16. The skin's outermost layer is fully keratinized, giving it the name _____ corneum.
    a. vesicle
    b. alopecia
    c. stratum
    d. nevi

17. The eponychium can best be described as the _____.
    a. cuticle
    b. nail bed
    c. soft tissue surrounding the nail plate
    d. distal free edge

18. Leaking out of tissues is termed _____.
    a. rosacea
    b. epidermolysis
    c. excoriation
    d. exudative

19. _____ glands are important for _____.
    a. Biopsy; secreting fluids for mating purposes
    b. Keloid; producing oils to keep the skin soft and pliable
    c. Sweat; heat regulation
    d. Sudoriferous; vitamin regulation

20. A tissue injury that occurs by contact with thermal, radioactive, chemical, or electrical agents is termed a/an _____.
    a. bulla
    b. vesicle
    c. acne
    d. burn

21. Temperature homeostasis suggests that the _____.
    a. body's internal temperature is satisfactory relative to the outside temperature
    b. body cannot keep up with the demands placed on it
    c. skin is capable of producing chemicals
    d. body temperature never fluctuates

Word Parts Exercises

Define the following word parts.

22. lip- _____

23. dermato- _____

24. xero- _____

25. melano- _____

26. papulo- _____

Provide a word part for each meaning.

27. tissue = _____

28. yellow = _____

Matching Exercises

Match the following terms with the correct definition. Each term is used only once.

29. The _____ is the skin layer beneath the epidermis.

30. This layer below the dermis is also called the subcutaneous layer. _____

31. A dark pigment, _____, is produced by melanocytes.

32. Tissue injury that results from heat, radiation, chemical, or electrical agents is termed a _____.

33. The medical term for excessive hair is _____.

34. Pigment-producing cells are termed _____.

35. An unusually hard, elevated scar is termed a _____.

36. The _____ glands produce sebum.

37. Another term for swelling is _____.

38. When the _____ contract, goose bumps result.

39. The _____ is the white, moon-shaped growth area of nails.

40. A small, discolored skin spot is termed a _____.

a. burn
b. keloid
c. sebaceous
d. arrector pili muscles
e. melanocytes
f. lunula
g. hypodermis
h. edema
i. melanin
j. hypertrichosis
k. macule
l. dermis

Match the disorder with its description.

_____ 41. actinic keratosis

_____ 42. alopecia

_____ 43. clavus

_____ 44. carcinoma

_____ 45. decubitus ulcer

a. malignant tumor
b. premalignant warty lesion on the skin that results from chronic exposure to sunlight, a sebaceous gland
c. corn
d. bedsore
e. baldness

Match the sign or symptom with its description.

_____ 46. erythema

_____ 47. pruritus

_____ 48. crusts

_____ 49. bullae

_____ 50. onychia

_____ 51. cyanosis

a. hard coverings that result when exudate dries on the skin
b. patches of redness
c. inflammation of the nail matrix
d. itching
e. blisters
f. bluish skin resulting from a lack of oxygen in the blood

Definitions

Define the following terms.

52. autoimmune disorder = _____

53. cancer = _____

54. first-degree burn = _____

55. lipoma = _____

Provide a medical term for the following definitions.

56. a common wart that appears on the fingers = _____

57. bluish-red, brown tumor that often occurs in patients with AIDS = _____

58. nail biting = _____

59. benign tumor made up of a blood vessel mass = _____

Write the plural form for each term.

60. nevus _____

61. bulla _____

62. papule _____

Spelling

Identify the correctly spelled term in each set.

63. _____
   a. benign
   b. benine
   c. banign
   d. benighn

64. _____
   a. jawndice
   b. jaundice
   c. jaundis
   d. johndice

65. _____
   a. ulcurs
   b. ulcers
   c. ullcerz
   d. allcers

66. _____
   a. pappule
   b. papool
   c. papyule
   d. papule

67. _____
   a. abscess
   b. absess
   c. abcess
   d. absces

Unscramble

Unscramble the letters to form a medical term.

68. vrrauece _____

69. trop neiw aints _____

70. sleahw _____

71. cars _____

72. sshengli _____

Abbreviations

Provide the terms for the abbreviations and then define the terms.

73. bx = _____

74. ABCD = _____

75. I&D = _____

76. SLE = _____

77. UV = _____

Short Answer

. . . .

Answer the following questions.

78. Mrs. Jones appears weak and is thirsty. After her skin is pinched to test its turgor, it does not respond normally. What does this indicate?

_____

79. A family member cannot understand why he is not permitted to visit his brother in the burn unit unless he wears a gown and mask. You explain the reason is because _____.

80. Anna was born with albinism. This places her at increased risk of _____.

81. You have just learned that a friend was diagnosed with purpura urticans and another is cyanotic. You know from your medical terminology class that the person with purpura urticans has _____ dots on the skin, and the person with cyanosis has skin appearing _____ in coloration.

82. Noah has just visited Arizona, and he tells you that 90°F in the desert seems cooler than 90°F in the tropical rain forest. Provide a plausible explanation for this statement.

_____

Labeling

. . . .

Label the structures in the following diagram.

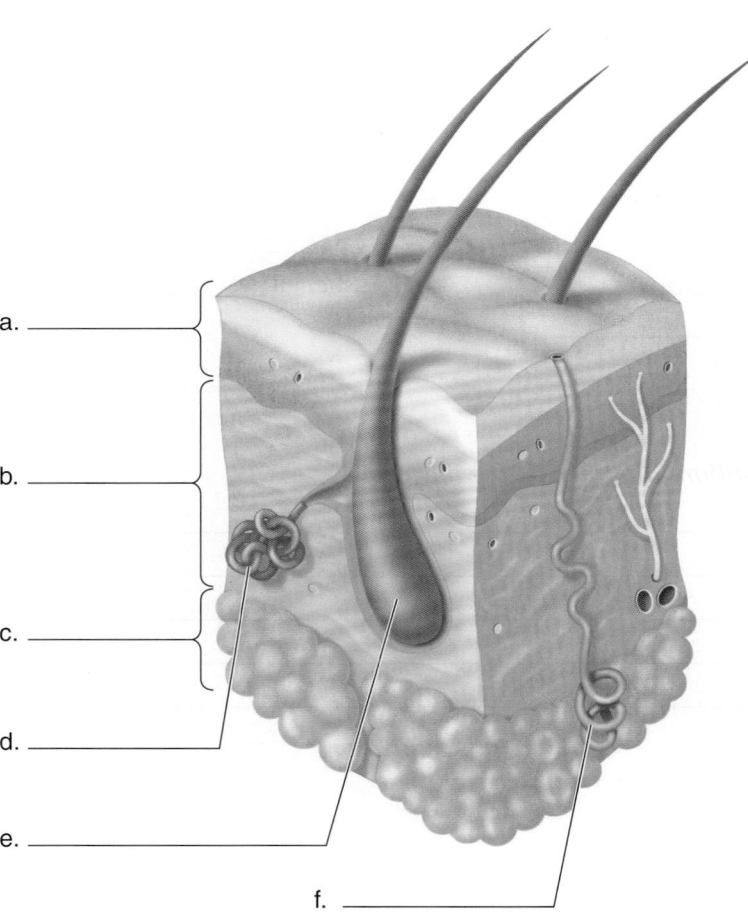

a. _____

b. _____

c. _____

d. _____

e. _____

f. _____

Word Search

Find the medical terms hidden in the puzzle.

X	G	G	M	I	N	Q	T	S	A	I	J	C	M	E	I	C	D
E	B	V	A	A	G	O	I	Q	D	B	O	W	L	J	R	A	E
Y	S	P	S	U	L	M	I	I	Q	L	S	C	E	R	L	Y	R
S	U	U	W	U	R	I	O	S	L	R	I	P	M	M	R	S	M
E	O	W	O	E	D	P	G	A	A	T	G	X	O	A	N	M	A
B	Z	G	D	E	A	O	G	N	U	R	G	H	T	S	V	M	T
A	Z	I	Y	T	N	E	R	C	A	N	B	N	A	Q	A	L	O
C	P	O	H	K	N	A	Y	I	B	N	E	A	M	V	S	F	L
E	S	I	D	E	G	C	T	F	F	M	T	Z	R	T	A	I	O
O	C	E	J	R	H	S	P	U	U	E	B	E	E	D	N	B	G
U	X	S	B	B	P	G	F	G	C	P	R	U	D	N	C	C	Y
S	H	O	A	U	Z	D	E	R	M	A	T	O	P	H	Y	T	E
S	A	P	M	P	M	T	J	N	N	G	J	X	U	O	B	O	R
I	I	I	U	K	N	E	L	C	I	L	L	O	F	S	E	D	P
J	R	D	L	I	P	O	C	Y	T	E	S	K	I	R	P	N	S
M	Q	A	K	E	R	A	T	I	N	N	R	X	K	D	G	C	M
E	E	V	I	T	A	I	L	L	A	P	K	A	S	V	W	S	T
M	V	O	J	N	F	V	L	V	A	P	R	V	B	S	H	O	O

abrasion
adipose
collagen
cutaneous
cuticle
dermatology
dermatome
dermatophyte
epidermis
follicle
hair
idiopathic
integumentary
keratin
lipocytes
malignant
palliative
sebaceous
sebum
sudoriferous

Vocabulary Review

Review the key terms from this chapter, study the spelling and pronunciation of each term, and write its definition in the space provided. Listen to the audio available for most terms at http://thepoint.lww.com/nath2e and pronounce each term for yourself. Then check the box when you feel confident that you know the definition and can pronounce the term correctly.

Key Term	Pronunciation	Definition
❏ **abrasion**	(uh-BRAY-zhun)	_____
❏ **abscess**	(ab-SES)	_____
❏ **acne**	(ACK-nee)	_____
❏ **actinic keratosis**	(ack-TIN-ick ker-uh-TOH-sis)	_____
❏ **adipose**	(AD-i-poce)	_____
❏ **albinism**	(AL-bi-niz-um)	_____
❏ **alopecia**	(al-oh-PEE-shee-uh)	_____
❏ **analgesics**	(an-al-JEE-zicks)	_____

Key Term	Pronunciation	Definition
❏ arrector pili muscles	(a-RECK-tur PYE-lye)	
❏ atopic dermatitis	(ay-TOP-ick dur-muh-TYE-tis)	
❏ atopic eczema	(ay-TOP-ick ECK-zuh-muh)	
❏ atopy	(ah-TUH-pee)	
❏ autoimmune disorder	(aw-toh-i-MEWN)	
❏ basal cell carcinoma	(BAY-sul SELL kahr-si-NOH-muh)	
❏ benign	(be-NINE)	
❏ biopsy	(BYE-op-see)	
❏ bullae	(BULL-ee)	
❏ burn		
❏ callus	(KAL-us)	
❏ cancer		
❏ carbuncle	(KAHR-bunk-ul)	
❏ carcinomas	(kahr-si-NOH-muhs)	
❏ causalgia	(kaw-SAL-jee-uh)	
❏ cellulitis	(sell-yoo-LYE-tis)	
❏ ceruminous glands	(se-ROO-mi-nus)	
❏ chloasma	(kloh-AZ-muh)	
❏ clavus	(KLAY-vus)	
❏ collagen	(KOL-uh-jin)	
❏ comedo	(KOM-ee-doh)	
❏ contact dermatitis	(dur-muh-TYE-tis)	
❏ contusion	(con-TEW-zhun)	
❏ corn		
❏ cradle cap		
❏ crusts		
❏ cryosurgery	(krye-oh-SUR-juh-ree)	
❏ curettage	(kewr-e-TAHZH)	
❏ cutaneous	(kew-TAY-nee-us)	
❏ cutaneous papillomas	(kew-TAY-nee-us pap-i-LOH-muhz)	
❏ cuticle	(KEW-ti-kul)	
❏ cyanosis	(sigh-uh-NOH-sis)	
❏ débridement	(dih-BREED-ment)	
❏ decubitus ulcers	(dee-KEW-bi-tus UL-surs)	
❏ dermatitis	(dur-muh-TYE-tis)	
❏ dermatologist	(dur-muh-TOL-uh-jist)	
❏ dermatology	(dur-muh-TOL-uh-jee)	
❏ dermatome	(DUR-muh-tome)	
❏ dermatomyositis	(dur-muh-toh-migh-oh-SIGH-tis)	

Key Term	Pronunciation	Definition
❑ **dermatophyte**	(der-MAT-oh-fite)	
❑ **dermatophytoses**	(dur-muh-toh-figh-TOH-seez)	
❑ **dermis**	(DUR-mis)	
❑ **ecchymosis**	(eck-i-MOH-sis)	
❑ **edema**	(e-DEE-muh)	
❑ **elephantiasis**	(el-e-fan-TYE-uh-sis)	
❑ **epidermis**	(ep-i-DER-mis)	
❑ **eponychium**	(ep-oh-NICK-ee-um)	
❑ **erythema**	(er-ih-THEE-mah)	
❑ **exfoliation**	(ecks-foh-lee-AY-shun)	
❑ **exudative**	(ig-zoo-DAY-tiv)	
❑ **first-degree burn**		
❑ **fissures**	(FISH-urz)	
❑ **follicle**	(FOL-i-kul)	
❑ **folliculitis**	(fol-ick-yoo-LYE-tis)	
❑ **free edge**		
❑ **furuncle**	(FEW-rung-kul)	
❑ **gangrene**	(GANG-green)	
❑ **hair**		
❑ **hemangioma**	(hee-man-jee-OH-muh)	
❑ **herpes zoster**	(HUR-peez ZOS-tur)	
❑ **hidrosis**	(high-DROH-sis)	
❑ **hirsutism**	(HER-soot-izm)	
❑ **hyperplasia**	(high-pur-PLAY-zhuh)	
❑ **hypertrichosis**	(high-pur-tri-KOH-sis)	
❑ **hypodermis**	(high-poh-DER-mis)	
❑ **ichthyosis**	(ick-thee-OH-sis)	
❑ **idiopathic**	(id-ee-OH-path-ick)	
❑ **impetigo**	(im-pe-TYE-goh)	
❑ **incision and drainage (I&D)**		
❑ **integumentary system**	(in-teg-yoo-MEN-tuh-ree SIS-tem)	
❑ **jaundice**	(JAWN-dis)	
❑ **Kaposi sarcoma**	(KAH-poh-zee sahr-KOH-muh)	
❑ **keloid**	(KEE-loid)	
❑ **keratin**	(KERR-uh-tin)	
❑ **keratinization**	(kerr-uh-tin-i-ZAY-shun)	
❑ **lesions**	(LEE-zhunz)	
❑ **leukoderma**	(lew-koh-DUR-muh)	
❑ **lipocytes**	(LIP-oh-sights)	

Key Term	Pronunciation	Definition
❏ lipoma	(li-POH-muh)	_____
❏ lunula	(LOO-new-luh)	_____
❏ macule	(MACK-yool)	_____
❏ malignant	(muh-LIG-nunt)	_____
❏ malignant melanoma	(muh-LIG-nunt mel-uh-NOH-muh)	_____
❏ melanin	(MEL-uh-nin)	_____
❏ melanocytes	(me-LAN-oh-sites)	_____
❏ melanoma	(mel-uh-NOH-muh)	_____
❏ Mohs surgery	(MOHZ)	_____
❏ nail bed		_____
❏ nail body		_____
❏ nail root		_____
❏ nails		_____
❏ necrosis	(ne-KROH-sis)	_____
❏ nevi	(NEE-vigh)	_____
❏ nodules	(NOD-yoolz)	_____
❏ onychia	(oh-NICK-ee-uh)	_____
❏ onychomycosis	(on-i-koh-migh-KOH-sis)	_____
❏ onychophagia	(on-i-koh-FAY-jee-uh)	_____
❏ pachyderma	(pack-i-DUR-muh)	_____
❏ palliative	(PAL-ee-uh-tiv)	_____
❏ papule	(PAP-yool)	_____
❏ pediculosis	(pe-dick-yoo-LOH-sis)	_____
❏ pediculosis capitis	(pe-dick-yoo-LOH-sis KAP-i-tis)	_____
❏ pemphigus	(PEM-fi-gus)	_____
❏ petechiae	(pee-TEE-kee-uh)	_____
❏ plantar wart		_____
❏ pores		_____
❏ port wine stain		_____
❏ premalignant	(PREE-muh-LIG-nunt)	_____
❏ pruritus	(proo-RYE-tus)	_____
❏ psoriasis	(soh-RYE-uh-sis)	_____
❏ purpura	(PUR-pew-ruh)	_____
❏ pustules	(PUS-tyoolz)	_____
❏ rhinophyma	(rye-noh-FIH-muh)	_____
❏ root (hair)		_____
❏ rosacea	(roh-ZAY-shee-uh)	_____
❏ rubella	(roo-BEL-uh)	_____
❏ scabies	(SKAY-beez)	_____

Key Term	Pronunciation	Definition
❏ scar		_____
❏ scleroderma	(skleer-oh-DUR-muh)	_____
❏ sebaceous cysts	(se-BAY-shus SISTS)	_____
❏ sebaceous glands	(se-BAY-shus)	_____
❏ seborrhea	(seb-oh-REE-uh)	_____
❏ seborrheic dermatitis	(seb-oh-REE-ick dur-muh-TYE-tis)	_____
❏ seborrheic keratosis	(seb-oh-REE-ick kerr-uh-TOH-sis)	_____
❏ sebum	(SEE-bum)	_____
❏ second-degree burn		_____
❏ shaft		_____
❏ shingles		_____
❏ squamous cell carcinoma	(SKWAY-mus SELL kahr-si-NOH-muh)	_____
❏ strata	(STRA-tuh)	_____
❏ strawberry hemangioma	(he-man-jee-OH-muh)	_____
❏ striae	(STRYE-ee)	_____
❏ subcutaneous layer	(sub-kew-TAY-nee-us)	_____
❏ sudoriferous glands	(sue-dur-IF-ur-us)	_____
❏ sweat glands		_____
❏ systemic lupus erythematosus (SLE)	(LOO-pus er-ih-thee-mah-TOH-sus)	_____
❏ third-degree burn		_____
❏ tinea	(TIN-ee-uh)	_____
❏ tinea capitis	(TIN-ee-uh KAP-i-tis)	_____
❏ tinea corporis	(TIN-ee-uh KOR-po-ris)	_____
❏ tinea pedis	(TIN-ee-uh PED-is)	_____
❏ tinea unguium	(TIN-ee-uh UNG-gwee-um)	_____
❏ turgor	(TUR-gur)	_____
❏ ulcers	(UL-surz)	_____
❏ urticaria	(ur-tih-KAHR-ee-ah)	_____
❏ varicella	(vair-i-SELL-uh)	_____
❏ verruca vulgaris	(ve-ROO-kuh vul-GAIR-us)	_____
❏ verrucae	(ve-ROO-kee)	_____
❏ vesicles	(VES-i-kuls)	_____
❏ vitiligo	(vit-i-LYE-go)	_____
❏ wheals	(WHEELZ)	_____
❏ xeroderma	(zeer-oh-DUR-muh)	_____

Answers

Word Grouping Exercises

Definition	Word Part	Definition	Word Part
beneath	sub-	hardness	sclera-, sclero-
black	melan-, melano-	horny tissue or cornea	kerat-, kerato-
blue	cyan-, cyano-	pimple, circumscribed solid elevation	papulo-
cell	cyt-, -cyte, cyto-	plants	phyt-, phyto-
cold	cry-, cryo-	pus accumulation	pyo-
color	chrom-, chromat-, chromato-, -chrome, chromo-	red or red blood cell	erythr-, erythro-
death	necr-, necro-	sebum (oil)	seb-, sebi-, sebo-
disease	path-, -pathy-, patho-	self	aut-, auto-
dry	xero-	skin	derm-, derma-, dermat-, dermato-, dermo-
epidermal scale	squamo-	sweat	A. hidr-, hidro B. sudor-
fat	adip-, adipo-	tissue	histio-, histo-
fatty	lip-, lipo-	tumor	-oma
fingernail or toenail	onych-, onycho-	vesicle, blister	vesic-, vesico-, vesiculo-
fish	ichthyo-	wax	cero-
flowing	-rrhea	white or white blood cell	leuc-, leuco-, leuk-, leuko-
formation	-plasia	yellow	xanth-, xantho-
fungus	myco-		
hair	A. pilo- B. trich-, trichi-, tricho-		

Word Building Exercises

Word Part	Meaning	Common or Known Word	Example Medical Term
adip-, adipo-	fat	adipose	adipocytes
aut-, auto-	self	automobile	autoimmune
cyt-, -cyte, cyto-	cell	cytoplast	erythrocyte
derm-, derma-, dermat-, -dermato-, dermo-	skin	dermis	epidermis
erythr-, erythro-	red or red blood cell	erythrocyte	erythrocyte
histio-, histo-	tissue	histology	histology
lip-, lipo-	fatty	lipid	liposuction
melan-, melano-	black	melanin	melanocyte

Word Part	Meaning	Common or Known Word	Example Medical Term
path-, patho-, -pathy	disease	pathology	pathophysiology
-rrhea	flowing	diarrhea	seborrhea
scler-, sclero-	hardness	sclera	scleroderma
sub-	beneath	submarine	subcutaneous
vesic-, vesico-, vesiculo-	vesicle, blister	vesicle	vesicle

Key Term Practice

Integumentary System Preview

1. keratin
2. cutaneous
3. sebaceous gland
4. dermatology
5. melanocytes; *melano-*; *-cyte*

Skin Layers

1. epidermis
2. subcutaneous
3. dermis
4. A. stratum; B. strata
5. adipocytes; *adipo-*; *-cytes*

Skin Color and Birthmarks

1. albinism
2. cyanosis
3. jaundice
4. papule
5. nevi

Hair

1. root; shaft; follicle
2. arrector pili

Glands

1. comedo
2. hidrosis; *hidro-*
3. ceruminous glands
4. pores

Nails

1. free edge
2. lunula
3. cuticle; onych-
4. onychophagia
5. nail root

Skin Conditions

1. causalgia
2. exfoliation
3. petechiae
4. edema
5. contusion

Burns

1. tissue injury as a result of contact with a thermal, radioactive, chemical, or electrical agent.
2. first-degree (superficial) burn; second-degree (partial-thickness) burn; third-degree (full-thickness) burn
3. scar

Alopecia

1. alopecia

Autoimmune Disorders

1. scleroderma
2. dermatomyositis
3. biopsy
4. psoriasis
5. autoimmune disorder

Noncancerous Tumors

1. benign
2. lipoma
3. actinic keratosis
4. keloid
5. hemangioma; *hemo-*

Cancerous Tumors

1. malignant melanoma
2. carcinomas
3. crusts
4. basal cell carcinoma
5. squamous cell carcinoma

Carbuncles and Furuncles

1. incision and drainage
2. furuncle
3. carbuncle
4. abscess

Corn (Clavus) and Callus

1. clavus or corn
2. calluse

Decubitus Ulcers

1. decubitus ulcer
2. débridement
3. ulcers
4. necrosis and gangrene

Dermatitis

1. dermatitis
2. idiopathic
3. cradle cap
4. atopic dermatitis
5. urticaria
6. wheal

Dermatophytosis

1. dermatophytoses
2. tinea
3. tinea capitis
4. tinea pedis
5. fissures

Cellulitis

1. cellulitis
2. analgesics

Hair, Follicle, and Gland Disorders

1. folliculitis
2. hypertrichosis
3. hirsutism
4. seborrhea
5. rosacea

Infectious Diseases

1. dermatome
2. scabies
3. capitis
4. verrucae
5. herpes zoster or shingles

Nail Disorders

1. onychomycosis
2. onychia

Pigment Disorders

1. vitiligo
2. leukoderma; *leuko-; -derma*
3. chloasma
4. ecchymosis

Common Abbreviations Exercises

1. ABCD = asymmetry, border, color, diameter
2. VZV = varicella-zoster virus
3. ultraviolet = UV
4. AIDS = acquired immunodeficiency syndrome
5. SLE = systemic lupus erythematosus

Case Study

1. a is the correct answer.
   - b is incorrect because the dermatologist is better trained in skin diseases.
   - c is incorrect because a pathologist's job is studying the actual tissue samples; patient care is reserved for the dermatologist.
   - d is incorrect because cytotechnologists are involved with the laboratory side of patient care and are not trained physicians.
2. c is the correct answer.
   - a, b, and d are incorrect because the shape, color, elevation, and irritation were all abnormal. Time is not necessarily a factor.
3. a is the correct answer.
   - b is incorrect because cyanosis refers to a blue color.
   - c is incorrect because small, fluid-filled raised areas are termed pustules.
   - d is incorrect because erythematous refers to a structure that is red, not hard.
4. c is the correct answer.
   - a, b, and d are all incorrect because sun-exposed skin should be protected. There is an increased risk of nonmalignant and malignant tumors in individuals who regularly engage in outdoor activities without applying skin protection.
5. a is the correct answer.
   - b is incorrect because it describes squamous cell carcinoma.
   - c is incorrect because it describes Kaposi sarcoma.
   - d is incorrect because basal cell carcinoma does require medical treatment for its excision.
6. d is the correct answer.
   - a is incorrect because cultures will be viewed microscopically.
   - b is incorrect because *excision* means it will be removed.
   - c is incorrect. Although cell cultures may be grown on agar in a Petri plate, the "pathological examination" portion of the question indicates that the cells will be professionally evaluated.

Real World Report

1. A new growth of abnormal cells. The word part *neo-* means "new."
2. a. excessive or above normal; b. horn or hard; c. diseased condition of; d. hypertrophy (excessive cells) of the horny layer of skin
3. atrophic
4. The outer epidermis and the inner dermis are joined together by a polysaccharide gel that "glues" the epidermis to the dermis. This is called the dermal–epidermal junction.
5. b is the correct answer.

Review and Application

1. b	6. c	11. a	16. c
2. a	7. a	12. c	17. a
3. d	8. b	13. b	18. d
4. b	9. d	14. b	19. c
5. c	10. d	15. a	20. d

21. a

22. fat

23. skin

24. dry

25. black

26. pimple

27. histio-, histo-

28. xanth-, xantho-

29. L

30. g

31. i

32. a

33. j

34. e

35. b

36. c

37. h

38. d

39. f

40. k

41. b

42. e

43. c

44. a

45. d

46. b

47. d

48. a

49. e

50. c

51. f

52. autoimmune disorder = a condition in which the immune response is directed against the body

53. cancer = malignant tumor that can lead to death

54. first-degree burn = superficial burn with damage to the epidermis

55. lipoma = benign, fatty tumor

56. verruca vulgaris

57. Kaposi sarcoma

58. onychophagia

59. hemangioma

60. nevi

61. bullae

62. papules

63. a

64. b

65. b

66. d

67. a

68. verrucae

69. port wine stain

70. wheals

71. scar

72. shingles

73. bx = biopsy; excision of live tissue for diagnostic study

74. ABCD = asymmetry, border, color, diameter; system to evaluate a mole's physical appearance to check for skin cancer

75. I&D = incision and drainage; surgical cut to drain fluid from tissue

76. SLE = systemic lupus erythematosus; autoimmune disease of connective tissue; also called lupus

77. UV = ultraviolet; type of radiation that comes from the sun

78. Mrs. Jones is dehydrated and her skin has lost some elastic properties as a result.

79. the skin is the body's first line of defense, and this patient is severely compromised

80. sunburn

81. purple; bluish

82. Sweat evaporates more quickly in the dry, arid desert than in the wet, humid tropics, thus cooling the body faster.

Labeling

a. Epidermis

b. Dermis

c. Subcutaneous layer

d. Sweat gland (in dermis)

e. Hair follicle

f. Sweat gland (in subcutaneous tissue)

Word Search

```
+  +  +  M  +  N  +  +  S  +  I  +  C  +  E  +  +  D
+  +  +  +  A  +  O  I  +  D  +  O  +  L  +  +  +  E
+  S  +  S  +  L  M  I  I  +  L  +  C  E  +  +  Y  R
S  +  U  +  U  R  I  O  S  L  +  I  +  M  +  R  +  M
E  +  +  O  E  D  P  G  A  A  T  +  +  O  A  +  +  A
B  +  +  D  E  A  O  G  N  U  R  +  +  T  +  +  +  T
A  +  I  +  T  N  E  R  C  A  +  B  N  A  +  +  +  O
C  P  +  H  +  N  A  +  I  +  N  E  A  M  +  +  +  L
E  S  I  +  +  +  T  +  F  M  T  +  R  +  +  +  +  O
O  C  E  +  +  +  +  +  U  U  E  +  +  E  +  +  +  G
U  +  S  B  +  +  +  +  G  C  +  R  +  D  +  +  +  Y
S  H  O  +  U  +  D  E  R  M  A  T  O  P  H  Y  T  E
+  A  P  +  +  M  T  +  +  +  +  +  +  U  +  +  +  +
+  I  I  +  +  N  E  L  C  I  L  L  O  F  S  +  +  +
+  R  D  L  I  P  O  C  Y  T  E  S  +  +  +  +  +  +
+  +  A  K  E  R  A  T  I  N  +  +  +  +  +  +  +  +
+  E  V  I  T  A  I  L  L  A  P  +  +  +  +  +  +  +
+  +  +  +  +  +  +  +  +  +  +  +  +  +  +  +  +  +
```

abrasion
adipose
collagen
cutaneous
cuticle
dermatology
dermatome
dermatophyte
epidermis
follicle
hair
idiopathic
integumentary
keratin
lipocytes
malignant
palliative
sebaceous
sebum
sudoriferous

Vocabulary Review

Key Term	Definition	Key Term	Definition
abrasion	damaged skin caused by scraping or rubbing	**atopic dermatitis**	a genetically determined inflammatory allergic skin disorder characterized by itching; also called atopic eczema
abscess	furuncle involving hair follicles and adjacent tissue		
acne	inflammation of the hair follicle and associated sebaceous glands	**atopic eczema**	a genetically determined inflammatory allergic skin disorder characterized by itching; also called atopic dermatitis
actinic keratosis	premalignant warty lesion on the skin that results from chronic exposure to sunlight		
		atopy	genetically determined
adipose	fat	**autoimmune disorder**	condition in which the immune response is directed against the body
albinism	hereditary absence of melanin		
alopecia	baldness or hair loss		
analgesics	drugs that relieve pain	**basal cell carcinoma**	cancer of the basal cell layer
arrector pili muscles	bundles of smooth muscle cells attached to hair follicles that cause goose bumps when contracted	**benign**	not malignant; noncancerous
		biopsy	excision of live tissue for diagnostic study

Key Term	Definition	Key Term	Definition
bullae	blisters	débridement	removal of dead tissue to expose healthy tissue and allow the wound to heal
burn	tissue reaction as a result of thermal, radioactive, chemical, or electrical exposure	decubitus ulcers	pressure sores or bedsores
callus	thickening of epithelial tissue resulting from overuse	dermatitis	skin inflammation
		dermatologist	physician specializing in skin and the integumentary system
cancer	malignant tumor that can lead to death	dermatology	the study of skin
carbuncle	large furuncle	dermatome	area of skin supplied by a peripheral nerve
carcinomas	malignant tumors arising from the epithelial layer of the skin (or other organs)	dermatomyositis	autoimmune disease characterized by inflammation of skin and muscles
causalgia	persistent burning sensation caused by nerve damage	dermatophyte	pathogenic fungus
cellulitis	inflammation of the skin and subcutaneous tissue caused by a bacterial infection	dermatophytoses	skin infections caused by fungi
		dermis	middle layer of skin, below the epidermis
ceruminous glands	glands that secrete cerumen (earwax)	ecchymosis	discoloration because of a ruptured blood vessel
chloasma	hyperpigmentation caused by hormonal factors	edema	swelling
		elephantiasis	abnormally thick skin and edema caused by a filarial worm infection
clavus	small, painful area of thickened skin, usually on the toe; also called a corn	epidermis	superficial skin layer
collagen	fibrous protein	eponychium	fold of skin near the nail root; also called the cuticle
comedo	blackhead	erythema	redness on the skin
contact dermatitis	skin inflammation caused by an irritant coming in contact with the skin	exfoliation	peeling and shedding of the epidermis
contusion	bruise	exudative	leaking out of tissues
corn	small, painful area of thickened skin, usually on the toe; also called a clavus	first-degree burn	superficial burn with damage to the epidermis
		fissures	cracks in the skin
cradle cap	seborrheic dermatitis in infants	follicle	tube-like depression containing the hair root
crusts	hard coverings that result when exudate dries on the skin	folliculitis	inflammation of the hair follicles that produces small boils
cryosurgery	localized freezing of diseased tissues for surgical removal	free edge	portion of the nail growing beyond the tips of fingers or toes
curettage	surgical procedure in which tissue is scraped away using a curet	furuncle	a boil
		gangrene	necrosis due to obstruction or diminished blood supply; also called mortification
cutaneous	relating to the skin		
cutaneous papillomas	skin tags	hair	keratinized filaments covering the body
cuticle	fold of skin near the nail root; also called the eponychium	hemangioma	benign tumor made up of a blood vessel mass
cyanosis	bluish skin resulting from a lack of oxygen in the blood		

Key Term	Definition	Key Term	Definition
herpes zoster	disease caused by reactivation of the varicella-zoster virus (VZV); also called shingles	nail bed	epithelial tissue on which the nail rests
hidrosis	sweating	nail body	main part of the nail
hirsutism	excessive body hair, especially in women	nail root	nail part beneath the cuticle
hyperplasia	excessive cell growth	nails	protective coverings on the fingers and toes
hypertrichosis	excessive growth of normal hair	necrosis	death of one or more cells, or of a portion of tissue or organ, resulting from irreversible damage
hypodermis	innermost skin layer; also called the subcutaneous layer	nevi	medical term for moles
ichthyosis	hereditary skin condition giving the appearance of scales	nodules	deep, boil-like structures
idiopathic	of unknown cause	onychia	inflammation of the nail matrix
impetigo	contagious skin condition caused by streptococcal or staphylococcal bacteria	onychomycosis	fungal infection of the nail
		onychophagia	nail biting
		pachyderma	abnormally thick skin
incision and drainage (I&D)	surgical cut to drain fluid from tissue	palliative	relieving or soothing without eliminating the cause
integumentary system	skin and its associated hair, nails, and glands	papule	solid, round skin elevation
		pediculosis	skin disease caused by lice
jaundice	yellowish skin resulting from bilirubin accumulation	pediculosis capitis	lice infestation on the head
Kaposi sarcoma	bluish-red, brown tumor occurring often in patients with AIDS	pemphigus	nonspecific term for blistering skin diseases
keloid	an area of irregular fibrous tissue that develops at the site of a scar	petechiae	spots on skin that result from bleeding
keratin	tough protein associated with hair and nails	plantar wart	wart on the foot
		pores	openings
keratinization	formation of keratin and the horny layer	port wine stain	large, reddish birthmark
		premalignant	precancerous
lesions	structural or functional alterations	pruritus	itching
leukoderma	absence of pigment	psoriasis	chronic, inflammatory autoimmune skin disease characterized by red, itchy, scaly patches
lipocytes	fat cells		
lipoma	benign, fatty tumor	purpura	condition with purple skin hemorrhages
lunula	white, moon-shaped growth area of nail near the root	pustules	skin elevations containing pus
		rhinophyma	form of rosacea affecting the nose
macule	small, discolored skin spot	root	hair portion embedded in the hair follicle that attaches the hair to the skin
malignant	having a tendency to spread, endangering health or life		
malignant melanoma	cancer of the melanocytes, typically rapidly spreading	rosacea	recurring inflammatory disorder characterized by redness on the cheeks, forehead, nose, and chin that results from dilation of capillaries and follicles
melanin	dark brown to black pigment produced by cells called melanocytes		
melanocytes	cells that produce the pigment melanin	rubella	a contagious infection caused by the rubella virus; also called German measles
melanoma	cancer of melanocytes		
Mohs surgery	microscopically controlled surgery using zinc oxide paste to remove skin layers	scabies	skin disease with itching caused by mites

Key Term	Definition	Key Term	Definition
scar	a permanent mark that forms where a wound heals	systemic lupus erythematosus (SLE)	autoimmune disease of connective tissue; also called lupus
scleroderma	autoimmune disease characterized by increased collagen formation in connective tissues	third-degree burn	full-thickness burn, with damage to epidermis and dermis and some underlying muscle and nerves
sebaceous cysts	fluid-filled sebaceous glands	tinea	fungal infection; commonly called ringworm
sebaceous glands	structures that secrete oil		
seborrhea	disease of the sebaceous glands involving excessive sebum secretion	tinea capitis	ringworm of the scalp
		tinea corporis	ringworm anywhere on the body
seborrheic dermatitis	inflammation of the skin at the sebaceous glands	tinea pedis	ringworm of the foot; commonly called athlete's foot
seborrheic keratosis	benign purple-brown skin tumor	tinea unguium	ringworm of the nails
sebum	oil	turgor	normal skin tension
second-degree burn	partial-thickness burn with damage to the epidermis and dermis	ulcers	sores that result from destruction of epithelial tissue
shaft	visible portion of the hair	urticaria	rash of round, red welts on the skin that itch; also called hives
shingles	disease caused by reactivation of the varicella-zoster virus (VZV); also called herpes zoster	varicella	contagious disease caused by the varicella-zoster virus; also called chickenpox
squamous cell carcinoma	cancer that develops in the epidermis	verruca vulgaris	common wart that occurs on the fingers
strata	layers	verrucae	warts caused by the human papillomavirus
strawberry hemangioma	raised, reddish purple birthmark that usually disappears without treatment around age 7	vesicles	blisters that leak fluid
striae	stretch marks	vitiligo	skin disease characterized by white patches on otherwise normal pigmented skin
subcutaneous layer	innermost skin layer; also called the hypodermis		
sudoriferous glands	glands that secrete sweat; also called sweat glands	wheals	rash of round, red welts
		xeroderma	extremely dry skin
sweat glands	glands that secrete sweat; also called sudoriferous glands		

CHAPTER 5

Skeletal System: Bones and Joints

OBJECTIVES

After completing this chapter, you should be able to:

1. State the meanings of word parts related to bones and joints.

2. Identify the parts of a typical long bone correctly.

3. Describe the classifications and types of bones.

4. Identify the major bones of the human skeleton.

5. State the structural and functional classifications of articulations.

6. Use terms describing movements at joints correctly.

7. Describe various signs, symptoms, clinical tests, diagnostic procedures, and treatments of common bone and joint disorders.

8. Specify anatomic and physiological alterations in the bones and joints throughout the lifespan.

9. Define common abbreviations related to bones and joints.

10. Define, spell, and pronounce the chapter's medical terms correctly.

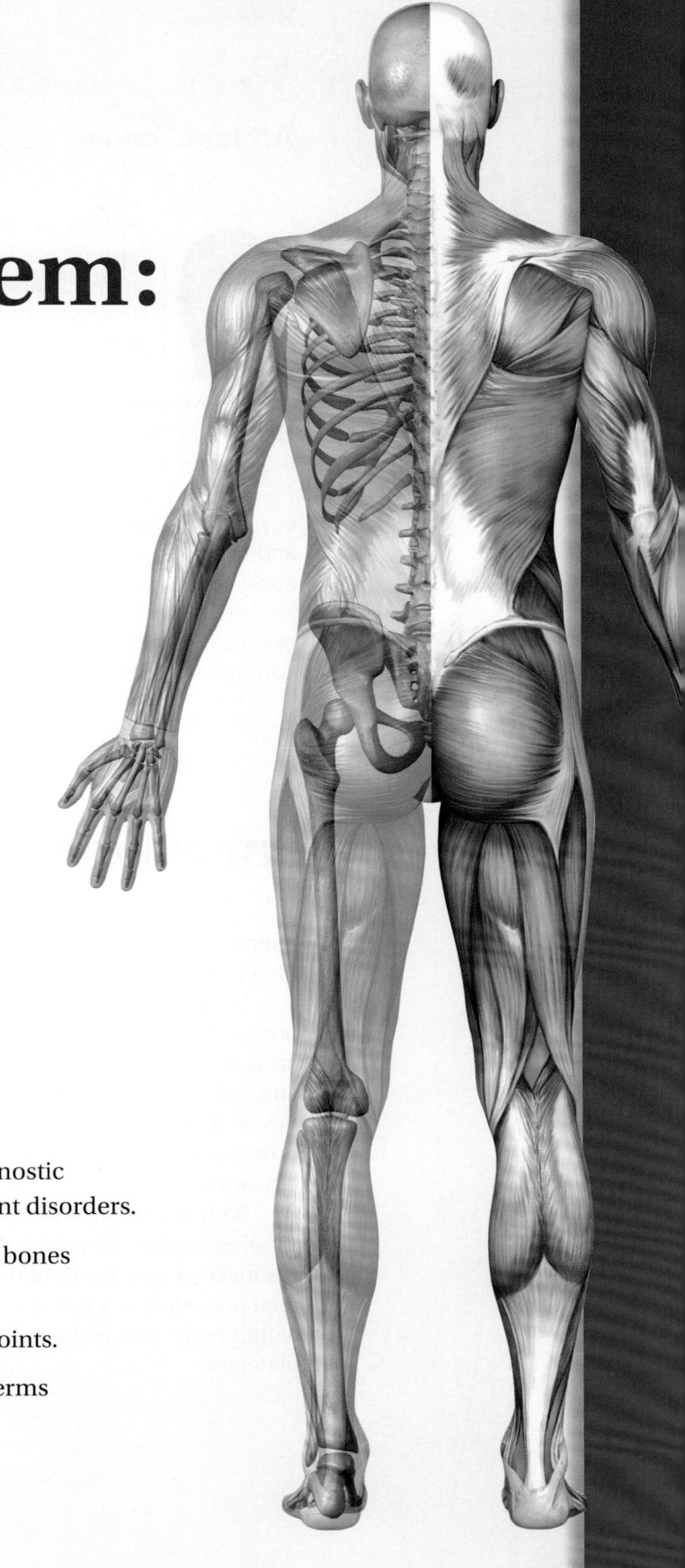

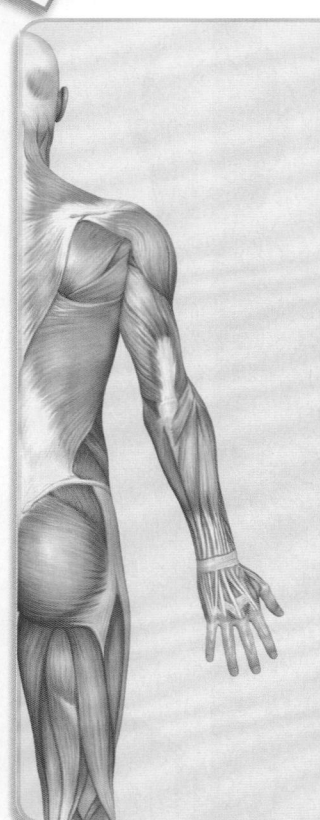

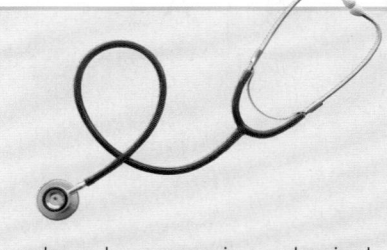

Professional Profile

Athletic Trainer

Paul is an athletic trainer at a university, where he supervises physical sports. He has been a trainer for 5 years, providing first aid; treating minor injuries; supporting medical services; and developing comprehensive nutritional, exercise, and postrehabilitation programs for his school's athletes.

To be an athletic trainer, Paul completed a 4-year undergraduate degree in exercise science. After graduating with a bachelor's degree, he became certified by the National Athletic Trainers Association. His university's internal policy also requires certification in cardiopulmonary resuscitation (CPR).

Working with athletes is exciting because the athletic trainer is called into action any time a player sustains an injury. On-the-job training provides valuable experience, and wrapping ankles, wrists, arms, and legs; using gauze and tape; cleaning wounds; applying therapeutic wraps; and operating braces and guards all become second nature.

Physical damage to the body, especially to the joints, is expected for football players during their season. In fact, injuries to the tibiofemoral articulation (knee joint) commonly occur on the field of play and are assessed first by the athletic trainer.

INTRODUCTION TO THE SKELETAL SYSTEM

The skeletal system plays several important roles in the body. Its functions include maintaining posture, protecting organs, moving the body, storing minerals, and producing blood cells (hemopoiesis). These functions also support other body systems.

Made of osseous (bone) tissue, bones create the body's fundamental framework. The bones of the feet, legs, pelvis, and backbone carry the weight of the body. The bones of the arms help with balance. Bones also provide stiff attachment points for muscles, soft tissues, and organs. The skeletal system protects many vital organs by encasing them. For example, the skull and vertebrae enclose the brain and spinal cord, the rib cage and shoulder girdle protect the organs in the chest, and the pelvic girdle shields the reproductive organs and other structures.

Body movement results from the contraction of muscles anchored to bones at joints. Another key function of the skeletal system is mineral storage. In fact, calcium and phosphorus make up two-thirds of bone by weight. Moreover, 95% of calcium and 90% of the body's total phosphorus is found in our bones and teeth. Finally, blood cell production takes place within bone tissue: The red bone marrow produces red blood cells, white blood cells, and platelets.

The interconnectedness of the body's systems is particularly evident when we consider the skeletal system. For example, bone is dynamic. In a cyclic process called remodeling, bone is resorbed and formed at the same time. This process works with the endocrine system to regulate the body's hormonal and mineral balance.

MEDICAL TERM PARTS: BONES

Word Parts: Bones

Medical term prefixes, suffixes, and combining forms related to the skeletal system are introduced in this section.

Word Part	Meaning
-blast	immature precursor cell
calc-, calci-	calcium
calcaneo-	calcaneus
carpo-	carpus (wrist), carpal
chondrio-, chondro-	cartilage
-clast	something that breaks; to break
costo-	rib
crani-, cranio-	cranium
ethmo-	ethmoid bone
femor-	thigh
hyo-	U-shaped
ilio-	ilium
meato-	passage
myel-, myelo-	bone marrow
orth-, ortho-	straight
osseo-, ossi-	bone
ost-, oste-, osteo-	bone
pelvi-, pelvio-, pelvo-	pelvis
pubo-	pubic
scapulo-	scapula, scapular, shoulder blade
spondyl-, spondylo-	vertebrae
stern-, sterno-	sternum, sternal, chest
tars-, tarso-	tarsus
tibio-	tibia, shin bone
vertebro-	vertebra, vertebral

Word Grouping Exercises: Bones

Using the *Medical Term Parts* table, identify the prefix, suffix, or combining form for each of the following definitions. The first one has been done as an example.

Definition	Word Part
tibia, shin bone	*tibio-*
bone	A.
	B.
bone marrow	
calcaneus	
calcium	
carpus (wrist), carpal	
cartilage	
cranium	
ethmoid bone	
ilium	
immature precursor cell	
passage	
pelvis	
pubic	
rib	
scapula, scapular, shoulder blade	
something that breaks; to break	
sternum, sternal, chest	
straight	
tarsus	
thigh	
tibia, shin bone	
U-shaped	
vertebra, vertebral	
vertebrae	

Word Building Exercises: Bones

Word parts introduced in the *Medical Term Parts* section are listed in the following table. For this exercise, first supply the meaning of each word part, then use the word part to build a word you already know. The word you list under *Common or Known Word* does not have to be a medical term; a commonly used word is fine. Be sure, however, that the word correctly reflects the intended meaning. The first one has been done as an example. Check your answers in a dictionary.

Word Part	Meaning	Common or Known Word	Example Medical Term
calc-, calci-	*calcium*	*calcium*	calcitonin
carpo-			carpal tunnel syndrome
crani-, cranio-			cranial cavity
orth-, ortho-			orthopedics
osseo-, ossi-			ossification
ost-, oste-, osteo-			osteoblast
vertebro-			vertebral column

ANATOMY AND PHYSIOLOGY: BONES

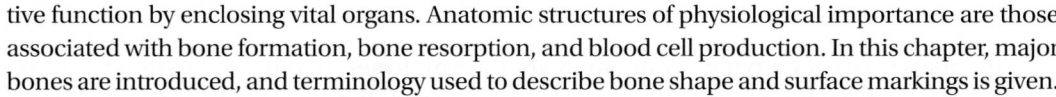

The skeletal system is involved with the movement of the body because it provides attachment sites for muscles at joints. It further serves a protective function by enclosing vital organs. Anatomic structures of physiological importance are those associated with bone formation, bone resorption, and blood cell production. In this chapter, major bones are introduced, and terminology used to describe bone shape and surface markings is given.

Many structures of the skeletal system are known by eponyms or other common names. Such terms are in regular use in the medical fields.

Bone Anatomy

One way bones can be classified is according to their morphology (shape). Different types of bones are shown in **Figure 5-1**. **Long bones**, such as those of the arms and legs, have longitudinal axes and expanded ends. The **short bones** of the wrists and ankles are somewhat cube-like, roughly equal in length and width. Ribs, scapulae, and bones of the skull are **flat bones**, which have a plate-like structure and broad surfaces. The **irregular bones** of the vertebrae and face have a variety of shapes and are often connected to several other bones. Round bones, or **sesamoid bones**, such as the patella (kneecap) are small and develop in a joint. The word *sesamoid* comes from the Greek language and means *shaped like a sesame seed*, whereas the term *patella* is a Latin word that means *small, flat dish*.

After birth, the skull bones grow together and close. During that time, small, irregularly shaped bony sections called **sutural bones** develop between the skull bones. Sutural bones are about the size of a quarter and they resemble jigsaw-puzzle pieces.

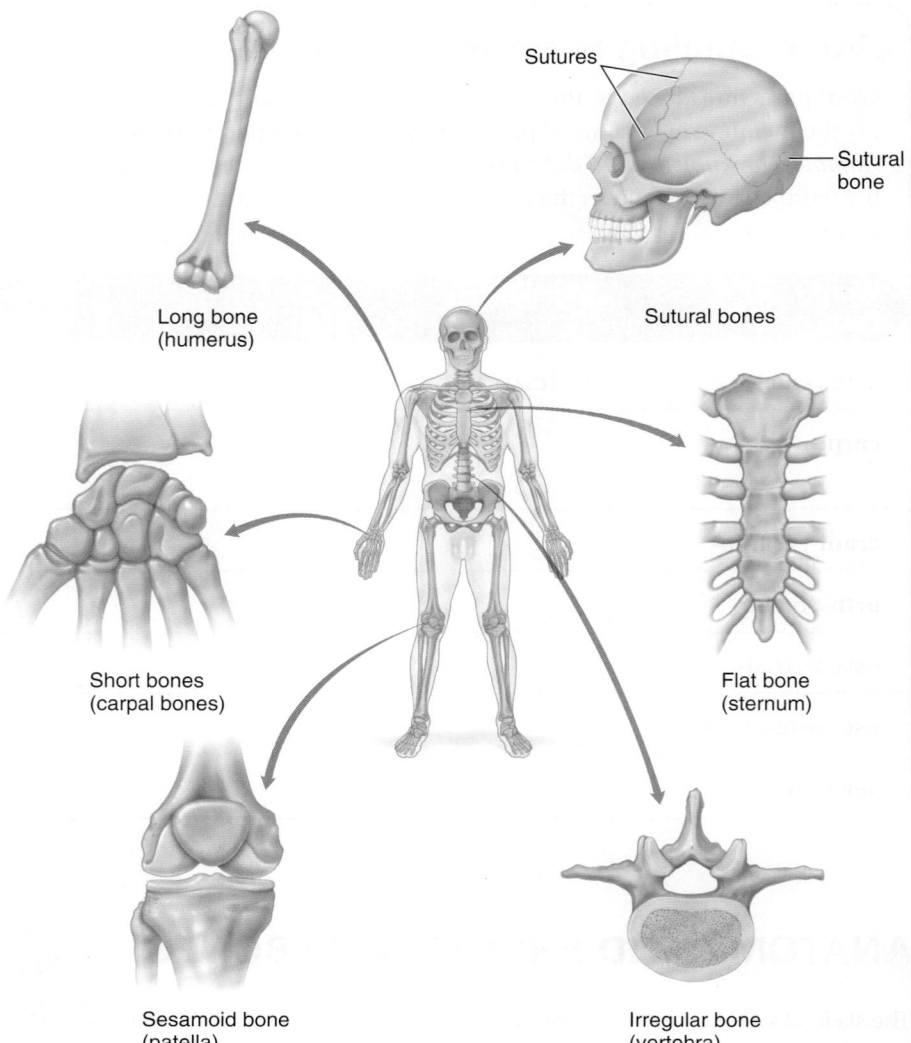

Figure 5-1 Classification of bones.

Long bone
(humerus)

Sutures

Sutural
bone

Sutural bones

Short bones
(carpal bones)

Flat bone
(sternum)

Sesamoid bone
(patella)

Irregular bone
(vertebra)

The major parts of a typical long bone are the epiphyses, diaphysis, medullary cavity, periosteum, and articular cartilage (**Figure 5-2**). (A medullary cavity and periosteum are also found in other bones.) The proximal **epiphysis** is the expanded end of the bone closer to the body's trunk. The shaft of a long bone, providing strong support, is the **diaphysis**. The distal epiphysis is the expanded end of bone farther from the trunk. In essence, the epiphyses cap the ends of long bones. The epiphyses provide attachments for muscle and are the contact points at joints.

The narrow bony region between the diaphysis and the epiphysis is the **metaphysis**. The central cavity within the diaphysis of a long bone, which is occupied by red bone marrow, is called the **medullary cavity**. The **periosteum** is the fibrous membrane that covers the surface of a bone. This membrane covers the bone except where tendons and ligaments attach. Instead of periosteum, the articular (joint) surfaces of bone are protected by articular cartilage.

Articular means pertaining to an articulation, or joint, and **cartilage** is tough connective tissue that lacks a blood supply. It is found throughout the body, notably at joints. **Articular cartilage** is a kind of cartilage that covers the ends of bones at certain joints to help movement and cushion impact.

Based on tissue characteristics, two types of bone exist: compact and spongy. Solid, strong **compact** (or dense) **bone** is found on the bone surface. The walls of diaphyses are composed of this tightly packed tissue. (Tooth enamel is the hardest substance in the body, and compact

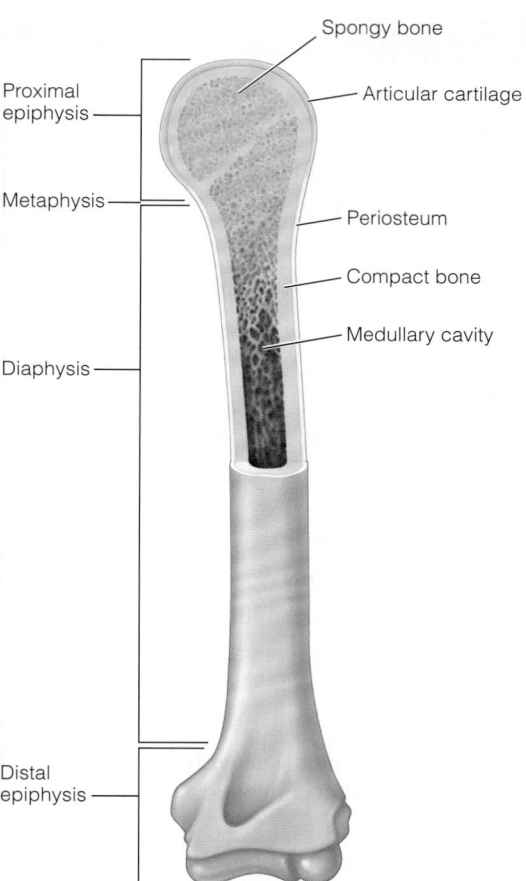

Spongy bone

Proximal
epiphysis

Articular cartilage

Metaphysis

Periosteum

Compact bone

Medullary cavity

Diaphysis

Distal
epiphysis

Figure 5-2 Major parts of a long bone.

bone is the second hardest.) **Spongy bone**, also called cancellous or trabecular bone, consists of a network of struts and plates called **trabeculae**. The branching, lattice-looking trabeculae separate irregular spaces within the spongy portion. These spaces help reduce the weight of the bone and provide strength. Epiphyses are composed largely of spongy bone with thin layers of compact bone on the surface (**Figure 5-3**).

Red bone marrow is blood cell–forming tissue located in spaces of spongy bone and within the medullary cavities of long bones. This marrow is called "red" because of the hemoglobin (the oxygen-carrying pigment) contained within red blood cells.

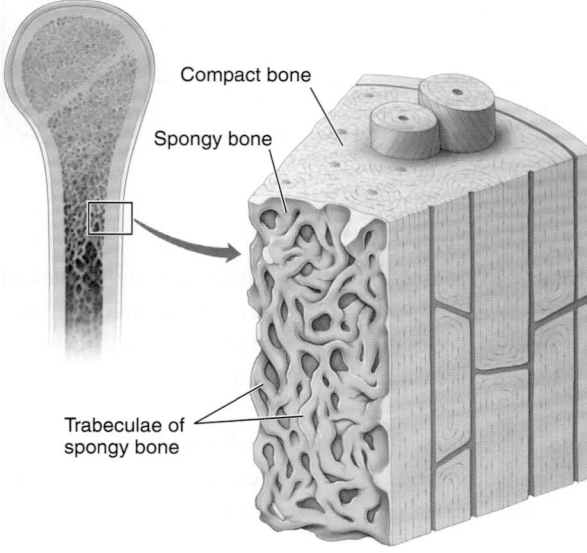

Compact bone

Spongy bone

Trabeculae of
spongy bone

Figure 5-3 Spongy and compact bone.

KEY TERM	Definition
long bones	bones found in arms and legs
short bones	cube-like bones found in wrists and ankles
flat bones	bones found in ribs, scapulae, and skulls
irregular bones	bones found in vertebrae and faces
sesamoid (SES-uh-moid) **bones**	small bones that develop in joints
sutural (SUE-chur-ul) **bones**	irregularly shaped bones between the flat bones of the skull
epiphysis (e-PIF-i-sis)	expanded end of a long bone
diaphysis (dye-AF-i-sis)	shaft of a long bone
metaphysis (me-TAF-i-sis)	section of bone between the epiphysis and the diaphysis of long bones
medullary (MED-yoo-lerr-ee) **cavity**	central canal of a long bone
periosteum (perr-ee-OS-tee-um)	fibrous membrane covering a bone
articular (ahr-TICK-yoo-lur)	pertaining to an articulation (joint)
cartilage (KAHR-ti-lij)	tough connective tissue that lacks a blood supply
articular cartilage	a kind of connective tissue that covers the ends of bones at certain joints
compact bone	solid bone tissue
spongy bone	bone made of a network of bone tissue with irregular spaces in it; also called cancellous bone or trabecular bone
trabeculae (tra-BECK-yoo-lee)	slender columns of bone in spongy bone
red bone marrow	blood cell–forming tissue in bone

KEY TERM PRACTICE: *Bone Anatomy*

1. Name the six classes of bone. _____

2. The term *periosteum* literally means _____.

3. Write the singular and plural forms for the term that means the expanded end of a long bone.

   _____

4. Write the singular and plural forms for the term that means the shaft of a bone. _____

5. Name the two types of bone. _____

Bone Formation

Bone formation is a continuous lifelong process. Bone begins to form during the sixth week of embryonic development. Most of the bones of the skeleton begin as cartilage, which is subsequently replaced by bone tissue. **Ossification** is the conversion of cartilage tissue into bone. Newborns have about 300 separated bones, which later ossify into 206. Square inch per square inch, bone is five times stronger than steel.

   Bone remodeling is a normal, lifelong physiological process in which old bone is destroyed and new bone is formed. It takes place through the combined actions of bone-forming cells called **osteoblasts** and bone-destroying cells called **osteoclasts**. Osteoblasts build bone by depositing a bony matrix around themselves. Osteoclasts destroy bone by breaking down bone and resorbing it. Regulation of bone mass is accomplished by the dual action of osteoclasts and osteoblasts. Mature bone cells are referred to as **osteocytes**.

The **epiphyseal plate** is a disc of cartilage between the metaphysis and epiphysis of an immature long bone that permits the bone to grow longer. This is also called the *growth plate* because it serves as a growing region (**Figure 5-4**). After long bone growth has stopped, a remnant of the plate, called the **epiphyseal line**, is evident.

Thickening or widening of long bones results from the deposition of compact bone on the outside, just beneath the periosteum. Periosteal osteoblasts add new bone to the region to create a bone-widening effect. As compact bone is forming on the surface, other bone tissue is being eroded away on the inside. This action creates the space for the medullary cavity in the diaphysis, which is filled with red bone marrow. Bone growth is similar to tree growth in that growth is upward, downward, and outward.

Throughout life, bone remodeling takes place as osteoclasts are stimulated to resorb bone tissue at specific sites, and osteoblasts are activated to replace the bone. This bone remodeling process of resorption and replacement is a well-regulated balancing act and is a classic example of homeostasis. Remodeling occurs throughout life as a means of maintaining bone tissue.

Vitamins play a pivotal role in bone maintenance. For example, vitamin D is necessary for proper absorption of calcium in the small intestine. The mineral **calcium** is needed for bone strength. In cases of vitamin D deficiency, calcium is poorly absorbed, resulting in deformed bones. Vitamin A is necessary for the bone resorption that occurs during normal development. Vitamin A deficiency may result in retardation of bone development. Vitamin C (ascorbic acid) is necessary for the synthesis of collagen, a substance of bone. Humans and guinea pigs are the only mammals incapable of synthesizing vitamin C; they must instead obtain it from the diet.

Under the direction of hormones, bone mineralization and resorption occur. Hormones are chemical messengers critical to many processes in the body, including bone development. Through hormonal actions, bones either store calcium or release it into the blood. In this way, bone activity also regulates blood calcium concentration. When blood calcium is low, osteoclasts are stimulated to break down bone tissue, releasing calcium into the bloodstream. When circulating blood calcium is high, osteoclast activity is inhibited, and osteoblasts are stimulated to form bone tissue.

Physical exercise affects bone structure. When skeletal muscles contract, they pull on bones, stimulating the bone tissue to thicken and strengthen in what is commonly known as bone **hypertrophy** (an increase in size). Lack of exercise causes bone tissue to waste away, and bones become thinner and weaker or **atrophy** (a reduction in size).

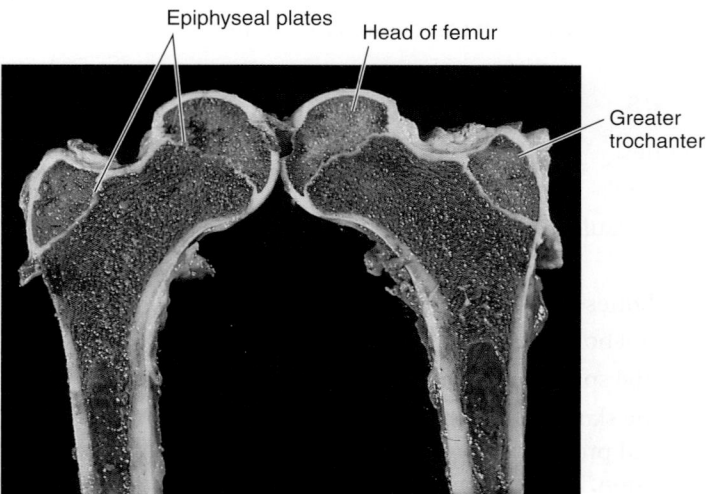

Figure 5-4 Anatomy of a long bone showing the epiphyseal plates, which are separating the head of the femur and the greater trochanter from the metaphysis.

KEY TERM	Definition
ossification (os-i-fi-KAY-shun)	conversion of cartilage tissue into bone
bone remodeling	process of breaking down and building up bone tissue
osteoblasts (OS-tee-oh-blasts)	bone-forming cells
osteoclasts (OS-tee-oh-klasts)	bone-destroying cells
osteocytes (OS-tee-oh-sites)	mature bone cells
epiphyseal (ep-i-FIZ-ee-ul) **plate**	site of long bone growth located between the metaphysis and epiphysis; also called the growth plate
epiphyseal (ep-i-FIZ-ee-ul) **line**	mark left at the site of the epiphyseal plate after the long bone has stopped growing
calcium	mineral essential to bone formation and strength
hypertrophy (high-PUR-truh-fee)	an increase in size
atrophy (AT-ruh-fee)	a reduction in size

KEY TERM PRACTICE: *Bone Formation*

1. Mature bone cells are called _____.

2. Bone-forming cells are termed _____, and bone-destroying cells are known as _____.

3. The medical term for the growth plate is the _____.

4. Which mineral is necessary for bone formation? _____

5. Conversion of cartilage tissue into bone is termed _____.

6. Write the term that means the opposite of *hypertrophy*. _____

Surface Markings

Surface markings are identifiable landmarks on the exterior of bones. Each is designed for a specific purpose, which demonstrates that structure and function are complementary. **Figure 5-5** shows surface markings and their associated bones. The markings occur for joint formation, muscle attachment, and passage of nerves and blood vessels. **Table 5-1** lists common surface marking terms along with their definitions and an example location. **Table 5-2** matches selected surface markings with their associated bones.

Cranial and Facial Bones

The **cranium**, or skull, has eight bones:

- 1 **occipital bone** or back head bone
- 2 **parietal bones** or superior lateral skull bones
- 1 **frontal bone** or forehead bone
- 2 **temporal bones** or lateral skull bones
- 1 **sphenoid** or butterfly-shaped skull bone
- 1 **ethmoid** or skull bone between the sphenoid and nasal bones.

Easily identifiable features on the skull include the mastoid process, styloid process, and external acoustic meatus. The mastoid process is found behind the ear. The styloid process is a slender needle-like pointed projection. The external acoustic meatus is the passage leading inward through the ear (**Figure 5-6**).

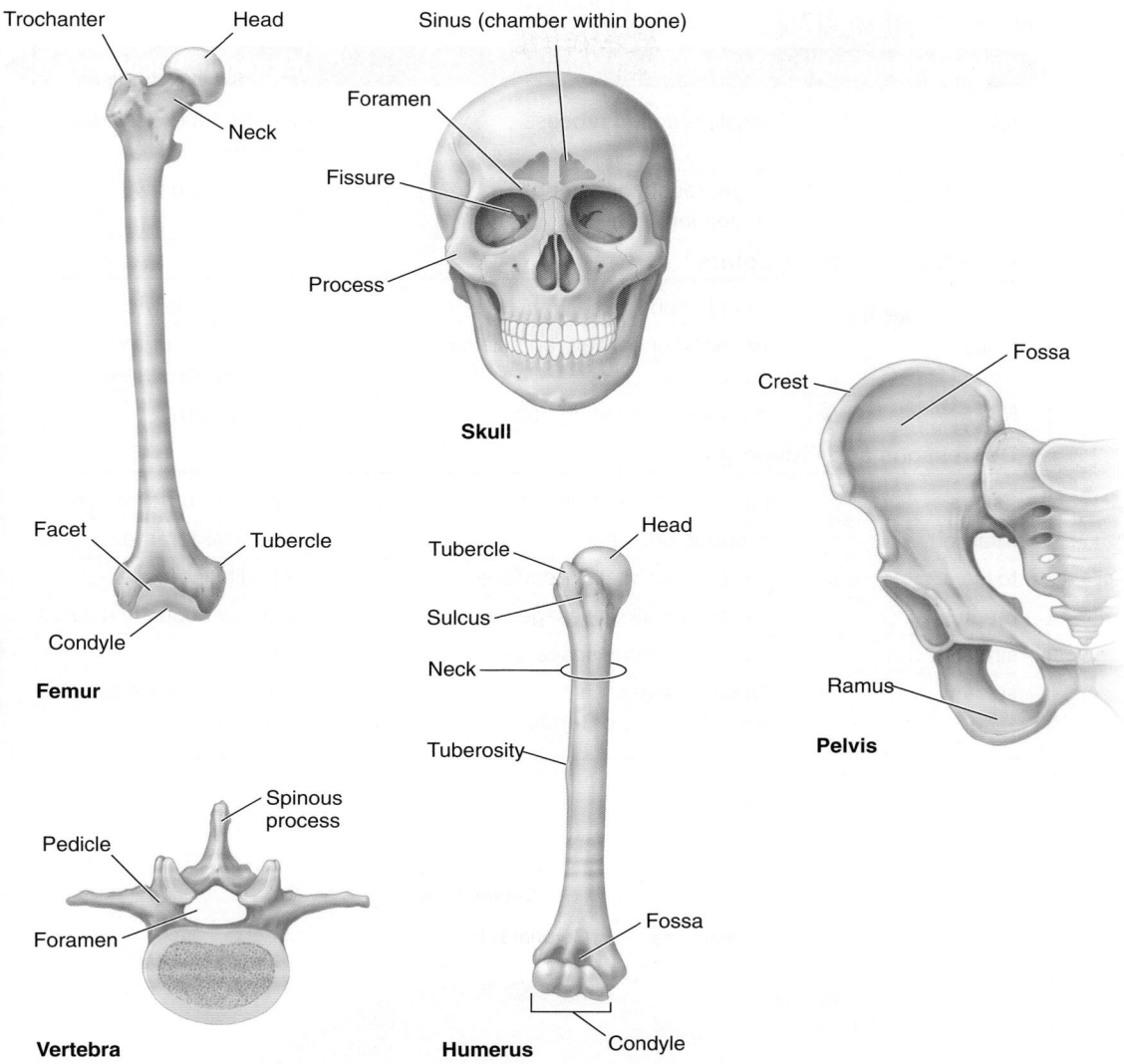

Figure 5-5 Surface markings and associated bones.

TABLE 5-1	BONE SURFACE MARKINGS	
Surface Marking	**Definition**	**Example Location**
Projections		
crest	narrow, ridge-like projection	iliac crest
epicondyle	projection superior to a condyle	medial epicondyle of the femur
process	bony prominence	mastoid process
ramus	branching part of bone	ramus of mandible
trochanter	large process found only on the femur	greater trochanter of the femur

continued

continued from page 217

Surface Marking	Definition	Example Location
tubercle	small, rounded process	greater tubercle of the humerus
tuberosity	large, roughened knob-like projection	radial tuberosity
Projections Forming Joints		
condyle	round knob	occipital condyle
facet	flattened or shallow articulating surface	costal facet of the thoracic vertebrae
head	rounded articulating end	head of femur
Depressons and Openings		
fissure	narrow, slit-like opening	superior orbital fissure
foramen	rounded opening	obturator foramen
fossa	flattened or shallow surface	mandibular fossa
meatus	canal; tube-like passageway	external acoustic meatus
sinus	cavity or hollow space	frontal sinus
sulcus	linear groove for a vessel, nerve, or tendon	intertubercular sulcus of the humerus

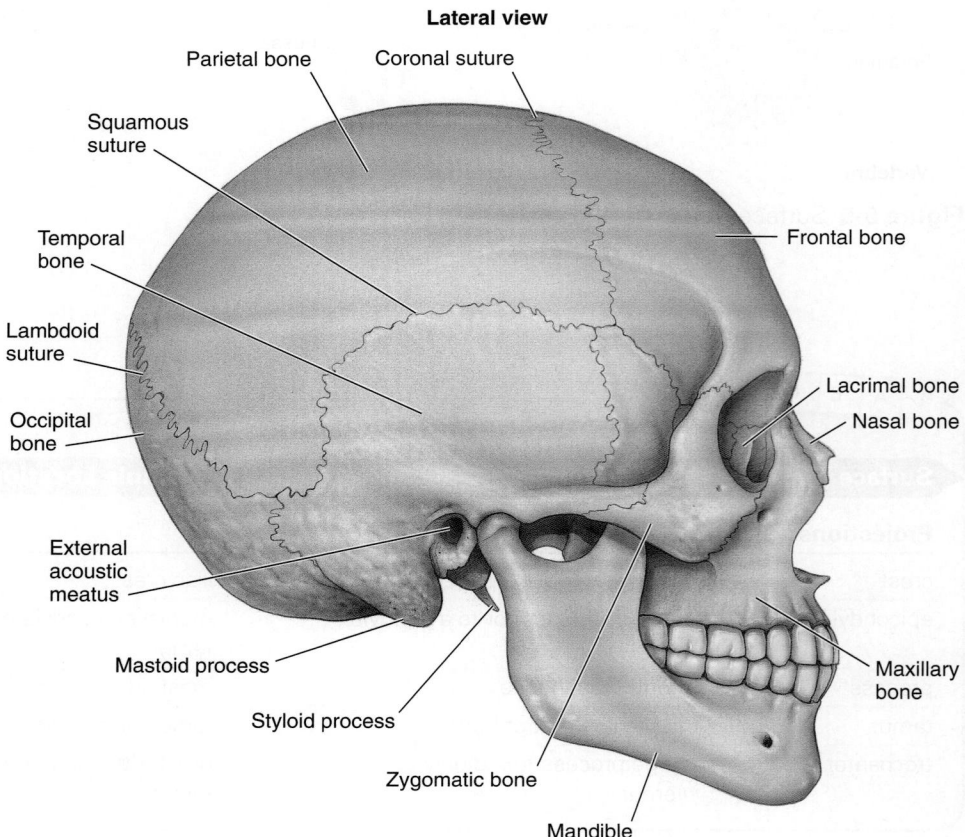

Figure 5-6 Skull bones.

TABLE 5-2	SELECTED SURFACE MARKINGS MATCHED WITH ASSOCIATED BONES	
Marking	**Bone**	
acetabulum	coxal bone	
greater sciatic notch	coxal bone	
acromion process	scapula	
glenoid cavity	scapula	
greater trochanter	femur	
transverse process	vertebra	
atlas	vertebra	
pedicle	vertebra	
xiphoid process	sternum	

Special skull features include fontanelles and sutures. **Fontanelles** (sometimes spelled fontanels) are membranous regions located between certain cranial bones in the skull of a fetus or infant (**Figure 5-7**). They are not ossified at birth and are commonly called the *soft spots*. They permit movement between bones so that the developing skull can change size and shape to allow for brain growth and to enable the head to pass easily through the birth canal during childbirth. The immovable joints that result when the fontanelles ossify are termed *sutures*. The skull sutures include the lambdoid suture, coronal suture, sagittal suture, and squamous suture (**Figure 5-8**).

The 14 facial bones are shown in **Figure 5-9** and include:

- 2 **maxillary bones** or upper jawbones
- 2 **palatine bones** or L-shaped bones
- 2 **nasal bones** or nose bones
- 2 **inferior nasal conchae (turbinates)** or curved nasal cavity bones
- 2 **zygomatic bones** or cheek bones
- 2 **lacrimal bones** or fingernail-shaped facial bones
- 1 **vomer**
- 1 **mandible** or lower jawbone

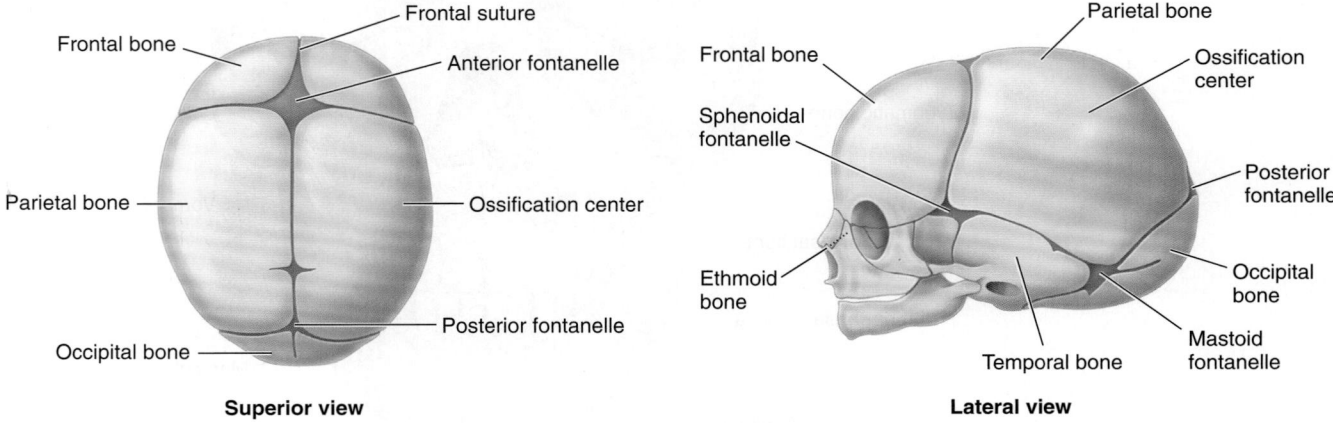

Figure 5-7 Fontanelles in an infant skull.

Posterior view

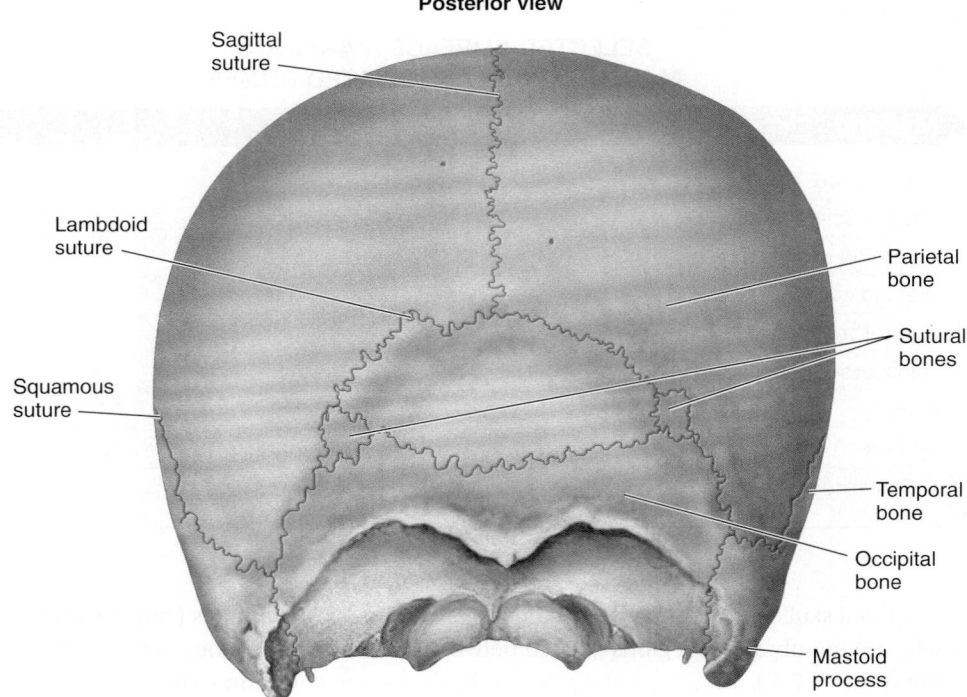

Sagittal suture

Lambdoid suture

Squamous suture

Parietal bone

Sutural bones

Temporal bone

Occipital bone

Mastoid process

Figure 5-8 Skull sutures.

Anterior view

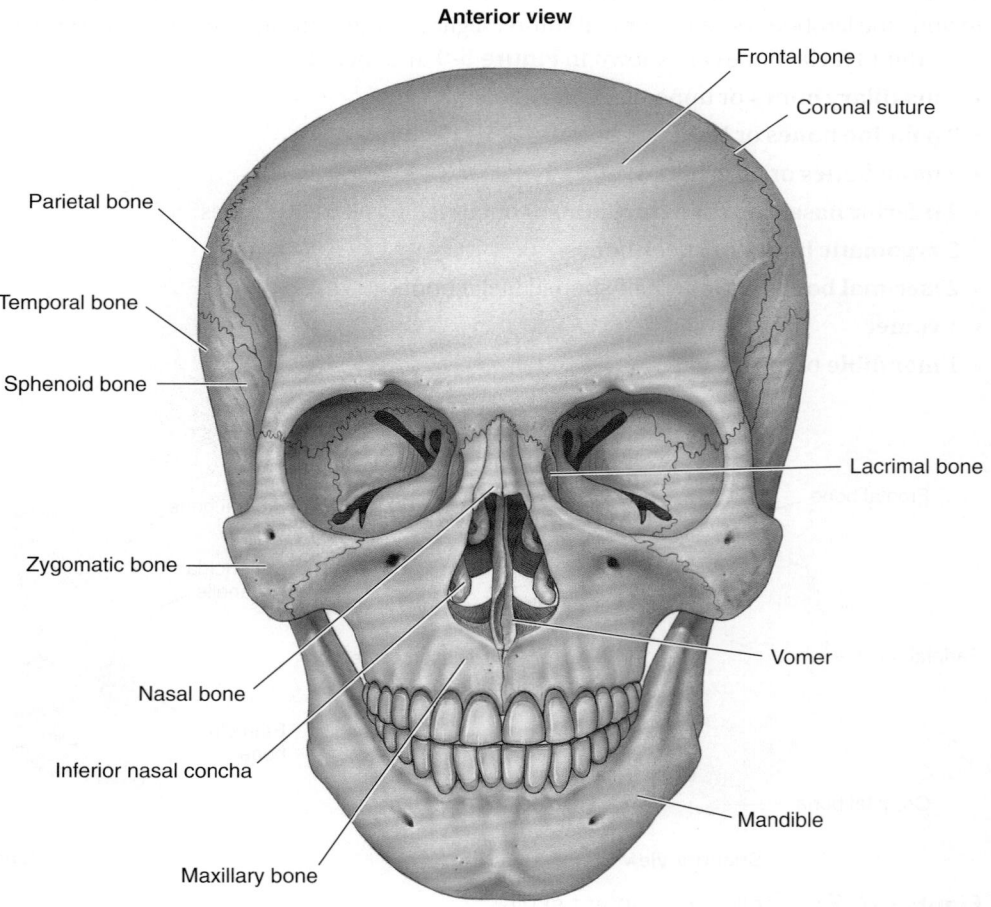

Frontal bone

Coronal suture

Parietal bone

Temporal bone

Sphenoid bone

Lacrimal bone

Zygomatic bone

Vomer

Nasal bone

Inferior nasal concha

Mandible

Maxillary bone

Figure 5-9 Facial bones.

Sinuses are cavities or hollow spaces in bones. The frontal, sphenoid, ethmoid, and maxillary bones contain mucous membrane–lined spaces (**Figure 5-10**). These sinuses reduce the weight of the skull and provide an area of mucous epithelium to the nasal cavity.

The U-shaped **hyoid bone**, also known as the "neck bone" in everyday terms, is unique because it is the only bone in the body that does not articulate with any other bone (**Figure 5-11**). It supports the tongue and provides attachment for some muscles.

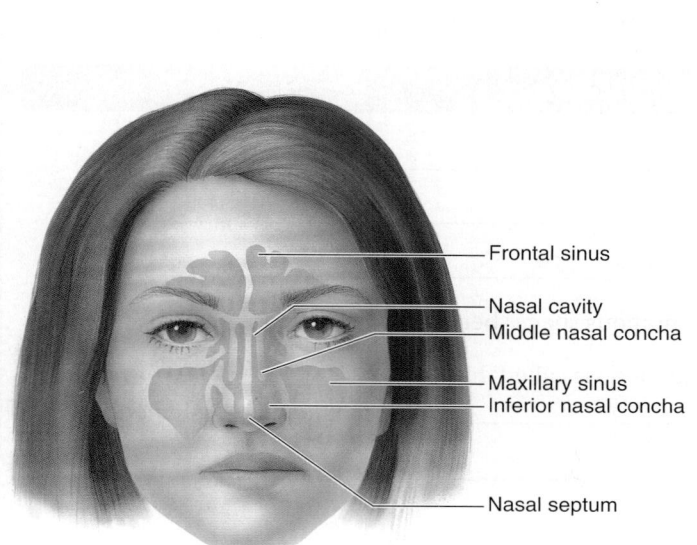

Frontal sinus

Nasal cavity
Middle nasal concha

Maxillary sinus
Inferior nasal concha

Nasal septum

Figure 5-10 The paranasal sinuses.

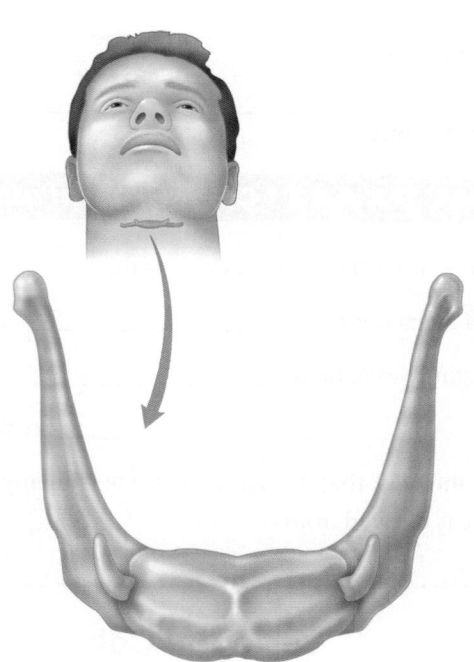

Figure 5-11 The U-shaped hyoid bone.

KEY TERM	Definition
cranium (KRAY-nee-um)	the bones of the head; also called the skull
occipital (ock-SIP-i-tul) **bone**	back head bone
parietal (pur-RYE-e-tul) **bones**	superior lateral skull bones
frontal (FRUN-tul) **bone**	forehead bone
temporal (TEM-puh-rul) **bones**	lateral skull bones
sphenoid (SFEE-noid) **bone**	butterfly-shaped skull bone
ethmoid (ETH-moid) **bone**	skull bone between sphenoid and nasal bones
fontanelles (fon-tuh-NELZ)	membranous space between cranial bones; also called soft spots
maxillary (mack-sih-LAIR-ee) **bones**	upper jawbones
palatine (PAL-uh-tine) **bones**	L-shaped facial bones
nasal (NAY-zul) **bones**	bones of the nose
inferior nasal conchae (KON-kee)	scroll-shaped bones in the nasal passages; also called inferior nasal turbinates

continued

continued from page 221

KEY TERM	Definition
turbinates (TUR-bin-ates)	scroll-shaped bones in the nasal passages; also called conchae
zygomatic (zye-goh-MAT-ick) **bones**	cheek bones
lacrimal (LACK-ri-mul) **bones**	fingernail-shaped facial bones
vomer (VOH-mur)	thin, vertically positioned bone forming a portion of the septum
mandible (MAN-di-bul)	lower jawbone
sinuses	cavities or hollow space in bones
hyoid (HIGH-oid) **bone**	U-shaped bone that supports the tongue

KEY TERM PRACTICE: *Cranial and Facial Bones*

1. The skull bones are collectively known as the _____.

2. Name the 14 facial bones. _____

3. Name the eight cranial bones. _____

4. _____ are membranous spaces between nonossified skull bones.

5. The bone in the neck that does not articulate with any other bone is called the _____; and its name is derived from the word part _____ that means "U-shaped."

Vertebral Column

The vertebral column, sternum, and ribs make up the skeleton of the trunk. Vertebrae support the head and trunk and protect the spinal cord. The main, thick part of the vertebra is called the **vertebral body**. Projecting posteriorly are two short stalks called **pedicles**, which form sides of an opening called the **vertebral foramen**. The spinal cord passes through this opening. Two plates form each **lamina**, and the laminae fuse in the back to become a spine-like projection called the **spinous process**. Crosswise projections called the **transverse processes** extend laterally from the vertebral body (**Figure 5-12**). Vertebrae have different shapes and sizes along the vertebral column.

Bones of the vertebral column include cervical, thoracic, and lumbar vertebrae, plus the sacrum and coccyx. The seven vertebrae closest to the head are the **cervical vertebrae**, designated by the letter C and numbered C_1–C_7. They make up the bony axis of the neck and are the

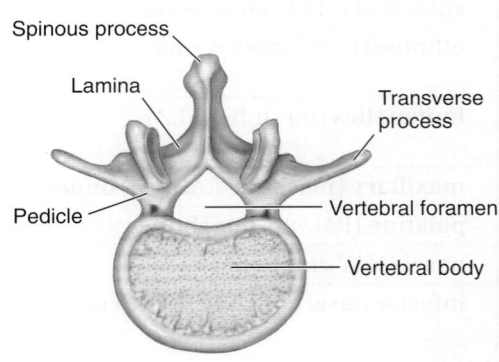

Figure 5-12 Anatomy of a typical vertebra.   **Superior view**

smallest vertebrae, yet have the densest bone tissue. The first cervical vertebra (C_1) is called the *atlas* and allows the head to nod. The second cervical vertebra (C_2) is the *axis*, which enables the head to rotate.

The 12 **thoracic vertebrae**, designated by the letter *T* and numbered T_1–T_{12}, are larger than the cervical vertebrae and are adapted to withstand stress. The thoracic vertebrae articulate with ribs posteriorly.

The five **lumbar vertebrae**, designated by the letter *L* and numbered L_1–L_5, are adapted to support body weight. To help you remember the number of vertebrae in each division from superior to inferior, think about the times of the day when you eat: breakfast at 7, lunch at 12, and dinner at 5 (**Figure 5-13**).

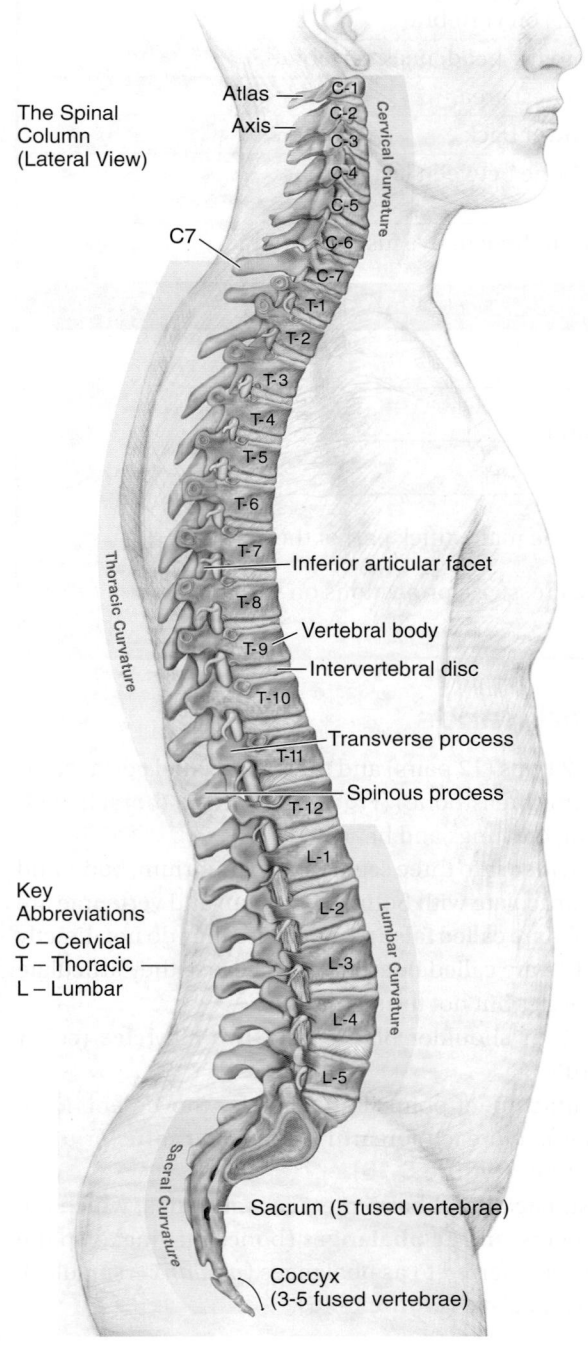

The Spinal Column (Lateral View)

Atlas — C-1
Axis — C-2
C-3
C-4
C-5
C7 — C-6
C-7

Cervical Curvature

T-1
T-2
T-3
T-4
T-5
T-6
T-7 — Inferior articular facet
T-8
T-9 — Vertebral body
— Intervertebral disc
T-10
T-11 — Transverse process
— Spinous process
T-12

Thoracic Curvature

L-1
L-2
L-3
L-4
L-5

Lumbar Curvature

Key Abbreviations
C – Cervical
T – Thoracic
L – Lumbar

Sacral Curvature

— Sacrum (5 fused vertebrae)
Coccyx (3-5 fused vertebrae)

Figure 5-13 The normal spinal column.

The **sacrum** is made up of five fused vertebrae that serve as the attachment for the pelvic girdle. The **coccyx** or tailbone is made up of three to five fused vertebrae. The shape of the sacrum and coccyx forms the sacral curve. The structure of the sacrum and coccyx can be seen in **Figure 5-13**.

KEY TERM	Definition
vertebral (VUR-te-brul) **body**	the main, thick part of a vertebra
pedicles (PED-i-kuls)	short narrow stalks that form the sides of the vertebral foramen
vertebral foramen (VUR-te-brul foh-RAY-mun)	opening through which the spinal cord passes
lamina (LAM-i-nuh)	thin plate on vertebra
spinous (SPYE-nus) **process**	spine-like projection on vertebra
transverse (trans-VERCE) **processes**	crosswise projections on vertebra
cervical vertebrae (C_1–C_7)	7 vertebrae closest to the head; neck vertebrae
thoracic vertebrae (T_1–T_{12})	12 vertebrae of the chest area
lumbar vertebrae (L_1–L_5)	5 vertebrae of the lower back
sacrum (SAY-krum)	curved, triangular bone between last lumbar vertebra and coccyx
coccyx (KOCK-siks)	tailbone formed from three to five fused vertebrae

KEY TERM PRACTICE: *Vertebral Column*

1. The spine-like process on a typical vertebra is called the _____.

2. Identify the vertebrae by name and number for the five vertebral regions. _____

3. The opening through which the spinal cord passes is termed the _____.

4. The _____ is the main, thick part of the vertebra.

5. _____ are crosswise projections on vertebrae.

Bones of the Chest, Arms, and Hands

The thoracic cage, or rib cage, is made up of 24 ribs (12 pairs) and their associated costal cartilages, the thoracic vertebrae, and the sternum (breastbone) (**Figure 5-14**). The thoracic skeleton protects the vital chest organs, including the lungs and heart.

Superiorly to inferiorly, the sternum is divided into three segments: manubrium, body, and xiphoid process. The seven pairs of ribs that articulate with both the sternum and vertebrae are called **true ribs.** The remaining five pairs of ribs are called **false ribs** because they do not directly attach to the sternum. Of these, pairs 11 and 12 are called **floating ribs** because they articulate with the thoracic vertebrae and posterior muscles but not the sternum.

The two **scapulae** (*scapula* = singular), or shoulder blades, and two **clavicles** (collar bones), make up the pectoral (shoulder) girdle.

The two upper limbs provide muscle attachment points and allow for movement. Each upper arm has a **humerus** (upper arm bone), and each forearm contains a **radius** or outer forearm bone and an **ulna** or inner forearm bone (**Figure 5-15**).

There are 8 **carpal bones** in each wrist. Each hand has 5 **metacarpal bones**, which are bones of the hand between the wrist and fingers, and 14 **phalanges** (bones that make up the fingers). The bones of both fingers and toes are referred to as phalanges (*phalanx* = singular). Phalanx parts are labeled proximal, middle, and distal (**Figure 5-16**).

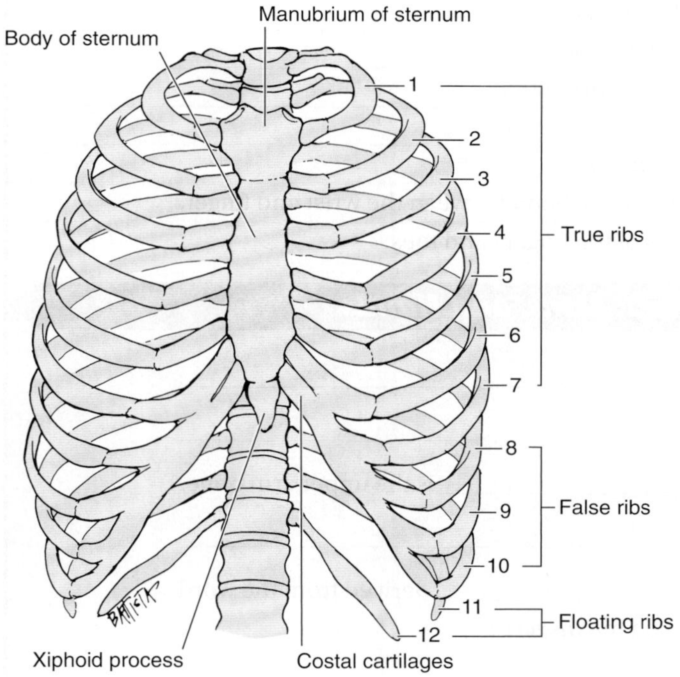

Figure 5-14 (The thoracic cage)

Body of sternum

Manubrium of sternum

1
2
3
4 — True ribs
5
6
7

8
9 — False ribs
10

11
12 — Floating ribs

Xiphoid process

Costal cartilages

Figure 5-14 The thoracic cage.

Figure 5-15 (Regions and bones of the upper limb)

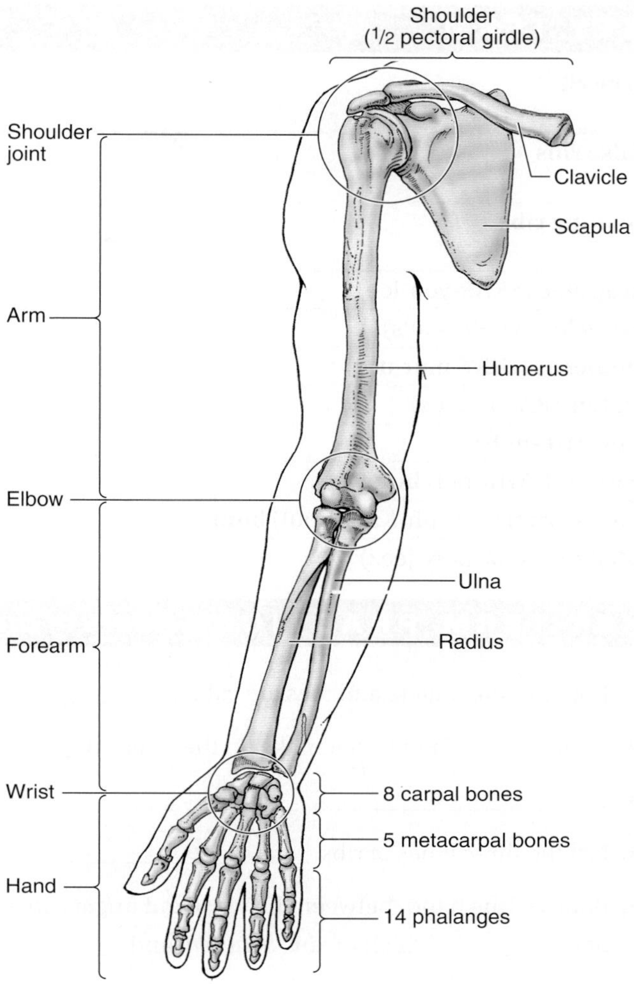

Shoulder
(½ pectoral girdle)

Shoulder joint

Arm

Clavicle

Scapula

Humerus

Elbow

Forearm

Ulna

Radius

Wrist

8 carpal bones

5 metacarpal bones

Hand

14 phalanges

Figure 5-15 Regions and bones of the upper limb.

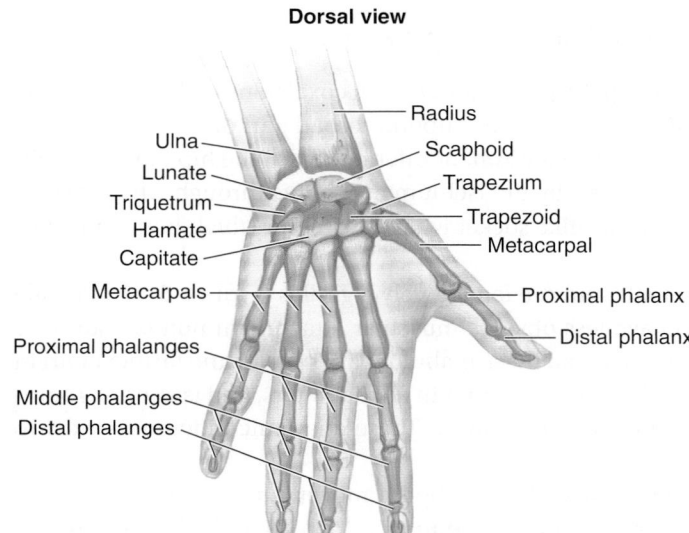

Dorsal view

Ulna

Radius

Lunate

Scaphoid

Triquetrum

Trapezium

Hamate

Trapezoid

Capitate

Metacarpal

Metacarpals

Proximal phalanx

Proximal phalanges

Distal phalanx

Middle phalanges

Distal phalanges

Figure 5-16 Wrist and hand bones: The pisiform is not visible in this view.

KEY TERM	Definition
true ribs	rib pairs 1–7; the ribs that articulate with both the sternum and the vertebrae
false ribs	rib pairs 8–10; the ribs that articulate with the vertebrae and the sternum by the costal cartilage of the last true rib
floating ribs	rib pairs 11 and 12; the ribs that articulate with the thoracic vertebrae and posterior muscles but not the sternum
scapulae (SKAP-yoo-lee)	triangular bones of the back; also called shoulder blades
clavicles (KLAV-i-kuls)	collar bones
humerus (HEW-mur-us)	upper arm bone
radius (RAY-dee-us)	outer forearm bone
ulna (UL-nuh)	inner forearm bone
carpal (KAHR-pul) **bones**	wrist bones
metacarpal (met-uh-KAHR-pul) **bones**	bones of the hand between the wrist and fingers
phalanges (fa-LAN-jeez)	bones of the fingers and toes

KEY TERM PRACTICE: *Bones of the Chest, Arms, and Hands*

1. Bones of the fingers and toes are called _____.

2. Name the two bones that make up the forearm. _____

3. The _____ is the upper arm bone.

4. List the three types of ribs. _____

5. Bones of the hand, between the wrist and fingers are called _____, derived from the word part _____, which means *between*, and _____, which means *wrist*.

Bones of the Pelvic Girdle, Legs, and Feet

The two coxal bones (hip bones) make up the pelvic girdle. Each coxal bone of the pelvic girdle consists of three fused bones: the **ilium**, which is the superior broad part of the hip bone; the **pubis**, or front part of the hip bone; and the **ischium**, or inferior part of the hip bone. The **obturator foramen** is a large opening formed by the ischium and pubis through which nerves and vessels pass. The **acetabulum** is a cup-like socket where the femur (thigh bone) attaches to the hip (**Figure 5-17**).

Differences exist between the male and the female pelvic girdles (**Figure 5-18**). Female hip bones are lighter, thinner, and have less obvious muscular attachment points than their male counterparts. The obturator foramen and the acetabulum are smaller and farther apart in females than in males. The female pelvic cavity is wider in all diameters, and is shorter, roomier, and less funnel-shaped than the male pelvic cavity. These anatomic differences exist to accommodate childbirth.

The lower extremities function to provide body support, movement, and muscle attachment. The proximal portion of each lower limb has a **femur** or thigh bone. At the knee joint is the **patella** or kneecap, and the distal portion of the lower limb is made up of the **tibia** (shin

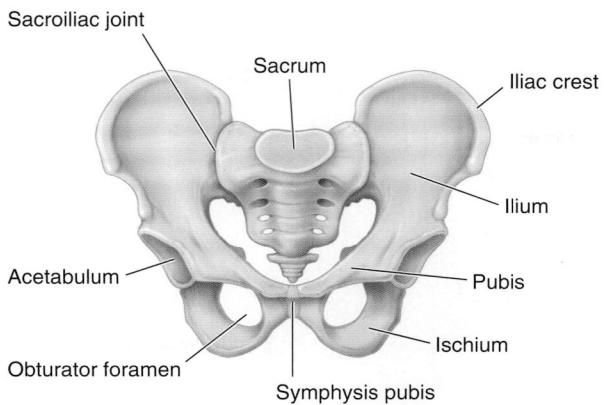

Sacroiliac joint

Sacrum

Iliac crest

Ilium

Acetabulum

Pubis

Obturator foramen

Ischium

Symphysis pubis

Anterior view

Figure 5-17 The pelvic girdle.

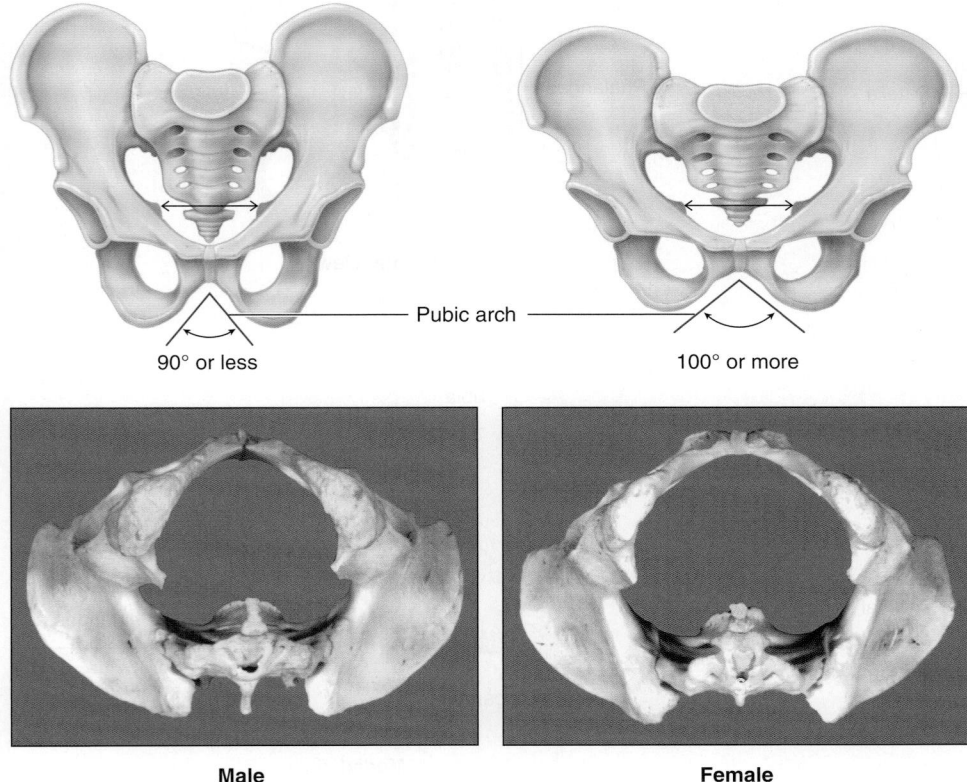

Pubic arch

90° or less

100° or more

Male

Female

Figure 5-18 The male and the female pelvic girdles.

bone) and **fibula** or slender lower leg bone (**Figure 5-19**). To help you remember the difference between the tibia and the fibula, keep in mind that the *fib*ula is *small*er than the tibia, and "to tell a small lie is to fib."

Each ankle is made up of 7 **tarsal bones**. They include the **talus**, the ankle bone that connects to the tibia, and the **calcaneus** or heel bone. Each foot contains 10 **metatarsal bones**, which are the bones between the ankle and toes, and 14 phalanges, or bones that make up the toes (**Figure 5-20**).

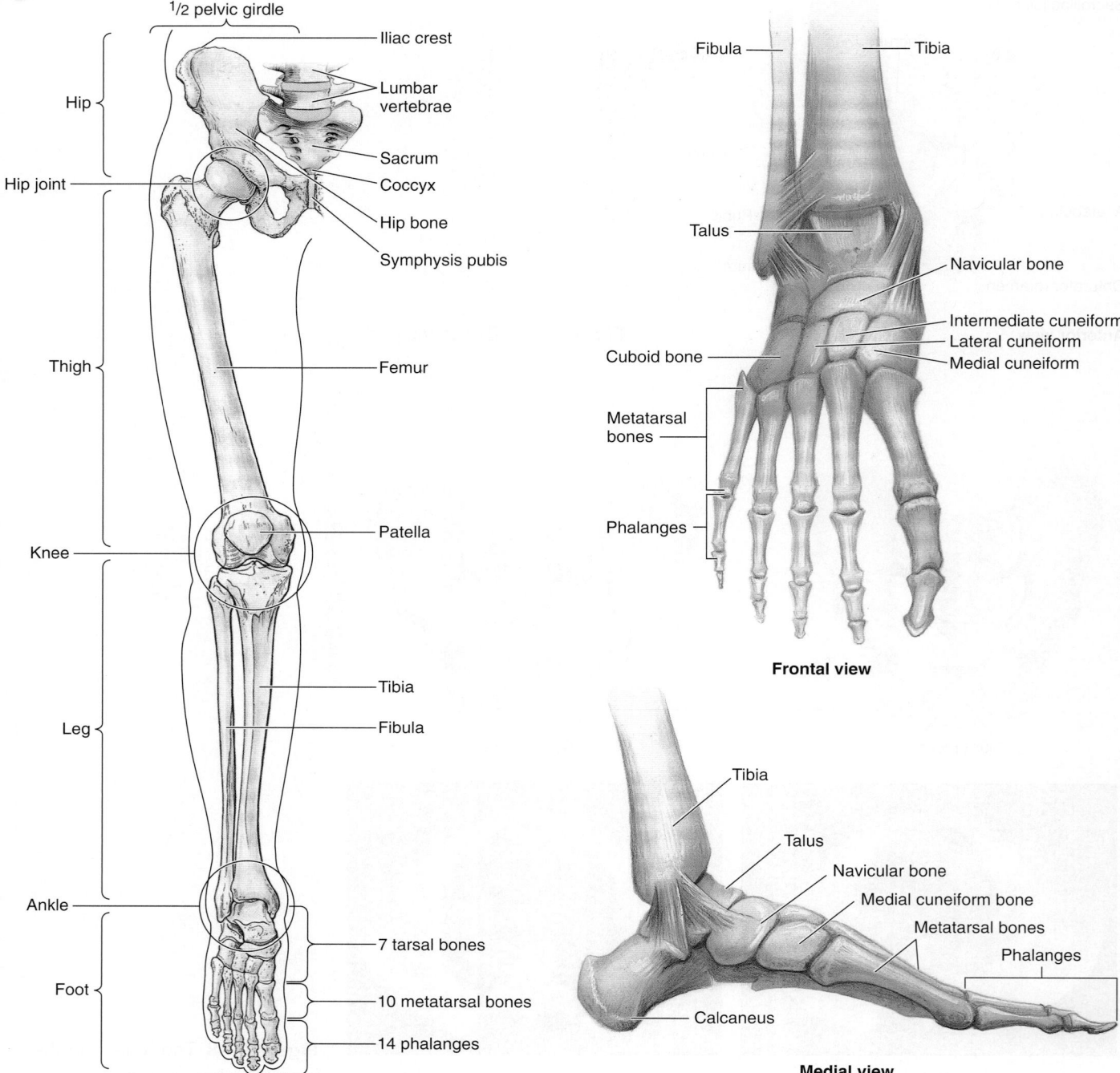

Figure 5-19 Regions and bones of the lower limb.

Figure 5-20 Ankle and foot bones.

KEY TERM	Definition
ilium (IL-ee-um)	superior broad part of the hip bone
pubis (PEW-bis)	front part of the hip bone, forming anterior pelvic girdle
ischium (IS-kee-um)	inferior part of the hip bone
obturator foramen (OB-tew-ray-tur foh-RAY-mun)	oval opening between the ischium and pubis
acetabulum (as-e-TAB-yoo-lum)	the socket of the hip bone into which the head of the femur fits
femur (FEE-mur)	thigh bone
patella (pa-TEL-uh)	kneecap
tibia (TIB-ee-uh)	shin bone; larger of two lower leg bones
fibula (FIB-yoo-luh)	slender lower leg bone
tarsal (TAHR-sul) **bones**	ankle bones
talus (TAY-lus)	ankle bone that connects to the tibia
calcaneus (kal-KAY-nee-us)	heel bone
metatarsal (met-uh-TAHR-sul) **bones**	bones of the foot between the ankle and toes

KEY TERM PRACTICE: *Bones of the Pelvic Girdle, Legs, and Feet*

1. Name the three bones that make up the pelvic girdle. _____

2. The bones of the feet between the ankle and toes are termed _____ bones, derived from the word part _____, which means *between*, and the word part, _____, which means _____ *ankle*.

3. _____ is the medical term for kneecap.

4. The _____ is the anatomic term for the thigh bone, and is derived from the word part _____, which means *thigh*.

5. The socket of the hip bone into which the head of the femur fits is termed the _____.

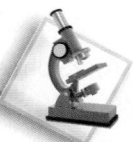

THE CLINICAL DIMENSION: BONES

Signs and symptoms of pathologic conditions in bone are often similar to those associated with other body disorders. Those specific to osseous disorders are discussed in this section. Common disorders of the skeletal system are also introduced.

Abnormal Spinal Curvatures

Abnormal curvatures of the spine include kyphosis, lordosis, and scoliosis. Attempts should be made to correct these abnormalities so that they do not progress to stages that compromise respiratory or cardiac function.

kyphosis   **Kyphosis** is an exaggeration of the thoracic curve (**Figure 5-21A**). Commonly referred to as hunchback or humpback, it is often caused by poor posture or tuberculosis. The person with kyphosis generally has rounded shoulders, and back pain is a regular symptom. Physical examination and x-rays give a definitive diagnosis. Treatment consists of exercises and physical therapy to strengthen the involved muscles.

lordosis   **Lordosis** is an abnormal anterior concavity of the lumbar curve (**Figure 5-21B**). It is frequently called swayback. It is generally caused by excessive abdominal weight from obesity or pregnancy. The person with lordosis makes a postural adjustment to compensate for the extra girth. Individuals with lordosis typically have a protruding abdomen and experience back pain as a result of muscle strain. Diagnosis is made by physical examination of the spine in various postures and x-ray evaluation. Treatment is aimed at weight reduction and exercise to strengthen abdominal and back muscles.

scoliosis   **Scoliosis** is an abnormal lateral curvature of the spine that appears S-shaped (**Figure 5-21C**). A sign of scoliosis is having one shoulder and hip higher than the other. The cause of scoliosis is either genetic or idiopathic (unknown). Physical examination and radiographic studies confirm the diagnosis and determine the degree of curvature. For mild cases, treatment involves exercises to strengthen muscles. Severe scoliosis with a curvature of 40 degrees or more can be treated by surgery or bracing.

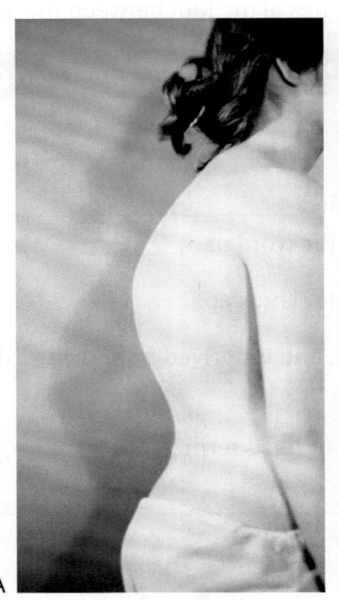 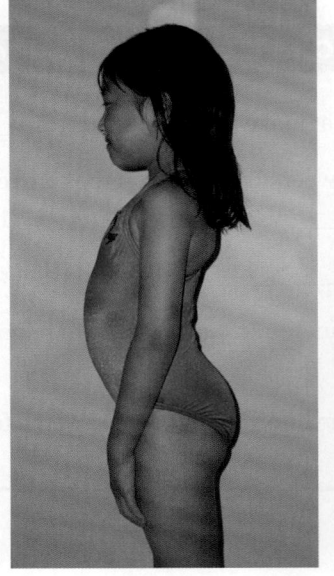 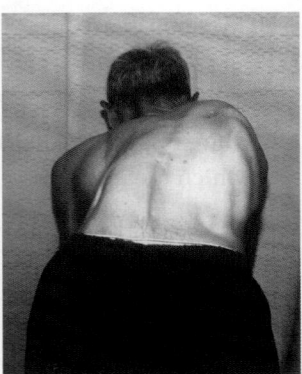

A   B   C

Figure 5-21 (A) Kyphosis. **(B)** Lordosis. **(C)** Scoliosis.

KEY TERM	Definition
kyphosis (kigh-FOH-sis)	angular curve of the thoracic spine; hunchback
lordosis (lor-DOH-sis)	forward curve of the lumbar spine; swayback
scoliosis (skoh-lee-OH-sis)	lateral curve of the spine

KEY TERM PRACTICE: *Abnormal Spinal Curvatures*

1. _____ is abnormal lateral curvature of the spine.

2. Supply the medical term for *hunchback*. _____

3. _____ is the medical term for *swayback*.

Fractures

fracture (Fx)   A **fracture (Fx)** is a break in a bone or tooth. **Table 5-3** identifies and describes several types of fractures, and **Figure 5-22** illustrates the more common examples. Broken bones are frequently accompanied by **crepitus**, the harsh, grating sound heard when broken bone ends rub together. Without proper treatment of fractures, the patient risks having one limb shorter than the other.

Whenever there is a disruption in bone integrity, the body repairs itself by forming a fracture hematoma (blood clot) and then a callus (a mass of tissue that establishes bone continuity) at the site of injury. Remodeling then completes the task of forming new bone at the fracture area. Fractures in an epiphyseal plate can be serious because this is the area of greatest cell division in a growing bone.

Options for treating fractures include skeletal traction, closed and open reduction, and fixation. **Skeletal traction** is the mechanism used to straighten broken bones and involves pulling on a bone structure by a pin or wire inserted into the bone. **Reduction** is the restoration of a part to its normal anatomical position by surgery or manipulation. **Closed reduction** refers to bone manipulation without

TABLE 5-3   FRACTURES

Fracture Type	Description
Colles fracture	fracture of the distal end of the radius and ulna with displacement of the hand backward and upward
comminuted fracture	complete break with bony fragments
complete fracture	break across the entire bone
compound (open) fracture	bone is exposed through injured (open) skin
compression fracture	fracture of vertebrae as a result of severe stress; may impinge the spinal cord
greenstick fracture	incomplete break on a convex bone surface (bends like a green tree twig)
partial (incomplete) fracture	fracture in which bony fragments remain partially joined
simple (closed) fracture	break is protected by uninjured (closed) skin
spiral fracture	excessive bone twisting for description of spiral fracture
stress fracture	tiny fractures caused by excessive mechanical strain
transverse fracture	complete break occurring at a right angle to the bone axis

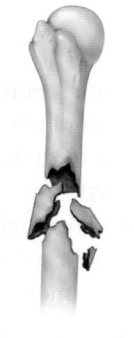 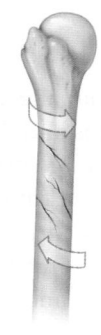 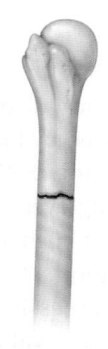 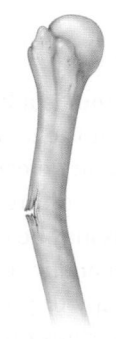 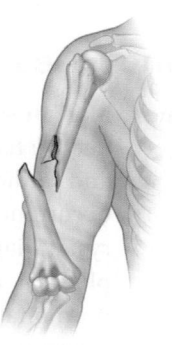 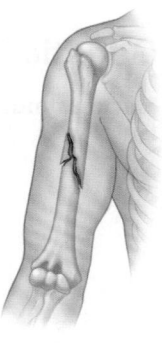

Comminuted   **Spiral**   **Transverse**   **Greenstick**   **Compound**   **Simple**

Figure 5-22 Types of bone fractures.

skin incision. When skin incision is necessary to restore a dislocated bone to its anatomical position, it is termed an **open reduction.** Two types of **fixation,** the immobilization of a fractured bone, are external and internal. With **external fixation,** splints, plastic dressings, or pins immobilize the fractured bone, whereas **internal fixation** involves the stabilization of fractured bony parts by directly attaching the fragments with surgical wires, screws, pins, rod, or plates.

KEY TERM	Definition
fracture (Fx)	break in a bone or tooth
crepitus (KREP-i-tus)	grating sound heard when broken bone ends rub together
skeletal traction	process of pulling on a broken bone to straighten it
reduction	restoration of a bone to its normal anatomic position by surgical or manipulative procedures
closed reduction	restoration of a dislocated joint or fractured bone to its normal anatomic position by surgical or manipulative procedures without skin incision
open reduction	restoration of a dislocated joint or fractured bone to its normal anatomic position by surgical or manipulative procedures with skin incision
fixation	immobilization of a fracture
external fixation	immobilization of a fracture by splints, plastic dressings, or pins
internal fixation	stabilization of a fracture by directly attaching the bony fragments together with surgical wires, screws, pins, rods, or plates

KEY TERM PRACTICE: *Fractures*

1. A break in a bone is termed a _____.

2. _____ refers to fracture immobilization.

3. Stabilizing a fracture by directly attaching the bony fragments together with surgical wires, screws, pins, rods, or plates is termed _____.

4. _____ is the grating sound heard when broken bone ends rub together.

5. Bone pulling mediated by internal fixation with pins or wires inserted into the bone to reduce a fracture is known as _____.

Genetic Bone Diseases

Marfan syndrome   **Marfan syndrome** is a hereditary disorder that affects the body's connective tissues. It is characterized by long limbs and fingers, joint laxity, and cardiovascular defects (**Figure 5-23**). It may go undetected until the occurrence of a life-threatening event such as a ruptured aortic aneurysm. Diagnosis may be made at birth or during early childhood through physical and genetic evaluation. Treatment involves prepubescent hormonal therapy to prevent excessive growth and therapies aimed at preventing hypertension. Cardiac evaluations are continuous.

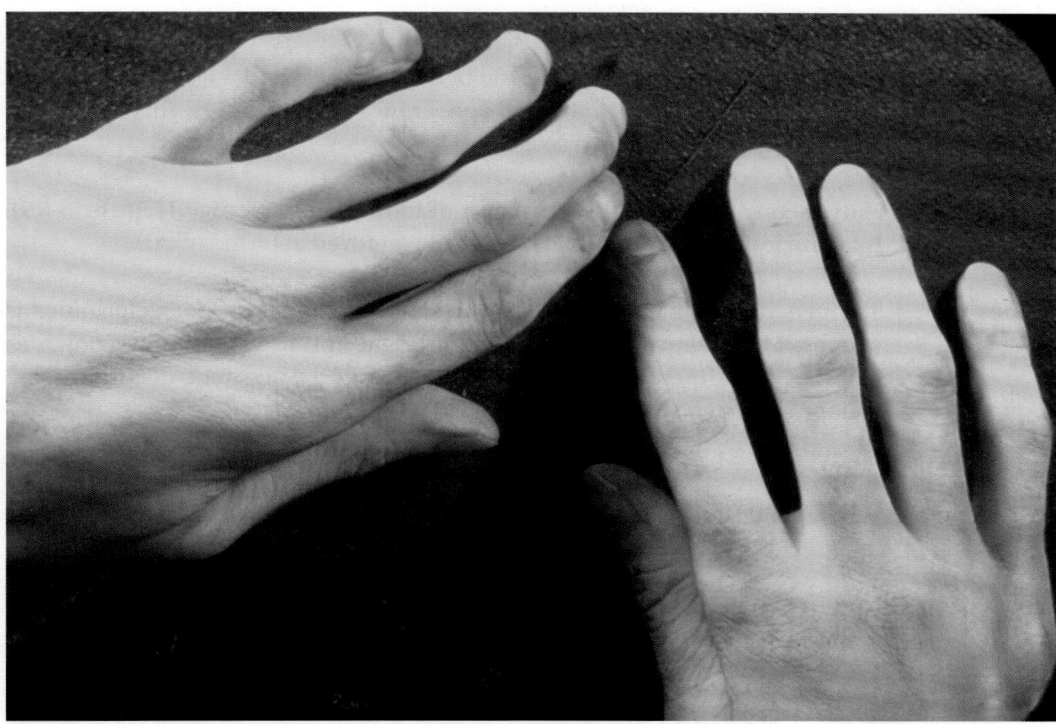

Figure 5-23 Long, slender fingers in a patient with Marfan syndrome.

osteogenesis imperfecta (OI)   Another genetic bone disease, characterized by bone fragility and hearing loss, is **osteogenesis imperfecta (OI)**. It is commonly known as brittle bone disease. This disease is marked by bone fractures resulting from minimal trauma, and individuals with this disease suffer multiple fractures throughout life. Several types of OI exist, and diagnosis is based on clinical manifestations and serologic tests. Research is advancing in this area. However, options are still limited and include surgical placement of rods to encourage bone growth and strengthen tissue and chemical therapies such as the use of bisphosphonate drugs to stimulate osteoblasts.

KEY TERM	Definition
Marfan (mahr-FAHN) **syndrome**	genetic disorder affecting connective tissues that is characterized by abnormal skeletal changes such as long limbs and fingers
osteogenesis imperfecta (OI) (os-tee-oh-JEN-e-sis im-pur-FECK-tuh)	genetic brittle bone disease

KEY TERM PRACTICE: *Genetic Bone Diseases*

1. Give the medical term for *brittle bone disease.* _____

2. _____ is a genetic disorder affecting connective tissues that is characterized by abnormally long limbs and fingers and joint laxity.

Hand and Foot Disorders

syndactyly   The term used to describe adhesion between fingers and toes is **syndactyly**. It refers to digits that have a webbed appearance (**Figure 5-24**). This is a feature common to some genetic diseases.

polydactyly   **Polydactyly** describes the condition of having an extra digit (**Figure 5-25**). Extra fingers or toes are usually surgically removed at birth.

talipes   The general medical term used to describe a variety of foot deformities is **talipes**. Most talipes are congenital in origin and are commonly known as clubfoot or **talipes equinovarus** (**Figure 5-26**). Such foot distortions are usually corrected surgically in infancy.

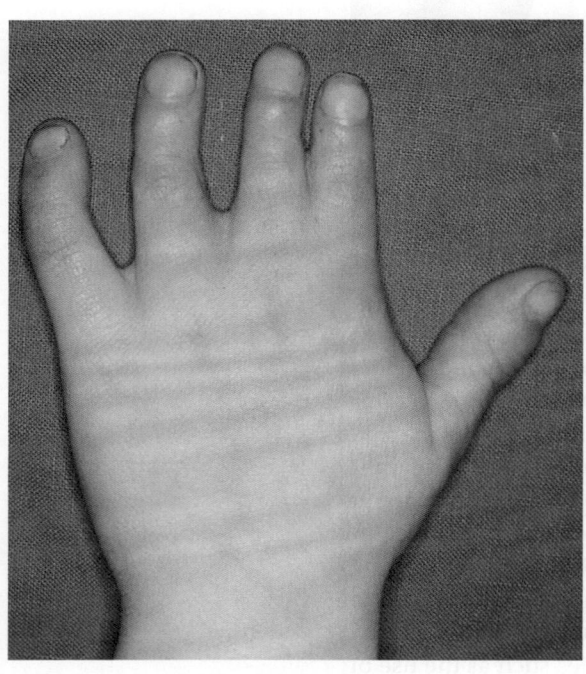

Figure 5-24 Syndactyly. Note the webbed fingers.

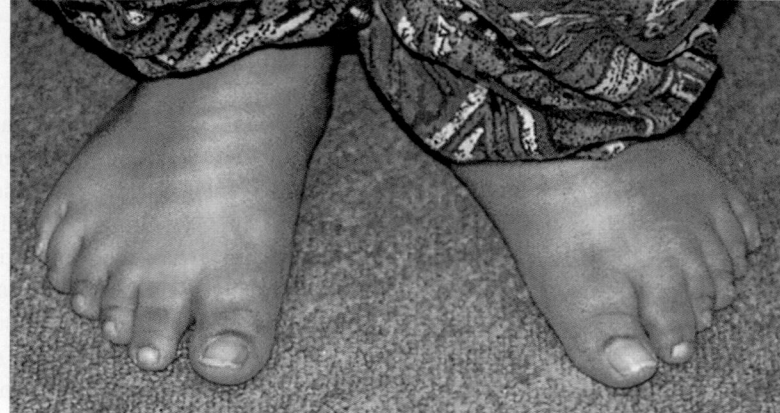

Figure 5-25 Polydactyly. Note the extra toe on each foot.

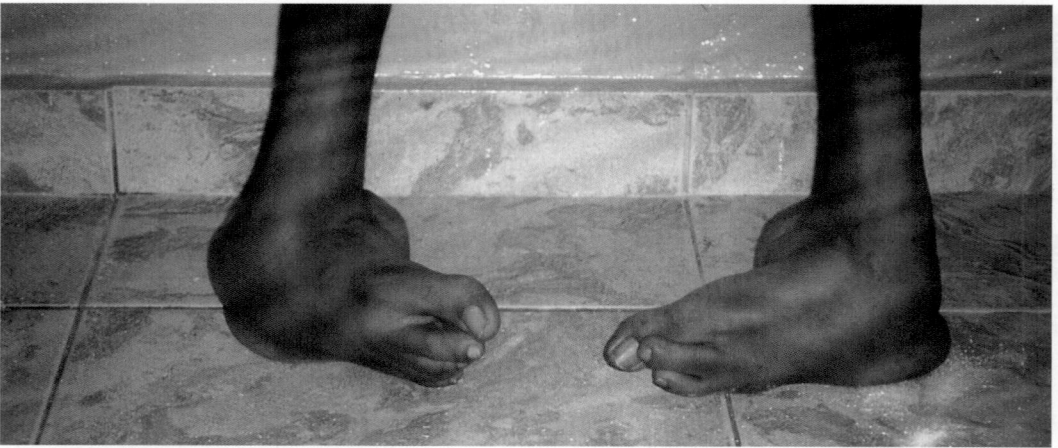

Figure 5-26 Talipes.

KEY TERM	Definition
syndactyly (sin-DACK-tih-lee)	webbed fingers or toes
polydactyly (pol-ee-DACK-tih-lee)	having extra fingers or toes
talipes (TAL-ih-peez)	human foot deformity
talipes equinovarus (TAL-ih-peez eh-kwigh-noh-VAIR-us)	clubfoot

KEY TERM PRACTICE: *Hand and Foot Disorders*

1. _____ refers to webbed fingers.

2. The general medical term that describes foot deformities is _____.

3. _____ is the medical term for *clubfoot*.

Vitamin Imbalances

Vitamin intake is essential for normal bone development, and vitamin D is especially critical.

Osteomalacia and rickets In both osteomalacia and rickets, there is inadequate mineralization of bone as a result of vitamin D deficiency. This condition is called **osteomalacia** if it occurs during adulthood, but it is referred to as **rickets** when it occurs in children. The lack of proper bone formation in children causes the bones to soften and bend under the body's weight (**Figure 5-27**). If vitamin D intake is inadequate or if the body cannot use it effectively, calcium absorption is hindered, leading to these disorders. Inadequate amounts of sunlight may also cause the condition because sunlight stimulates natural vitamin D synthesis. Treatment consists of vitamin D and calcium supplements, administration of the hormone calcitonin (which causes the absorption of calcium into bone tissue), and/or sunlight exposure.

scurvy **Scurvy** is a condition caused by a deficiency of vitamin C, which is evidenced by abnormal bone and teeth development and gum ulceration. Treatment involves ingesting vitamin C.

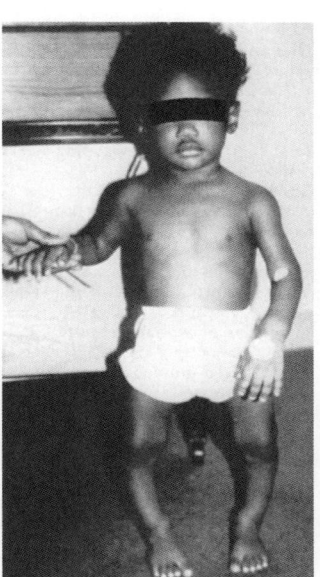

Figure 5-27 Rickets in a 3-year-old boy. Note the severe bowing of the legs.

KEY TERM	Definition
osteomalacia (os-tee-oh-muh-LAY-shee-uh)	vitamin D deficiency disease in adulthood
rickets	vitamin D deficiency disease in children
scurvy (SKUR-vee)	disorder resulting from a diet lacking vitamin C

KEY TERM PRACTICE: *Vitamin Imbalances*

1. Insufficient amounts of vitamin D and calcium in adults is termed _____.

2. Inadequate calcification and amounts of vitamin D in children leads to this disease. _____

3. _____ is a disorder resulting from a diet lacking vitamin C.

Other Bone Disorders

craniostenosis

Premature ossification of infant fontanelles is referred to as **craniostenosis.** Cranial sutures form too quickly, before the brain has matured. Its cause is not known, but surgical intervention is necessary to prevent brain damage and mental impairment.

osteitis deformans or **Paget disease**

A disease of unknown origin, **osteitis deformans**, also known as **Paget disease**, is characterized by increased bone resorption and formation leading to thickening and softening of bones. Signs and symptoms can include pain, edema, and bending of weight-bearing bones. Diagnosis is made by physical examination, patient history, blood tests, urinalysis (analysis of urine), and x-rays. Symptomatic disease is treated with analgesics; anti-inflammatory drugs; cytotoxic (cell-killing) agents; and diet therapy consisting of a high-protein, high-calcium, and high-vitamin D intake.

osteomyelitis

Osteomyelitis is an infection of bone characterized by an inflammation of the bone marrow and adjacent bone tissue. It is usually caused by *Staphylococcus aureus*. Symptoms include pain, tenderness at the site, and malaise. Children with the condition generally are just recovering from a streptococcal infection. Classic signs of advanced infection include bone **abscesses** (pus-filled cavities created by infection and inflammation). Treatment involves long-term antibiotic use, vitamin therapy, analgesics (painkillers), and immobilization to reduce fracture risk. Surgical draining of the abscess may also be required.

osteoporosis

Osteoporosis is a decrease in bone density and strength. It occurs when bone loss is greater than bone gain. This occurs when osteoclast activity outpaces osteoblast activity. A photograph of osteoporotic bone is shown in **Figure 5-28**. It is generally asymptomatic,

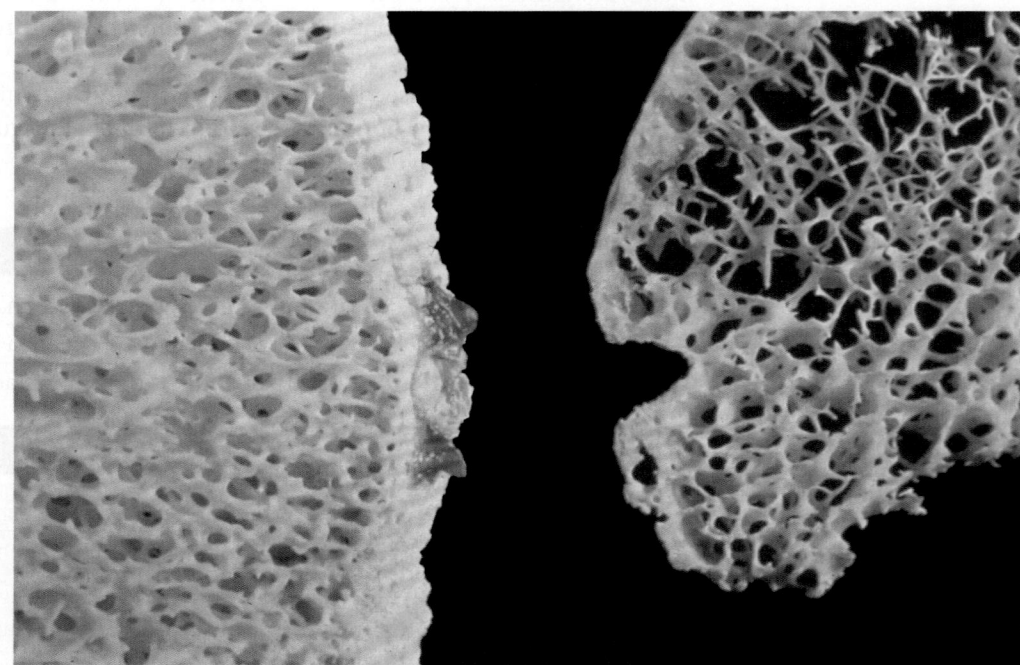

Figure 5-28 Osteoporosis. Femoral head of an 82-year-old female with osteoporosis (right) compared with a normal femoral head cut to the same thickness (left).

unless the bone loss happens in vertebrae or weight-bearing bones. It occurs more frequently in women than in men, and the first indication is often a bone fracture. Hormonal and dietary factors influence the development of osteoporosis.

Blood tests, x-rays, computed tomography (CT) scans, and bone densitometry make the definitive diagnosis. A bone **densitometer** is an instrument that uses x-rays to measure the thickness and mineral density of bone tissue. Through computer analysis, densitometry identifies individuals at risk for osteoporosis.

Treatment options depend on the severity of disease. Increased dietary calcium, vitamin D, and exercise are viable options. Pharmaceutical measures include drugs such as Fosamax (alendronate) and hormone replacement therapy for postmenopausal women to assist with bone building. Estrogen is an important hormone for bone building. In postmenopausal women, estrogen levels decline, and replacing the lost estrogen through **estrogen replacement therapy (ERT)** is often beneficial for stimulating bone growth. The term **hormone replacement therapy (HRT)** is frequently used to describe ERT, but note that the word hormone implies that estrogen is used in combination with another hormone such as progesterone.

osteochondroma	The most common benign cartilaginous tumor is an **osteochondroma**. It frequently causes bone spurs at the ends of long bones. Their cause is unknown.
osteosarcoma or **osteogenic sarcoma**	An **osteosarcoma**, also called an **osteogenic sarcoma**, is the most common malignant bone tumor that arises from osteoblasts. It primarily affects the ends of long bones and its greatest incidence is in the age group between 10 and 25 years. Treatment options include surgical removal and chemotherapy.
Ewing sarcoma	**Ewing sarcoma** is a malignant bone tumor that occurs usually before the age of 20 and is twice as common in males. In nearly 75% of patients, the tumors affect the bones of the extremities.

KEY TERM	Definition
craniostenosis (KRAY-nee-oh-stuh-NOH-sis)	premature ossification of the fontanelles and fusion of the cranial sutures
osteitis deformans (os-tee-EYE-tis de-FOR-manz)	bone disease characterized by increased bone resorption and formation resulting in thickening and softening of bones; also called Paget disease
Paget (PAJ-et) **disease**	bone disease characterized by increased bone resorption and formation resulting in thickening and softening of bones; also called osteitis deformans
osteomyelitis (os-tee-oh-migh-eh-LYE-tis)	bacterial infection of bone marrow and adjacent bone tissue
abscesses (AB-ses-ez)	pus-filled cavities created by infection and inflammation

continued

continued from page 237

KEY TERM	Definition
osteoporosis (os-tee-oh-poh-ROH-sis)	disorder characterized by a decrease in bone density and strength
densitometer (den-si-TOM-e-tur)	instrument used to measure bone density
estrogen (ES-troh-jen) **replacement therapy** (**ERT**)	administration of the hormone estrogen
hormone replacement therapy (HRT)	administration of hormones, notably estrogen and progesterone
osteochondroma (os-tee-oh-kon-DROH-muh)	benign tumor of cartilage
osteosarcoma (os-tee-oh-sahr-KOH-muh)	most common malignant bone tumor that arises from osteoblasts; also called osteogenic sarcoma
osteogenic sarcoma (os-tee-oh-JEN-ick sahr-KOH-muh)	most common malignant bone tumor that arises from osteoblasts; also called osteosarcoma
Ewing sarcoma (YOO-ing sahr-KOH-muh)	malignant bone tumor that occurs usually before the age of 20 and is twice as common in males

KEY TERM PRACTICE: *Other Bone Disorders*

1. The medical term for the most common malignant bone tumor that arises from osteoblasts is _____.

2. _____ is a bacterial infection of bone marrow and adjacent bone tissue.

3. An instrument used to measure bone density is called a _____.

4. _____are pus-filled cavities created by infection and inflammation.

5. Premature ossification of the fontanelles and fusion of the cranial sutures is termed _____.

INTRODUCTION TO JOINTS

Movement of the body is made possible through the interaction of muscles and bones operating at an articulation, or joint. A joint is simply the union of two or more bones. Well-known articulations include the elbow, shoulder, foot, ankle, knee, hip, and vertebral column, but there are actually 230 joints in the body!

Diagnosis of joint disease is made through patient history and physical examination, and laboratory and x-ray data provide supplemental assistance. Joint disorders result from autoimmune diseases, trauma, genetic influences, infection, and the aging process.

Articulations are classified according to the type of tissue that binds the bones together at each joint, the joint's function, or the amount of movement possible at the joint. Joints are designed to withstand stress placed on the body while providing leverage, stability, and assistance with balance. Fibrous, cartilaginous, and synovial joints make various movements possible.

MEDICAL TERM PARTS: JOINTS

Word Parts: Joints

Medical term prefixes, suffixes, and combining forms related to joints are introduced in this section.

Word Part	Meaning
amph-, amphi-, ampho-	on both sides
ankylo-	bent, crooked
arthr-, arthro-	joint
capsul-, capsulo-	capsule
chondrio-, chondro-	cartilage
-ectomy	surgical removal
hyal-, hyalo-	glassy, transparent
orth-, ortho-	straight
-plasty	molding or shaping
spondyl-, spondylo-	vertebrae
sym-, syn-	together, with, joined
tendo-, teno-	tendon

Word Grouping Exercises: Joints

Using the *Medical Term Parts* table, identify the prefix, suffix, or combining form for each of the following definitions. The first one has been done as an example.

Definition	Word Part
bent, crooked	*ankylo-*
cartilage	
glassy, transparent	
joint	
molding or shaping	
on both sides	
straight	
surgical removal	
tendon	
together, with, joined	
vertebrae	

Word Building Exercises: Joints

Word parts introduced in the *Medical Term Parts* section are listed in the following table. For this exercise, first supply the meaning of each word part, then use the word part to build a word you already know. The word you list under *Common or Known Word* does not have to be a medical term; a commonly used word is fine. Be sure, however, that the word correctly reflects the intended meaning. The first one has been done as an example. Check your answers in a dictionary.

Word Part	Meaning	Common or Known Word	Example Medical Term
amph-, amphi-, ampho-	*on both sides*	*amphibian*	amphiarthrosis
arthr-, arthro-			arthroscopy
-ectomy			bunionectomy
orth-, ortho-			orthopedics
sym-, syn-			syndesmoses
tendo-, teno-, tenon-			tendonitis

ANATOMY AND PHYSIOLOGY: JOINTS

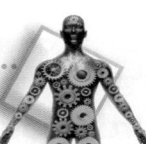

A **joint**, or **articulation**, is a point of close contact between two or more bones. Articulations (joints) work with the musculoskeletal system and make body movements, such as standing, sitting, and walking, possible.

Articulations can be classified according to their function or structure, which determines the type of movement possible. Functional classification is based on the degree of movement and groups the joints as immovable, slightly movable, and freely movable. Structural classification is based on the type of connective tissue found at the joint. Based on structure, articulations may be fibrous, cartilaginous, or synovial.

Cartilage, ligaments, and tendons are key components of joints. Recall that cartilage is tough, nonvascular, connective tissue found throughout the body, notably at joints. The sheath of cartilage capping the ends of bones is called articular cartilage and reduces friction and absorbs shock. For example, between the femur and the tibia, the band of articular cartilage prevents the bone ends from rubbing together and absorbs the shock of walking.

Ligaments are bands of tough, fibrous connective tissue that connect bones or cartilage at a joint. They help bind the articular ends of the bones together while preventing excess movement at the joint. By the way, there is no such thing as being *double jointed*; rather, a person simply has loose ligaments. **Tendons** are bands of fibrous connective tissue that attach muscles to bones. They assist motion at joints by attaching to articular structures.

KEY TERM	Definition
joint	point of close contact between two or more bones; also called an articulation
articulation (ahr-tick-yoo-LAY-shun)	point of close contact between two or more bones; also called a joint
ligaments (LIG-uh-munts)	bands of tough, fibrous connective tissue that connect bones or cartilage at a joint
tendons (TEN-dunz)	bands of fibrous connective tissue that attach muscles to bones

KEY TERM PRACTICE: *Joints*

1. Supply two terms that mean "point of close contact between two or more bones." _____

2. _____ are bands of tough, fibrous connective tissue that connect bones or cartilage at a joint.

3. _____ are bands of fibrous connective tissue that attach muscles to bones.

Types of Joints

The structural classification of joints describes several types, including the following:

- **Fibrous joints** are found between bones coming into close contact with one another, such as the bones of the skull, between the teeth and jaw, and at the junction of the tibia (shin bone) and fibula (smaller lower leg bone) (**Figure 5-29A**). Structurally, the bones are fastened tightly together with a thin layer of fibrous connective tissue, and functionally, little or no appreciable movement occurs there. **Sutures** are a kind of fibrous, immovable joint. Sutures create seams in the skull when the cranial bones ossify (**Figure 5-29B**).

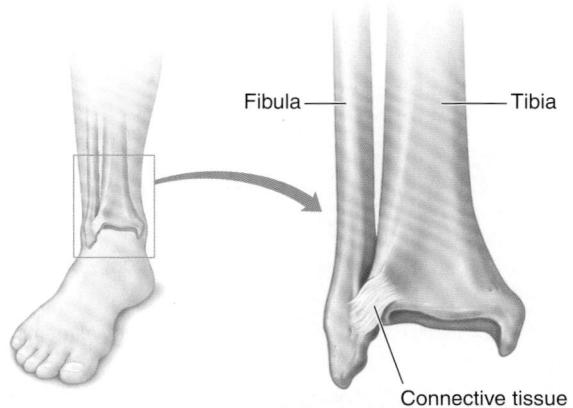

Fibula — — Tibia

Connective tissue

A

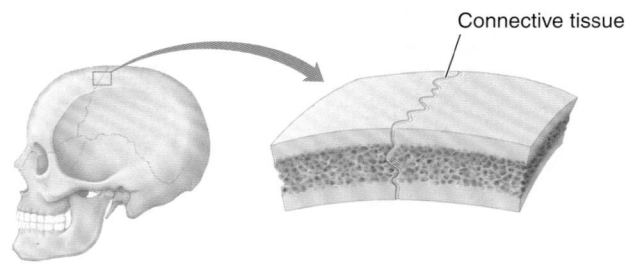

Connective tissue

B

Figure 5-29 (A) Example of a fibrous joint found at the articulation between the tibia and fibula. **(B)** Example of a suture, a type of fibrous joint.

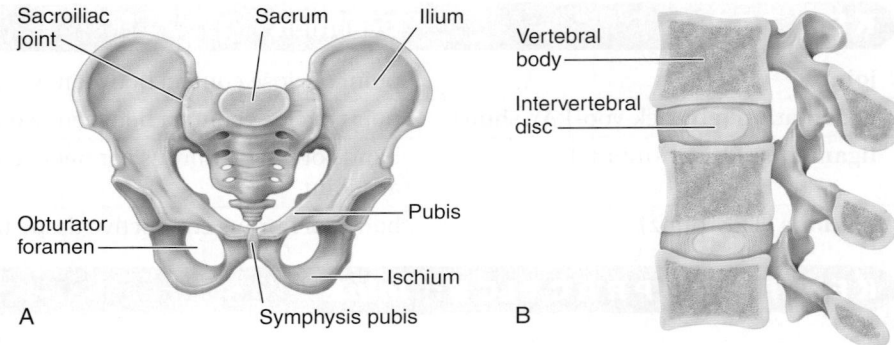

Figure 5-30 (A) The symphysis pubis is an example of a cartilaginous joint. **(B)** Example of cartilaginous joint formed by two adjacent vertebrae.

- **Cartilaginous joints** are primarily composed of nonvascular connective tissue known as cartilage. Cartilaginous joints are either slightly movable or immovable. A **symphysis** is a slightly movable cartilaginous joint. An example in the pelvic girdle is the **symphysis pubis**, the anterior union of the pubic bones, which are separated by a pad of fibrocartilage (**Figure 5-30A**). Another example is the joint formed by two adjacent vertebrae, which are separated by an intervertebral disc (**Figure 5-30B**). Each **intervertebral disc** is composed of an outer band of fibrocartilage and an inner core of soft gelatinous material that allows the disc to act as a shock absorber. Because each disc is slightly flexible, the combined movement of all of the joints in the vertebral column allows limited motion when the back is bent forward, or to the side, or is twisted. These joints are classified as cartilaginous instead of fibrous because they do allow for *some* movement, whereas fibrous joints are basically nonmovable.

- **Synovial joints** are freely movable, and most joints in the skeletal system are of this type. **Figure 5-31** illustrates the structures of synovial joints: articular cartilage, joint capsule, menisci, synovial membranes, and bursae.

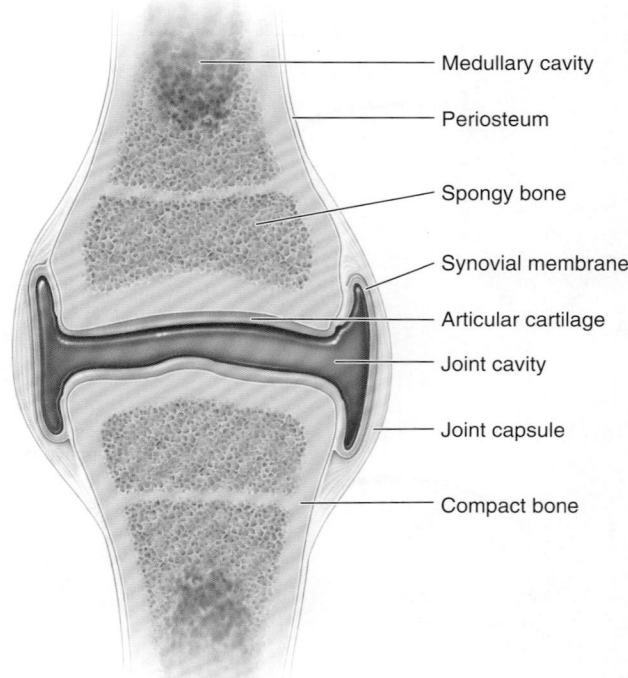

Figure 5-31 Structures of a synovial joint.

Joints have several associated structures that lend support to their form and function, including ligaments and tendons. Articular cartilage covers the ends of the bones. The fibrous sheet enclosing a synovial joint is called the **joint capsule**. Joint capsules are reinforced by bundles of ligaments. **Menisci** (*meniscus* = singular) are crescent-shaped discs of fibrocartilage that separate and cushion the articulating surfaces of bones. Menisci are found in the knee and in the shoulder joints. The synovial membrane forms the inner lining of the joint capsule and surrounds a closed sac called the synovial (joint) cavity. The clear viscous fluid secreted by the synovial membrane is called synovial fluid. This fluid moistens and lubricates surfaces within the joint. It also helps supply articular cartilage with nutrients obtained from the blood vessels of the synovial membrane. **Bursae** (*bursa* = singular) are fluid-filled sacs that reduce friction around joints. They act as cushions and aid the movement of tendons that glide over bony parts (**Figure 5-32**).

Several types of synovial joints are found in the human body. They permit various movements. One type, the **ball-and-socket joint**, is located in the hip and shoulder. Ball-and-socket joints allow motion and rotational movement in all planes. **Hinge joints** are found at the elbows, knees, and phalanges. The hinge joint has movement in one plane only, much like the hinge on a door.

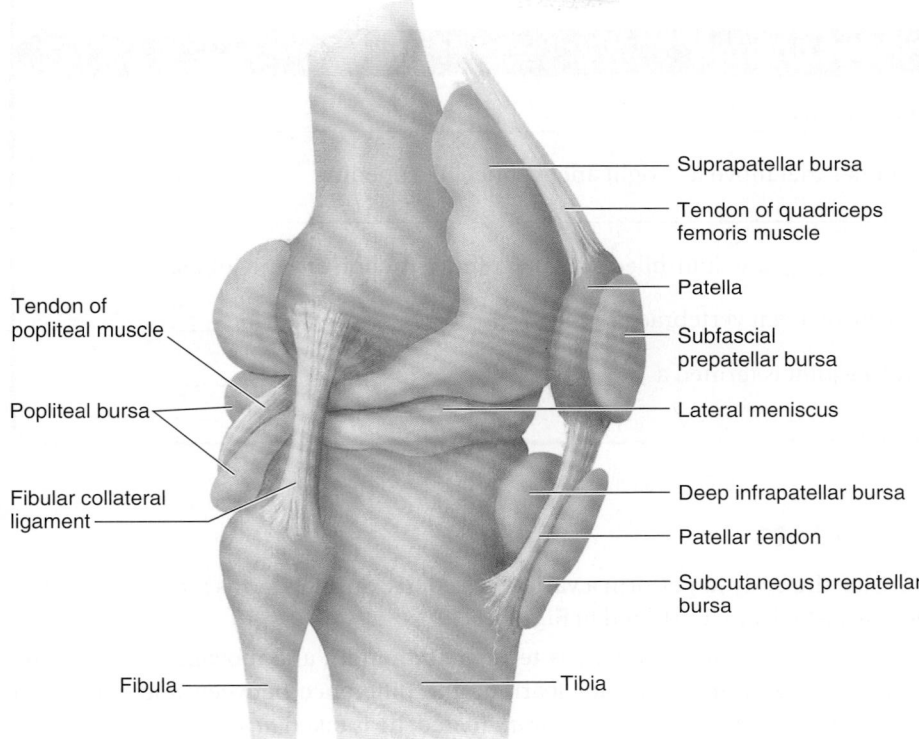

Figure 5-32 Bursae and the lateral meniscus in the knee.

KEY TERM	Definition
fibrous (FIGH-brus) **joints**	articulation made of fibrous connective tissue found between bones in close contact
sutures (SUE-churz)	joint type found in the skull in which the bones are bound together by fibrous connective tissue
cartilaginous (kahr-ti-LAJ-i-nus) **joints**	articulations made of cartilage
symphysis (SIM-fi-sis)	slightly movable joint in which the bones are connected by a pad of fibrocartilage
symphysis pubis (SIM-fi-sis PEW-bis)	the fibrocartilaginous union of the anterior pubic bones
intervertebral (in-tur-VUR-te-brul) **disc**	mass of fibrocartilage between adjacent vertebrae
synovial (si-NOH-vee-ul) **joints**	freely movable articulations
joint capsule	fibrous sheet enclosing a freely movable joint
menisci (me-NIS-kee)	crescent-shaped discs of fibrocartilage that separate and cushion the articulating surfaces of bones
bursae (BUR-see)	fluid-filled sacs that reduce friction around joints
ball-and-socket joint	joint in which the rounded head of one bone fits in the concave surface of another
hinge joints	joints formed by two bones that move in a right angle, much like opening or closing a door

KEY TERM PRACTICE: *Types of Joints*

1. List the three types of joints classified by structure. _____

2. Identify the type of joint formed by two bones that move in a right angle, much like opening or closing a door. _____

3. _____ are fluid-filled sacs that reduce friction around joints.

4. The masses of fibrocartilage found between adjacent vertebrae are called_____.

5. The fibrous sheet enclosing a freely movable joint is termed a _____.

Joint Movements

Articulations enable the body to perform a variety of actions. Specific terms are used for types of joint movements, which are illustrated in **Figure 5-33**.

- Movement away from the body's midline is termed **abduction**, and movement toward the body's midline is **adduction**. An aid for learning the difference between *ab*duction and *ad*duction is to remember that if somebody is *ab*ducted, he is taken *away*.

- Increasing the angle between two bones is referred to as **extension**, and decreasing the angle between two bones is **flexion**. Bringing the lower arm up to "flex" the upper arm muscles is an example of flexion. Moving the arm back to its original position is extension. **Hyperextension** is excessive extension of a body part beyond the 180-degree angle of the anatomic position. Tilting the head back to look up at the sky is an example of hyperextension.

- Circular movements are described as if the person were in the anatomic position. **Circumduction** is movement in a circular motion as when throwing a ball. In circumduction, the proximal end is fixed while the distal end moves in a circle. **Rotation** involves turning a bone on its own axis. The motion made while turning a key in a lock is a rotational movement.

- Turning the palm posteriorly or downward is termed **pronation**, and turning the palm anteriorly or upward is called **supination**. Movement of the forearm into the anatomic position involves pronation. As a tip, associate the *p* in *posterior* with the *p* in *pronation*. Another clue is to think about the position of a waiter's hand while carrying a bowl of *soup* as the same position as *sup*ination. You can only carry a bowl of soup if your hand is supinated!

- Several movement terms apply to the foot and lower leg. **Dorsiflexion** describes the movement of bending the foot toward the tibia. The opposite of dorsiflexion—bending the foot away from the tibia and pointing the toe while extending the ankle—is **plantar flexion.** Movement in which the sole of the foot is turned outward or laterally is **eversion**, and **inversion** is movement of the sole of the foot inward or medially.

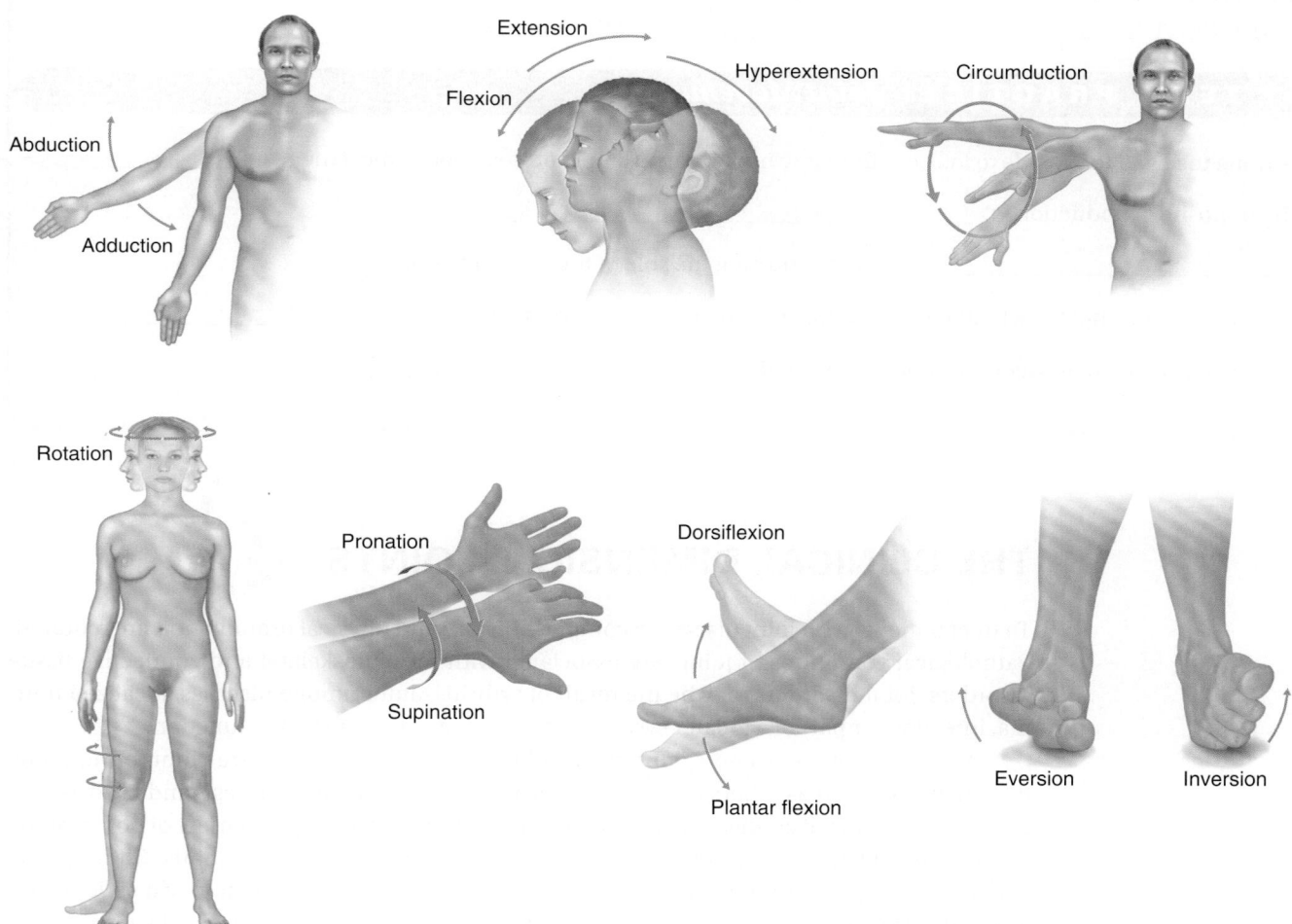

Figure 5-33 Movements at joints.

KEY TERM	Definition
abduction (ab-DUCK-shun)	movement away from the body's midline
adduction (ad-DUCK-shun)	movement toward the body's midline
extension	increasing the angle between two bones; making a flexed part straight
flexion (FLECK-shun)	decreasing the angle between two bones
hyperextension	excessive extension beyond the anatomic position
circumduction (sur-kum-DUCK-shun)	movement in which the proximal end is fixed while the distal end moves in a circle as when throwing a ball
rotation	turning around on an axis or fixed point as when turning a key in a lock
pronation (proh-NAY-shun)	turning the palm posteriorly or downward
supination (soo-pi-NAY-shun)	turning the palm anteriorly or upward
dorsiflexion (dor-si-FLECK-shun)	bending the foot so the toes move upward toward the tibia
plantar flexion (PLAN-tahr FLECK-shun)	bending the foot so the toes move downward and the ankle is extended
eversion (e-VUR-zhun)	turning the sole of the foot outward
inversion (in-VUR-zhun)	turning the sole of the foot inward

KEY TERM PRACTICE: *Joint Movements*

1. Turning the head to the side to look out the car window is an example of what type of movement? _____

2. The opposite of abduction is _____.

3. _____ describes turning the sole of the foot outward.

4. Standing on your tiptoes would be an example of which type of movement? _____

5. Increasing an angle between two bones is termed _____.

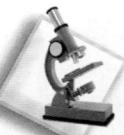

THE CLINICAL DIMENSION: JOINTS

To treat patients with joint disease, a complete history and physical examination are required. Pathological conditions of joints are associated with musculoskeletal and connective tissue disorders. Joint disorders may be the result of arthritis, autoimmune diseases, localized trauma, infection, or part of a greater systemic disease that can disturb joint function.

As with other signs and symptoms exhibited by the body, some are common to many dysfunctions, whereas others are specific to articulations. Edema, tiredness, and fibrosis (abnormal thickening of connective tissue) are common descriptions for a variety of homeostatic imbalances. Others, such as the various types of arthritis, are specific to joints. Clinical tests and diagnostic procedures supplement the history and physical examination of a patient with a joint disorder. Definitive diagnoses often require laboratory data and diagnostic tests.

Arthritis

arthritis

Arthritis refers to several disorders characterized by inflammation of the joints, often accompanied by stiffness of adjacent structures. Mineral deposits (calcification) may form on bone tissue causing joint inflexibility.

gouty arthritis or **gout**

Gouty arthritis, also called **gout**, is a condition in which uric acid crystals are deposited in the soft tissues of joints, eventually destroying them. Its cause is thought to be a metabolic or renal disorder causing excessive uric acid production. Gout usually affects toe joints, typically the first metatarsal joint of the great toe (hallux), but can affect finger joints as well. It generally appears in bouts with acute attacks. Signs and symptoms include pain, edema, fever, chills, and headache; however, the person is symptom free between attacks. **Figure 5-34** illustrates the **edema** (swelling) associated with gout. The inflammation is the result of excessive fluid accumulation between the tissue cells.

For diagnostic and/or therapeutic purposes it may be necessary to extract liquid from the synovial space. Puncturing the joint capsule with a needle to remove the fluid is termed **arthrocentesis**. Arthrocentesis is a diagnostic tool when the fluid is extracted for analysis and it is a treatment when the fluid is removed to reduce inflammation. Treatment of gout involves joint immobilization, ice to reduce edema, anti-inflammatory drugs, a low-protein/high-fluid diet, and medications to reduce uric acid production.

Lyme arthritis

Lyme arthritis, also known as Lyme disease, is an infectious disease transmitted to humans from the bite of a tick infected with *Borrelia burgdorferi*. Signs and symptoms are overall malaise, flu-like symptoms, joint pain, and a skin lesion with a target or bull's-eye pattern. **Malaise** is the term for general weakness, fatigue, and lethargy, which are common symptoms of infection. The disease mimics rheumatoid arthritis.

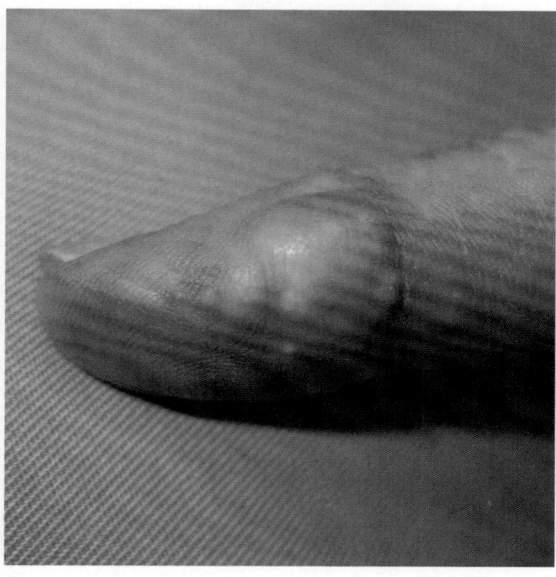

Figure 5-34 Gout of the finger.

Most cases are diagnosed on the basis of the clinical picture, but a definitive diagnosis is made through a positive blood antibody test identifying specific antibodies (proteins that fight specific foreign substances or invaders) to Lyme disease. A bull's-eye rash around the tick bite is often seen in patients (**Figure 5-35**). Unfortunately, symptoms may not appear for weeks or months after infection. Treatment begins by removing the tick if still evident, followed by prompt administration of antibiotics.

osteoarthritis

Osteoarthritis is an age-related degenerative joint disease (DJD) characterized by deterioration of articular cartilage and formation of **osteophytes** (bone spurs), which are bony outgrowths that develop around the joint (**Figure 5-36**). Affecting mainly large, weight-bearing joints, this form of arthritis results from normal wear and tear on the articulations. The surgical removal of bone spurs and degenerative changes by chiseling away at the bony irregularities is termed **cheilectomy**. When the hands are involved, osteoarthritis often leads to characteristic bony overgrowths that form knobby fingers. Signs and symptoms include achiness and stiffness in the joints, deformity, and a crackling sound that is heard when bones rub together. It can be either a primary (main) condition or a secondary (result of another disease) condition. Autoimmune factors may be involved.

Diagnosis is made through the history and physical examination, CT scan, and/or magnetic resonance imaging (MRI) scans. Treatment includes anti-inflammatory medicines, analgesics (painkillers), and physical therapy (PT) to increase range of motion (ROM) at articulations. Total joint replacement (TJR) and other surgical options may be used in severe cases.

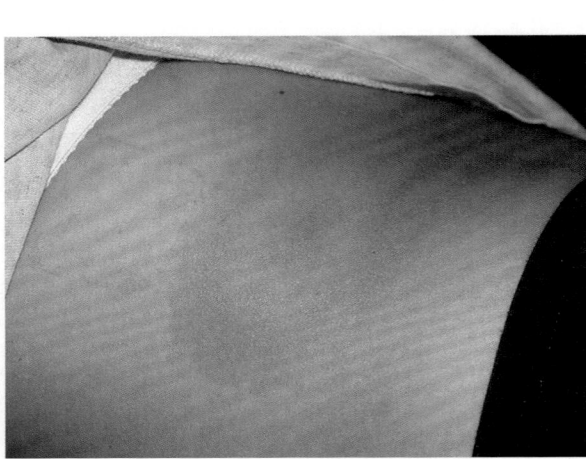

Figure 5-35 Bull's-eye rash seen in Lyme disease.

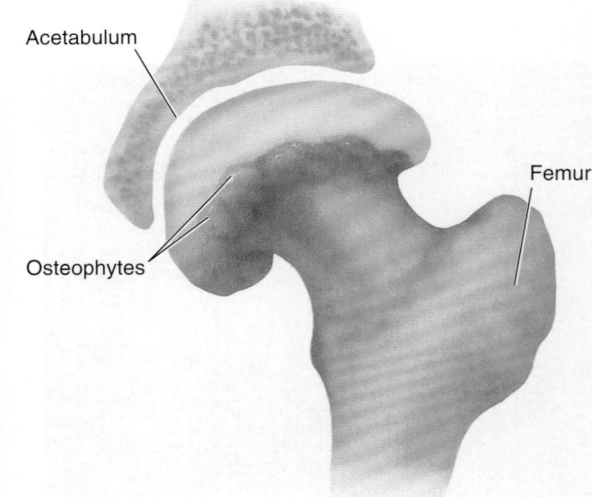

Figure 5-36 Osteophytes on the hip joint.

KEY TERM	Definition
arthritis (ahr-THRIGH-tis)	joint inflammation
gouty arthritis (GOW-tee ahr-THRIGH-tis)	metabolic disorder causing excessive uric acid production and deposition in joints, often in the great toe; also called gout
gout (gowt)	metabolic disorder causing excessive uric acid production and deposition in joints, often in the great toe; also called gouty arthritis
edema (e-DEE-muh)	swelling; tissue inflammation with fluid accumulation
arthrocentesis (ahr-throh-sen-TEE-sis)	needle puncture into a joint capsule to extract synovial fluid
Lyme arthritis (lime ahr-THRIGH-tis)	joint inflammation as a result of the bite of a tick infected with *Borrelia burgdorferi*; also called Lyme disease
malaise (mal-AIZ)	general weakness, tiredness, and discomfort
osteoarthritis (os-tee-oh-ahr-THRIGH-tis)	degenerative joint disease characterized by deterioration of articular cartilage and formation of bone spurs
osteophytes (OS-tee-oh-fights)	abnormal bony outgrowths at joints, commonly called bone spurs
cheilectomy (kye-LECK-toh-mee)	chiseling away of bony outgrowths that interfere with joint mobility

KEY TERM PRACTICE: *Arthritis*

1. Give the two terms for the metabolic disorder that causes excessive uric acid production and deposition in joints, often in the great toe. _____

2. Another term for bone spurs is _____.

3. Joint inflammation as a result of the bite of a tick infected with *Borrelia burgdorferi* is termed _____.

4. An _____ is a needle puncture into a joint capsule to extract synovial fluid and is derived from the word part _____ for *joint* and the word part _____ for *puncture*.

5. _____ is a medical term used to describe general weakness, tiredness, and discomfort.

Autoimmune Diseases

Autoimmune diseases are caused by the reaction of antibodies (proteins that the body produces to destroy foreign substances) to naturally occurring substances in the body. Several autoimmune diseases affect the joints.

ankylosing spondylitis   **Ankylosing spondylitis** is a chronic, progressive inflammatory disease of the intervertebral spaces that causes abnormal fusion (growing together) of the vertebrae. The vertebral fusion results in a solid, inflexible spinal column. Joint immobility or fixation is referred to as **ankylosis.** Ankylosis is a sign that there is some sort of joint disorder. Edematous joints, fibrosis, kyphosis, and osteoporosis characterize it. Abnormal thickening and scarring of connective tissue is called **fibrosis.** Symptoms of ankylosing spondylitis include back pain and morning stiffness. Diagnosis is made through the physical examination, x-rays, and MRI evaluations (which use electromagnetic radiation to obtain images of body tissues).

Treatment is supportive and includes physical therapy, acetylsalicylic acid (ASA; commonly known as aspirin), and nonsteroidal anti-inflammatory drugs. **Nonsteroidal anti-inflammatory drugs** (**NSAID**s; pronounced "EN saids") are medicines such as ibuprofen and aspirin that have both analgesic and anti-inflammatory properties.

rheumatism

Rheumatism is the general term used to describe diseases of muscle, tendon, joint, or bone that share characteristics of musculoskeletal pain and stiffness.

rheumatoid arthritis (RA)

An example of a rheumatic disease is **rheumatoid arthritis (RA)**, a chronic autoimmune disease causing joint inflammation and deformity (**Figure 5-37**). It is a degenerative joint disease characterized by deterioration of articular cartilage and bone spur formation. Remissions and exacerbations causing progressive damage are common. There is generally symmetrical inflammation of peripheral joints as well as the temporomandibular joint (TMJ). Hallmark signs and symptoms include malaise, synovitis, fibrosis, cartilage erosion, and ankylosis.

Synovitis means inflammation of the synovial membrane. Diagnosis is made through the history, physical examination, and analysis of synovial fluid. Treatment is supportive and includes rest during periods of flare-ups and physical therapy at other times. Anti-inflammatory analgesics such as ASA and ibuprofen (Motrin and Advil) also prove beneficial.

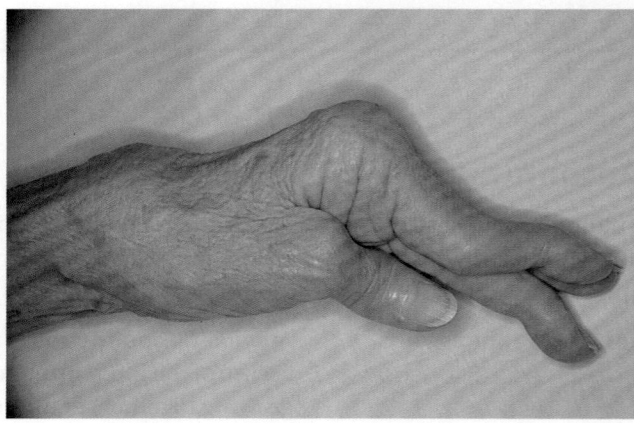

Figure 5-37 "Swan-neck" deformity of the index finger in a patient with rheumatoid arthritis.

systemic lupus erythematosus (SLE)   **Systemic lupus erythematosus (SLE)** is a chronic inflammatory connective tissue disorder of unknown origin that primarily affects women. This disorder involves several systems because connective tissue is widely dispersed throughout the body. Articular symptoms are observed in 90% of cases of SLE. Early-stage SLE is difficult to differentiate from rheumatoid arthritis and other connective tissue disorders.

Initial diagnosis is made by the clinical picture and confirmed by SLE antibody tests, which identify markers specific to SLE. Management of SLE depends on its manifestations and severity. Mild SLE is treated with NSAIDs and physical therapy. Corticosteroids and immunosuppressive drugs that dampen the immune response are used to treat severe disease. **Corticosteroids** are synthetic drugs similar to the body's natural steroid hormones produced by the adrenal gland. They are generally injected directly into the joint area to reduce swelling and inflammation.

KEY TERM	Definition
ankylosing spondylitis (ang-i-LOH-sing spon-di-LYE-tis)	fusion and inflammation of the vertebrae
ankylosis (ang-i-LOH-sis)	joint immobility or fixation
fibrosis (figh-BROH-sis)	abnormal thickening and scarring of connective tissue
nonsteroidal (non-STEER-oid-ul) **anti-inflammatory drugs (NSAIDs)**	medicines that reduce tissue inflammation and pain
rheumatism (ROO-muh-tiz-um)	general term for diseases characterized by musculoskeletal pain and stiffness
rheumatoid arthritis (RA) (ROO-muh-toid ahr-THRIGH-tis)	systemic autoimmune disease characterized by joint inflammation and deformity
synovitis (sin-oh-VYE-tis)	inflammation of the synovial membrane
systemic lupus erythematosus (SLE) (LEW-pus er-ih-thee-mah-TOH-sus)	chronic inflammatory connective tissue disease
corticosteroids (kor-ti-koh-STEER-oidz)	synthetic drugs similar to the steroid hormones produced by the adrenal glands that are used to reduce inflammation

KEY TERM PRACTICE: *Autoimmune Diseases*

1. _____ is the general term for diseases characterized by musculoskeletal pain and stiffness.

2. The term for fusion and inflammation of the vertebrae is _____ and is derived from the word part _____, which means *bent, crooked,* and the word part _____, which means *the vertebrae.*

3. The medical term for inflammation of the synovial membrane is _____.

4. _____ is the medical term for abnormal thickening and scarring of connective tissue.

5. Synthetic drugs similar to the natural steroids produced by the adrenal glands that are used to reduce inflammation are termed _____.

Foot, Ankle, and Knee Disorders

Articular foot disorders are associated with cartilage, whereas other problems involve tendons, nerves, ligaments, or bones. The knee joint is formed by the articulation between the femur and tibia and the articulation between the femur and patella. A complete dislocation of the knee is rare because the joint contains many stabilizing ligaments and tendons.

bunion   A **bunion** is a protrusion from a metatarsophalangeal (MTP) joint caused by inflammation of the bursa around the joint of the great toe (hallux). The resultant abnormal bending of the hallux toward the little toe is termed **hallux valgus** (**Figure 5-38**). The condition is associated with flat-footedness and rheumatoid arthritis. Signs and symptoms are pain and joint displacement. Diagnosis is made by physical examination and radiographic studies. Treatment options include analgesics, corticosteroid injections, and surgical removal of the bunion, termed **bunionectomy**.

sprain   A **sprain** is a painful injury to the ligaments of a joint caused by wrenching or overstretching. The ankle is a common site for sprains. Signs and symptoms of mild to moderate sprains include tenderness, swelling, and difficulty moving the joint. Complete ligamentous tears cause swelling and hemorrhage. Treatments for mild to moderate sprains are immobilization and strapping with elastic bandages, followed by light exercise of the affected part. Severe sprains may require cast immobilization or surgery.

torn meniscus   A tear in the crescent-shaped cartilage disc in the knee as a result of twisting the knee is termed a **torn meniscus**. Often involved is one of the ligaments found inside the joint capsule, the anterior cruciate ligament (ACL), which attaches the tibia to the femur. A torn meniscus is characterized by acute pain, crepitus, and flexion impairment. The injury is usually sports related and caused by twisting or external rotation while the knee is flexed.

To obtain an image of the joint interior, **arthrography** may be performed. This involves obtaining a radiograph of the joint space after it has been injected with a contrast medium. Physical examination, x-ray, MRI, or arthrography confirms the diagnosis.

Visual inspection of the joint interior using an **arthroscope** (fiberoptic camera) is termed **arthroscopy** (**Figure 5-39**). Clinicians use these tests to

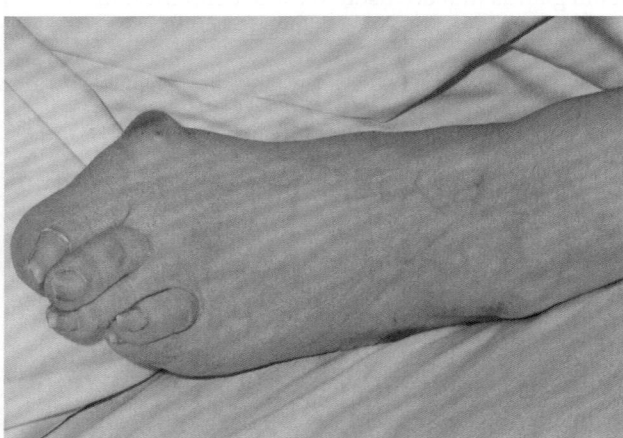

Figure 5-38 Bunion with hallux valgus.

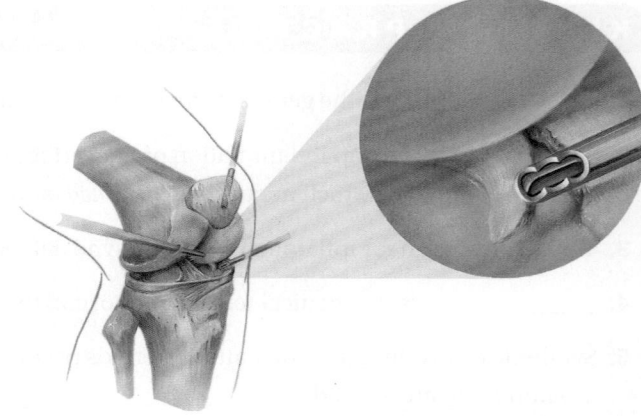

Figure 5-39 During arthroscopy, the joint interior can be inspected with an arthroscope.

assess the extent of damage, if any, in an articulation. Treatment involves arthroscopic surgery and physical therapy.

Severe trauma, disease, or joint deterioration may necessitate the reconstruction or creation of an artificial joint, as in a hip or knee replacement. This is called **arthroplasty** (**Figure 5-40**).

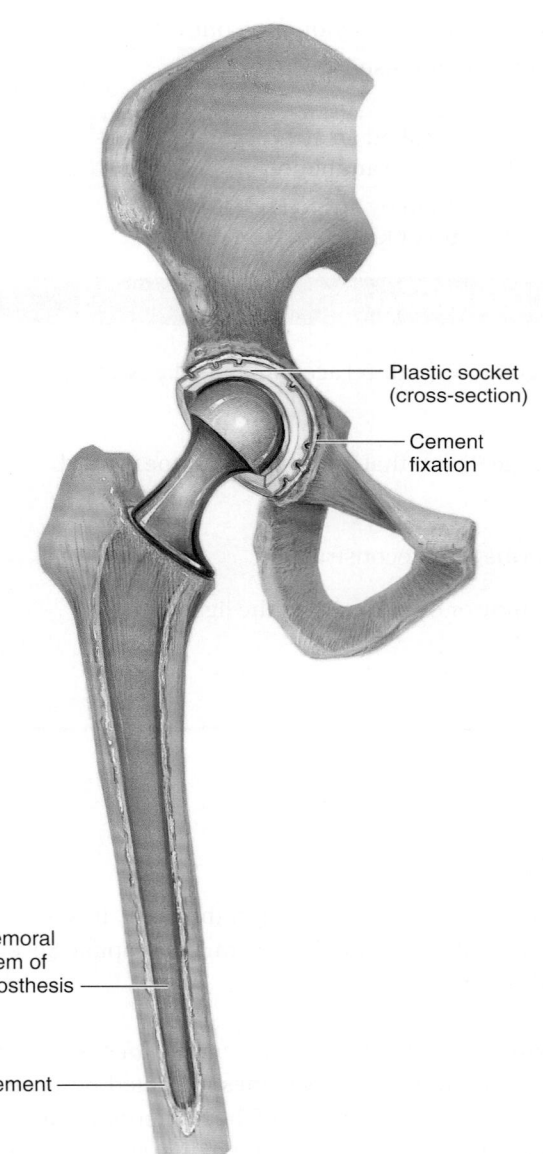

Plastic socket (cross-section)

Cement fixation

Femoral stem of prosthesis

Cement

Figure 5-40 Arthroplasty. Total hip replacement.

KEY TERM	Definition
bunion (BUN-yun)	inflammation of the bursa around the great toe (hallux) accompanied by swelling and sideways displacement of the joint
hallux valgus (HAL-ucks VAL-gus)	a deformity at the metatarsophalangeal joint that forces the great toe toward the other toes
bunionectomy (bun-yun-ECK-tuh-mee)	removal of a bunion

continued

USING MEDICAL TERMINOLOGY

continued from page 253

KEY TERM	Definition
sprain	painful injury to the joint ligaments caused by wrenching or overstretching
torn meniscus (me-NIS-kus)	meniscus abnormality that results from twisting the joint
arthrography (ahr-THROG-ruh-fee)	x-ray of the joint space after introduction of a contrast dye
arthroscope (ahr-THROH-skope)	fiberoptic instrument (camera) used to view a joint's interior
arthroscopy (ahr-THROS-kuh-pee)	insertion of a fiberoptic lens called an arthroscope directly into the joint for visual examination
arthroplasty (AHR-throh-plas-tee)	joint removal with replacement by artificial joints or prostheses, as in hip or knee replacements

KEY TERM PRACTICE: *Foot, Ankle, and Knee Disorders*

1. A _____ is inflammation of the bursa around the great toe (hallux) accompanied by swelling and sideways displacement of the joint.

2. _____ describes a deformity at the metatarsophalangeal joint that forces the great toe toward the other toes

3. _____ is the medical term used to describe joint reconstruction.

4. A _____ is a painful injury caused by wrenching or overstretching the ligaments.

5. A meniscus abnormality that results from twisting a joint is called a _____.

Shoulder and Wrist Disorders

The shoulder joint, or *glenohumeral joint,* is the most movable joint in the body. It is formed by the union between the head of the humerus with the glenoid cavity on the scapula. Several important ligaments and muscles stabilize this joint.

adhesive capsulitis

Adhesive capsulitis, commonly called *frozen shoulder,* is a condition in which the joint movement becomes restricted because of inflammatory thickening of the capsule of the humerus. It is a common cause of shoulder stiffness. Physical therapy, analgesics, and anti-inflammatory drugs are common treatments.

carpal tunnel syndrome

Carpal tunnel syndrome is caused by unceasing pressure on the median nerve passing through the tunnel in carpal bones. It results from repetitive movements of the hands and wrists and is characterized by numbness, weakness, and tingling. The physical examination and a positive Tinel sign are generally enough to diagnose the condition. For the Tinel sign test, the patient's arms are outstretched while the clinician taps the inside affected wrist over the median nerve with a reflex hammer. If the person experiences a "pins and needles" sensation, he or she has tested positive for carpal tunnel syndrome (**Figure 5-41**). Treatment involves physical therapy, splinting, or surgery that divides the carpal ligament to relieve median nerve pressure.

ganglion   A **ganglion** is a benign growth filled with colorless fluid arising from the joint capsule or tendon sheath. Ganglia commonly develop on the wrist (**Figure 5-42**). The underlying cause is not known, but fortunately they are painless, creating only an unsightly bump. Treatment often is not necessary because they disappear on their own. When treatment is warranted, a needle aspiration to reduce the ganglion's size or a ganglionectomy (surgical excision of a ganglion) may be performed.

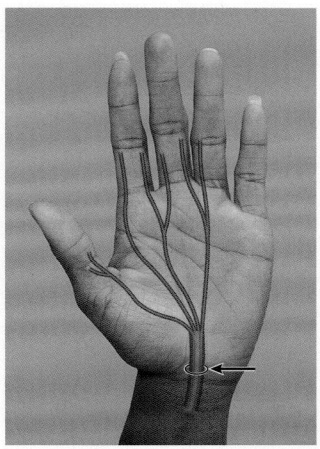

Figure 5-41 Tingling in the distribution of the median nerve constitutes a positive Tinel sign, suggesting carpal tunnel syndrome.

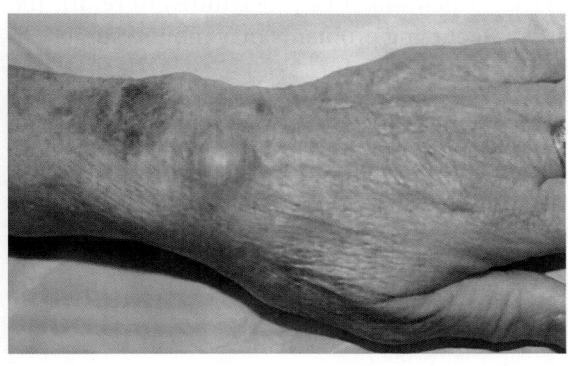

Figure 5-42 Ganglion on the wrist.

KEY TERM	Definition
adhesive capsulitis (ad-HEE-siv kap-soo-LIGH-tis)	condition characterized by restricted joint mobility because of inflammatory thickening of the capsule of the humerus; also called frozen shoulder
carpal (KAHR-pul) **tunnel syndrome**	wrist affliction caused by pressure on the median nerve in the carpal bones
ganglion (GANG-glee-un)	benign growth in or around a tendon sheath or joint capsule

KEY TERM PRACTICE: *Shoulder and Wrist Disorders*

1. A wrist affliction caused by pressure on the median nerve in the carpal bones that results from repetitive movements is termed _____.

2. A _____ is a benign growth in or around a tendon sheath or joint capsule.

3. _____ is a condition characterized by restricted joint mobility because of inflammatory thickening of the capsule of the humerus.

Trauma

bursitis

Bursitis is an acute or chronic inflammation of the bursae. Signs and symptoms are pain, tenderness, edema, and limited ROM. It results from overuse injuries such as those occurring in tennis players and baseball pitchers whose bursae are subjected to excessive friction. Calcified deposits form in advanced disease. Diagnosis is made through the history and physical examination, ROM as measured by a goniometer, x-rays, and MRI studies.

dislocation or **luxation**

A **dislocation**, or **luxation**, is a displacement of a bone from its normal joint position. A partial or incomplete dislocation is called a **subluxation**. A dislocation is usually caused by trauma or a sports injury. Typically, the affected joint has an abnormal appearance, is immobile, and shows signs of edema, and the patient generally complains of pain. Diagnosis is made through history and physical examination and is confirmed by x-rays. Treatment involves joint reduction (surgical or manipulative procedures) to return the bones to their normal position. Recurring problems may require surgery to tighten the associated joint ligaments.

herniated disc

A **herniated disc** occurs when the gelatinous center of the intervertebral disc protrudes through the surrounding fibrocartilage (**Figure 5-43**). The protruding material may press on nerves and cause pain. Treatments include anti-inflammatories for pain or surgery.

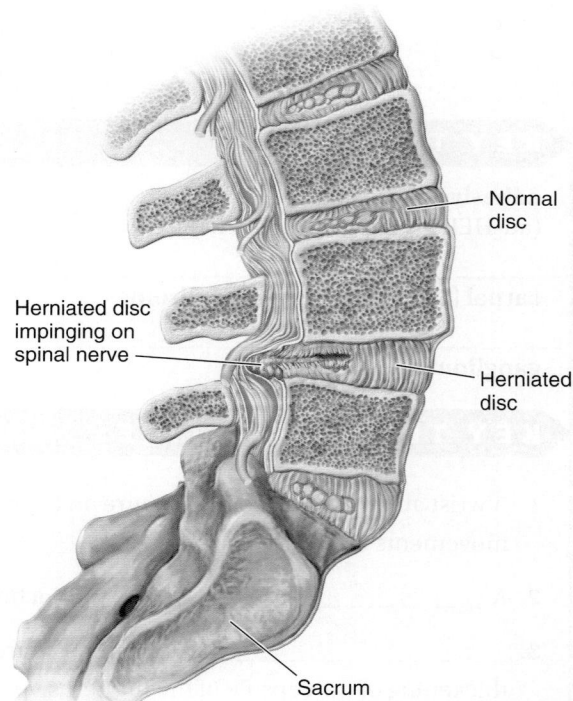

Normal disc

Herniated disc impinging on spinal nerve

Herniated disc

Sacrum

Figure 5-43 Herniated disc in the lumbar region.

KEY TERM	Definition
bursitis (bur-SIGH-tis)	inflammation of the bursae
dislocation	displacement of a joint; also called a luxation
luxation (luck-SAY-shun)	displacement of a joint; also called a dislocation
subluxation (sub-luck-SAY-shun)	partial or incomplete dislocation of a joint
herniated (HUR-nee-ate-ed) **disc**	condition in which the center of an intervertebral disc protrudes through the fibrocartilage

KEY TERM PRACTICE: *Trauma*

1. Give the medical term for each of the following terms.

a. dislocation _____

b. partial dislocation _____

2. _____ is the medical term for bursae inflammation.

3. A _____ is a condition in which the center of an intervertebral disc protrudes through the fibrocartilage.

LIFE SPAN

Bone formation begins around the eighth week in utero. Because the skeletal system develops in a specific time frame, fetal age can be determined by looking at bone development through x-rays or sonograms. At birth, the head is disproportionately large, and the spine of a newborn appears kyphotic, or concave. At 3 months after birth, the cervical spine becomes lordotic (convex) and has an increased ability to hold the head. As the infant matures, normal lordotic curvature of the lumbar region develops. The ability to sit enhances this developmental change.

The bones are essentially ossified at birth, but the epiphyseal plates are present until long bone growth stops, typically around adolescence. At birth, infant legs are bowed as a result of confinement in the womb. As the child ages, the arms and legs undergo rotational and alignment changes. It is common for children to appear "bowlegged" until 2.5 years of age or "knock-kneed" until 6 years. If either condition persists beyond these ages, it is considered pathologic and should be treated. During childhood, the arms and legs grow at a greater rate than the spine. By age 1, the spine reaches 50% of its total growth.

During childhood and adolescence, bone formation exceeds bone resorption. By age 25, bones are completely ossified. A balance between osteoblastic and osteoclastic activity characterizes adulthood. Osteoclastic activity outpaces osteoblastic activity during late adulthood. Bone mass, except cranial bone mass, begins declining around age 40. Calcium loss appears to be the main effect on the aging process. Furthermore, decreased production of organic matter makes bones more susceptible to fracture. Exercise and proper nutrition can strengthen bones and increase osteoblastic activity at any time during a person's life. In this way, osteoporosis can be prevented.

Joint disorders generally do not appear until advanced age, with the exception of congenital defects (present at birth), autoimmune diseases, and injuries. Congenital articular disorders, possibly resulting from intrauterine positioning, include hip and knee dislocation. However, joint abuse as a result of overtraining or traumatic exercise can lead to early degenerative diseases or dysfunction. Surgery on articular tissue is also known to hasten the onset of generalized arthritis.

As a person ages, fibrous protein strands of collagen form differently, resulting in decreased tissue elasticity and increased joint stiffening. Osteoarthritis appears to be a normal part of aging. Individuals ages 70 years and older typically exhibit some degree of degenerative joint disease. Fortunately, with the use of anti-inflammatory drugs coupled with lifelong ROM exercises, arthritis does not have to be totally debilitating.

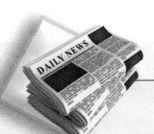

IN THE NEWS: Lyme Arthritis

In November 1975, Lyme arthritis, also known as Lyme disease, was first observed in the United States in the towns of Lyme and Old Lyme, Connecticut. Its identification began when a woman in Lyme decided to keep a personal journal to track the disease when she realized that neighbors in her community were exhibiting common symptoms of malaise, a bull's-eye rash, (see **Figure 5-35**) and severe joint pain. Between June and September of that same year, 59 cases were observed. Eventually, rheumatologist Dr. Allen Steere and his research group affiliated with Yale University traced the bizarre finding to a tick-borne bacterial infection.

Two years later, the deer tick *Ixodes scapularis* was identified as the vector of disease transmission (**Figure 5-44**). It was not until 1982 that Dr. Willy Burgdorfer of the National Institutes of Health (NIH) discovered that the disease was caused by a bacterium living inside the tick. Today, that microbe is known as *Borrelia burgdorferi*.

The cycle of disease transmission to humans involves bacteria, ticks, and tick bites. Two types of ticks carry Lyme disease: deer ticks (in the Northeast and Midwest) and western black-legged ticks (northern California and Oregon). Ticks normally feed on wildlife, and the bacteria are often harbored in the ticks. Animals do not become ill when bitten by affected ticks but spread the disease to humans who are bitten by the tick. The classic sign is a round, red rash at the site of the tick bite, but this is not always present and people often do not realize they have been bitten by a tick. Other signs and symptoms include general malaise, headaches, sore muscles and joints, and fever.

Infected ticks usually do not spread the disease until they have been attached to the human for at least 36 hours. For this reason, it is important that you remove ticks as soon as you notice them. The symptoms can start any time from 3 days up to 1 month after being bitten. Treatment includes antibiotics. Untreated Lyme disease can lead to arthritis, trouble focusing your thoughts, poor memory, and weakness or paralysis of your facial muscles.

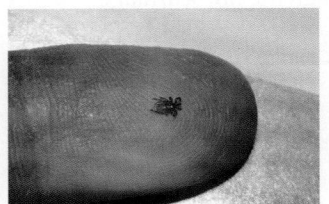

Figure 5-44 An adult tick is the size of the head of a matchstick.

COMMON Abbreviations

Abbreviation	Term
ACL	anterior cruciate ligament
ASA	acetylsalicylic acid (aspirin)
C_1–C_7	cervical vertebrae 1–7
CPR	cardiopulmonary resuscitation
CT	computed tomography
DJD	degenerative joint disease
ERT	estrogen replacement therapy
Fx	fracture
HRT	hormone replacement therapy
L_1–L_5	lumbar vertebrae 1–5
MRI	magnetic resonance imaging
MTP	metatarsophalangeal
NSAIDs	nonsteroidal anti-inflammatory drugs
OI	osteogenesis imperfecta
PT	physical therapy
RA	rheumatoid arthritis
ROM	range of motion
SLE	systemic lupus erythematosus
T_1–T_{12}	thoracic vertebrae 1–12
TJR	total joint replacement
TMJ	temporomandibular joint

COMMON ABBREVIATIONS EXERCISES

1. ROM is the abbreviation for _____.

2. Write the abbreviation for acetylsalicylic acid. _____

3. Fx is the abbreviation for _____.

4. When discussing joints, TJR refers to _____.

5. Write the abbreviation for physical therapy. _____

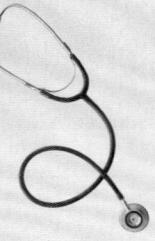

Case Study

Justin Miller is a wide receiver on his college football team. A conscientious athlete, he has strictly adhered to his conditioning plan, which includes weightlifting four times per week, practice six days per week, and nutritious meals. Justin began playing tackle football in grade school. Since that time he has sustained no serious sports-related injuries.

During a Saturday afternoon game, Justin took an unusually hard hit from behind. Justin heard a "crunching" sound and thought something "popped." While he lay immobile on the field, Paul, the athletic trainer, rushed to his side. Justin was conscious, able to talk, and had little difficulty moving his extremities. Two other players assisted Justin to his feet. While standing erect, Justin experienced excruciating pain radiating from his cervical and lumbar regions. He also had slight pain while walking.

On the sidelines, the athletic trainer assessed Justin's physical strength, range of motion, and balance, which were unremarkable in all joints except the cervical and lumbar spine and the left tibiofemoral. Joint tenderness was evident in these areas, and edema was noted in the patellar region. Tibiofemoral flexion was slight, and complete extension was not possible. Extension and flexion at the coxal articulation caused considerable pain. Paul administered a therapeutic dosage of an NSAID and recommended that Justin undergo radiographic studies.

Case Study Questions

Select the best answer to each of the following questions.

1. **During his assessment of Justin's injuries, Paul noted edema at the** _____.
   a. knee
   b. shin
   c. hip
   d. neck

2. **The tibiofemoral joint is also known as the** _____ **joint.**
   a. shoulder
   b. hip
   c. knee
   d. elbow

3. **Normal knee joint movements include** _____.
   a. flexion
   b. extension
   c. hyperextension
   d. a and b

4. **NSAIDs were administered to** _____.
   a. reduce swelling
   b. relieve pain
   c. assist with the cartilage growth
   d. a and b

5. **The cervical and lumbar regions refer to the** _____.
   a. head and neck
   b. shoulder and leg
   c. neck and lower back
   d. lower back and knee

6. **Radiographic studies involve the use of** _____.
   a. magnetic fields
   b. sound waves
   c. x-rays
   d. sonograms

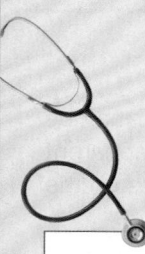

Real World Report

CENTRAL IMAGING DEPARTMENT

NAME: Justin Miller
ORDPHYS: M. A. Johnson, MD
TEST: Lumbar, routine, 6 views
REFERRING: D. Brindly, MD
EXAM DATE: 09/13/2011

DATEORD: 09/10/2011
DOB: 10/13/1992
ATTENDING: G. G. Timmons, MD
CLINIC: SM

CLINICAL INFORMATION

Back pain; injured in football game.

LUMBAR SPINE

Multiple views of the lumbar spine were obtained and show no fracture or subluxation. There is moderate degenerative disc narrowing at L_5–S_1, which shows degenerative vacuum phenomenon. No spondylolysis or spondylolisthesis is shown.

IMPRESSION

1. No fracture.
2. Moderate degenerative disc narrowing and degenerative vacuum phenomenon at L_5–S_1.

CERVICAL SPINE

Multiple views of the cervical spine were obtained and show no fracture or subluxation. The intervertebral disc spaces and neuroforamina are maintained. The prevertebral soft tissues are unremarkable.

IMPRESSION

No fracture or subluxation.

TIBIOFEMORAL

Multiple views of the knee were obtained and show no fracture or subluxation. Effusion is evident.

IMPRESSION

No fracture or subluxation.
DICTATED BY: Jack D. O'Henry, MD
This document has been reviewed and electronically approved by Jack D. O'Henry, MD 09/14/2011

continued

continued from page 261

Real World Report Questions

The following exercises review the medical terms used in the preceding medical report. Two terms may be unfamiliar: *Vacuum phenomenon* means that there is a stripe on an intervertebral disc that becomes apparent on an x-ray. The stripe is a sign of disc degeneration. *Prevertebral tissue* refers to the fascia and muscles on the anterior aspect of the vertebral column.

1. **Degenerative disc narrowing was noted. The term *disc* refers to _____.**

   a. the vertebral lamina

   b. vertebrae

   c. the intervertebral pad of fibrocartilage

   d. the spinal column

2. ***Degenerative disc narrowing* means _____.**

   a. the intervertebral discs are showing deterioration

   b. there is bone damage

   c. the vertebrae are normal

   d. a subluxation is present

3. **Subluxation refers to a/an _____.**

   a. fracture

   b. strain

   c. dislocation

   d. abrasion

4. **The report referred to spondylolysis.**

   a. The word part *spondylo-* means _____.

   b. The word part *lys-* means _____.

   c. So *spondylolysis* means _____.

5. **The report referred to spondylolisthesis.**

   a. The word part *spondylo-* means _____.

   b. The word part *-esis* means _____.

   c. So *spondylolisthesis* means _____.

6. **The report referred to neuroforamina. The word part *neuro-* means "nerve or nerve tissue," and the word *foramen* means "opening."**

   a. What is the plural form of foramen? _____

   b. So *neuroforamina* means _____.

Review and Application

Multiple-Choice Questions

Select the best response to each of the following questions.

1. Functions of the skeletal system include _____.
   a. mineral storage   b. protection   c. hemopoiesis   d. all of these

2. Most of the body's phosphorous and calcium is stored in _____.
   a. bones and teeth   b. bones and blood   c. muscle and bone   d. none of these

3. Which word part means cartilage? _____
   a. osteo-   b. chondro-   c. myelo-   d. peroneo-

4. What does the word part *spondylo-* mean? _____
   a. pelvis   b. bone   c. vertebrae   d. straight

5. The _____ is the shaft of a long bone.
   a. diaphysis   b. epiphysis   c. metaphysis   d. head

6. The ends of long bones are called _____.
   a. diaphyses   b. epiphyses   c. sutures   d. metaphyses

7. The medullary cavity can be found _____.
   a. on a bone's exterior   b. at an articulation   c. in the bone's interior   d. in conjunction with hyaline cartilage

8. Sutural bones are found in this location _____.
   a. cervical region   b. in the knee   c. within the hip bone   d. in the skull

9. Cancellous bone is also known as _____.
   a. cortical bone   b. compact bone   c. osteonic bone   d. spongy bone

10. _____ is the conversion of cartilage tissue into bone.
    a. Blastogenesis   b. Ossification   c. Clastogenesis   d. Histogenesis

11. _____ are mature bone cells, whereas _____ are bone-forming cells.
    a. Osteocytes; osteoblasts   b. Osteoblasts; osteocytes   c. Osteoclasts; osteoblasts   d. Osteoclasts; osteocytes

12. Long bone growth occurs at the _____.
    a. epiphyseal plate   b. subchondral plate   c. appositional line   d. diaphysis

13. Vitamins essential for bone growth include _____.
    a. vitamin B   b. vitamin E   c. vitamin D   d. vitamin B_{12}

14. Metatarsal refers to the _____ between the _____ and _____.
    a. hand; wrist; fingers   b. knee; hip; foot   c. foot; ankle; toes   d. elbow; shoulder; wrist

15. Anatomic terminology referring to identifiable landmarks on bone is best described as _____.
    a. surface markings   b. exterior formations   c. surface definitions   d. morphology lines

16. A break in a bone is called a _____.
    a. strain   b. sprain   c. fracture   d. compression

17. Cervical vertebrae are _____.
    a. numbered T_1–T_{12} b. identified as C_1–C_7 c. inferior to the sacral region   d. between the thoracic and lumbar vertebrae

18. Epiphyseal plates are present until _____.
    a. birth   b. adolescence   c. long bone growth ceases   d. puberty

19. The combining form *arthro-* means _____.
    a. anthropology   b. anthrax   c. cartilage   d. joint

20. The combining form *amphi-* means _____.
    a. amphibian   b. anthrax   c. cartilage   d. on both sides

21. Articulations are classified according to _____.
    a. structure   b. function   c. position   d. a and b

22. Synarthrosis means that the joint bones are _____.
    a. close together   b. far apart   c. freely movable   d. none of these

23. A suture is a type of _____ joint.
    a. fibrous   b. freely movable   c. synovial   d. cartilaginous

24. The symphysis pubis is a type of _____ joint.
    a. synovial   b. cartilaginous   c. intervertebral   d. fibrous

25. Synovial joints are _____ movable.
    a. not   b. slightly   c. freely   d. somewhat

26. Fluid-filled sacs that reduce friction in a synovial joint are termed _____.
    a. vursae.   b. bursae.   c. menisci.   d. capsules.

27. This disease is caused by the bite of a tick infected with *Borrelia burgdorferi* _____.
    a. Legionnaires' disease   b. West Nile virus   c. Lyme arthritis   d. kennel cough

Word Parts Exercises

Using the following word parts, form a medical term for each definition. Each group of word parts may be used more than once.

-blast
chondrio-, chondro-
-cyte
-malacia
ost-, oste-, osteo-

28. bone-forming cell = _____

29. bone softening = _____

30. cartilage cell = _____

Matching Exercises

Match the disorder with its description.

31. _____ is abnormal lateral curvature of the vertebral column.

32. _____ is an exaggeration of the thoracic curve.

33. _____ is concavity of the lumbar curve.

a. Scoliosis
b. Kyphosis
c. Lordosis

Match the sign or symptom with its description.

_____ 34. ankylosis

_____ 35. synovitis

_____ 36. malaise

a. inflammation of synovial membrane
b. joint fixation
c. general fatigue

Match the bone with its location.

_____ 37. ulna

_____ 38. humerus

_____ 39. tibia

_____ 40. femur

_____ 41. scapula

a. upper leg bone
b. forearm
c. upper arm bone
d. lower leg bone
e. back; forms part of shoulder

Match the surface marking with its description.

_____ 42. crest

_____ 43. sinus

_____ 44. condyle

_____ 45. tuberosity

_____ 46. tubercle

a. cavity or hollow space
b. round knob
c. narrow, ridge-like projection
d. small, rounded process
e. large, roughened knob-like protuberance

Match the surface marking with its associated bone.

_____ 47. acetabulum

_____ 48. foramen magnum

_____ 49. xiphoid process

_____ 50. greater trochanter

_____ 51. transverse process

a. femur
b. coxal bone
c. vertebra
d. occipital bone of skull
e. sternum

Match the description with the fracture type.

_____ 52. fracture of vertebrae as a result of severe stress

_____ 53. broken bone; skin intact

_____ 54. incomplete break; bone bends

_____ 55. fractured distal radius and ulna

_____ 56. broken bone; skin cut

a. simple fracture
b. Colles fracture
c. greenstick fracture
d. compound fracture
e. compression fracture

Match the movement with its correct description.

_____ 57. extension

_____ 58. abduction

_____ 59. pronation

_____ 60. plantar flexion

_____ 61. inversion

a. movement away from the body's midline
b. increasing the angle between bones
c. turning sole of foot inward
d. turning palm downward
e. pointing toes

Singular and Plural Forms

Write the singular form for each term.

62. laminae = _____

63. vertebrae = _____

64. sacra = _____

65. humeri = _____

Write the plural form for each term.

66. ulna = _____

67. phalanx = _____

68. fibula = _____

69. patella = _____

Spelling

Identify the correctly spelled term in each set.

70. _____
  a. ziphoid
  b. zifoid
  c. xiphoid
  d. xifoid

71. _____
  a. humerous
  b. humerus
  c. humurus
  d. humurous

72. _____
  a. forramen
  b. foramen
  c. foraman
  d. foremon

73. _____
  a. acetabulm
  b. acetabelum
  c. asatabulum
  d. acetabulum

74. _____
  a. ilium bone
  b. illium bone
  c. illeum bone
  d. ileum bone

75. _____
  a. spinus process
  b. spinnus process
  c. spinous process
  d. spineous process

76. _____
  a. ankalosis
  b. ankylosis
  c. ankyelosis
  d. anckylosis

77. _____
  a. burcitis
  b. bursitis
  c. bursitus
  d. bersitus

78. _____
  a. lucksation
  b. luxashun
  c. luxtion
  d. luxation

79. _____
  a. rheumatizm
  b. rumatism
  c. rheumatism
  d. rhumatizm

80. _____
  a. abduction
  b. abducsion
  c. abduckshun
  d. abbducshun

Opposites

For each of the following directional terms, write the term that has the opposite meaning.

81. adduction / _____

82. pronation / _____

83. flexion / _____

84. eversion / _____

85. supination / _____

Unscramble

Unscramble the letters to form a medical term.

86. tsalcesoot _____

87. yiodh noeb _____

88. ginhe notisj _____

89. xyccco _____

90. caimrnu _____

Abbreviations

Provide the term for the abbreviations and then define the terms.

91. OI = _____

92. TMJ = _____

93. T_1–T_{12} = _____

94. ACL = _____

95. NSAID = _____

Analogies

Provide a medical term to complete a meaningful analogy.

96. Dislocation is to luxation as joints are to _____.

97. Subluxation is to partial dislocation as great toe is to _____.

Short Answer

Answer the following questions.

98. Iva is an 80-year-old woman who was hospitalized for a broken hip. This was her first experience with a fracture. Her history and physical (H&P) examination revealed that since the death of her spouse she remained homebound, got very little exercise, and began to experience back pain. Her diet evaluation indicated that she was not eating properly and lacked appropriate dietary intake of calcium, phosphorus, and vitamin D. Without performing any other diagnostic procedure or clinical test, the physician told her she suspected a very common porous bone disorder. What bone disease did the doctor suspect and why?

_____

99. A patient was brought to the emergency department with a compound fracture. After the initial set of x-rays, the radiologist and orthopedic surgeon diagnosed an epiphyseal fracture of the femur and sent the patient to the pediatric ward for surgical treatment. What prompted the pediatric assignment?

_____

100. What types of movement are possible at the shoulder joint?

_____

101. Which articulation is also known as the glenohumeral joint?

_____

102. Mike is playing in a football game. The pigskin is thrown directly at him, but slightly above his head. He plants his feet firmly on the ground, twists, and extends his arms to make the catch. As he is making this tremendous play, an opposing player hits him on the anterior knee and tackles him. After the down, Mike experiences acute pain and has difficulty walking. Identify a possible knee injury, and cite the bones that make up the tibiofemoral articulation.

_____

Labeling

Label the structures in the following diagram.

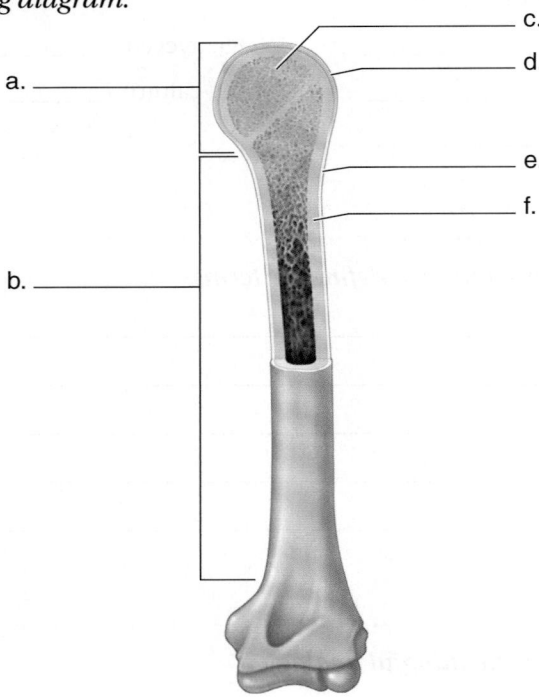

Word Search

Find the medical terms hidden in the puzzle.

R	S	L	P	N	E	N	O	W	M	R	N	M	N	S	F
M	U	E	T	S	O	I	R	E	P	O	S	O	W	E	O
V	O	M	E	R	U	I	T	N	I	B	I	P	H	L	N
L	O	Z	E	D	G	A	L	T	H	S	B	S	N	C	T
H	M	U	Q	F	P	G	C	G	N	C	U	S	Y	I	A
S	E	R	G	H	T	U	Q	E	N	L	P	E	C	D	N
I	W	A	Y	V	D	W	T	M	A	A	C	T	W	E	E
N	Y	S	L	D	Q	X	U	T	U	V	G	A	Z	P	L
U	I	J	A	U	E	I	I	C	C	I	A	N	O	H	L
S	H	C	I	R	C	U	M	D	U	C	T	I	O	N	E
E	I	G	E	L	N	E	Z	M	F	L	O	B	P	X	S
S	O	P	A	Y	E	V	B	U	K	E	P	R	L	U	H
P	Y	C	W	I	J	M	W	A	O	S	D	U	V	I	D
H	A	R	T	I	C	U	L	A	R	W	K	T	H	D	L
M	U	R	C	A	S	Q	G	M	X	T	Y	M	S	U	P
S	T	N	E	M	A	G	I	L	I	S	C	H	I	U	M

adduction
articular
calcium
circumduction
clavicles
femur
fontanelles
ganglion
hyperextension
ischium
ligaments
metaphysis
pedicles
periosteum
pubis
sacrum
sinuses
talus
trabeculae
turbinates
vomer

Vocabulary Review

Review the key terms from this chapter, study the spelling and pronunciation of each term, and write its definition in the space provided. Listen to the audio available for most terms at http://thepoint.lww.com/nath2e and pronounce each term for yourself. Then check the box when you feel confident that you know the definition and can pronounce the term correctly.

Key Term	Pronunciation	Definition
☐ abduction	(ab-DUCK-shun)	_____
☐ abscess	(AB-ses)	_____
☐ acetabulum	(as-e-TAB-yoo-lum)	_____
☐ adduction	(ad-DUCK-shun)	_____
☐ adhesive capsulitis	(ad-HEE-siv kap-soo-LIGH-tis)	_____
☐ ankylosing spondylitis	(ang-i-LOH-sing spon-di-LYE-tis)	_____
☐ ankylosis	(ang-i-LOH-sis)	_____
☐ arthritis	(ahr-THRIGH-tis)	_____
☐ arthrocentesis	(ahr-throh-sen-TEE-sis)	_____
☐ arthrography	(ahr-THROG-ruh-fee)	_____
☐ arthroplasty	(AHR-throh-plas-tee)	_____
☐ arthroscope	(ahr-THROH-skope)	_____
☐ arthroscopy	(ahr-THROS-kuh-pee)	_____
☐ articular	(ahr-TICK-yoo-lur)	_____
☐ articular cartilage		_____
☐ articulation	(ahr-tick-yoo-LAY-shun)	_____
☐ atrophy	(AT-ruh-fee)	_____
☐ ball-and-socket joint		_____
☐ bone remodeling		_____
☐ bunion	(BUN-yun)	_____
☐ bunionectomy	(bun-yun-ECK-tuh-mee)	_____
☐ bursae	(BUR-see)	_____
☐ bursitis	(bur-SIGH-tis)	_____
☐ calcaneus	(kal-KAY-nee-us)	_____
☐ calcium		_____
☐ carpal bones	(KAHR-pul)	_____
☐ carpal tunnel syndrome	(KAHR-pul)	_____
☐ cartilage	(KAHR-ti-lij)	_____
☐ cartilaginous joints	(kahr-ti-LAJ-i-nus)	_____
☐ cervical vertebrae (C_1–C_7)		_____
☐ cheilectomy	(kye-LECK-toh-mee)	_____
☐ circumduction	(sur-kum-DUCK-shun)	_____

Key Term	Pronunciation	Definition
❑ clavicles	(KLAV-i-kuls)	
❑ closed reduction		
❑ coccyx	(KOCK-siks)	
❑ compact bone		
❑ corticosteroids	(kor-ti-koh-STEER-oidz)	
❑ craniostenosis	(KRAY-nee-oh-stuh-NOH-sis)	
❑ cranium	(KRAY-nee-um)	
❑ crepitus	(KREP-i-tus)	
❑ densitometer	(den-si-TOM-e-tur)	
❑ diaphysis	(dye-AF-i-sis)	
❑ dislocation		
❑ dorsiflexion	(dor-si-FLECK-shun)	
❑ edema	(e-DEE-muh)	
❑ epiphyseal line	(ep-i-FIZ-ee-ul)	
❑ epiphyseal plate	(ep-i-FIZ-ee-ul)	
❑ epiphysis	(e-PIF-i-sis)	
❑ estrogen replacement therapy (ERT)	(ES-troh-jen)	
❑ ethmoid bone	(ETH-moid)	
❑ eversion	(e-VUR-zhun)	
❑ Ewing sarcoma	(YOO-ing sahr-KOH-muh)	
❑ extension		
❑ external fixation		
❑ false ribs		
❑ femur	(FEE-mur)	
❑ fibrosis	(figh-BROH-sis)	
❑ fibrous joints	(FIGH-brus)	
❑ fibula	(FIB-yoo-luh)	
❑ fixation		
❑ flat bones		
❑ flexion	(FLECK-shun)	
❑ floating ribs		
❑ fontanelles	(fon-tuh-NELZ)	
❑ fracture (Fx)		
❑ frontal bone	(FRUN-tul)	
❑ ganglion	(GANG-glee-un)	
❑ gout	(gowt)	
❑ gouty arthritis	(GOW-tee ahr-THRIGH-tis)	

Key Term	Pronunciation	Definition
❏ hallux valgus	(HAL-ucks VAL-gus)	_____
❏ herniated disc	(HUR-nee-ate-ed)	_____
❏ hinge joints		_____
❏ hormone replacement therapy (HRT)		_____
❏ humerus	(HEW-mur-us)	_____
❏ hyoid bone	(HIGH-oid)	_____
❏ hyperextension		_____
❏ hypertrophy	(high-PUR-truh-fee)	_____
❏ ilium	(IL-ee-um)	_____
❏ inferior nasal conchae	(KON-kee)	_____
❏ internal fixation		_____
❏ intervertebral disc	(in-tur-VUR-te-brul)	_____
❏ inversion	(in-VUR-zhun)	_____
❏ irregular bones		_____
❏ ischium	(IS-kee-um)	_____
❏ joint		_____
❏ joint capsule		_____
❏ kyphosis	(kigh-FOH-sis)	_____
❏ lacrimal bones	(LACK-ri-mul)	_____
❏ lamina	(LAM-i-nuh)	_____
❏ ligaments	(LIG-uh-munts)	_____
❏ long bones		_____
❏ lordosis	(lor-DOH-sis)	_____
❏ lumbar vertebrae (L_1–L_5)		_____
❏ luxation	(luck-SAY-shun)	_____
❏ Lyme arthritis	(lime ahr-THRIGH-tis)	_____
❏ malaise	(mal-AIZ)	_____
❏ mandible	(MAN-di-bul)	_____
❏ Marfan syndrome	(mahr-FAHN)	_____
❏ maxillary bones	(mack-sih-LAIR-ee)	_____
❏ medullary cavity	(MED-yoo-lerr-ee)	_____
❏ menisci	(me-NIS-kee)	_____
❏ metacarpal bones	(met-uh-KAHR-pul)	_____
❏ metaphysis	(me-TAF-i-sis)	_____
❏ metatarsal bones	(met-uh-TAHR-sul)	_____
❏ nasal bone	(NAY-zul)	_____
❏ nonsteroidal anti-inflammatory drugs (NSAIDs)	(non-STEER-oid-ul)	_____

Key Term	Pronunciation	Definition
❏ obturator foramen	(OB-tew-ray-tur foh-RAY-mun)	_____
❏ occipital bone	(ock-SIP-i-tul)	_____
❏ open reduction		_____
❏ ossification	(os-i-fi-KAY-shun)	_____
❏ osteitis deformans	(os-tee-EYE-tis de-FOR-manz)	_____
❏ osteoarthritis	(os-tee-oh-ahr-THRIGH-tis)	_____
❏ osteoblasts	(OS-tee-oh-blasts)	_____
❏ osteochondroma	(os-tee-oh-kon-DROH-muh)	_____
❏ osteoclasts	(OS-tee-oh-klasts)	_____
❏ osteocytes	(OS-tee-oh-sites)	_____
❏ osteogenesis imperfecta (OI)	(os-tee-oh-JEN-e-sis im-pur-FECK-tuh)	_____
❏ osteogenic sarcoma	(os-tee-oh-JEN-ick sahr-KOH-muh)	_____
❏ osteomalacia	(os-tee-oh-muh-LAY-shee-uh)	_____
❏ osteomyelitis	(os-tee-oh-migh-eh-LYE-tis)	_____
❏ osteophytes	(OS-tee-oh-fights)	_____
❏ osteoporosis	(os-tee-oh-poh-ROH-sis)	_____
❏ osteosarcoma	(os-tee-oh-sahr-KOH-muh)	_____
❏ Paget disease	(PAJ-et)	_____
❏ palatine bones	(PAL-uh-tine)	_____
❏ parietal bones	(pur-RYE-e-tul)	_____
❏ patella	(pa-TEL-uh)	_____
❏ pedicles	(PED-i-kuls)	_____
❏ periosteum	(perr-ee-OS-tee-um)	_____
❏ phalanges	(fa-LAN-jeez)	_____
❏ plantar flexion	(PLAN-tahr FLECK-shun)	_____
❏ polydactyly	(pol-ee-DACK-tih-lee)	_____
❏ pronation	(proh-NAY-shun)	_____
❏ pubis	(PEW-bis)	_____
❏ radius	(RAY-dee-us)	_____
❏ red bone marrow		_____
❏ reduction		_____
❏ rheumatism	(ROO-muh-tiz-um)	_____
❏ rheumatoid arthritis (RA)	(ROO-muh-toid ahr-THRIGH-tis)	_____
❏ rickets		_____
❏ rotation		_____
❏ sacrum	(SAY-krum)	_____
❏ scapulae	(SKAP-yoo-lee)	_____

Key Term	Pronunciation	Definition
❑ scoliosis	(skoh-lee-OH-sis)	
❑ scurvy	(SKUR-vee)	
❑ sesamoid bones	(SES-uh-moid)	
❑ short bones		
❑ sinuses		
❑ skeletal traction		
❑ sphenoid bone	(SFEE-noid)	
❑ spinous process	(SPYE-nus)	
❑ spongy bone		
❑ sprain		
❑ subluxation	(sub-luck-SAY-shun)	
❑ supination	(sue-pi-NAY-shun)	
❑ sutural bones	(SUE-chur-ul)	
❑ sutures	(SUE-churz)	
❑ symphysis	(SIM-fi-sis)	
❑ symphysis pubis	(SIM-fi-sis PEW-bis)	
❑ syndactyly	(sin-DACK-tih-lee)	
❑ synovial joints	(si-NOH-vee-ul)	
❑ synovitis	(sin-oh-VYE-tis)	
❑ systemic lupus erythematosus (SLE)	(LEW-pus er-ih-thee-mah-TOH-sus)	
❑ talipes	(TAL-ih-peez)	
❑ talipes equinovarus	(TAL-ih-peez eh-kwigh-noh-VAIR-us)	
❑ talus	(TAY-lus)	
❑ tarsal bones	(TAHR-sul)	
❑ temporal bones	(TEM-puh-rul)	
❑ tendons	(TEN-dunz)	
❑ thoracic vertebrae (T_1–T_{12})		
❑ tibia	(TIB-ee-uh)	
❑ torn meniscus	(me-NIS-kus)	
❑ trabeculae	(tra-BECK-yoo-lee)	
❑ transverse processes	(trans-VERCE)	
❑ true ribs		
❑ turbinates	(TUR-bin-ates)	
❑ ulna	(UL-nuh)	
❑ vertebral body	(VUR-te-brul)	
❑ vertebral foramen	(VUR-te-brul foh-RAY-mun)	
❑ vomer	(VOH-mur)	
❑ zygomatic bones	(zye-goh-MAT-ick)	

Answers

Word Grouping Exercises: Bones

Definition	Word Part	Definition	Word Part
tibia, shin bone	tibio-	pubic	pubo-
bone	A. osseo-, ossi- B. ost-, oste-, osteo-	rib	costo-
bone marrow	myel-, myelo-	scapula, scapular, shoulder blade	scapulo-
calcaneus	calcaneo-	something that breaks; to break	-clast
calcium	calc-, calci-,	sternum, sternal, chest	stern-, sterno-
carpus (wrist), carpal	carpo-	straight	orth-, ortho-
cartilage, cartilaginous	chondrio-, chondro-	tarsus	tars-, tarso-
cranium	crani-, cranio-	thigh	femor-
ethmoid bone	ethmo-	tibia, shin bone	tibio-
ilium	ilio-	U-shaped	hyo-
immature precursor cell	-blast	vertebra, vertebral	vertebro-
passage	meato-	vertebrae	spondyl-, spondylo-
pelvis	pelvi-, pelvio-, pelvo		

Word Building Exercises: Bones

Word Part	Meaning	Common or Known Word	Example Medical Term
calc-, calci-, calco-	calcium	calcium	calcitonin
carpo-	carpus (wrist), carpal	carpal	carpal tunnel syndrome
crani-, cranio-	cranium	cranium	cranial cavity
orth-, ortho-	straight	orthodontist	orthopedics
osseo-, ossi-	bone	ossification	ossification
ost-, oste-, osteo-	bone	osteocytes	osteoblast
vertebro-	vertebra, vertebral	vertebrae	vertebral column

Key Term Practice: Bones

Bone Anatomy

1. long; short; flat; irregular; sesamoid; sutural
2. around (*peri-*) the bony (*ost-*) membrane
3. epiphysis; epiphyses
4. diaphysis; diaphyses
5. compact bone and spongy bone

Bone Formation

1. osteocytes
2. osteoblasts; osteoclasts
3. epiphyseal plate
4. calcium
5. ossification
6. atrophy

Cranial and Facial Bones

1. cranium
2. maxillary bones, palatine bones, nasal bones, inferior nasal conchae, zygomatic bones, lacrimal bones, vomer, and mandible.
3. occipital bone, parietal bones, frontal bone, temporal bones, sphenoid, ethmoid
4. Fontanelles
5. hyoid bone; hyo-

Vertebral Column

1. spinous process
2. cervical vertebrae (7), thoracic vertebrae (12), lumbar vertebrae (5), sacrum (5 fused), and coccyx (3 to 5 fused vertebrae)
3. vertebral foramen
4. vertebral body
5. Transverse processes

Bones of the Chest, Arms, and Hands

1. phalanges
2. radius and ulna
3. humerus
4. true ribs, false ribs, and floating ribs
5. metacarpal bones; meta-, carpo-

Bones of the Pelvic Girdle, Legs, and Feet

1. ilium, ischium, pubis
2. metatarsal; meta-, tars-
3. Patella
4. femur; femor-
5. acetabulum

Abnormal Spinal Curvatures

1. Scoliosis
2. kyphosis
3. Lordosis

Fractures

1. fracture (Fx)
2. Fixation
3. internal fixation
4. Crepitus
5. skeletal traction

Genetic Bone Diseases

1. osteogenesis imperfecta (OI)
2. Marfan syndrome

Hand and Foot Disorders

1. Syndactyly
2. talipes
3. Talipes equinovarus

Vitamin Imbalances

1. osteomalacia
2. rickets
3. Scurvy

Other Bone Disorders

1. osteosarcoma
2. Osteomyelitis
3. densitometer
4. Abscesses
5. craniostenosis

Word Grouping Exercises: Joints

Definition	Word Part	Definition	Word Part
bent, crooked	ankylo-	straight	orth-, ortho-
cartilage	chondr-, chondri-, chondro-	surgical removal	-ectomy
glassy, transparent	hyal-, hyalo-	tendon	tendo-, teno-
joint	arthr-, arthro-	together, with, joined	sym-, syn-
molding or shaping	-plasty	vertebrae	spondyl-, spondylo-
on both sides	amph-, amphi-, ampho-		

Word Building Exercises: Joints

Word Part	Meaning	Common or Known Word	Example Medical Term
amph-, amphi-, ampho-	on both sides	amphibian	amphiarthrosis
arthr-, arthro-	joint	arthritis	arthroscopy
-ectomy	surgical removal	appendectomy	bunionectomy
orth-, ortho-	straight	orthodontist	orthopedics
sym-, syn-	together, with, joined	synergy	syndesmoses
tendo-, teno-	tendon	tendon	tendonitis

Key Term Practice: Joints

Joints

1. joint and articulation
2. Ligaments
3. Tendons

Types of Joints

1. fibrous joints, cartilaginous joints, and synovial joints
2. hinge joint
3. Bursae
4. intervertebral discs
5. joint capsule

Joint Movements

1. rotation
2. adduction
3. Eversion
4. plantar flexion
5. extension

Arthritis

1. gouty arthritis and gout
2. osteophytes
3. Lyme arthritis
4. arthrocentesis; arthro-; -centesis
5. Malaise

Autoimmune Diseases

1. Rheumatism
2. ankylosing spondylitis; ankylo-; spondyl-
3. synovitis
4. Fibrosis
5. corticosteroids

Foot, Ankle, and Knee Disorders

1. bunion
2. Hallux valgus
3. Arthroplasty
4. sprain
5. torn meniscus

Shoulder and Wrist Disorders

1. carpal tunnel syndrome
2. ganglion
3. Adhesive capsulitis

Trauma

1. a. luxation; b. subluxation
2. Bursitis
3. herniated disc

Common Abbreviations Exercises

1. ROM = range of motion
2. acetylsalicylic acid = ASA
3. Fx = fracture
4. TJR = total joint replacement
5. physical therapy = PT

Case Study

1. a is the correct answer.
   - b is incorrect because that region is tibial.
   - c is incorrect because that region is coxal.
   - d is incorrect because that region is cervical.
2. c is the correct answer.
   - a is incorrect because the shoulder joint is known as the glenohumeral joint.
   - b is incorrect because the hip joint is also known as the coxal joint.
   - d is incorrect because the elbow joint is also known as the humeroulnar joint.
3. d is the correct answer.
   - c is incorrect because hyperextension is not a normal knee joint movement and would indicate a disorder.
4. d is the correct answer.
   - c is incorrect because NSAIDs do not assist with cartilage growth.
5. c is the correct answer.
   - a is incorrect because the head and neck regions are called cranial and cervical.
   - b is incorrect because the shoulder region is called acromial, femoral describes the upper leg, and tibial refers to the lower leg.
   - d is incorrect because the lumbar region describes the lower back and the patellar region describes the knee.
6. c is the correct answer.
   - a is incorrect because magnetic fields are used in MRI studies.
   - b is incorrect because sound waves are used for ultrasound.
   - d is incorrect because sonograms are the images obtained from ultrasonography.

Real World Report

1. c
2. a
3. c
4. a. vertebra; b. lysis, destruction; c. degeneration or destruction of a vertebra
5. a. vertebra; b. condition or process; c. a condition of the vertebra. Specifically, it refers to forward movement of the body of one of the lower lumbar vertebrae on the vertebra below it, or on the sacrum.
6. a. foramina; b. the openings through which the spinal nerves pass

Review and Application

1. d	6. b	11. a	16. c
2. a	7. c	12. a	17. b
3. b	8. d	13. c	18. c
4. c	9. d	14. c	19. d
5. a	10. b	15. a	20. d

21. d
22. a
23. a
24. b
25. c
26. b
27. c
28. osteoblast
29. osteomalacia
30. chondrocyte
31. a
32. b
33. c
34. b
35. a
36. c
37. b
38. c
39. d
40. a
41. e
42. c
43. a
44. b
45. e
46. d
47. b
48. d
49. e
50. a
51. c

52. e
53. a
54. c
55. b
56. e
57. b
58. a
59. d
60. e
61. c
62. lamina
63. vertebra
64. sacrum
65. humerus
66. ulnae
67. phalanges
68. fibulae
69. patellae
70. c
71. b
72. b
73. d
74. a
75. c
76. b
77. b
78. d
79. c
80. a
81. abduction
82. supination

83. extension
84. inversion
85. pronation
86. osteoclasts
87. hyoid bone
88. hinge joints
89. coccyx
90. cranium
91. OI = osteogenesis imperfecta; genetic brittle bone disease
92. TMJ = temporomandibular joint; the joint in the jaw at the junction of the temporal bone and the mandible
93. T_1–T_{12} = thoracic vertebrae 1–12; location of the 12 thoracic vertebrae
94. ACL = anterior cruciate ligament; important stabilizing ligament of the knee
95. NSAID = nonsteroidal anti-inflammatory drugs; medicine used to reduce swelling and pain
96. articulations
97. hallux
98. The doctor suspected osteoporosis because Iva's history fit the classic profile of this degenerative bone disease.
99. The assignment to the pediatric ward was based on the evidence of an epiphyseal fracture. Because children are still growing, they would still have an epiphyseal plate; only a remnant epiphyseal line is present in adults. Thus, the patient was a child.
100. abduction, adduction, circumduction, rotation, pronation, and supination
101. shoulder joint
102. Mike may have a torn meniscus or an injury to his ACL. Bones comprising the tibiofemoral joint include the femur, patella, and tibia.

Labeling

a. proximal epiphysis   **b.** diaphysis   **c.** spongy bone
d. articular cartilage   **e.** periosteum   **f.** compact bone

Word Search

```
R  +  +  +  N  +  +  +  +  M  +  N  +  N  S  F
M  U  E  T  S  O  I  R  E  P  O  S  O  +  E  O
V  O  M  E  R  +  I  T  +  I  +  I  +  +  L  N
+  +  +  E  +  +  A  L  T  +  S  B  S  +  C  T
+  +  +  +  F  P  +  C  G  N  C  U  S  +  I  A
S  E  +  +  H  +  U  +  E  N  L  P  E  +  D  N
I  +  A  Y  +  D  +  T  M  A  A  +  T  +  E  E
N  +  S  L  D  +  X  U  T  +  V  G  A  +  P  L
U  I  +  A  U  E  I  +  +  +  I  +  N  +  +  L
S  +  C  I  R  C  U  M  D  U  C  T  I  O  N  E
E  +  +  E  L  +  E  +  +  +  L  +  B  +  +  S
S  +  P  A  +  +  +  B  +  +  E  +  R  +  +  +
+  Y  C  +  +  +  +  +  A  +  S  +  U  +  +  +
H  A  R  T  I  C  U  L  A  R  +  +  T  +  +  +
M  U  R  C  A  S  +  +  +  +  T  +  +  +  +  +
S  T  N  E  M  A  G  I  L  I  S  C  H  I  U  M
```

adduction
articular
calcium
circumduction
clavicles
femur
fontanelles
ganglion
hyperextension
ischium
ligaments
metaphysis
pedicles
periosteum
pubis
sacrum
sinuses
talus
trabeculae
turbinates
vomer

Vocabulary Review

Key Term	Definition
abduction	movement away from the body's midline
abscesses	pus-filled cavities due to infection and inflammation
acetabulum	the socket of the hip bone into which the head of the femur fits
adduction	movement toward the body's midline
adhesive capsulitis	condition characterized by restricted joint mobility because of inflammatory thickening of the capsule of the humerus; also called frozen shoulder
ankylosing spondylitis	fusion and inflammation of the vertebrae
ankylosis	joint immobility or fixation
arthritis	joint inflammation
arthrocentesis	needle puncture into a joint capsule to extract synovial fluid
arthrography	x-ray of the joint space after introduction of a contrast dye

Key Term	Definition
arthroplasty	joint removal with replacement by artificial joints or prostheses, as in hip or knee replacements
arthroscope	fiberoptic instrument (camera) used to view a joint's interior
arthroscopy	insertion of a fiberoptic lens called an arthroscope directly into the joint for visual examination
articular	pertaining to an articulation (joint)
articular cartilage	a kind of connective tissue that covers the ends of bones at certain joints
articulation	point of close contact between two or more bones; also called a joint
atrophy	a reduction in size
ball-and-socket joint	joint in which the rounded head of one bone fits in the concave surface of another
bone remodeling	process of breaking down and building up bone tissue

Key Term	Definition
bunion	inflammation of the bursa around the great toe (hallux) accompanied by swelling and sideways displacement of the joint
bunionectomy	removal of a bunion
bursae	fluid-filled sacs that reduce friction around joints
bursitis	inflammation of the bursae
calcaneus	heel bone
calcium	mineral essential to bone formation and strength
carpal bones	wrist bones
carpal tunnel syndrome	wrist affliction caused by pressure on the median nerve in the carpal bones
cartilage	tough connective tissue that lacks a blood supply
cartilaginous joints	articulations made of cartilage
cervical vertebrae (C_1–C_7)	7 vertebrae closest to the head; neck vertebrae
cheilectomy	chiseling away of bony outgrowths that interfere with joint mobility
circumduction	movement in which the proximal end is fixed while the distal end moves in a circle as when throwing a ball
clavicles	collar bones
closed reduction	restoration of a dislocated joint or fractured bone to its normal anatomic position by surgical manipulative procedures without skin incision
coccyx	tailbone formed from three to five fused vertebrae
compact bone	solid bone tissue
corticosteroids	synthetic drugs similar to the steroid hormones produced by the adrenal glands that are used to reduce inflammation
craniostenosis	premature ossification of the fontanelles and fusion of the cranial sutures
cranium	the bones of the head; also called the skull
crepitus	grating sound heard when broken bone ends rub together
densitometer	instrument used to measure bone density
diaphysis	shaft of a long bone
dislocation	displacement of a joint; also called a luxation
dorsiflexion	bending the foot so the toes move upward toward the tibia
edema	swelling; tissue inflammation with fluid accumulation
epiphyseal line	mark left at the site of the epiphyseal plate after the long bone has stopped growing
epiphyseal plate	site of long bone growth located between the metaphysis and epiphysis; also called the growth plate
epiphysis	expanded end of a long bone
estrogen replacement therapy (ERT)	administration of the hormone estrogen
ethmoid bone	skull bone between sphenoid and nasal bones
eversion	turning the sole of the foot outward
Ewing sarcoma	malignant bone tumor that occurs usually before the age of 20 and is twice as common in males
extension	increasing the angle between two bones; making a flexed part straight
external fixation	immobilization of a fracture by splints, plastic dressings, or pins
false ribs	rib pairs 8–10; the ribs that articulate with vertebrae and the sternum by the costal cartilage of the last true rib
femur	thigh bone
fibrosis	abnormal thickening and scarring of connective tissue
fibrous joints	articulation made of fibrous connective tissue found between bones in close contact
fibula	slender lower leg bone
fixation	immobilization of a fracture
flat bones	bones found in ribs, scapulae, and skulls
flexion	decreasing the angle between two bones
floating ribs	rib pairs 11 and 12; ribs that articulate with the thoracic vertebrae and posterior muscles but not the sternum
fontanelles	membranous space between cranial bones; also called soft spots
fracture (Fx)	break in a bone or tooth
frontal bone	forehead bone
ganglion	benign growth in or around a tendon sheath or joint capsule
gout	metabolic disorder causing excessive uric acid production and deposition in joints, often in the great toe; also called gouty arthritis
gouty arthritis	metabolic disorder causing excessive uric acid production and deposition in joints, often in the great toe; also called gout

Key Term	Definition	Key Term	Definition
hallux valgus	a deformity at the metatarsophalangeal joint that forces the great toe toward the other toes	**Lyme arthritis**	joint inflammation as a result of the bite of a tick infected with *Borrelia burgdorferi*; also called Lyme disease
herniated disc	condition in which the center of an intervertebral disc protrudes through the fibrocartilage	**malaise**	general weakness, tiredness, and discomfort
hinge joints	joints formed by two bones that move in a right angle like opening or closing a door	**mandible**	lower jawbone
		Marfan syndrome	genetic disorder affecting connective tissues that is characterized by abnormal skeletal changes such as long limbs and fingers
hormone replacement therapy (HRT)	administration of hormones, notably estrogen and progesterone	**maxillary bones**	upper jawbones
humerus	upper arm bone	**medullary cavity**	central canal of a long bone
hyoid bone	U-shaped bone that supports the tongue	**menisci**	crescent-shaped discs of fibrocartilage that separate and cushion the articulating surfaces of bones
hyperextension	excessive extension beyond the anatomic position	**metacarpal bones**	bones of the hand between the wrist and fingers
hypertrophy	an increase in size	**metaphysis**	section of bone between the epiphysis and the diaphysis of long bones
ilium	superior broad part of the hip bone		
inferior nasal conchae	scroll-shaped bones in the nasal passages; also called inferior nasal turbinates	**metatarsal bones**	bones of the foot between the ankle and toes
		nasal bones	bones of the nose
internal fixation	stabilization of a fracture by directly attaching the bony fragments together with surgical wires, screws, pins, rods, or plates	**nonsteroidal anti-inflammatory drugs**	medicines that reduce tissue inflammation and pain
		obturator foramen	oval opening between the ischium and pubis
intervertebral disc	mass of fibrocartilage between adjacent vertebrae	**occipital bone**	back head bone
inversion	turning the sole of the foot inward	**open reduction**	restoration of a dislocated joint or fractured bone to its normal anatomic position by surgical or manipulative procedures with skin incision
irregular bones	bones found in vertebrae and faces		
ischium	inferior, rearmost part of the hip bone	**ossification**	conversion of cartilage tissue into bone
joint	point of close contact between two or more bones; also called an articulation	**osteitis deformans**	bone disease characterized by increased bone resorption and formation resulting in thickening and softening bones; also called Paget disease
joint capsule	fibrous sheet enclosing a freely movable joint		
kyphosis	angular curve of the thoracic spine; hunchback	**osteoarthritis**	degenerative joint disease characterized by deterioration of articular cartilage and formation of bone spurs
lacrimal bones	fingernail-shaped facial bones		
lamina	thin plate on vertebra	**osteoblasts**	bone-forming cells
ligaments	bands of tough, fibrous connective tissue that connect bones or cartilage at a joint	**osteochondroma**	benign tumor of cartilage
		osteoclasts	bone-destroying cells
		osteocytes	mature bone cells
long bones	bones found in arms and legs	**osteogenesis imperfecta (OI)**	genetic brittle bone disease
lordosis	forward curve of the lumbar spine; swayback		
lumbar vertebrae (L_1–L_5)	5 vertebrae of the lower back	**osteogenic sarcoma**	most common malignant bone tumor that arises from osteoblasts; also called osteosarcoma
luxation	displacement of a joint; also called a dislocation	**osteomalacia**	vitamin D deficiency disease in adulthood

Key Term	Definition	Key Term	Definition
osteomyelitis	bacterial infection of bone marrow and adjacent bone tissue	sinuses	cavities or hollow space in bones
osteophytes	abnormal bony outgrowths at joints, commonly called bone spurs	skeletal traction	pulling on a broken bone to straighten it
osteoporosis	disorder characterized by a decrease in bone density and strength	sphenoid bone	butterfly-shaped skull bone
		spinous process	spine-like projection on vertebra
osteosarcoma	most common malignant bone tumor that arises from osteoblasts; also called osteogenic sarcoma	spongy bone	bone made of a network of bone tissue with irregular spaces in it; also called cancellous bone or trabecular bone
Paget disease	bone disease characterized by increased bone resorption and formation resulting in thickening and softening bones; also called osteitis deformans	sprain	painful injury to the joint ligaments caused by wrenching or overstretching
palatine bones	L-shaped facial bones	subluxation	partial or incomplete dislocation of a joint
parietal bones	superior lateral skull bones	supination	turning the palm anteriorly or upward
patella	kneecap		
pedicles	short narrow stalks that form the sides of the vertebral foramen	sutural bones	irregularly shaped bones between the flat bones of the skull
periosteum	fibrous membrane covering a bone	sutures	joint type found in the skull in which the bones are bound together by fibrous connective tissue
phalanges	bones of the fingers and toes		
plantar flexion	bending the foot so the toes move downward and the ankle is extended	symphysis	slightly movable joint in which the bones are connected by a pad of fibrocartilage
polydactyly	having extra fingers or toes	symphysis pubis	the fibrocartilaginous union of the anterior pubic bones
pronation	turning the palm posteriorly or downward		
		syndactyly	webbed fingers or toes
pubis	front part of the hip bone, forming anterior pelvic girdle	synovial joints	freely movable articulations
		synovitis	inflammation of the synovial membrane
radius	outer forearm bone		
red bone marrow	blood-forming tissue in bone	systemic lupus erythematosus (SLE)	chronic inflammatory connective tissue disease
reduction	restoration of a bone to its normal anatomic position by surgical or manipulative procedures		
		talipes	human foot deformity
rheumatism	general term for diseases characterized by musculoskeletal pain and stiffness	talipes equinovarus	clubfoot
		talus	ankle bone that connects to the tibia
rheumatoid arthritis (RA)	systemic autoimmune disease characterized by joint inflammation and deformity	tarsal bones	ankle bones
		temporal bones	lateral skull bones
		tendons	bands of fibrous connective tissue that attach muscles to bones
rickets	vitamin D deficiency disease in children		
rotation	turning around on an axis or fixed point as when turning a key in a lock	thoracic vertebrae (T$_1$-T$_{12}$)	12 vertebrae of the chest area
sacrum	curved, triangular bone between last lumbar vertebra and coccyx	tibia	shin bone; larger of two lower leg bones
scapulae	triangular bones of the back; also called shoulder blades	torn meniscus	meniscus abnormality that results from twisting the joint
scoliosis	lateral curve of the spine	trabeculae	slender columns of bone found in spongy bone
scurvy	disorder resulting from a diet lacking vitamin C	transverse processes	crosswise projections on vertebra
sesamoid bones	small bones that develop in joints	true ribs	rib pairs 1–7; the ribs that articulate with both the sternum and the vertebrae
short bones	cube-like bones found in wrists and ankles		

Key Term	Definition	Key Term	Definition
turbinates	scroll-shaped bones in the nasal passages; also called conchae	**vomer**	thin, vertically positioned bone forming a portion of the septum
ulna	inner forearm bone	**zygomatic bones**	cheek bones
vertebral body	the main, thick part of a vertebra		
vertebral foramen	opening through which the spinal cord passes		

Muscular System

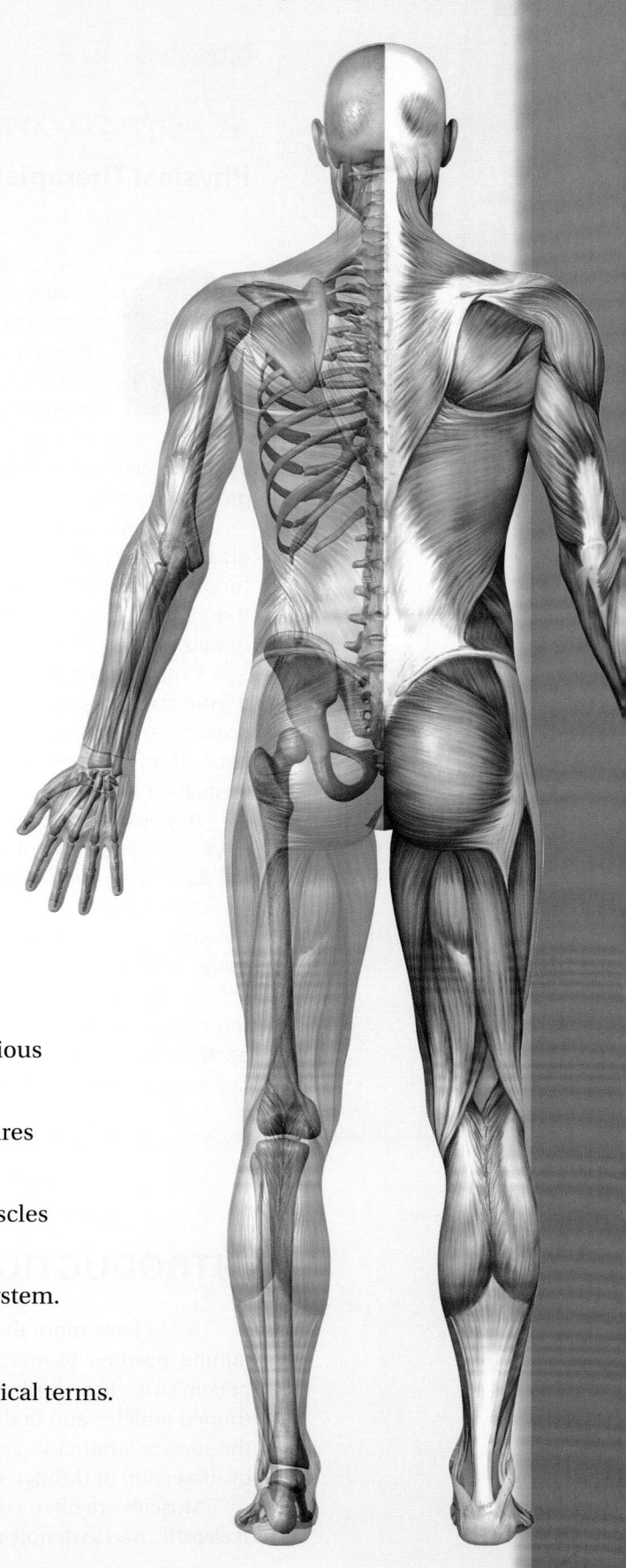

O B J E C T I V E S

After completing this chapter, you should be able to:

1. State the meanings of word parts related to the muscular system.

2. Describe the basis for naming muscles.

3. Identify common superficial and deep muscles and their locations.

4. List the common signs, symptoms, and treatments of various muscular system diseases.

5. Recognize common clinical tests and diagnostic procedures related to the muscular system.

6. Describe anatomical and physiological alterations of muscles throughout the lifespan.

7. Define common abbreviations related to the muscular system.

8. Define terms used in medical reports involving muscles.

9. Correctly define, spell, and pronounce the chapter's medical terms.

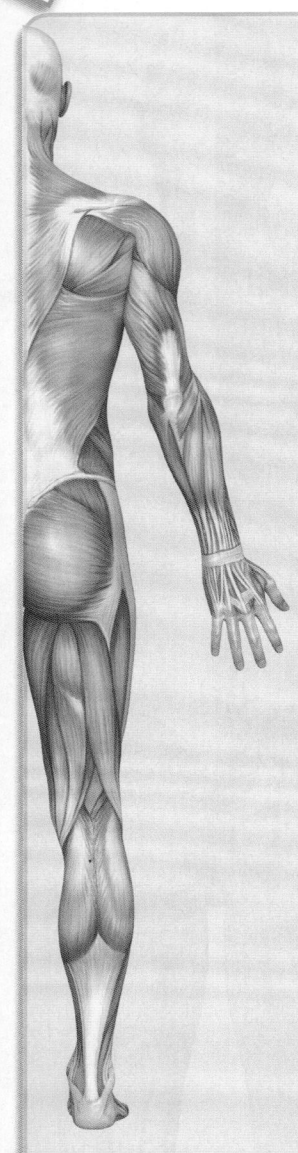

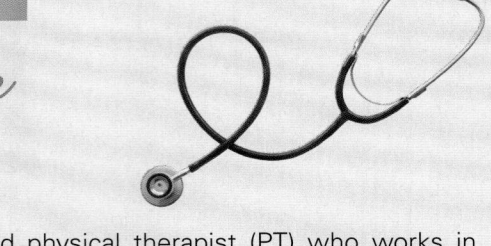

Professional Profile

Physical Therapist

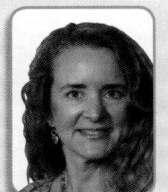

I'm Cindy, and I'm a licensed physical therapist (PT) who works in private practice. In addition to a master of science (MS) degree in physical therapy, I also hold a doctor of philosophy (PhD) in biomechanics. Physical therapy programs in the United States are now all doctoral-level courses because the bachelor of science (BS) degree has been phased out of existence in these programs. A strong science background is critical to acceptance into a PT program. Once admitted to a program, coursework includes classes in biology, chemistry, physics, biomechanics, neuroanatomy, and gross anatomy.

As a physical therapist, I evaluate and provide treatment to people who have been disabled by injury, pain, disease, physical condition, or medical procedure. PTs restore function, improve mobility, and relieve pain by nonsurgical methods, using physiotherapy. For example, after undergoing a sports injury or fracture repair, a patient often requires physical therapy to regain normal function.

While working in the field for more than 10 years, I've encountered a vast array of musculoskeletal disorders, including those requiring postsurgery rehabilitation. This practice employs a physical therapy assistant (PTA), who works closely under my guidance. The PTA prepares patients for treatment and performs selected therapeutic and evaluative tests.

A major focus of physical therapy is to help patients regain function, develop new physical skills, and enhance their quality of life. As a PT, I undertake many tasks. My duties in a typical workweek include evaluating patients using appropriate tests and clinical observation, developing individual treatment plans, discussing patient goals, and prescribing therapeutic activities. The therapy programs devised for individual patients range from exercise and massage to yoga and myofascial release.

A fair amount of client interaction deals with instruction. A PT must also develop the necessary skills to plan and implement a therapy program to match the needs of each patient. In addition, I convey information effectively using both oral and written communication, and I must maintain accurate, detailed records and documentation.

INTRODUCTION

We have more than 700 muscles, which are responsible for moving the body, maintaining posture, producing heat, and assisting lymph transport. Approximately 40% of a person's weight is attributed to muscle mass, although this percentage can be much higher in trained athletes and body builders. Muscles are arranged in layers. Superficial muscles form the surface landmarks easily identified when viewing exposed skin. Deep muscles are visible by dissection or through imaging techniques.

Muscles are often considered with the skeletal system. For this reason the term *musculoskeletal* is used to denote the interaction of bones with muscles. There are three types of muscle tissue, each in specific locations. All muscular movement is made possible through nerve impulses that act on the tissue, causing contraction, another term for muscle fiber shortening. Muscles, tendons, ligaments, bones, and nerves work together to achieve optimal functioning.

Key alterations related to the muscular system are considered in this chapter. Pathological conditions result from infection, trauma, inheritance, and tumors or are secondary to (the result of some other) existing disease. Age-related disorders are greatly influenced by physical activity.

MEDICAL TERM PARTS

Word Parts

Medical term prefixes, suffixes, and combining forms related to the muscular system are introduced in this section.

Word Part	Meaning
brachio-	arm
brachy-	short
bucco-	cheek
cardi-, cardio-	heart
fascio-	fascia, a band
fibr-, fibro-	fiber
kin-, kine-, kino-	movement, motion
kinesi-, kinesio-, kineso-	motion
muscul-, musculo-	muscle
my-, myo-	muscle
platy-	flat, broad
pter-, ptero-	wing, feather
pterygo-	wing shaped
rhabd-, rhabdo-	rod shaped
sarco-	muscle, flesh
tendo-, teno-	tendon
-troph, troph-, tropho-, -trophic	food, nutrition

Word Grouping Exercises

Using the *Medical Term Parts* table, identify the prefix, suffix, or combining form for each of the following definitions. The first one has been done as an example.

Definition	Word Part
arm	*brachio-*
cheek	
fascia, a band	
fiber	
flat, broad	
food, nutrition	
heart	
movement, motion	A. B.
muscle	
muscle, flesh	
rod shaped	
short	
tendon	
wing, feather	
wing shaped	

Word Building Exercises

Word parts introduced in the *Medical Term Parts* section are listed in the following table. For this exercise, first supply the meaning of each word part, then use the word part to build a word you already know. The word you list under *Common or Known Word* does not have to be a medical term; a commonly used word is fine. Be sure, however, that the word correctly reflects the intended meaning. The first one has been done as an example. Check your answers in a dictionary.

Word Part	Meaning	Common or Known Word	Example Medical Term
cardi-, cardio-	*heart*	*cardiac*	cardiomyopathy
fibr-, fibro-			fibromyalgia
kinesi-, kinesio-, kineso-			kinesiology
tendo-, teno-			tendinitis

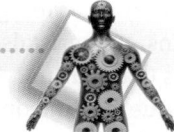

ANATOMY AND PHYSIOLOGY

Muscular System Preview

The key characteristic of muscles is their ability to contract to produce movement when stimulated by nerves. When a nerve impulse travels to muscle tissue, it excites the muscle to contract. **Muscle cells**, also called **muscle fibers**, are microscopic thread-like structures that form from several fused cells. Muscle fibers contract to move muscles, and **muscle tissue** consists of these contractile fibers.

KEY TERM	Definition
muscle cells	microscopic thread-like structures that contract to move muscles; also called muscle fibers
muscle fibers	microscopic thread-like structures that contract to move muscles; also called muscle cells
muscle tissue	tissue composed of contractile muscle fibers

KEY TERM PRACTICE: *Muscular System Preview*

1. Give the alternate name for muscle cells. _____

2. Which type of tissue is made of contractile fibers? _____

Muscle Tissue: Skeletal, Smooth, and Cardiac

The three types of muscle tissue are skeletal, smooth, and cardiac. **Skeletal muscle** tissue attaches to the bones of the skeletal system. Band-like masses of tough fibrous connective tissue, called **tendons**, attach the muscles to bones. Because skeletal muscle attaches to bones, we can move. It is also called *striated muscle* because it has a striped appearance when viewed under the microscope (**Figure 6-1**). This muscle type is under voluntary control, giving it its alternate name of voluntary tissue.

Located in the organs, **smooth muscle** tissue is nonstriated and is involuntarily controlled. Under a microscope, smooth muscle lacks the stripes of skeletal muscle (**Figure 6-2**). Hollow organs and blood vessels are lined with smooth muscle, which contracts and relaxes slowly to produce the rhythmic squeezing action of these structures.

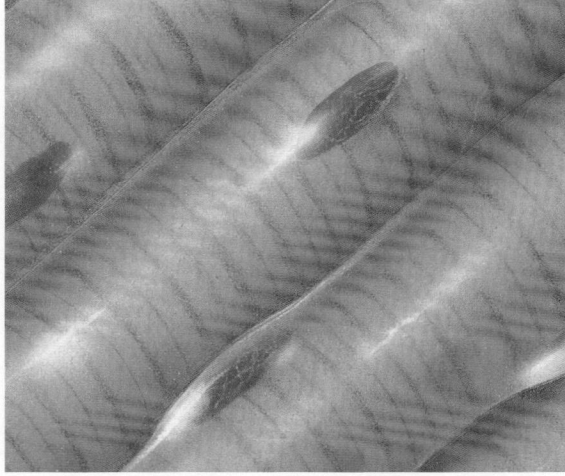

Figure 6-1 Skeletal muscle tissue is voluntary and attaches to bones.

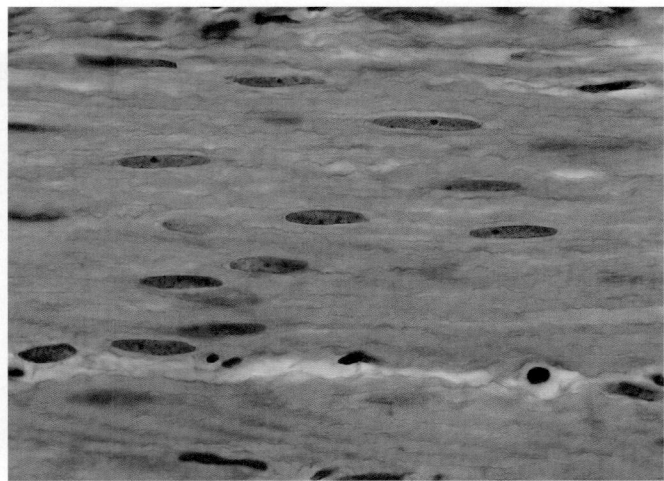

Figure 6-2 Smooth muscle is involuntary and lines blood vessels and organs.

Peristalsis is the term describing rhythmic waves of muscular contractions that occur in various tubular organs. By peristalsis, contents are moved through the intestines, urine is moved from the kidneys to the urinary bladder, and blood is forced through blood vessels.

Cardiac muscle tissue is found only in the heart. It produces the constant pumping action necessary for circulation. Its appearance is striated, yet it is involuntary muscle (**Figure 6-3**). Cardiac muscle contraction is unique because the fibers contract as a rhythmic unit and are self-stimulated.

A sheet of fibrous tissue that takes the place of a tendon is called an **aponeurosis**. An aponeurosis is found in areas with a wide area of attachment, such as between two muscles. **Fascia** is a thin sheet of fibrous connective tissue that envelops the body beneath the skin (**Figure 6-4**). Fascia also encloses muscles and groups of muscles.

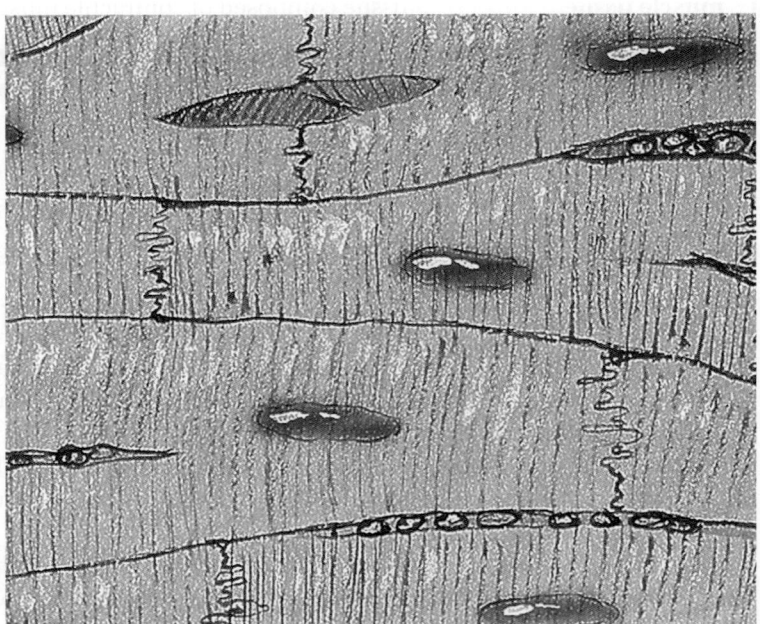

Figure 6-3 Cardiac muscle tissue is striated and involuntary and is found in the heart.

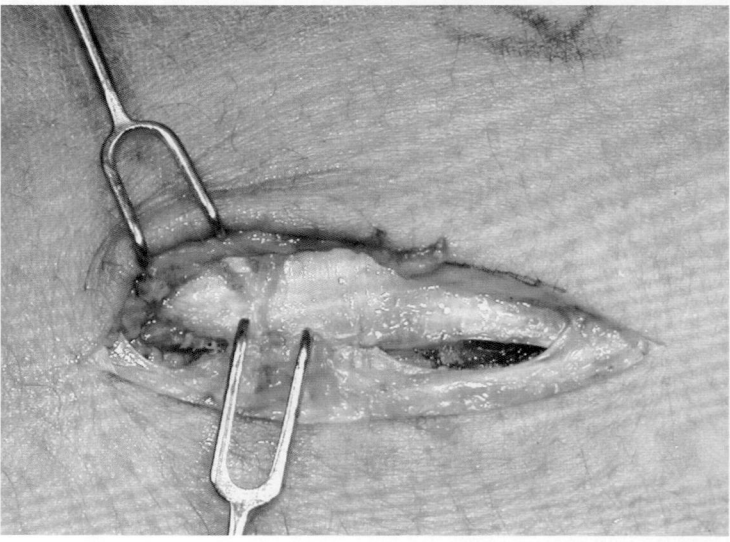

Figure 6-4 Closing the fascia over the joint.

KEY TERM	Definition
skeletal muscle	striated, voluntary muscle tissue attached to bones
tendons	tough, fibrous connective tissues that connect muscles to bones
smooth muscle	nonstriated, involuntary muscle tissue found lining organs and blood vessels
peristalsis (perr-i-STAHL-sis)	rhythmic waves of muscular contraction
cardiac muscle	striated, involuntary muscle found only in the heart
aponeurosis (ap-oh-new-ROH-sis)	a sheet of fibrous tissue that connects a muscle to another muscle
fascia (FASH-uh)	a thin sheet of fibrous connective tissue that envelops the body beneath the skin or encloses muscles or groups of muscles

KEY TERM PRACTICE: *Muscle Tissue: Skeletal, Smooth, and Cardiac*

1. The word parts *cardi-* and *cardio-* mean _____; so _____ tissue is found in the heart.

2. The term for rhythmic, wave-like contractions that propel food through the digestive tract is _____.

3. A thin sheath of fibrous connective tissue that encloses a muscle is termed _____.

4. Name the three types of muscle tissue _____.

5. _____ are tough, fibrous connective tissues that attach muscles to bones.

Muscle Movement

Skeletal muscles produce movement by pulling on bones. The end of the muscle that is attached to a relatively immovable part is the **origin**. Origins are attached to the more fixed part of the skeleton and *do not* move when contraction occurs. The **insertion** is the end of the muscle that is attached to a movable part. When contraction occurs, the insertion *does* move.

Muscles often work in pairs. One muscle typically produces movement in one direction, and another muscle produces movement in the opposite direction. You can see an example of the opposing actions of two different muscles on the same body part in your arm: The biceps brachii muscle flexes the arm, whereas the triceps brachii extends the arm. When one muscle in the pair contracts, the other muscle in the pair relaxes.

Atrophy is a term describing muscle wasting or a decrease in muscle size as a result of injury, disease, or lack of use. The opposite of atrophy is **hypertrophy**, or growth in size of muscle tissue. Hypertrophic muscles are seen in well-defined body builders. Doing repetitive weight-bearing exercises causes muscle tissue to enlarge because more blood and nutrients are delivered to the fibers in response to the greater workload demands.

KEY TERM	Definition
origin	muscle end that remains fixed during contraction
insertion	muscle end that moves during contraction
atrophy (AT-roh-fee)	decrease in muscle size
hypertrophy (high-PUR-troh-fee)	increase in muscle size

continued

continued from page 291

KEY TERM PRACTICE: *Muscle Movement*

1. The _____ is the immovable muscle attachment, and the _____ moves during a muscle contraction.

2. Exercising with weights will cause muscle _____, or an increase in muscle size.

3. _____ is a reduction in muscle size.

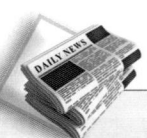

IN THE NEWS: Botox

Botulism is a serious form of food poisoning caused by eating food contaminated with *Clostridium botulinum* bacteria, which thrive in anaerobic conditions. The toxin produced by these bacteria is the most potent poison known. People become infected with the toxin by eating food that has not been canned or cooked appropriately.

Yet botulinum toxin is increasing in popularity. It has made its way into mainstream America as a cosmetic treatment for facial wrinkles. People once considered it a poison to avoid at all cost, but now some people are anxiously awaiting their injections.

Foodborne botulism cases in the United States have been linked to peppers, potato salad, sautéed onions, canned tuna, smoked fish, and cold soups. Symptoms appear within 36 hours of eating contaminated food. Antibiotic treatment is of no use because microbial growth does not cause the disease, rather the toxin produced by the bacteria does. Treatment is supportive and may involve pulmonary ventilation. Despite the disease severity, the mortality rate is approximately 10%.

This same toxin is being used to lessen frown furrows in the forehead, crow's feet (lines at the temples), and other forehead wrinkles. The trade name is Botox, short for botulinum toxin. Botulinum toxin is injected in very low doses into certain facial muscles, causing muscle paralysis and relaxation. This, in turn, eliminates wrinkles because without movement of underlying muscles, the skin does not form the deep creases. The treatment lasts any where from 3 to 6 months and must be repeated to retain the effects. The toxin is also used to treat other neuromuscular (NM) conditions such as multiple sclerosis and muscle spasms (involuntary, sudden contractions).

Naming Skeletal Muscles

The names of skeletal muscles are based on several factors. The names of very small muscles may contain the word *minimi*, and of very large muscles, the word *vastus*. Names indicating a muscle's shape include terms for broad, narrow, long, tapering, short, blunt, triangular, quadrilateral, irregular, flat sheets, or bulky masses. Many muscles have Latin names related to size, function, appearance, or shape.

Action names correspond to directional movements of the muscle. **Abductors** are muscles that pull a limb away from the midline, and **adductors** pull the limb toward the body's midline. Muscles that straighten or extend an arm or leg are termed **extensors**, and muscles that bend an arm or leg at a joint are termed **flexors**. Tables **6-1**, **6-2**, **6-3**, and **6-4** list the names, pronunciations, and functions of common skeletal muscles. **Figures 6-5**, **6-6**, **6-7**, and **6-8** show the corresponding muscles in the body.

TABLE 6-1	MUSCLES OF THE FACE, HEAD AND NECK (see Figure 6-5)	
Muscle	**Pronunciation**	**Action**
buccinator	(BUK-si-nay-tur)	muscle of smiling; compresses cheeks
frontalis	(frun-TAY-lis)	raises eyebrows
masseter	(ma-SEE-tur)	involved in mastication (chewing)
occipitalis	(ock-sip-i-TAL-is)	retracts and tenses scalp
orbicularis oculi	(or-bick-yoo-LAIR-is OCK-yoo-lye)	closes eyelid
orbicularis oris	(or-bick-yoo-LAIR-is OR-is)	compresses lips
platysma	(pla-TIZ-muh)	stretches neck from chest to face
pterygoid	(TEER-i-goid)	involved in opening and closing the jaw; grates teeth during mastication (chewing)
sternocleidomastoid	(ster-noh-klye-doh-MAS-toid)	flexes head; prayer muscle
sternohyoid	(ster-noh-IGH-oid)	depresses hyoid bone and larynx
temporalis	(tem-poh-RAY-lis)	closes jaw
zygomaticus	(zye-goh-MAT-ih-kus)	draws corner of mouth upward

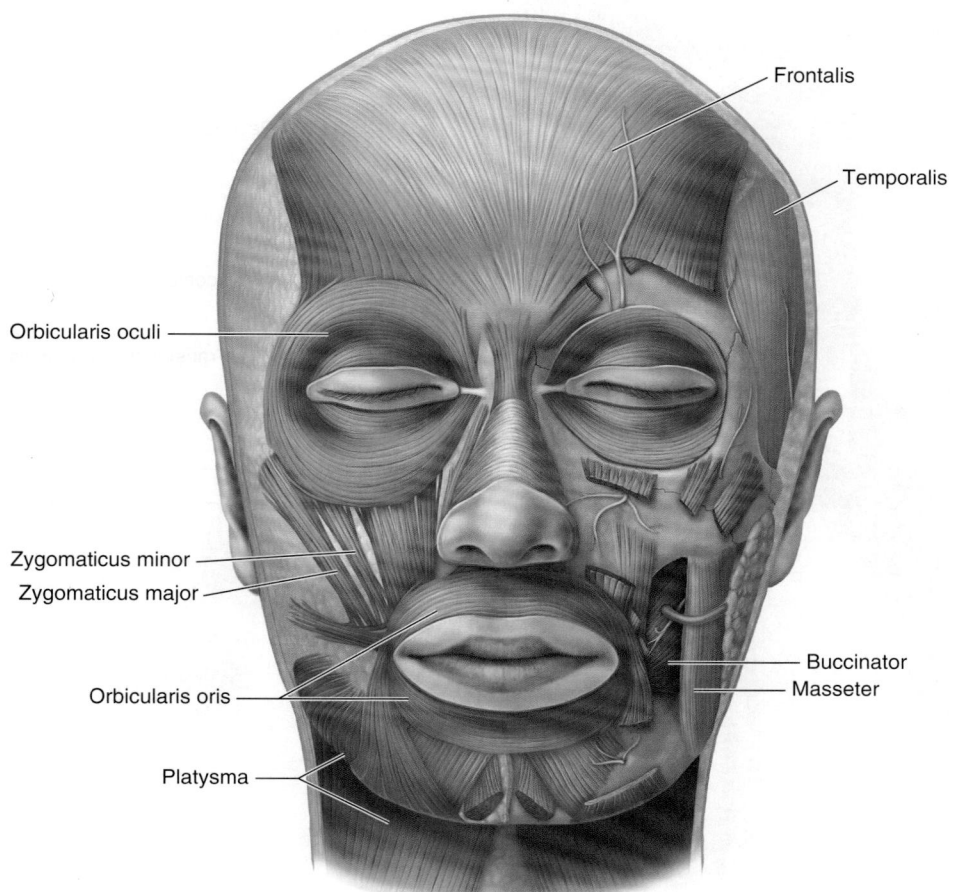

Figure 6-5 Muscles of the face, head, and neck.

T A B L E 6-2	MUSCLES OF THE TRUNK (see Figure 6-6)	
Muscle	**Pronunciation**	**Action**
diaphragm	(DYE-uh-fram)	enlarges thoracic cavity
external oblique		compresses abdomen; aids in posture
intercostal	(in-tur-KOS-tul)	contracts and relaxes rib cage
internal oblique		compresses abdomen
latissimus dorsi	(la-TIS-i-mus DOR-see)	extends and adducts upper arm
pectoralis major	(peck-toh-RAH-lis)	pulls arm forward and across chest
pectoralis minor	(peck-toh-RAH-lis)	moves scapula against chest
rectus abdominis	(RECK-tus ab-DOM-i-nis)	flexes trunk
rhomboideus major	(rom-BOY-dee-us)	raises and adducts scapula
transversus abdominis	(trans-VUR-sus ab-DOM-i-nis)	compresses abdomen; aids in posture
trapezius	(tra-PEE-zee-us)	shrugs shoulders

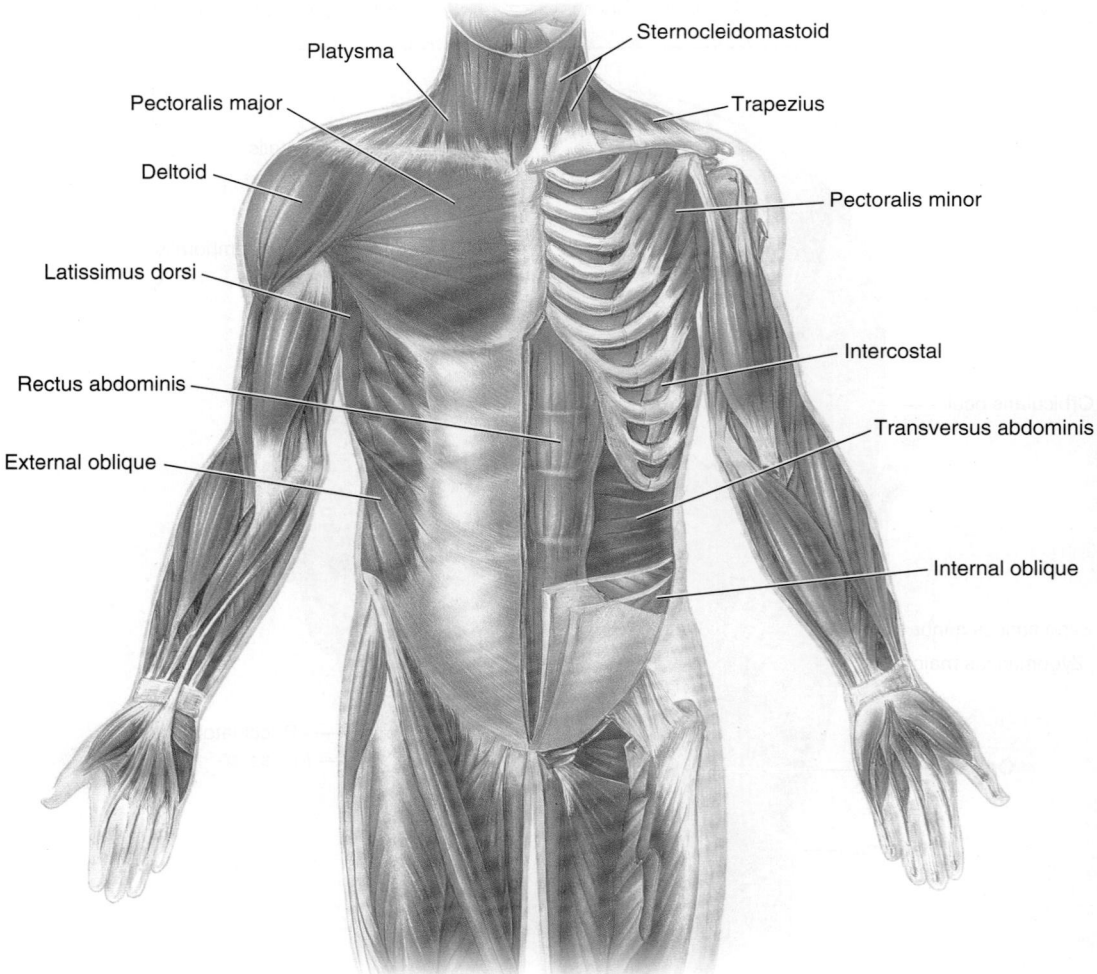

Figure 6-6 Muscles of the trunk.

MUSCLES OF THE ARM AND FOREARM (see Figure 6-7)

Muscle	Pronunciation	Action
biceps brachii	(BYE-seps BRAY-kee-eye)	supinates forearm; flexes forearm
brachialis	(bray-kee-AY-lis)	flexes forearm
brachioradialis	(BRAY-kee-oh-ray-dee-AY-lis)	flexes forearm
deltoid	(DEL-toid)	abducts upper arm
infraspinatus	(in-fruh-spye-NAY-tus)	laterally rotates shoulder
pronator teres	(proh-NAY-tur TEER-eez)	medial arm rotation
rotator cuff		rotates arm muscles; includes supraspinatus, infraspinatus, teres minor, subscapularis (SITS)
subscapularis	(sub-SKAP-yoo-lahr-ris)	medially rotates shoulder
supinator	(SUE-pi-nay-tur)	supinates forearm
supraspinatus	(sue-pruh-spye-NAY-tus)	abducts shoulder
teres major	(TEER-eez)	extends, adducts, and medially rotates shoulder
teres minor	(TEER-eez)	rotates arm laterally
triceps brachii	(TRYE-seps BRAY-kee-eye)	extends forearm

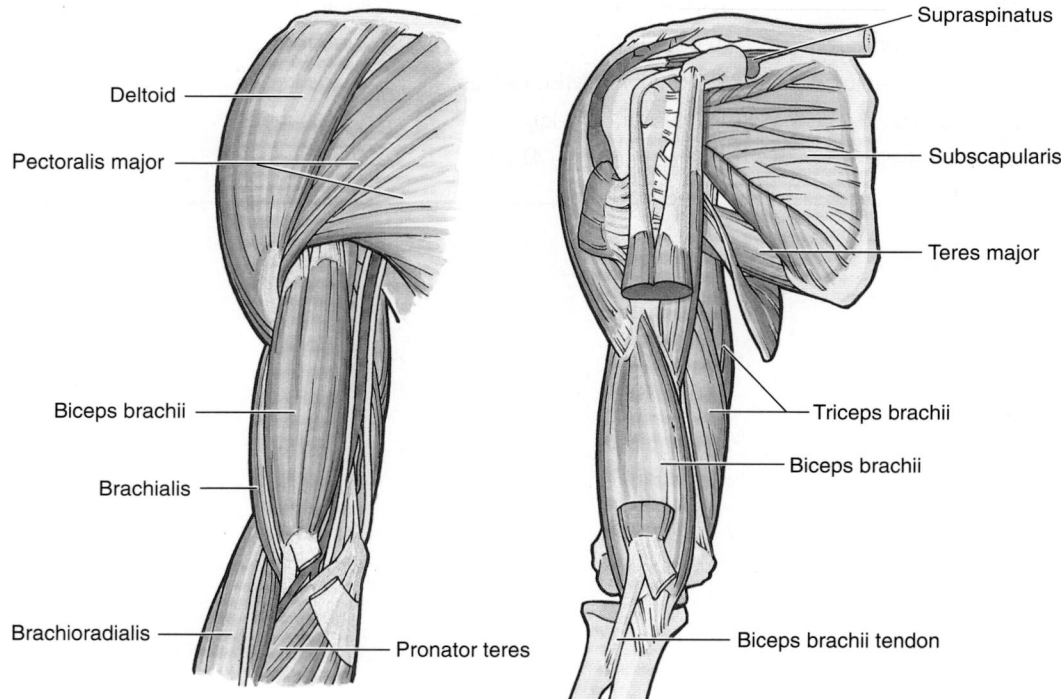

Figure 6-7 Muscles of the arm and forearm.

TABLE 6-4

MUSCLES OF THE THIGH AND LEG (see Figure 6-8)

Muscle	Pronunciation	Action
adductor magnus	(a-DUCK-tur MAG-nus)	adducts hip; flexes and rotates leg
biceps femoris	(BYE-seps FEM-oh-ris)	moves leg
fibularis longus	(fib-yoo-LAIR-is LONG-us)	eversion of foot and plantar flexion
gastrocnemius	(gas-trock-NEE-mee-us)	plantar flexion
gluteus maximus	(gloo-TEE-us MACKS-ih-mus)	extends thigh
gluteus medius	(gloo-TEE-us MEE-dee-us)	abducts thigh
gracilis	(GRAS-i-lis)	adducts thigh; flexes and adducts leg
hamstring group		flexes leg muscles; includes biceps femoris, semimembranosus, and semitendinosus
quadriceps group	(KWAH-dri-seps)	extends leg muscles; includes rectus femoris, vastus intermedius, vastus lateralis, and vastus medialis
rectus femoris	(RECK-tus FEM-oh-ris)	moves thigh
sartorius	(sahr-TOH-ree-us)	flexes knee; rotates hip
semimembranosus	(sem-ee-mem-bruh-NOH-sus)	flexes knee; extends and rotates hip
semitendinosus	(SEM-ee-ten-di-NOH-sus)	flexes knee; extends and rotates hip
soleus	(SOH-lee-us)	plantar flexion
tibialis anterior	(tib-ee-A-lis)	inverts foot
vastus intermedius	(VAS-tus in-tur-MEE-dee-us)	extends knee
vastus lateralis	(VAS-tus lat-ur-AL-is)	extends knee
vastus medialis	(VAS-tus mee-dee-AL-is)	extends knee

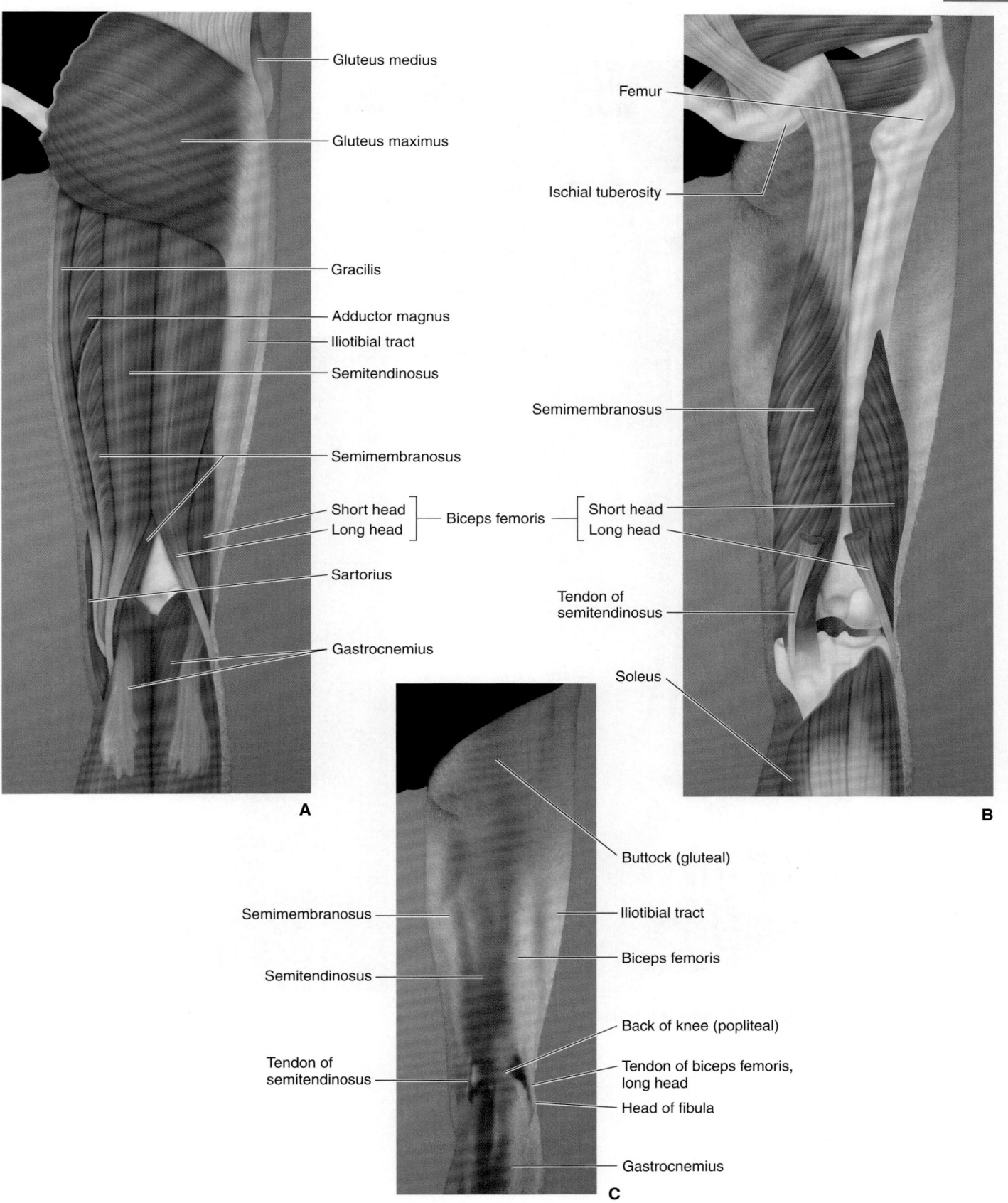

FIGURE 6-8 (A) (B) (C) Muscles of the thigh.

continued

continued from page 297

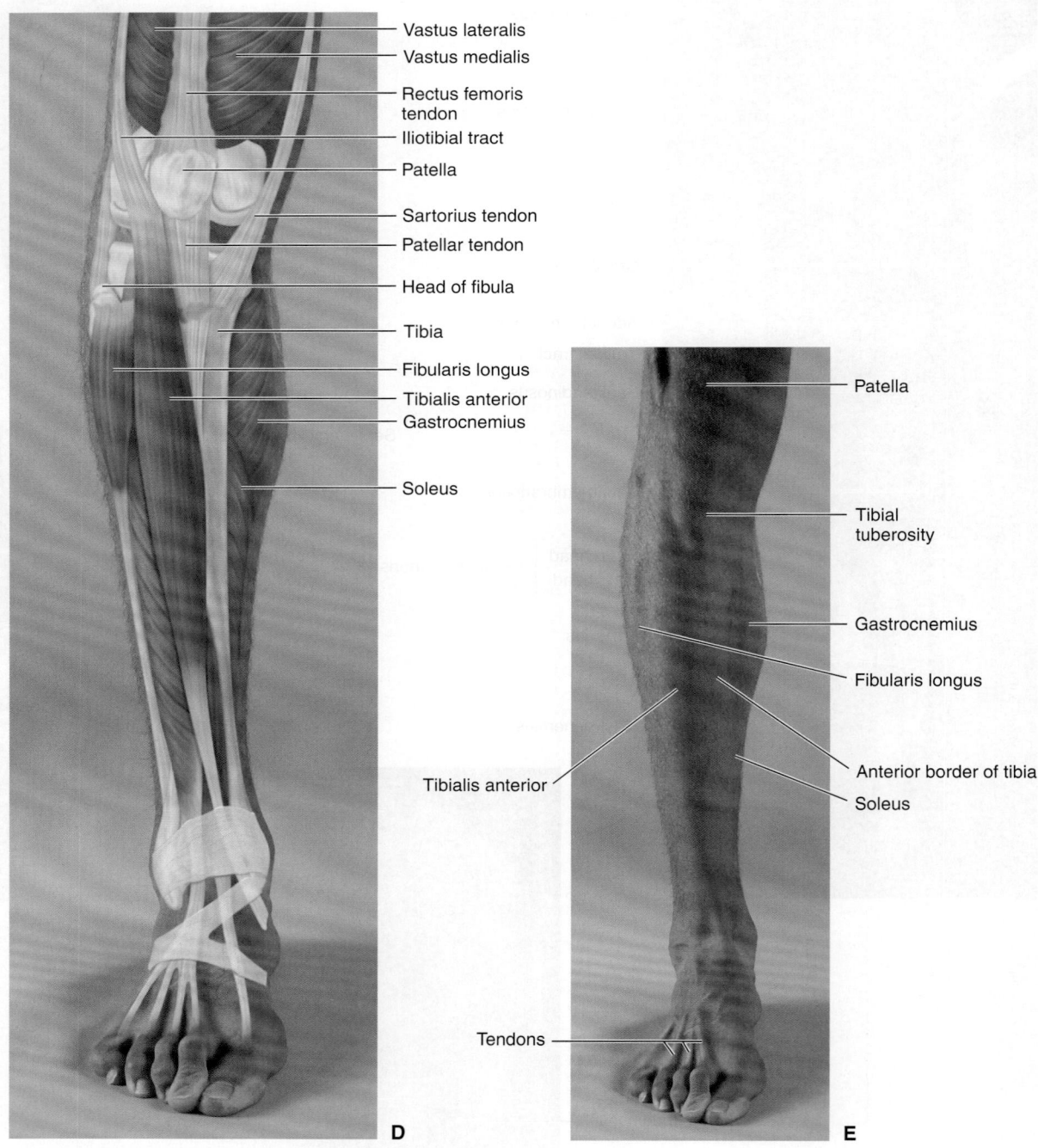

FIGURE 6-8 (D) and (E) Muscles of the leg.

KEY TERM	Definition
abductors (ab-DUCK-turz)	muscles that pull a body part away from the midline when contracted
adductors (a-DUCK-turz)	muscles that pull a body part toward the midline when contracted
extensors (eck-STEN-surz)	muscles that extend or straighten a limb when contracted
flexors (FLECK-surz)	muscles that bend a limb when contracted

KEY TERM PRACTICE: *Naming Skeletal Muscles*

1. _____ are muscles that would cause the biceps brachii to bulge while "making a muscle."

2. These muscles enable you to move the legs laterally as if doing the splits. _____

3. These muscles allow you to stretch out your arms to carry something. _____

4. _____ are muscles that bring a body part toward the midline.

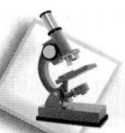

THE CLINICAL DIMENSION

Signs of muscle disorder are often evident during a physical examination and may provide clues to underlying neurological pathology. Muscle pain and weakness are common signs and symptoms of muscular system disorders. Terms describing signs and symptoms of the muscular system are often built from the combining form *my-* or *myo-*. Medical terms pertaining to muscles and tendons are often built from the combining form *fibr-* or *fibro-*, which refers to fiber.

The causes of muscle disorders are numerous. They may result from trauma, tumors, autoimmunity, underlying nervous system dysfunction, genetics, or infection.

Treatments for many muscle disorders involve physical therapy (PT), occupational therapy (OT), rehabilitative exercise, or surgery. The aim of physical therapy is to gain and/or restore function and range of motion in body parts. Occupational therapy helps individuals overcome medical disability and live a quality life in all aspects of their lives despite existing disease. A goal of OT is to provide alternative methods, utensils, or skills to assist the activities of daily living (ADLs). Exercise often helps physical and emotional well-being.

Myopathies

Myopathy describes any disease of muscles that is either inherited, such as muscular dystrophy, or acquired, such as polio.

fibromyalgia	**Fibromyalgia** is a syndrome of unknown origin characterized by diffuse **myalgia** (muscle pain), stiffness, and tenderness at joints. Signs include fibrosis and fibrositis. **Fibrosis** is the formation of fibrous tissue where it normally does not exist, and **fibrositis** is

inflammation of fibrous tissue causing pain and stiffness. Diagnosis is made through patient history and physical examination. Patients usually experience fatigue; sensitivity to noise, light, and odors; and irregular sleep patterns. Treatment includes analgesics, aspirin, and nonsteroidal anti-inflammatory drugs (NSAIDs); stress reduction; and exercise. Drugs reduce inflammation, alleviate pain, or interfere with the immune response. NSAIDs are used to reduce swelling. Aspirin and analgesics work to lessen pain.

muscular dystrophies (MDs)

Muscular dystrophies (MDs) are inherited diseases of muscles characterized by degeneration of individual muscle cells causing progressive muscle weakness. The genetic disorder causes muscle atrophy and muscle tissue to be replaced by fat and connective tissue, both of which cannot contract. Duchenne muscular dystrophy (DMD) is the most common form. It usually affects boys and is characterized by rapid progression and weakness, and death by approximately age 21 years.

Progression of other dystrophies is usually slow, taking decades unless cardiac muscle is involved. Blood tests are used to establish muscle tissue damage. Because there is no cure, treatment is limited and involves PT, OT, and orthopedic procedures.

polymyositis (PM)

Polymyositis (PM) is an autoimmune disease that causes **myositis** (muscle inflammation), muscle tissue softening, and atrophy. Nearly 67% of those afflicted are women. It is called dermatomyositis (DM) when the skin is also involved. The initial signs and symptoms are malaise (a general feeling of sickness) and fatigue, which progress to an inability to raise the arms above the head and difficulty walking. The preliminary diagnosis is made through the history and physical examination, blood tests to rule out other disorders with similar characteristics, and electromyography.

Electromyography is the procedure used to record the electrical activity of muscle tissue using electrodes attached to the skin or inserted into the muscle. The record produced by electromyography is called an **electromyogram**. Electromyography and electromyogram are both abbreviated EMG. Neurologists generally administer an EMG. Elevated levels of a particular enzyme, creatine phosphokinase (CPK), indicate the presence of polymyositis, but the definitive test to confirm a diagnosis is a muscle biopsy. Creatine phosphokinase is also known as creatine kinase (CK). In a **muscle biopsy** procedure, muscle tissue specimens are excised for evaluation. This often is the only method for obtaining an accurate diagnosis of some myopathies.

Treatment is aimed at controlling symptoms and impeding the immune response. Steroids such as prednisone are prescribed to minimize inflammation, immunosuppressants are often used to treat the immune component, and physical therapy helps preserve muscle function and prevent further atrophy. There is no known cure, but the disease can be managed fairly successfully.

KEY TERM	Definition
myopathy (migh-OP-uh-thee)	any disease of the muscles that is inherited or acquired
fibromyalgia (figh-broh-migh-AL-juh)	widespread muscle and joint pain of unknown origin
myalgia (migh-AL-jee-uh)	muscle pain
fibrosis (figh-BROH-sis)	abnormal formation of fibrous tissue
fibrositis (figh-broh-SIGH-tis)	inflammation of fibrous tissue causing pain and stiffness
muscular dystrophies (DIS-troh-feez) (MDs)	hereditary diseases marked by muscle cell degeneration
polymyositis (pol-ee-migh-oh-SIGH-tis)	autoimmune disease characterized by muscle inflammation and atrophy
myositis (migh-oh-SIGH-tis)	muscle inflammation
electromyography (ee-leck-troh-migh-OG-ruh-fee) (EMG)	procedure using electrodes attached to the skin or inserted into the muscle to record the electrical activity of muscle tissue
electromyogram (ee-leck-troh-MIGH-oh-gram) (EMG)	record produced by electromyography
muscle biopsy (BYE-op-see)	muscle tissue sample taken for evaluation

KEY TERM PRACTICE: *Myopathies*

1. Identify the autoimmune disease characterized by muscle atrophy and inflammation. _____

2. The medical term for muscle pain is _____.

3. EMG is the abbreviation for _____ or _____.

4. A _____ is a muscle tissue sample taken for evaluation.

5. _____ is widespread muscle and joint pain of unknown origin.

Trauma

hernia

A protrusion of an organ through an opening is termed a **hernia** or *rupture*. Hernias can occur when forceful muscle contractions increase abdominopelvic pressure considerably, forcing organ bulging. There are numerous types, but common forms are inguinal and umbilical hernias. When an organ extends through the inguinal canal (groin) into the scrotum or labia, it is called an inguinal hernia. Inguinal hernias are more common in males than females. An umbilical hernia involves the intestines bulging through the abdominal wall under the skin as a result of increased abdominal pressure (**Figure 6-9**).

rotator cuff injury

A **rotator cuff injury** involves a group of four shoulder muscles and their tendons. This type of injury is a consequence of acute trauma, degenerative changes, or overuse as is seen with baseball pitchers. A snapping sound is usually heard when the surrounding tendons tear. There is immediate pain and inability to abduct the arm. Physical evaluation, computed tomography (CT) scan, or magnetic resonance imaging (MRI)

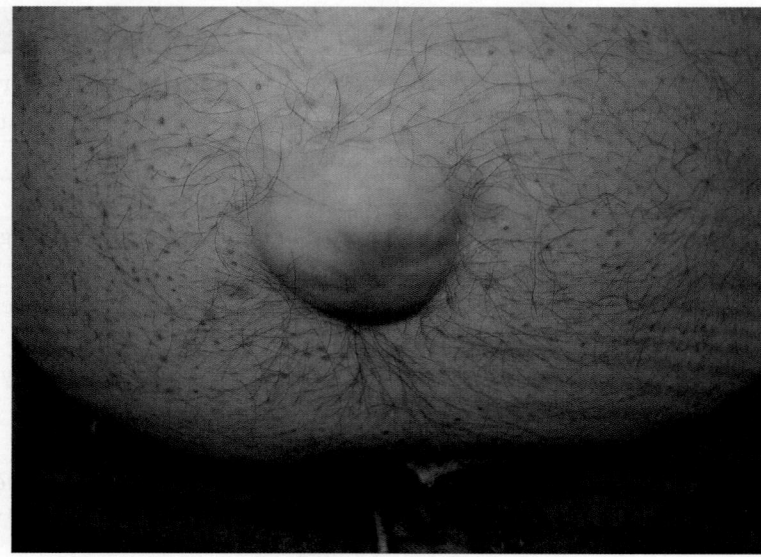

FIGURE 6-9 An umbilical hernia.

studies make the diagnosis. Surgery is required to repair damaged tissue and preserve muscle integrity. Drugs may also be used to manage pain.

shin splints

Shin splints are a painful inflammation of the muscles surrounding the tibia (shin bone), often caused by running or jogging on hard surfaces. Athletic overexertion in untrained individuals can also cause shin splints. Diagnosis is made by physical examination and radiographic studies. The diagnosis is usually confirmed when pain occurs while exercising but disappears during rest. Alternate heat and ice treatments (cold packs) alleviate some symptoms. Analgesics, NSAIDs, rest, good-fitting shoes, and proper exercise techniques are prescribed. When using the term shin splints, it can be treated as either a singular or plural noun.

severed tendon

Severed tendon injuries result from trauma or laceration. When severed, the elastic fibrous cord, like a thick rubber band, snaps. The signs and symptoms include pain, inflammation, and immobility of the affected structure. Diagnosis is made through the patient's history, physical examination, and radiographic studies. Treatment involves **tenoplasty**, which is surgery to repair and attach the cleaved part (**Figure 6-10**).

strain

A **strain** is an injury to muscle resulting from overexertion or trauma. Strains involve stretching or tearing of muscle fibers.

sprain

Similar to strains, a **sprain** is an injury to the ligaments of a joint caused by excessive forces applied to the joint, but without dislocation or fracture. Edema (swelling), muscle and tendon inflammation, and myalgia are signs and symptoms of both. Diagnosis is made by physical examination and radiographic studies to differentiate between a sprain, strain, and bone fracture.

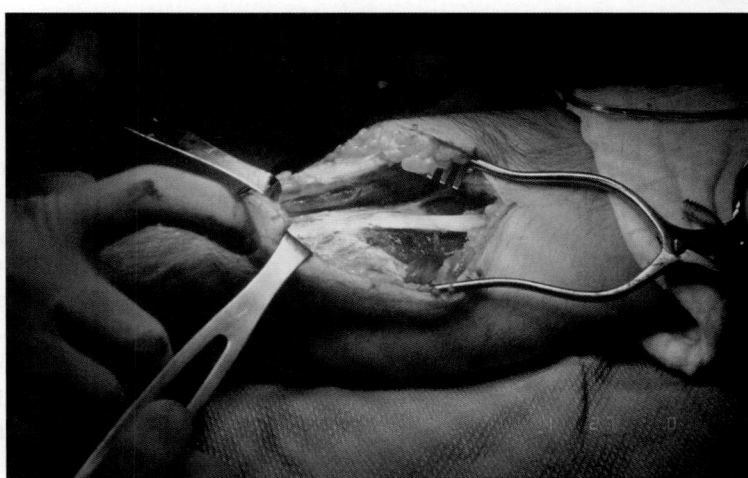

FIGURE 6-10 Insertion of the pronator teres tendon into the radius.

Treatment involves limb elevation, rest, analgesics, and NSAIDs. Because ligaments have no direct blood supply, these injuries are slow healing and can take up to 6 weeks for complete recovery.

tendinitis

Tendinitis is inflammation of a tendon. It is often painful, usually occurs after excessive use, and is generally cured by rest.

KEY TERM	Definition
hernia (HUR-nee-uh)	abnormal protrusion of an organ as a result of pressure; also called a rupture
rotator cuff injury	injury to the four muscles of the shoulder and their associated tendons
shin splints	a painful inflammation of the muscles surrounding the tibia as a result of running or jogging on hard surfaces
severed tendon (TEN-dun)	lacerated tendon
tenoplasty (TEN-oh-plas-tee)	surgical repair of a tendon
strain	injury from overexertion or trauma that involves the stretching or tearing of muscle fibers
sprain	injury to the ligaments of a joint caused by excessive forces on the joint
tendinitis (ten-din-EYE-tis)	tendon inflammation

KEY TERM PRACTICE: *Trauma*

1. An abnormal protrusion of an organ as a result of increased pressure is termed a rupture or _____.

2. _____ is the surgical repair of a tendon.

3. Injury to four muscles of the shoulder and the associated tendons is termed a _____.

4. A _____ is an overexertion or trauma injury that involves the stretching or tearing of muscle fibers.

5. A painful inflammation of the muscles surrounding the tibia as a result of running on hard surfaces is called _____.

LIFE SPAN

Muscle tissue is derived from embryonic stem cells. Cardiac muscle is already operating in 3-week-old embryos. By week 7 in utero, skeletal muscle tissue begins functioning.

Approximately 25% of the body weight of infants is attributed to muscle mass. This proportion increases to approximately 40% in the adult. Most infant muscle mass is contained in the musculature of the head, neck, and trunk. In the adult, 55% of muscle weight is located in lower limbs.

Satellite cells (stem cells that repair damaged tissue) in skeletal muscle allow for limited muscle regeneration. Cardiac satellite cells promote heart tissue regeneration, but damaged tissue is replaced primarily by scar tissue. Smooth muscle tissue remains capable of dividing and regenerating throughout life.

A normal response to aging in skeletal muscle tissue is a progressive deterioration of tissue. As a person ages, skeletal muscles become less elastic, and the reflexes are diminished. An active lifestyle that includes regular exercise can help to counteract these changes.

Muscle tissue can grow all through life. Exercise exerts its effect by increasing the size of existing muscle fibers. Exercise promotes blood flow to muscle tissue, helps to control body weight, and enhances the quality of life. It also increases stability and balance in all life stages.

COMMON Abbreviations

Abbreviation	Term
ACL	anterior cruciate ligament
ADLs	activities of daily living
BS	bachelor of science
CK	creatine kinase
CPK	creatine phosphokinase
CT	computed tomography
DM	dermatomyositis
DMD	Duchenne muscular dystrophy
EMG	electromyogram, electromyography
MCL	medial collateral ligament
MDs	muscular dystrophies
MRI	magnetic resonance imaging
MS	master of science
NM	neuromuscular
NSAID	nonsteroidal anti-inflammatory drug
OT	occupational therapy
PhD	doctor of philosophy
PM	polymyositis

continued

continued from page 304

Abbreviation	Term
PT	physical therapy
PTA	physical therapy assistant
ROM	range of motion
SITS	supraspinatus, infraspinatus, teres minor, subscapularis muscles (four rotator cuff muscles)
WFL	within functional limits
WNL	within normal limits

COMMON ABBREVIATIONS EXERCISES

1. SITS is the abbreviation for which four muscles comprising the rotator cuff? _____

2. ADLs refer to _____ .

3. The abbreviation for neuromuscular is _____ .

4. PTA is the abbreviation for _____ .

5. CK is the abbreviation for _____ .

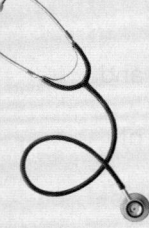

Case Study

Mrs. Lee, a 45-year-old tax clerk, presented in Cindy's physical therapy office for evaluation and therapy. Her orthopedic surgeon referred her for rehabilitative services after she had been involved in an automobile accident.

Subjective Findings

Mrs. Lee's chief complaints were pain in the right leg and inability to walk. During the casting period, her activity level declined and she engaged in no physical pursuits beyond going to work. Mrs. Lee was able to ambulate using a wheelchair and walker. She noted pain in her right lower extremity of 4 on a 0–10 pain scale. Her goal for physical therapy was to regain mobility.

Objective Findings

Her initial diagnosis was fractured right lateral malleolus, torn right anterior cruciate ligament (ACL), and torn right medial collateral ligament (MCL). Her right fibula was casted inferior to the patella for 7 weeks. There was disruption of the deep fibers of the medial collateral ligament complex. Edema and hemorrhage within the substance of the components of the medial collateral ligament were evident. She supported her weight through her left lower extremity and bilateral upper extremities. Patient's range of motion (ROM) was severely restricted. Several measurements were taken.

continued from page 305

Range of Motion

Measure	Right	Left
Knee extension	−40°	0°
Knee flexion	55°	145°
Hip extension	−17°	WFL[a]
Plantar flexion	49°	WNL[b]
Dorsiflexion	−25°	WFL

[a]WFL = within functional limits; [b]WNL = within normal limits.

Circumference Measurements

Location	Right	Left
Thigh	45 cm	50 cm
Calf	30 cm	35 cm

Case Study Questions

Select the best answer to each of the following questions.

1. **ROM refers to _____.**
   a. range of motion
   b. restriction of motion
   c. range of muscle
   d. reading on measurement

2. **The circumferential measurements revealed that the right leg is smaller than the left. Which of the following is a plausible explanation? _____**
   a. One leg is usually considerably smaller than the other.
   b. Mrs. Lee is experiencing some atrophy in the muscle tissue due to disuse.
   c. The physical therapist probably made an error in charting.

3. **The goal of Mrs. Lee's therapy is to _____.**
   a. increase flexion of left knee
   b. decrease flexion of left knee
   c. increase flexion of right knee
   d. decrease flexion of right knee

4. **Other therapy options for Mrs. Lee are _____.**
   a. warm packs to reduce swelling and active exercise to alleviate pain
   b. moist hot packs to reduce swelling and passive exercise to reduce pain
   c. home instruction to increase range of motion and isometric (muscle tension without contraction) exercises to strengthen the shoulder girdle
   d. cold packs to reduce swelling and pain, and range-of-motion exercises to increase strength

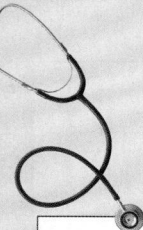

Real World Report

Cindy assessed Mrs. Lee and developed a physical therapy plan. The physical therapy report follows.

PATIENT ASSESSMENT

Patient: Annabelle Lee
Date: August 15, 2011

STRENGTH

Patient demonstrates 5/5 strength for left lower extremity and 2/5 strength throughout right lower extremity, grossly secondary to an inability to move through ROM. Significant atrophy is noted throughout right lower extremity.

GAIT

Patient ambulates only very short distances with the walker and with no weight bearing on the right lower extremity; she uses a "hop-to" gait pattern with the walker.

OTHER

Patient demonstrates significant fear of trying to weight bear on the right lower extremity although minimal to no pain is present when attempting to bear weight.

PROBLEMS

Inability to walk; decreased strength; hip, knee, and ankle contractures; decreased ADLs and mobility; lack of home-exercise program.

EXERCISES

EXERCISE 1: STRETCH GASTROCNEMIUS—SITTING WITH TOWEL
- Perform 1 set of 3 repetitions, twice a day.
- Hold exercise for 30s.
- Rest 15s between sets.

EXERCISE 2: STRETCH GASTROCNEMIUS—STANDING
- Perform 1 set of 4 repetitions, twice a day.
- Hold exercise for 30s.
- Rest 15s between sets.

EXERCISE 3: STRETCH SOLEUS—STANDING
- Perform 1 set of 4 repetitions, twice a day.
- Hold exercise for 30s.
- Rest 15s between sets.

continued

continued from page 307

GOALS

SHORT-TERM—AFTER 10 TREATMENTS

- Increase extension of right knee to $-10°$
- Increase flexion of right knee to $75°$
- Patient able to ambulate independently with weight bearing of right lower extremity using walker or appropriate assistive device
- Patient independent with beginning home-exercise program
- Increase hip extension to $10°$
- Increase dorsiflexion of right ankle to $-5°$
- Patient to note 50% improvement in ADLs

LONG-TERM—AFTER 20 TREATMENTS

- Increase right knee ROM to minimum of $3°$ to $120°$
- Increase dorsiflexion right ankle to minimum of $5°$
- Patient able to ambulate independently without use of assistive device with full weight bearing on right lower extremity
- Increase strength of right lower extremity to 5/5
- Independent with advanced home-exercise program

PLAN

Patient to be seen two to three times per week for a total of 10 treatments per prescription and reevaluated at that time. Patient has significant limitations secondary to muscle contracture and expresses fear; additional visits will be required to return the patient to function and normal gait pattern.
Cindy Hartsel, PT, PhD

Real World Report Questions

The following exercises review the medical terms used in the preceding medical report.

1. Flexion, accomplished by flexor muscles, refers to _____.

a. increasing the angle between body parts

b. decreasing the angle between body parts

c. moving the foot in a circular fashion

d. standing with the feet facing forward

2. Mrs. Lee has limitations that are secondary to muscle contracture. This means that the muscle contracture _____.

a. caused her limitations

b. is the result of her limitations

c. is going to heal after she can walk

d. has nothing to do with her range-of-motion limitations

3. Gastrocnemius stretching exercises were prescribed. These will strengthen muscles in the _____.

a. hip

b. thigh

c. calf

d. ankle

4. Soleus exercises while standing were given as part of the rehabilitation plan. The action of this muscle is _____.

a. leg extension

b. plantar flexion

c. leg flexion

d. thigh adduction

Review and Application

Multiple-Choice Questions

Select the best answer to each of the following questions.

1. Functions of the muscular system include _____.
   a. movement   b. heat production   c. posture maintenance   d. all of these

2. Skeletal muscle tissue is also known as _____.
   a. striated   b. unstriated   c. involuntary   d. cardiac

3. Smooth muscle tissue is also known as _____.
   a. striated   b. unstriated   c. involuntary   d. cardiac

4. Heart muscle tissue is also known as _____.
   a. voluntary   b. unstriated   c. involuntary   d. cardiac

5. This type of muscle tissue is found lining blood vessels _____.
   a. skeletal   b. smooth   c. voluntary   d. cardiac

6. Skeletal muscles are named according to _____.
   a. size   b. location   c. action   d. all of these

7. Most muscles have _____ names.
   a. Latin   b. Spanish   c. English   d. German

Word Parts Exercises

Match the word part with its meaning.

_____ 8. brachy-

_____ 9. platy-

_____ 10. -trophic, troph-, tropho-

_____ 11. my-, myo-

_____ 12. fascio-

a. fascia, a band
b. food, nutrition
c. muscle
d. short
e. flat, broad

Using the following word parts, form a medical term for each definition. Each word part is used only once.

kinesio-
-logy
-logy
my-, myo-
my-, myo-
-pathy
-plasty ·
teno-

13. the study of muscles = _____

14. the study of movement = _____

15. repair of a tendon = _____

16. any disease of muscle = _____

Matching

Match the disorder with its description.

_____ 17. strain

_____ 18. sprain

_____ 19. muscular dystrophy

_____ 20. fibromyalgia

_____ 21. shin splints

a. hereditary muscle disease marked by muscle cell degeneration
b. widespread muscle and joint pain of unknown origin
c. torn muscle
d. ligament injury at a joint
e. painful inflammation of the muscles in the tibial region

Match the muscle with its location.

_____ 22. rectus abdominis

_____ 23. diaphragm

_____ 24. latissimus dorsi

_____ 25. biceps brachii

_____ 26. masseter

_____ 27. rectus femoris

_____ 28. tibialis anterior

a. upper arm
b. lower leg
c. upper leg
d. thoracic region
e. abdominal region
f. back
g. face

Definitions

Define the following word parts.

29. fascio- _____

30. sarco- _____

31. -trophic, troph-, tropho- _____

32. pterygo- _____

Define the following terms.

33. abductors = _____

34. tendons = _____

35. peristalsis = _____

Spelling

Identify the correctly spelled term in each set.

36. _____
   a. elecktromyogram
   b. electromiogram
   c. electromyogram
   d. electromighogram

37. _____
   a. insersion
   b. insertion
   c. ensertion
   d. insershun

38. _____
   a. atrofee
   b. atrophee
   c. atrophie
   d. atrophy

39. _____
   a. delltoid
   b. deltod
   c. deltoid
   d. deltowd

40. _____
   a. aponeurosis
   b. aponewrosis
   c. appleneurosis
   d. apponeurossis

Unscramble

Unscramble the letters to form a medical term.

41. tenrossex _____

42. ductsorda _____

43. toohms slecum _____

44. aaicsf _____

Abbreviations

Provide the terms for the abbreviations and then define the terms.

45. PM = _____

46. MDs = _____

47. OT = _____

Analogies

Provide a medical term to complete a meaningful analogy.

48. Origin is to immovable as _____ is to movable.

Naming Muscles

Identify the criterion used to name each of the following muscles. Answers may be used more than once.

_____ 49. pterygoids

_____ 50. triceps brachii

_____ 51. adductor longus

_____ 52. quadriceps femoris

_____ 53. rectus abdominis

_____ 54. gluteus maximus

a. size
b. location
c. number of heads/origins
d. action
e. appearance

Short Answer

Answer the following questions.

55. Jack's physician sent him to the physical therapist for an evaluation. The physical examination revealed that Jack is unable to extend at the knee and cannot flex or laterally rotate his leg. Identify the muscles involved with these actions.

_____

56. Which muscle has the following origin and insertion?
    a. Origin: distal lateral end of humerus
    b. Insertion: lateral surface of radius
    c. Muscle: _____

Labeling

....

Label the muscles in the following diagram.

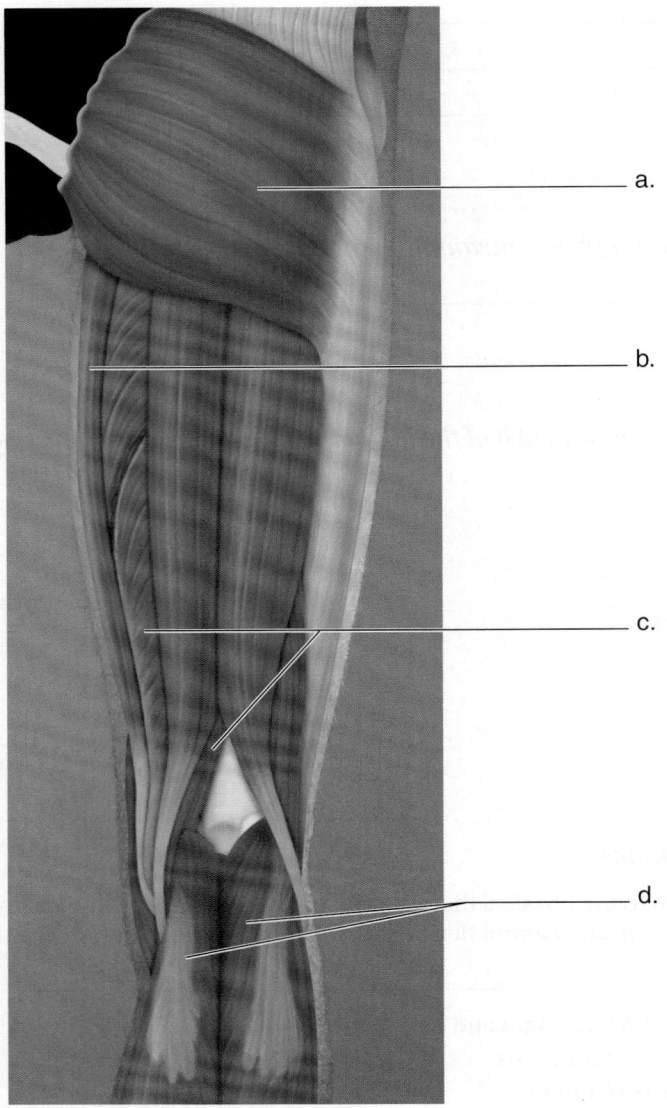

a.

b.

c.

d.

Word Search

Find the medical terms hidden in the puzzle.

```
E  D  U  J  R  T  P  E  S  F  N  A  F  U  Q
M  L  M  D  L  P  B  L  N  A  O  T  F  Y  Z
F  U  C  S  J  C  A  C  O  S  I  R  A  V  K
E  L  S  S  L  L  F  S  D  C  T  O  S  L  L
Y  I  E  C  U  L  I  U  N  I  R  P  V  W  A
S  B  H  X  L  M  E  M  E  A  E  H  W  Y  P
Z  C  B  M  O  E  L  C  T  E  S  Y  D  C  O
E  S  U  T  Q  R  T  A  E  M  N  N  S  M  N
A  I  N  R  E  H  S  I  T  L  I  W  M  R  E
A  I  G  L  A  Y  M  D  S  E  C  M  M  H  U
A  B  D  U  C  T  O  R  S  S  L  S  S  F  R
X  H  V  O  D  A  S  A  D  X  U  E  U  O  O
O  R  I  G  I  N  Z  C  B  I  S  E  K  M  S
M  U  S  C  L  E  F  I  B  E  R  S  H  S  I
Y  H  P  O  R  T  R  E  P  Y  H  A  B  A  S
```

abductors
aponeurosis
atrophy
cardiac muscle
fascia
flexors
hernia
hypertrophy
insertion
muscle cells
muscle fibers
muscle tissue
myalgia
origin
skeletal muscle
tendons

Vocabulary Review

Review the key terms from this chapter, study the spelling and pronunciation of each term, and write its definition in the space provided. Listen to the audio available for most terms at http://thepoint.lww.com/nath2e and pronounce each term for yourself. Then check the box when you feel confident that you know the definition and can pronounce the term correctly.

Key Term	Pronunciation	Definition
❏ **abductors**	(ab-DUCK-turz)	_____
❏ **adductors**	(a-DUCK-turz)	_____
❏ **aponeurosis**	(ap-oh-new-ROH-sis)	_____
❏ **atrophy**	(AT-roh-fee)	_____
❏ **cardiac muscle**		_____
❏ **electromyogram (EMG)**	(ee-leck-troh-MIGH-oh-gram)	_____
❏ **electromyography (EMG)**	(ee-leck-troh-migh-OG-ruh-fee)	_____
❏ **extensors**	(eck-STEN-surz)	_____
❏ **fascia**	(FASH-uh)	_____
❏ **fibromyalgia**	(figh-broh-migh-AL-juh)	_____
❏ **fibrosis**	(figh-BROH-sis)	_____
❏ **fibrositis**	(figh-broh-SIGH-tis)	_____
❏ **flexors**	(FLECK-surz)	_____

Key Term	Pronunciation	Definition
❏ hernia	(HUR-nee-uh)	_____
❏ hypertrophy	(high-PUR-troh-fee)	_____
❏ insertion		_____
❏ muscle biopsy	(BYE-op-see)	_____
❏ muscle cells		_____
❏ muscle fibers		_____
❏ muscle tissue		_____
❏ muscular dystrophies	(DIS-troh-feez)	_____
❏ myalgia	(migh-AL-jee-uh)	_____
❏ myopathy	(migh-OP-uh-thee)	_____
❏ myositis	(migh-oh-SIGH-tis)	_____
❏ origin		_____
❏ peristalsis	(perr-i-STAHL-sis)	_____
❏ polymyositis	(pol-ee-migh-oh-SIGH-tis)	_____
❏ rotator cuff injury		_____
❏ severed tendon	(TEN-dun)	_____
❏ shin splints		_____
❏ skeletal muscle		_____
❏ smooth muscle		_____
❏ sprain		_____
❏ strain		_____
❏ tendinitis	(ten-din-EYE-tis)	_____
❏ tendons		_____
❏ tenoplasty	(TEN-oh-plas-tee)	_____

Answers

Word Grouping Exercises

Definition	Word Part	Definition	Word Part
arm	brachio-	muscle	my-, myo-
cheek	bucco-	muscle, flesh	sarco-
fascia, a band	fascio-	rod shaped	rhabd-, rhabdo-
fiber	fibr-, fibro-	short	brachy-
flat, broad	platy-	tendon	tendo-, teno-
food, nutrition	troph-, tropho-, -trophic	wing, feather	pter-, ptero-
heart	cardi-, cardio-	wing shaped	pterygo-
movement, motion	A. kin-, kine-, kino - B. - kinesi-, kinesio-, kineso		

Word Building Exercises

Word Part	Meaning	Common or Known Word	Example Medical Term
cardi-, cardio-	heart	cardiac	cardiomyopathy
fibr-, fibro-	fiber	fibrous	fibromyalgia
kinesi-, kinesio-, kineso-	motion	kinesiologist	kinesiology
tendo-, teno-	tendon	tendon	tendonitis

Key Term Practice

Muscular System Preview

1. muscle fibers
2. muscle tissue

Muscle Tissue: Skeletal, Smooth, and Cardiac

1. heart; cardiac
2. peristalsis
3. fascia
4. skeletal muscle, smooth muscle, and cardiac muscle
5. Tendons

Muscle Movement

1. origin; insertion
2. hypertrophy
3. Atrophy

Naming Skeletal Muscles

1. Flexors
2. abductors
3. extensors
4. Adductors

Myopathies

1. polymyositis
2. myalgia
3. electromyography; electromyogram
4. muscle biopsy
5. Fibromyalgia

Trauma

1. hernia
2. Tenoplasty
3. rotator cuff injury
4. strain
5. shin splints

Common Abbreviations Exercises

1. SITS = supraspinatus, infraspinatus, teres minor, subscapularis
2. ADLs = activities of daily living
3. neuromuscular = NM
4. PTA = physical therapy assistant
5. CK = creatine kinsase

Case Study

1. a is the correct answer.
   - b, c, and d are incorrect because the abbreviation ROM does not stand for these terms.
2. b is the correct answer.
   - a is incorrect because in the absence of disease, there is little difference in circumference measurements between legs.
   - c is incorrect because the report states that Mrs. Lee injured her right leg, thus the measurements seem to be correct.

3. c is the correct answer.
 - a and b are incorrect because the left leg was not affected.
 - d is incorrect because the goal is to increase the range of motion.

4. d is the correct answer.
 - a and b are incorrect because warm or moist hot packs would not reduce swelling. They would increase circulation to the area and perhaps alleviate pain.
 - c is incorrect because the shoulder girdle was not injured.

Real World Report

1. b
2. a
3. c
4. b

Review and Application

1. d
2. a
3. c
4. d
5. b
6. d
7. a
8. d
9. e
10. b
11. c
12. a
13. myology
14. kinesiology
15. tenoplasty
16. myopathy
17. c
18. d
19. a
20. b
21. e
22. e
23. d
24. f
25. a
26. g
27. c
28. b

29. fascio- = fascia, a band
30. sarco- = muscle, flesh
31. -trophic, troph-, tropho- = nutrition
32. pterygo- = wing shaped
33. abductors = muscles that pull a body part away from the midline when contracted
34. tendons = tough, fibrous connective tissues that connect muscles to bones
35. peristalsis = rhythmic waves of muscular contraction
36. c
37. b
38. d
39. c
40. a
41. extensors
42. adductors
43. smooth muscle

44. fascia
45. PM = polymyositis; autoimmune disease characterized by muscle inflammation and atrophy
46. MDs = muscular dystrophies; hereditary diseases marked by muscle degeneration
47. OT = occupational therapy; the use of regular periods of suitable productive activity as part of the treatment of illness or medical condition
48. insertion
49. e
50. b, c
51. a, d
52. b, c
53. b, e
54. a, b
55. The muscles involved are the quadriceps femoris and biceps femoris.
56. brachioradialis

Labeling

a. gluteus maximus

b. gracilis

c. semimembranosus

d. gastrocnemius

Word Search

E	+	+	+	+	+	+	E	S	F	N	A	+	+	+
M	L	+	+	+	+	+	L	N	A	O	T	+	+	+
F	U	C	S	+	+	+	C	O	S	I	R	+	+	+
+	L	S	S	L	+	+	S	D	C	T	O	+	+	+
+	+	E	C	U	L	+	U	N	I	R	P	+	+	A
+	+	+	X	L	M	E	M	E	A	E	H	+	+	P
+	+	+	+	O	E	L	C	T	+	S	Y	+	+	O
+	+	+	+	+	R	T	A	E	+	N	+	+	+	N
A	I	N	R	E	H	S	I	T	L	I	+	+	+	E
A	I	G	L	A	Y	M	D	S	E	C	+	+	+	U
A	B	D	U	C	T	O	R	S	S	L	S	+	+	R
+	+	+	+	+	+	+	A	+	+	U	E	U	+	O
O	R	I	G	I	N	+	C	+	+	+	E	K	M	S
M	U	S	C	L	E	F	I	B	E	R	S	+	S	I
Y	H	P	O	R	T	R	E	P	Y	H	+	+	+	S

abductors
aponeurosis
atrophy
cardiac muscle
fascia
flexors
hernia
hypertrophy
insertion
muscle cells
muscle fibers
muscle tissue
myalgia
origin
skeletal muscle
tendons

Vocabulary Review

Key Term	Definition	Key Term	Definition
abductors	muscles that pull a body part away from the midline when contracted	**fascia**	a thin sheet of fibrous connective tissue that envelops the body beneath the skin or encloses muscles or groups of muscles
adductors	muscles that pull a body part toward the midline when contracted		
aponeurosis	a sheet of fibrous tissue that connects a muscle to another muscle	**fibromyalgia**	widespread muscle and joint pain of unknown origin
atrophy	decrease in muscle size	**fibrosis**	abnormal formation of fibrous tissue
cardiac muscle	striated, involuntary muscle found only in the heart	**fibrositis**	inflammation of fibrous tissue causing pain and stiffness
electromyogram (EMG)	record produced by electromyography	**flexors**	muscles that bend a limb when contracted
electromyography (EMG)	procedure using electrodes attached to the skin or inserted into the muscle to record the electrical activity of muscle tissue	**hernia**	abnormal protrusion of an organ as a result of pressure; also called a rupture
		hypertrophy	increase in muscle size
extensors	muscles that extend or straighten a limb when contracted	**insertion**	muscle end that moves during contraction

Key Term	Definition	Key Term	Definition
muscle biopsy	muscle tissue sample taken for evaluation	rotator cuff injury	injury to the four muscles of the shoulder and their associated tendons
muscle cells	microscopic thread-like structures that contract to move muscles; also called muscle fibers	severed tendon	lacerated tendon
		shin splints	a painful inflammation of the muscles surrounding the tibia as a result of running or jogging on hard surfaces
muscle fibers	microscopic thread-like structures that contract to move muscles; also called muscle cells		
muscle tissue	tissue composed of contractile muscle fibers	skeletal muscle	striated, voluntary muscle tissue attached to bones
muscular dystrophies	hereditary diseases marked by muscle cell degeneration	smooth muscle	nonstriated, involuntary muscle tissue found lining organs and blood vessels
myalgia	muscle pain		
myopathy	any disease of the muscles that is inherited or acquired	sprain	injury to the ligaments of a joint caused by excessive forces on the joint
myositis	muscle inflammation	strain	injury from overexertion or trauma that involves the stretching or tearing of muscle fibers
origin	muscle end that remains fixed during contraction		
peristalsis	rhythmic waves of muscular contraction	tendinitis	tendon inflammation
		tendons	tough, fibrous connective tissues that connect muscles to bones
polymyositis	autoimmune disease characterized by muscle inflammation and atrophy	tenoplasty	surgical repair of a tendon

Nervous System

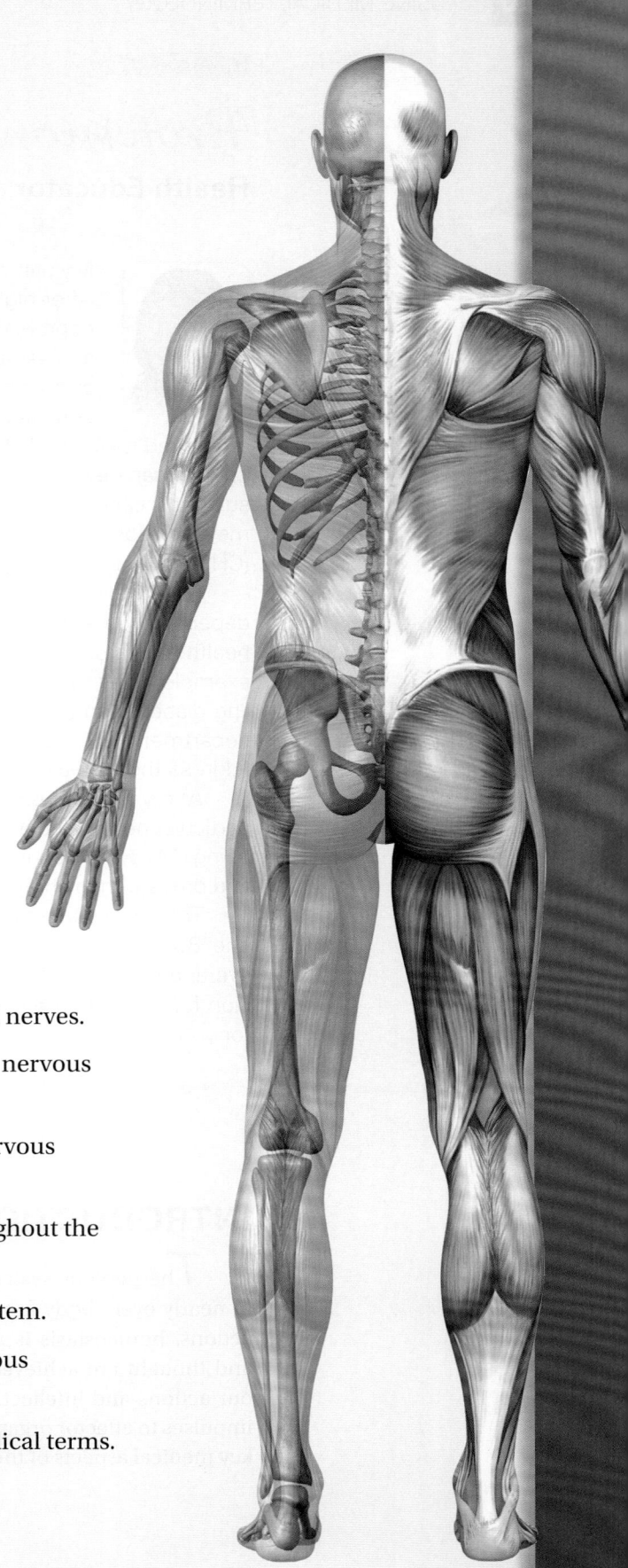

O B J E C T I V E S

After completing this chapter, you should be able to:

1. Define the meanings of word parts related to the nervous system.

2. Identify major structures of the brain, spinal cord, and nerves.

3. Describe primary functions of the brain, spinal cord, and nerves.

4. List different signs, symptoms, and treatments of various nervous system diseases.

5. Recognize clinical tests and procedures related to the nervous system.

6. Describe anatomical and physiological alterations throughout the life span.

7. Define common abbreviations related to the nervous system.

8. Define terms used in medical reports involving the nervous system.

9. Correctly define, spell, and pronounce the chapter's medical terms.

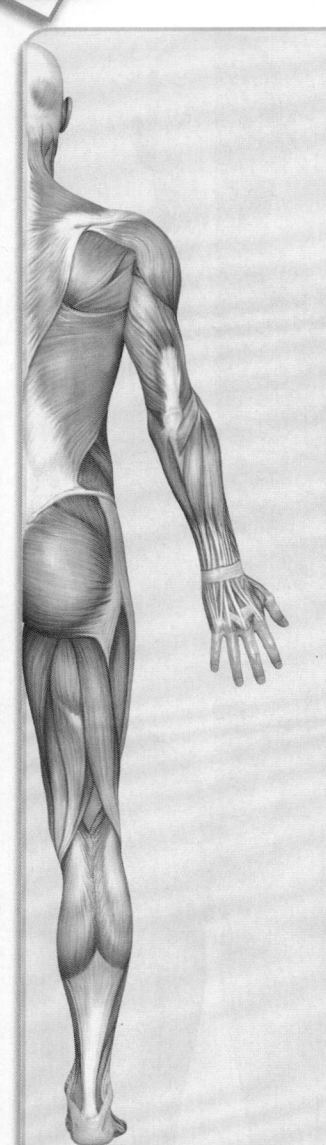

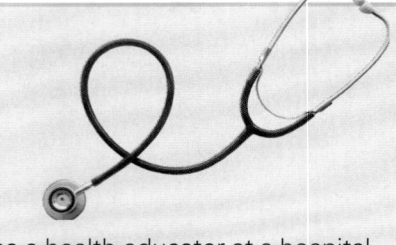

Professional Profile

Health Educator

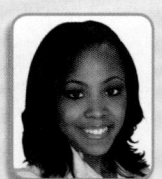

My name is Karen and I am employed as a health educator at a hospital. After high school I entered college and earned my bachelor of science degree. When I could not find a fulfilling career, I entered nursing school and earned my RN. The nursing school's faculty stressed the importance of continuing my education. While investigating my options for further education, the possibility of a degree in the area of health education presented itself and I chose that path. I took courses in biology, anatomy and physiology, human development, statistics, and psychology—all of which are essential in pursuing this career. Successful completion of my college's public health program allowed me to sit for the exam to get credentialed as a Certified Health Education Specialist (CHES) through the National Commission for Health Education Credentialing (NCHEC).

Health education is a career that has a wide range of possibilities and applications depending on someone's personality, chosen area, and education level. In general, health educators educate patients or the community about health-related topics. For example, I talk to people about diet and exercise, measures for preventing or controlling diabetes and/or obesity, and ways to stop smoking. I work with the local health department to collect data on specific local health issues, develop local programs to address those health issues, and to do more to promote health.

At my job I generally work with patients and their families to educate them about particular health issues that they have and how to manage them for their general well-being. My work also involves educating the community on how to lead healthier lives and prevent many major illnesses.

The job prospects for health educators are quite favorable as the United States. The Bureau of Labor Statistics forecasts job growth in this area to be higher than average for the next decade. If you love learning, can communicate well, have a passion for helping others, and are a caring, understanding person, this may be a career for you.

INTRODUCTION

The nervous system is one of the most complex systems in the body. It plays a role in nearly every body function and acts as the primary means of self-protection. Through its actions, homeostasis is maintained and distinctly human characteristics such as emotion and thought are achieved. Nerves and their associated structures bring about nearly all of our actions and intellect. The nervous system receives and interprets stimuli and transmits impulses to effector organs. This chapter focuses on specific anatomy, general physiology, and key medical aspects of the nervous system.

MEDICAL TERM PARTS

Word Parts

Medical term prefixes, suffixes, and combining forms related to the nervous system are introduced in this section.

Word Part	Meaning
astro-	star-like
cephal-, cephalo-	head
cerebr-, cerebri-, cerebro-	cerebrum
chem-, chemo-	chemistry
dendro-	tree-like
encephal-, encephalo-	brain
glio-	glue, glue-like
gloss-, glosso-	tongue
hemi-	half
mening-, meningo-	meninges
myel-, myelo-	myelin sheath of nerve fibers
neur-, neuri-, neuro-	nerve, nerve tissue
polio-	gray matter
-tome	section, part

Word Grouping Exercises

Using the *Medical Term Parts* table, identify the prefix, suffix, or combining form for each of the following definitions. The first one has been done as an example.

Definition	Word Part
section, part	-tome
brain	
cerebrum	
chemical	
glue, glue-like	
gray matter	
half	
head	
meninges	
myelin sheath of nerve fibers	
nerve, nerve tissue	
star-like	
tongue	
tree-like	

Word Building Exercises

Word parts introduced in the *Medical Term Parts* section are listed in the following table. For this exercise, first supply the meaning of each word part, then use the word part to build a word you already know. The word you list under *Common or Known Word* does not have to be a medical term; a commonly used word is fine. Be sure, however, that the word correctly reflects the intended meaning. The first one has been done as an example. Check your answers in a dictionary.

Word Part	Meaning	Common or Known Word	Example Medical Term
cerebr-, cerebri-, cerebro-	*cerebrum*	*cerebral*	cerebrum
chem-, chemo-			chemoreceptor
neur-, neuri-, neuro-			neuron
polio-			poliomyelitis

ANATOMY AND PHYSIOLOGY

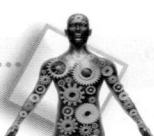

Nervous System Preview

The nervous system has two main divisions, the **central nervous system (CNS)** and the **peripheral nervous system (PNS)**. The CNS consists of the brain and spinal cord, and the PNS consists of the supporting cranial and spinal nerves that connect the CNS to other body parts.

The brain and spinal cord are the only components of the central nervous system. The peripheral nervous system has two divisions: the **somatic nervous system (SNS)** and the **autonomic nervous system (ANS)**. The SNS is under voluntary control, but the ANS is entirely automatic and cannot be consciously controlled. There are two divisions of the ANS: sympathetic and parasympathetic. The **sympathetic nervous system** prepares the body for stressful and emergency conditions and is involved in the "fight-or-flight" response. Another term is the thoracolumbar nervous system because thoracic and lumbar nerve fibers are involved. The **parasympathetic nervous system** is most active under ordinary conditions and is involved in the "rest-and-digest" or "rest-and-repair" response. An alternate term is the craniosacral nervous system because cranial and sacral nerve fibers are involved (**Figure 7-1**).

The nervous system has three general functions: sensory, integrative, and motor. The **sensory function** involves the use of receptors that detect (sense) changes in internal and external body conditions to regulate homeostasis, a state of balance in the body. The integrative function coordinates the sensory information with internal activity and motor function. Motor function implies skeletal muscle activity in which effectors like muscles respond when they are stimulated by motor impulses. The **special senses** are olfaction (smelling), gustation (tasting), vision, equilibrium (physical balance), and hearing. Because the nose, tongue, eyes, and ears are sensory organs of the nervous system involved with the special senses, they are often considered as an integrated whole. For this reason, the eyes and ears are discussed in the next chapter.

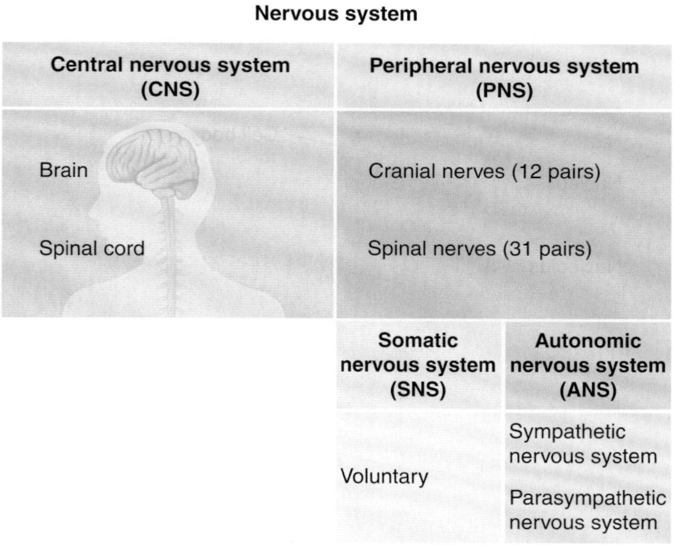

Nervous system

Central nervous system (CNS)	Peripheral nervous system (PNS)	
Brain	Cranial nerves (12 pairs)	
Spinal cord	Spinal nerves (31 pairs)	
	Somatic nervous system (SNS)	Autonomic nervous system (ANS)
	Voluntary	Sympathetic nervous system
		Parasympathetic nervous system

Figure 7-1 Organization of the nervous system.

KEY TERM	Definition
central nervous system (CNS)	the brain and spinal cord
peripheral nervous system (PNS)	all neural tissue outside the central nervous system
somatic nervous system (SNS)	division of the peripheral nervous system that controls skeletal muscle contractions
autonomic (aw-tuh-NOM-ick) **nervous system (ANS)**	division of the peripheral nervous system that is controlled subconsciously
sympathetic (sim-puh-THET-ick) **nervous system**	the division of the autonomic nervous system involved in the "fight-or-flight" response; also called the thoracolumbar nervous system
parasympathetic (par-uh-sim-puh-THET-ick) **nervous system**	the division of the autonomic nervous system involved in the "rest-and-digest" response; also called the craniosacral nervous system
sensory (SEN-suh-ree) **function**	using receptors to detect changes and respond in order to maintain homeostasis
special senses	the five senses of olfaction, gustation, vision, equilibrium, and hearing

KEY TERM PRACTICE: *Nervous System Preview*

1. Name the two main divisions of the nervous system. _____

2. Name the two divisions of the autonomic nervous system. _____

3. The _____ is composed of the brain and spinal cord.

4. The _____ is made up of all neural tissue outside the central nervous system.

5. The five senses of olfaction, gustation, vision, equilibrium, and hearing make up the _____.

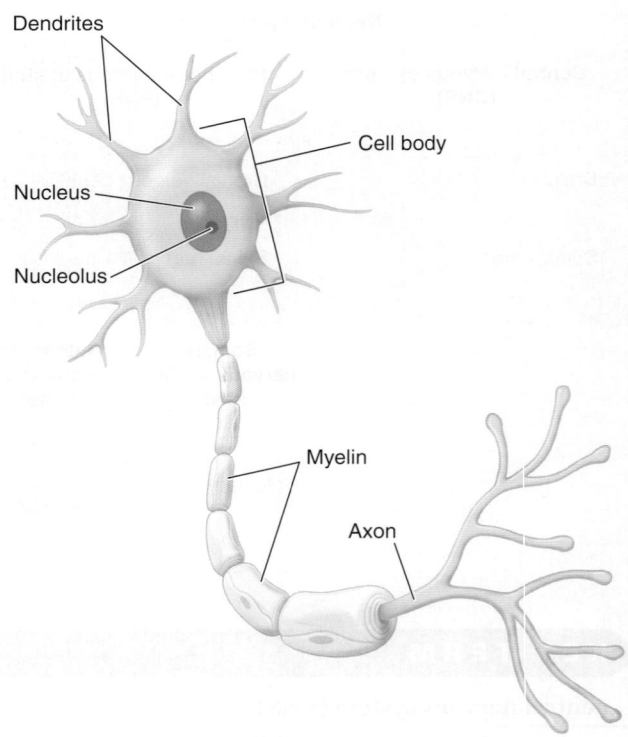

Dendrites

Cell body

Nucleus

Nucleolus

Myelin

Axon

Figure 7-2 Neurons are the basic functional units of the nervous system.

Neurons and Neuroglia

Neurons, or nerve cells, are the basic functional units of the nervous system. They are the structural components that react to physical and chemical changes by sending, receiving, and conducting nerve impulses. There are about 100 billion neurons in the body.

The basic neuron structure consists of a single cell body, an axon, and multiple dendrites. The **cell body** is the main part of a neuron. Within the cell body are the nucleus (where DNA is located) and the nucleolus (the site of RNA). It has slim branches or extensions, also called nerve fibers. The extension that conducts impulses, called *action potentials,* away from the cell body is an **axon**. (As a memory aid, associate the *a* in *a*xon with the *a* in *a*way.) **Dendrites** are sensitive branching extensions that receive information and transmit impulses toward the neuron cell body. **Myelin** is a white, fatty substance that forms an insulating sheath around axons (**Figure 7-2**). It increases the speed of nerve impulses.

Adjacent neurons communicate with one another at sites called **synapses**, which are junctions between two neurons. Neurons communicate through the release of **neurotransmitters**, which are chemical messengers between different neurons or between neurons and muscles. A neurotransmitter is released at the end of one neuron by the arrival of a nerve impulse. The chemical then crosses the synapse, causing the transfer of the impulse to another neuron or muscle cell.

The networks of nourishing **neuroglia**, or glial cells, are supporting cells within the CNS and PNS. These accessory cells function as connective tissue by filling spaces and surrounding and supporting parts. Four types of neuroglia in the CNS are astrocytes, which form the protective blood–brain barrier (BBB); ependymal cells, which line the brain ventricles (spaces) and spinal cord central canals; microglia, which engulf debris; and oligodendrocytes, which form myelin around CNS axons. Neuroglia of the PNS include satellite cells and Schwann cells. Satellite cells surround neuron cell bodies, and Schwann cells surround peripheral nerve axons.

KEY TERM	Definition
neurons (NEW-ronz)	nerve cells that send and receive nerve impulses
cell body	the main part of a neuron
axon (ACKS-on)	nerve cell extension that carries impulses away from the cell body
dendrites (DEN-drites)	branched nerve extensions that carry impulses toward the cell body
myelin (MIGH-e-lin)	white, fatty substance that forms an insulating sheath around axons
synapses (sih-NAP-sez)	sites where adjacent neurons communicate
neurotransmitters (new-roh-TRANS-mit-urz)	chemical messengers between neurons or between neurons and muscles
neuroglia (new-ROG-lee-uh)	supporting cells of the CNS and PNS

KEY TERM PRACTICE: *Neurons and Neuroglia*

1. Name the three basic parts of a typical neuron. _____

2. _____ is the white, fatty insulating substance that surrounds axons.

3. The sites where adjacent neurons communicate are termed _____.

4. _____ are the supporting cells found within the CNS and PNS.

5. Nerve cells are also known as _____.

Spinal Cord and Spinal Nerves

The spinal cord is attached to the brain and extends to the first lumbar vertebra. The spinal cord is slightly shorter than the vertebral column and has 31 segments. Each segment gives rise to a pair of spinal nerves.

Gray matter and white matter are characteristics of central nervous system tissue. **White matter** is considered to be those regions that are dominated by myelinated axons. **Gray matter** is considered to be those regions made up primarily of the cell bodies, neuroglia, and unmyelinated axons. Anatomically, the position of the gray matter and white matter in the spinal cord gives it a "butterfly (gray matter) on a background (white matter)" appearance. The passageway through the spinal cord that contains cerebrospinal fluid (CSF) is the **central canal** (**Figure 7-3**). **Cerebrospinal fluid** bathes the internal and external surfaces of the central nervous system.

Spinal nerves arise from the spinal cord and branch to supply peripheral body regions. Spinal nerves are grouped in a numbered sequence according to their level on the spinal column. Accordingly, there are 8 pairs of cervical nerves, 12 pairs of thoracic nerves, 5 pairs

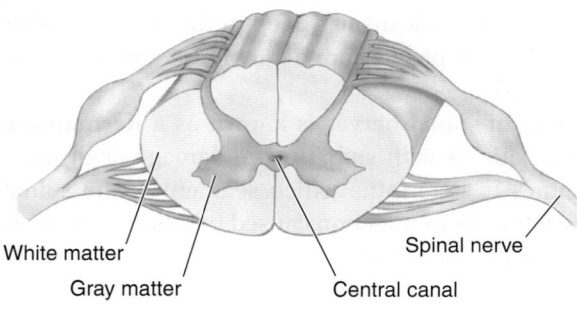

White matter
Gray matter
Spinal nerve
Central canal

Figure 7-3 A cross-section of the spinal cord.

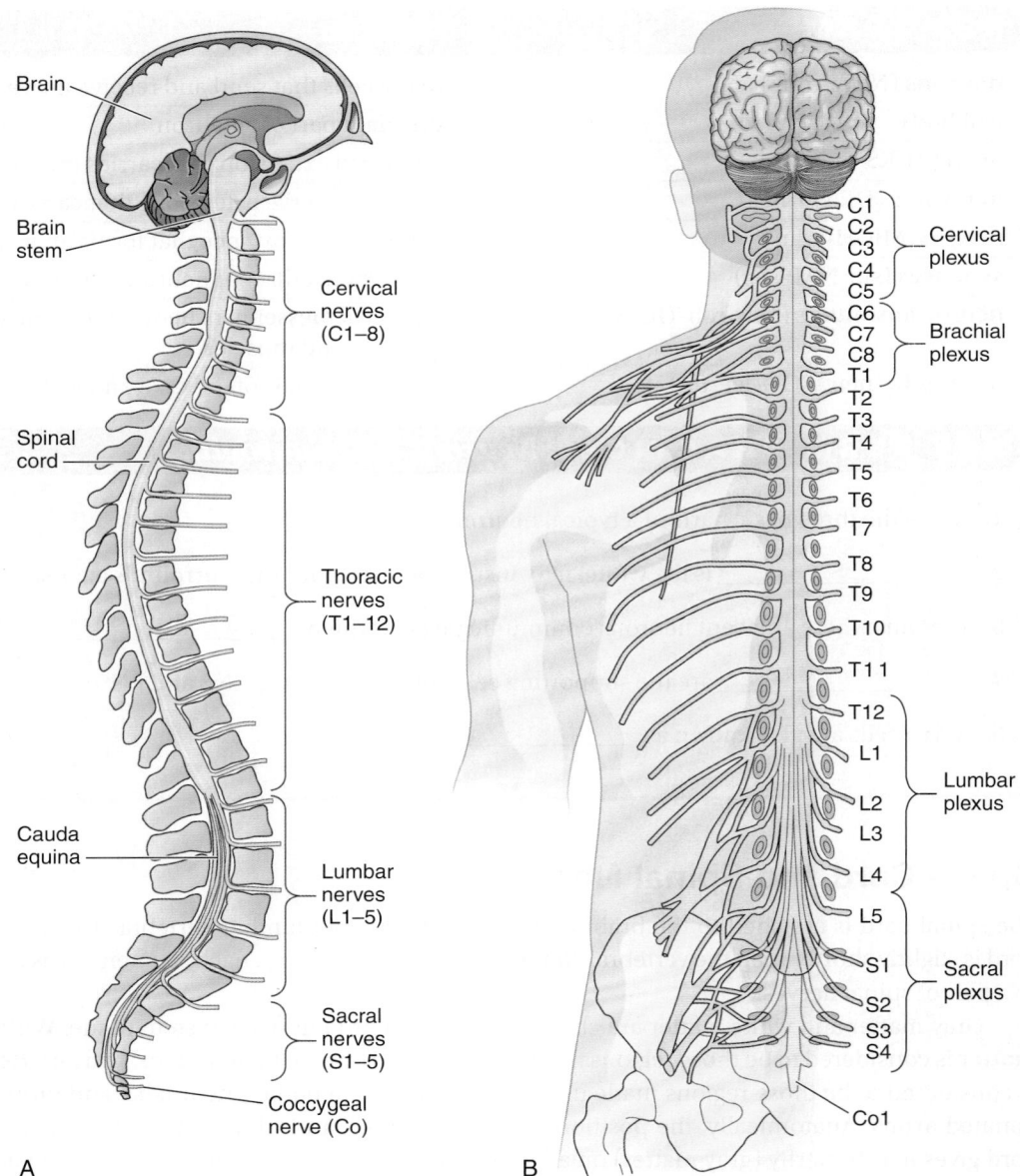

Figure 7-4 (A) Spinal nerves branch to supply peripheral body regions. **(B)** The plexuses of the spinal cord.

of lumbar nerves, 5 pairs of sacral nerves, and 1 pair of coccygeal nerves. A group of spinal nerves called the **cauda equina** (horse's tail) extends below the distal end of the spinal cord (**Figure 7-4A**).

Associated with the spinal nerves is a nerve network referred to as a **plexus** (*plexuses* = plural). The interlacing nerve networks of each plexus enable motor functioning in regions of the body. There are four major plexuses. The cervical plexus lies deep in the neck on either side. The brachial plexus serves the arms. The lumbar plexus and sacral plexus serve the lumbar and sacral regions, respectively (**Figure 7-4B**).

An area of skin supplied by a single pair of spinal nerves is known as a **dermatome** (**Figure 7-5**). When examining and treating patients with spinal nerve damage or disease, clinicians use their knowledge of dermatomes to determine which segment of the spinal cord is malfunctioning or affected. Shingles, which is an infection caused by a herpes virus, is characterized by skin eruptions that follow a dermatome (**Figure 7-6**).

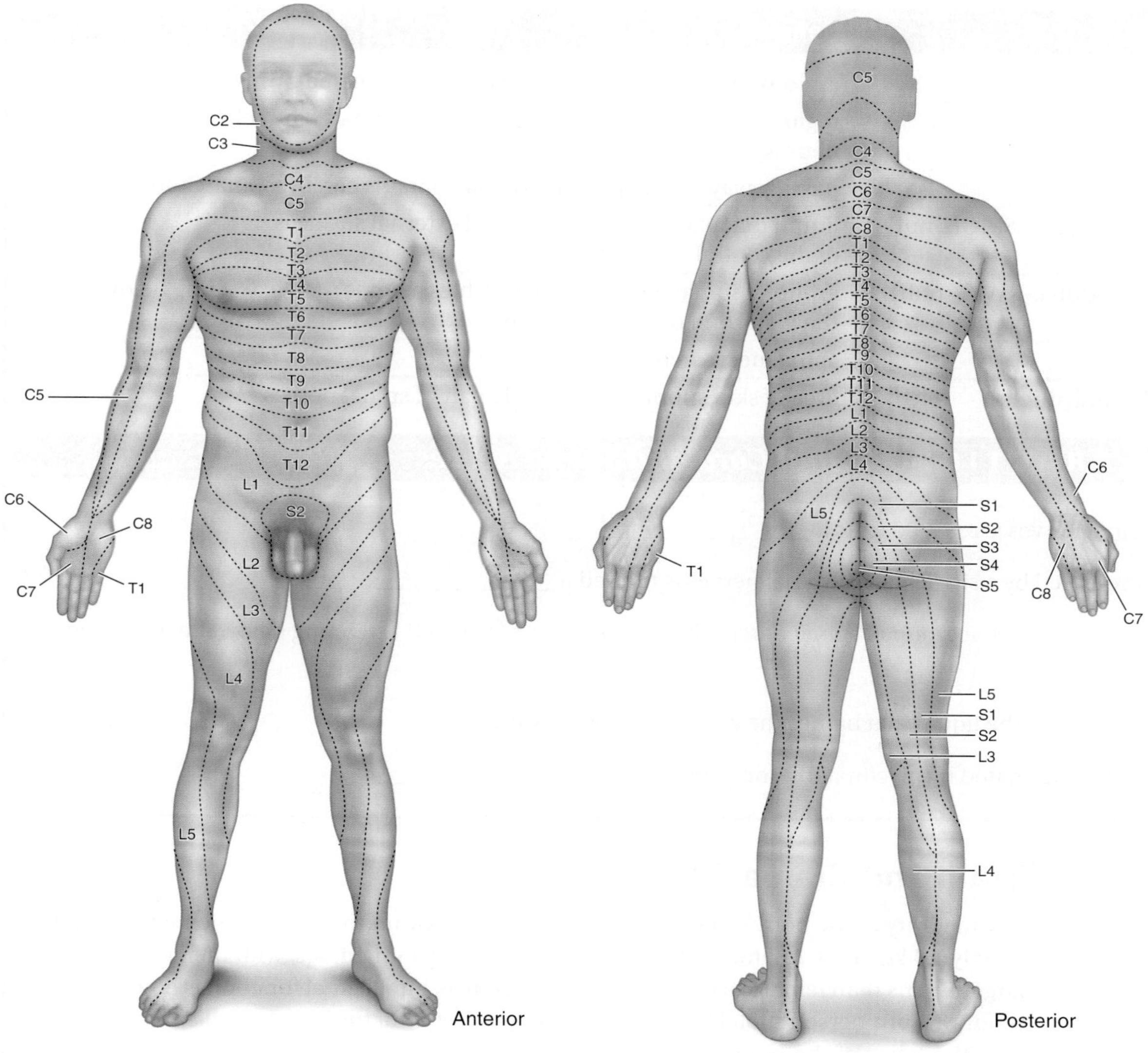

C2
C3
C4
C5
T1
T2
T3
T4
T5
T6
T7
T8
T9
T10
T11
T12
L1
S2
L2
L3
L4
L5
C5
C6
C8
C7
T1

Anterior

C5
C4
C5
C6
C7
C8
T1
T2
T3
T4
T5
T6
T7
T8
T9
T10
T11
T12
L1
L2
L3
L4
L5
S1
S2
S3
S4
S5
C6
C8
C7
T1
L5
S1
S2
L3
L4

Posterior

Figure 7-5 Anterior and posterior dermatomes.

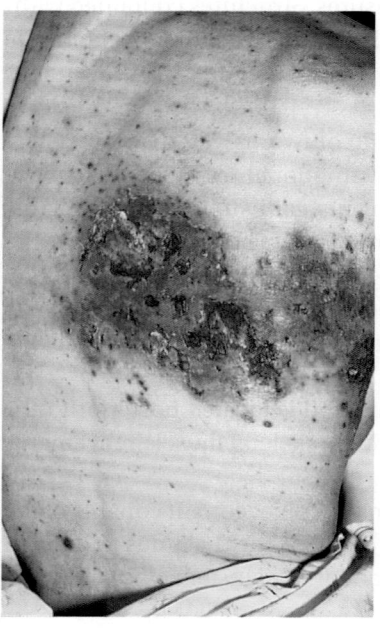

Figure 7-6 Primary skin lesions of shingles following the path of a dermatome.

KEY TERM	Definition
white matter	regions in the central nervous system dominated by myelinated axons
gray matter	regions in the central nervous system dominated by cell bodies, neuroglia and unmyelinated axons
central canal	passageway in the spinal cord that contains cerebrospinal fluid
cerebrospinal (se-ree-broh-SPIGH-nul) fluid (CSF)	liquid that bathes the internal and external surfaces of the central nervous system
cauda equina (KAW-duh e-KWYE-nuh)	group of spinal nerves that resembles a horse's tail extending below the distal end of the spinal cord
plexus (PLECK-sus)	spinal nerve network
dermatome (DUR-muh-tome)	area of skin supplied by a single pair of spinal nerves

KEY TERM PRACTICE: *Spinal Cord and Spinal Nerves*

1. A network of spinal nerves is referred to as a _____.

2. An area of skin supplied by a single pair of spinal nerves is termed a _____.

3. The _____ is a group of spinal nerves that resembles a horse's tail extending below the distal end of the spinal cord.

4. _____ is the liquid that bathes the central nervous system.

5. Regions in the CNS dominated by myelinated axons are termed _____.

Brain and Cranial Nerves

The majority of the body's neural tissue is contained within the brain, which weighs approximately 1.4 kg (3 lb). Anatomical variations exist among individuals, with men typically having larger brains than females. Despite the size difference, intellectual function is equal. The brain is only 2% of a person's total body weight, but it uses 20% of the body's total energy.

The lobes of the brain—frontal, parietal, occipital, and temporal—are named the same as their overlying bones. The principal parts of the brain are the cerebrum, cerebellum, and brainstem. Other major landmarks include gyri, sulci, and fissures. Structures contained within the deep portions of the brain include the thalamus, hypothalamus, and pituitary gland. The pituitary gland is a small, oval-shaped gland at the base of the brain that produces hormones and will be discussed in Chapter 9.

The **cerebrum** is the largest part of the brain, consisting of two halves called **cerebral hemispheres**. Reasoning, learning, sensory perception, and emotional responses take place in the cerebrum. The hemispheres are connected by the **corpus callosum**, which is a large bundle of axons that looks like a broad band of white matter when the brain is dissected. The **cerebral cortex** is an outer layer of gray matter that covers the entire surface of the cerebral hemispheres. The cerebral cortex covers a series of elevated ridges known as **gyri** (*gyrus* = singular), which increase the surface area of the brain. Shallow depressions called **sulci** (*sulcus* = singular) and deeper grooves called **fissures** separate gyri.

The **cerebellum** is the second-largest region of the brain and is located posterior to the pons and medulla. Its main function is to control and coordinate skeletal muscle movements and maintain balance.

The **brainstem** extends from the base of the cerebrum to the spinal cord. It consists of the midbrain, pons, and medulla oblongata. The **diencephalon** contains the thalamus and hypothalamus and is the link between the cerebral hemispheres and the brainstem. The **thalamus**

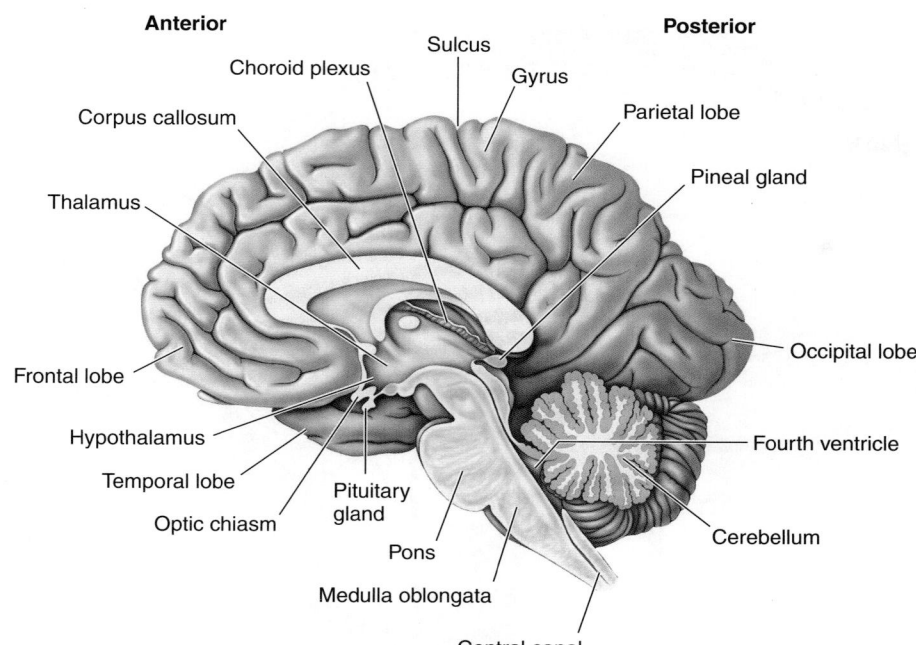

Anterior

Posterior

Sulcus

Choroid plexus

Gyrus

Corpus callosum

Parietal lobe

Pineal gland

Thalamus

Frontal lobe

Occipital lobe

Hypothalamus

Fourth ventricle

Temporal lobe

Pituitary gland

Optic chiasm

Pons

Cerebellum

Medulla oblongata

Central canal

Figure 7-7 A sagittal section of the brain.

serves as a central relay station for incoming sensory impulses, and the **hypothalamus** plays a role in homeostasis such as regulating body temperature and releasing hormones.

The reflex centers associated with eye and head movements are in the **midbrain**. The **pons** separates the midbrain from the medulla oblongata and transmits impulses between the cerebrum and other parts of the nervous system by serving as a relay station for sensory impulses from the peripheral nerves to the brain. It also contains centers that aid in regulating the rate and depth of breathing. The **medulla oblongata** is an enlarged continuation of the spinal cord that transmits all ascending and descending impulses. It also contains reflex centers such as the cardiac center for responding to heart function; the vasomotor center, which is involved with blood vessel constriction and dilation; and the respiratory center, which regulates breathing (**Figure 7-7**).

The surrounding bones, meninges, and cerebrospinal fluid (CSF) protect the brain and spinal cord. The choroid plexus is a membrane with many small vessels in the fluid-filled spaces of the brain that secretes CSF. Three membranes called **meninges** (*meninx* = singular) are the dura mater, arachnoid mater, and pia mater. The **dura mater**, whose name literally means "tough mother," is the strong outer layer. The **arachnoid mater** is the delicate, spider web–like middle layer of the meninges that spreads over the brain and spinal cord. The last membrane, the **pia mater**, is the inner layer of meninges that encloses the brain and spinal cord. The pia mater contains many nerves as well as blood vessels that nourish underlying brain and spinal cord cells.

There are three meningeal spaces: epidural, subdural, and subarachnoid. The **epidural space** is located between the bony covering of the brain and spinal cord and the dura mater. The **subdural space** is found between the dura mater and the arachnoid mater. It secretes lubricating serous fluid. The **subarachnoid space** is situated between the arachnoid mater and the pia mater, and CSF flows through this space (**Figure 7-8**). The brain has four fluid-filled chambers called **ventricles**. Cerebrospinal fluid circulates to cushion structures, support the brain, and serve as a transport medium for nutrients, hormones, and waste products.

Peripheral nerves originating at the brain are called **cranial nerves**. There are 12 pairs of cranial nerves that connect directly to the brain but not the spinal cord. Cranial nerves are designated by the abbreviation CN and are numbered with Roman numerals. Each cranial nerve is numbered according to its position on the brain, beginning at the cerebrum, and each name is related to its function or appearance (**Figure 7-9**). The cranial nerves and their functions

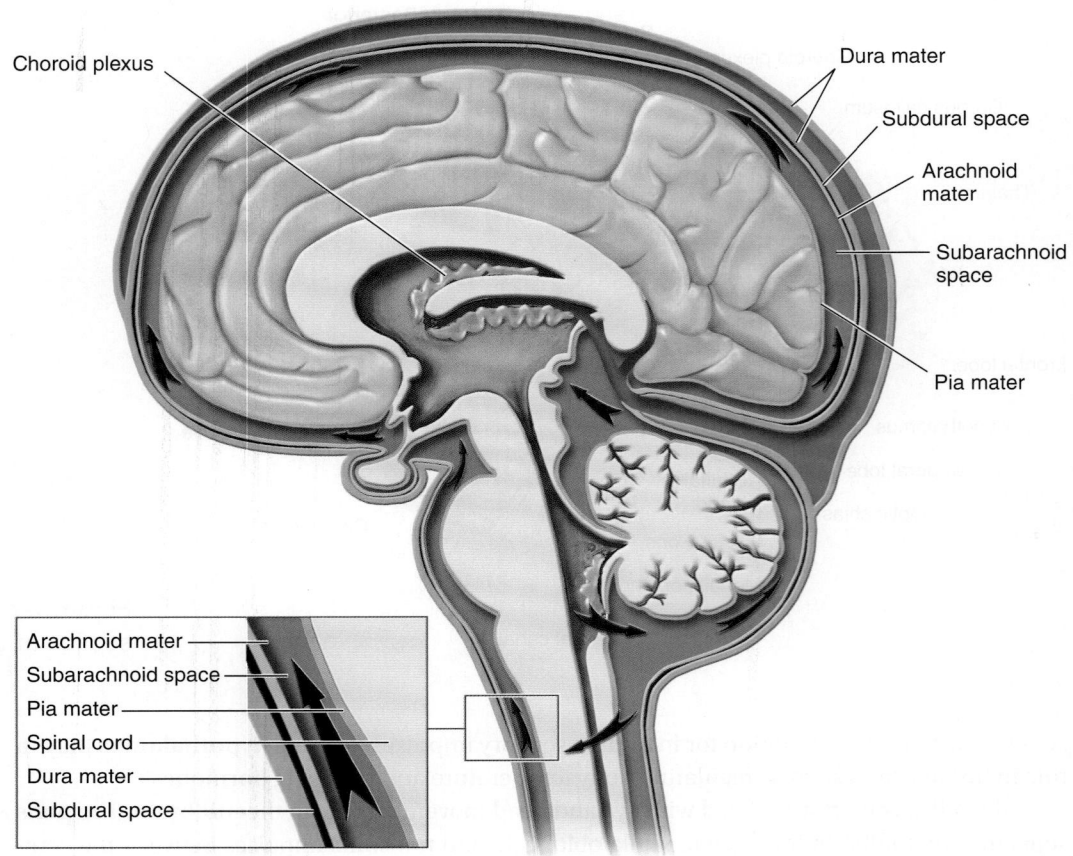

Choroid plexus

Dura mater

Subdural space

Arachnoid mater

Subarachnoid space

Pia mater

Arachnoid mater
Subarachnoid space
Pia mater
Spinal cord
Dura mater
Subdural space

Figure 7-8 Meninges and the flow of cerebrospinal fluid.

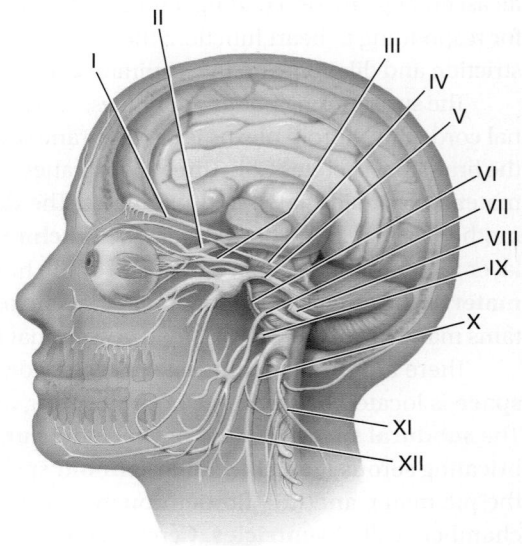

Figure 7-9 The distribution of the cranial nerves.

Key

Cranial nerves

I	Olfactory nerve	VII	Facial nerve
II	Optic nerve	VIII	Vestibulocochlear nerve
III	Oculomotor nerve	IX	Glossopharyngeal nerve
IV	Trochlear nerve	X	Vagus nerve
V	Trigeminal nerve	XI	Accessory nerve
VI	Abducens nerve	XII	Hypoglossal nerve

TABLE 7-1

CRANIAL NERVES AND THEIR MAIN FUNCTIONS

Cranial Nerve	Function
CN I Olfactory	Smell
CN II Optic	Vision
CN III Oculomotor	Eye movements
CN IV Trochlear	Eye movements
CN V Trigeminal	Facial movements
CN VI Abducens	Eye movements
CN VII Facial	Facial movements
CN VIII Vestibulocochlear	Balance
CN IX Glossopharyngeal	Tongue and neck movements
CN X Vagus	Serves thoracic and abdominal organs such as the diaphragm, heart, lungs, stomach, and intestines
CN XI Accessory	Serves muscles of the neck and upper back
CN XII Hypoglossal	Tongue movements

are listed in **Table 7-1**. There are several mnemonic devices, or memory aids, for the cranial nerves. For example, the first letter of each word in the following sentence corresponds to the first letter of each cranial nerve, in order: "*O*h, *o*h, *o*h, *t*o *t*ouch *a*nd *f*eel *v*ery *g*reen *v*egetables, *a*h, *h*eaven."

KEY TERM	Definition
cerebrum (se-REE-brum)	largest portion of the brain that functions in reasoning, learning, sensory perception, and emotions
cerebral (se-REE-brul) **hemispheres**	two symmetrical halves of the cerebrum
corpus callosum (KOR-pus kuh-LOH-sum)	broad band of white matter connecting the cerebral hemispheres
cerebral cortex (se-REE-brul KOR-tecks)	outer layer of the cerebrum
gyri (JYE-rye)	elevated ridges of the brain surface
sulci (SUL-sigh)	shallow depressions in the brain surface
fissures (FISH-urz)	deep grooves in the brain that separate gyri (elevated ridges)
cerebellum (serr-e-BEL-um)	second-largest region of the brain that functions to coordinate skeletal muscle activity and to maintain balance
brainstem	brain part remaining outside of the cerebrum and cerebellum consisting of the midbrain, pons, and medulla oblongata
diencephalon (dye-en-CEF-uh-lon)	brain part that contains the thalamus and hypothalamus and is the link between the cerebral hemispheres and the brainstem
thalamus (THAL-uh-mus)	brain part that serves as a central relay station for incoming sensory impulses
hypothalamus (high-poh-THAL-uh-mus)	brain part that plays a role in homeostasis, such as regulating body temperature and releasing hormones

continued

continued from page 331

KEY TERM	Definition
midbrain	part of the brainstem that houses reflex centers associated with eye and head movements
pons (PONZ)	portion of the brainstem between the medulla and midbrain that serves as a relay station from the peripheral nerves to the brain
medulla oblongata (me-DUL-uh ob-long-GAH-tuh)	enlarged continuation of the spinal cord that contains important reflex centers for the heart, blood vessels, and breathing
meninges (me-NIN-jeez)	three membrane layers covering the brain and spinal cord
dura mater (DEW-ruh MAH-tur)	the tough, outermost membrane that covers the brain and spinal cord
arachnoid mater (uh-RACK-noid MAH-tur)	the middle membrane that covers the brain and spinal cord
pia mater (PEE-uh MAH-tur)	the delicate, innermost membrane that surrounds the brain and spinal cord
epidural (ep-i-DEW-rul) **space**	space between the overlying bone and dura mater
subdural (sub-DEW-rul) **space**	space between the dura mater and arachnoid mater
subarachnoid (sub-uh-RACK-noid) **space**	space between the arachnoid mater and pia mater, filled with CSF
ventricles (VEN-trih-kulz)	4 fluid-filled chambers in the brain
cranial nerves	12 pairs of peripheral nerves originating at the brain that connect to the brain but not the spinal cord

KEY TERM PRACTICE: *Brain and Cranial Nerves*

1. List the three structures comprising the brainstem. _____

2. Elevated ridges of the brain surface are termed _____.

3. The structure that connects the two cerebral hemispheres is known as the _____.

4. Give the names for the three cranial meninges. _____

5. Give the names of the three spaces associated with the cranial meninges. _____

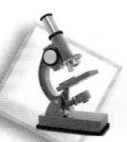

THE CLINICAL DIMENSION

The following sections outline common signs, symptoms, clinical tests, diagnostic procedures, pathological conditions, and treatments pertinent to the brain, spinal cord, and peripheral nerves.

Clinicians working in the neurological field are varied because the nervous system is so diverse. Neurologists (physicians specializing in the nervous systems), neurosurgeons (surgeons specializing in the nervous system), and physical therapists often see nervous system cases.

General Brain Disorders

cephalalgia

Pain in the head is termed **cephalalgia**, or *headache*. There are no pain receptors in the brain, but they do exist in the meninges. Therefore, the pain can be isolated to this region. (This also explains why brain surgery can be performed while the patient is wide awake.) Common types of cephalalgia are tension and vascular. Tension headaches result from strain on facial, neck, and scalp muscles. Vascular headaches result from edema in arterial vessels. Initial diagnosis is made through history and physical examination.

To rule out underlying pathology, electroencephalography and computed tomography scans are performed. **Electroencephalography (EEG)** is the recording of the electrical potentials in the brain obtained by an electroencephalograph (EEG). The electroencephalograph is a machine that uses electrodes placed on the scalp to monitor the electrical activity of different parts of the brain. It records the activity as complex tracings (**Figure 7-10A**). The record itself is termed an electroencephalogram (EEG) (**Figure 7-10B**). A technique for producing images of cross-sections of the body using a computer that processes data from radiographs (x-rays) is termed **computed tomography (CT)**.

migraine

A **migraine** is a recurrent, throbbing, very painful vascular headache. Migraines commonly occur on one side and are associated with vomiting, nausea, visual disturbances, and **photophobia** (sensitivity to light). Sufferers may experience an **aura**, a distinctive sensation that signals the beginning of a migraine headache. Other common symptoms include flashes appearing as heat waves, jagged lines, flashing lights, and striped vision. Migraines are usually familial and affect women twice as frequently as men. History and physical examination are used for initial diagnosis. Other tests such as MRI and CT scans are given to rule out pathology.

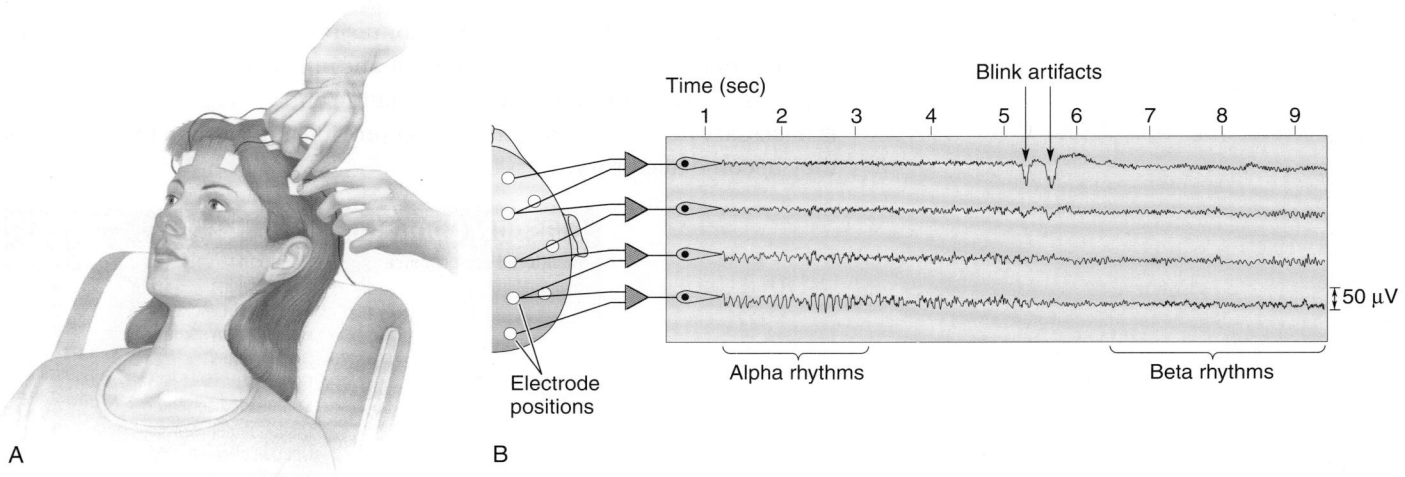

Figure 7-10 (A) Using an electroencephalograph to monitor brain activity. **(B)** A normal EEG.

Treatment is aimed at making the person comfortable and includes bed rest in a dark, quiet room and prescription medications. Vasoconstrictors to reduce vascular spasms and antiemetics to control vomiting are administered. An agent for preventing or relieving vomiting is called an **antiemetic**. The prescription drug Imitrex (sumatriptan) may also be prescribed. Biofeedback, acupuncture, and Botox (onabotulinumtoxinA) are complementary treatments for migraines. Biofeedback is a training technique that enables a patient to gain some voluntary control over autonomic body functions.

concussion

The immediate loss of consciousness, orientation, or memory resulting from a traumatic head injury is called a **concussion**. The word is derived from the Latin term *concutere,* which means "to shake violently." It is also referred to as being "knocked out" for seconds to a few minutes. Brain electrical activity is altered. Concussions generally resolve, but **amnesia** (loss of memory) may persist for up to 24 hours. Signs and symptoms after regaining consciousness are headache, vomiting, blurred vision, and photophobia. Neurological examination and history of the injury confirm the diagnosis. Concussions are treated with bed rest and pain medications. There is mounting evidence that repeated concussions—as often happens with high school and professional football players—lead to other brain disorders later in life.

coma

Coma is a state of deep unconsciousness from which a person cannot be roused. Some causes include ingesting a toxic substance, lack of oxygen, trauma, or disease. Ruling out hypoglycemia (low blood glucose level) is the first step in the diagnosis, followed by a complete neurologic examination that includes an EEG. The **Glasgow Coma Scale (GCS)** is used to assess the patient's level of consciousness (LOC) (**Figure 7-11**).

brain contusion

Bruising of brain tissue without rupture of the pia mater and arachnoid mater is termed a **brain contusion**. Headache, loss of consciousness, hemiparesis, and drowsiness are typical signs and symptoms. **Paresis** means there is muscular weakness or slight paralysis, and **hemiparesis** is muscle weakness or paralysis affecting one side of the body. Loss of consciousness may be temporary or result in coma. Contusions may be more serious than concussions and often result from traumatic injury such as a skull fracture. Diagnosis is made by neurological evaluation and CT scan. Hospitalization is necessary to monitor the patient and provide appropriate treatments as they become necessary.

Glasgow Coma Scale	Best possible total score 15	Worst possible total score 3
Monitored performance	**Reaction**	**Score**
Eye opening	Spontaneous	4
	Open when spoken to	3
	Open at pain stimulus	2
	No reaction	1
Verbal performance	Coherent	5
	Confused, disoriented	4
	Disconnected words	3
	Unintelligible sounds	2
	No verbal reaction	1
Motor responsiveness	Follows instructions	6
	Intentional pain-avoidance	5
	Large motor movement	4
	Flexor synergism	3
	Extensor synergism	2
	No reaction	1

Figure 7-11 The Glasgow Coma Scale (GCS). The GCS is scored between 3 and 15, with 3 being the worst score, and 15 the best. It is composed of three parameters: Best Eye Response, Best Verbal Response, Best Motor Response. A coma score of 13 or higher correlates with a mild brain injury, 9 to 12 is a moderate injury, and 8 or less is a severe brain injury.

epilepsy

Epilepsy is a chronic brain disorder involving episodes of abnormal electrical discharge in the brain and is characterized by periodic sudden loss or impairment of consciousness, often accompanied by convulsions. It results from irregular electrical discharges of neurons. Two common types of seizures are experienced by people with epilepsy. **Cerebral seizures** (formerly known as *petit mal seizures*) are recurrent convulsions with blank stares and temporary loss of awareness. **Generalized tonic–clonic seizures** (also called *grand mal seizures*) are characterized by a loud cry, falling to the floor, sudden onset of intermittent muscle contractions and relaxations, and loss of consciousness. The cause is either idiopathic or the result of a known brain pathology. An EEG and medical history are used to diagnose epilepsy. Treatment includes patient and family education and the administration of anticonvulsant drugs.

Parkinson disease (PD)

Parkinson disease (PD) is an incurable nervous disorder marked by progressive degeneration of the dopamine-producing neurons in a region of the brain called the substantia nigra. This results in insufficient dopamine (DA) in the area known as the basal ganglia. Its cause is unknown. Other symptoms include trembling hands and a "pill-rolling" tremor of the thumb and index finger; lifeless face; monotone voice; and a slow, shuffling gait.

The disease affects more men than women. The typical age of onset is around 60 years. Physical examination, neurological evaluation, and history confirm the diagnosis. There is no cure, but drugs such as levodopa, antidepressants, and anticholinergics (drugs that interfere with the neurotransmitter acetylcholine) are used.

transient ischemic attack (TIA)

Transient refers to something being "present for a short period of time." A **transient ischemic attack (TIA)** is the sudden loss of neurological function with complete recovery usually within 24 hours. Most TIAs last only 15 to 20 minutes. They result from an interruption of blood supply to the brain for a brief period of time. The person experiences blurred vision, hemiparesis, and speech difficulty. A TIA is often a signal of an impending stroke (brain blockage that leads to a clinical event lasting longer than 24 hours) and is frequently caused by a plaque fragment that interrupts vascular flow in the brain. Diagnosis is made through physical examination, MRI, CT scan, and EEG, although these studies may not always confirm a TIA. Administration of anticoagulants (blood thinners) is the treatment of choice.

cerebrovascular accident (CVA) or stroke

A **cerebrovascular accident (CVA),** or **stroke**, involves irreversible brain damage as a result of blood flow interruption to a particular brain region (**Figure 7-12**). It is sometimes called a "brain attack." Signs and symptoms vary, depending on the area affected by occlusion. Headache, blurred vision, slurred speech, dysphasia, hemiparesis, and facial paralysis are common. Strokes rank third as a cause of death in adults in the United States, after ischemic heart disease and cancer.

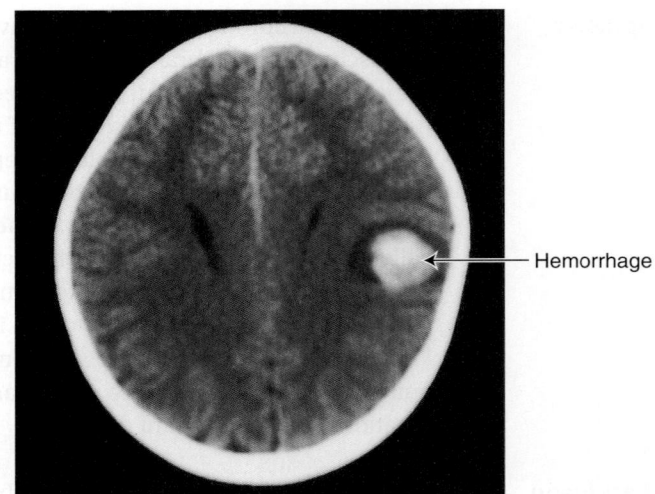

Figure 7-12 Cerebrovascular accident (stroke). This is a CT scan showing a large hemorrhage in the brain of a 4-year-old boy.

dysphasia

Dysphasia is difficulty in speaking and understanding spoken or written language caused by brain injury or disease. The initial diagnosis is made by history and physical examination and confirmed by MRI, CT scan, cerebral angiography, or EEG. With **cerebral angiography**, blood vessels are radiographically mapped after introduction of a dye. Treatment involves the prompt administration of tissue plasminogen activator or anticoagulants to prevent blood clotting. **Tissue plasminogen activator (TPA** or **tPA)** is an anticlotting enzyme that is produced naturally in blood vessel linings and is also genetically engineered for use in dissolving blood clots. It is also used for the treatment of stroke, heart attack, and peripheral vascular clotting. Follow-up care in the form of speech therapy and physical rehabilitation is often necessary.

KEY TERM	Definition
cephalalgia (sef-uhl-AL-jee-uh)	pain in the head; another term for headache
electroencephalography (EEG) (ee-leck-troh-en-sef-uh-LOG-ruh-fee)	method of graphically recording the electrical activity of the brain
computed tomography (CT) (toh- MOG-ruh-fee)	imaging method that uses a computer to reconstruct the anatomical features obtained by x-ray
migraine (MIGH-grain)	recurrent, severe vascular headache
photophobia (foh-toh-FOH-bee-uh)	eye sensitivity to light
aura (AW-ruh)	distinctive sensation that signals the onset of a migraine headache
antiemetic (an-tee-e-MET-ick)	agent for preventing or relieving vomiting
concussion (kun-KUSH-un)	immediate loss of consciousness, orientation, or memory caused by head injury
amnesia (am-NEE-zhuh)	loss of memory
coma (KOH-muh)	prolonged state of deep unconsciousness
Glasgow (GLAS-goh) **Coma Scale (GCS)**	scale used to assess the level of consciousness
brain contusion (kon-TEW-zhun)	brain tissue bruise

continued

continued from page 336

KEY TERM	Definition
paresis (puh-REE-sis)	muscle weakness or slight paralysis
hemiparesis (hem-ee-puh-REE-sis)	muscle weakness or paralysis on one side
epilepsy (EP-i-lep-see)	brain disorder resulting from an irregular electrical discharge of neurons
cerebral seizures (se-REE-brul SEE-zhurz)	recurrent convulsions with blank stares and temporary loss of awareness
generalized tonic-clonic (TON-ick-KLO-nick) **seizure**	seizure characterized by collapse, loss of consciousness, and intermittent muscle contractions and relaxations
Parkinson disease (PD)	disorder resulting from progressive degeneration of dopamine-producing neurons in the brain
transient ischemic (TRAN-zee-unt is-KEE-mick) **attack (TIA)**	brain disorder that is not permanent resulting from blood flow interruption
cerebrovascular (se-ree-broh-VAS-kew-lur) **accident (CVA)**	destruction of brain tissue due to the disruption of blood flow to a particular brain region; also called a stroke or brain attack
stroke	destruction of brain tissue due to the disruption of blood flow to a particular brain region; also called a cerebrovascular accident or brain attack
dysphasia (dis-FAY-zhuh)	difficulty in speaking and understanding written or spoken language as a result of brain injury
cerebral angiography (se-REE-brul an-jee-and-OG-ruh-fee)	mapping of the cerebral blood vessels using dye and x-rays
tissue plasminogen (plaz-MIN-oh-jen) **activator (TPA or tPA)**	substance that dissolves blood clots

KEY TERM PRACTICE: *General Brain Disorders*

1. Which disease is associated with the loss of dopamine-producing neurons in the brain? _____

2. _____ refers to difficulty in speaking and understanding written or spoken language as a result of brain injury.

3. Give the two terms that refer to the destruction of brain tissue as a result of blood flow interruption. _____

4. The medical term for a *headache* is _____, which is derived from the word part _____ for "head" and the word part _____ for "ache."

5. Muscle weakness or slight paralysis on one side is called _____; the word part _____ means "half."

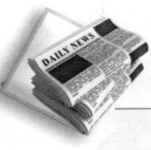

IN THE NEWS: Bicycling Alleviates the Symptoms of Parkinson Disease

Can tandem bicycle riding really alleviate the symptoms of Parkinson disease (PD)? Amazingly it can! Tandem bicycle riding is one of the Cleveland Clinic's Top 10 Medical Innovations for 2010.

People with Parkinson disease slowly lose the ability to control their body's movements. Tremors, shaking, loss of balance, and changes in speech are among the common symptoms of this disease that has no known cure. Some medications ease the symptoms for short periods of time, but extended relief has eluded researchers so far.

And then there was a serendipitous event that occurred when a scientist rode a tandem bike with a friend, an avid cyclist who also has PD. They rode vigorously for about 1 hour and mysteriously the friend's symptoms of the disorder diminished.

Did this side effect of riding contain a medical possibility? Could motor control in the arms and hands be improved by exercising only the legs? Was some change taking place in the central nervous system and triggering the release of biochemicals that improved global motor function?

Clinical tests indicated that a solo bicycle rider who has Parkinson disease could achieve only about 50 to 60 revolutions per minute (rpm) on the bicycle—which did not cause the symptoms to decrease. However, a person with PD riding in tandem with a person leading a workout at 80 to 90 rpm did achieve diminished symptoms. In fact, there was as much as a 35% improvement that lasted for up to 4 months. Further studies are currently being conducted to determine the link between cycling and diminished symptoms in PD patients.

Dementia

dementia

Dementia is a general term used to describe the progressive loss of intellectual functions, such as memory, while other brain functions such as those controlling movement and senses are retained. Senile dementia is a form of brain disorder marked by progressive and irreversible mental deterioration, memory loss, and disorientation. It usually affects people ages 65 or older.

Alzheimer disease (AD)

Alzheimer disease (AD) is a disabling dementia, primarily of the elderly, that involves widespread intellectual impairment, personality changes, and sometimes delirium. The disorder is named after the German neurologist, Alois Alzheimer, who first described the disease in 1906. It causes characteristic lesions in the cortex. It has an unknown cause, although some research suggests a genetic basis. It is the most common cause of premature senility. Diagnosis is made by family history and performance on specific cognitive function tests. Definitive diagnosis is possible only after death, when examination of brain tissue at autopsy reveals brain changes such as β-amyloid plaques, neurofibrillary tangles, atrophy, slender gyri, and widened sulci and ventricles (**Figure 7-13**). Treatment is palliative; however, newer drug therapies targeting the behavioral aspects are available. Early diagnosis and intervention may delay disease progression. AD currently ranks fourth as a cause of death in the United States.

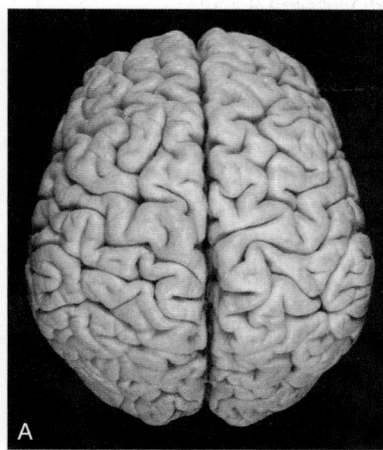 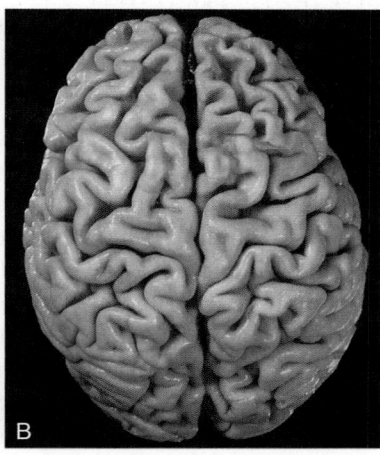

Figure 7-13 Alzheimer disease: **(A)** Normal brain. **(B)** The brain of a patient with Alzheimer disease shows cortical atrophy, characterized by slender gyri and widened sulci.

Huntington chorea	**Huntington chorea**, also called *Huntington disease (HD),* is an inherited form of dementia and the Huntington gene is found on chromosome 4. George Huntington was a U.S. physician who first described the condition in 1872. Chorea refers to "widespread involuntary, jerky movements of brief duration." Symptoms appear between 30 and 40 years of age. It is characterized by progressive atrophy of regions of the brain known as the putamen and caudate nucleus. Neurological examination and family history suggest the disease. Brain scans can demonstrate anatomical brain changes. There is no cure, and drug treatment is provided as a supportive measure.

KEY TERM	Definition
dementia (de-MEN-shuh)	loss of intellectual and cognitive functions while other brain functions are maintained
Alzheimer (AWLTZ-hye-mur) **disease** (**AD**)	degenerative brain disorder that causes a disabling dementia with an onset typically later in life and is characterized by β-amyloid plaques and neurofibrillary tangles in the brain
Huntington chorea (koh-REE-uh)	inherited form of dementia accompanied by atrophy of particular brain regions; also called Huntington disease (HD)

KEY TERM PRACTICE: *Dementia*

1. The medical term for the progressive deterioration of intellectual functions while other brain functions remain intact is _____.

2. An inherited form of dementia accompanied by atrophy of particular brain regions and named for physician George Huntington is known as _____.

3. _____ is a degenerative brain disorder that causes a disabling dementia with an onset typically later in life and is characterized by β-amyloid plaques and neurofibrillary tangles.

Brain Neoplasms

A brain neoplasm is an abnormal growth in the brain.

glioma   A brain neoplasm derived from neuroglial cells is termed a **glioma**. More specifically, a tumor originating from an astrocyte, oligodendrocyte, or ependymal cell is termed an **astrocytoma**, **oligodendroglioma**, or **ependymoma**, respectively. An astrocytoma occurs anywhere in the brain or spinal cord and is typically slow growing. An oligodendrocytoma is relatively avascular and most commonly occurs in the frontal lobes, although it may arise from the brainstem, cerebellum, or spinal cord. An ependymoma is found in the brain ventricles (fluid-filled spaces) and is more common in children than in adults. Early signs and symptoms of astrocytomas and oligodendrogliomas are usually headaches or seizures. Signs and symptoms of ependymomas include uncoordinated muscle movement, visual changes, and headache. Gliomas are diagnosed by CT scan and treated by surgery and/or radiation therapy.

KEY TERM	Definition
glioma (glye-OH-muh)	tumor composed of cells derived from neuroglia
astrocytoma (as-troh-sigh-TOH-muh)	tumor derived from astrocytes
oligodendroglioma (ol-i-goh-den-droh-OH-muh)	tumor derived from oligodendrocytes
ependymoma (ep-en-digh-MOH-muh)	tumor derived from ependymal cells

KEY TERM PRACTICE: *Brain Neoplasms*

1. A _____ is a tumor composed of cells derived from neuroglia.

2. Identify the glioma derived from each of the following cell types.

   a. astrocyte _____

   b. ependymal cell _____

   c. oligodendrocyte _____

Pediatric Disorders

cerebral palsy (CP)   A group of motor disorders caused by damage to motor centers of the cerebral cortex, cerebellum, or basal ganglia (four deep masses of gray matter in each hemisphere) during fetal development, childbirth, or early infancy is termed **cerebral palsy (CP)**. The word palsy means "paralysis or weakness." The disease may result from inadequate oxygen supply while in utero or by an interruption of oxygen-rich blood to the brain during birth. It is characterized by lack of muscle control, especially in the limbs. Diagnosis is made by neurological examination. Treatment options depend on the level of severity. Physical therapy and occupational therapy are often prescribed. Antispasmodic and anticonvulsant drugs are indicated in some cases.

Reye syndrome   **Reye syndrome** is an acute illness generally of young children that occurs after a viral infection such as influenza or varicella (chickenpox). Fever, vomiting, brain dysfunction, and liver damage are characteristic signs and symptoms. It can progress from loss of consciousness to coma. There are also fatty deposits on the liver and swelling of the kidneys and brain. The cause is unknown, but there is a link between aspirin ingestion and its onset when a fever is present. Patients are hospitalized so cerebral edema can be monitored.

KEY TERM	Definition
cerebral palsy (se-REE-brul PAWL-zee) **(CP)**	group of motor function diseases present at birth or in infancy that may be the result of interrupted blood flow to the brain during fetal development, childbirth, or infancy
Reye (RYE) **syndrome**	complex of symptoms with liver damage and brain dysfunction that occurs after a viral infection; has been linked to aspirin use

KEY TERM PRACTICE: *Pediatric Disorders*

1. A rare and serious childhood disease that usually occurs following a respiratory infection and is associated with aspirin ingestion is termed _____.

2. _____ is a group of motor function diseases present at birth or in infancy that may be the result of interrupted blood flow to the brain during fetal development, childbirth, or infancy.

Cranial Nerve Disorders

Bell palsy

Bell palsy is a condition of probable viral infection involving the facial nerve (CN VII). It is characterized by paralysis of the muscles on one side of the face, causing a distorted facial expression (**Figure 7-14**). Its usual onset occurs while sleeping, so the person wakes up with the condition. Men and women, usually between 20 and 60 years, are equally affected. Bell palsy is normally transient, but occasionally it can be permanent. It is diagnosed on the basis of the signs and symptoms, neurological evaluation, and case history. Analgesics; warm, moist heat; and corticosteroids (immunosuppressive anti-inflam-

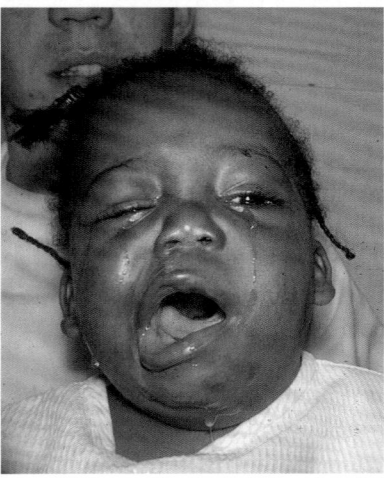

Figure 7-14 Bell palsy caused by peripheral paralysis of the facial nerve. The palsy weakens the muscles on the affected side, causing facial drooping.

matory drugs) are recommended. Avoidance of extreme temperature variation is also suggested. Most patients can expect complete recovery if treated early.

trigeminal neuralgia or tic douloureux

Trigeminal neuralgia, or **tic douloureux**, is a condition of unknown cause marked by sudden, severe pain in the face along the branches of the trigeminal nerve (CN V). Depending on the branch involved, there is pain in the eye and forehead; nose, upper lip, and cheek; or lower lip and tongue. The condition is an occasional sequela of herpes zoster or it accompanies multiple sclerosis. A **sequela** (sequelae = plural) is a disorder that is caused by a preceding disorder in the same person. It can be thought of as an "aftereffect." The disorder may persist from months to years, but it normally subsides. Patient observation and pain mapping are used to make the diagnosis. For mild episodes, analgesics (pain relievers) are given. Severe cases may require surgery.

KEY TERM	Definition
Bell palsy (PAWL-zee)	paralysis of the muscles on one side of the face innervated by the facial nerve (CN VII)
trigeminal neuralgia (trye-JEM-i-nul new-RAL-juh)	condition characterized by pain in parts of the face served by one or more branches of the trigeminal nerve (CN V); also called tic douloureux
tic douloureux (TIC doo-loo-RUH)	condition characterized by pain in parts of the face served by one or more branches of the trigeminal nerve (CN V); also called trigeminal neuralgia
sequela (se-KWEL-uh)	disorder that is caused by a preceding disorder in the same person

KEY TERM PRACTICE: *Cranial Nerve Disorders*

1. The term _____ refers to a disorder that is caused by a preceding disorder in the same person.

2. A condition characterized by pain in parts of the face served by one or more branches of the trigeminal nerve (CN V) is known as _____ or _____.

Spinal Cord and Spinal Nerve Disorders

amyotrophic lateral sclerosis (ALS)

Amyotrophic lateral sclerosis (ALS) is a fatal degenerative disease of the nervous system marked by progressive muscle weakness and atrophy. It affects both upper and lower motor neurons. It is commonly known as Lou Gehrig disease after the New York Yankees baseball player who was afflicted with the disorder. Amyotrophy means "muscular atrophy." The onset is between the ages of 40 and 70 years, and it affects more men than women. The underlying pathology demonstrates neuronal loss and degeneration in certain parts of the spinal cord. Neurological evaluation and electromyogram (EMG) studies confirm nerve involvement. Treatment is supportive because there is no cure. Death usually occurs within 2 to 5 years of onset.

multiple sclerosis (MS)

Multiple sclerosis (MS) is a serious progressive autoimmune disease of the CNS, occurring mainly in young adults. The disease may result from a previous viral infection that leads to destruction of the myelin sheaths of the CNS neurons, thereby causing an interruption of nerve impulse transmission. There are four major classifications of MS, and general signs and symptoms of its associated syndromes include optic neuritis, weakness, motor difficulty, **vertigo** (the sensation of whirling, tilting, or dizziness that causes balance loss), and faulty speech. Diagnosis is made by physical examination, history, clinical picture, CT scans, and MRI studies. There is no cure. Treatment is supportive and rehabilitative and may include immunosuppressive drugs.

sciatica

Sciatica is pain in the lower back and hip that radiates down the back of the thigh into the leg. Sciatica was initially attributed to sciatic nerve dysfunction (hence its name), but is now known to be caused by a herniated lumbar disc that compresses on a nerve in the L_5 or S_1 region (**Figure 7-15**). Typical signs and symptoms are numbness, pain, tingling, and tenderness extending from the hip down to the calf. History and physical examination confirm

Sagittal view of lower spine

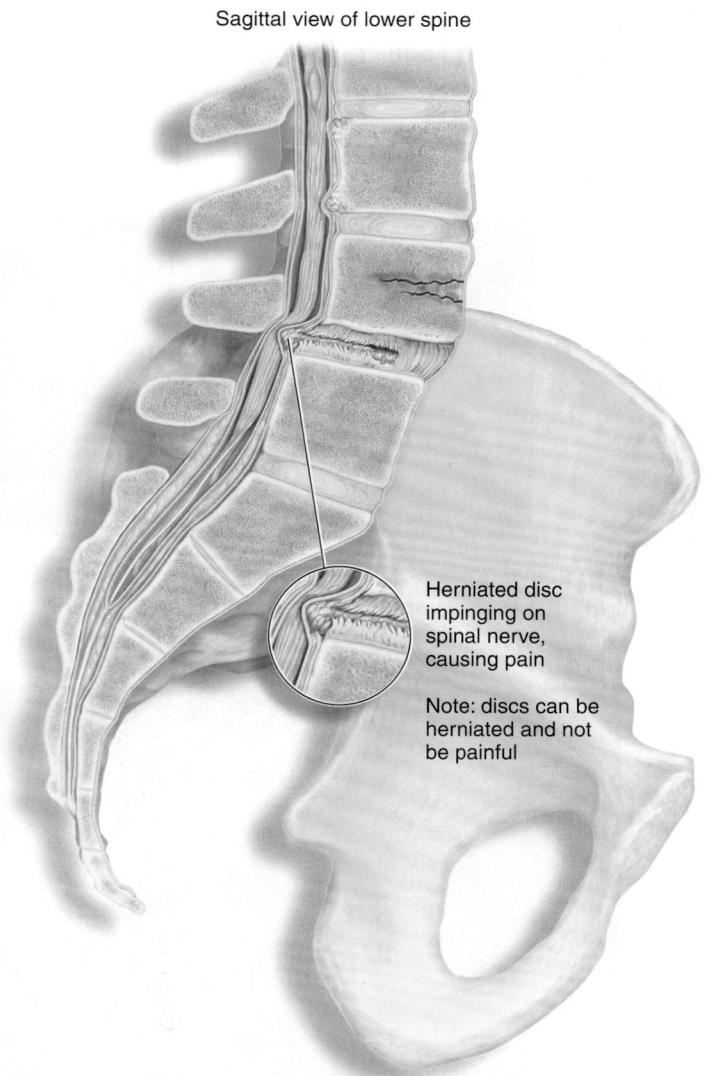

Herniated disc impinging on spinal nerve, causing pain

Note: discs can be herniated and not be painful

Figure 7-15 Herniated disc causing sciatica.

the diagnosis. Rest, massage therapy, analgesics, muscle relaxants, nonsteroidal anti-inflammatory drugs (NSAIDs), and physical therapy are prescribed. Narcotics are given for severe pain; and in some cases, surgery is an option.

spina bifida

Spina bifida is a congenital defect resulting from incomplete closure of the vertebral arch that allows the spinal cord or meninges to protrude. It is usually located in the lumbosacral region and causes partial to total paralysis of the lower body. Two types exist: spina bifida occulta and spina bifida cystica. **Spina bifida occulta** is caused by the incomplete fusion of the vertebral posterior arch. There is no protrusion of the cord, and the lesion is covered by skin and generally evident only on x-ray evaluation. **Spina bifida cystica** is a severe type characterized by increased intracranial pressure (ICP). Meningocele, hydrocephalus, paraplegia, and the inability to control the urinary bladder and rectum are common. A **meningocele** is a protrusion of the meninges through bone that forms a cyst filled with cerebrospinal fluid (CSF) (**Figure 7-16**).

Hydrocephalus

Hydrocephalus ("water on the brain") is an accumulation of CSF on the brain (**Figure 7-17**). The CSF is not absorbed, causing it to pool. Surgery is the only form of treatment.

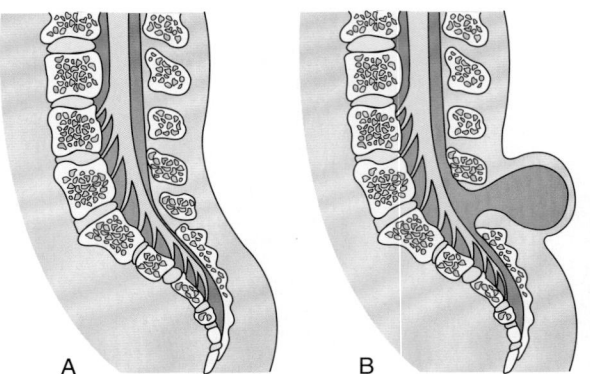 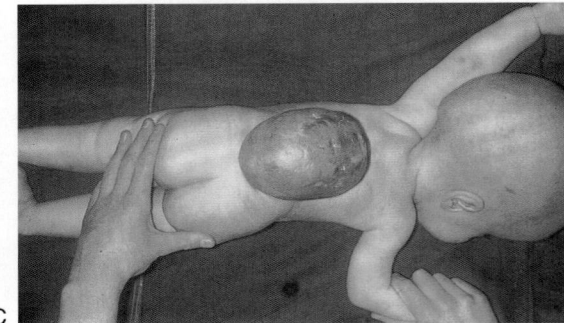

A   B   C

Figure 7-16 Spina bifida is incomplete closure of the spinal cord. **(A)** Normal spinal cord. **(B)** Spina bifida with protrusion of the meninges (meningocele). **(C)** Protrusion of the spinal cord and meninges.

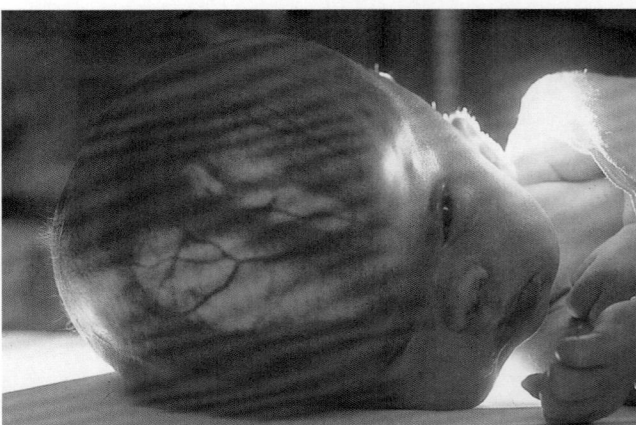

Figure 7-17 An infant with hydrocephalus.

KEY TERM	Definition
amyotrophic (am-migh-oh-TROH-fick) **lateral sclerosis** (skle-ROH-sis) (**ALS**)	fatal degenerative disease of the motor neurons marked by muscle weakness and atrophy; also called Lou Gehrig disease
multiple sclerosis (skle-ROH-sis) (**MS**)	autoimmune disorder that causes destruction of the myelin sheaths of neurons
vertigo (VUR-ti-goh)	the sensation of dizziness while not moving that causes loss of balance
sciatica (sigh-AT-i-kuh)	pain in the lower back that radiates from the back of the thigh and down to the leg
spina bifida (SPYE-nuh BIF-i-duh)	congenital defect of incomplete vertebral closure that allows the spinal cord or meninges to protrude
spina bifida occulta (SPYE-nuh BIF-duh ock-UL-tuh)	incomplete fusion of the posterior arch of vertebrae
spina bifida cystica (SPYE-nuh BIF-i-duh SIS-ti-kuh)	severe type of congenital vertebral defect characterized by increased intracranial pressure
meningocele (me-NING-goh-seel)	protrusion of the meninges through bone, forming a CSF-filled cyst
hydrocephalus (high-droh-SEF-uh-lus)	accumulation of CSF on the brain; commonly known as "water on the brain"

KEY TERM PRACTICE: *Spinal Cord and Spinal Nerve Disorders*

1. Lou Gehrig disease is also known as _____.

2. _____ is a congenital birth defect in which there is incomplete closure of a vertebra, allowing for the spinal cord or meninges to protrude.

3. A protrusion of the meninges through bone that forms a CSF-filled cyst is termed a _____.

4. _____ is a dizzy sensation while a person is still that causes a loss of balance.

5. An accumulation of CSF on the brain is called _____ and is derived from the word part _____ for "water" and the word part _____ for "head."

Infectious Diseases of the Central Nervous System

encephalitis

Brain inflammation is termed **encephalitis**. Viral toxins associated with chickenpox, measles, or mumps may cause the inflammation. Confusion, lethargy, headache, fever, muscle weakness, and visual disturbances are ordinary signs and symptoms. The clinical picture, abnormal EEG, and a lumbar puncture are useful for making the diagnosis. A **lumbar puncture** (also called a spinal tap) is a procedure in which CSF is extracted through a needle inserted into the subarachnoid space of the spinal cord. A lumbar puncture is usually performed between the L_3 and L_4 vertebrae. An epidural is a local anesthetic injected into the epidural space and is often used to inject medication during childbirth (**Figure 7-18**). Evidence of the

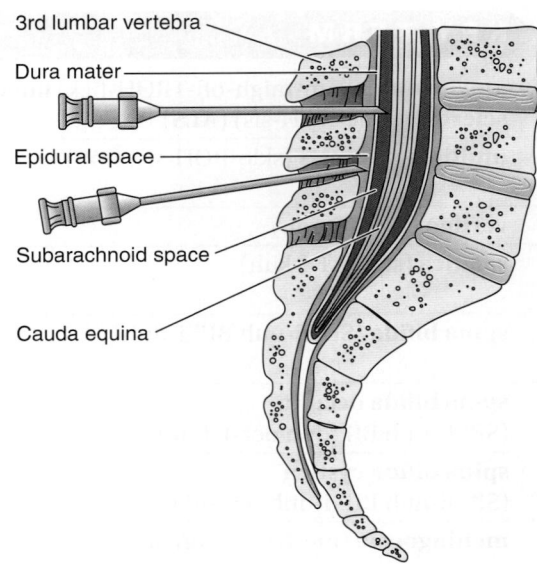

Figure 7-18 Showing the locations for a lumbar puncture and epidural anesthesia.

virus in the blood and CSF indicates encephalitis. Treatment options include antiviral agents, analgesics, and antipyretics to reduce fever.

Guillain-Barré syndrome

Guillain-Barré syndrome is an acute, symmetrical, lower motor neuron paralysis of unknown cause. It is thought to be an autoimmune disorder. Advanced cases have trunk and cranial involvement with progression to respiratory failure. It results from demyelinization of the affected nerves. The syndrome often follows a respiratory infection or gastroenteritis. Diagnosis is made by physical examination, patient history, and elevated protein level in the CSF. Treatment is supportive. If the diaphragm and respiratory muscles are involved, pulmonary ventilation may be necessary. Plasmapheresis, a procedure in which whole blood is extracted and the antibodies are removed, lessens the time of duration. Recovery is usually complete.

meningitis

Meningitis is inflammation of the meninges. It is caused by a bacterial or viral infection. The bacterial form is typically more severe than the viral type. *Haemophilus influenzae, Neisseria meningitides,* and *Streptococcus pneumoniae* are common bacteria associated with its onset. Signs and symptoms include vomiting, severe headache, high fever, and stiff neck. Neck stiffness and impaired neck flexion resulting from muscle spasms and meningeal irritation are termed **nuchal rigidity**. The word nucha means "back of the neck." Diagnosis is made through physical and clinical examination. Physical findings that demonstrate meningeal inflammation are the Kernig sign and Brudzinski sign. With the Kernig sign, the patient is supine and the thighs and knees are flexed, but leg extension at the knee joint is impossible because of pain. When passive flexion of the leg on one side causes a similar movement in the opposite side, Brudzinski sign is present. Aggressive treatment with antibiotics for the bacterial form is essential. Analgesics can be given for pain. Vaccines to prevent meningitis are available in the United States, and college-age students are routinely immunized. In 2001, the Bill & Melinda Gates Foundation awarded the World Health Organization $70 million to launch the Meningitis Vaccine Project to eliminate meningitis as a public health problem in sub-Saharan Africa.

poliomyelitis or **polio**

Poliomyelitis, commonly called *polio,* is a severe infectious viral disease, usually affecting children or young adults, that inflames gray matter of the spinal cord, sometimes leading to paralysis and muscular wasting (**Figure 7-19**). Two forms exist: nonparalytic and paralytic. The disease is preventable through immunization. Malaise, muscle weakness, neck stiffness, vomiting, and flaccid (limp) paralysis are common. Isolation of poliovirus from sputum culture, feces, or CSF confirms the diagnosis. Treatment is supportive for mild cases, but pulmonary ventilation may be required for severe cases. Physical therapy may be appropriate after recovery. Post-polio syndrome (PPS) is a condition that affects 25% to 50% of people who previously contracted poliomyelitis. Most of these individuals contracted polio before the vaccine was routinely administered. The symptoms include muscle weakness, myalgia, and fatigue and generally appear 15 to 30 years after recovery.

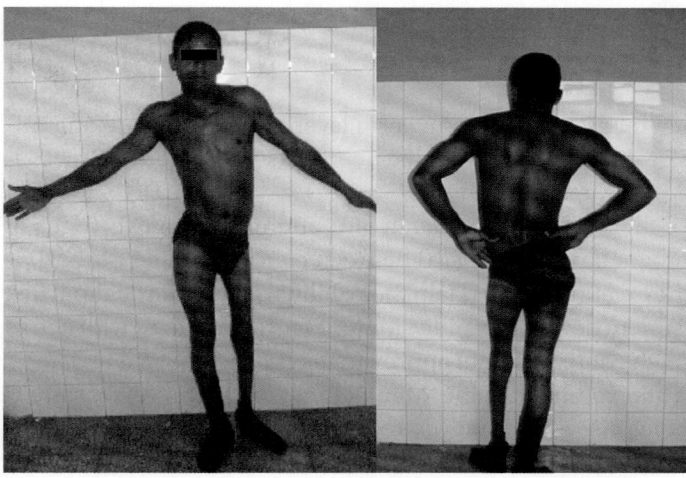

Figure 7-19 The deformed leg of the boy is due to poliomyelitis.

KEY TERM	Definition
encephalitis (en-sef-uh-LYE-tis)	brain inflammation
lumbar puncture	procedure using a needle inserted into the subarachnoid space of the lumbar region to remove CSF; also called a spinal tap
Guillain-Barré (gee-yan-bahr-RAY) **syndrome**	acute symmetrical lower motor neuron paralysis of unknown cause
meningitis (men-in-JYE-tis)	inflammation of the meninges
nuchal (NEW-kul) **rigidity**	stiffness of the neck and impaired neck flexion as a result of meningeal irritation
poliomyelitis (poh-lee-oh-migh-e-LYE-tis)	severe infectious viral disease that inflames the gray matter of the spinal cord and sometimes leads to paralysis and muscle wasting; also called polio

KEY TERM PRACTICE: *Infectious Diseases of the Central Nervous System*

1. _____ is the medical term for brain inflammation and is derived from the word part _____ for "brain" and the word part _____ for "inflammation."

2. _____ is the term describing meningeal inflammation.

3. A severe infectious viral disease that inflames the gray matter of the spinal cord and sometimes leads to paralysis and muscle wasting is termed _____ and is derived from the word part _____ for "gray matter" and the word part _____ for "inflammation."

4. Stiffness of the neck with impaired neck flexion as a result of meningeal irritation is called _____.

5. A _____ is a procedure in which a needle is inserted into the subarachnoid space in the lumbar region to extract CSF.

LIFE SPAN

Nervous tissue is derived from the embryonic ectoderm germ layer. Cells proliferate and migrate to determined positions before differentiating into the neuroblasts that ultimately transform into the various components of the nervous system.

As neurons mature, most lose their ability to divide. In fact, approximately two-thirds of nerve cells engage in apoptosis (programmed cell death) between conception and birth. Hippocampus and olfaction cells are the exceptions and retain their ability to divide throughout life.

During infancy, the nervous system develops rapidly. Motor control improves with age as myelination takes place. Brain growth continues until approximately age 18.

During old age, brain weight and volume decline. Mental functioning, however, can remain when there is no neurovascular disease. Moreover, recent research indicates that individuals who maintain intellectual stimulation preserve normal brain function throughout life. Due to brain plasticity and the ability to learn new information and skills, elderly persons can have high cognitive function, but the rate at which they learn novel tasks, along with their reflex activity, diminishes with age. Other autonomic functions also decline with age.

COMMON *Abbreviations*

Abbreviation	Term
AD	Alzheimer disease
ALS	amyotrophic lateral sclerosis
ANS	autonomic nervous system
BBB	blood–brain barrier
CN	cranial nerve
CNS	central nervous system
CP	cerebral palsy
CSF	cerebrospinal fluid
CT	computed tomography
CVA	cerebrovascular accident
DA	dopamine
EEG	electroencephalogram; electroencephalograph; electroencephalography
EMG	electromyogram
GCS	Glasgow Coma Scale
HD	Huntington disease
ICP	intracranial pressure
LOC	level of consciousness
MRI	magnetic resonance imaging
MS	multiple sclerosis
NSAIDs	nonsteroidal anti-inflammatory drugs
PD	Parkinson disease
PNS	peripheral nervous system
PPS	post-polio syndrome
SNS	somatic nervous system
TIA	transient ischemic attack
TPA or tPA	tissue plasminogen activator

COMMON ABBREVIATIONS EXERCISES

1. Give the term for SNS. _____

2. PPS is the abbreviation for _____.

3. LOC stands for _____.

4. The abbreviation for dopamine is _____.

5. The abbreviation for a cerebrovascular accident is _____.

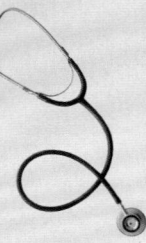

Case Study

Mr. Lind, 45 years old, had been complaining of headaches, dizziness, and confusion. He went to his family physician when he thought he might have an internal ear infection. When Mr. Lind told the physician about the "knot on the back of his skull," visual inspection demonstrated a bump about 1.5 inches in diameter on the right parietal bone.

Mr. Lind did not remember hitting his head, and stated that the bump had been there for as long as he could remember. Mr. Lind has a family history of heart disease and diabetes mellitus. He is a smoker, and smokes about one pack of cigarettes per day. He also was just diagnosed with sleep apnea.

A neurological examination was performed and included assessment in several key areas: general appearance and vital signs, mental status, cranial nerves, motor system, sensory system, reflexes, and the Romberg test. When performing the Romberg test, the patient stands with his heels together and closes his eyes. If he loses his balance, the test is positive. Otoscopic evaluation of the internal ear also revealed an ear canal with cerumen accumulation, but no inflammation. Blood pressure was slightly elevated at 144/90. The Romberg test was negative.

Mr. Lind was sent to a neurologist for follow-up evaluation and to a health educator for assistance with smoking cessation. A CT scan of the brain was ordered.

Case Study Questions

Answer the following questions related to this case study.

1. **Which lobe of the brain is directly beneath (deep to) the parietal bone?**

   _____

2. **What does the Romberg test assess? Mr. Lind tested negative on the Romberg test. What does this mean?**

   _____

3. **Does the cranial nerve test evaluate the central nervous system or the peripheral nervous system?**

   _____

4. **During the cranial nerve assessment, the physician had the patient stick out his tongue and move it side to side.**

   a. What cranial nerve is being assessed?

   _____

   b. What is the word part for tongue?

5. **What is the purpose of a motor system examination?** _____

6. **Mr. Lind's mental status was evaluated. Does this assess the central nervous system or the peripheral nervous system?**

   _____

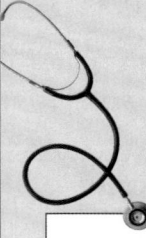

Real World Report

Name: Eric Lind

DOB: 04/01/1966

Date Ordered: 05/23/2011

Ordering Physician: Dr. Hammond

Exam Date: 05/23/2011

REASON FOR EXAMINATION: Change in mental status.

CT BRAIN

Multiple transverse images of the brain were obtained without contrast dye followed by the IV injection of 100 mL of Omniscan 300 contrast media. Soft tissue, bone window, and subdural windows were utilized for the exam. Preliminary scout film demonstrates a lytic appearing lesion involving the high parietal bone. On the transaxial images, a large expansile mass is identified within the calvarium of the high right parietal bone. It is expansile with thinning of the inner and outer tables, with more pronounced thinning involving the inner table. It measures approximately 4.1 × 2.3 cm in size. It does not demonstrate any contrast enhancement. There is associated compression of adjacent brain parenchyma. There is no shift of the midline structures of the brain. The ventricular system is normal. No contrast enhancing lesions are identified. There is displacement of the dura mater. A sharply defined area of low attenuation involving the right frontal lobe is seen consistent with an old area of infarction.

IMPRESSION

An expansile bone destructive mass involving the high right parietal bone is seen. There is erosion of both the inner and outer tables. More pronounced involving the inner table, as well as compression of the adjacent brain. Differential considerations would include epidermoid, hemangioma, eosinophilic granuloma, or sarcoma. Old right frontal lobe infarct is noted. Moderate focal atrophy is shown at the right frontal lobe probably from old infarct or old injury. Mild age-related cortical atrophy is shown.

Real World Report Questions

Answer the following questions related to this medical report.

1. **According to the CT scan, where is the mass located?**

   _____

2. **The report states that the ventricular system was normal. Explain this statement.**

   _____

3. **The report indicated displacement of the dura mater. What is the dura mater?**

   _____

4. **Describe what is meant by cortical atrophy.**

   _____

Review and Application

Multiple-Choice Questions

Select the best answer to each of the following questions.

1. The CNS consists of _____.
   a. the brain and spinal cord
   b. the spinal cord and peripheral nerves
   c. CSF and PMS
   d. PNS and motor pathways

2. Supporting cells of the CNS are termed _____.
   a. collaterals
   b. Schwann cells
   c. neuroglia
   d. dendrites

3. Special senses refer to _____.
   a. olfaction
   b. gustation
   c. vision and hearing
   d. all of these

4. A plexus is best described as _____.
   a. tangled auditory tubes
   b. a vision abnormality
   c. a spinal nerve network
   d. a hearing disorder

5. Identify the three meninges of the CNS _____.
   a. dura mater, pia mater, and subdural mater
   b. dura mater, arachnoid mater, and pia mater
   c. arachnoid mater, pia mater, and subdural mater
   d. epidural mater, subdural mater, and pia mater

6. The largest part of the brain is the _____.
   a. cerebrum
   b. cerebellum
   c. brainstem
   d. pons

7. Loss of memory is termed _____.
   a. amnesia
   b. dermatome
   c. stroke
   d. concussion

8. Elevated ridges of the brain surface are _____.
   a. gyri and fissures
   b. pons and gyri
   c. gyri
   d. sulci and fissures

9. A_____ is an area of skin supplied by a single pair of spinal nerves.
   a. somatotype
   b. fibroderm
   c. epidome
   d. dermatome

10. Jill is standing in her room and experiences dizziness. This describes _____.
    a. tinnitus
    b. reflexia
    c. photophobia
    d. vertigo

Word Parts Exercises

Match the word part with its correct definition.

11. _____ encephalo-

12. _____ myelo-

13. _____ neur-

14. _____ polio-

15. _____ astro-

a. star-like
b. nerve
c. myelin sheath of nerve fibers
d. brain
e. gray matter

Using the following word parts, form a medical term for each definition. Each word part is used only once.

-phasia
cerebro-
cerebro-
-spinal
dys-
-vascular

16. pertaining to the cerebrum and spinal cord _____

17. pertaining to the blood vessels in the cerebrum _____

18. impaired speech _____

Match the brain disorder with its chief characteristics.

_____ 19. cerebral palsy

_____ 20. Alzheimer disease

_____ 21. Huntington disease

_____ 22. Parkinson disease

_____ 23. transient ischemic attack

a. mini-stroke; nonpermanent brain disorder
b. progressive degeneration of dopamine-producing neurons
c. dementia with neurofibrillary tangles
d. inherited form of dementia; atrophy of cerebral cortex
e. group of motor function diseases

Definitions

Identify the test or diagnostic procedure described by each of the following definitions.

24. mapping of cerebral blood _____

25. spinal tap to remove CSF _____

Identify the disorder or disease described by each of the following key characteristics.

26. peripheral paralysis of facial nerve _____

27. inflammation of meninges _____

Provide the medical term for the following definitions.

28. nerve inflammation _____

29. nerve pain _____

30. disease of the nervous system _____

Write the adjective form for each given term.

31. dura _____

32. meninges _____

Spelling

Identify the correctly spelled term in each set.

33. _____	34. _____	35. _____	36. _____	37. _____
a. cerrebrum	a. demensha	a. mighgraine	a. polymyelitis	a. vurtigo
b. serebrum	b. dimentia	b. migraine	b. poleomyelitis	b. vertigo
c. cerebrum	c. dementea	c. migrane	c. poliomyelitis	c. vertego
d. cerebrem	d. dementia	d. meigraine	d. poleymyelitis	d. vurtego

Unscramble

Unscramble the letters to form a medical term.

38. noxa _____

39. thiew rattem _____

40. eialcps ssseen _____

41. suxple _____

Abbreviations

Provide the terms for the abbreviations and then define the terms.

42. MS = _____

43. CSF = _____

44. CVA = _____

45. ALS = _____

Short Answer

Answer the following questions.

46. Patient Smith presents with a TIA affecting his vision. Using medical and common terminology, describe what the patient is experiencing.

_____

47. Dr. Xenon orders an EEG on patient Smith to obtain an EEG. Spell out each abbreviation correctly so the sentence makes sense.

_____

Labeling

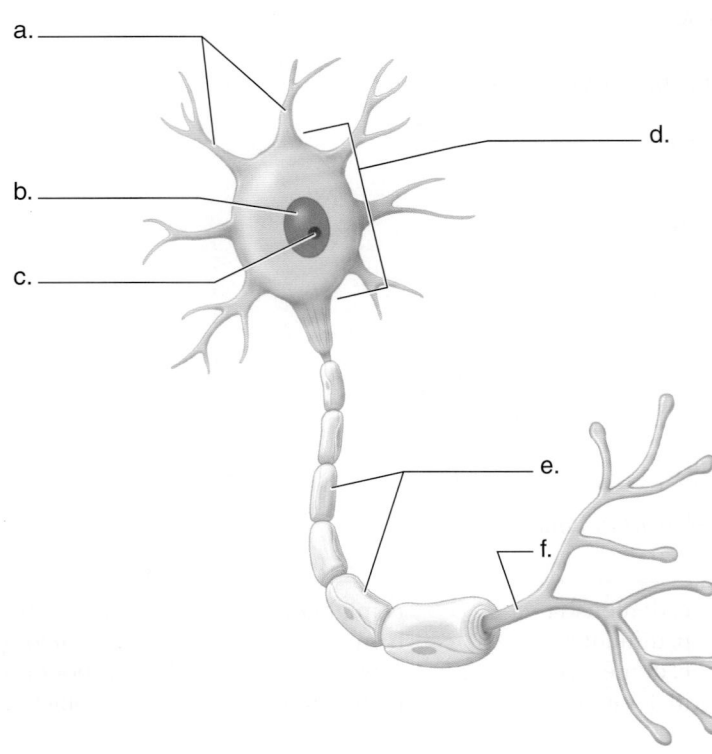

a.

b.

c.

d.

e.

f.

Word Search

Find the medical terms hidden in the puzzle.

```
D  F  S  K  S  V  M  C  M  M  U  S  L  A  M  P
N  E  D  U  Y  E  E  Y  E  X  E  N  R  I  U  L
E  F  R  Y  M  R  G  T  E  S  W  A  E  A  L  E
J  P  Y  M  E  A  S  N  P  L  C  D  T  H  L  X
E  Q  G  B  A  N  L  A  I  H  I  R  A  B  E  U
X  M  R  A  I  T  N  A  N  N  L  N  M  V  B  S
W  U  V  A  H  Y  O  O  H  S  E  I  A  F  E  W
M  Z  R  S  S  P  I  M  M  T  B  M  I  Z  R  D
S  B  M  G  Z  D  Y  I  E  N  O  E  P  T  E  U
C  U  R  N  M  H  B  R  N  Q  J  P  Z  E  C  R
J  J  T  A  S  E  R  U  S  S  I  F  Y  Q  Q  A
V  V  T  N  E  U  R  O  N  S  L  H  O  H  T  M
S  E  U  O  N  E  I  M  K  V  L  C  B  G  T  A
R  N  J  Q  Z  A  M  R  X  K  H  T  Y  R  T  T
X  E  T  R  O  C  L  A  R  B  E  R  E  C  X  E
D  E  N  D  R  I  T  E  S  M  I  Z  I  P  B  R
```

arachnoid mater
brainstem
cerebellum
cerebral cortex
cerebrum
dendrites
dermatome
dura mater
fissures
gyri
hypothalamus
meninges
myelin
neurons
pia mater
plexus
synapses

Vocabulary Review

Review the key terms from this chapter, study the spelling and pronunciation of each term, and write its definition in the space provided. Listen to the audio available for most terms at http://thepoint.lww.com/nath2e and pronounce each term for yourself. Then check the box when you feel confident that you know the definition and can pronounce the term correctly.

Key Term	Pronunciation	Definition
❏ **Alzheimer disease (AD)**	(AWLTZ-hye-mur)	_____
❏ **amnesia**	(am-NEE-zhuh)	_____
❏ **amyotrophic lateral sclerosis (ALS)**	(am-migh-oh-TROH-fick) (skle-ROH-sis)	_____
❏ **antiemetic**	(an-tee-e-MET-ick)	_____
❏ **arachnoid mater**	(uh-RACK-noid MAH-tur)	_____
❏ **astrocytoma**	(as-troh-sigh-TOH-muh)	_____
❏ **aura**	(AW-ruh)	_____
❏ **autonomic nervous system (ANS)**	(aw-tuh-NOM-ick)	_____
❏ **axon**	(ACKS-on)	_____
❏ **Bell palsy**	(PAWL-zee)	_____

Key Term	Pronunciation	Definition
❑ brain contusion	(kon-TEW-zhun)	_____
❑ brainstem		_____
❑ cauda equina	(KAW-duh e-KWYE-nuh)	_____
❑ cell body		_____
❑ central canal		_____
❑ central nervous system (CNS)		_____
❑ cephalalgia	(sef-uhl-AL-jee-uh)	_____
❑ cerebellum	(serr-e-BEL-um)	_____
❑ cerebral angiography	(se-REE-brul an-jee-and-OG-ruh-fee)	_____
❑ cerebral cortex	(se-REE-brul KOR-tecks)	_____
❑ cerebral hemispheres	(se-REE-brul)	_____
❑ cerebral palsy (CP)	(se-REE-brul PAWL-zee)	_____
❑ cerebral seizures	(se-REE-brul SEE-zhurz)	_____
❑ cerebrospinal fluid (CSF)	(se-ree-broh-SPIGH-nul)	_____
❑ cerebrovascular accident (CVA)	(se-ree-broh-VAS-kew-lur)	_____
❑ cerebrum	(se-REE-brum)	_____
❑ coma	(KOH-muh)	_____
❑ computed tomography (CT)	(toh-MOG-ruh-fee)	_____
❑ concussion	(kun-KUSH-un)	_____
❑ corpus callosum	(KOR-pus kuh-LOH-sum)	_____
❑ cranial nerves		_____
❑ dementia	(de-MEN-shuh)	_____
❑ dendrites	(DEN-drites)	_____
❑ dermatome	(DUR-muh-tome)	_____
❑ diencephalon	(dye-en-CEF-uh-lon)	_____
❑ dura mater	(DEW-ruh-MAH-tur)	_____
❑ dysphasia	(dis-FAY-zhuh)	_____
❑ electroencephalography (EEG)	(ee-leck-troh-en-sef-uh-LOG-ruh-fee)	_____
❑ encephalitis	(en-sef-uh-LYE-tis)	_____
❑ ependymoma	(ep-en-digh-MOH-muh)	_____
❑ epidural space	(ep-i-DEW-rul)	_____
❑ epilepsy	(EP-i-lep-see)	_____
❑ fissures	(FISH-urz)	_____
❑ generalized tonic-clonic seizure	(TON-ick-KLO-nick)	_____
❑ Glasgow Coma Scale (GCS)	(GLAS-goh)	_____
❑ glioma	(glye-OH-muh)	_____
❑ gray matter		_____
❑ Guillain-Barré syndrome	(gee-yan-bahr-RAY)	_____

Key Term	Pronunciation	Definition
❏ gyri	(JYE-rye)	_____
❏ hemiparesis	(hem-ee-puh-REE-sis)	_____
❏ Huntington chorea	(koh-REE-uh)	_____
❏ hydrocephalus	(high-droh-SEF-uh-lus)	_____
❏ hypothalamus	(high-poh-THAL-uh-mus)	_____
❏ lumbar puncture		_____
❏ medulla oblongata	(me-DUL-uh ob-long-GAH-tuh)	_____
❏ meninges	(me-NIN-jeez)	_____
❏ meningitis	(men-in-JYE-tis)	_____
❏ meningocele	(me-NING-goh-seel)	_____
❏ midbrain		_____
❏ migraine	(MIGH-grain)	_____
❏ multiple sclerosis (MS)	(skle-ROH-sis)	_____
❏ myelin	(MIGH-e-lin)	_____
❏ neuroglia	(new-ROG-lee-uh)	_____
❏ neurons	(NEW-ronz)	_____
❏ neurotransmitters	(new-roh-TRANS-mit-urz)	_____
❏ nuchal rigidity	(NEW-kul)	_____
❏ oligodendroglioma	(ol-i-goh-den-droh-OH-muh)	_____
❏ parasympathetic nervous system	(par-uh-sim-puh-THET-ick)	_____
❏ paresis	(puh-REE-sis)	_____
❏ Parkinson disease (PD)		_____
❏ peripheral nervous system (PNS)		_____
❏ pia mater	(PEE-uh MAH-tur)	_____
❏ plexus	(PLECK-sus)	_____
❏ poliomyelitis	(poh-lee-oh-migh-e-LYE-tis)	_____
❏ pons	(PONZ)	_____
❏ Reye syndrome	(RYE)	_____
❏ sciatica	(sigh-AT-i-kuh)	_____
❏ sequela	(se-KWEL-uh)	_____
❏ somatic nervous system		_____
❏ special senses		_____
❏ spina bifida	(SPYE-nuh BIF-i-duh)	_____
❏ spina bifida cystica	(SPYE-nuh BIF-i-duh SIS-ti-kuh)	_____
❏ spina bifida occulta	(SPYE-nuh BIF-duh ock-UL-tuh)	_____
❏ stroke		_____
❏ subarachnoid space	(sub-uh-RACK-noid)	_____
❏ subdural space	(sub-DEW-rul)	_____

Key Term	Pronunciation	Definition
❏ sulci	(SUL-sigh)	_____
❏ sympathetic nervous system	(sim-puh-THET-ick)	_____
❏ synapses	(sih-NAP-sez)	_____
❏ thalamus	(THAL-uh-mus)	_____
❏ tic douloureux	(TIC doo-loo-RUH)	_____
❏ tissue plasminogen activator (TPA or tPA)	(plaz-MIN-oh-jen)	_____
❏ transient ischemic attack (TIA)	(TRAN-zee-unt is-KEE-mick)	_____
❏ trigeminal neuralgia	(trye-JEM-i-nul new-RAL-juh)	_____
❏ ventricles	(VEN-trih-kulz)	_____
❏ vertigo	(VUR-ti-goh)	_____
❏ white matter		_____

Answers

Word Grouping Exercises

Definition	Word Part	Definition	Word Part
section, part	-tome	head	cephal-, cephalo-
brain	encephal-, encephalo-	meninges	mening-, meningo-
cerebrum	cerebr-, cerebri-, cerebro-	myelin sheath of nerve fibers	myel-, myelo-
chemistry	chem-, chemo-	nerve, nerve tissue	neur-, neuri-, neuro-
force, energy	dynamo-	star-like	astro-
glue, glue-like	glio-	tongue	gloss-, glosso-
gray matter	polio-	tree-like	dendro-
half	hemi-		

Word Building Exercises

Word Part	Meaning	Common or Known Word	Example Medical Term
cerebr-, cerebri-, cerebro-	cerebrum	cerebral	cerebrum
chem-, chemo-	chemistry	chemotherapy	chemoreceptor
neur-, neuri-, neuro-	nerve, nerve tissue	neuron	neuron
polio-	gray matter	polio	poliomyelitis

Key Term Practice

Nervous System Preview

1. central nervous system (CNS) and peripheral nervous system (PNS)
2. sympathetic nervous system and parasympathetic nervous system
3. central nervous system (CNS)
4. peripheral nervous system (PNS)
5. special senses

Neurons and Neuroglia

1. cell body, axon, and dendrites
2. Myelin
3. synapses
4. Neuroglia
5. neurons

Spinal Cord and Spinal Nerves

1. plexus
2. dermatome
3. cauda equina
4. Cerebrospinal fluid (CSF)
5. white matter

Brain and Cranial Nerves

1. midbrain, pons, and medulla oblongata
2. gyri
3. corpus callosum
4. dura mater, arachnoid mater, and pia mater
5. epidural space, subdural space, and subarachnoid space

General Brain Disorders

1. Parkinson disease (PD)
2. Dysphasia
3. cerebrovascular accident (CVA) and stroke
4. cephalgia; *cephal-*; *-algia*
5. hemiparesis; *hemi-*

Dementia

1. dementia
2. Huntington chorea
3. Alzheimer disease (AD)

Brain Neoplasms

1. glioma
2. a. astrocytoma; b. ependymoma; c. oligodendroglioma

Pediatric Disorders

1. Reye syndrome
2. Cerebral palsy

Cranial Nerve Disorders

1. sequela
2. trigeminal neuralgia; tic douloureux

Spinal Cord and Spinal Nerve Disorders

1. amyotrophic lateral sclerosis (ALS)
2. Spina bifida
3. meningocele
4. Vertigo
5. hydrocephalus; *hydro-*; *cephal-*

Infectious Diseases of the Central Nervous System

1. Encephalitis; *encephal-*; *-itis*
2. Meningitis
3. Poliomyelitis; *polio-*; *-itis*
4. nuchal rigidity
5. lumbar puncture

Common Abbreviations Exercises

1. SNS = somatic nervous system
2. PPS = post-polio syndrome
3. LOC = level of consciousness
4. dopamine = DA
5. cerebrovascular accident = CVA

Case Study

1. The parietal lobe of the brain is beneath the parietal bone.
2. The Romberg test is done to assess a patient's balance. The negative test finding indicates that on this day, Mr. Lind's balance was fine.
3. The cranial nerve test evaluates the peripheral nervous system, because cranial nerves are part of the PNS.
4. a. The hypoglossal nerve, CN XII, was being assessed. This nerve controls tongue movement.
    b. *gloss-, glosso-*
5. The motor system examination assesses body movements, muscle tone, and muscle strength.
6. Mental status involves the brain, so this test assesses the central nervous system.

Real World Report

1. The mass is located on the right parietal bone.
2. The ventricles are a series of four interconnected cavities in the brain through which CSF circulates. These appear to be fine (normal).
3. The dura mater is the tough outermost membrane of the three membranes that cover the brain.
4. The cerebral cortex is the wrinkled outer layer of the front parts of the brain known as the cerebral hemispheres. Its functions include learning, reasoning, and memory. Atrophy refers to the shrinking in size of the brain. In this patient, the brain has lost some of its mass.

Review and Application

1. a
2. c
3. d
4. c
5. b
6. a
7. a
8. c
9. d
10. d
11. d
12. c
13. b
14. e
15. a
16. cerebrospinal
17. cerebrovascular
18. dysphasia
19. e
20. c
21. d
22. b
23. a
24. cerebral angiography
25. lumbar puncture
26. Bell palsy
27. meningitis
28. neuritis
29. neuralgia
30. neuropathy
31. dural
32. meningeal
33. c
34. d
35. b
36. c
37. b
38. axon
39. white matter
40. special senses
41. plexus
42. MS = multiple sclerosis; autoimmune disorder that causes destruction of the myelin sheaths of neurons
43. CSF = cerebrospinal fluid; liquid that bathes the internal and external surfaces of the central nervous system
44. CVA = cerebrovascular accident; destruction of brain tissue due to the disruption of blood flow to a particular brain region; also called a stroke or brain attack
45. ALS = amyotrophic lateral sclerosis; fatal degenerative disease of the motor neurons marked by muscle weakness and atrophy; also called Lou Gehrig disease
46. The patient is experiencing a transient ischemic attack (TIA) or mini-stroke with visual disturbances.
47. Dr. Xenon orders an electroencephalograph or electroencephalography to obtain an electroencephalogram.

Labeling

a. dendrites   **b.** nucleus   **c.** nucleolus
d. cell body   **e.** myelin   **f.** axon

Word Search

D	F	S	K	S	V	M	C	M	M	U	S	L	A	M	P
N	E	D	U	Y	E	E	Y	E	X	E	N	R	I	U	L
E	F	R	Y	M	R	G	T	E	S	W	A	E	A	L	E
J	P	Y	M	E	A	S	N	P	L	C	D	T	H	L	X
E	Q	G	B	A	N	L	A	I	H	I	R	A	B	E	U
X	M	R	A	I	T	N	A	N	N	L	N	M	V	B	S
W	U	V	A	H	Y	O	O	H	S	E	I	A	F	E	W
M	Z	R	S	S	P	I	M	M	T	B	M	I	Z	R	D
S	B	M	G	Z	D	Y	I	E	N	O	E	P	T	E	U
C	U	R	N	M	H	B	R	N	Q	J	P	Z	E	C	R
J	J	T	A	S	E	R	U	S	S	I	F	Y	Q	Q	A
V	V	T	N	E	U	R	O	N	S	L	H	O	H	T	M
S	E	U	O	N	E	I	M	K	V	L	C	B	G	T	A
R	N	J	Q	Z	A	M	R	X	K	H	T	Y	R	T	T
X	E	T	R	O	C	L	A	R	B	E	R	E	C	X	E
D	E	N	D	R	I	T	E	S	M	I	Z	I	P	B	R

arachnoid mater
brainstem
cerebellum
cerebral cortex
cerebrum
dendrites
dermatome
dura mater
fissures
gyri
hypothalamus
meninges
myelin
neurons
pia mater
plexus
synapses

Vocabulary Review

Key Term	Definition	Key Term	Definition
Alzheimer disease (AD)	degenerative brain disorder that causes a disabling dementia with an onset typically later in life and is characterized by β-amyloid plaques and neurofibrillary tangles in the brain	**aura**	distinctive sensation that signals the onset of a migraine headache
amnesia	loss of memory	**autonomic nervous system (ANS)**	division of the peripheral nervous system that is controlled subconsciously
amyotrophic lateral sclerosis (ALS)	fatal degenerative disease of the motor neurons marked by muscle weakness and atrophy; also called Lou Gehrig disease	**axon**	nerve cell extension that carries impulses away from the cell body
antiemetic	agent for preventing or relieving vomiting	**Bell palsy**	paralysis of the muscles on one side of the face innervated by the facial nerve (CN VII)
arachnoid mater	the middle membrane that covers the brain and spinal cord	**brain contusion**	brain tissue bruise
astrocytoma	tumor derived from astrocytes	**brainstem**	brain part remaining outside of the cerebrum and cerebellum consisting of the midbrain, pons, and medulla oblongata

Key Term	Definition
cauda equina	group of spinal nerves that resembles a horse's tail extending below the distal end of the spinal cord
cell body	the main part of a neuron
central canal	passageway in the spinal cord that contains cerebrospinal fluid
central nervous system (CNS)	the brain and spinal cord
cephalalgia	pain in the head; another term for headache
cerebellum	second-largest region of the brain that functions to coordinate skeletal muscle activity and to maintain balance
cerebral angiography	mapping of the cerebral blood vessels using dye and x-rays
cerebral cortex	outer layer of the cerebrum
cerebral hemispheres	two symmetrical halves of the cerebrum
cerebral palsy (CP)	group of motor function diseases present at birth or in infancy that may be the result of interrupted blood flow to the brain during fetal development, childbirth, or infancy
cerebral seizures	recurrent convulsions with blank stares and temporary loss of awareness
cerebrospinal fluid (CSF)	liquid that bathes the internal and external surfaces of the central nervous system
cerebrovascular accident (CVA)	destruction of brain tissue due to the disruption of blood flow to a particular brain region; also called a stroke or brain attack
cerebrum	largest portion of the brain that functions in reasoning, learning, sensory perception, and emotions
coma	prolonged state of deep unconsciousness
computed tomography (CT)	imaging method that uses a computer to reconstruct the anatomical features obtained by x-ray
concussion	immediate loss of consciousness, orientation, or memory caused by head injury
corpus callosum	broad band of white matter connecting the cerebral hemispheres
cranial nerves	12 pairs of peripheral nerves originating at the brain that connect to the brain but not the spinal cord
dementia	loss of intellectual and cognitive functions while other brain functions are maintained
dendrites	branched nerve extensions that carry impulses toward the cell body

Key Term	Definition
dermatome	area of skin supplied by a single pair of spinal nerves
diencephalon	brain part that contains the thalamus and hypothalamus and is the link between the cerebral hemispheres and the brainstem
dura mater	the tough, outermost membrane that covers the brain and spinal cord
dysphasia	difficulty in speaking and understanding written or spoken language as a result of brain injury
electroencephalography (EEG)	method of graphically recording the electrical activity of the brain
encephalitis	brain inflammation
ependymoma	tumor derived from ependymal cells
epidural space	space between the overlying bone and dura mater
epilepsy	brain disorder resulting from an irregular electrical discharge of neurons
fissures	deep grooves in the brain that separate gyri (elevated ridges)
generalized tonic-clonic seizure	seizure characterized by collapse, loss of consciousness, and intermittent muscle contractions and relaxations
Glasgow Coma Scale (GCS)	scale used to assess the level of consciousness
glioma	tumor composed of cells derived from neuroglia
gray matter	regions in the central nervous system dominated by cell bodies, neuroglia, and unmyelinated axons
Guillain-Barré syndrome	acute symmetrical lower motor neuron paralysis of unknown cause
gyri	elevated ridges of the brain surface
hemiparesis	muscle weakness or paralysis on one side
Huntington chorea	inherited form of dementia accompanied by atrophy of particular brain regions; also called Huntington disease (HD)
hydrocephalus	accumulation of CSF on the brain; commonly known as "water on the brain"
hypothalamus	brain part that plays a role in homeostasis, such as regulating body temperature and releasing hormones
lumbar puncture	procedure using a needle inserted into the subarachnoid space of the lumbar region to remove CSF; also called a spinal tap
medulla oblongata	enlarged continuation of the spinal cord that contains important reflex centers for the heart, blood vessels, and breathing

Key Term	Definition	Key Term	Definition
meninges	three membrane layers covering the brain and spinal cord	sequela	disorder that is caused by a preceding disorder in the same person
meningitis	inflammation of the meninges	somatic nervous system	division of the peripheral nervous system that controls skeletal muscle contractions
meningocele	protrusion of the meninges through bone, forming a CSF-filled cyst		
midbrain	part of the brainstem that houses reflex centers associated with eye and head movements	special senses	the five senses of olfaction, gustation, vision, equilibrium, and hearing
migraine	recurrent, severe vascular headache	spina bifida	congenital defect of incomplete vertebral closure that allows the spinal cord or meninges to protrude
multiple sclerosis (MS)	autoimmune disorder that causes destruction of the myelin sheaths of neurons	spina bifida cystica	severe type of congenital vertebral defect characterized by increased intracranial pressure
myelin	white, fatty substance that forms an insulating sheath around axons	spina bifida occulta	incomplete fusion of the posterior arch of vertebrae
neuroglia	supporting cells of the CNS and PNS	stroke	destruction of brain tissue due to the disruption of blood flow to a particular brain region; also called a cerebrovascular accident or brain attack
neurons	nerve cells that send and receive nerve impulses		
neurotransmitters	chemical messengers between neurons or between neurons and muscles		
nuchal rigidity	stiffness of the neck and impaired neck flexion as a result of meningeal irritation	subarachnoid space	space between the arachnoid mater and pia mater, filled with CSF
oligodendroglioma	tumor derived from oligodendrocytes	subdural space	space between the dura mater and arachnoid mater
parasympathetic nervous system	the division of the autonomic nervous system involved in the "rest-and-digest" response; also called the craniosacral nervous system	sulci	shallow depressions in the brain surface
		sympathetic nervous system	the division of the autonomic nervous system involved in the "fight-or-flight" response; also called the thoracolumbar nervous system
paresis	muscle weakness or slight paralysis		
Parkinson disease (PD)	disorder resulting from progressive degeneration of dopamine-producing neurons in the brain	synapses	sites where adjacent neurons communicate
peripheral nervous system (PNS)	all neural tissue outside the central nervous system	thalamus	brain part that serves as a central relay station for incoming sensory impulses
pia mater	the delicate innermost membrane that surrounds the brain and spinal cord	tic douloureux	condition characterized by pain in parts of the face served by one or more branches of the trigeminal nerve (CNV); also called trigeminal neuralgia
plexus	spinal nerve network		
poliomyelitis	severe infectious viral disease that inflames the gray matter of the spinal cord and sometimes leads to paralysis and muscle wasting; also called polio	tissue plasminogen activator (TPA or tPA)	substance that dissolves blood clots
pons	portion of the brainstem between the medulla and midbrain that serves as a relay station from the peripheral nerves to the brain	transient ischemic attack (TIA)	brain disorder that is not permanent resulting from blood flow interruption
		trigeminal neuralgia	condition characterized by pain in parts of the face served by one or more branches of the trigeminal nerve (CNV); also called tic douloureux
Reye syndrome	complex of symptoms with liver damage and brain dysfunction that occurs after a viral infection; has been linked to aspirin use	ventricles	4 fluid-filled chambers in the brain
		vertigo	the sensation of dizziness while not moving that causes loss of balance
sciatica	pain in the lower back that radiates from the back of the thigh and down to the leg	white matter	regions in the central nervous system dominated by myelinated axons

CHAPTER 8

Special Senses

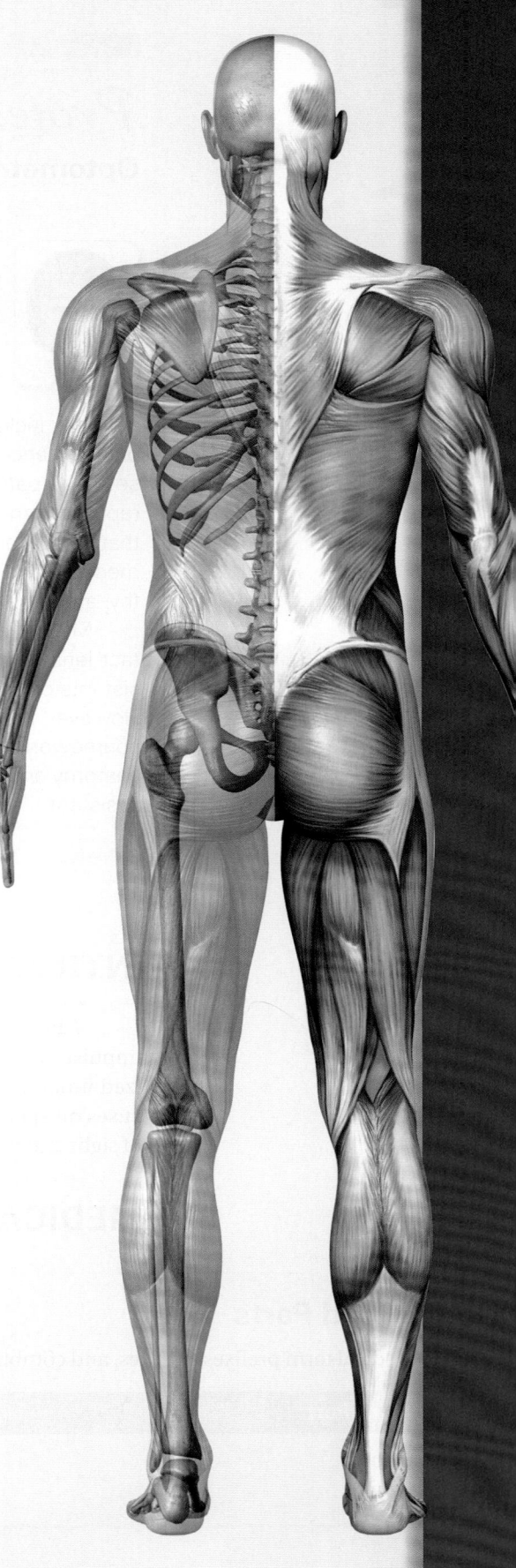

OBJECTIVES

After completing this chapter, you should be able to:

1. Define the meanings of word parts related to the special senses.

2. Identify major structures of the eye and ear.

3. Describe primary functions of eye and ear parts.

4. List different signs, symptoms, and treatments of diseases of the special senses.

5. Recognize clinical tests and procedures related to the special senses.

6. Describe anatomical and physiological alterations throughout the lifespan.

7. Define common abbreviations related to special senses.

8. Define terms used in medical reports involving the special senses.

9. Correctly define, spell, and pronounce the chapter's medical terms.

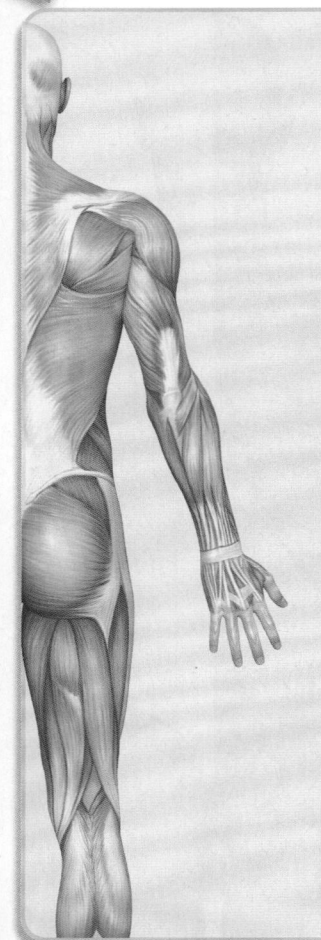

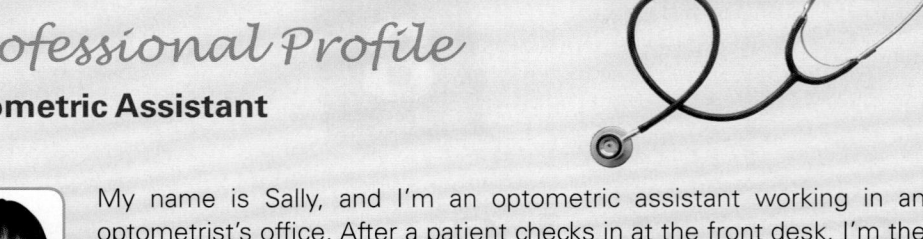

Professional Profile

Optometric Assistant

My name is Sally, and I'm an optometric assistant working in an optometrist's office. After a patient checks in at the front desk, I'm the next person he or she encounters in the office. My job is to collect the patient's history, perform preliminary tests, and orchestrate the flow of services. In addition to preparing and replenishing supplies in the examination and screening rooms, I perform the preliminary tests on patients, including the following: color vision, keratometry, autorefraction, visual fields, pupil distance (PD), visual acuities, and blood pressure. I do all of this before the doctor sees the patient, so accurate charting is crucial. I also file all the charts and preview reports from ophthalmologists and neurologists, checking to be sure that any reports that need immediate attention by the optometrist are placed on her desk. Common medical conditions seen in the office include cataracts, macular degeneration, retinopathy, and other sight-related disorders.

My job involves a good deal of interaction with patients because I also teach contact lens insertion, removal, and care. The employer commonly trains optometric assistants on the job. We are frequently cross-trained to perform minor eyeglass repairs. However, I recently completed a 1-year optometric assistant program, which included coursework in dispensing, office skills, lens fabrication, contact lens modification, anatomy and physiology, and medical terminology. I am now certified as an optometric assistant.

INTRODUCTION

The nervous system and special sense organs receive and interpret stimuli and transmit impulses to effector organs. Because sight, hearing, smell, taste, and equilibrium are specialized functions of the nervous system, they are referred to as special senses. This chapter focuses on specific anatomy, general physiology, and key medical aspects of the special senses of sight and hearing.

MEDICAL TERM PARTS

Word Parts

Medical term prefixes, suffixes, and combining forms related to the special senses are introduced in this section.

Word Part	Meaning
ambly-	dullness, dimness
audio-	sense of hearing

continued

continued from page 366

Word Part	Meaning
auri-	ear
blephar-, blepharo-	eyelid
choroido-	the choroid
cry-, cryo-	cold
dextr-, dextro-	right side, toward the right
dynamo-	force, energy
irid-, irido-	iris
kerat-, kerato-	cornea
meato-	passage
myring-, myringo-	tympanic membrane (eardrum)
neur-, neuri-, neuro-	nerve, nerve tissue
oculo-	eye or ocular
ophthalm-, ophthalmo-	pertaining to the eye
-opia	vision
optico-, opto-	optical, eye
ot-, oto-	ear
phot-, photo-	light
oculo-	eye or ocular
presby-, presbyo-	old age
retin-, retino-	the retina
rhod-, rhodo-	red color
scler-, sclero-	hardness
sinistro-	left side, toward the left
stereo-	three-dimensionality perception
tympan-, tympani-, tympano-	tympanum, drum
vasculo-	blood vessel

Word Grouping Exercises

Using the *Medical Term Parts* table, identify the prefix, suffix, or combining form for each of the following definitions. The first one has been done as an example.

Definition	Word Part
blood vessel	*vasculo-*
the choroid	
cold	
cornea	
dullness, dimness	
ear	A. B.
eye or ocular	

continued

continued from page 367

Definition	Word Part
eyelid	
hardness	
iris	
left side, toward the left	
light	
nerve, nerve tissue	
old age	
optical, eye	
passage	
pertaining to the eye	
red color	
the retina	
right side, toward the right	
sense of hearing	
three-dimensionality	
tympanic membrane (eardrum)	
tympanum, drum	
vision	

Word Building Exercises

Word parts introduced in the *Medical Term Parts* section are listed in the following table. For this exercise, first supply the meaning of each word part, then use the word part to build a word you already know. The word you list under *Common or Known Word* does not have to be a medical term; a commonly used word is fine. Be sure, however, that the word correctly reflects the intended meaning. The first one has been done as an example. Check your answers in a dictionary.

Word Part	Meaning	Common or Known Word	Example Medical Term
audio-	*sense of hearing*	*audio*	audiologist
auri-			auricle
dynamo-			dynamic equilibrium
irid-, irido-			iridectomy
neur-, neuri-, neuro-			neuron
optico-, opto-			optometry

continued

continued from page 368

Word Part	Meaning	Common or Known Word	Example Medical Term
ot-, oto-			otoscope
phot-, photo-			photoreceptor
retin-, retino-			retina
scler-, sclero-			sclera
stereo-			stereopsis
vasculo-			vascular tunic

ANATOMY AND PHYSIOLOGY

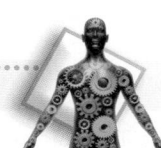

Special Senses Preview

There are five **special senses**: olfaction (smell), gustation (taste), vision, equilibrium (balance), and hearing. Anatomy and generalized functions of the nervous system were discussed in Chapter 7. The same basic principles apply to the special senses. This chapter focuses on the eyes (vision) and the ears (hearing and equilibrium).

KEY TERM	Definition
special senses	the five senses of olfaction, gustation, vision, equilibrium, and hearing

KEY TERM PRACTICE: *Special Senses Preview*

1. Name the five senses collectively referred to as special senses. _____

Eye and Vision

The eyes are important to both sight and maintaining equilibrium. The eyes can detect changes in posture that result from body movements. Such visual information is so important that even if a person suffers damage to the organs of equilibrium in the ear, he or she may be able to maintain normal balance by keeping the eyes open and moving slowly.

The eye is a complex, fascinating organ. We begin our discussion with the accessory structures. The eyelids, or **palpebrae**, protect the eye. While a person is awake, the eyelids blink every 2 to 10 seconds, sweeping debris from the surface. The mucous membrane called the **conjunctiva** lines the inner surfaces of eyelids and supplies fluid to keep the surface moist. **Lacrimal glands** secrete tears for lubrication and the enzyme **lysozyme** for destroying bacteria. Extrinsic muscles move the eyes.

Three layers—fibrous, vascular, and inner—make up the walls of each eye. The outer *fibrous layer* includes the cornea and sclera. The clear **cornea** is the window of the eye that

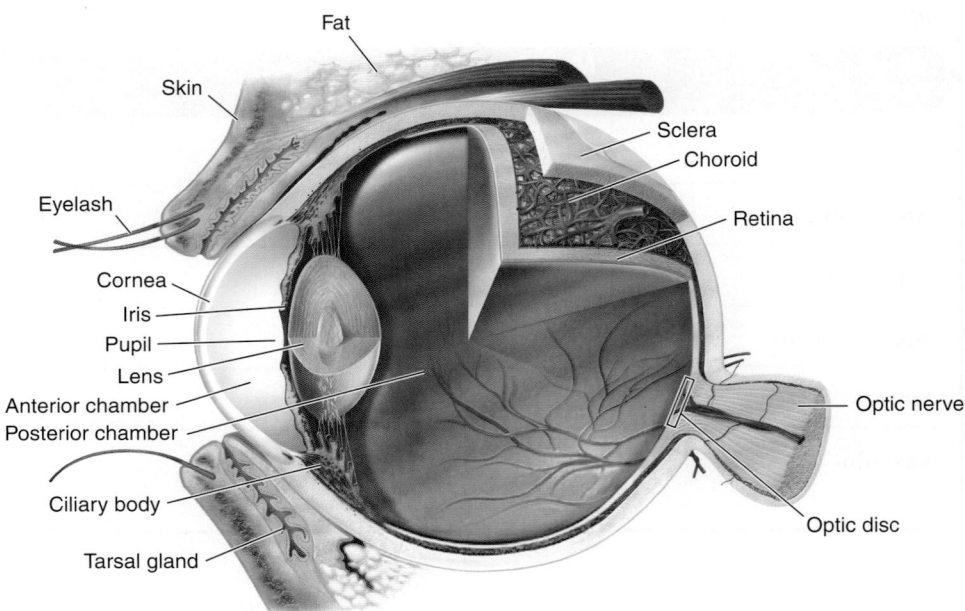

Figure 8-1 The structures of the eye.

helps focus entering light. The **sclera** is the white portion, which protects and serves as an attachment for extrinsic eye muscles.

The *vascular layer* of the eye includes the choroid, ciliary body, and iris. The nourishing tissue that contains melanocytes (pigment-producing cells), which absorb excess light and keep the inside of the eye dark, is called the **choroid**. The **ciliary body** is a thickened part of the choroid that encircles the lens of the eye and connects the choroid to the iris. The colored portion of the eye is termed the **iris**. The iris contains muscles that control the amount of light entering the eye through an opening in its center called the **pupil**. The **lens** lies posterior to the cornea and is an elastic, transparent structure that changes its shape and refracts (bends) light to allow the eye to focus (**Figure 8-1**).

Refraction, the bending of light rays, is the ability of the eye to change the direction of light in order to focus it on the retina. When adjusting for a close object, the lens becomes more convex (curving outward rather than inward), and when focusing on a distant object, the lens becomes more concave (curving inward rather than outward). Light rays are refracted primarily by the cornea and lens to focus an image on the retina. **Accommodation** is the automatic adjustment of the eye to focus an object to give clear vision. During accommodation, the lens changes shape.

The *inner layer* includes the retina and the optic nerve. The **retina** is a light-sensitive membrane in the back of the eye that contains photoreceptors (rods and cones) that receive an image from the lens and send it to the brain through the optic nerves. The **optic nerves** are paired cranial nerves (CN II) whose fibers transmit visual light signals from each eye to the brain. The **macula** is a small spot in the middle of the retina containing the fovea centralis. The region of greatest visual acuity (sharpness) is found within the **fovea centralis**, a depression in the central region of the macula. The **optic disc** is the location where nerve fibers from the retina converge to form the optic nerve. The optic disc is also referred to as the *blind spot*, because it has no photoreceptors (**Figure 8-2**).

The eyeball has anterior and posterior chambers, each containing a different fluid, termed a humor. **Aqueous humor** is a watery, nourishing fluid located in the anterior chamber between the back of the cornea and front of the iris and pupil. The **vitreous humor** of the posterior chamber is a transparent, gelatinous (semisolid) fluid, found between the lens and retina. It functions to support internal eye parts while helping the eye maintain its shape.

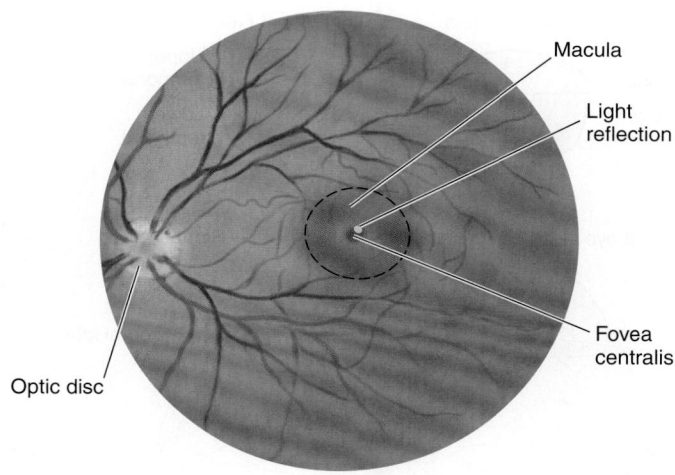

Macula

Light
reflection

Optic disc

Fovea
centralis

Figure 8-2 The internal
right eye.

Rods and cones are important photoreceptors in the retina. **Rods** are rod-shaped photo-receptors that are sensitive to dim light but not color. **Cones** are cone-shaped photoreceptors responsible for color vision. (Think of *c*ones for *c*olor.) The eye has 125 million rods and about 6 million cones.

The human eye is capable of adapting to both light and dark through the interaction of rods, cones, and pigments. One pigment responsible for this is a reddish light-sensitive pig-ment in rods called **rhodopsin**. This pigment decomposes in the presence of light and triggers a complex series of reactions that initiate nerve impulses on the optic nerve.

Cone vision is more acute than rod vision because impulses originating from the cones are often transmitted to the brain on separate nerve fibers, allowing for sharper vi-sion. Impulses from several rods may be combined and transmitted to the brain on a single sensory nerve fiber. For this reason, images from these cells are not nearly as precise. The structural pathway light passes begins at the cornea. Mapping the pathway for *light rays* looks like this:

cornea → anterior chamber and aqueous humor → pupil → lens → posterior chamber and vitreous humor → retina (rods & cones)

In order to actually *see*, the physiological system that is activated is known as the visu-al pathway. The visual pathway begins with the photoreceptors in the retina (**Figure 8-3**). Mapping the *visual pathway* looks like this:

1. Light stimulates the nerve fibers in the retina that form the optic nerves (CN II).

2. From the optic nerves, impulses are transmitted to the optic chiasm, which is the intersec-tion of the optic nerves.

3. From the optic chiasm, the impulses travel along the optic tracts, which are a continuation of the optic nerve fibers that pass into the brain.

4. Finally, the impulses reach a part of the cerebral cortex called the visual cortex, where the information is processed and interpreted.

Abbreviations for eye terms are O.S., O.D., and O.U. The letter *O* stands for the word *ocu-lus,* referring to the eye. The letter *S* stands for *sinister*, or left; the letter *D*, stands for *dexter*, or right; and the letter *U* stands for *uterque*, for each or both. So, *oculus sinister* (O.S.) means *left eye*. *Oculus dexter* (O.D.) describes the *right eye*, and *oculus uterque* (O.U.) refers to *each eye* or *both eyes*. Although you may still see O.S., O.D., and O.U used, they are listed as error-prone abbreviations that should no longer be used in medical practice.

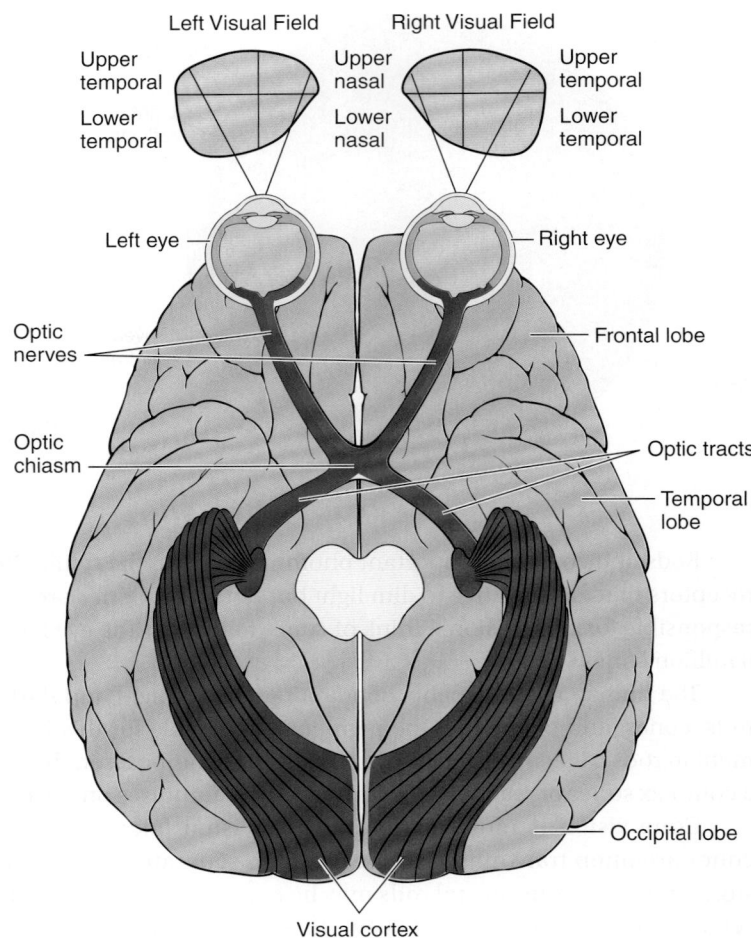

Figure 8-3 Visual pathway from the retina to the visual cortex.

KEY TERM	Definition
palpebrae (pal-PEE-bree)	eyelids
conjunctiva (kon-junk-TYE-vuh)	mucous membrane covering the inner surfaces of the eyelids
lacrimal (LACK-ri-mul) **glands**	tear-secreting glands
lysozyme (LYE-soh-zime)	antibacterial enzyme of tears
cornea (KOR-nee-uh)	transparent anterior part of the eye
sclera (SKLEER-uh)	whitish, outer layer of the eyeball
choroid (KOR-oid)	pigmented vascular layer that keeps the eye dark
ciliary (SIL-ee-err-ee) **body**	thickened region of the choroid that encircles the lens of the eye and connects the choroid to the iris
iris (EYE-ris)	colored portion of the eye that regulates the amount of light entering the pupil
pupil (PEW-pil)	opening in the iris
lens (LENZ)	elastic, transparent portion of the eye that changes shape and refracts light
refraction (ree-FRACK-shun)	bending of light rays to focus on the retina
accommodation	the automatic adjustment of the eye to focus an object to give clear vision

continued

continued from page 372

KEY TERM	Definition
retina (RET-i-nuh)	light-sensitive membrane containing rods and cones that receives images from the lens and sends them to the brain
optic (OP-tick) **nerves (CN II)**	cranial nerves that connect the eye to the brain
macula (MACK-yoo-luh)	a small spot in the middle of the retina that contains the fovea centralis
fovea centralis (FOH-vee-uh sen-TRAY-lis)	region of greatest visual acuity
optic (OP-tick) **disc**	circular area of the retina where nerve fibers converge to form the optic nerve; also called the blind spot
aqueous (AY-kwee-us) **humor**	watery, nourishing eye secretion in the anterior chamber
vitreous (VIT-ree-us) **humor**	semisolid fluid of the eye between the lens and retina
rods	rod-shaped photoreceptors that provide vision in dim light
cones	cone-shaped photoreceptors that provide color vision
rhodopsin (roh-DOP-sin)	reddish light-sensitive pigment in rods that decomposes in the presence of light

KEY TERM PRACTICE: *Eye and Vision*

1. _____ are photoreceptors for color vision.

2. The _____ is a light-sensitive membrane containing rods and cones that receives images from the lens and sends them to the brain.

3. _____ are photoreceptors that provide vision in dim light.

4. The colored portion of the eye that regulates the opening of the pupil is termed the _____.

5. _____ is the semisolid fluid of the eye between the lens and retina.

Ear, Hearing, and Equilibrium

Hearing and equilibrium are two of the special senses and both involve the ear. Anatomically, the ear has three main regions: the external ear, the middle ear, and the internal ear. The parts of the **external ear** are the auricle, external acoustic meatus, and ceruminous glands. The **auricle** is the external cartilaginous structure that projects from the head to direct sound waves. The **external acoustic meatus** is a passageway that transmits these sound waves to the **tympanic membrane** (eardrum), which in turn transmits the waves to the middle ear. The **ceruminous glands** line the external acoustic meatus and secrete cerumen, commonly called earwax. Cerumen keeps the tympanic membrane soft and pliable.

The **middle ear** houses the **auditory ossicles**, the three small bones called the **malleus** (hammer-shaped bone), **incus** (anvil-shaped bone), and **stapes** (stirrup-shaped bone). The stapes is about the size of a rice grain and is connected to the **oval window**, which is a membranous opening between the middle and internal ear. Ossicles transmit sound vibrations (waves) from the tympanic membrane to the internal ear.

The **internal ear** is the fluid-filled part of the ear, including the cochlea, which is responsible for hearing, and the semicircular canals, which control balance. The **bony labyrinth** is a complex system of interconnected tubes and chambers. Structures within the bony labyrinth include the semicircular canals, vestibule, and cochlea. The **semicircular canals** are interconnected bony tubes situated in three different planes, and the **vestibule** is the bony chamber between them. These two structures have to do with maintaining balance and equilibrium. The **membranous labyrinth** is a fluid-filled tube that lies within the bony labyrinth and conforms to its shape. The fluid within the membranous labyrinth is endolymph. The fluid between the bony and membranous labyrinths is perilymph. The **cochlea**, a structure shaped like a coiled snail's shell, is the spiral portion of the bony labyrinth that houses the **spiral organ** (organ of Corti). The cochlea contains the hearing receptors.

Skeletal muscles attached to the auditory ossicles act in the tympanic reflex to protect the internal ear from the effects of loud sounds. When the reflex occurs, muscles contract, and the malleus and stapes are moved. This results in rigidity of the ossicle bridges in the middle ear, thereby reducing its effectiveness in transmitting vibrations to the internal ear.

The **auditory tube**, or Eustachian tube, connects the middle ear cavity to the pharynx (throat). Because of the shared connection, bacterial and viral infections sometimes migrate between the ear and the throat cavities. The auditory tube also helps maintain equal pressure on both sides of the tympanic membrane. This structure creates the characteristic ear "pop" experienced when changing altitudes (**Figure 8-4**).

The internal ear contains the receptors of hearing called **hair cells**. There are approximately 15,000 hair cells in each ear. Different frequencies of vibrations stimulate different sets of these receptor cells. Hearing receptors then stimulate sensory neurons along a pathway.

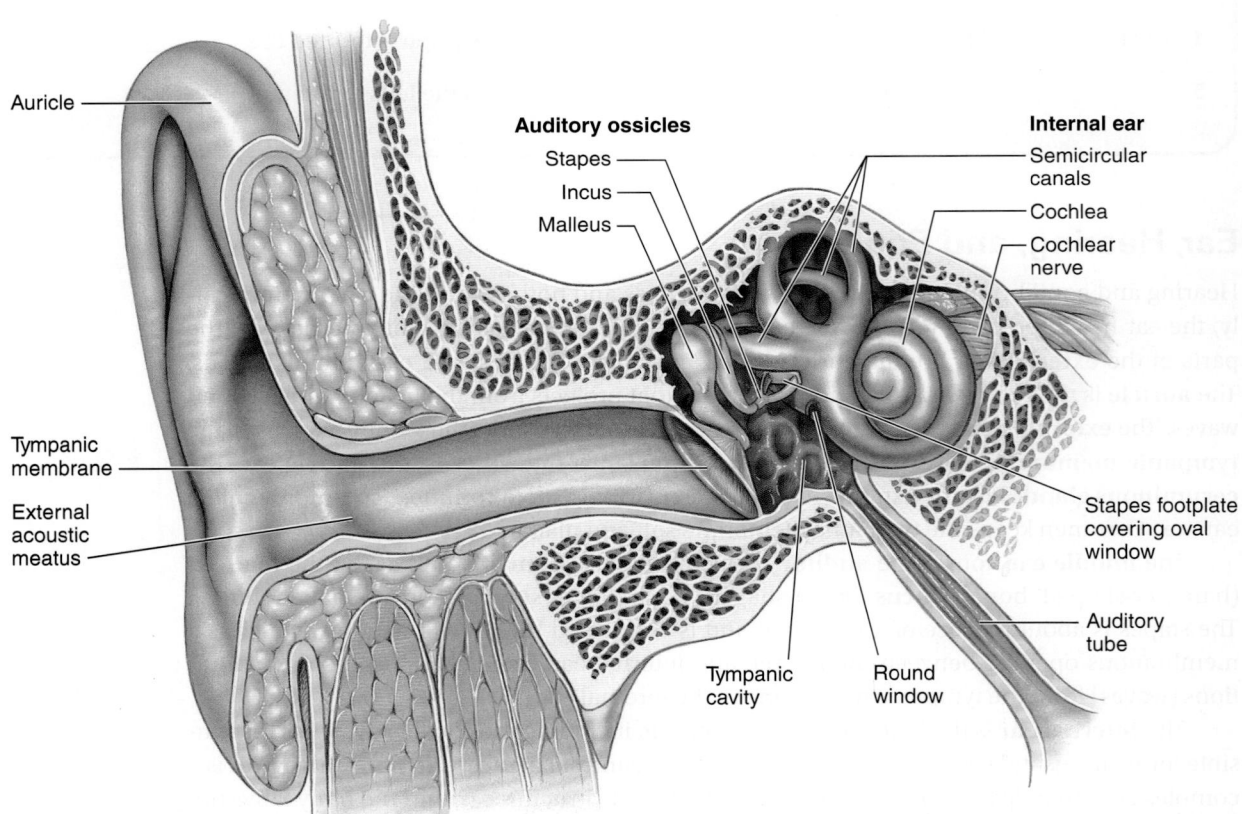

Figure 8-4 The structures of the ear.

The pattern of sound wave transmission is as follows:

1. Directed by the auricle, sound waves enter the external acoustic meatus.
2. The tympanic membrane reproduces the sound vibrations.
3. The vibrations move to the auditory ossicles (malleus, incus, and stapes), the oval window, and eventually to the hair cells.
4. Information is relayed to the brain by the cochlear branch of the vestibulocochlear nerve (CN VIII).
5. A part of the brain called the auditory cortex interprets the information.

Several abbreviations associated with the ear are derived from Latin words. For example, the medical abbreviation for ear is the letter *A*, which stands for the word *auris*. *Auris dextra* (A.D.) means the *right ear*, *auris sinistra* (A.S.) refers to the *left ear*. In Latin, *auris uterque* (A.U.) can be translated to mean *each ear* or *both ears*. Although you may still see A.D., A.S., and A.U. used, they are listed as error-prone abbreviations that should no longer be used in medical practice.

Ears also play an important role in equilibrium, whether the body is moving or not. Static equilibrium is concerned with maintaining the stability of the head and body when they are motionless. Dynamic equilibrium is stability while in motion. Equilibrium sensations enable balance by monitoring head position, acceleration, and rotation. Organs of static and dynamic equilibrium are located in the vestibule and the semicircular canals.

KEY TERM	Definition
external (ecks-TUR-nul) **ear**	outer ear that contains the auricle, external acoustic meatus, and ceruminous glands
auricle (AW-ri-kul)	external cartilaginous structure that projects from the head to direct sound waves
external acoustic meatus (ecks-TUR-nul uh-KOOS-tick mee-AY-tus)	passageway between the auricle and tympanic membrane (eardrum)
tympanic (tim-PAN-ick) **membrane**	membrane separating the external ear from the middle ear; also called the eardrum
ceruminous (se-ROO-mi-nus) **glands**	glands that secrete cerumen (earwax) in the external acoustic meatus
middle ear	space between the external ear and internal ear that houses the auditory ossicles (malleus, incus, and stapes)
auditory ossicles (AW-di-tor-ee OS-i-kulz)	three small bones (malleus, incus, and stapes) of the middle ear
malleus (MAL-ee-us)	hammer-shaped middle ear bone
incus (ING-kus)	anvil-shaped middle ear bone between the malleus and the stapes
stapes (STAY-peez)	stirrup-shaped middle ear bone connected to the oval window
oval window	membranous opening between the middle ear and the internal ear
internal ear	fluid-filled part of the ear that contains the cochlea and semicircular canals
bony labyrinth	complex of tubes and chambers that includes the semicircular canals, vestibule, and cochlea
semicircular canals (sem-i-SIRR-kew-lur kuh-NALS)	bony tubes situated in three planes that are involved with equilibrium
vestibule	chamber between the semicircular canals that is involved with equilibrium
membranous (MEM-bruh-nus) **labyrinth**	fluid-filled tube that lines the bony labyrinth
cochlea (KOCK-lee-uh)	internal ear structure that houses the essential organs of hearing
spiral organ	location of the hearing receptors in the cochlea; also called organ of Corti
auditory (AW-di-tor-ee) **tube**	canal connecting the middle ear to the pharynx (throat)
hair cells	receptors of hearing in the internal ear

continued

continued from page 375

KEY TERM PRACTICE: *Ear, Hearing, and Equilibrium*

1. The membranous opening between the middle ear and the internal ear is called the _____.

2. The _____ is a canal that connects the middle ear to the pharynx.

3. The membrane that separates the external ear from the middle ear is termed the _____, which is commonly called the eardrum.

4. _____ are receptors of hearing located in the internal ear.

5. The medical term for the external cartilaginous structure projecting from the head that directs sound waves is _____.

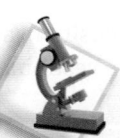

THE CLINICAL DIMENSION

The following sections outline common signs, symptoms, clinical tests, diagnostic procedures, pathological conditions, and treatments pertinent to the eyes and ears.

Clinicians working in this area include ophthalmologists (physicians—doctors of medicine [MDs] or doctors of osteopathy [DO]—specializing in the eyes), optometrists (doctors of optometry [OD]), and audiologists (practitioners with specialized degrees and training in the area of audiology).

General Eye Disorders

An **ophthalmoscope** is an instrument used to examine the interior of the eye (**Figure 8-5**). It consists of a light source and a mirror with a hole in it, through which the observer looks. The eye is illuminated by the light reflected from the mirror into the eye through the pupil. The reflected rays enable visualization of the back of the eyeball.

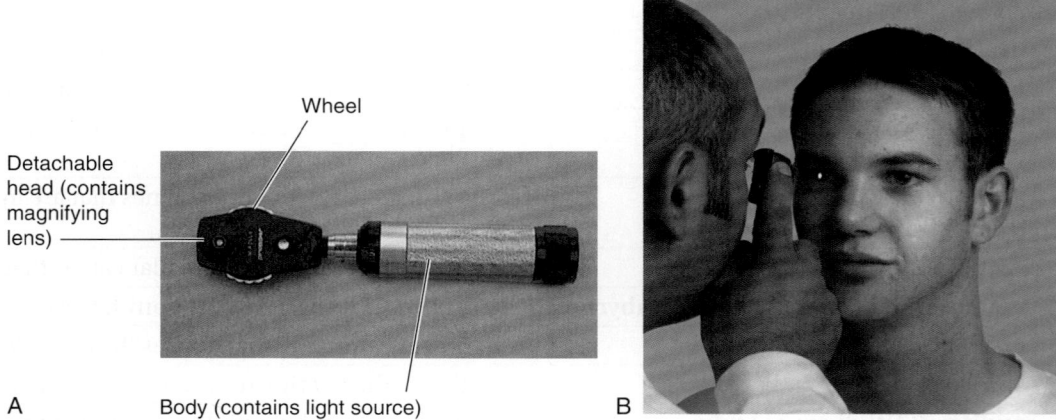

Wheel

Detachable head (contains magnifying lens)

A   Body (contains light source)   B

Figure 8-5 (A) An ophthalmoscope. **(B)** Using an ophthalmoscope to view the interior of the eye.

cataract   A **cataract** is a condition in which the lens becomes progressively cloudy, resulting in blurred vision (**Figure 8-6**). The clouding results from the breakdown of the lens protein. Cataracts appear to be a normal consequence of aging, but they may also result from congenital defects, diabetes mellitus, trauma, corticosteroid toxicity, or long-term exposure to ultraviolet radiation. Some research has shown that pilots are three times more likely to develop cataracts than are individuals in nonflying occupations and cataracts are common among glass blowers, who are exposed to infrared radiation. Signs and symptoms include blurred vision and a milky appearance on the lens. Patients often see halos around objects.

Eye care professionals diagnose the condition with a slit-lamp examination. A **slit lamp** is an instrument consisting of a microscope combined with a high-intensity rectangular light source in which the beam can be narrowed into a small stream (slit) (**Figure 8-7**).

Surgery to remove the lens is the only effective means of treating vision loss associated with cataracts. Two types of surgery are commonly performed: phacoemulsification (the most common type) and standard extracapsular cataract extraction (ECCE). With phacoemulsification surgery, small incisions are made and sound waves (ultrasound) are used to break up the lens into small pieces. With extracapsular cataract extraction, the lens and anterior portion of the lens capsule (which is wrapped around the lens) is opened, and the lens is removed in one piece. At the time of treatment, an intraocular lens (IOL) may be implanted to replace the faulty one. Otherwise, eyeglasses or contact lenses can compensate for the absent lens.

conjunctivitis   **Conjunctivitis** is inflammation of the conjunctiva caused by viral or bacterial infectionor allergy (**Figure 8-8**). Redness, swelling, itching, and tearing commonly occur. Diagnosed by visual examination, it is treated with warm compresses. The eye care professional may prescribe antibiotics if it is the result of a bacterial infection. The condition usually resolves within 2 weeks.

glaucoma   **Glaucoma** is an eye disorder characterized by increased intraocular pressure (IOP), degeneration of the optic nerve, and visual impairment. If not treated, it

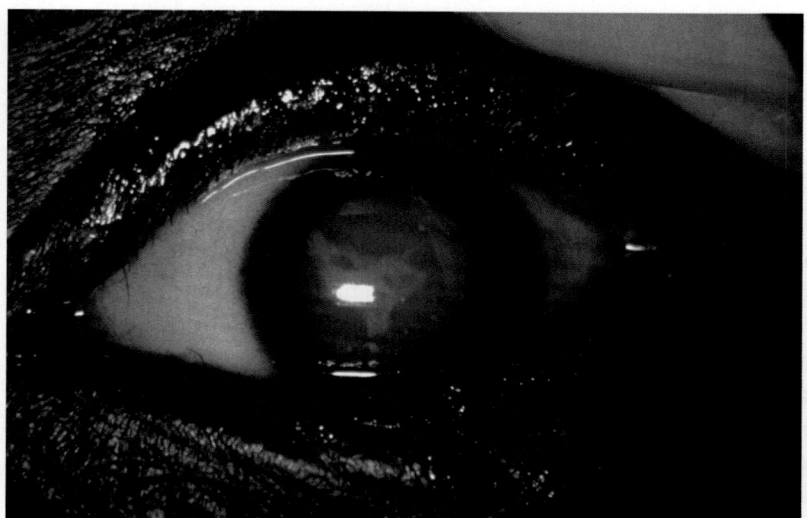

Figure 8-6 Cataract. The white appearance of the pupil in the eye is due to complete clouding of the lens.

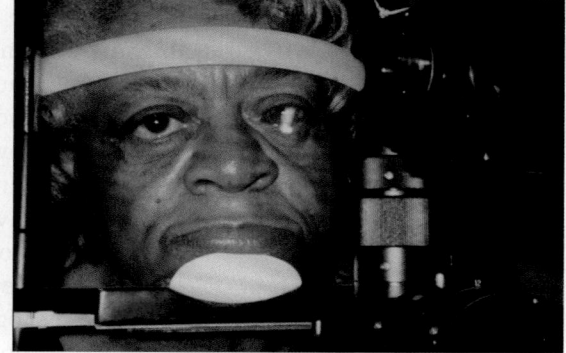

Figure 8-7 Technique for examining the anterior chamber of the eye using a slit lamp.

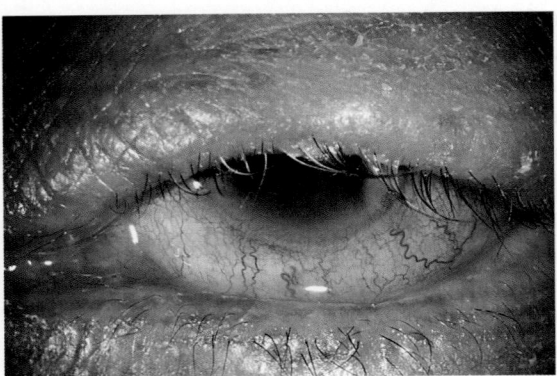

Figure 8-8 Acute bacterial conjunctivitis.

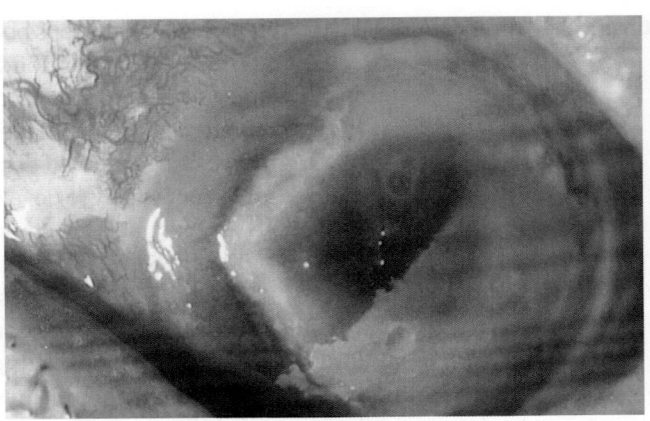

Figure 8-9 Keratitis.

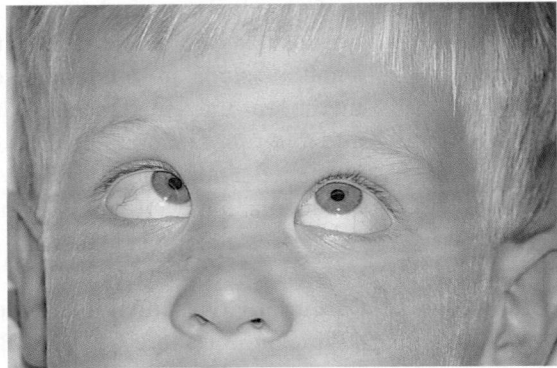

Figure 8-10 Congenital esotropia.

can lead to blindness and is a leading cause of blindness in people over 60 years of age. It is caused by an accumulation of aqueous humor. History, eye examination, and **tonometry** (measurement of intraocular pressure using a tonometer, which is an instrument that measures pressure in the eyeball) are used to make a diagnosis. Eyedrops and laser surgery are viable treatment options.

keratitis

The medical term for inflammation of the cornea is **keratitis** (**Figure 8-9**). It is usually caused by infection or corneal trauma. Visual disturbances, tearing, and photophobia are key characteristics. An eye examination using a slit lamp confirms the diagnosis. Available treatments include ointments, eyedrops, and possibly antibiotics to prevent secondary infection.

strabismus

An eye abnormality in which both eyes cannot focus on a desired object simultaneously is termed **strabismus** (crossed eyes). Two forms of strabismus include esotropia and exotropia. *Esotropia* is characterized by one eye turning inward (**Figure 8-10**), whereas *exotropia* is characterized by one eye turning outward. In esotropia, the visual axes converge and in exotropia the visual axes diverge. **Amblyopia**, or lazy eye, is the loss or lack of development of central vision in one eye that is unrelated to any eye health problem. Amblyopia usually develops before the age of 6 and can result from the inability to use both eyes together. These visual disorders are diagnosed by comprehensive eye examination. Treatment options include corrective lenses and vision therapy (orthoptic training). **Vision therapy** is a sequence of activities that are individually prescribed to develop ocular muscles, visual skills, and visual processing.

uveitis   Inflammation of the uvea (made up of the iris, ciliary body, and choroid) is termed **uveitis**. It may be idiopathic or caused by infection. It is characterized by pain, blurred vision, and extreme photophobia. A slit-lamp exam provides diagnosis. Treatment consists of managing the underlying cause.

KEY TERM	Definition
ophthalmoscope (off-THAL-muh-skope)	medical instrument with a light source and mirror used to examine the eye's interior through the pupil
cataract (KAT-uh-rakt)	partial or complete opacity of the lens
slit lamp	instrument used to examine the eye while aiming a light beam directly into it
conjunctivitis (kun-junk-ti-VYE-tis)	inflammation of the conjunctiva
glaucoma (glaw-KOH-muh)	eye disease caused by increased intraocular pressure
tonometry (toh-NOM-e-tree)	measurement of eye pressure using a tonometer
keratitis (kehr-uh-TYE-tis)	inflammation of the cornea
strabismus (stra-BIZ-mus)	problem related to abnormal alignment of the eyes; also called crossed eyes
amblyopia (am-blee-OH-pee-uh)	loss or lack of development of central vision in one eye that is unrelated to any eye health problem; also called lazy eye
vision therapy	sequence of activities that are individually prescribed to develop ocular muscles, visual skills, and visual processing; also called orthoptic training
uveitis (yoo-vee-EYE-tis)	inflammation of the uvea (iris, ciliary body, and lens)

KEY TERM PRACTICE: *General Eye Disorders*

1. Give the medical term for partial or complete opacity of the lens. _____

2. An _____ is an instrument with a light source and mirror used to examine the interior of the eye through the pupil.

3. Measurement of eye pressure using a tonometer is termed _____.

4. _____ is inflammation of the cornea.

5. _____ is an eye disease caused by increased intraocular pressure.

IN THE NEWS: Bionic Eyes ····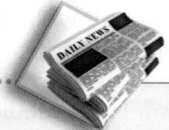

The Argus II system, first used by humans in 2007, is the concept behind bionic eyes. The Argus II system uses special glasses with built-in cameras, which are connected to a small computer (about the size of a deck of cards) that the blind person carries. The computer sends wireless signals to electrodes implanted in the blind person's eyes. The electrodes then pass electronic impulses to the brain. Currently, such retinal implants are only able to partially restore black-and-white vision.

The typical Argus II user has a disease such as macular degeneration (discussed later) or retinitis pigmentosa. Retinitis pigmentosa is a progressive retinal degeneration disorder. Worldwide about 1.5 million people have retinitis pigmentosa. Nearly 10% of all people over the age of 55 have age-related macular degeneration. These diseases affect the retinal cells and gradually cause the cells to die, thus preventing the processing of light into signals to be sent to the brain.

continued

continued from page 379

IN THE NEWS: Bionic Eyes

Retinal implants comprise an array of tiny electrodes placed into the back of the retina. Early versions resulted in the patient being able to see a highly pixelated black-and-white image. Advanced models are becoming more complex with much better "picture" resolution. Whereas the first-generation "bionic eye" only had 60 electrodes in each array, today's version has 2,000 electrodes per implant.

However, the Argus II system faces two stumbling blocks in the United States. Number one is that the Federal Drug Administration, or FDA, has yet to approve the newest implants as it waits for further assurances of patient safety. The second obstacle is cost. Currently the device costs about $100,000.

The implant creators warn that there are limits to what they can achieve because nature is the ultimate engineer. The Argus II system has technological limitations and is only applicable to people with certain types of visual impairments.

Refractive Problems

In normal eyes, light rays are bent to focus on the retina, forming a sharp image. When the eyes focus the light rays in front of or behind the retina, refractive problems occur. Refractive problems include myopia, hyperopia, presbyopia, and astigmatism, and are described in this section. Blurred vision and squinting are common to all these disorders. Diagnosis is made by physical eye examination. Corrective lenses are used to treat the conditions.

myopia (M)	In **myopia (M)**, or *nearsightedness,* the light rays focus in front of the retina. It occurs because the eyeball is too deep or the resting curvature of the lens is too great.
hyperopia (H)	A refractive problem in which light rays focus behind the retina is termed **hyperopia (H)**, commonly called *farsightedness.* If the eyeball is too shallow or the lens is too flat, hyperopia results. It affects near vision; distant vision is not normally affected.
presbyopia (Pr)	**Presbyopia (Pr)** is a vision disorder resulting from diminished accommodation due to impaired lens elasticity. Accommodation refers to the lens changing shape to focus a near object. Presbyopia has an onset around age 40-45. Individuals with presbyopia have difficulty focusing on near objects and reading fine print.
astigmatism	**Astigmatism** is the medical term for an irregular curvature of the cornea or lens. Its cause is unknown. Light rays are not focused at one point on the retina, but rather the rays spread, producing an imperfect image. Blurred vision is the most common complaint. Examination by an optometrist or ophthalmologist reveals its existence.

Figure 8-11 illustrates common refractive problems. Treatment involves corrective lenses, contact lenses, or radial keratotomy. Radial keratotomy and LASIK surgery are available for the treatment of myopia. **Radial keratotomy** is an invasive surgical procedure for correcting vision in which incisions are made in the cornea (**Figure 8-12**). The incisions cause the cornea to flatten to the prescriptive cure for visual acuity (VA). The instrument used to measure the corneal curve is a keratometer.

LASIK surgery is an acronym for *las*er-assisted *in* situ *k*eratomileusis. This eye surgery to correct vision uses a laser to reshape the inner cornea.

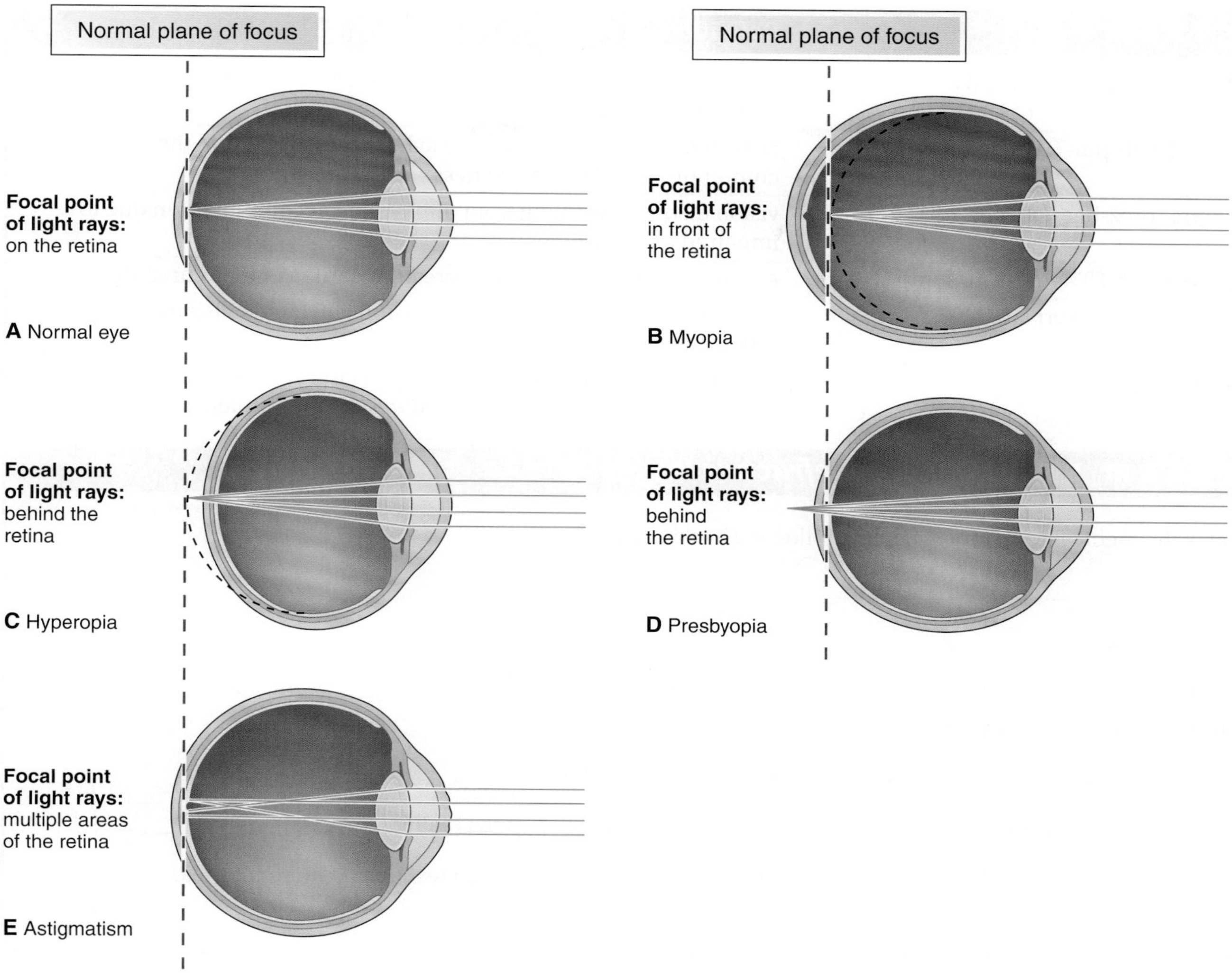

Normal plane of focus

Focal point of light rays: on the retina

A Normal eye

Normal plane of focus

Focal point of light rays: in front of the retina

B Myopia

Focal point of light rays: behind the retina

C Hyperopia

Focal point of light rays: behind the retina

D Presbyopia

Focal point of light rays: multiple areas of the retina

E Astigmatism

Figure 8-11 Common refractive problems.

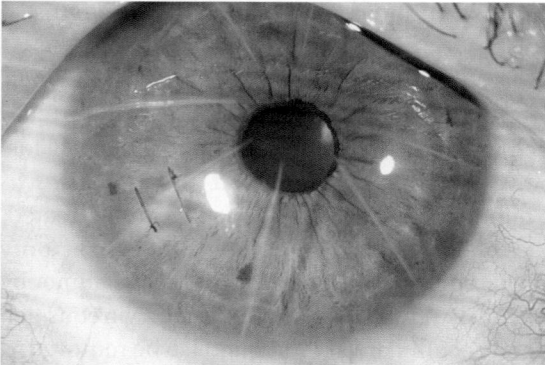

Figure 8-12 Radial keratotomy showing two sutures in the 8 o'clock incision.

KEY TERM	Definition
myopia (migh-OH-pee-uh) **(M)**	refractive problem in which light rays focus in front of the retina; commonly called nearsightedness
hyperopia (high-pur-OH-pee-uh) **(H)**	refractive problem in which the light rays focus behind the retina; commonly called farsightedness
presbyopia (prez-bee-OH-pee-uh) **(Pr)**	vision disorder resulting from diminished accommodation due to impaired lens elasticity
astigmatism (uh-STIG-muh-tiz-um)	eye disorder that results from irregular cornea or lens curvature
radial keratotomy (kerr-uh-TOM-e-tree)	surgical procedure for correcting vision in which incisions are made into the cornea
LASIK surgery	eye surgery to correct vision in which a laser reshapes the inner cornea; acronym for *las*er-assisted *in* situ *k*eratomileusis

KEY TERM PRACTICE: *Refractive Problems*

1. What is the medical term for each of the following eye disorders?

   a. farsightedness _____

   b. nearsightedness _____

2. The word part *presby-* means _____; and the word part _____ means *vision*; thus, the term refers to *age-related vision loss.*

3. This condition is caused by irregular curvature of the cornea or lens. _____

4. A surgical procedure for correcting vision that involves cutting the cornea is called _____.

5. _____ is an eye surgery to correct vision that uses a laser to reshape the inner cornea.

Retina Disorders

retinopathy

Retinopathy is a noninflammatory degenerative disease of the retina that is usually associated with damage to the blood vessels of the retina. Diagnosis of retinopathy is made by complete eye examination and fluorescein angiography. With **fluorescein angiography**, a yellow dye called fluorescein is injected into a peripheral vein, which allows the clinician to observe and map the vascular eye patterns.

diabetic retinopathy

Diabetic retinopathy is a retinal change secondary to diabetes mellitus (**Figure 8-13**). The underlying microvascular disease is the main culprit. Capillary microaneurysms, hemorrhages, and abnormal formation of new blood vessels from existing blood vessels (*neovascularization*) result in blindness. Diabetic retinopathy can be treated, but not cured, by laser photocoagulation or vitrectomy. **Vitrectomy** is a surgical operation to remove some or all of the vitreous humor by suction and simultaneously replace it with a synthetic vitreous gel. Adjacent scar tissue and accumulated blood may also be removed.

detached retina

The separation of the retina from the posterior of the eyeball is called a **detached retina**. It usually begins with a retinal tear as the result of

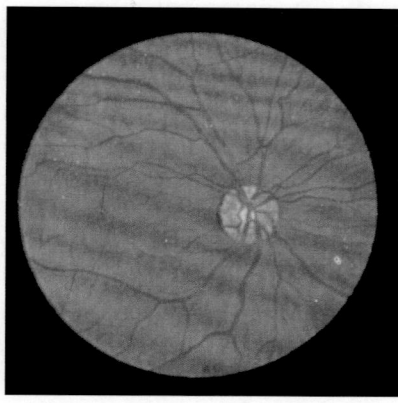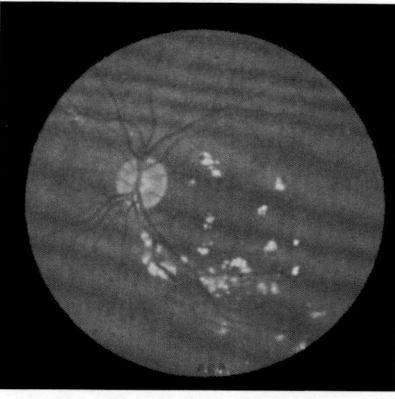

Figure 8-13 Photograph showing examples of a normal eye (left) and one with diabetic retinopathy (right).

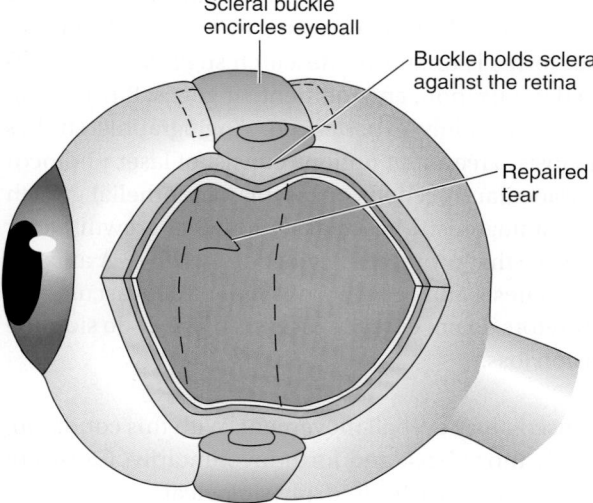

Scleral buckle encircles eyeball

Buckle holds sclera against the retina

Repaired tear

Figure 8-14 A scleral buckle.

eye trauma or vitreous detachment. The retina peels away from the back of the eyeball much like wallpaper comes off a wall. It is characterized by loss of vision, floaters, and flashes. **Floaters** are tiny clumps of gel or cellular debris within the vitreous. They are experienced as small specks seen moving across the visual field (VF). The illusion of flashing lights resulting from vitreous gel pulling on the retina is referred to as **flashes**. Retinal evaluation provides confirmation.

Treatment includes surgery aimed at closing the tear to return the retina to its normal position. Other treatment options include cryotherapy, intraocular gas bubble, laser, scleral buckle, and vitrectomy. **Cryotherapy** involves the freezing of tissue to prevent further damage, and the **intraocular gas bubble** treatment involves the injection of a gas bubble into the vitreous cavity. The pressure from the gas bubble holds the retina in place until the retinal tear is healed. The body absorbs the gas within several weeks. A **scleral buckle** is a permanent silicone band that attaches to the sclera periphery behind the eye, pulling the retina together (**Figure 8-14**).

macular degeneration　Pathological changes of the macula are termed **macular degeneration**. These changes often occur bilaterally, reducing central vision, although peripheral vision remains intact. The cause may be genetic, traumatic, age related, or atherosclerotic. Eye examination and fluorescein angiography provide information for accurate diagnosis. Laser photocoagulation is used to treat the condition. In **laser photocoagulation**, a concentrated light beam is focused on the retina to cauterize blood vessels. Recent research suggests zinc supplementation may also be beneficial.

Age-related macular degeneration (AMD) is the leading cause of poor vision in the United States. The two forms are wet and dry, and both are characterized by a decrease in the central vision (**Figure 8-15**). The dry form accounts for nearly 90% of AMD cases. Photoreceptors in the macula break down, causing loss of central vision. It usually affects one eye first, and the other eye may be affected later. The wet form results from neovascularization in the retina with vessels growing toward the macula. These delicate new vessels leak blood and fluid under the retina, causing the central vision loss. The cause of both forms is unknown. Research suggests the condition may be linked to nutrition, environment, or genes. Blurred and distorted vision is commonly experienced. Angiographic studies confirm the diagnosis. Treatment options consist of laser photocoagulation and intraocular injections of vascular endothelial growth factor A (VEGF-A) antagonists. Vascular endothelial growth factor is a peptide in the eye that promotes angiogenesis. VEGF-A antagonists inhibit angiogenesis and prevent subsequent neovascularization. VEGF-A inhibitors do not cure the disease, but they do slow the rate of central vision loss.

nystagmus

Nystagmus is an oscillatory eyeball movement. With this condition, the eyes continually move back and forth involuntarily. Causes of nystagmus can be congenital, acquired, physiological, or pathological. Blurred vision is the main symptom. Eye examination and visual inspection lead to the diagnosis. Correction of the underlying cause is the best treatment, but surgery may be an option for some.

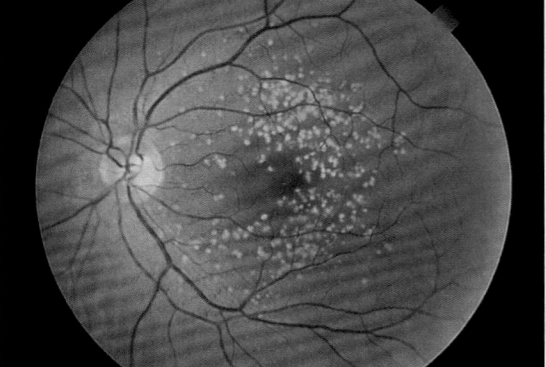

Figure 8-15 Multiple, hard bright structures seen in the retina and in the optic disc in early-stage age-related macular degeneration.

KEY TERM	Definition
retinopathy (ret-i-NOP-uh-thee)	noninflammatory degenerative disease of the retina
fluorescein angiography (floo-uh-RES-ee-in an-jee-OG-ruh-fee)	x-ray mapping of the vascular eye pattern after introduction of a yellow dye into a peripheral vein
diabetic retinopathy (dye-uh-BET-ick ret-i-NOP-uh-thee)	retinal disease resulting from diabetes mellitus
vitrectomy (vi-TRECK-toh-mee)	surgical removal of vitreous humor and simultaneous replacement with a synthetic vitreous gel
detached retina (RET-i-nuh)	separation of the retina from its normal position on the posterior eye
floaters	abnormal small specks seen in the field of vision
flashes	illusion of flashing lights seen in the field of vision
cryotherapy (krye-oh-THERR-uh-pee)	tissue freezing
intraocular (in-truh-OCK-yoo-lur) **gas bubble**	introduction of a gas bubble into the vitreous cavity
scleral (SKLEER-ul) **buckle**	a silicone band that is placed on the scleral periphery to tighten the retina
macular (MACK-yoo-lair) **degeneration**	pathological changes of the macula
laser photocoagulation (foh-toh-koh-ag-yoo-LAY-shun)	treatment technique that cauterizes blood vessels with a laser
age-related macular (MACK-yoo-lair) **degeneration (AMD)**	disease affecting the macula of the eye as a result of aging
nystagmus (nis-TAG-mus)	involuntary oscillatory eyeball movement

KEY TERM PRACTICE: *Retina Disorders*

1. Small abnormal flecks seen in the field of vision are termed _____; and the term _____ describes the illusion of flashing lights in the visual field.

2. A surgical operation to remove some or all of the vitreous humor of the eye is called a _____.

3. Involuntary oscillatory eyeball movement is known as _____.

4. _____ is a noninflammatory disease of the retina.

5. Separation of the retina from its normal position on the posterior eye is termed _____.

Eyelid Disorders

blepharitis   Inflammation of the eyelid is termed **blepharitis** (Figure 8-16). Itching, redness, and crusting around eyelids typify the condition, which is usually caused by allergies or a staphylococcal infection. Diagnosis is based on a visual examination. Saline solution eye washes, ointments, and good eyelid hygiene are recommended. Antibiotics are prescribed in some instances of bacterial infection.

blepharoptosis   The word for upper eyelid drooping is **blepharoptosis**. It is caused by eyelid muscle weakness that tends to be secondary to diabetes mellitus, muscular dystrophy, myasthenia gravis, tumor, or nerve damage. Diagnosis is made by history, physical examination, and visual inspection. Surgery is the only treatment option to correct a sagging eyelid. Any underlying disease also requires attention.

hordeolum

Hordeolum is an inflammation of a gland of the eyelid. It is commonly called a sty and is derived from the Latin word *hordeolus,* which means *a sty in the eye* (**Figure 8-17**). The infectious agent is usually Staphylococcus. Signs and symptoms include pain, swelling, and pus at the site. Visual examination confirms the diagnosis. Treatment involves applying hot compresses to the area and antibiotics in severe cases.

chalazion

Inflammation of the eyelid resulting from a blocked tarsal gland is called **chalazion** (**Figure 8-18**). Tarsal glands, also known as meibomian glands, are sebaceous glands found in the eyelids. Redness, pain, swelling, and cyst formation are common. The cysts are often referred to as meibomian cysts. Chalazia are diagnosed by visual examination. Treatment is not usually necessary, but if the condition persists, surgery may be required.

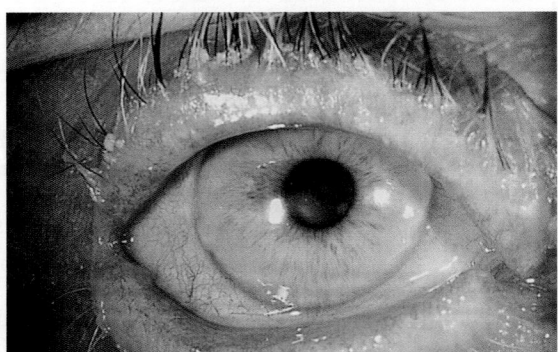

Figure 8-16 Blepharitis.

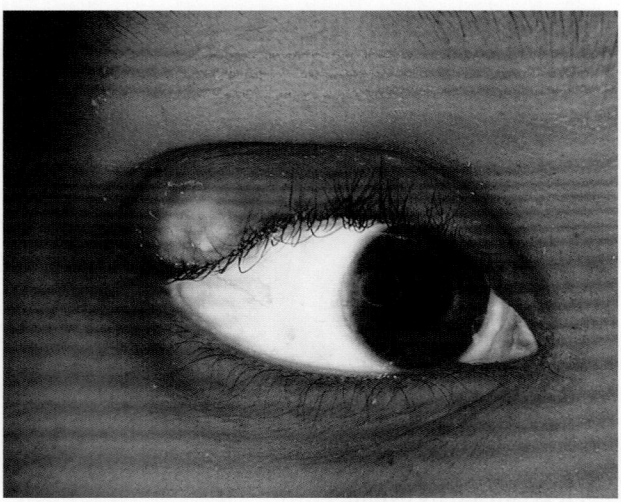

Figure 8-17 A hordeolum on the upper eyelid.

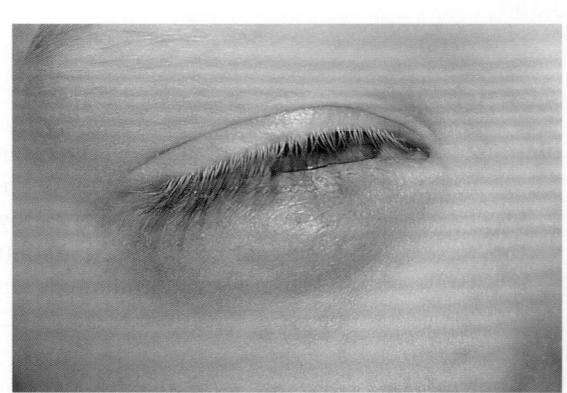

Figure 8-18 A chalazion in a 7-year-old boy.

KEY TERM	Definition
blepharitis (blef-uh-RYE-tis)	inflammation of the eyelid
blepharoptosis (blef-uh-rop-TOH-sis)	upper eyelid drooping
hordeolum (hor-DEE-oh-lum)	a sty
chalazion (kay-LAY-zee-on)	inflammation of the eyelid from a blocked tarsal gland

KEY TERM PRACTICE: *Eyelid Disorders*

1. The medical term for a sty is _____.

2. The word part *blephar-* means _____, and the word part *-ptosis* means "drooping"; therefore, the term _____ means "upper eyelid drooping. "

3. The word part _____ means "eyelid" and the word part _____ means "inflammation"; so, the medical term for "inflammation of the eyelid" is _____.

4. Inflammation of the eyelid caused by a blocked tarsal gland is termed _____.

External Ear Disorders and Deafness

otitis externa

Otitis externa is inflammation of the external acoustic meatus caused by an infection. It is also known as swimmer's ear. Cerumen mixing with water creates an environment rich for microbial growth. Signs and symptoms include pain, redness, swelling, hearing loss, and pruritus (itching). Otological examination and cell culture provide the diagnosis. Treatment consists of washing the ear canal. Antibiotics are given if necessary.

deafness

Deafness is partial or complete hearing impairment in one or both ears. Two types of deafness include conduction and sensorineural. It is diagnosed by **audiometry**, an examination using an audiometer to test the ability of the human ear to detect sounds over a range of frequencies and intensities. The record of auditory acuity measured by an audiometer is an **audiogram**.

conduction deafness

Conduction deafness is the loss of hearing as a result of improper sound passage through the ossicles.

sensorineural deafness

Sensorineural deafness is hearing loss caused by damage to the cochlea or auditory nerve. Sound waves reach the internal ear, but nerve impulses are not transmitted to the brain. Aging, side effects of some medications, and loud noise are causes. It may be the result of occupational exposure to noise. The aim of treatment is to reduce environmental noise. Hearing aids may provide some assistance. Sensorineural deafness is irreversible if the cochlea is damaged.

presbycusis

Presbycusis is sensorineural hearing loss associated with aging. It results from loss of hair cells in the organ of Corti.

KEY TERM	Definition
otitis externa (oh-TYE-tis ecks-TUR-nuh)	inflammation of the external acoustic meatus caused by an infection; also called swimmer's ear
deafness	partial or complete hearing loss
audiometry (aw-dee-OM-e-tree)	evaluation using an audiometer to test a person's ability to hear a range of sounds
audiogram (AW-dee-oh-gram)	record of auditory acuity as measured by an audiometer
conduction deafness	hearing loss with ossicle involvement
sensorineural (sen-suh-ri-NEW-rul) **deafness**	hearing loss involving a damaged cochlea or auditory nerve
presbycusis (prez-bee-KEW-sis)	hearing loss associated with old age

KEY TERM PRACTICE: *External Ear Disorders and Deafness*

1. The type of hearing loss associated with a damaged auditory nerve is termed _____.

2. _____ is the medical term for *inflammation of the external acoustic meatus* and is caused by an infection.

3. Hearing loss associated with age is called _____ and is derived from the word part _____ for "old age."

4. Partial or complete hearing loss is termed _____.

5. An _____ is a record of auditory acuity as measured by an audiometer.

Middle Ear and Tympanic Membrane Disorders

otitis media   Painful inflammation of the middle ear is called **otitis media**. Associated fluid accumulation, hearing loss, and dizziness are common. Infections are the most common cause. Diagnosis is made by otoscopy. **Otoscopy** is the visualization of the external acoustic meatus and tympanic membrane with an otoscope (**Figure 8-19**). Audiometry reveals hearing loss.

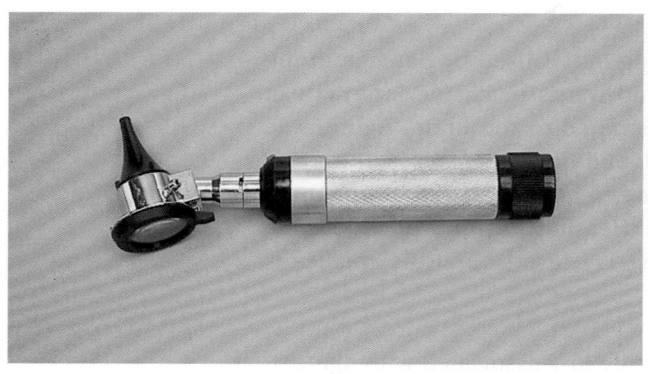

A

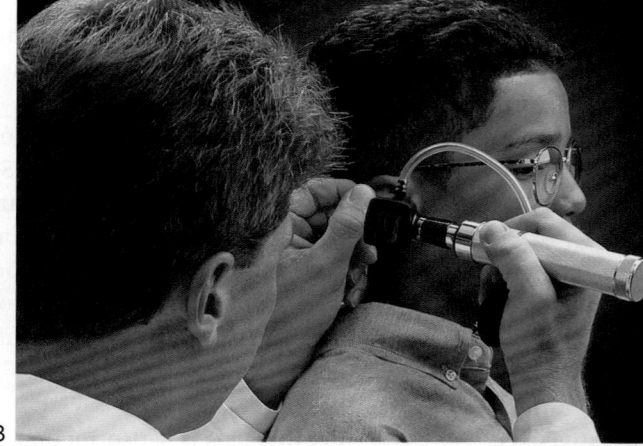

B

Figure 8-19 (A) An otoscope. **(B)** Using an otoscope to view the external ear.

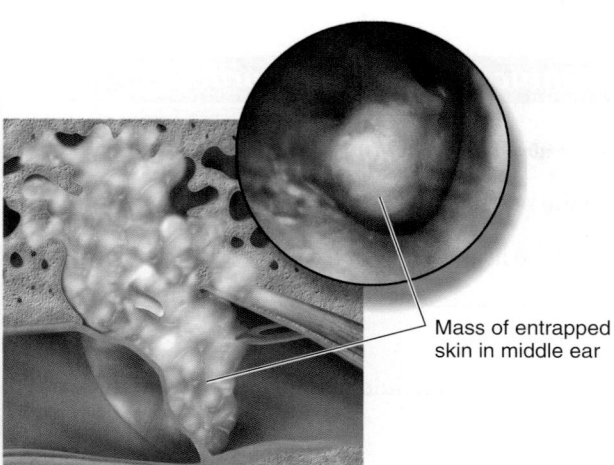

Mass of entrapped skin in middle ear

Figure 8-20 A cholesteatoma in the middle ear.

Analgesics, decongestants, and antibiotics are conservative treatments. Myringotomy or tympanostomy tubes may be required. A **myringotomy** is an incision through the tympanic membrane to drain fluid or pus buildup. (The alternate term for the tympanic membrane is myringa.) **Tympanostomy tubes** are tubes that are inserted through the tympanic membrane to create a passageway for fluid drainage.

cholesteatoma   A **cholesteatoma**, an epidermal cyst of the middle ear, creates a potentially dangerous condition in which a mass of cholesterol and skin scales forms, grows, and invades the bone (**Figure 8-20**). Cholesteatomas may develop in infancy as a result of recurrent otitis media that causes a pocket of skin cells to develop. Vertigo and earache are common. Treatment consists of ear washings and surgical removal of the cyst.

mastoiditis   Inflammation of mastoid cells (intercommunicating cavities) in the mastoid process of the temporal bone is called **mastoiditis**. (Recall from chapter 5 that the temporal bones are lateral skull bones.) It is generally the result of untreated otitis media. Pain and edema occur around the mastoid process. Diagnosis is made by an ear examination and otoscopy. Antibiotics are usually prescribed, but severe cases may require mastoidectomy. A mastoidectomy is the surgical removal of an infected mastoid process to allow pus to drain off and prevent infection from spreading to the meninges.

KEY TERM	Definition
otitis media (oh-TYE-tis MEE-dee-uh)	acute inflammation of the middle ear cavity, usually due to an infection
otoscopy (oh-TOS-kuh-pee)	visualization of the external acoustic meatus and tympanic membrane with an otoscope
myringotomy (mirr-in-GOT-uh-mee)	incision through the tympanic membrane (myringa) to drain fluid
tympanostomy tubes (tim-puh-NOS-tuh-mee)	tubes placed as a passageway for fluid drainage through the tympanic membrane
cholesteatoma (koh-les-tee-uh-TOH-muh)	cyst in the middle ear that grows into the bone
mastoiditis (mas-toid-EYE-tis)	inflammation of mastoid cells in the mastoid process of the temporal bone

continued

continued from page 389

K E Y   T E R M   P R A C T I C E : *Middle Ear and Tympanic Membrane Disorders*

1. _____ is the visualization of the external acoustic meatus and tympanic membrane with an otoscope

2. A _____ is a cyst in the middle ear that grows into the bone.

3. Inflammation of the middle ear, usually caused by an infection, is known as _____, derived from the word part _____ for "ear," the word part _____ for "inflammation," and the word _____ for "middle."

4. A _____ is an incision through the tympanic membrane to drain fluid and is derived from the word part _____ for "tympanic membrane."

5. Inflammation of mastoid cells in the mastoid process of the temporal bone is called _____.

Internal Ear Disorders

tinnitus

Tinnitus is a continual perception of sound in the absence of any environmental noise. The sound can be ringing, whistling, hissing, roaring, or booming. It is usually caused by damage to the hair cells of the internal ear.

otosclerosis

Otosclerosis is a disease of the internal ear in which new bone growth around the oval window and/or cochlea leads to progressive hearing loss. The onset is between puberty and age 35 years. The primary sign is conduction deafness. Otoscopic evaluation, history, and audiogram provide a diagnosis. **Stapedectomy**, the surgical removal of the stapes and replacement with a metal or plastic prosthesis (artificial stapes), is the available treatment.

labyrinthitis

Labyrinthitis is an inflammation of the internal ear labyrinth that causes nausea and loss of balance. It is sometimes called otitis interna. It is caused by a viral or bacterial infection and is marked by fever and extreme vertigo. Ear examination and audiometry provide the diagnosis. Treatment involves rest, antibiotics, and an antiemetic, if necessary, for the nausea.

Ménière disease

Ménière disease is an ear disorder caused by an accumulation of fluid in the labyrinth in the internal ear and is characterized by deafness, tinnitus, and vertigo. Nausea, vomiting, and nystagmus commonly occur. The onset is usually between the ages of 40 and 50 years. The signs and symptoms along with electronystagmography confirm the diagnosis. **Electronystagmography (ENG)** is a method of recording eye movement in response to stimuli. Antinausea and antivomiting medications are prescribed. A nutrition plan that includes the restriction of both salts and fluids is effective for some people. Surgical destruction of the labyrinth may be necessary.

KEY TERM	Definition
tinnitus (ti-NIGH-tus)	perception of sound, such as ringing or hissing in the ears, in the absence of any environmental noise
otosclerosis (oh-toh-skle-ROH-sis)	ear disorder in which new bone is deposited in the internal ear
stapedectomy (stay-pe-DECK-tuh-mee)	surgical removal of the stapes
labyrinthitis (lab-i-rin-THIGH-tis)	inflammation of the internal ear labyrinth that causes nausea and loss of balance
Ménière (mey-NYEHR) **disease**	disease of the internal ear caused by fluid accumulation in the labyrinth; it is characterized by deafness, tinnitus, and vertigo
electronystagmography (ENG) (ee-leck-troh-nigh-stag-MOG-ruh-fee)	method of recording eye movements in response to stimuli

KEY TERM PRACTICE: *Internal Ear Disorders*

1. An illness in which the internal ear labyrinth becomes inflamed, causing balance loss and nausea, is termed
   _____.

2. _____ is a method of recording eye movements in response to stimuli.

3. _____ is a disease of the internal ear caused by fluid accumulation in the labyrinth and is characterized by deafness, tinnitus, and vertigo.

4. The perception of sound, such as ringing in the ears, when there is no environmental noise is called
   _____.

5. The surgical removal of the stapes is termed _____.

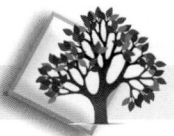

LIFE SPAN

The nervous system is derived from the embryonic ectoderm germ layer. Eye development continues until around age 9, when the eyes reach their adult size. Visual acuity gradually declines in aging persons, and it appears that no one is exempt from needing corrective lenses later in life. Age-related hearing loss is also prevalent beginning in the sixth or seventh decade of life.

COMMON Abbreviations

Abbreviation	Term
A.D.	right ear
AMD	age-related macular degeneration
A.S.	left ear
A/V ratio	artery to vein ratio
A.U.	each ear; both ears
CN	cranial nerve
CS	cortical spokes
CT	computed tomography
ECCE	extracapsular cataract extraction
ENG	electronystagmography
H	hyperopia
IOL	intraocular lens
IOP	intraocular pressure
LASIK	*las*er-assisted *in* situ *k*eratomileusis
MD	medical doctor
M	myopia
NS	nuclear sclerosis
O.D.	right eye
OD	doctor of optometry
O.S.	left eye
O.U.	each eye; both eyes
PD	pupil distance
Pr	presbyopia
VA	visual acuity
VF	visual field

COMMON ABBREVIATIONS EXERCISES

1. Give the term for Pr. _____

2. IOL is the abbreviation for _____.

3. PD stands for _____.

4. The abbreviation for electronystagmography is _____.

5. The abbreviation for visual field is _____.

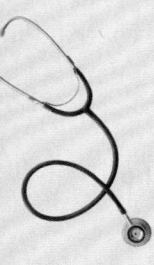

Case Study

Mr. Treeton, a 61-year-old male, visited his optometrist for his annual eye examination. Sally met him and began the initial procedures, including color vision testing, keratometry, autorefraction, visual fields, measuring pupil distance (PD) and visual acuities, and taking his blood pressure. Mr. Treeton's chief complaint was decreased vision in the right eye for approximately 3 weeks. The diminished visual acuity was gradual.

Upon examination, the optometrist discovered that Mr. Treeton had a history of diabetic retinopathy. His medical history indicated that he has had insulin-dependent diabetes mellitus for 13 years, hypertension for 15 years, myocardial infarction, and cardiac arrhythmia. His social history indicated no alcohol or tobacco use. There is a family history of heart disease and hypertension. The following results were obtained.

Visual Acuity

Eye	With Correction	Pinhole	Near
right	20/70	20/40−1	J8
left	20/25−2		J1

Other Measures

Measure	Value
Applanation tensions	18 right eye; 20 left eye at 9:20 AM
PD	68 mm
Pupils	Both pupils are 4 mm in size with brisk response
Blood pressure	170/110
Color vision	7/14 right eye; 8/14 left eye

Slit-Lamp Examination

Measure	Right Eye	Left Eye
Conjunctiva	1+ injection	1+ injection
Cornea	Clear	Clear
Anterior chamber	Deep and quiet	Deep and quiet
Iris	Within normal limits	Within normal limits
* Lens	2+ NS; 1+ CS	2+ NS

*NS = nuclear sclerosis; CS = cortical spokes. Both NS and CS are types of cataracts.

Recommendation

• Fluorescein angiogram to further define.

continued from page 393

Case Study Questions

Select the best answer to each of the following questions.

1. **Applanation tensions (the force required to flatten a small area of the cornea) are measured by tonometry, which indicates the intraocular pressure. Mr. Treeton's results show _____.**

   a. 18 in the left eye and 20 in the right eye
   b. 18 in the right eye and 20 in the left eye
   c. 25 in the left eye and 70 in the right eye
   d. 20 in the left eye and 20 in the right eye

2. **The test results for the cornea _____.**

   a. are normal
   b. are abnormal
   c. indicate cataracts

3. **The PD is 68 mm. This means that the _____ is 68 mm.**

   a. average size of each pupil
   b. primary distance between the eyes
   c. distance between the centers of each pupil
   d. photodensity

4. **Explain the recommended test. Why was this test suggested? _____**

5. **The instrument used to view various parts of the eye is called a _____.**

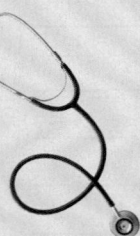

Real World Report

Sally just received Mr. Treeton's fluorescein angiography report.

PATIENT NAME: Randolph Treeton   DATE: July 30, 2011
REFERRED BY: Dr. Vanden   ATTENDING: Dr. Nolen
COLOR VISION: 7/14 right eye; 8/14 left eye   CONFRONTATION FIELDS: Full, each eye

INDIRECT OPHTHALMOSCOPY/BIOMICROSCOPY

RIGHT EYE

The optic nerve head is pink with sharp disc borders. The artery to vein (A/V) ratio is 1:2. The mid and far periphery shows an occasional intraretinal hemorrhage. There are some fine scattered intravitreal condensations. Views of the macula show scattered microaneurysms with a question of some mild intraretinal thickening adjacent to the fovea. There is no evidence of active neovascularization.

LEFT EYE

The optic nerve head is pink with sharp disc borders. The A/V ratio is 1:2. The mid and far periphery show an occasional intraretinal hemorrhage. Views of the posterior pole show one to two cotton-wool spots nasal to the optic nerve head. There are scattered perimacular microaneurysms but no definite evidence of active neovascularization.

continued

continued from page 394

IMPRESSION

- Background diabetic retinopathy.
- Bilateral vitreous degeneration.
- Rule out clinically significant macular edema.
- Nuclear sclerotic and cortical cataractous changes.
- Mild intraretinal ischemia.
- Essential hypertension.

Real World Report Questions

The following exercises review the medical terms used in the preceding medical report.

1. **The term *intraretinal hemorrhage* was used for both the right and the left eye.**

   a. *Intra-* means

   _____.

   b. *Retinal* refers to the

   _____.

   c. *Hem-* means

   _____.

   d. Thus *intraretinal hemorrhage* means

   _____.

2. **The report noted that there was no evidence of neovascularization. *Neovascularization* means _____.**

3. **Perimacular microaneurysms would be located _____ the macula.**

   a. around or adjacent to
   b. behind
   c. on
   d. in

4. **Macular edema is the medical term for macular**

   _____.

5. **Define the following medical terms used in the report.**

   a. intraretinal ischemia

   _____

   b. vitreous degeneration

   _____

   c. cortical cataractous changes

   _____

Review and Application

Multiple-Choice Questions

....

Select the best answer to each of the following questions.

1. Special senses refer to _____.
   a. olfaction   b. gustation   c. vision and hearing   d. all of these

2. The three anatomical regions of the ear are the _____.
   a. external ear, middle ear, and internal ear   b. malleus, incus, and stapes   c. arachnoid mater, pia mater, and dura mater   d. anterior cavity, posterior cavity, and anteroposterior cavity

3. The myringa is also known as the _____.
   a. pinna   b. tympanic membrane   c. auditory tube   d. cochlea

4. A patient presents with constant "ringing white noise" in her ears. This ringing is termed _____.
   a. reflexia   b. aphonia   c. tinnitus   d. areflexia

Word Parts Exercises

....

Match the word part with its correct definition.

_____ 5. oto-

_____ 6. ambly-

_____ 7. photo-

_____ 8. sinistro-

_____ 9. dextro-

a. dullness, dimness
b. ear
c. left side, toward the left
d. light
e. right side, toward the right

Using the following word parts, form a medical term for each definition. Each word part is used only once.

blephar-
hyper-
-itis
retino-
-opia
-pathy

10. visual image focused behind the retina; farsightedness _____

11. disease of the retina _____

12. eyelid inflammation _____

Matching

Match the ear part with its correct description.

_____ 13. auditory ossicles

_____ 14. auricle

_____ 15. external ear

_____ 16. semicircular canals

_____ 17. auditory tube

a. auricle, external acoustic meatus, and ceruminous glands
b. malleus, incus, and stapes
c. outer, cartilaginous structure projecting from head
d. bony tubes positioned in three planes that are involved with equilibrium
e. connecting tube between middle ear and pharynx

Match the eye part with its correct description.

_____ 18. choroid

_____ 19. pupil

_____ 20. sclera

_____ 21. retina

_____ 22. opticnerve

_____ 23. iris

a. cranial nerve II
b. whitish, outer layer of eyeball
c. opening
d. pigmented vascular layer that keeps the eye dark
e. colored portion visible to exterior
f. light-sensitive membrane containing rods and cones

Match the eye disorder with its correct definition.

_____ 24. strabismus

_____ 25. macular degeneration

_____ 26. myopia

_____ 27. nystagmus

_____ 28. blepharitis

_____ 29. chalazion

a. involuntary, oscillatory eyeball movement
b. problem related to abnormal alignment of the eyes
c. pathological changes of the macula
d. nearsightedness
e. inflammation of the eyelid caused by a blocked tarsal gland
f. inflammation of the eyelid caused by allergy or infection

Match the ear disorder with its correct definition.

_____ 30. presbycusis

_____ 31. cholesteatoma

_____ 32. Ménière disease

a. cyst of the middle ear that grows into the bone
b. specific disease of the internal ear
c. age-related hearing loss

Definitions

Identify the test or diagnostic procedure described by each of the following definitions.

33. measurement of intraocular pressure _____

34. visualization of the external acoustic meatus _____

35. record of auditory acuity _____

Identify the disorder or disease described by each of the following key characteristics.

36. inflammation of the conjunctiva _____

37. eye disorder that results from irregular cornea or lens curvature _____

Provide the medical term for the following definitions.

38. antibacterial enzyme of tears _____

39. eye sensitivity to light _____

40. chamber between the semicircular canals that is involved with equilibrium _____

For each of the following, indicate whether the treatment involves the eye or the ear.

41. scleral buckle _____

44. stapedectomy _____

42. vitrectomy _____

45. extracapsular cataract extraction _____

43. myringotomy _____

46. tympanostomy _____

Write the adjective form for each given term.

47. cornea _____

48. pupil _____

Spelling

Identify the correctly spelled term in each set.

49. _____
   a. astigmatism
   b. assitigmatism
   c. assigmatizm
   d. astimetism

50. _____
   a. koroid
   b. choroid
   c. coroid
   d. coroyd

51. _____
   a. labyrinthitis
   b. labirinthitis
   c. laberinthitis
   d. labarinthitis

52. _____
   a. fakoemulsification
   b. phakoemulsification
   c. phacoemulsification
   d. phackoemulsification

Unscramble

Unscramble the letters to form a medical term.

53. tipoc scid _____

56. llamsue _____

54. eialcps ssseen _____

57. pastes _____

55. splari gonra _____

Abbreviations

Provide the term for the abbreviations and then define the terms.

58. ENG = _____

59. LASIK surgery = _____

60. CN II = _____

Analogies

Provide a medical term to complete a meaningful analogy.

61. Pinna is to auricle as eardrum is to _____.

62. Rods are to dim vision as _____ are to color vision.

Short Answer

Answer the following questions.

63. Patient Russell presents with a stroke affecting vision in his left eye. Using medical and common terminology, describe what the patient is experiencing. _____

Labeling

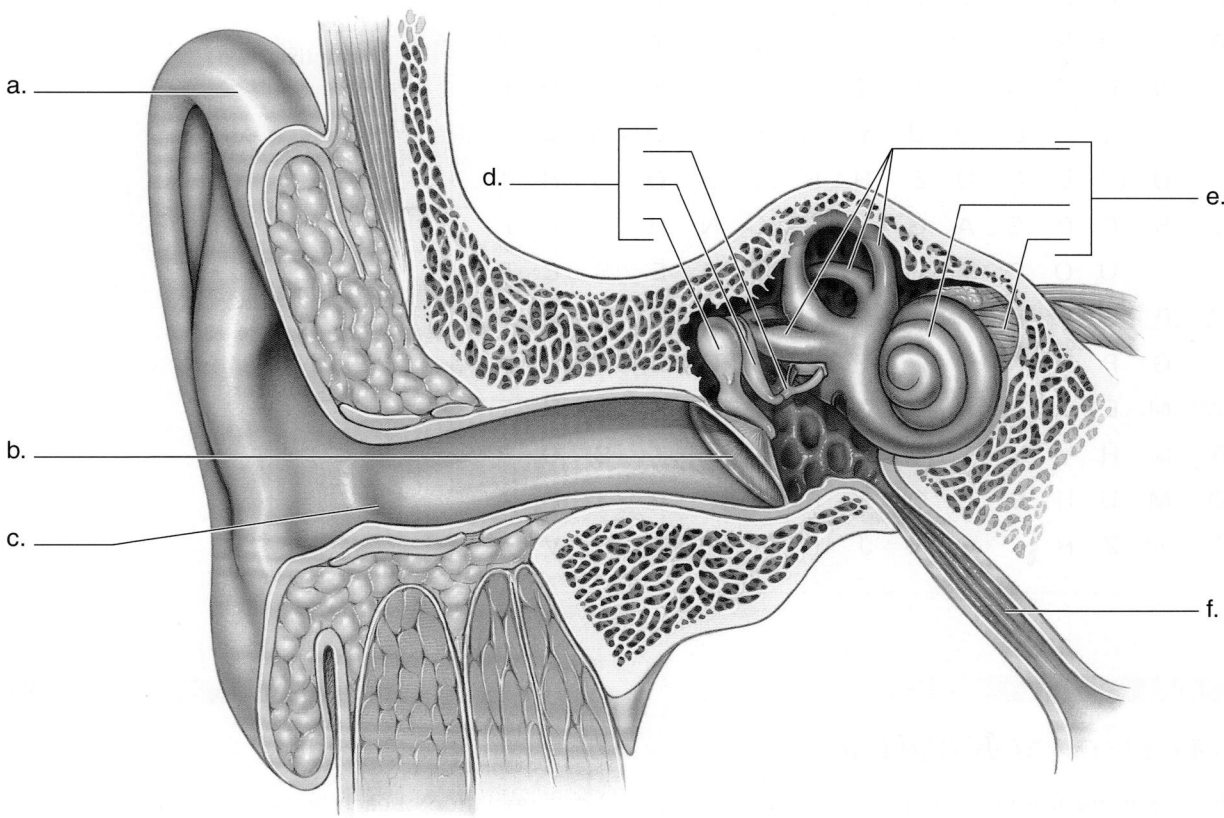

Word Search

Find the medical terms hidden in the puzzle.

```
R  Z  K  F  R  P  A  K  E  F  F  H  H  L  A  E
E  E  Q  S  J  N  C  S  U  K  R  U  J  E  R  B
F  L  T  G  E  L  C  I  R  U  A  Z  N  V  O  U
R  B  K  I  R  S  O  L  D  E  L  R  Q  N  R  T
A  A  I  Q  N  O  M  P  X  I  O  C  Y  F  R  Y
C  E  N  R  C  A  M  T  T  C  O  L  M  H  G  R
T  L  C  E  G  E  O  U  V  I  A  R  O  W  Z  O
I  H  U  T  D  D  Z  H  B  C  D  O  Q  H  T
O  C  S  P  P  G  A  G  Y  S  O  N  H  H  H  I
N  O  J  U  O  P  T  R  X  P  U  D  E  S  C  D
B  C  P  S  I  R  I  A  S  P  B  O  Z  R  R  U
L  I  G  P  H  N  O  I  H  V  S  Q  E  Q  V  A
L  W  M  E  T  X  N  M  A  C  U  L  A  U  V  E
Q  R  M  H  Y  Y  C  M  N  S  N  J  T  S  Q  P
R  O  M  U  H  S  U  O  E  R  T  I  V  Z  O  A
L  C  W  Z  H  C  O  N  J  U  N  C  T  I  V  A
```

accommodation
aqueous humor
auditory tube
auricle
bony labyrinth
choroid
cochlea
conjunctiva
cornea
incus
iris
macula
optic nerve
pupil
refraction
retina
rhodopsin
vitreous humor

Vocabulary Review

Review the key terms from this chapter, study the spelling and pronunciation of each term, and write its definition in the space provided. Listen to the audio available for most terms at http://thepoint.lww.com/nath2e and pronounce each term for yourself. Then check the box when you feel confident that you know the definition and can pronounce the term correctly.

Key Term	Pronunciation	Definition
❏ **accommodation**		_____
❏ **age-related macular degeneration (AMD)**	(MACK-yoo-lair)	_____
❏ **amblyopia**	(am-blee-OH-pee-uh)	_____
❏ **aqueous humor**	(AY-kwee-us)	_____
❏ **astigmatism**	(uh-STIG-muh-tiz-um)	_____
❏ **audiogram**	(AW-dee-oh-gram)	_____
❏ **audiometry**	(aw-dee-OM-e-tree)	_____
❏ **auditory ossicles**	(AW-di-tor-ee OS-i-kulz)	_____
❏ **auditory tube**	(AW-di-tor-ee)	_____
❏ **auricle**	(AW-ri-kul)	_____

Key Term	Pronunciation	Definition
❏ blepharitis	(blef-uh-RYE-tis)	_____
❏ blepharoptosis	(blef-uh-rop-TOH-sis)	_____
❏ bony labyrinth		_____
❏ cataract	(KAT-uh-rakt)	_____
❏ ceruminous glands	(se-ROO-mi-nus)	_____
❏ chalazion	(kay-LAY-zee-on)	_____
❏ cholesteatoma	(koh-les-tee-uh-TOH-muh)	_____
❏ choroid	(KOR-oid)	_____
❏ ciliary body	(SIL-ee-err-ee)	_____
❏ cochlea	(KOCK-lee-uh)	_____
❏ conduction deafness		_____
❏ cones		_____
❏ conjunctiva	(kon-junk-TYE-vuh)	_____
❏ conjunctivitis	(kun-junk-ti-VYE-tis)	_____
❏ cornea	(KOR-nee-uh)	_____
❏ cryotherapy	(krye-oh-THERR-uh-pee)	_____
❏ deafness		_____
❏ detached retina	(RET-i-nuh)	_____
❏ diabetic retinopathy	(dye-uh-BET-ick ret-i-NOP-uh-thee)	_____
❏ electronystagmography (ENG)	(ee-leck-troh-nigh-stag-MOG-ruh-fee)	_____
❏ external acoustic meatus	(ecks-TUR-nul uh-KOOS-tick mee-AY-tus)	_____
❏ external ear	(ecks-TUR-nul)	_____
❏ flashes		_____
❏ floaters		_____
❏ fluorescein angiography	(floo-uh-RES-ee-in an-jee-OG-ruh-fee)	_____
❏ fovea centralis	(FOH-vee-uh sen-TRAY-lis)	_____
❏ glaucoma	(glaw-KOH-muh)	_____
❏ hair cells		_____
❏ hordeolum	(hor-DEE-oh-lum)	_____
❏ hyperopia	(high-pur-OH-pee-uh)	_____
❏ incus	(ING-kus)	_____
❏ internal ear		_____
❏ intraocular gas bubble	(in-truh-OCK-yoo-lur)	_____
❏ iris	(EYE-ris)	_____
❏ keratitis	(kehr-uh-TYE-tis)	_____
❏ labyrinthitis	(lab-i-rin-THIGH-tis)	_____

Key Term	Pronunciation	Definition
❏ lacrimal glands	(LACK-ri-mul)	
❏ laser photocoagulation	(foh-toh-koh-ag-yoo-LAY-shun)	
❏ LASIK surgery		
❏ lens	(LENZ)	
❏ lysozyme	(LYE-soh-zime)	
❏ macula	(MACK-yoo-luh)	
❏ macular degeneration	(MACK-yoo-lair)	
❏ malleus	(MAL-ee-us)	
❏ mastoiditis	(mas-toid-EYE-tis)	
❏ membranous labyrinth	(MEM-bruh-nus)	
❏ Ménière disease	(mey-NYEHR)	
❏ middle ear		
❏ myopia (M)	(migh-OH-pee-uh)	
❏ myringotomy	(mirr-in-GOT-uh-mee)	
❏ nystagmus	(nis-TAG-mus)	
❏ ophthalmoscope	(off-THAL-muh-skope)	
❏ optic disc	(OP-tick)	
❏ optic nerves (CN II)	(OP-tick)	
❏ otitis externa	(oh-TYE-tis ecks-TUR-nuh)	
❏ otitis media	(oh-TYE-tis MEE-dee-uh)	
❏ otosclerosis	(oh-toh-skle-ROH-sis)	
❏ otoscopy	(oh-TOS-kuh-pee)	
❏ oval window		
❏ palpebrae	(pal-PEE-bree)	
❏ photophobia	(foh-toh-FOH-bee-uh)	
❏ presbycusis	(prez-bee-KEW-sis)	
❏ presbyopia (Pr)	(prez-bee-OH-pee-uh)	
❏ pupil	(PEW-pil)	
❏ radial keratotomy	(kerr-uh-TOM-e-tree)	
❏ refraction	(ree-FRACK-shun)	
❏ retina	(RET-i-nuh)	
❏ retinopathy	(ret-i-NOP-uh-thee)	
❏ rhodopsin	(roh-DOP-sin)	
❏ rods		
❏ sclera	(SKLEER-uh)	
❏ scleral buckle	(SKLEER-ul)	
❏ semicircular canals	(sem-i-SIRR-kew-lur kuh-NALS)	
❏ sensorineural deafness	(sen-suh-ri-NEW-rul)	
❏ slit lamp		

Key Term	Pronunciation	Definition
❑ special senses		_____
❑ spiral organ		_____
❑ stapedectomy	(stay-pe-DECK-tuh-mee)	_____
❑ stapes	(STAY-peez)	_____
❑ strabismus	(stra-BIZ-mus)	_____
❑ tinnitus	(ti-NIGH-tus)	_____
❑ tonometry	(toh-NOM-e-tree)	_____
❑ tympanic membrane	(tim-PAN-ick)	_____
❑ tympanostomy tubes	(tim-puh-NOS-tuh-mee)	_____
❑ uveitis	(yoo-vee-EYE-tis)	_____
❑ vestibule		_____
❑ vision therapy		_____
❑ vitrectomy	(vi-TRECK-toh-mee)	_____
❑ vitreous humor	(VIT-ree-us)	_____

Answers

Word Grouping Exercises

Definition	Word Part	Definition	Word Part
blood vessel	vasculo-	old age	presby-, presbyo-
the choroid	choroido-	optical, eye	optico-, opto-
cold	cry-, cryo-	passage	meato-
cornea	kerat-, kerato-	pertaining to the eye	ophthalm-, ophthalmo-
dullness, dimness	ambly-	red color	rhod-, rhodo-
ear	A. auri- B. ot-, oto-	the retina	retin-, retino-
eye or ocular	ocul-, oculo-	right side, toward the right	dextr-, dextro-
eyelid	bleph-, blepharo-	sense of hearing	audio-
hardness	scler-, sclero-	three-dimensionality	stereo-
iris	irid-, irido-	tympanic membrane (eardrum)	myring-, myringo-
left side, toward the left	sinistro-	tympanum, drum	tympan-, tympani-, tympano-
light	phot-, photo-	vision	-opia,
nerve, nerve tissue	neur-, neuri-, neuro-		

Word Building Exercises

Word Part	Meaning	Common or Known Word	Example Medical Term
audio-	sense of hearing	audio	audiologist
auri-	ear	aural	auricle
dynamo-	force, energy	dynamite	dynamic equilibrium
irid-, irido-	iris	iridescent	iridectomy
neur-, neuri-, neuro-	nerve, nerve tissue	neuron	neuron
optico-, opto-	optical, eye	optical illusion	optometry
ot-, oto-	ear	otitis	otoscope
phot-, photo-	light	photograph	photoreceptor
retin-, retino-	the retina	retina	retina
scler-, sclero-	hardness	sclera	sclera
stereo-	three-dimensionality;	stereo	stereopsis
vasculo-	blood vessel	vascular	vascular tunic

Key Term Practice

Special Senses Preview

1. The five senses known collectively as the special senses are olfaction, gustation, vision, equilibrium, and hearing.

Eye and Vision

1. Cones
2. retina
3. Rods
4. iris
5. Vitreous humor

Ear, Hearing, and Equilibrium

1. oval window
2. auditory tube
3. tympanic membrane
4. Hair cells
5. auricle

General Eye Disorders

1. cataract
2. ophthalmoscope
3. tonometry
4. Keratitis
5. Glaucoma

Refractive Problems

1. a. hyperopia (H); b. myopia (M)
2. old age, -opia; presbyopia (Pr)
3. astigmatism
4. radial keratotomy
5. LASIK surgery

Retina Disorders

1. floaters; flashes
2. vitrectomy
3. nystagmus
4. Retinopathy
5. detached retina

Eyelid Disorders

1. hordeolum
2. eyelid; blepharoptosis
3. *blephar-; -itis*; blepharitis
4. chalazion

External Ear Disorders and Deafness

1. sensorineural
2. Otitis externa
3. Presbycusis; *presby-*
4. deafness
5. audiogram

Middle Ear and Tympanic Membrane Disorders

1. Otoscopy
2. cholesteatoma
3. otitis media; *ot-*; *-itis*; *media*
4. myringotomy; *myring-*
5. mastoiditis

Internal Ear Disorders

1. labyrinthitis
2. Electronystagmography
3. Ménière disease
4. tinnitus
5. stapedectomy

Common Abbreviations Exercises

1. Pr = presbyopia
2. IOL = intraocular lens
3. PD = pupil distance
4. electronystagmography = ENG
5. visual field = VF

Case Study

1. b is the correct answer.
   - a is incorrect because it is 18 in the right eye and 20 in the left eye.
   - c and d are incorrect because these numbers were obtained from the visual acuity test.
2. a is the correct answer.
   - b is incorrect because the cornea should be clear.
   - c is incorrect because the lens appears cloudy with cataracts; this question refers to the cornea.
3. c is the correct answer.
   - a is incorrect because the pupils are not that large, and PD stands for "papillary distance," or distance between the pupils.
   - b is incorrect because the measure *primary distance between the eyes* is not used in optometric medicine.
   - d is incorrect because *photodensity* is not used in optometric medicine.
4. A fluorescein angiogram was suggested because this test can provide a good picture of the retina. Mr. Treeton has diabetes and a history of diabetic retinopathy. The angiogram would give clear visualization of the retinal vessels.
5. slit lamp.

Real World Report

1. a. within, in; b. retina; c. blood; d. bleeding within the retina
2. new blood vessel growth where it should not be occurring
3. a
4. swelling
5. a. vascular obstruction within the retina; b. deterioration of the vitreous; c. opacity of the lens cortex (outer portion) is changing; cataract forming on lens cortex

Review and Application

1. d
2. a
3. b
4. c
5. b
6. a
7. d
8. c
9. e
10. hyperopia
11. retinopathy
12. blepharitis
13. b
14. c

15. a
16. d
17. e
18. d
19. c
20. b
21. f
22. a
23. e
24. b
25. c
26. d
27. a
28. f

29. e
30. c
31. a
32. b
33. tonometry
34. otoscopy
35. audiogram
36. conjunctivitis
37. astigmatism
38. lysozyme
39. photophobia
40. vestibule
41. eye
42. eye

43. ear
44. ear
45. eye
46. ear
47. corneal
48. pupillary
49. a
50. b
51. a
52. c
53. optic disc
54. special senses
55. spiral organ
56. malleus

57. stapes
58. ENG = electronystagmography; method of recording eye movements in response to stimuli
59. LASIK = *las*er-assisted *in* situ *k*eratomileusis; eye surgery to correct vision in which a laser reshapes the inner cornea

60. CN II = cranial nerve II, also called the optic nerve; cranial nerve that connects the eye to the brain
61. tympanic membrane or myringa
62. cones
63. The patient is experiencing a stroke (brain attack) with visual disturbances in the oculus sinister, or left eye.

Labeling

a. auricle
d. auditory ossicles
b. tympanic membrane
e. internal ear
c. external acoustic meatus
f. auditory tube

Word Search

```
R  Z  K  F  R  P  A  K  E  F  F  H  H  L  A  E
E  E  Q  S  J  N  C  S  U  K  R  U  J  E  R  B
F  L  T  G  E  L  C  I  R  U  A  Z  N  V  O  U
R  B  K  I  R  S  O  L  D  E  L  R  Q  N  R  T
A  A  I  Q  N  O  M  P  X  I  O  C  Y  F  R  Y
C  E  N  R  C  A  M  T  T  C  O  L  M  H  G  R
T  L  C  E  G  E  O  U  V  I  A  R  O  W  Z  O
I  H  U  T  D  D  D  Z  H  B  C  D  O  Q  H  T
O  C  S  P  P  G  A  G  Y  S  O  N  H  H  H  I
N  O  J  U  O  P  T  R  X  P  U  D  E  S  C  D
B  C  P  S  I  R  I  A  S  P  B  O  Z  R  R  U
L  I  G  P  H  N  O  I  H  V  S  Q  E  Q  V  A
L  W  M  E  T  X  N  M  A  C  U  L  A  U  V  E
Q  R  M  H  Y  Y  C  M  N  S  N  J  T  S  Q  P
R  O  M  U  H  S  U  O  E  R  T  I  V  Z  O  A
L  C  W  Z  H  C  O  N  J  U  N  C  T  I  V  A
```

accommodation
aqueous humor
auditory tube
auricle
bony labyrinth
choroid
cochlea
conjunctiva
cornea
incus
iris
macula
optic nerve
pupil
refraction
retina
rhodopsin
vitreous humor

Vocabulary Review

Key Term	Definition	Key Term	Definition
accommodation	the automatic adjustment of the eye to focus an object to give clear vision	auricle	external cartilaginous structure that projects from the head to direct sound waves
age-related macular degeneration (AMD)	disease affecting the macula of the eye as a result of aging	blepharitis	inflammation of the eyelid
		blepharoptosis	upper eyelid drooping
amblyopia	loss or lack of development of central vision in one eye that is unrelated to any eye health problem; also called lazy eye	bony labyrinth	complex of tubes and chambers that includes the semicircular canals, vestibule, and cochlea
		cataract	partial or complete opacity of the lens
aqueous humor	watery, nourishing eye secretion in the anterior chamber	ceruminous glands	glands that secrete cerumen (earwax) in the external acoustic meatus
astigmatism	eye disorder that results from irregular cornea or lens curvature	chalazion	inflammation of the eyelid from a blocked tarsal gland
audiogram	record of auditory acuity as measured by an audiometer	cholesteatoma	cyst in the middle ear that grows into the bone
audiometry	evaluation using an audiometer to test a person's ability to hear a range of sounds	choroid	pigmented vascular layer that keeps the eye dark
		ciliary body	thickened region of the choroid that encircles the lens of the eye and connects the choroid to the iris
auditory ossicles	three small bones (malleus, incus, stapes) of the middle ear		
auditory tube	canal connecting the middle ear to the pharynx (throat)	cochlea	internal ear structure that houses the essential organs of hearing

Key Term	Definition
conduction deafness	hearing loss with ossicle involvement
cones	cone-shaped photoreceptors that provide color vision
conjunctiva	mucous membrane covering inner surfaces of the eyelids
conjunctivitis	inflammation of the conjunctiva
cornea	transparent anterior part of the eye
cryotherapy	tissue freezing
deafness	partial or complete hearing loss
detached retina	separation of the retina from its normal position on the posterior eye
diabetic retinopathy	retinal disease resulting from diabetes mellitus
electronystagmography (ENG)	method of recording eye movements in response to stimuli
external acoustic meatus	passageway between the auricle and tympanic membrane (eardrum)
external ear	outer ear that contains the auricle, external acoustic meatus, and ceruminous glands
flashes	illusion of flashing lights seen in the field of vision
floaters	abnormal small specks seen in the field of vision
fluorescein angiography	x-ray mapping of the vascular eye pattern after introduction of a yellow dye into a peripheral vein
fovea centralis	region of greatest visual acuity
glaucoma	eye disease caused by increased intra-ocular pressure
hair cells	receptors of hearing in the internal ear
hordeolum	a sty
hyperopia	refractive problem in which the light rays focus behind the retina; commonly called farsightedness
incus	anvil-shaped middle ear bone between the malleus and the stapes
internal ear	fluid-filled part of the ear that contains the cochlea and semicircular canals
intraocular gas bubble	introduction of a gas bubble into the vitreous cavity
iris	colored portion of the eye that regulates the amount of light entering the pupil
keratitis	inflammation of the cornea
labyrinthitis	inflammation of the internal ear labyrinth that causes nausea and loss of balance
lacrimal glands	tear-secreting glands
laser photocoagulation	treatment technique that cauterizes blood vessels with a laser

Key Term	Definition
LASIK surgery	eye surgery to correct vision in which a laser reshapes the inner cornea; acronym for *las*er-assisted *in* situ *k*eratomileusis
lens	elastic, transparent portion of the eye that changes shape and refracts light
lysozyme	antibacterial enzyme of tears
macula	a small spot in the middle of the retina that contains the fovea centralis
macular degeneration	pathological changes of the macula
malleus	hammer-shaped middle ear bone
mastoiditis	inflammation of mastoid cells in the mastoid process of the temporal bone
membranous labyrinth	fluid-filled tube that lines the bony labyrinth
Ménière disease	disease of the internal ear caused by fluid accumulation in the labyrinth; it is characterized by deafness, tinnitus, and vertigo movements
middle ear	space between the external ear and internal ear that houses the auditory ossicles (malleus, incus, and stapes)
myopia (M)	refractive problem in which light rays focus in front of the retina; commonly called nearsightedness
myringotomy	incision through the tympanic membrane (myringa) to drain fluid
nystagmus	involuntary oscillatory eyeball movement
ophthalmoscope	medical instrument with a light source and mirror used to examine the eye's interior through the pupil
optic disc	circular area of the retina where nerve fibers converge to form the optic nerve; also called the blind spot
optic nerves (CN II)	cranial nerves that connect the eye to the brain
otitis externa	inflammation of the external acoustic meatus caused by an infection; also called swimmer's ear
otitis media	acute inflammation of the middle ear cavity, usually due to an infection
otosclerosis	ear disorder in which new bone is deposited in the internal ear
otoscopy	visualization of the external acoustic meatus and tympanic membrane with an otoscope
oval window	membranous opening between the middle ear and the internal ear
palpebrae	eyelids
photodynamic therapy with Visudyne	treatment procedure in which the interaction of the drug with a nonthermal laser closes the blood vessels in the retina
photophobia	eye sensitivity to light

Key Term	Definition	Key Term	Definition
presbycusis	hearing loss associated with old age	**stapedectomy**	surgical removal of the stapes
presbyopia (Pr)	vision disorder resulting from diminished accommodation due to impaired lens elasticity	**stapes**	stirrup-shaped middle ear bone connected to the oval window
pupil	opening in the iris	**strabismus**	problem related to abnormal alignment of the eyes; also called crossed eyes
radial keratotomy	surgical procedure for correcting vision in which incisions are made into the cornea	**tinnitus**	perception of sound, such as ringing or hissing in the ears, in the absence of any environmental noise
refraction	bending of light rays to focus on the retina	**tonometry**	measurement of eye pressure using a tonometer
retina	light-sensitive membrane containing rods and cones that receives images from the lens and sends them to the brain	**tympanic membrane**	membrane separating the external ear from the middle ear; also called the eardrum
retinopathy	noninflammatory degenerative disease of the retina	**tympanostomy tubes**	tubes placed as a passageway for fluid drainage through the tympanic membrane
rhodopsin	reddish light-sensitive pigment in rods that decomposes in the presence of light	**uveitis**	inflammation of the uvea (iris, ciliary body, and lens)
rods	rod-shaped photoreceptors that provide vision in dim light	**vertigo**	the sensation of dizziness while still that causes loss of balance
sclera	whitish, outer layer of the eyeball	**vestibule**	chamber between the semicircular canals that is involved with equilibrium
scleral buckle	a silicone band that is placed on the scleral periphery to tighten the retina	**vision therapy**	sequence of activities that are individually prescribed to develop ocular muscles, visual skills, and visual processing; also called orthoptic training
semicircular canals	bony tubes situated in three planes that are involved with equilibrium		
sensorineural deafness	hearing loss involving a damaged cochlea or auditory nerve	**vitrectomy**	surgical removal of vitreous humor and simultaneous replacement with a synthetic vitreous gel
slit lamp	instrument used to examine the eye while aiming a light beam directly into it	**vitreous humor**	semisolid fluid of the eye between the lens and retina
special senses	the five senses of olfaction, gustation, vision, equilibrium, and hearing		
spiral organ	location of the hearing receptors in the cochlea; also called organ of Corti		

CHAPTER 9

Endocrine System

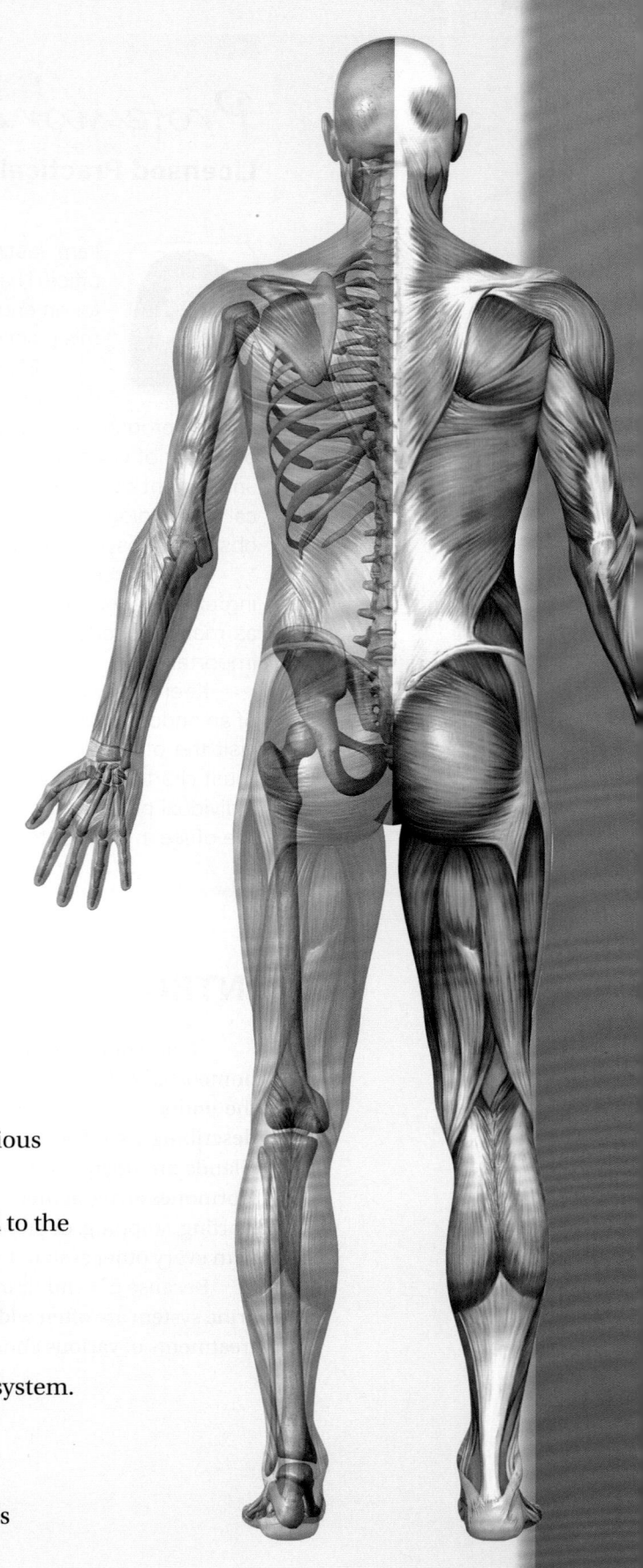

OBJECTIVES

After completing this chapter, you should be able to:

1. State the meanings of word parts related to the endocrine system.

2. Identify and locate organs and glands of the endocrine system.

3. Identify the endocrine glands, their hormones, and key actions of each.

4. Explain the role of the endocrine system in overall body functioning.

5. Define common signs, symptoms, and treatments of various endocrine system diseases.

6. Describe clinical tests and diagnostic procedures related to the endocrine system.

7. Describe anatomical and physiological alterations of the endocrine system throughout the life span.

8. Define common abbreviations related to the endocrine system.

9. Define terms used in medical reports involving the endocrine system.

10. Define, spell, and pronounce the chapter's medical terms correctly.

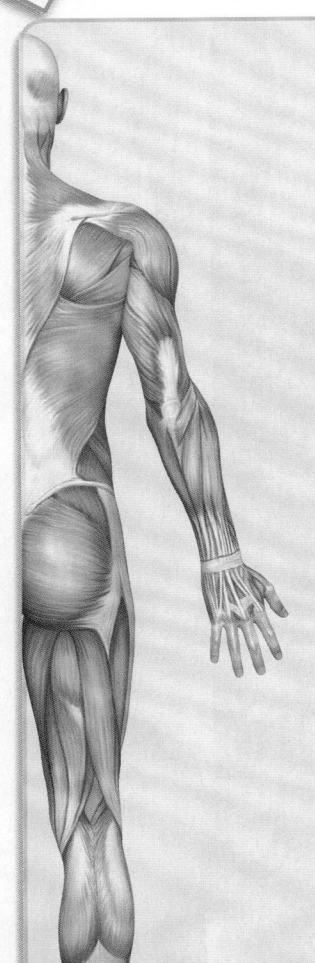

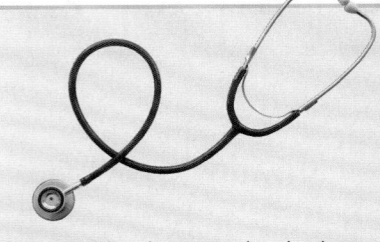

Professional Profile

Licensed Practical Nurse

I am Justina, a licensed practical nurse (LPN) working in an endocrinology office. I have been a nurse for 20 years. Most recently I have been working for an endocrinologist in private practice. The majority of patients seen in this practice have diabetes, but thyroid disorders are also common.

LPN educational programs require less time for completion than do registered nurse (RN) courses of study. The state-approved practical nursing program that I attended was offered by a local vocational school and consisted of 1 year of classroom study and supervised clinical practice. Basic nursing concepts and patient care–related subjects were covered during training. I took courses in medical terminology, basic anatomy and physiology, medical-surgical nursing, pediatrics, obstetrics, psychiatric nursing, drug administration, nutrition, and first aid.

After successful completion of the educational program, I had to pass a licensing examination before I could be called an LPN. LPNs are not permitted to perform as many procedures as are RNs, but our role in the health care setting is extremely important.

Keen observational skills are critical to the LPN profession. Patients under the care of an endocrinologist, a physician who specializes in disorders of glands, must routinely visit the office for follow-up and continuing care. For example, patients with diabetes must chart their daily blood glucose levels, which the staff reviews when determining individual patient protocols. Thyroid disorders often require iodine-uptake tests, which the office interprets to decide on the best treatment options.

INTRODUCTION

*T*he endocrine system is involved with complicated processes aimed at maintaining homeostasis, the state of body equilibrium. The nervous system operates in conjunction with the endocrine system. For this reason, the term *neuroendocrine system* is often used when describing its roles. Two components of the endocrine system are glands and hormones. Glands are organs or clusters of specialized cells, and hormones are chemical messengers. Hormones arrive at their destinations through the systemic circulation and are responsible for starting, stopping, or orchestrating some types of body activity. The endocrine system interacts with every other system to create balance in the body.

Because the endocrine system affects so many other body systems, disorders of the endocrine system are often widespread. Signs, symptoms, clinical tests, diagnostic procedures, and treatments of various endocrine diseases are discussed in this chapter.

MEDICAL TERM PARTS

Word Parts

Medical term prefixes, suffixes, and combining forms related to the endocrine system are introduced in this section.

Word Part	Meaning
acro-	extreme
aden-, adeno-	gland, glandular
adren-, adrenal-, adreno-	relating to the adrenal gland
calc-, calci-	relating to calcium
cortico-	cortex
end-, endo-	within, inner
gluc-, gluco-	glucose
glyco-	sugar
hypo-	deficient, below normal
lact-, lacti-, lacto-	milk
mel-, meli-, melo-	honey, sugar
myx-, myxo-	mucus
pancreat-, pancreatico-, pancreato-, pancreo-	involving the pancreas
para-	alongside, near
-phage, -phagia, -phagy	eating
thyr-, thyreo-, thyro-	thyroid gland
toco-	childbirth
-tropic	having an affinity for

Word Grouping Exercises

Using the *Medical Term Parts* table, identify the prefix, suffix, or combining form for each of the following definitions. The first one has been done as an example.

Definition	Word Part
glucose	*gluc-, gluco-*
alongside, near	
childbirth	
cortex	
deficient, below normal	
eating	
extreme	
gland, glandular	
having an affinity for	

continued

continued from page 413

Definition	Word Part
honey, sugar	
involving the pancreas	
milk	
mucus	
relating to calcium	
relating to the adrenal gland	
sugar	
thyroid gland	
within, inner	

Word Building Exercises

Word parts introduced in the *Medical Term Parts* section are listed in the following table. For this exercise, first supply the meaning of each word part, then use the word part to build a word you already know. The word you list under *Common or Known Word* does not have to be a medical term; a commonly used word is fine. Be sure, however, that the word correctly reflects the intended meaning. The first one has been done as an example. Check your answers in a dictionary.

Word Part	Meaning	Common or Known Word	Example Medical Term
aden-, adeno-	*gland, glandular*	*adenoid*	adenohypophysis
adren-, adrenal-, adreno-			adrenal gland
end-, endo-			endocrine
gluc-, gluco-			glucose
hypo-			hypoparathyroidism
lact-, lacti-, lacto-			prolactin
mel-, meli-, melo-			diabetes mellitus
pancreat-, pancreatico-, pancreato-, pancreo-			pancreas
para-			parathyroid glands
thyr-, thyreo-, thyro-			thyroid gland

ANATOMY AND PHYSIOLOGY

Endocrine System Preview

The **endocrine system** is composed of glands and organs that secrete hormones directly into the blood to ensure long-term regulation and internal balance. This regulation and balance is called *homeostasis*. A **gland** is an organized mass of cells that functions as a secreting or excreting organ. **Secretion** is the process by which substances are produced and discharged from the gland for a particular physiological function. **Excretion** refers to separating materials from the blood to be eliminated as waste. Exocrine glands, such as sweat glands, excrete a substance into a duct, but endocrine glands have no ducts, so the blood absorbs their products directly. For this reason, endocrine glands are sometimes referred to as *ductless glands*. The **hormones** that they release or secrete are chemical substances formed in one gland and transported in the blood to another site, termed target cells, where they exert their effects. The effects of hormones, such as changing the metabolic or functional activity of other cells, are slower to appear and longer lasting than those of neurotransmitters, supplied by the nervous system. Hormones exert their effects on numerous cells, body tissues, and organs. Hormonal effects are widespread and important for maintaining homeostatic balance.

Target cells play a critical role in the endocrine system. A **target cell** is a cell that responds to a particular hormone. It does so because it has specific receptors to which certain hormone molecules can bind. Think of the hormone and target cell as if they were a lock and key—only one particular hormone can interact with one type of receptor site, much like only one key can fit a specific lock. When the hormone combines with the binding site (receptor attachment) of the target cell, the interaction stimulates activity.

Tropic hormones and trophic hormones are chemical messengers released from one gland that stimulate another endocrine gland or organ to secrete its hormones. The word part *-tropic* is derived from the Greek and means "having an affinity for." Thus hormones with *-tropic, -trophic,* or *-tropin* in their names are attracted to, or target, other endocrine structures.

Figure 9-1 illustrates the major endocrine glands and organs: pineal gland, hypothalamus, pituitary gland, thyroid gland, parathyroid glands, thymus gland, adrenal glands, pancreas, and ovaries (in females) or testes (in males). Key glands and their particular hormones are discussed in general terms in the following sections.

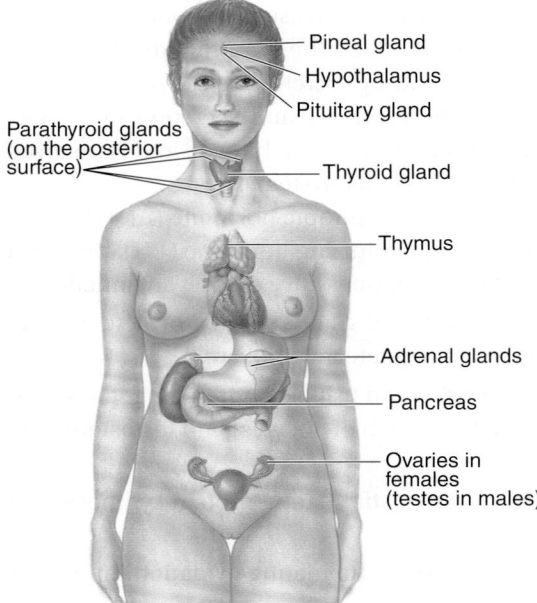

Pineal gland
Hypothalamus
Pituitary gland
Parathyroid glands (on the posterior surface)
Thyroid gland
Thymus
Adrenal glands
Pancreas
Ovaries in females (testes in males)

Figure 9-1 Organs and glands of the endocrine system.

KEY TERM	Definition
endocrine (EN-doh-krin) **system**	composed of glands and organs that secrete hormones directly into the blood to ensure long-term regulation and internal balance (homeostasis)
gland	an organized group of cells that functions as a secreting or excreting organ
secretion (se-KREE-shun)	process by which substances are produced and discharged from a gland for a particular physiological function
excretion (eck-SKREE-shun)	separating materials from the blood to be eliminated as waste
hormones (HOR-mohnz)	chemicals released by endocrine glands that are transported by blood to exert their effect at a site other than their origin
target cell	cell that responds to a particular hormone

KEY TERM PRACTICE: *Endocrine System Preview*

1. Ductless glands can be found in the _____ system.

2. Chemical messengers called _____ are part of the endocrine system.

3. Separating materials from the blood to be eliminated as waste is termed _____.

4. _____ is the process by which substances are produced and discharged from a gland for a particular physiological function.

5. A _____ is a cell that responds to a particular hormone.

Pituitary Gland

The **pituitary gland** (also called the hypophysis) is a small, oval endocrine gland about 1 cm (0.4 inch or the size of a pea) in diameter that is attached to the base of the brain. The pituitary gland is referred to as the master gland because it controls so many other endocrine glands. It has two main parts, each of which has two synonymous names. The pituitary gland as a whole is also referred to as the hypophysis. Its two lobes are the **anterior pituitary gland** (adenohypophysis) and the **posterior pituitary gland** (neurohypophysis). The anterior pituitary gland secretes hormones and the posterior pituitary gland stores and releases hormones.

A nearby region of the brain below the thalamus is called the **hypothalamus**. The hypothalamus coordinates the activity of the pituitary gland by secreting releasing hormones. Releasing hormones are substances that stimulate the synthesis and secretion of a given hormone. The hypothalamus also regulates body temperature, thirst, hunger, and is involved in sleep and emotions. The hormones are regulated by feedback systems.

Anterior pituitary gland hormones include adrenocorticotropic hormone (ACTH), follicle-stimulating hormone (FSH), growth hormone (GH), luteinizing hormone (LH), prolactin (PRL), and thyroid-stimulating hormone (TSH). These hormones have a variety of functions:

- Adrenocorticotropic hormone (ACTH) targets the adrenal gland, stimulating the adrenal cortex to produce corticosteroids, namely cortisol, to regulate metabolism.
- Follicle-stimulating hormone (FSH) targets the ovaries and testicles, stimulating the secretion of estrogen and progesterone in the ovaries (for growth of oocytes) and testosterone in the testes (for growth of sperm cells).
- Growth hormone (GH) targets bones and other tissues, stimulating protein synthesis and long bone growth.
- Luteinizing hormone (LH) targets the ovaries and testes, stimulating ovulation in females and the synthesis of testosterone in males.

- Prolactin (PRL) targets breast tissue, stimulating milk production (lactation).
- Thyroid-stimulating hormone (TSH) targets the thyroid gland, stimulating the production of thyroid hormones for regulating metabolism.

There is a narrow lobe between the anterior pituitary gland and the posterior pituitary gland called the *pars intermedia*. Melanocyte-stimulating hormone (MSH), secreted by this intermediate lobe, promotes melanin synthesis in the skin.

Only two hormones are associated with the posterior pituitary gland: antidiuretic hormone (ADH) and oxytocin (OXT). The posterior pituitary gland does not synthesize these hormones. Instead, it merely stores and releases them.

- Antidiuretic hormone (ADH), also called vasopressin, targets the kidneys. It promotes water retention by the kidneys and increases blood pressure.
- Oxytocin (OXT) targets the uterus and breasts, stimulating uterine contractions during labor and stimulating milk ejection into the ducts of the breasts. **Figure 9-2** shows the hypothalamus and pituitary gland, along with their secretions and target tissues.

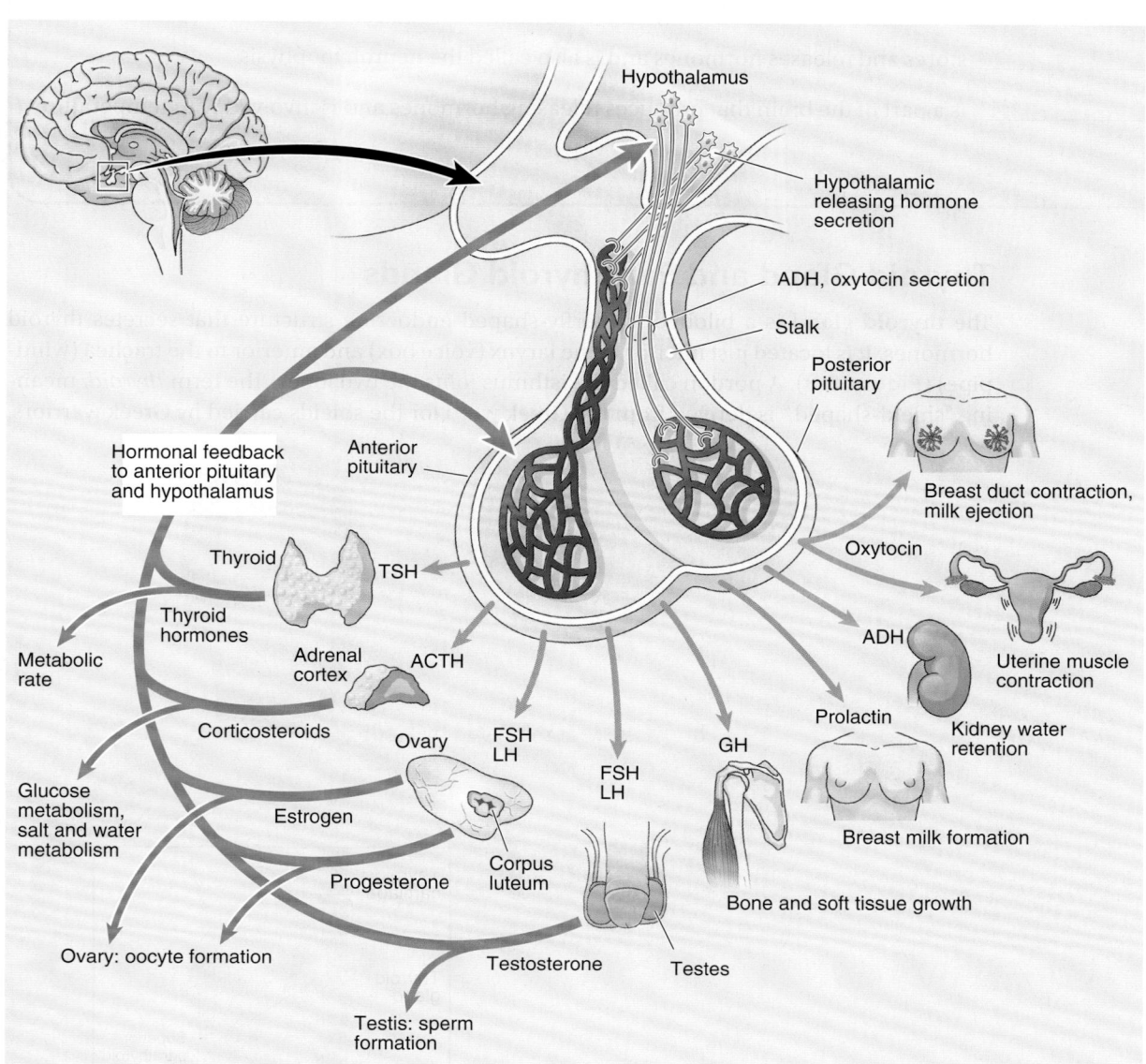

Figure 9-2 The hypothalamus, pituitary gland, and target organs and tissues. Arrows indicate targets and subsequent secretions.

KEY TERM	Definition
pituitary (pi-TEW-i-terr-ee) **gland**	master gland that orchestrates endocrine function; also called the hypophysis
anterior pituitary (pi-TEW-i-terr-ee) **gland**	part of the pituitary gland that secretes hormones; also called the adenohypophysis
posterior pituitary (pi-TEW-i-terr-ee) **gland**	part of the pituitary gland that stores and releases hormones; also called the neurohypophysis
hypothalamus (high-poh-THAL-uh-mus)	area of the brain that secretes releasing hormones and is involved with regulating temperature, thirst, and hunger

KEY TERM PRACTICE: *Pituitary Gland*

1. The master gland is known as the _____ or hypophysis.

2. The part of the pituitary gland that produces hormones and is also known as the adenohypophysis is termed the _____.

3. The _____ stores and releases hormones and is also called the neurohypophysis.

4. The _____ is a part of the brain that produces releasing hormones and is involved with temperature regulation.

Thyroid Gland and Parathyroid Glands

The **thyroid gland** is a bilobed, butterfly-shaped endocrine structure that secretes thyroid hormones. It is located just inferior to the larynx (voice box) and anterior to the trachea (windpipe) (**Figure 9-3**). A portion called the isthmus joins the two lobes. The term *thyroid*, meaning "shield-shaped," is derived from the Greek word for the shields carried by Greek warriors.

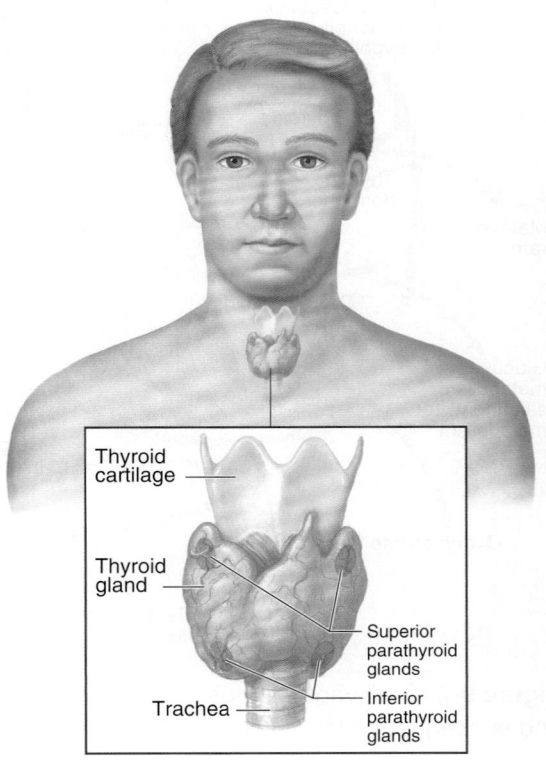

Figure 9-3 The thyroid gland and parathyroid glands.

Dietary iodine is essential for making thyroid hormones. Iodine can be obtained only by eating food that contains the mineral.

Three hormones are associated with this gland: thyroxine, triiodothyronine, and calcitonin. Thyroid hormones control metabolism and growth. Both **thyroxine (T$_4$)** (also called tetraiodothyronine) and **triiodothyronine (T$_3$)** increase metabolic rate, enhance protein synthesis, and stimulate the breakdown of lipids. Each gets its name from the number of iodine atoms found within its molecule. TSH from the anterior pituitary gland controls the secretion of hormones from the thyroid gland. **Calcitonin (CT)** *decreases* calcium ion concentrations in the blood. It does this by increasing the deposition of calcium in bones.

The **parathyroid glands** are four small endocrine glands that are embedded in the posterior surface of the thyroid gland (see **Figure 9-3**). These glands produce a calcium- and phosphorus-regulating hormone called **parathyroid hormone (PTH)**. Whereas calcitonin serves to lower blood calcium ion levels, PTH *increases* circulating blood calcium ion levels. It does this by mobilizing calcium from bone and enhancing reabsorption at the kidneys so that the calcium level in the blood rises. Through the combined actions of thyroid hormones and parathyroid hormones, calcium balance in the blood is achieved. PTH also causes a decrease in blood phosphate (phosphorus ion) concentration by causing the kidneys to conserve calcium and excrete phosphate.

KEY TERM	Definition
thyroid (THIGH-roid) **gland**	bilobed endocrine gland in the neck that secretes thyroid hormones responsible for growth and metabolism
thyroxine (thigh-ROCK-seen) **(T$_4$)**	a thyroid hormone that increases metabolic rate, enhances protein synthesis, and stimulates the breakdown of lipids; also called tetraiodothyronine
triiodothyronine (T$_3$) (trye-eye-oh-doh-THIGH-roh-neen)	a thyroid hormone that increases metabolic rate, enhances protein synthesis, and stimulates the breakdown of lipids
calcitonin (kal-si-TOH-nin) **(CT)**	a thyroid hormone that lowers blood calcium ion levels
parathyroid (pair-uh-THIGH-roid) **glands**	four small endocrine glands located on the posterior surface of the thyroid gland
parathyroid (pair-uh-THIGH-roid) **hormone (PTH)**	hormone that increases blood calcium ion levels

KEY TERM PRACTICE: *Thyroid Gland and Parathyroid Glands*

1. The hormone _____ lowers blood calcium levels, whereas the hormone _____ increases calcium ion levels.

2. Name the two hormones secreted by the thyroid gland that are involved with growth and metabolism. _____

3. The _____ are four small endocrine glands located on the posterior surface of the thyroid gland.

4. The bilobed endocrine gland located in the neck that secretes T$_3$ and T$_4$ is the _____.

Pancreas

The **pancreas** is a gland 20 to 25 cm (8 to 10 inches) long with both endocrine and exocrine functions. It is sandwiched between the stomach and the first portion of the small intestine (**Figure 9-4**). The exocrine portion secretes pancreatic juice (with digestive enzymes) directly into a duct, and the endocrine portion secretes hormones that enter the bloodstream.

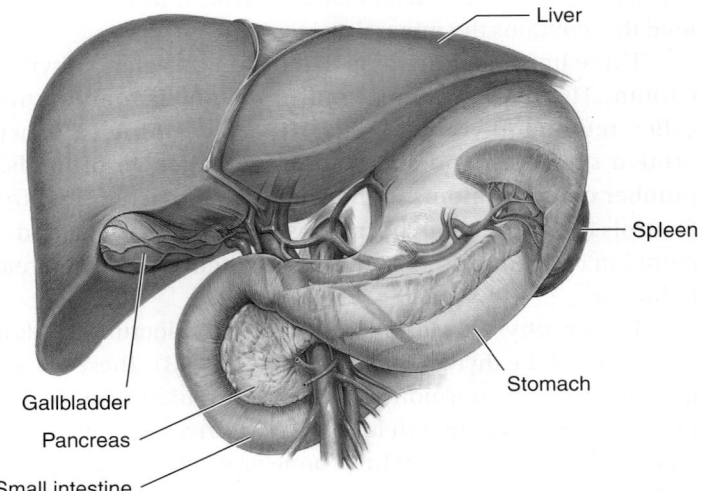

Figure 9-4 The pancreas is positioned between the stomach and the first portion of the small intestine.

Specialized cells in groups called **pancreatic islets** perform its endocrine functions. The pancreatic islets were once referred to as the islets of Langerhans, after the German pathologist Paul Langerhans, who discovered them. Each islet contains four types of cells: alpha cells, beta cells, delta cells, and F cells. Alpha cells and beta cells are discussed.

Alpha cells produce **glucagon**, a hormone that raises blood glucose (sugar) levels. It does this by increasing the rates of glycogen (the storage form of glucose) breakdown and glucose release from the liver, allowing glucose to enter the blood. The action of **insulin**, produced by beta cells, is opposite that of glucagon. Insulin lowers blood glucose levels by moving glucose from the blood into the cells. Insulin also promotes the formation of glycogen from glucose. When blood glucose levels rise, insulin is released to transport the sugar from the bloodstream into the cells, and when blood glucose levels fall, glucagon is secreted to stimulate the liver to release glucose into the blood.

KEY TERM	Definition
pancreas (PAN-kree-us)	glandular organ with endocrine and exocrine functions
pancreatic (pan-kree-AT-ick) **islets**	the endocrine cells of the pancreas that secrete hormones
glucagon (GLOO-kuh-gon)	pancreatic hormone from alpha cells that increases blood glucose levels
insulin (IN-suh-lin)	pancreatic hormone from beta cells that decreases blood glucose levels

KEY TERM PRACTICE: *Pancreas*

1. Identify the hormone that increases blood glucose levels. _____

2. Identify the hormone that lowers blood glucose levels. _____

3. The endocrine cells of the pancreas are known as _____.

4. The glandular organ with both exocrine and endocrine functions is the _____.

Adrenal Glands

The **adrenal glands** are pyramid-shaped structures positioned above each kidney, forming a cap on the superior borders. The word *adrenal* literally means "above the renal" or "above the kidney." The adrenal gland can be thought of as two glands in one because it is composed of cortical (outer) and medullary (inner) regions that each have different functions.

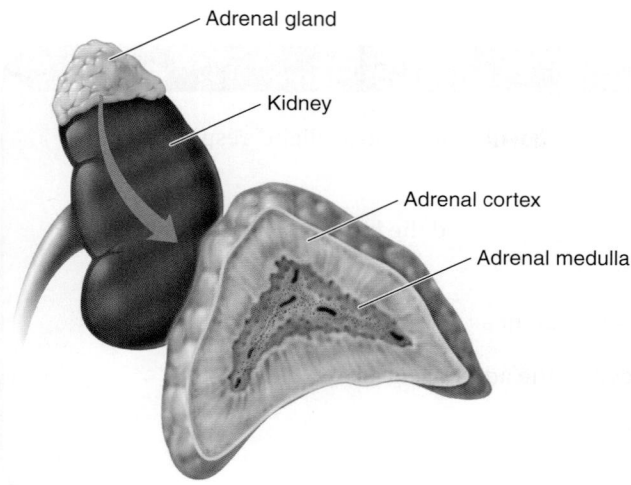

Adrenal gland

Kidney

Adrenal cortex

Adrenal medulla

Figure 9-5 The adrenal glands are positioned above each kidney and have an inner medulla and an outer cortex.

The **adrenal cortex** is the outer portion of the gland. It produces aldosterone, cortisol, and androgens. The **adrenal medulla** is the inner portion of the gland and secretes epinephrine and norepinephrine (**Figure 9-5**).

Aldosterone is a hormone that controls the balance of salt and water in the body. It causes the kidneys to conserve salt, or sodium ions (Na^+), and to excrete potassium ions (K^+). This helps maintain blood volume and pressure. As a memory aid, the letters of the word *salt* are found in *al*dos*t*erone.

Cortisol, also called hydrocortisone, is secreted in response to tissue damage and has anti-inflammatory effects. It also regulates blood sugar, fat deposition, and protein metabolism.

Androgens, sex hormones, are also produced in the adrenal cortex of both males and females. These hormones supplement the sex hormones already produced by the gonads (testes and ovaries) and are usually masculinizing in their effects.

Hormones of the adrenal medulla take part in nervous system functions such as the fight-or-flight response. The fight-or-flight response is the body's instinctive reaction to impending danger or other stress. **Epinephrine (E)**, also called adrenaline, increases heart rate, causes vasodilation, elevates blood pressure, dilates airways, increases blood glucose levels, and enhances the metabolic rate. **Norepinephrine (NE)**, also called noradrenaline, accelerates the heart rate, increases blood flow, increases blood pressure, and increases the metabolic rate.

KEY TERM	Definition
adrenal (uh-DREE-nul) **glands**	endocrine gland located above each kidney
adrenal cortex (uh-DREE-nul KOHR-tecks)	outer portion of the adrenal gland
adrenal medulla (uh-DREE-nul me-DEW-luh)	inner portion of the adrenal gland
aldosterone (al-DOS-te-rohn)	adrenal cortex hormone that regulates salt and water balance
cortisol (KOR-ti-sol)	adrenal cortex hormone that has anti-inflammatory effects; also called hydrocortisone
androgens (AN-droh-jinz)	supplemental sex hormones produced by the adrenal cortex
epinephrine (ep-i-NEF-rin) **(E)**	adrenal medulla hormone involved in the fight-or-flight response; also called adrenaline
norepinephrine (nor-ep-i-NEF-rin) **(NE)**	adrenal medulla hormone involved in the fight-or-flight response; also called noradrenaline

continued

continued from page 421

KEY TERM PRACTICE: *Adrenal Glands*

1. Name two hormones secreted by the adrenal medulla that are involved with the "fight-or-flight" response.

   _____ _____

2. The outer portion of the adrenal gland is termed the _____, and the inner region is known as the

   _____.

3. _____ is the hormone that regulates salt and water balance.

4. _____ are supplemental sex hormones produced by the adrenal cortex.

5. The adrenal cortex hormone that has anti-inflammatory effects is _____.

IN THE NEWS: DHEA

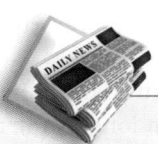

DHEA may be the snake oil medicine of the early 21st century. You have probably heard of it while watching baseball's home run record breakers or Sunday afternoon football. DHEA is the acronym for dehydroepiandrosterone (dee-HIGH-droh-ep-ee-an-DROS-tur-ohn), a hormone sold in health food stores to athletes as an alternative to anabolic steroids. The claimed benefits include improving energy, boosting strength, and serving as an aging remedy. Since 1994, it has been sold as a dietary supplement, but it is not a necessary food in the human diet. It is quite popular in the sports culture where athletes tout DHEA's ability to enhance their performance.

Unfortunately, these claims have not been borne out in the scientific research. In fact, what is known about the hormone is quite disturbing. Short-term effects of DHEA use include acne, oily skin, hirsutism, gynecomastia, hepatomegaly, heart arrhythmias, and aggressive behavior. About 20 milligrams of DHEA is secreted naturally by the adrenal cortex in both males and females, and DHEA is also secreted in the male testes. The compound is weakly androgenic (causing development of male characteristics), but once metabolized, it converts to another hormone—delta-5 androstenediol—that has both androgenic and estrogenic (causing development of female characteristics) effects. This second hormone is the precursor molecule (chemical that leads to) of testosterone.

Efficacy and safety studies are lacking. Because the U.S. Food and Drug Administration (FDA) does not regulate the supplement, labeling can be deceiving. Independent laboratory analyses have shown that the strength of DHEA supplements can range from 0% to 150% of the amount indicated on the bottle. To date, the therapeutic effects have not been realized, and alleged benefits have not been demonstrated in controlled studies. The International Olympic Committee and the National Collegiate Athletic Association have banned its use. The drug can be detected by the 17-ketosteroids urine test.

Research on DHEA is continuing but is still in its infancy. There is sufficient evidence supporting the use of DHEA for the treatment of systemic lupus erythematosus and adrenal insufficiency in women because of its androgenic–estrogenic actions. It can also be used to treat depression and induce labor. Until more is known, individuals should not use DHEA unless they are under the direct care of a physician who can monitor critical physiological and clinical outcomes.

Pineal Gland and Thymus

The **pineal gland** is a small structure named for its pine cone shape. It is attached to the thalamus in the brain (**Figure 9-6**). Cells in the pineal gland secrete the hormone **melatonin**, which may influence circadian rhythms. The **circadian rhythm** is a naturally recurring pattern of biological processes that repeats on a 24-hour cycle, even in the absence of light fluctuations (**Figure 9-7**).

The **thymus** is an organ located at the base of the neck, posterior to the sternum, and between the lungs (**Figure 9-8**). It secretes **thymosins**, a group of hormones involved in the development of immune system cells, particularly T cells.

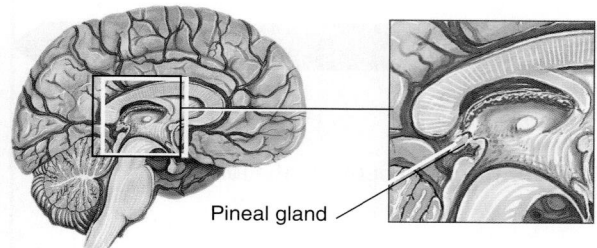

Pineal gland

Figure 9-6 The pineal gland is a very small structure located in the brain.

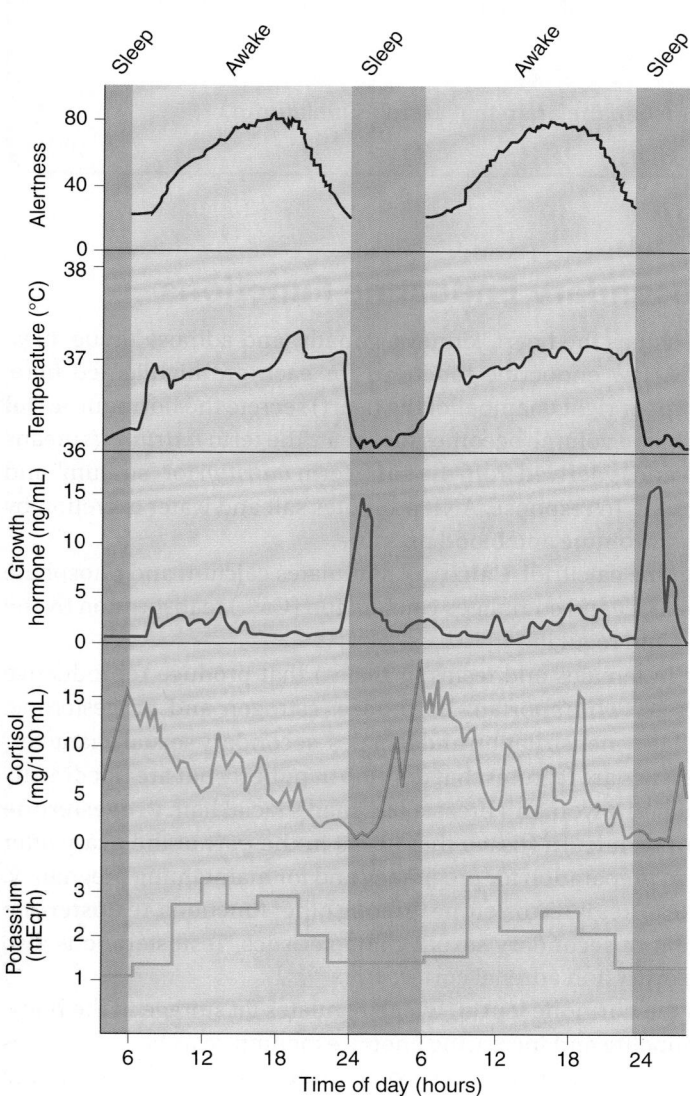

Figure 9-7 Circadian rhythms of physiological functions. Fluctuations over two consecutive days are shown.

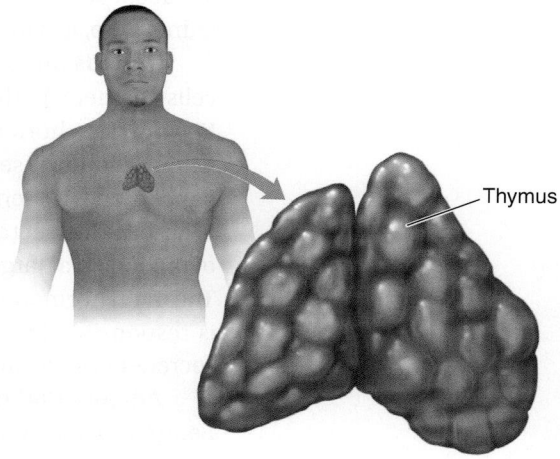

Thymus

Figure 9-8 The thymus, consisting of two irregularly shaped parts, is located just posterior to the sternum.

KEY TERM	Definition
pineal (PYE-nee-ul) gland	small pine cone-shaped organ in the brain that secretes melatonin
melatonin (mel-uh-TOH-nin)	hormone secreted by pineal gland cells that may influence circadian rhythms
circadian (sur-KAY-dee-un) rhythm	human biorhythm that repeats every 24 hours
thymus (THIGH-mus)	organ at the base of the neck, posterior to the sternum, and between the lungs that secretes thymosins
thymosins (THIGH-moh-sins)	group of hormones from the thymus gland involved in the development of immune system cells, particularly T cells

KEY TERM PRACTICE: *Pineal Gland and Thymus*

1. Hormones from the thymus are collectively termed _____.

2. Name the organ that is located at the base of the neck, posterior to the sternum, and between the lungs that secretes thymosins. _____

3. _____ is a hormone secreted by the pineal gland cells that may influence circadian rhythms.

4. The human biorhythm that repeats every 24 hours is termed the _____.

5. The _____ is a small, pine cone-shaped organ in the brain that secretes melatonin.

Other Organs with Secondary Endocrine Functions

Many other organs and tissues, such as the heart, kidneys, gonads, and adipose tissue, have secondary endocrine functions. A few endocrine functions for each are highlighted here. Cardiac cells in the right atrium (upper right chamber of the heart) secrete the hormone **atrial natriuretic peptide (ANP)** when blood volume becomes too great. The term *natriuresis* means "excretion of sodium in the urine" and is derived from the Latin term *natrium* for "sodium" and the Greek term *ouresis* for "urination." In response, ANP promotes salt and water excretion by the kidneys, thereby reducing blood volume and blood pressure.

The kidneys release the hormone calcitriol. **Calcitriol** stimulates calcium and phosphate ion absorption along the digestive tract and stimulates calcium ion (Ca^{2+}) reabsorption by the kidneys. So, it is important for calcium regulation.

Gonads are organs (ovaries in females and testes in males) that produce reproductive cells (gametes). The ovaries secrete two important hormones: estrogen and progesterone. **Estrogen** is a hormone that stimulates menstruation and females' secondary sexual characteristics. Secondary sexual characteristics are features that develop at puberty but are not directly concerned with reproduction, such as a woman's breasts or a man's facial hair. **Progesterone** is a hormone secreted by the corpus luteum (tissue that forms in the part of the ovary after ovulation) that targets the uterus in preparation for pregnancy and for maintaining pregnancy. The main hormone secreted by the testes is testosterone. Among other functions, **testosterone** is responsible for the development of secondary sexual characteristics. Testosterone is also secreted in small amounts by the ovary and adrenal cortex.

Adipose (fat) tissue secretes the hormone **leptin**, which regulates fat storage in the body. Leptin is involved with curbing appetite and increasing energy expenditure as body fat stores increase. Leptin levels are 40% higher in women, and show a further 50% rise just before the very first menstrual cycle (menarche), later returning to baseline levels. Levels are lowered by fasting and increased by inflammation.

KEY TERM	Definition
atrial natriuretic peptide (ANP) (AYE-tree-ul nay-tree-yoo-RET-ick PEP-tide)	hormone secreted by heart cells that promotes fluid loss and blood pressure reduction
calcitriol (kal-sih-TRY-ul)	hormone released by the kidneys that is important for calcium regulation
gonads (GOH-nadz)	organs (ovaries in females and testes in males) that produce reproductive cells
estrogen (es-TROH-jen)	hormone produced by the ovaries to stimulate secondary sexual characteristics
progesterone (proh-JES-ter-ohn)	hormone secreted by the corpus luteum that targets the uterus in preparation for, and maintenance of, pregnancy
testosterone (tes-TOS-teh-rohn)	hormone secreted by the testes to stimulate secondary sexual characteristics
leptin (LEP-tin)	hormone secreted by adipose tissue that regulates fat storage in the body

KEY TERM PRACTICE: *Other Organs with Secondary Endocrine Functions*

1. Name two hormones secreted by the ovaries. _____ _____

2. _____ is a hormone secreted by adipose tissue that regulates fat storage in the body.

3. Name the hormone secreted by the testes that stimulates secondary sexual characteristics. _____

4. _____ is a hormone secreted by heart cells in response to increasing blood volume that acts to decrease blood pressure.

5. _____ is a hormone released by the kidneys that is important for regulating calcium.

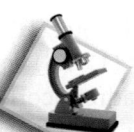

THE CLINICAL DIMENSION

This section identifies signs and symptoms, pathological conditions, and treatments related to the endocrine system. Endocrine disorders can be assessed through a variety of clinical tests and diagnostic procedures. Laboratory analyses used to evaluate endocrine function include plasma, serum, blood, urine, glucose tolerance, and glycosylated hemoglobin (A_{1c}) tests. Common disorders and treatments of the endocrine system are described.

Disorders of the endocrine system are generally the result of tumors or the hyperfunction (hypersecretion) or hypofunction (hyposecretion) of specific glands. They can also be secondary to some other primary condition. The pathological disorders discussed in this section are commonly associated with endocrine dysfunction.

Adrenal Gland Disorders

Addison disease

Addison disease is a wasting disorder characterized by decreased aldosterone concentration, bronzing of the skin, low blood pressure, and weakness. It results from underactivity of the adrenal glands (**Figure 9-9**). In many cases, the cause is unknown, but an

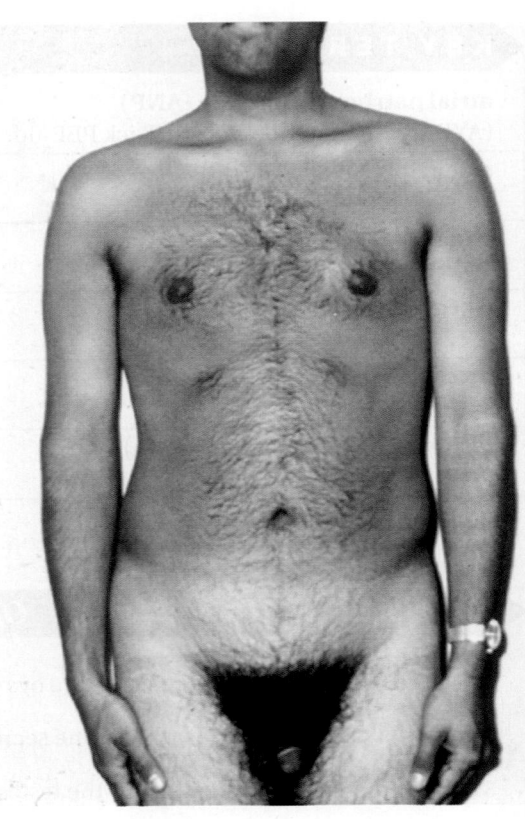

Figure 9-9 Bronze skin pigmentation of Addison disease.

autoimmune problem is suspected. In addition to idiopathic Addison disease, adrenal tumors and tuberculosis have been implicated.

Urine and blood tests show decreased cortisol levels, and adrenal calcification may be evident on x-rays. **Blood tests** are used to evaluate blood components, and the **urine ketosteroids test** is used to detect androgen metabolites (byproducts of metabolism). Types of urine ketosteroid tests include the hydroxycorticosteroid urine test, which detects the presence of cortisol byproducts, and the 17-ketosteroids (17-KS) test, which detects steroidal metabolites of androgenic and adrenocortical hormones. Treatment involves hormone replacement therapy with glucocorticoids (cortisol) and mineralocorticoids (aldosterone). **Hormone replacement therapy (HRT)** may be used to restore normal endocrine function or to alter the secretion of another hormone.

Cushing disease

Cushing disease is a condition caused by excessive production of cortisol by the adrenal cortex. It is characterized by adipose deposition in the face and trunk, a "buffalo hump" in the scapular region, hypertension (high blood pressure), fatigue, glycosuria (glucose in the urine), increased susceptibility to infection, muscle weakness, and a "moon face" appearance. Its cause can be an adrenal cortex tumor, pituitary tumor, ACTH-producing tumor, or overdose reaction to adrenocortical hormone administration. Physical evaluation and increased cortisol level in the urine lead to the diagnosis. The treatment depends on the cause. Options are tumor excision and drugs to suppress the pituitary gland's production of ACTH, which stimulates the adrenal cortex to produce cortisol.

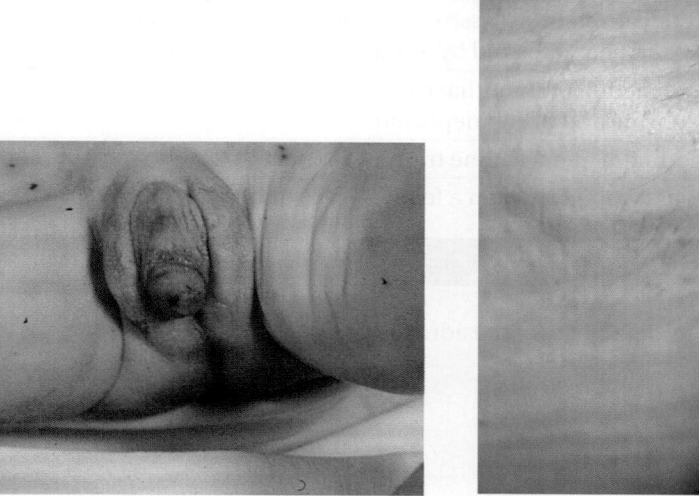

Figure 9-10 Congenital virilism in a female infant showing enlargement of the clitoris.

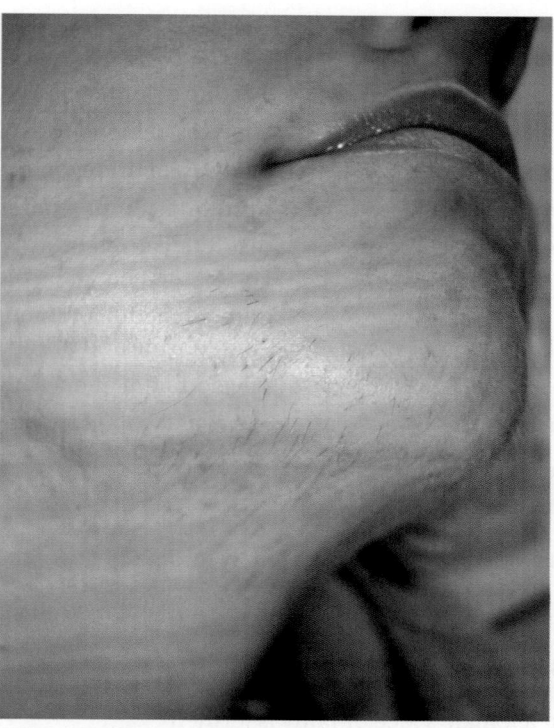

Figure 9-11 Hirsutism. Note the excessive hair growth on this female's chin.

pheochromocytoma A **pheochromocytoma** is a small vascular tumor of the adrenal medulla that causes irregular secretion of epinephrine and norepinephrine. It is characterized by an irregular heart rate, hypertension, and pounding headaches. Blood tests showing increased levels of epinephrine and norepinephrine or radiographic studies confirm the diagnosis. Surgical removal of the tumor is the best treatment.

virilism Excessive output of adrenal androgens leading to the development of masculine traits in females is termed adrenal **virilism** (Figure 9-10). Its underlying cause is usually adrenal hyperplasia (excessive tissue formation) or a tumor. Signs and symptoms include **hirsutism** (excessive hair growth in abnormal locations; *hirsutus* = shaggy; Figure 9-11), uterine atrophy, clitoris enlargement, decreased breast size, and increased masculinity. Diagnostic studies, including a computed tomography (CT) scan or magnetic resonance imaging (MRI), identify tumors. CT scans are cross-sectional body images produced using a computer and x-rays. MRI is a technique that uses electromagnetic radiation to obtain images. Treatment options are cortisol, tumor removal, and adrenalectomy.

KEY TERM	Definition
Addison disease	wasting disorder caused by underactivity of the adrenal glands
blood tests	analyses of blood to evaluate its components
urine ketosteroids (kee-toh-STEER-oidz) **test**	analyses of urine to detect androgen metabolites
hormone replacement therapy (HRT)	hormone administration to restore normal function
Cushing (KOOSH-ing) **disease**	disorder caused by excessive cortisol production by the adrenal cortex and characterized by a "moon face" appearance
pheochromocytoma (fee-oh-kroh-moh-sigh-TOH-muh)	adrenal medulla tumor that causes irregular secretion of epinephrine and norepinephrine
virilism (VEER-ih-liz-um)	development of masculine traits in a female
hirsutism (HUR-sewt-iz-um)	abnormal hair growth on a female's face or body

KEY TERM PRACTICE: *Adrenal Gland Disorders*

1. _____ is a wasting disorder caused by underactivity of the adrenal gland.

2. A _____ is a tumor associated with the adrenal medulla.

3. _____ is the development of masculine traits in females.

4. Abnormal hair growth on a female's face or body is termed _____.

5. _____ is a disorder caused by excessive cortisol production leading to a "moon face" appearance.

Pancreas Disorders

diabetes mellitus (DM)

Diabetes mellitus (DM) is a chronic disorder of carbohydrate metabolism. Carbohydrates are commonly known as sugars, with glucose being an important carbohydrate. The disease is so named because of the sugary urine that is excreted. The term literally means "sweetened with honey." The condition is characterized by inadequate insulin production (Type 1) or decreased cellular sensitivity to insulin (Type 2). Signs and symptoms include **hyperglycemia** (elevated blood glucose level), glycosuria (glucose in the urine), altered fat and protein metabolism, polyuria (excessive urination), polydipsia (excessive thirst), and polyphagia (excessive appetite or eating). Diabetes mellitus affects at least 16 million people in the United States and ranks seventh as a cause of death. It costs the national economy over $100 billion yearly. The increase in DM prevalence in the United States has been linked to a rise in the prevalence of obesity. About 95% of those with DM have Type 2 and the rest have Type 1.

Type 1 diabetes is a chronic disorder that begins before age 25. It is also known as juvenile-onset diabetes. In Type 1 DM, an autoimmune process causes beta cell destruction, which leads to inadequate insulin production. For this reason, individuals with Type 1 diabetes must take insulin injections.

Type 2 diabetes, or maturity-onset diabetes, has a gradual onset. It is caused by either a lack of insulin or the body's inability to use insulin efficiently. The disease generally begins after age 40 years and is managed initially with dietary measures. Research suggests that there may be a genetic predisposition for Type 2 diabetes, especially in obese individuals or those with excessive abdominal girth. Some research also suggests that type 2 diabetes should be redefined as an autoimmune disease rather than just a metabolic disorder.

Gestational diabetes mellitus (GDM) occurs only during pregnancy. Gestational diabetes has the same signs and symptoms as Types 1 and 2. It usually disappears after pregnancy, but 30% to 40% of women with GDM develop Type 2 diabetes mellitus within 10 years of giving birth. GDM may be caused by placental destruction of insulin when the level of human placental lactogen (hPL) is increased. The diagnosis is confirmed by glycosuria and the results of the glucose tolerance test and **postprandial** (after a meal) glucose test. The term postprandial is derived from the Latin term for breakfast, *prandium*.

The diagnosis of DM depends on measurement of plasma glucose concentration. The **glucose tolerance test (GTT)** measures blood glucose levels at 30-minute intervals up to 3 hours. The patient fasts for 12 hours and then ingests a glucose mixture. Blood is drawn before the patient drinks the glucose so clinicians can measure the fasting level, and blood is then drawn at half-hour intervals to measure the glucose level over time. The diagnosis is confirmed when any two measurements of blood glucose performed on different days yield levels at or above established thresholds: in the fasting state, 126 mg/dL; 2 hours postprandially (after a 75-g oral glucose load) or at random, 200 mg/dL. A fasting blood glucose of 100 to 125 mg/dL or a 2-hour postprandial glucose of 140 to 199 mg/dL is defined as impaired glucose tolerance. People with impaired glucose tolerance are at higher risk of developing DM within 10 years. For such people, lifestyle modification such as weight reduction and exercise may prevent or postpone the onset of DM.

The **glycosylated hemoglobin (A_{1c}) test** assists in evaluating blood glucose levels over a 3-month period. The average life span of a red blood cell is 120 days. During the life of a red blood cell, glucose molecules adhere to the cell's hemoglobin, forming glycosylated hemoglobin molecules (A_{1c}). Once formed, the glycosylated hemoglobin remains until red blood cell death. Therefore, evaluating this molecule assesses the effectiveness of the therapy of the patient with diabetes.

Current recommendations for the management of DM emphasize education and individualization of therapy. The goal of treatment for all types is to control blood glucose levels through exercise, insulin injections, diet, and/or oral drug therapy. Diabetes leads to systemic complications, such as kidney, eye, and nerve damage, so glucose management is lifelong and of great importance for preventing future complications.

hypoglycemia

Hypoglycemia is an abnormally low level of glucose in the blood. It is characterized by hunger, nervousness, sweating, and fatigue. If not treated, the signs could progress to convulsions. Hypoglycemia can be caused by fasting, increased insulin secretion, or a pancreatic tumor. A patient with diabetes may become hypoglycemic from an insulin overdose, not eating, or too much exercise. Hypoglycemia is diagnosed by abnormally low blood glucose (<40 mg/dL in men; <45 mg/dL in women). Eating food, ingesting glucose tablets, or removing the tumor are the usual treatments.

KEY TERM	Definition
diabetes mellitus (DM) (dye-uh-BEE-teez mel-EYE-tus)	chronic disorder of carbohydrate metabolism
hyperglycemia (high-pur-glye-SEE-mee-uh)	abnormally high blood glucose level
Type 1 diabetes (dye-uh-BEE-teez)	form of diabetes mellitus that occurs before age 25 as a result of beta cell destruction; also called juvenile-onset diabetes
Type 2 diabetes (dye-uh-BEE-teez)	form of diabetes mellitus that occurs after age 40 as a result of either a lack of insulin or the body's inability to use insulin efficiently
gestational diabetes mellitus (GDM) (jes-TAY-shun-ul dye-uh-BEE-teez mel-EYE-tus)	disorder of carbohydrate metabolism that occurs during pregnancy
postprandial (pohst-PRAN-dee-ul)	after a meal
glucose (GLOO-kose) **tolerance test (GTT)**	determination of blood glucose levels at different times after drinking a glucose syrup
glycosylated hemoglobin (A_{1c}) (GLYE-koh-si-lay-ted HEE-moh-gloh-bin) **test**	test used to measure circulating blood glucose levels over the life span of a red blood cell
hypoglycemia (high-poh-glye-SEE-mee-uh)	abnormally low blood glucose level

KEY TERM PRACTICE: *Pancreas Disorders*

1. _____ is the term used to describe abnormally low blood glucose levels.

2. The term _____ means "after a meal."

3. The _____ test is used to measure circulating blood glucose levels over the life span of a red blood cell.

4. This type of diabetes mellitus is referred to as juvenile-onset diabetes because it typically occurs early in life. _____

5. This type of diabetes mellitus occurs during pregnancy. _____

Parathyroid Gland Disorders

hyperparathyroidism

Hyperparathyroidism is an abnormally high level of parathyroid hormone (PTH) in the blood caused by overactive parathyroid glands. The elevated PTH causes weakening of bones through calcium loss. This in turn leads to elevated calcium ion levels in the blood, a condition called **hypercalcemia**. The hypercalcemia initiates a cascade of events affecting the functioning of other systems. The cause may be idiopathic or the result of an adenoma (benign tumor). Signs and symptoms are muscle weakness, gastrointestinal upset, nausea, cardiac arrhythmia, renal calculi (kidney stones), and fragile bones that fracture easily.

Elevated PTH levels on radioimmunoassay, blood studies that show increased calcium ion concentration and decreased potassium ion levels, and urinalysis that demonstrates excessive calcium ion level confirm the diagnosis. **Radioimmunoassay (RIA)** is a method used for detecting antigens, antibodies, enzymes, and

CHAPTER **9**   Endocrine System   **431**

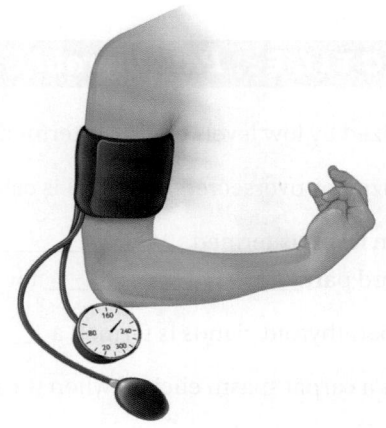

Figure 9-12 Right arm of patient showing positive Trousseau sign (carpal spasm) that is induced by occluding circulation in the arm with a blood pressure cuff.

hormones in the blood using radioactive tracers. Treating the underlying cause (tumor removal or parathyroidectomy) alleviates the condition. Surgical removal of one or more of the parathyroid glands is called **parathyroidectomy.**

hypoparathyroidism Diminished concentration of PTH in the blood results in **hypoparathyroidism.** The condition is caused by a tumor or by injury to the parathyroid glands. It may be autoimmune induced or a congenital disorder. Hypoparathyroidism causes calcium deficiency (hypocalcemia) and results in muscular spasms. It can progress to seizures and tetany (sustained muscle contractions). Diagnosis is made by the clinical picture, physical examination, and clinical test results. Decreased serum calcium ion level, increased bone density, and decreased PTH level show on an RIA. The **Trousseau sign,** muscle tetany in which carpal spasm is elicited by compressing the brachial region, is also evident (**Figure 9-12**). Treatment is a high-calcium, low-phosphorus diet supplemented with calcium and vitamin D tablets. (Vitamin D enhances calcium ion absorption.)

KEY TERM	Definition
hyperparathyroidism (high-pur-pair-uh-THIGH-roid-iz-um)	abnormally high level of parathyroid hormone (PTH) in the blood caused by overactive parathyroid glands
hypercalcemia (high-pur-kal-SEE-mee-uh)	abnormally high blood calcium levels
radioimmunoassay (RIA) (RAY-dee-oh-im-yoo-noh-as-say)	test using radioactive tracers to detect antigens, antibodies, enzymes, and hormones in the blood
parathyroidectomy (pair-uh-thigh-roy-DECK-tuh-mee)	surgical removal of one or more of the parathyroid glands
hypoparathyroidism (high-poh-pair-uh-THIGH-roid-iz-um)	inadequate secretion of parathyroid hormone
Trousseau (true-SOH) **sign**	carpal spasm elicited when the brachial region is compressed, suggesting hypoparathyroidism

continued from page 431

K E Y T E R M P R A C T I C E : *Parathyroid Gland Disorders*

1. The condition characterized by low levels of PTH is termed _____.

2. The condition characterized by oversecretion of PTH is called _____.

3. Abnormally high calcium levels is termed _____, derived from the word part _____ for "calcium" and the word part _____ for "blood."

4. Surgical removal of the parathyroid glands is termed a _____.

5. _____ is a carpal spasm elicited when the brachial region is compressed and is suggestive of hypoparathyroidism.

Pituitary Gland Disorders

acromegaly

Acromegaly is a disease of adults resulting from overproduction of growth hormone (GH) from the anterior pituitary gland. It is characterized by overgrowth of bone in the hands, feet, jaw, nose, and ribs. The cause is a pituitary tumor, and diagnosis is made through physical and clinical examination. RIA studies reveal an elevated GH level. Radiographic and MRI studies show a pituitary tumor. Treatment includes radiation or surgery to remove the tumor.

gigantism

Like acromegaly, **gigantism** (or giantism) is the result of oversecretion of GH by the anterior pituitary gland, but in this case, the excessive production takes place before puberty. The underlying cause is a tumor. Signs include very long bones and an arched mouth palate. Diagnosis is made by physical examination, elevated GH levels, and evidence of bone thickening. Radiographic studies, CT scans, and MRI scans expose a pituitary tumor. **Figure 9-13** shows gigantism in one twin compared to his identical brother.

pituitary dwarfism

Pituitary dwarfism is characterized by abnormal underdevelopment. The disorder is caused by the absence of a functional anterior pituitary gland and may be present at birth or develop during early childhood. Signs and symptoms include a small body with disproportionate limbs, delayed secondary sexual characteristics, and possible mental retardation (**Figure 9-14**). Physical examination demonstrates lipid deposition in the lower trunk. Blood studies show low GH level. Lifelong treatment of the chronic condition is aimed at correcting the hormonal imbalance and involves administration of GH.

diabetes insipidus

In contrast to diabetes mellitus, which is a pancreatic disorder, **diabetes insipidus** is related to the posterior pituitary gland and results from a deficiency of ADH (vasopressin). This causes the body to produce large amounts of urine. (Remember, ADH regulates kidney function.) It is characterized by polyuria and compensatory polydipsia. The sequence of urinating and drinking sets up a continuous

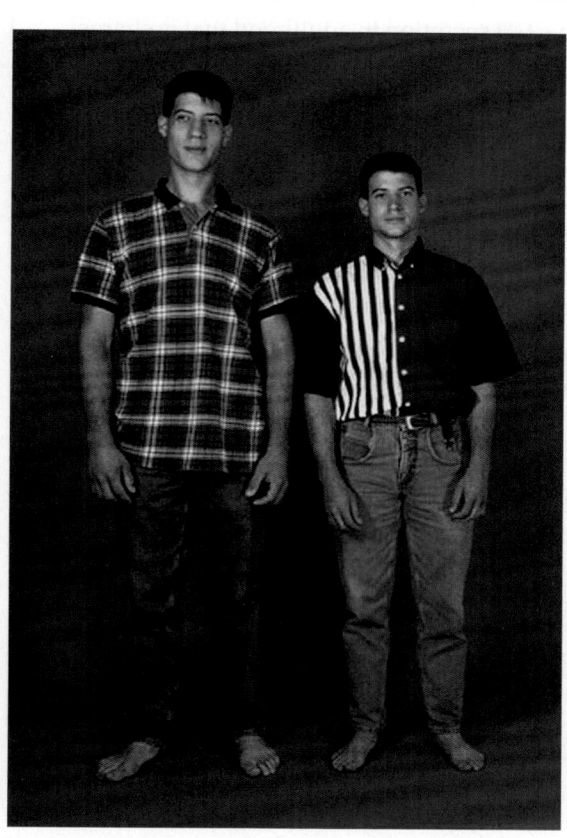

Figure 9-13 A 22-year-old man with gigantism due to excess growth hormone is shown to the left of his identical twin.

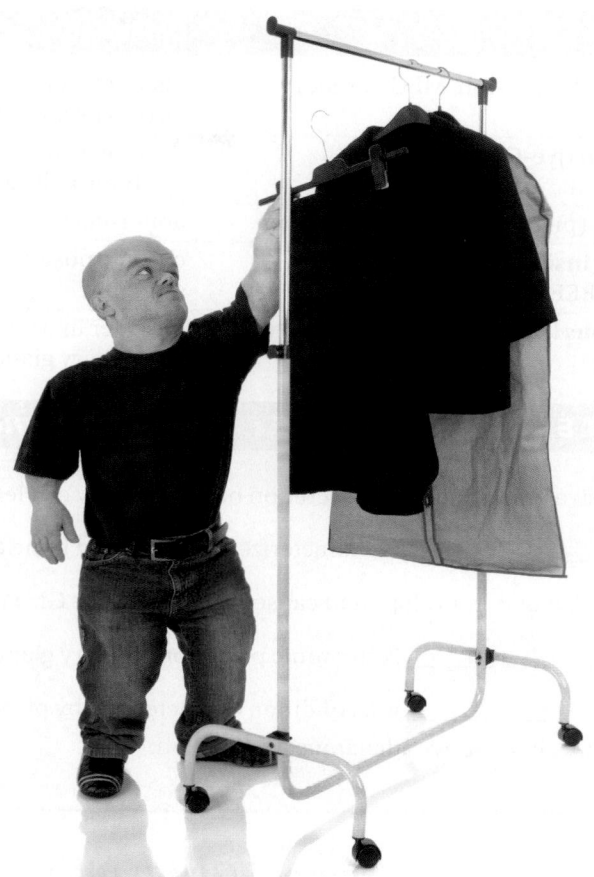

Figure 9-14 Photo of a man with pituitary dwarfism.

cycle of attempting to balance the body's water level. The cause is unknown. Diagnosis is made by patient history of symptoms and a urinalysis that demonstrates extremely dilute urine. Confirmation of diabetes insipidus is made if the urine output diminishes and becomes less dilute after administration of ADH. Treatment includes vasopressin (ADH) injections or nasal spray to increase the hormone level.

precocious puberty   Developing signs of physical maturity at an unusually early age is termed **precocious puberty**. In girls, it is manifested by pubic and axillary hair, along with breast development before age 8. In boys, it is marked by pubic and facial hair with increased gonad size before age 9. The cause is pituitary gland or hypothalamus dysfunction, tumor of the pituitary gland or hypothalamus, or a testicular tumor in boys. Physical examination and increased hormone levels in the blood and urine provide an accurate diagnosis. Girls also have increased blood levels of the anterior pituitary hormones FSH and LH. Treatment depends on the cause. Tumor removal and hormone therapy to suppress the overactive gland are options.

KEY TERM	Definition
acromegaly (ack-roh-MEG-uh-lee)	disorder caused by excessive GH secretion in adulthood that is characterized by abnormally thick bones
gigantism (jye-GAN-tiz-um)	disorder caused by excessive GH secretion before puberty characterized by abnormally long bones; also called giantism
pituitary (pi-TEW-i-terr-ee) **dwarfism**	abnormal underdevelopment caused by inadequate GH secretion
diabetes insipidus (dye-uh-BEE-teez in-SIP-i-dus)	chronic posterior pituitary gland disorder that causes inadequate ADH secretion
precocious (pree-KOH-shus) **puberty**	disorder in which physical maturity occurs at an unusually early age due to pituitary gland dysfunction or hypothalamus dysfunction

KEY TERM PRACTICE: *Pituitary Gland Disorders*

1. Excessive growth hormone secretion before puberty can lead to this disorder. _____

2. _____ is characterized by increased bone thickness in the hands and face during adulthood.

3. Abnormal underdevelopment caused by inadequate GH levels leads to _____.

4. _____ is a chronic posterior pituitary gland problem that results from inadequate secretion of ADH.

5. _____ is a condition characterized by physical maturity occurring at an unusually early age due to pituitary gland or hypothalamus dysfunction.

Thyroid Gland Disorders

hypothyroidism   **Hypothyroidism** is a condition of diminished thyroid hormone production characterized by low metabolic rate, weight gain, and sluggishness. Thyroid hormone can be assessed by a simple blood test that evaluates TSH, T_3, and T_4 levels. Hypothyroidism is treated with thyroid hormone medication.

Thyroid function can be evaluated by a **radioactive iodine uptake (RIU) test**, which uses radioactive iodine as a tracer. Radioiodine (^{131}I), a radioactive form of iodine, can be delivered intravenously or orally. Its dosage is measured in a unit called a microcurie (μCi). ^{131}I is ingested and taken up (absorbed) by the thyroid. A special detector determines the amount taken up over a period of time. This value is then used to assess thyroid function.

myxedema   **Myxedema** occurs in adulthood as an impaired ability of the thyroid gland to produce T_4 hormones. The condition is characterized by water retention, sluggishness, and weight gain. A blood test reveals decreased T_4 and TSH levels. It is treated with administration of synthetic T_4 (levothyroxine or Synthroid).

infantile hypothyroidism   **Infantile hypothyroidism**, a congenital form of hypothyroidism, is caused by a number of factors including failure of the thyroid to position properly, autoimmune disease, and maternal ingestion of medication that interfered with fetal development. In some cases, the thyroid gland may be absent or fail to produce hormones. Common characteristics are a large, protruding tongue and abdomen, hoarse cry, mental retardation, and depressed muscle tone. It is diagnosed by thyroid gland absence on a CT scan or by a low T_4 level that is accompanied by an increased thyroid-stimulating hormone (TSH) level. It can be successfully treated with thyroid hormones. If treatment begins early, the individual will have no physiological manifestations. Thyroid hormone replacement therapy is necessary throughout life.

goiter

A simple **goiter** is an enlargement of the thyroid gland that presents as a large, outwardly obvious swollen mass on the neck (**Figure 9-15**). It results from inadequate iodine ingestion. The lack of iodine causes an increased release of TSH to stimulate the thyroid gland to produce more thyroid hormone. The thyroid gland hypertrophies to compensate. Physical examination and blood tests showing an increase in TSH and a decrease in thyroid hormone (T_3 and T_4) levels confirm the diagnosis. In addition to the swollen neck, other signs include cough, hoarseness, and swallowing difficulties. Administration of iodine as potassium iodide or eating iodine-rich foods alleviates the signs. In some cases, a partial **thyroidectomy** (surgical removal of the thyroid gland) may be performed.

Hashimoto thyroiditis

Hashimoto thyroiditis (Hashimoto disease) is an autoimmune disease that causes chronic inflammation of the thyroid (thyroiditis) and consequential failure of the thyroid gland. As with most autoimmune diseases, women are more affected than men. The inflammatory response causes diffuse thyroid enlargement. The disease advances to a stage in which the glandular tissue is replaced by fibrous connective tissue. Signs and symptoms include hypothyroidism, cold sensitivity, weight gain, and fatigue. Diagnosis is confirmed by the presence of autoantibodies in the blood and a radioactive iodine uptake (RIU) test. Lifelong treatment involves the administration (usually orally) of synthetic thyroid hormone.

hyperthyroidism or thyrotoxicosis

Overproduction of thyroid hormone is called **hyperthyroidism** or **thyrotoxicosis**. It is characterized by a hypermetabolic state, usually with weight loss, and sometimes **exophthalmos** (abnormal eye protrusion) (**Figure 9-16**). If not treated, hyperthyroidism results in **thyroid storm**.

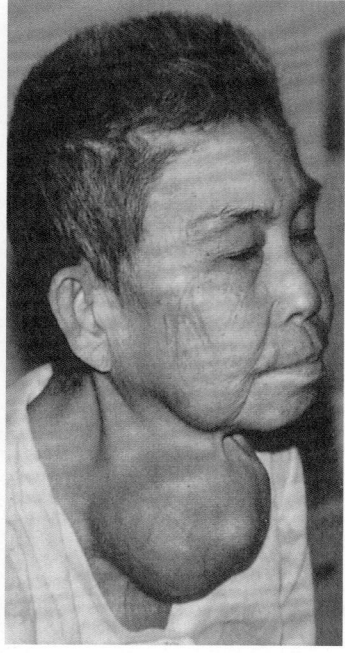

Figure 9-15 Goiter in a middle-aged woman.

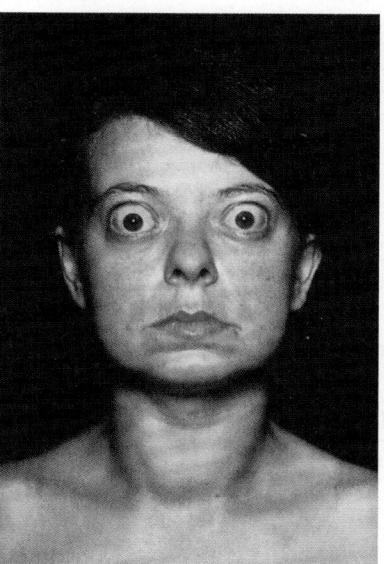

Figure 9-16 A young woman with hyperthyroidism presented with an enlarged thyroid gland and exophthalmos.

Thyroid storm, also termed thyrotoxic crisis, is marked by acute hyperthyroidism that can lead to tachycardia (accelerated heart rate), high fever, and muscle weakness. If the crisis does not resolve, coma and possibly death ensue. Administering antithyroid drugs to decrease thyroid hormone output or radioactive iodine therapy to ablate (remove or destroy unwanted tissue) the thyroid treats hyperthyroidism.

Graves disease

Graves disease, an autoimmune disorder with a familial link, is a form of hyperthyroidism. Signs and symptoms include weight loss, sweating, and exophthalmos. Diagnosis is based on the clinical manifestations, increased blood T_3 and T_4 levels, and increased uptake of radioiodine as indicated on thyroid function tests. Treatment options include antithyroid medications or radioactive iodine therapy.

thyroid cancer

Thyroid cancer is a malignant growth of the thyroid gland. It can occur in all age groups, and people who have had radiation therapy to the neck are at higher risk. Signs and symptoms include a lump in the neck, cough, hoarseness, and difficulty swallowing. Ultrasound of the thyroid and needle aspiration biopsy (tissue excision through a needle for evaluative purposes) are used for diagnosing. Treatments include lobectomy (removal of a thyroid lobe), thyroidectomy (excision of thyroid gland), and radioiodine ablation (destruction of unwanted tissue).

KEY TERM	Definition
hypothyroidism (high-poh-THIGH-roid-izm)	condition of decreased thyroid hormone production characterized by weight gain and sluggishness
radioactive iodine uptake (RIU) test	test used to evaluate thyroid gland function by measuring the rate of radioactive iodine absorption in the thyroid gland
myxedema (mick-seh-DEE-muh)	condition caused by decreased thyroid hormone production; a form of hypothyroidism
infantile hypothyroidism (high-poh-THIGH-roid-izm)	congenital form of hypothyroidism
goiter (GOY-tur)	enlargement of the thyroid gland
thyroidectomy (thigh-roid-ECK-tuh-mee)	partial or complete surgical removal of the thyroid gland
Hashimoto thyroiditis (hah-shee-MOH-toh thigh-roid-EYE-tis)	autoimmune disease that causes an inflamed thyroid gland, resulting in hypothyroidism; also called Hashimoto disease
hyperthyroidism (high-pur-THIGH-roid-izm)	condition of excessive thyroid hormone production; also called thyrotoxicosis
thyrotoxicosis (thigh-roh-tock-si-KOH-sis)	condition of excessive thyroid hormone production; also called hyperthyroidism
exophthalmos (eck-sof-THAL-mus)	protrusion of the eyes from their sockets
thyroid (THIGH-roid) **storm**	exacerbation of the signs and symptoms of hyperthyroidism; also called thyrotoxic crisis
Graves disease	autoimmune condition caused by excessive thyroid hormone production; a form of hyperthyroidism
thyroid (THIGH-roid) **cancer**	malignant neoplasm of the thyroid gland

continued

continued from page 436

KEY TERM PRACTICE: *Thyroid Gland Disorders*

1. The form of hyperthyroidism that is an autoimmune disease and characterized by exophthalmos is known as

   _____.

2. Surgical removal of the thyroid gland is termed _____, which is derived from the word part

   _____, meaning "thyroid," and the word part *-ectomy,* meaning _____.

3. The condition of decreased thyroid hormone production is termed _____.

4. _____ is the medical term for abnormal eyeball protrusion.

5. An enlargement of the thyroid gland is termed a _____.

LIFE SPAN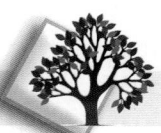

Endocrine function remains relatively stable throughout life in the absence of overlying disease. Exceptions to this involve the thymus and reproductive glands. The thymus reaches its greatest size at a weight of about 40 g (1.4 oz) just before puberty. After puberty it begins to atrophy and may be no larger than a walnut during the elderly years. This decrease may be linked to diminished immune response in later years. The decline in female ovary function in the late 40s results in menopause, but testicular testosterone production in males does not decrease until very old age.

Some hormone production declines with age, yet endocrine glands continue to perform throughout life. Growth hormone secretion diminishes with age, causing muscle atrophy. Thyroid hormone output decreases, leading to a decline in metabolic rate and fat mobilization.

Epinephrine and norepinephrine levels remain unchanged throughout the aging process. Cortisol and aldosterone levels decrease as the adrenal glands become more fibrous after 50 years of age.

Although the pancreas is capable of functioning until death, it becomes slower at insulin release. Furthermore, there is reduced glucose sensitivity, resulting in slower glucose regulation with advancing years.

COMMON *Abbreviations*

Abbreviation	Term
ACTH	adrenocorticotropic hormone; corticotropin
ADH	antidiuretic hormone; vasopressin
ANP	atrial natriuretic peptide
A$_{1c}$	glycosylated hemoglobin
CT	calcitonin

continued

continued from page 437

Abbreviation	Term
CT scan	computed tomography scan
DHEA	dehydroepiandrosterone
DM	diabetes mellitus
E	epinephrine
FDA	Food and Drug Administration
FSH	follicle-stimulating hormone
GH	growth hormone
GDM	gestational diabetes mellitus
GTT	glucose tolerance test
hPL	human placental lactogen
HRT	hormone replacement therapy
^{131}I	radioisotope of iodine
K^+	potassium ion
17-KS	17-ketosteroids test
LH	luteinizing hormone
LPN	licensed practical nurse
μCi	microcurie
MRI	magnetic resonance imaging
MSH	melanocyte-stimulating hormone
Na^+	sodium ion
NE	norepinephrine
OXT	oxytocin
PRL	prolactin
PTH	parathyroid hormone
RIA	radioimmunoassay
RIU test	radioactive iodine uptake test
RN	registered nurse
T_3	triiodothyronine
T_4	tetraiodothyronine; thyroxine
TSH	thyroid-stimulating hormone

COMMON ABBREVIATIONS EXERCISES

1. Give the abbreviation for radioimmunoassay. _____

2. OXT is the abbreviation for _____.

3. ANP is the abbreviation for _____.

4. T_3 is the abbreviation for _____.

5. Give the abbreviation for norepinephrine. _____

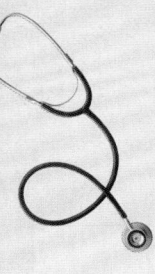

Case Study

Mr. Cleveland presented in Nurse Justina's endocrinology office complaining of weight loss and general malaise. Mr. Cleveland is 50 years old with no medical history of thyroid disease. His vital signs were within normal limits. Over the last 6 months, he had lost 35 pounds without dieting. A routine thyroid palpation—in which the patient swallows water while the clinician applies pressure to the anterior cervical region—indicated a thyroid abnormality. A thyroid ¹³¹I uptake and thyroid scan provided the following results:

- Enlarged bilateral lobes. The right thyroid lobe measured 5.6 × 1.8 × 3.0 cm. The left thyroid lobe measured 4.6 × 2.0 × 2.0 cm.
- Abnormal uptake of 78% at 25 h.

Case Study Questions

Select the best answer to each of the following questions.

1. **The physician palpated which region of Mr. Cleveland's body?**

   _____

   a. shoulder
   b. throat
   c. chest
   d. groin

2. **A thyroid scan is best described as a**

   _____.

   a. procedure in which x-ray images of the thyroid gland are produced after the patient ingests a radioactive ion
   b. test in which the patient fasts for 12 h and then drinks a glucose mixture
   c. method used for detecting antigens, antibodies, enzymes, and hormones using radiolabeled reactants
   d. test that can determine circulating levels of ACTH, CT, LH, and cortisol

3. **The ¹³¹I test is best described as**

   _____.

   a. a urine test to determine cortisol and androgen excretions
   b. a measure of serum glucose levels at intervals up to 3 h
   c. the test used to determine hyperactivity or hypoactivity of the thyroid gland after the patient ingests radioactive iodine
   d. a blood test used to detect iodine

4. **Mr. Cleveland's thyroid uptake was measured at 78%. The normal value for thyroid uptake at 24 h is between 9% and 36%. Mr. Cleveland's value suggests**

   _____.

   a. hyperthyroidism
   b. hypothyroidism
   c. hyperparathyroidism
   d. hypoparathyroidism

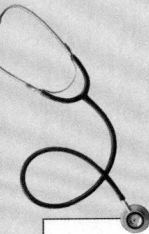

Real World Report

SOUTHWEST IMAGING DEPARTMENT

NAME: Elmer Cleveland
DOB: 02/18/61   AGE: 50 years
DATEORD: 06/06/11   EXAM DATE: 06/13/11
TEST: Localize tumor; whole body   CLINIC: Nuclear Medical Department
ATTENDING: K. L. Lindau, MD   ORDPHYS: K. L. Lindau, MD

CLINICAL DATA

Hyperthyroidism, thyroid carcinoma

^{131}I WHOLE-BODY SCAN

A whole-body thyroid scan was obtained 7 days after the patient had been given 105 μCi of iodine-131 orally. This study was compared with previous RIU and scan examination of November 7, 2008.

There is abnormal increased uptake in the region of the thyroid, consistent with thyroid carcinoma. Physiological uptake is noted in the regions of the pharynx and liver. No abnormal areas of increased uptake seen in the remaining study to suggest metastasis.

IMPRESSION

- Abnormal increased uptake in the region of the thyroid consistent with the thyroid carcinoma
- No metastasis seen

Dictated by: J. R. Waterville, MD

Real World Report Questions

The following exercises review the medical terms used in the preceding medical report.

1. **Mr. Cleveland was given 105 μCi of ^{131}I orally.**

   a. What does 105 μCi mean?

   _____

   b. What is ^{131}I and why is it used?

   _____

2. **Define the abbreviation RIA. What is an RIA scan?** _____

3. **Define hyperthyroidism.**

   _____

4. **Identify the targeted organ for the ^{131}I uptake test in this report.**

   _____

Review and Application

Multiple-Choice Questions

Select the best answer to each of the following questions.

1. In the endocrine system, which gland is referred to as the master gland? _____
   a. hypothalamus   b. thymus   c. thyroid gland   d. pituitary gland

2. A _____ cell is one with a specific receptor for a particular hormone.
   a. target   b. hormone   c. substrate   d. precursor

3. This type of diabetes has an onset during pregnancy. _____
   a. Type 1   b. Type 2   c. gestational diabetes   d. Type 1 and Type 2

4. A disorder resulting from excessive growth hormone secretion before puberty is known as _____.
   a. acromegaly   b. gigantism   c. dwarfism   d. virilism

5. Endocrine glands secrete their hormones _____
   a. directly into the   b. into ducts exposed   c. into ducts on the   d. directly into cells.
      bloodstream.   to the surface.   body's interior.

6. Which hormone is *not* secreted by the anterior pituitary gland? _____
   a. ACTH   b. MSH   c. ADH   d. LH

7. The pituitary gland is divided into _____ and _____ portions.
   a. primary; secondary   b. proximal; distal   c. anterior; posterior   d. dorsal; ventral

8. Which area of the pituitary gland is merely a storage and releasing site? _____
   a. posterior pituitary   b. adrenal cortex   c. adrenal medulla   d. anterior pituitary

9. The anterior pituitary gland is directed by hormones from the _____.
   a. hypothalamus   b. posterior pituitary gland   c. pineal gland   d. thyroid gland

10. What is another name for the neurohypophysis? _____
    a. anterior pituitary   b. adrenal gland   c. parathyroids   d. posterior pituitary
       gland   gland

11. Human biorhythms of 24-hour cycles are termed _____ rhythms in the medical field.
    a. cyclical   b. melatonin   c. circadian   d. pineal

12. The parathyroid glands are located on the _____.
    a. anterior surface   b. posterior surface   c. anterior surface   d. posterior surface of
       of the thyroid gland   of the thymus   of the pituitary gland   the thyroid gland

13. Tetraiodothyronine is also called _____.
    a. T_3 b. T_4 c. thyroxine   d. b and c

14. The pancreas is located adjacent to the _____ and _____.
    a. anterior pituitary   b. stomach; small   c. thyroid gland;   d. thymus;
       gland; posterior   intestine   parathyroids   pineal gland
       pituitary gland

15. The _____ and _____ are the two portions of the adrenal gland.

   a. outer; cortex   b. inner; medulla   c. medulla; cortex   d. anterior; posterior

16. Polydipsia, polyuria, and polyphagia mean _____, respectively.

   a. excessive thirst, excessive urination, and excessive hunger   b. excessive urination, excessive thirst, and excessive hunger   c. excessive hunger, excessive thirst, and excessive urination   d. excessive appetite, excessive hunger, and excessive thirst

17. The glucose tolerance test is useful for diagnosing _____.

   a. thyroid disorders   b. pancreatic disorders   c. parathyroid gland disorders   d. pituitary gland disorders

18. After eating supper, which hormone is likely to be secreted in greater amounts than while fasting?
   _____

   a. insulin   b. glucagon   c. ACTH   d. epinephrine

19. Upon rising in the morning after a good night's sleep, your body secretes this hormone to prevent hypoglycemia.
   _____

   a. insulin   b. glucagon   c. glucose   d. glycogen

Word Parts Exercises

Using the following words and word parts, form a medical term for each definition. Each word or word part is used only once.

acro-	-ectomy	epi-
hyper-	-ism	-ine
megal-	nephr-	parathyroid
-sis	thyro-	thyroid
toxico-	-y	

20. removal of thyroid gland _____

21. disorder characterized by oversecretion of growth hormone in an adult _____

22. disorder characterized by excessive activity of the parathyroid glands _____

23. toxic disorder of thyroid gland caused by hyperactivity of the gland _____

24. hormone of the adrenal medulla _____

Matching Exercises

Match the disorder with its description.

_____ 25. diabetes mellitus

_____ 26. diabetes insipidus

_____ 27. Addison disease

_____ 28. Cushing disease

_____ 29. pheochromocytoma

a. tumor of the adrenal medulla
b. excessive cortisol production by the adrenal cortex; "moon face"
c. disorder of carbohydrate metabolism
d. disorder of posterior pituitary gland
e. wasting disorder caused by underactivity of the adrenal glands

Match the hormone with its primary target.

_____ 30. GH

_____ 31. TSH

_____ 32. ADH

_____ 33. glucagon

_____ 34. LH

a. kidneys
b. bones
c. liver
d. thyroid
e. ovaries

Match the hormone with its primary action.

_____ 35. ACTH

_____ 36. androgens

_____ 37. thymosins

_____ 38. OXT

_____ 39. GH

a. supplement sex hormones
b. development of immune system cells
c. hypertrophy of body cells
d. stimulates uterine contractions
e. stimulates cortex of adrenal gland to produce cortisol

Definitions

Define the following terms.

40. hyperthyroidism _____

41. hypothyroidism _____

42. hypophysectomy _____

43. hypoglycemia _____

Provide a medical term for the following definitions.

44. adrenal cortex hormone that regulates salt and water balance _____

45. hormone secreted by heart cells that promotes fluid loss and blood pressure reduction _____

46. glands and organs that secrete directly into the bloodstream; also called ductless glands _____

47. process by which substances are produced and discharged from a gland for a particular physiological function _____

48. small pine cone-shaped organ in the brain that secretes melatonin _____

Alternative Terms

Give an alternative term for each of the following terms.

49. ADH _____

50. neurohypophysis _____

51. adenohypophysis _____

52. juvenile-onset diabetes _____

53. hydrocortisone _____

54. adrenaline _____

55. Hashimoto disease _____

56. noradrenaline _____

Spelling

Identify the correctly spelled term in each set.

57. _____

a. addrenal medulla
b. adrenal medulla
c. adrenal medula
d. addrenal meddula

58. _____

a. adrennocorticotropic
b. adrenocorticotroppic
c. adrenocorticotropick
d. adrenocorticotropic

59. _____

a. kortisol
b. cortisol
c. cortesol
d. kortesol

60. _____

a. pinneal
b. pineul
c. pineal
d. peneal

61. _____
    a. gloocagon
    b. glucagun
    c. glycagon
    d. glucagon

Unscramble

. . . .

Unscramble the letters to form a medical term.

62. xymeedam _____

63. spancrae _____

64. absteeid _____

65. nitpel _____

66. greatt ellc _____

Abbreviations

. . . .

Provide the term for the abbreviations and then define the terms.

67. E = _____

68. TSH = _____

69. T_3 = _____

70. OXT = _____

71. PRL = _____

Analogies

. . . .

Provide a medical term to complete a meaningful analogy.

72. The exocrine system is to glands with ducts as the _____ system is to ductless glands.

73. The anterior pituitary gland is to FSH as the _____ is to OXT.

74. Calcitonin is to PTH as _____ is to glucagon.

Short Answer

. . . .

Answer the following questions.

75. Wendy is highly allergic to bee stings, so when she got stung at a family picnic, her reaction was immediate. She gave herself an injection with an EpiPen. Upon arrival at the emergency room, she presented with increased heart rate, increased blood pressure, airway dilation, and a rise in blood glucose as a result of her EpiPen injection. Given this information, what hormone was probably in her pen? _____

76. Tom went to his physician complaining of polyuria and polydipsia. He said he was constantly thirsty and could not seem to drink enough water. His urine is very pale, and he excretes large volumes. The physician prescribed a short course of vasopressin therapy. What disorder did the physician suspect? _____

Labeling

Label the structures in the following diagram.

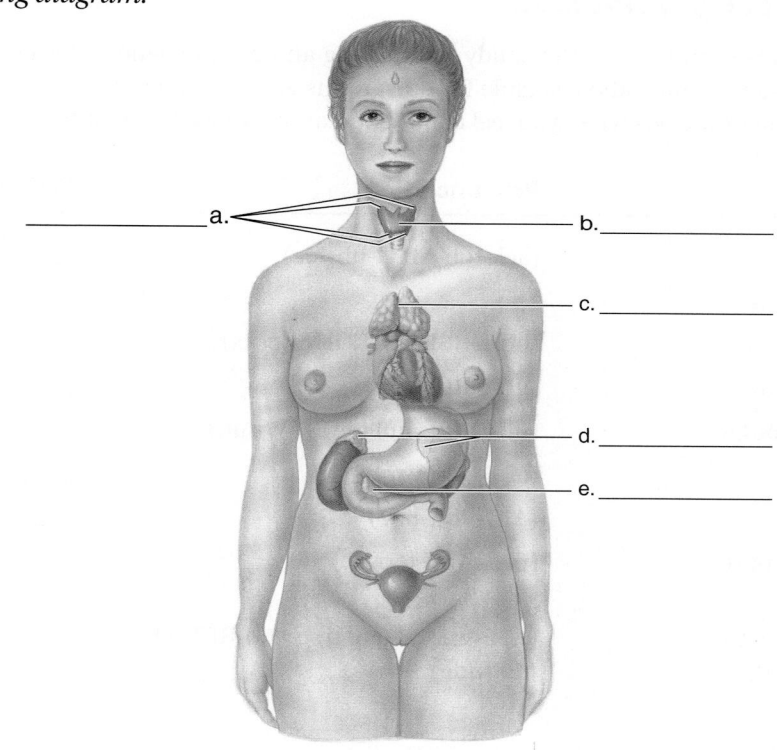

a. _____

b. _____

c. _____

d. _____

e. _____

Word Search

Find the medical terms hidden in the puzzle.

A	U	S	D	G	B	M	X	E	S	P	A	T	L	Z	I
L	D	N	E	R	O	M	X	N	T	L	E	H	O	B	T
C	G	R	I	N	U	N	E	Z	D	C	S	Y	I	Y	H
M	O	N	E	N	O	G	A	O	E	P	T	R	R	C	L
F	C	R	S	N	O	M	S	D	H	U	R	O	T	M	T
X	Z	T	T	R	A	T	R	M	S	N	O	I	I	S	D
S	S	R	D	I	E	L	I	O	G	T	G	D	C	A	S
S	H	N	Q	R	S	I	C	C	H	E	E	G	L	E	F
Y	A	H	O	W	S	O	H	O	L	A	N	L	A	R	T
Q	U	N	E	J	Y	W	L	V	R	A	V	A	C	C	H
M	E	L	A	T	O	N	I	N	L	T	C	N	C	N	Y
E	N	I	R	H	P	E	N	I	P	E	E	D	O	A	M
Y	O	N	O	G	A	C	U	L	G	R	B	X	W	P	U
I	N	S	U	L	I	N	W	X	E	H	G	Y	X	S	S
L	G	M	P	A	A	Z	E	J	X	W	I	A	D	A	P
F	S	Z	T	U	Z	I	J	J	F	I	M	O	Z	G	M	K

adrenal cortex
aldosterone
androgens
calcitonin
calcitriol
cortisol
epinephrine
estrogen
glucagon
gonads
hormones
insulin
melatonin
pancreas
thymus
thyroid gland

Vocabulary Review

Review the key terms from this chapter, study the spelling and pronunciation of each term, and write its definition in the space provided. Listen to the audio available for most terms at http://thepoint.lww.com/nath2e and pronounce each term for yourself. Then check the box when you feel confident that you know the definition and can pronounce the term correctly.

Key Term	Pronunciation	Definition
❏ acromegaly	(ack-roh-MEG-uh-lee)	
❏ Addison disease		
❏ adrenal cortex	(uh-DREE-nul KOHR-tecks)	
❏ adrenal glands	(uh-DREE-nul)	
❏ adrenal medulla	(uh-DREE-nul me-DEW-luh)	
❏ aldosterone	(al-DOS-te-rohn)	
❏ androgens	(AN-droh-jinz)	
❏ anterior pituitary gland	(pi-TEW-i-terr-ee)	
❏ atrial natriuretic peptide (ANP)	(AYE-tree-ul nay-tree-yoo-RET-ick PEP-tide)	
❏ blood tests		
❏ calcitonin (CT)	(kal-si-TOH-nin)	
❏ calcitriol	(kal-sih-TRY-ul)	
❏ circadian rhythm	(sur-KAY-dee-un)	
❏ cortisol	(KOR-ti-sol)	
❏ Cushing disease	(KOOSH-ing)	
❏ diabetes insipidus	(dye-uh-BEE-teez in-SIP-i-dus)	
❏ diabetes mellitus (DM)	(dye-uh-BEE-teez mel-EYE-tus)	
❏ endocrine system	(EN-doh-krin)	
❏ epinephrine (E)	(ep-i-NEF-rin)	
❏ estrogen	(es-TROH-jen)	
❏ excretion	(eck-SKREE-shun)	
❏ exophthalmos	(eck-sof-THAL-mus)	
❏ gestational diabetes mellitus (GDM)	(jes-TAY-shun-ul dye-uh-BEE-teez mel-EYE-tus)	
❏ gigantism	(jye-GAN-tiz-um)	
❏ gland		
❏ glucagon	(GLOO-kuh-gon)	
❏ glucose tolerance test (GTT)	(GLOO-kose)	
❏ glycosylated hemoglobin (A_{1c}) test	(GLYE-koh-si-lay-ted HEE-moh-gloh-bin)	

Key Term	Pronunciation	Definition
❑ goiter	(GOY-tur)	_____
❑ gonads	(GOH-nadz)	_____
❑ Graves disease		_____
❑ Hashimoto thyroiditis	(hah-shee-MOH-toh thigh-roid-EYE-tis)	_____
❑ hirsutism	(HUR-sewt-iz-um)	_____
❑ hormone replacement therapy (HRT)		_____
❑ hormones	(HOR-mohnz)	_____
❑ hypercalcemia	(high-pur-kal-SEE-mee-uh)	_____
❑ hyperglycemia	(high-pur-glye-SEE-mee-uh)	_____
❑ hyperparathyroidism	(high-pur-pair-uh-THIGH-roid-iz-um)	_____
❑ hyperthyroidism	(high-pur-THIGH-roid-izm)	_____
❑ hypoglycemia	(high-poh-glye-SEE-mee-uh)	_____
❑ hypoparathyroidism	(high-poh-pair-uh-THIGH-roid-iz-um)	_____
❑ hypothalamus	(high-poh-THAL-uh-mus)	_____
❑ hypothyroidism	(high-poh-THIGH-roid-izm)	_____
❑ infantile hypothyroidism	(high-poh-THIGH-roid-izm)	_____
❑ insulin	(IN-suh-lin)	_____
❑ leptin	(LEP-tin)	_____
❑ melatonin	(mel-uh-TOH-nin)	_____
❑ myxedema	(mick-seh-DEE-muh)	_____
❑ norepinephrine (NE)	(nor-ep-i-NEF-rin)	_____
❑ pancreas	(PAN-kree-us)	_____
❑ pancreatic islets	(pan-kree-AT-ick)	_____
❑ parathyroid glands	(pair-uh-THIGH-roid)	_____
❑ parathyroid hormone (PTH)	(pair-uh-THIGH-roid)	_____
❑ parathyroidectomy	(pair-uh-thigh-roy-DECK-tuh-mee)	_____
❑ pheochromocytoma	(fee-oh-kroh-moh-sigh-TOH-muh)	_____
❑ pineal gland	(PYE-nee-ul)	_____
❑ pituitary dwarfism	(pi-TEW-i-terr-ee)	_____
❑ pituitary gland	(pi-TEW-i-terr-ee)	_____
❑ posterior pituitary gland	(pi-TEW-i-terr-ee)	_____
❑ postprandial	(pohst-PRAN-dee-ul)	_____
❑ precocious puberty	(pree-KOH-shus)	_____
❑ progesterone	(proh-JES-ter-ohn)	_____

Key Term	Pronunciation	Definition
❑ radioactive iodine uptake test (RIU)		_____
❑ radioimmunoassay (RIA)	(RAY-dee-oh-im-yoo-noh-as-say)	_____
❑ secretion	(se-KREE-shun)	_____
❑ target cell		_____
❑ testosterone	(tes-TOS-teh-rohn)	_____
❑ thymosins	(THIGH-moh-sins)	_____
❑ thymus	(THIGH-mus)	_____
❑ thyroid cancer	(THIGH-roid)	_____
❑ thyroid gland	(THIGH-roid)	_____
❑ thyroid storm	(THIGH-roid)	_____
❑ thyroidectomy	(thigh-roid-ECK-tuh-mee)	_____
❑ thyrotoxicosis	(thigh-roh-tock-si-KOH-sis)	_____
❑ thyroxine (T$_4$)	(thigh-ROCK-seen)	_____
❑ triiodothyronine (T$_3$)	(trye-eye-oh-doh-THIGH-roh-neen)	_____
❑ Trousseau sign	(true-SOH)	_____
❑ Type 1 diabetes	(dye-uh-BEE-teez)	_____
❑ Type 2 diabetes	(dye-uh-BEE-teez)	_____
❑ urine ketosteroids tests	(kee-toh-STEER-oidz)	_____
❑ virilism	(VEER-ih-liz-um)	_____

Answers

Word Grouping Exercises

Definition	Word Part	Definition	Word Part
glucose	gluc-, gluco-	involving the pancreas	pancreat-, pancreatico-, pancreato-, pancreo-
alongside, near	para-	milk	lact-, lacti-, lacto-
childbirth	toco-	mucus	myx-, myxo-
cortex	cortico-	relating to calcium	calc-, calci-
deficient, below normal	hypo-	relating to the adrenal gland	adren-, adrenal-, adreno-
eating	-phage, -phagia, -phagy	sugar	glyco-
extreme	acro-	thyroid gland	thyr-, thyreo-, thyro-
gland, glandular	aden-, adeno-	within, inner	end-, endo-
having an affinity for	-tropic		
honey, sugar	mel-, meli-, melo-		

Word Building Exercises

Word Part	Meaning	Common or Known Word	Example Medical Term
aden-, adeno-	gland, glandular	adenoid	adenohypophysis
adren-, adrenal-, adreno-	adrenal	adrenaline	adrenal gland
end-, endo-	within, inner	endoderm	endocrine
gluc-, gluco-	glucose	glucose	glucose
hypo-	deficient, below normal	hypoglycemic	hypoparathyroidism
lact-, lacti-, lacto-	milk	lactose	prolactin
mel-, meli-, melo-	honey, sugar	mellifluous	diabetes mellitus
pancreat-, pancreatico-, pancreato-, pancreo-	involving the pancreas	pancreas	pancreas
para-	alongside, near	parasail	parathyroid glands
thyr-, thyreo-, thyro-	thyroid gland	thyroid	thyroid gland

Key Term Practice

Endocrine System Preview

1. endocrine
2. hormones
3. excretion
4. Secretion
5. target cell

Pituitary Gland

1. pituitary gland
2. anterior pituitary gland
3. posterior pituitary gland
4. hypothalamus

Thyroid Gland and Parathyroid Glands

1. calcitonin (CT); parathyroid hormone (PTH)
2. thyroxine (T_4) and triiodothyronine (T_3)
3. parathyroid glands
4. thyroid gland

Pancreas

1. glucagon
2. insulin
3. pancreatic islets
4. pancreas

Adrenal Glands

1. epinephrine (E) and norepinephrine (NE)
2. adrenal cortex; adrenal medulla
3. Aldosterone
4. Androgens
5. cortisol

Pineal Gland and Thymus

1. thymosins
2. thymus
3. Melatonin
4. circadian rhythm
5. pineal gland

Other Organs with Secondary Endocrine Functions

1. estrogen and progesterone
2. Leptin
3. testosterone
4. Atrial natriuretic peptide (ANP)
5. Calcitriol

Adrenal Gland Disorders

1. Addison disease
2. pheochromocytoma
3. Virilism
4. hirsutism
5. Cushing disease

Pancreas Disorders

1. Hypoglycemia
2. postprandial
3. glycosylated hemoglobin (A_{1c})
4. Type 1 diabetes
5. gestational diabetes mellitus (GDM)

Parathyroid Gland Disorders

1. hypoparathyroidism
2. hyperparathyroidism
3. hypercalcemia; *calc-*; *-emia*
4. parathyroidectomy
5. Trousseau sign

Pituitary Gland Disorders

1. gigantism
2. Acromegaly
3. pituitary dwarfism
4. Diabetes insipidus
5. Precocious puberty

Thyroid Gland Disorders

1. Graves disease
2. thyroidectomy; *thyro-*; removal of an anatomical structure
3. hypothyroidism
4. Exophthalmos
5. goiter

Common Abbreviations Exercises

1. Radioimmunoassay = RIA
2. OXT = oxytocin
3. ANP = atrial natriuretic peptide
4. T_3 = triiodothyronine
5. Norepinephrine = NE

Case Study

1. b is the correct answer.
   - a is incorrect because the shoulder is the acromial region.
   - c is incorrect because the chest is the pectoral region.
   - d is incorrect because the groin is the inguinal region.
2. a is the correct answer.
   - b is incorrect because it describes a glucose tolerance test.
   - c is incorrect because it describes a radioimmunoassay.
   - d is incorrect because these levels are determined by a blood test.
3. c is the correct answer.
   - a is incorrect because urine tests do not require the ingestion of radioactive iodine.
   - b is incorrect because this test describes a glucose tolerance test.
   - d is incorrect because it is not a blood test used to detect iodine.
4. a is the correct answer.
   - b is incorrect because the gland is undergoing hypertrophy and increased thyroid activity, not atrophy and decreased thyroid activity.
   - c and d are incorrect because the thyroid gland was evaluated using this test, not the parathyroid gland, which would require a different testing procedure.

Real World Report

1. a. 105 microcuries.

   b. ^{131}I is a radioactive isotope of iodine that is used as a tracer in thyroid studies.

2. Radioactive iodine uptake; a test that measures the amount of ^{131}I taken up by the thyroid gland.

3. A condition in which excessive thyroid hormones are produced.

4. Thyroid gland.

Review and Application

1. d
2. a
3. c
4. b
5. a
6. c
7. c
8. a
9. a
10. d
11. c
12. d
13. d
14. b
15. c
16. a
17. b
18. a
19. b
20. thyroidectomy
21. acromegaly
22. hyperparathyroidism
23. thyrotoxicosis
24. epinephrine
25. c
26. d
27. e
28. b
29. a
30. b

31. d
32. a
33. c
34. e
35. e
36. a
37. b
38. d
39. c
40. disorder caused by excessive secretion of thyroid hormone
41. disorder caused by inadequate secretion of thyroid hormone
42. surgical excision of the hypophysis (pituitary gland)
43. low blood glucose levels
44. aldosterone
45. atrial natriuretic peptide (ANP)
46. endocrine system
47. secretion
48. pineal gland
49. vasopressin
50. posterior pituitary gland
51. anterior pituitary gland
52. Type 1 diabetes
53. cortisol
54. epinephrine
55. Hashimoto thyroiditis
56. norepinephrine
57. b

58. d
59. b
60. c
61. d
62. myxedema
63. pancreas
64. diabetes
65. leptin
66. target cell
67. E = epinephrine; adrenal medulla hormone involved in the fight-or-flight response
68. TSH = thyroid-stimulating hormone; stimulates the production of thyroid hormones
69. T$_3$ = triiodothyronine; thyroid hormone involved with metabolism
70. OXT = oxytocin; stimulates uterine contractions and milk ejection into breast ducts
71. PRL = prolactin; stimulates milk production (lactation)
72. endocrine
73. posterior pituitary gland
74. insulin
75. Hormones of the adrenal medulla—epinephrine and/or norepinephrine—were probably in the injection.
76. The physician suspected diabetes insipidus.

Labeling

a. parathyroid glands

b. thyroid gland

c. thymus

d. adrenal glands

e. pancreas

Word Search

A	U	S	D	G	B	M	X	E	S	P	A	T	L	Z	I
L	D	N	E	R	O	M	X	N	T	L	E	H	O	B	T
C	G	R	I	N	U	N	E	Z	D	C	S	Y	I	Y	H
M	O	N	E	N	O	G	A	O	E	P	T	R	R	C	L
F	C	R	S	N	O	M	S	D	H	U	R	O	T	M	T
X	Z	T	T	R	A	T	R	M	S	N	O	I	I	S	D
S	S	R	D	I	E	L	I	O	G	T	G	D	C	A	S
S	H	N	Q	R	S	I	C	C	H	E	E	G	L	E	F
Y	A	H	O	W	S	O	H	O	L	A	N	L	A	R	T
Q	U	N	E	J	Y	W	L	V	R	A	V	A	C	C	H
M	E	L	A	T	O	N	I	N	L	T	C	N	C	N	Y
E	N	I	R	H	P	E	N	I	P	E	E	D	O	A	M
Y	O	N	O	G	A	C	U	L	G	R	B	X	W	P	U
I	N	S	U	L	I	N	W	X	E	H	G	Y	X	S	S
L	G	M	P	A	A	Z	E	J	X	W	I	A	D	A	P
F	S	Z	T	U	Z	I	J	F	I	M	O	Z	G	M	K

adrenal cortex
aldosterone
androgens
calcitonin
calcitriol
cortisol
epinephrine
estrogen
glucagon
gonads
hormones
insulin
melatonin
pancreas
thymus
thyroid gland

Vocabulary Review

Key Term	Definition	Key Term	Definition
acromegaly	disorder caused by excessive GH secretion in adulthood that is characterized by abnormally thick bones	**anterior pituitary gland**	part of the pituitary gland that secretes hormones; also called the adenohypophysis
Addison disease	wasting disorder caused by underactivity of the adrenal glands	**atrial natriuretic peptide (ANP)**	hormone secreted by heart cells that promotes fluid loss and blood pressure reduction
adrenal cortex	outer portion of the adrenal gland	**blood tests**	analyses of blood to evaluate its components
adrenal glands	endocrine gland located above each kidney		
adrenal medulla	inner portion of the adrenal gland	**calcitonin (CT)**	a thyroid hormone that lowers blood calcium ion levels
aldosterone	adrenal cortex hormone that regulates salt and water balance	**calcitriol**	hormone released by the kidneys that is important for calcium regulation
androgens	supplemental sex hormones produced by the adrenal cortex	**circadian rhythm**	human biorhythm that repeats every 24 hours

Key Term	Definition	Key Term	Definition
cortisol	adrenal cortex hormone that has anti-inflammatory effects; also called hydrocortisone	hormone replacement therapy (HRT)	hormone administration to restore normal function
Cushing disease	disorder caused by excessive cortisol production by the adrenal cortex and characterized by a "moon face" appearance	hormones	chemicals released by endocrine glands that are transported by blood to exert their effect at a site other than their origin
diabetes insipidus	chronic posterior pituitary gland disorder that causes inadequate ADH secretion	hypercalcemia	abnormally high blood calcium levels
diabetes mellitus (DM)	chronic disorder of carbohydrate metabolism	hyperglycemia	abnormally high blood glucose level
endocrine system	composed of glands and organs that secrete hormones directly into the blood to ensure long-term regulation and internal balance (homeostasis)	hyperparathyroidism	abnormally high level of parathyroid hormone (PTH) in the blood caused by overactive parathyroid glands
		hyperthyroidism	condition of excessive thyroid hormone production; also called thyrotoxicosis
epinephrine (E)	adrenal medulla hormone involved in the fight-or-flight response; also called adrenaline	hypoglycemia	abnormally low blood glucose level
estrogen	hormone produced by the ovaries to stimulate secondary sexual characteristics	hypoparathyroidism	inadequate secretion of parathyroid hormone
		hypothalamus	area of the brain that secretes releasing hormones and is involved with regulating temperature, thirst, and hunger
excretion	separating materials from the blood to be eliminated as waste	hypothyroidism	condition of decreased thyroid hormone production characterized by weight gain and sluggishness
exophthalmos	protrusion of the eyes from their sockets	infantile hypothyroidism	congenital form of hypothyroidism
gestational diabetes mellitus (GDM)	disorder of carbohydrate metabolism that occurs during pregnancy	insulin	pancreatic hormone from beta cells that decreases blood glucose levels
gigantism	disorder caused by excessive GH secretion before puberty characterized by abnormally long bones; also called giantism	leptin	hormone secreted by adipose tissue that regulates fat storage in the body
gland	an organized group of cells that functions as a secreting or excreting organ	melatonin	hormone secreted by pineal gland cells that may influence circadian rhythms
glucagon	pancreatic hormone from alpha cells that increases blood glucose levels	myxedema	condition caused by decreased thyroid hormone production; a form of hypothyroidism
glucose tolerance test (GTT)	determination of blood glucose levels at different times after drinking a glucose syrup	norepinephrine (NE)	adrenal medulla hormone involved in the fight-or-flight response; also called noradrenaline
glycosylated hemoglobin (A$_{1c}$) test	test used to measure circulating blood glucose levels over the life span of a red blood cell	pancreas	glandular organ with endocrine and exocrine functions
goiter	enlargement of the thyroid gland	pancreatic islets	the endocrine cells of the pancreas that secrete hormones
gonads	organs (ovaries in females and testes in males) that produce reproductive cells	parathyroid glands	four small endocrine glands located on the posterior surface of the thyroid gland
Graves disease	autoimmune condition caused by excessive thyroid hormone production; a form of hyperthyroidism	parathyroid hormone (PTH)	hormone that increases blood calcium ion levels
Hashimoto thyroiditis	autoimmune disease that causes an inflamed thyroid gland, resulting in hypothyroidism; also called Hashimoto disease	parathyroidectomy	surgical removal of one or more of the parathyroid glands
hirsutism	abnormal hair growth on a female's face or body	pheochromocytoma	adrenal medulla tumor that causes irregular secretion of epinephrine and norepinephrine

Key Term	Definition	Key Term	Definition
pineal gland	small pine cone-shaped organ in the brain that secretes melatonin	thymus	organ at the base of the neck, posterior to the sternum, and between the lungs that secretes thymosins
pituitary dwarfism	abnormal underdevelopment caused by inadequate GH secretion	thyroid cancer	malignant neoplasm of the thyroid gland
pituitary gland	master gland that orchestrates endocrine function; also called the hypophysis	thyroid gland	bilobed endocrine gland in the neck that secretes thyroid hormones responsible for growth and metabolism
posterior pituitary gland	part of the pituitary gland that stores and releases hormones; also called the neurohypophysis	thyroid storm	exacerbation of the signs and symptoms of hyperthyroidism; also called thyrotoxic crisis
postprandial	after a meal	thyroidectomy	partial or complete surgical removal of the thyroid gland
precocious puberty	disorder in which physical maturity occurs at an unusually early age due to pituitary gland dysfunction or hypothalamus dysfunction	thyrotoxicosis	condition of excessive thyroid hormone production; also called hyperthyroidism
progesterone	hormone secreted by the corpus luteum that targets the uterus in preparation for, and maintenance of, pregnancy	thyroxine (T_4)	a thyroid hormone that increases metabolic rate, enhances protein synthesis, and stimulates the breakdown of lipids; also called tetraiodothyronine
radioactive iodine uptake (RIU) test	test used to evaluate thyroid gland function by measuring the rate of radioactive iodine absorption in the thyroid gland	triiodothyronine (T_3)	a thyroid hormone that increases metabolic rate, enhances protein synthesis, and stimulates the breakdown of lipids
radioimmunoassay (RIA)	test using radioactive tracers to detect antigens, antibodies, enzymes, and hormones in the blood	Trousseau sign	carpal spasm elicited when the brachial region is compressed, suggesting hypoparathyroidism
secretion	process by which substances are produced and discharged from a gland for a particular physiological function	Type 1 diabetes	form of diabetes mellitus that occurs before age 25 as a result of beta cell destruction; also called juvenile-onset diabetes
target cell	cell that responds to a particular hormone	Type 2 diabetes	form of diabetes mellitus that occurs after age 40 as a result of either a lack of insulin or the body's inability to use insulin efficiently
testosterone	hormone secreted by the testes to stimulate secondary sexual characteristics	urine ketosteroids tests	analyses of urine to detect androgen metabolites
thymosins	group of hormones from the thymus gland involved in the development of immune system cells, particularly T cells	virilism	development of masculine traits in a female

CHAPTER 10

Blood

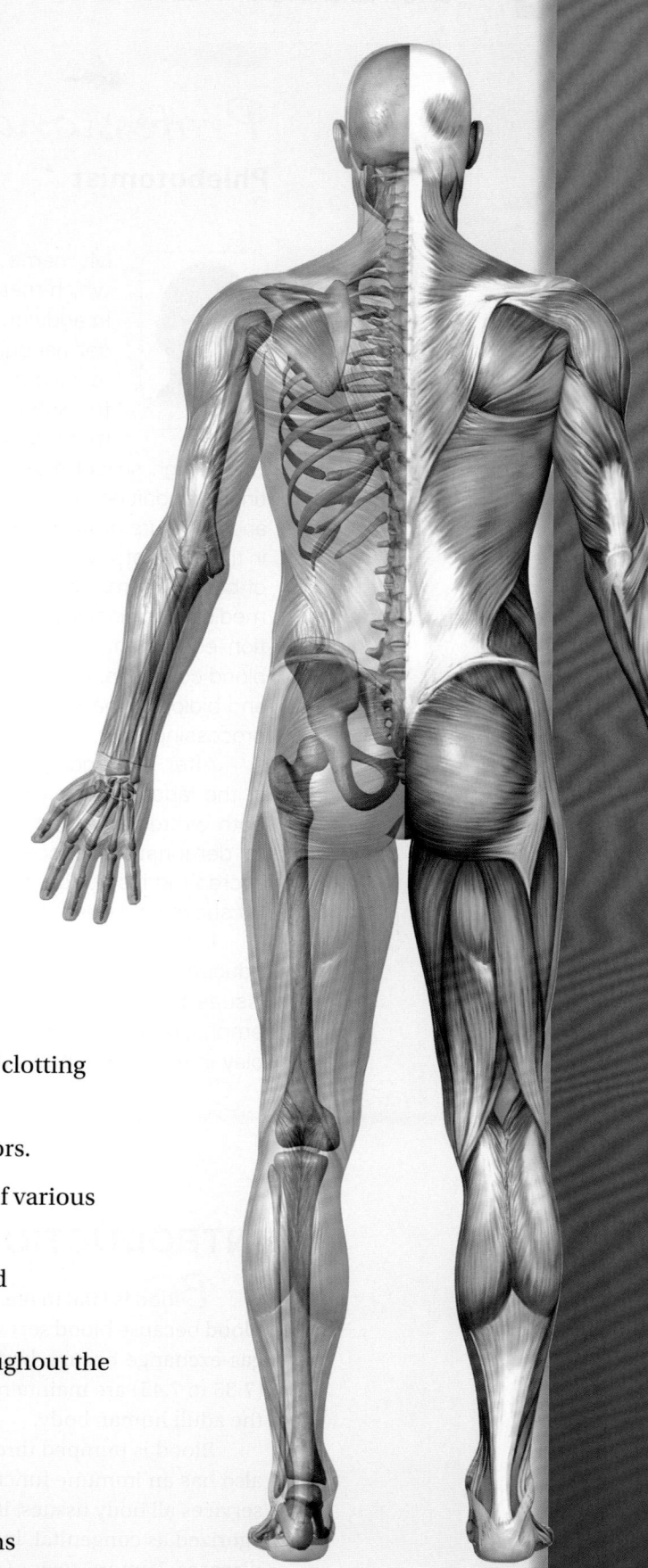

OBJECTIVES

After completing this chapter, you should be able to:

1. State the meanings of word parts related to blood.

2. Explain the importance of blood to normal physiological functioning.

3. Identify blood components.

4. List the various types of blood cells.

5. Describe the significance of lipoproteins and the role of clotting proteins and enzymes.

6. Summarize the basis for ABO blood groups and Rh factors.

7. Distinguish different signs, symptoms, and treatments of various blood diseases.

8. Describe clinical tests and diagnostic procedures related to blood.

9. Describe anatomical and physiological alterations throughout the life span.

10. Define abbreviations related to blood.

11. Define terms used in medical reports involving blood.

12. Define, spell, and pronounce the chapter's medical terms correctly.

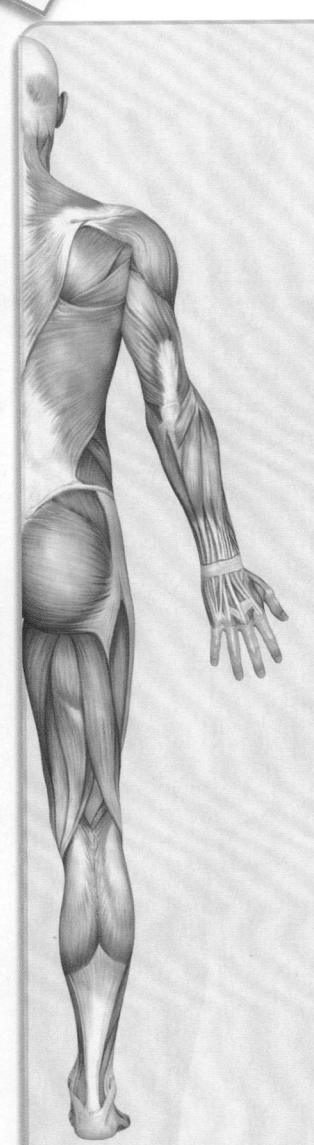

Professional Profile

Phlebotomist

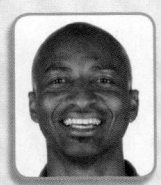

My name is John. I am a phlebotomist working in a hospital clinic, which means I collect blood samples from adult and pediatric patients. In addition to performing venipuncture (drawing blood from a vein) and dermal puncture (drawing blood through the skin), as a phlebotomist I receive and organize requests for blood collection, prepare the blood for distribution to the laboratory, clean laboratory glassware and equipment, and record blood collection statistics.

A high school diploma or equivalency is necessary for employment in many settings. In addition, phlebotomy-training programs generally require 40 hours of instruction and 20 hours of hands-on phlebotomy practice. Basic phlebotomy includes knowledge in the areas of infection control, universal precautions and safety, anatomy and physiology of body systems with special emphasis on the blood and circulatory system, appropriate medical terminology, patient and specimen identification, selection of blood collection equipment, skin preparation, and disposal of instruments and materials used in blood collection. It is also helpful to have advanced training in infectious disease control and biological hazards; anticoagulation theory; and specimen collection, transport, and processing.

After undergoing classroom instruction, phlebotomists may work a short time in the laboratory before taking a licensing examination. The examination consists of both written and practical portions. Some states do not require such licensure. I had to demonstrate successful completion of a phlebotomy-training program from an accredited institution and had to complete at least 100 successful venipunctures and 20 successful dermal punctures.

I sharpen my skills by attending seminars, update sessions, and continuing education workshops. These programs cover topics such as legal, moral, and ethical issues related to blood collection. Hospitals usually have training on health issues, emphasizing the significance of bloodborne pathogens and the role phlebotomists play in ensuring blood safety.

INTRODUCTION

Blood is vital to life. Homeostasis (internal balance) of the human body depends on the blood because blood serves as the medium by which nutrients and hormones are transported, gas exchange occurs, body temperature is regulated at a constant 37°C (98.6°F), pH levels (7.35 to 7.45) are maintained, and immunity is provided. There are about 10 pints of blood in the adult human body.

Blood is pumped through blood vessels to the body by the cardiovascular system. Blood also has an immune function through interaction with the lymphatic system. Because blood services all body tissues, its disorders often have systemic effects. Blood disorders can be categorized as congenital, infectious, coagulation (clotting), nutritional, and secondary to other diseases. Tumors, toxins (poisons), and trauma can also adversely affect blood delivery.

As a result of its systemic effects, blood can be tested to identify and assess a variety of conditions. This chapter focuses on the significance of blood to human physiology and identifies signs and symptoms, clinical tests and diagnostic procedures, and treatments pertaining to various blood-related problems.

MEDICAL TERM PARTS

Word Parts

Medical term prefixes, suffixes, and combining forms related to blood are introduced in this section.

Word Part	Meaning
basi-, basio-, baso-	base, basis
bili-	bile
chrom-, chromat-, chromato-, chromo-	color
cyan-, cyano-	blue
-cyte	cell
-emia	condition of blood
erythr-, erythro-	red, red blood cell
fibr-, fibro-	fiber
fibrino-	fibrin
granulo-	granular
hem-, hema-	blood
hemat-, hemato-, hemo-	blood
leuk-, leuko-	white, white blood cell
lymph-, lympho-	lymph (tissue fluid in a lymphatic vessel)
-lytic	causing lysis (disintegration)
myel-, myelo-	bone marrow
neutr-, neutro-	neutral
nucle-, nucleo-	nucleus
oxy-	presence of oxygen
-penia	deficiency
-phage, -phagia, -phagy	eating, devouring
phago-	eating, devouring
phen-, pheno-	denoting appearance
phil-, -phile, -philia, -philic	affinity for, craving for
phleb-, phlebo-	vein
plasma-, plasmat-, plasmato-, plasmo-	plasma (liquid part of blood)
pluri-	several
-poiesis	production, producing
-rrhagia	excessive discharge, hemorrhage
septic-, septico-	sepsis, septic (blood infection)
sero-	serum, serous
sidero-	iron
thromb-, thrombo-	blood clot, coagulation, thrombin

Word Grouping Exercises

Using the *Medical Term Parts* table, identify the prefix, suffix, or combining form for each of the following definitions. The first one has been done as an example.

Definition	Word Part
base, basis	*basi-, basio-, baso-*
affinity for, craving for	
bile	
blood	A. B.
blood clot, coagulation, thrombin	
blue	
bone marrow	
causing lysis (destruction)	
cell	
color	
condition of blood	
deficiency	
denoting appearance	
eating, devouring	A. B.
excessive discharge, hemorrhage	
fiber	
fibrin	
granular	
iron	
lymph (tissue fluid in a lymphatic vessel)	
neutral	
nucleus	
plasma (liquid part of blood)	
presence of oxygen	
production, producing	
red, red blood cell	
sepsis, septic (blood infection)	
serum, serous	
several	
vein	
white, white blood cell	

📖 Word Building Exercises

Word parts, introduced in the *Medical Term Parts* section, are listed in the following table. For this exercise, first supply the meaning of each word part, then use the word part to build a word you already know. The word you list under *Common or Known Word* does not have to be a medical term; a commonly used word is fine. Be sure, however, that the word correctly reflects the intended meaning. The first one has been done as an example. Check your answers in a dictionary.

Word Part	Meaning	Common or Known Word	Example Medical Term
leuk-, leuko-	*white, white blood cell*	*leukemia*	leukocyte
cyan-, cyano-			cyanosis
-emia			anemia
fibr-, fibro-			fibrosis
hem-, hema-			hemostasis
hemat-, hemato-, hemo-			hematopoiesis
neutr-, neutro-			neutrophil
oxy-			oxygen
phleb-, phlebo-			phlebotomy
phil-, -phile, -philia, -philic			hemophilia
pluri-			pluripotent
septic-, septico-			septicemia
sero-			serum
thromb-, thrombo-			thrombocyte

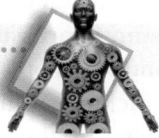

ANATOMY AND PHYSIOLOGY

Blood preview

The body has over 75 trillion cells that rely on blood to deliver nutrients and oxygen and to remove carbon dioxide and wastes. The blood also transports immune cells to protect against infection. In short, it is a vital component of life—so much so that cells deprived of blood die within a matter of minutes. **Hematology** is the branch of medicine devoted to the study of blood and diseases of the blood.

Whole blood that courses through blood vessels is a viscous (thick and sticky) liquid that consists of two major portions: formed elements and plasma. Formed elements include three

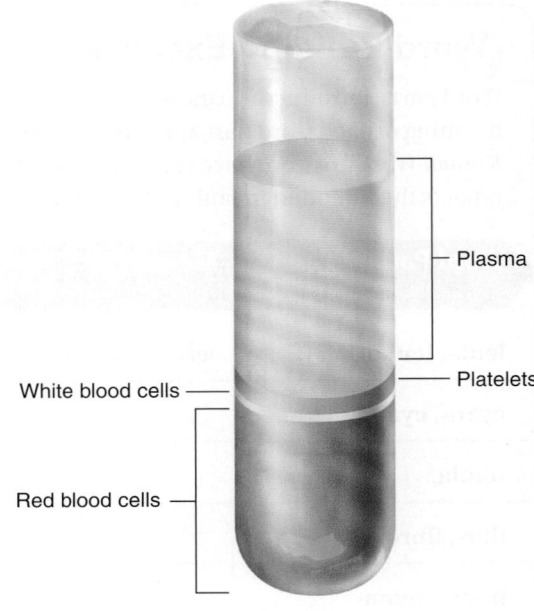

Plasma

Platelets

White blood cells

Red blood cells

Blood sample

Figure 10-1 Typical sample of whole blood.

types of blood cells: red blood cells (RBCs) or erythrocytes, white blood cells (WBCs) or leuko-cytes, and platelets. Red blood cells make up about 99.9% of formed elements, while WBCs and platelets make up less than 0.1% each. The other portion, plasma, is the liquid part of whole blood and it plays a role in blood clotting (**Figure 10-1**).

The fraction of whole blood that is made up of RBCs is known as the **packed cell volume (PCV)** or **hematocrit (Hct)**. The hematocrit of normal whole blood is approximately 45%, and the remaining 55% is plasma. Hematocrit values are important for assessing human blood disorders, and are discussed in greater detail later in this chapter.

Red blood cells, white blood cells, and platelets are formed by a process termed **hemopoiesis**, which is also called **hematopoiesis**. Hemopoiesis occurs in the red bone marrow. Recall that *blast* cells are early precursor cells. All blood cells begin as a **pluripotential hemopoietic stem cell (PHSC)**, a stem cell that changes (differentiates) into the various blood cell types (**Figure 10-2**). These cells were formerly known as hemocytoblasts.

Red blood cells make up the bulk of the formed elements. The remaining components are platelets and white blood cells. There are five types of white blood cells: neutrophils, lympho-cytes, monocytes, eosinophils, and basophils.

Plasma is the noncellular, pale yellow liquid part of whole blood and is made up mostly of water. It transports nutrients and hormones, regulates fluid and electrolytes, maintains a constant blood pH, and contains several proteins. Antibodies are also found in plasma. Plasma electrolytes (such as sodium and chloride) are important for maintaining both osmotic pressure and blood pH. **Osmotic pressure** is the pressure of fluid in the blood vessels, and it is important to maintaining blood pressure.

Plasma proteins include albumin, globulin, and fibrinogen. **Albumin** is a white-colored protein produced by the liver that provides blood with its viscosity, which is a factor in maintaining blood pressure and blood volume. It makes up about 60% of plasma. Approximately 36% of the plasma protein is globulin, a protein group with an immune function. Antibodies are an example of globulins. **Fibrinogen** makes up 4% of plasma proteins and plays an essential role in blood clotting (**Figure 10-3**). **Serum** is plasma without the clotting protein fibrinogen. Serum is often considered the fluid portion of coagulated (clotted) blood.

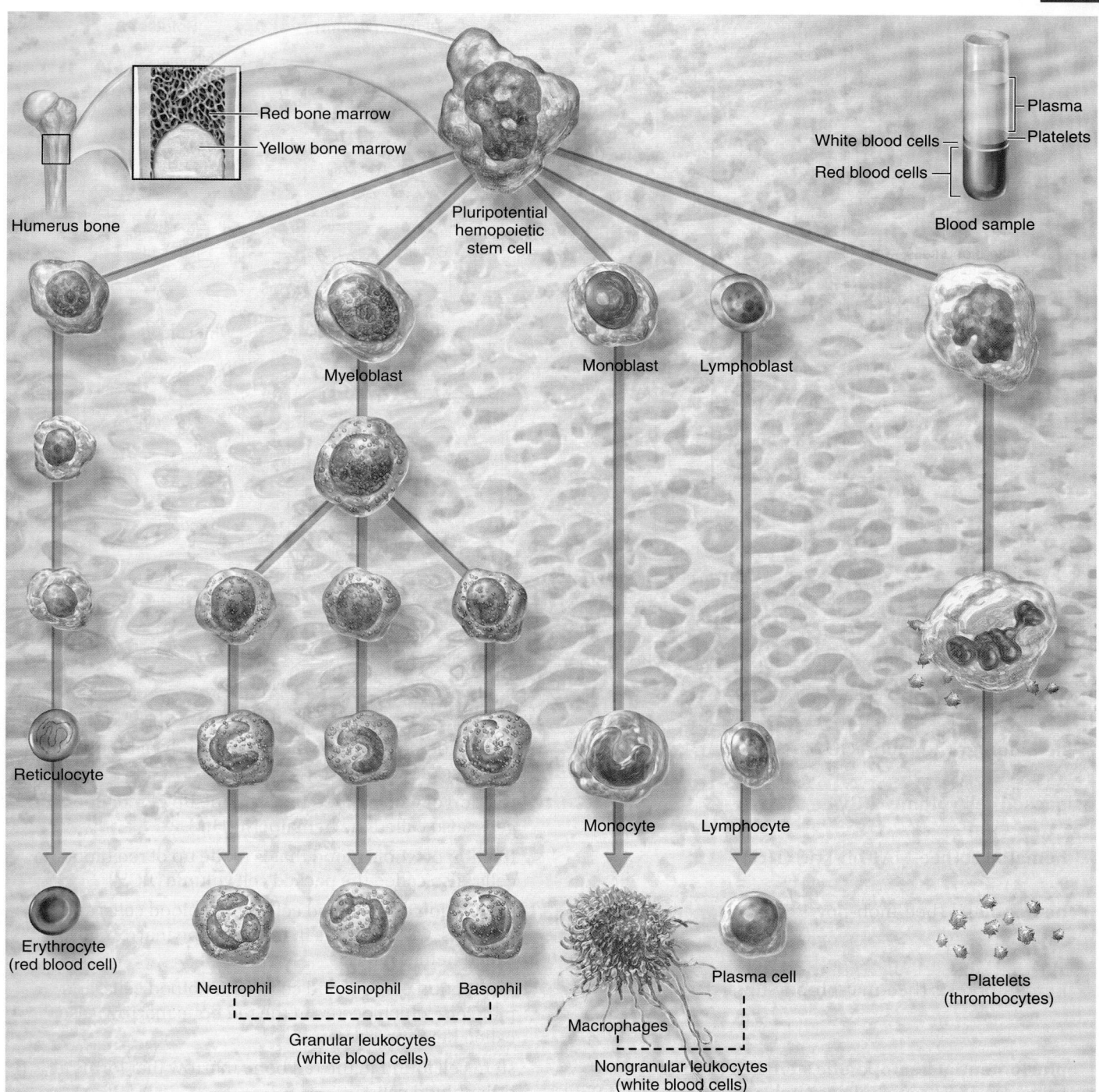

Figure 10-2 Development of blood cells.

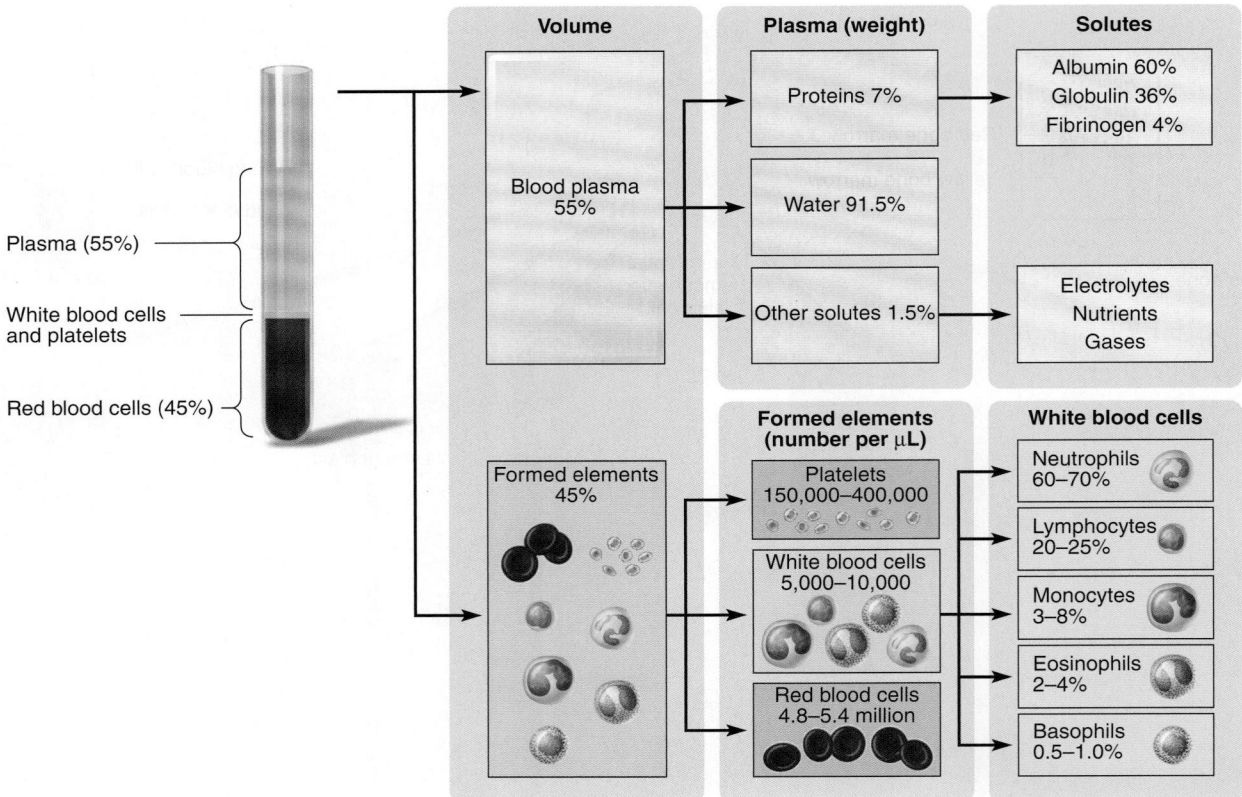

Figure 10-3 The major components of whole blood.

KEY TERM	Definition
hematology (he-muh-TOL-oh-jee)	branch of medicine devoted to the study of blood and diseases of the blood
packed cell volume (PCV)	fraction of whole blood that is made up of red blood cells; also called the hematocrit (Hct)
hematocrit (hee-MAT-oh-krit) **(Hct)**	fraction of whole blood that is made up of red blood cells; also called the packed cell volume (PCV)
hemopoiesis (hee-moh-poy-EE-sis)	production of red blood cells, white blood cells, and platelets, which occurs in the red bone marrow; also called hematopoiesis
hematopoiesis (hee-mat-oh-poy-EE-sis)	production of red blood cells, white blood cells, and platelets, which occurs in the red bone marrow; also called hemopoiesis
pluripotential hemopoietic stem cell (PHSC) (ploo-ree-POH-ten-shul hee-moh-poy-ET-ick STEM SELL)	stem cell found in the red bone marrow that forms all other blood cells
plasma (PLAZ-muh)	liquid, noncellular portion of whole blood
osmotic (oz-MOT-ick) **pressure**	fluid pressure in the blood vessels
albumin (al-BEW-min)	white-colored protein found in plasma that gives blood its viscosity
globulin (GLOB-yoo-lin)	protein group found in the plasma that has an immune function
fibrinogen (figh-BRIN-oh-jen)	protein found in plasma that plays an essential role in blood clotting
serum (SEER-um)	blood plasma without the clotting protein fibrinogen

continued

continued from page 462

KEY TERM PRACTICE: *Blood Preview*

1. The two terms that refer to the production of blood cells and platelets are _____ and _____, which are derived from the word parts _____ and _____ for "blood" and _____ for "production."

2. Plasma without the clotting protein fibrinogen is called _____.

3. Name the three main proteins found in plasma. _____

4. The stem cell found in the red bone marrow that forms all the other blood cells is called a _____, derived from the word part _____ for "several," _____ for "blood," and _____ for "production."

5. _____ is the liquid, noncellular portion of whole blood.

Red Blood Cells (RBCs) or Erythrocytes

Red blood cells (RBCs), which are also called **erythrocytes**, are oxygen-carrying cells. RBCs are the most abundant cells in whole blood and are shaped like biconcave discs that are thinner near their centers and thicker toward their edges (**Figure 10-4**). Erythrocyte formation, **erythropoiesis**, is a process that begins with stem cells in the red bone marrow and ends with the release of mature red blood cells. This process is influenced by the endocrine system, when the kidneys release the hormone **erythropoietin (EPO)**, which promotes erythropoiesis.

Mature erythrocytes do not have nuclei or mitochondria (energy-producing organelles) and are formed from reticulocytes. A **reticulocyte** is an immature RBC. Just before its final stage of development, the reticulocyte loses its nucleus and eventually becomes a fully developed red blood cell. The loss of the nucleus as the cell matures is important because the space that it previously occupied can now be filled with oxygen-rich hemoglobin. **Hemoglobin (Hb, Hgb)** is a protein that is responsible for transporting oxygen and carbon dioxide to and from the tissues.

Red blood cells can travel easily through blood vessel walls to transport oxygen, carbon dioxide, and nutrients. The respiratory system replenishes the blood's oxygen supply. Within the lungs, carbon dioxide is exchanged for oxygen. Red blood cells carry **oxyhemoglobin (HbO_2)**, a bright red compound formed when oxygen combines with hemoglobin. This form of hemoglobin is present in arterial blood.

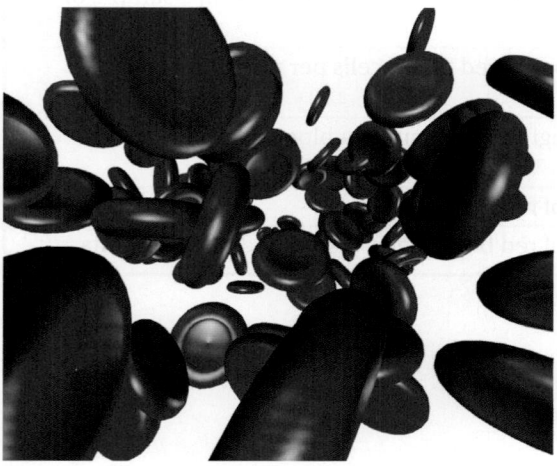

Figure 10-4 Three-dimensional shape of red blood cells showing thin centers and thick edges.

Red blood cells have a life span of approximately 120 days. Within this time, cells in the liver and spleen called macrophages phagocytize (eat) old or damaged cells. About 2 million erythrocytes are destroyed every second. In the liver, the hemoglobin is broken down into heme (an iron-containing compound) and globin (protein), with heme breaking down further into an orange-yellow bile pigment called **bilirubin**. This pigment is excreted in feces, and the iron is recycled for future hemopoiesis.

The blood is often considered the "window on health" because so much can be learned about health status by evaluating the blood. A **complete blood count (CBC)** is a diagnostic test used to identify blood cell types and levels. These tests identify types, shapes, and numbers of RBCs, WBCs, and platelets. The **red blood cell count** measures the number of red blood cells per microliter (mcL; one millionth of a liter) of whole blood, while the **hemoglobin count** measures the concentration of hemoglobin in blood. As noted earlier, the measure of the percentage of red blood cells in whole blood is called the hematocrit. The difference between hemoglobin count and hematocrit is that one measures absolute numbers (hemoglobin count) and the other measures the percentage volume of RBCs (hematocrit).

A deficiency in the number of red blood cells is termed **erythropenia**, and an abnormally high number of red blood cells is called **erythrocytosis** or polycythemia.

KEY TERM	Definition
red blood cells (RBCs)	mature cells shaped like biconcave discs without a nucleus that contain hemoglobin for the transport of oxygen and carbon dioxide; also called erythrocytes
erythrocytes (e-RITH-roh-sites)	mature cells shaped like biconcave discs without a nucleus that contain hemoglobin for the transport of oxygen and carbon dioxide; also called red blood cells
erythropoiesis (e-rith-roh-poy-EE-sis)	formation of red blood cells that begins in the red bone marrow and ends with the release of mature cells
erythropoietin (EPO) (e-rith-roh-POY-e-tin)	hormone released from kidneys that promotes red blood cell production
reticulocyte (re-TICK-yoo-loh-site)	immature red blood cell
hemoglobin (HEE-muh-gloh-bin) **(Hg, Hgb)**	protein found in red blood cells that reversibly binds and transports oxygen and carbon dioxide
oxyhemoglobin (HbO$_2$) (ock-se-HEE-muh-gloh-bin)	bright red compound formed when oxygen combines with hemoglobin
bilirubin (bil-i-ROO-bin)	orange-yellow bile pigment formed from the breakdown of hemoglobin
complete blood count (CBC)	diagnostic test that measures blood cell types and levels in a sample of blood
red blood cell count	measurement of the number of red blood cells per microliter (mcL) of whole blood
hemoglobin (HEE-muh-GLOH-bin) **count**	test used to measure hemoglobin content in a blood sample
erythropenia (e-rith-roh-PEE-nee-uh)	deficiency in the number of red blood cells
erythrocytosis (e-rith-roh-sigh-TOH-sis)	abnormally high number of red blood cells; also called polycythemia

continued

continued from page 464

KEY TERM PRACTICE: *Red Blood Cells (RBCs) or Erythrocytes*

1. The formation of red blood cells is called _____, and is derived from the word part _____ for "red blood cell" and _____ for "production."

2. When oxygen combines with hemoglobin, _____ is formed.

3. _____ is the orange-yellow pigment formed from the breakdown of hemoglobin.

4. A _____ is an immature red blood cell.

5. _____ is the protein found in red blood cells that reversibly binds and transports oxygen and carbon dioxide.

White Blood Cells (WBCs) or Leukocytes

White blood cells (WBCs), also called **leukocytes**, circulate in the blood and body fluids and help protect the body against infection. They also play a role in inflammation and allergic reactions. White blood cells lack hemoglobin, but they do have a nucleus. There are five types of WBCs, divided into two categories, depending on whether the cytoplasm contains granules (granulocytes) or lacks granules (agranulocytes). The granulocytes include neutrophils, eosinophils, and basophils. The agranulocytes are monocytes and lymphocytes (**Figure 10-5**). The formation of leukocytes is termed **leukopoiesis**.

Neutrophils are the most numerous (50% to 70% of WBC population) and mobile of the white blood cells. They are called neutrophils because they can be stained with a neutral dye for microscopic examination. They contain lysosomes (enzyme-containing organelles) and antibiotic-like proteins called defensins, which increase in number during bacterial infections. Associate the *n* in *n*umerous with the *n* in *n*eutrophils to remember that these "blood hounds" seek out invaders in great force. The life span of a neutrophil is about 1 week.

Eosinophils make up 2% to 4% of the circulating leukocytes. They are called eosinophils because they can be stained with eosin dye for microscopic examination. Eosinophils reduce inflammation and increase in number during parasitic infections and allergic reactions. They also secrete enzymes that break down blood clots. The life span of an eosinophil is 10 to 12 days.

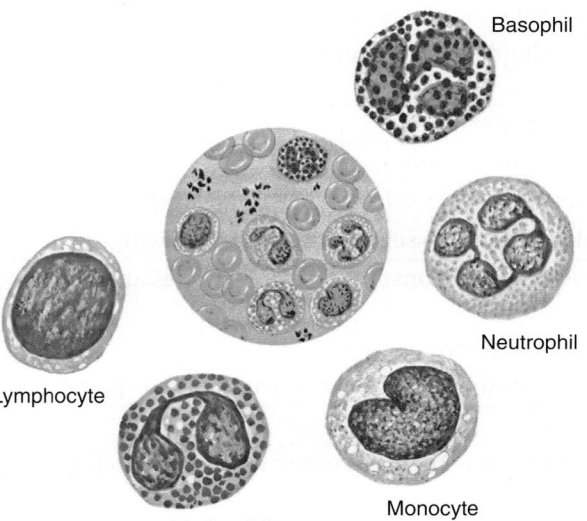

Figure 10-5 The population of white blood cells.

Basophils are similar to eosinophils and make up less than 1% of the white blood cell count. They are called basophils because they can be stained by a basic dye for microscopic examination. Basophils release three potent substances: heparin, histamine, and serotonin. During allergic reactions, basophils release **heparin**, an anticoagulant or antiplatelet factor. An **anticoagulant** is a substance that prevents blood clotting. **Histamine**, an inflammation mediator, causes blood vessels to expand, resulting in increased blood flow to injured tissues. **Serotonin** acts as a vasoconstrictor, causing blood vessels to tighten. The life span of a basophil is from a few hours to 3 days.

The largest agranular white blood cells found in blood are the **monocytes**, which make up 2% to 8% of the WBC count. Some monocytes differentiate into **macrophages**, which either remain fixed (in one location) or wander. The wandering macrophages are phagocytic warriors arising from red bone marrow. The term *macrophage* literally means "big eater," and these cells play an important role in infection resistance and the immune response. They have a life span of several weeks to several months.

Agranular white blood cells called **lymphocytes** comprise 20% to 30% of the WBCs and have a life span of up to several years. Lymphocytes are derived from lymphoid organs, such as the thymus, bone marrow, spleen, lymph nodes, tonsils, and nodules in the small intestine. Lymphocytes provide specific immune responses by differentiating into T cells, B cells, and natural killer (NK) cells. T cells combat viral infections and cancers, whereas B cells differentiate into antibody-producing plasma cells. Antibodies are substances that battle infection and provide **immunity**, or protection against disease. Natural killer cells attack foreign cells, virus-infected cells, and cancer cells.

White blood cell counts are useful in clinical diagnosing. Determining the number of each type of WBC is called a **differential white blood count**. It is called a differential test because it serves to discriminate (differentiate) the various types of white blood cells and then enumerate (count) them. This value is significant for diagnosis because disorders cause characteristic changes in circulating levels of WBCs.

KEY TERM	Definition
white blood cells (WBCs)	granular and agranular cells of whole blood that play a role in immunity; also called leukocytes
leukocytes (LEW-koh-sites)	granular and agranular cells of whole blood that play a role in immunity; also called white blood cells
leukopoiesis (lew-koh-poy-EE-sis)	formation of white blood cells
neutrophils (NEW-truh-filz)	most common type of granular white blood cell that contains antibiotic-like proteins
eosinophils (ee-oh-SIN-uh-fils)	type of granular white blood cell that increases in number during parasitic infections and allergic reactions
basophils (BAY-soh-fils)	type of granular white blood cell that releases heparin, histamine, and serotonin
heparin (HEP-uh-rin)	an anticoagulant or antiplatelet factor
anticoagulant (an-tee-koh-AG-yoo-lunt)	substance that prevents blood clotting
histamine (HIS-tuh-meen)	chemical that stimulates blood vessel dilation (expansion)
serotonin (seer-oh-TOH-nin)	chemical that stimulates blood vessel constriction (narrowing)
monocytes (MON-oh-sites)	agranular white blood cells that consume foreign particles and cellular debris
macrophage (MACK-roh-faij)	phagocytic cell derived from a monocyte
lymphocytes (LIM-foh-sites)	agranular white blood cells that are active in the immune response
immunity (i-MEW-ni-tee)	protection against disease
differential (dif-ur-EN-shul) **white blood count**	test that determines the number of each type of white blood cell in a blood sample

continued

continued from page 466

KEY TERM PRACTICE: *White Blood Cells (WBCs) or Leukocytes*

1. The most numerous type of white blood cell circulating in blood is a _____.

2. What are the two types of agranular white blood cells? _____

3. _____ is the term for protection against disease.

4. The formation of white blood cells is termed _____, which is derived from the word part _____ for "white blood cell" and _____ for "production."

5. This test determines the percentage of each type of white blood cell in a blood sample. _____

Platelets or Thrombocytes

Platelets, also known as **thrombocytes**, are irregularly shaped, colorless structures without a nucleus that play a role in blood clotting and controlling blood loss (**Figure 10-6**). They are not complete cells, but rather are cellular fragments, and they represent the smallest of the formed elements in whole blood. When you have a cut, platelets release serotonin, which causes contraction of the smooth muscle in vessel walls, thereby reducing blood flow within the vessel. Platelets also prevent germs from entering the body through open wounds by forming scabs, and they prevent blood loss by developing clots. They have a life span of approximately 10 days. Old platelets are destroyed in the liver and spleen.

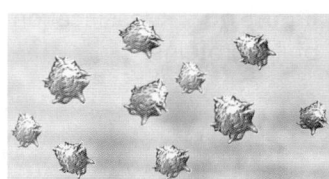
Figure 10-6 Platelets.

KEY TERM	Definition
platelets (PLAIT-lits)	cellular fragments found in whole blood that play a role in controlling blood loss and in blood clotting; also called thrombocytes
thrombocytes (THROM-boh-sites)	cellular fragments found in whole blood that play a role in controlling blood loss and in blood clotting; also called platelets

KEY TERM PRACTICE: *Platelets or Thrombocytes*

1. Cellular fragments found in whole blood that help control blood loss are termed _____ or _____.

2. The term *thrombocyte* is derived from the word part _____, which means "blood clot," and the word part _____, which means "cell."

Lipoproteins

Another important example of a globulin is a lipoprotein. A **lipoprotein** is a complex that contains both lipid (fat) and soluble proteins and transports lipids in the blood plasma. Lipoproteins are biologically important for maintaining cell membranes on cells and myelin sheaths on neurons. Two main lipoproteins in the blood are low-density lipoproteins (LDLs) and high-density lipoproteins (HDLs).

Low-density lipoproteins (LDLs), or LDL cholesterol, are plasma complexes that have a relatively high cholesterol content and low protein content and transport cholesterol to body

Classification of Lipoproteins

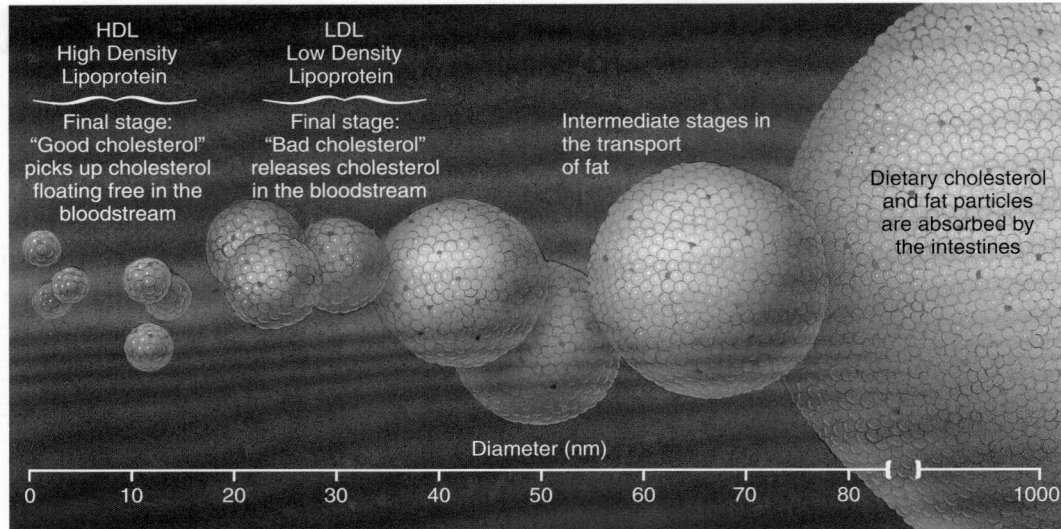

Figure 10-7 Classification of lipoproteins.

cells and tissues. LDLs are referred to as "bad cholesterol" because high levels are correlated with disease. **High-density lipoproteins (HDLs)**, or HDL cholesterol, are complexes composed of fat and protein molecules that transport cholesterol to the liver for excretion in bile. A high circulating level of LDLs is linked with cardiovascular disease, but a high circulating level of HDLs is not. Over time, LDLs can accumulate in your blood and build up in vessel walls, creating plaques that block blood flow. HDLs are referred to as "good cholesterol" because they prevent the accumulation of blood cholesterol by acting as scavengers, soaking up the cholesterol, and transporting it to the liver for breakdown. The higher the HDL level, the better for boosting heart health (**Figure 10-7**).

KEY TERM	Definition
lipoprotein (lip-oh-PROH-teen)	blood plasma complex that contains both lipid (fat) and soluble proteins
low-density lipoprotein (LDL) (lip-oh-PROH-teen)	lipoprotein that transports cholesterol to the cells and tissues; also referred to as LDL cholesterol or "bad cholesterol"
high-density lipoprotein (HDL) (lip-oh-PROH-teen)	lipoprotein that transports cholesterol to the liver for excretion in bile; also referred to as HDL cholesterol or "good cholesterol"

KEY TERM PRACTICE: *Lipoproteins*

1. A blood plasma complex that contains both lipid and protein components is termed a _____.

2. The lipoprotein complex that transports cholesterol to the liver for excretion in bile is known as _____.

3. The lipoprotein complex that transports cholesterol to the cells and tissues is called _____.

Blood Clotting

It is critical for the body to prevent blood loss after tissue injury. **Hemostasis** is the stoppage of uncontrolled bleeding. Uncontrolled, profuse bleeding is known as **hemorrhage**. Hemostasis takes place when blood vessels are stimulated to spasm (undergo involuntary contractions) after an injury. Then **coagulation**, or blood clotting, occurs when blood thickens to form clots,

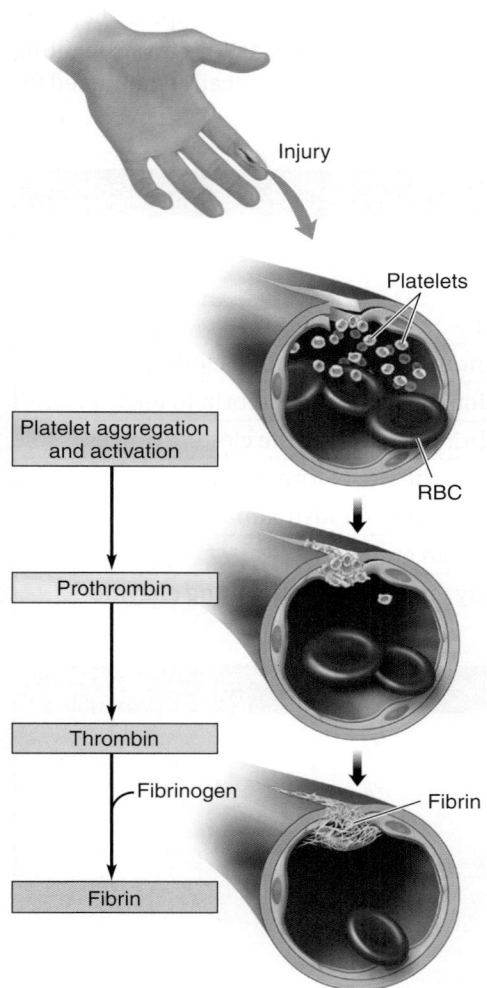

Injury

Platelets

Platelet aggregation
and activation

RBC

Prothrombin

Thrombin

Fibrinogen

Fibrin

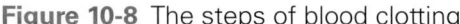

Fibrin

Figure 10-8 The steps of blood clotting.

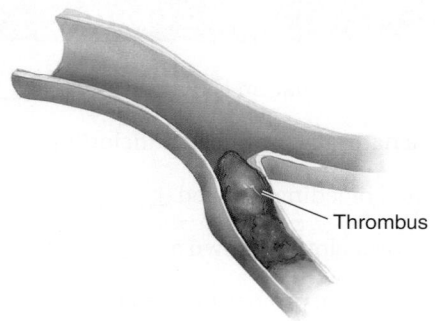

Thrombus

Figure 10-9 A thrombus in a blood vessel.

which halt bleeding. There are several phases of blood clotting. The first involves vascular spasm in which smooth muscles in vessel walls contract to decrease the diameter of the vessel. The second phase is the platelet phase in which platelets stick together and form a platelet plug that seals off the break. The third phase is the coagulation phase in which clotting factors form a blood clot. Clotting factors are substances in the blood that assist in blood clotting. There are 12 clotting factors.

During the coagulation phase, four plasma proteins take part in a chain of events that leads to blood clotting: prothrombin, thrombin, fibrinogen, and fibrin. **Prothrombin** is a plasma protein formed in the liver through the action of vitamin K. (This is why it is important to have enough vitamin K in your diet.) Prothrombin is converted to thrombin during the clotting of blood. **Thrombin** induces clotting by causing the conversion of fibrinogen to fibrin. The key event in blood clot formation is the conversion of the soluble (easily dissolved) plasma protein fibrinogen into the insoluble (not easily dissolved) plasma protein **fibrin**. **Figure 10-8** illustrates blood clotting.

Two types of abnormal clots are a thrombus and an embolus. A **thrombus** is a blood clot that forms in a vessel and remains at the formation site (**Figure 10-9**). An **embolus** is a blood clot that dislodges from its original site and is carried away in the blood, forming an obstruction that blocks blood flow. An **embolism** is a blood vessel obstruction (occlusion) caused by an embolus.

Anticoagulants are substances that prevent blood clotting. They include aspirin, heparin, and tissue plasminogen activator. **Tissue plasminogen activator (TPA, tPA)** is an anticlotting enzyme that is produced naturally in blood vessel linings and is also genetically engineered for use in dissolving blood clots.

KEY TERM	Definition
hemostasis (hee-moh-STAY-sis)	stoppage of uncontrolled bleeding
hemorrhage (HEM-ur-rij)	uncontrolled, profuse bleeding
coagulation (koh-ag-yoo-LAY-shun)	thickening of blood to form a clot
prothrombin (proh-THROM-bin)	plasma protein that converts to thrombin during blood clotting
thrombin (THROM-bin)	protein that induces the conversion of fibrinogen to fibrin to form a clot
fibrin (FIGH-brin)	insoluble protein formed from fibrinogen during the clotting process
thrombus (THROM-bus)	abnormal blood clot that remains at the site of formation
embolus (EM-boh-lus)	thrombus that migrates and lodges in the bloodstream
embolism (EM-boh-liz-um)	blood vessel obstruction caused by an embolus
tissue plasminogen (plaz-MIN-oh-jen) **activator (TPA, tPA)**	naturally produced and genetically engineered anticlotting enzyme

KEY TERM PRACTICE: *Blood Clotting*

1. A clot that remains at the site of formation is termed a _____.

2. _____ is a naturally produced anticlotting enzyme.

3. The stoppage of uncontrolled bleeding is called _____.

4. Thickening of the blood to form clots is known as _____.

5. The medical term for uncontrolled, profuse bleeding is _____.

Blood Types

Blood is divided into types or groups based on the presence or absence of genetically determined antigens (specific proteins). Blood types are meaningful for blood transfusions, transplants, genetic and anthropological studies, and paternity/maternity legal cases. Typing and cross-matching (testing the compatibility of a donor's and a recipient's blood) must be done before a patient receives a transfusion.

A **transfusion** is the transfer of whole blood, blood components, or bone marrow from a healthy donor into the bloodstream of somebody who has lost blood or who has a blood disorder. Transfused blood must be compatible with the patient's blood. If the blood types are not compatible, **agglutination**, or clumping of the blood cells, will take place, thereby clogging vessels.

Two terms important to the understanding of blood transfusions are agglutinogen and agglutinin. An **agglutinogen** is an **antigen (Ag)** on the red blood cell membrane that determines the blood type and is also responsible for the formation of a specific agglutinin (antibody). An **agglutinin** is a substance, such as an **antibody (Ab)**, dissolved in plasma that causes cells to clump together when it reacts with a foreign (not your own or incompatible) antigen. Blood types are identified as A, B, AB, and O, and the antigens present (or absent) on a person's red blood cells are the basis of the ABO blood groups. The two major antigens are A and B. People with Type A blood have antigen A and will form antibody B (which will work against Type B blood). Type B blood has antigen B and antibody A (which will work against Type A blood). Individuals with

	BLOOD TYPE			
	Type A	**Type B**	**Type AB**	**Type O**
Red blood cells	A antigen	B antigen	Both A and B antigens	Neither A nor B antigens
Plasma	Antibody B	Antibody A	Neither antibody	Both antibody A and antibody B

Figure 10-10 Blood types are determined by antigens on the surface of red blood cells.

blood Type AB have both A and B antigens present and will form neither antibody A nor antibody B. Type O blood has no antigens and forms both antibody A and antibody B (**Figure 10-10**). In the United States, 46% of the population is Type O, 40% Type A, 10% Type B, and 4% Type AB.

A person with Type AB blood is called a universal recipient because the blood lacks both antibody A and antibody B. For this reason, a person with Type AB blood could receive a transfusion of blood of any type. A person with Type O blood is referred to as a universal donor because his or her blood lacks antigens A and B, so this type can be transfused into people with blood of any type.

In addition to blood types, another antigen must be considered in the medical setting. The **Rh factor** is an antigen on the red blood cells. The Rh factor was discovered when a group of researchers were performing scientific studies on rhesus monkeys. Thus the *Rh* from *rh*esus remains as the medical term.

Rh positive (Rh⁺) indicates that Rh antigens are present on the membrane of the red blood cells. Individuals with Rh negative (Rh⁻) blood do not have Rh antigens on the cell membrane. Interestingly, 85% of the world's population is Rh⁺. If an Rh⁻ person receives a transfusion of Rh⁺ blood, the recipient's antibody-producing cells would be stimulated and agglutination could result. When the blood type is written, Rh is usually eliminated, so a person with blood Type A who is Rh⁺ is denoted as A⁺. A person with blood Type B who is Rh⁻ is marked as B⁻.

KEY TERM	Definition
transfusion (trans-FYOO-zhun)	transfer of blood from one person to another
agglutination (uh-gloo-ti-NAY-shun)	clumping of blood cells
agglutinogen (uh-GLOO-tin-oh-jen)	protein (antigen) on the surface of the red blood cell that determines the blood type; an antigen
antigen (AN-ti-jen) **(Ag)**	protein on the surface of the red blood cell that determines the blood type; an agglutinogen
agglutinin (uh-GLOO-ti-nin)	substance in blood plasma that causes clumping when it reacts with a foreign antigen; an antibody
antibody (AN-tee-bod-ee) **(Ab)**	substance in blood plasma that causes clumping when it reacts with a specific antigen; an agglutinin
Rh factor	a specific antigen found on the surface of red blood cells; those with the Rh factor are Rh⁺ and those without it are Rh⁻

continued

continued from page 471

KEY TERM PRACTICE: *Blood Types*

1. The medical term for blood cell clumping is _____.

2. The protein on the surface of a red blood cell that determines the blood type is called an _____ or _____.

3. A _____ is a transfer of blood from one person to another.

4. An _____ or _____ is a substance found in plasma that causes clumping when it reacts with a foreign antigen.

5. Name the antigen on the surface of red blood cells named after Rhesus monkeys._____

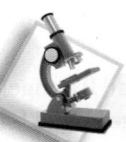

THE CLINICAL DIMENSION

Pathology, signs and symptoms, clinical tests and diagnostic procedures, and treatments pertaining to the blood are described in this section. A blood disorder is known as a **dyscrasia**.

Anemia

anemia	**Anemia** is a blood condition in which there are not enough red blood cells or the red blood cells are deficient in hemoglobin. This results in poor health, because the blood can no longer carry sufficient oxygen to meet the body's demands. Anemia is caused by inadequate erythropoiesis, excessive hemolysis (bursting red blood cells), or a combination of these factors, resulting in overlapping signs and symptoms. Several forms of anemia exist and all are marked by pale complexion and tiredness. Most forms are characterized by erythropenia and deficient hemoglobin caused by blood loss. Defective hemoglobin synthesis, which causes deficient levels, occurs with hereditary anemias.
hemorrhagic anemia	Anemia caused by excessive blood loss is **hemorrhagic anemia**.
aplastic anemia	Anemia that results from decreased formation of red blood cells is **aplastic anemia.** It occurs when the red bone marrow is not productive.
hemolytic anemia	**Hemolytic anemia** results from the destruction of red blood cells. Causes of hemolysis include transfusion reaction, autoimmune disease, infection, or toxic chemicals. Blood transfusions usually correct the problem.

Transfusions involve the introduction of whole blood or blood components from one person into another individual whose blood volume is diminished or deficient in some way. During an **exchange transfusion**, a person's blood is removed and simultaneously replaced with whole blood from another source. An **autologous transfusion** occurs when an individual has his or her own blood removed and stored for later use. This is also called predonation.

Two hereditary forms of anemia caused by defective hemoglobin synthesis are sickle cell anemia and thalassemia.

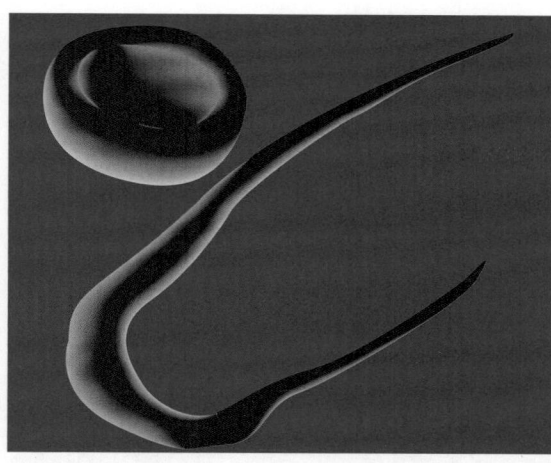

Figure 10-11 A normal red blood cell and a sickled cell.

sickle cell anemia	**Sickle cell anemia**, an inherited chronic disease that occurs almost exclusively in people of African descent, is characterized by sickle-shaped red blood cells (**Figure 10-11**). This abnormal shape inhibits the cells from passing easily through the blood vessels. Distorted erythrocytes cause plugging of vessels, and these fragile RBCs cannot withstand the mechanical trauma of circulation and eventually lyse (burst). This hereditary form of hemolytic anemia is caused by defective hemoglobin synthesis. Blood of individuals with the disease contains a form of hemoglobin called hemoglobin S (HbS). People who only carry the trait for sickle cell anemia, but do not have the disease, show resistance to malaria.
	General signs and symptoms include impaired growth and development, chronic marrow hyperactivity, arthralgia (joint pain), and fever, but these vary, depending on the severity of the disease. Treatment focuses on symptoms because no antisickling drugs have been developed. Individuals develop "crisis" episodes of severe pain due to vessel blockage. Crises are managed by blood transfusions, oral hydration, and pain medications.
thalassemia	**Thalassemia** is a chronic, inherited anemia characterized by an inability to produce adequate amounts of hemoglobin. As a result, RBC production is slowed and these cells are short lived, preventing adequate numbers of cells to deliver oxygen to tissues. It is prevalent in individuals of Mediterranean, African, and Southeast Asian ancestry. Signs and symptoms include **jaundice** (skin yellowness due to a buildup of bilirubin) and splenomegaly (enlarged spleen). Blood tests show hypochromic (pale colored) and small erythrocytes. Treatments vary and blood transfusions to replenish RBC numbers are necessary.
nutritional anemia	**Nutritional anemia** results from a dietary deficiency of nutrients essential to red blood cell formation. These nutrients include iron, vitamin B_{12}, thiamin, folate, and protein. Iron-deficiency anemia is common in premenopausal women. Blood tests confirm the diagnosis. Treatment involves eating a balanced diet.
pernicious anemia	**Pernicious anemia** results from the body's inability to absorb vitamin B_{12}, an essential nutrient for manufacturing red blood cells. It rarely occurs before age 30 and is often caused by a lack of intrinsic factor. Intrinsic factor is manufactured in the stomach and is required

for the absorption of vitamin B_{12}. The term pernicious means harmful and potentially fatal. Signs and symptoms include fatigue, impaired pain and temperature sensitivity, and confusion.

The Schilling test is used for diagnosis. The **Schilling test** is a diagnostic tool to determine whether the body absorbs vitamin B_{12} by determining the amount of radioactive vitamin B_{12} excreted in the urine. For the test, radioactive vitamin B_{12} is administered orally. Urine samples are then collected and analyzed for the presence of radioactive B_{12} over a 24-hour period. If the body is absorbing the B_{12} normally, at least 5% of the radioactive B_{12} will appear in the urine. If there is impaired absorption, less than 5% will be detected. Pernicious anemia is treated with a lifetime regimen of vitamin B_{12} injections.

KEY TERM	Definition
dyscrasia (dis-KRAY-zee-uh)	general term for a blood disorder
anemia (uh-NEE-mee-uh)	condition characterized by red blood cell deficiency or hemoglobin deficiency
hemorrhagic anemia (hem-uh-RAJ-ick uh-NEE-mee-uh)	anemia caused by excessive bleeding
aplastic anemia (ay-PLAS-tick uh-NEE-mee-uh)	anemia caused by failure of the red bone marrow to produce enough red blood cells
hemolytic anemia (hee-moh-LIT-ick uh-NEE-mee-uh)	anemia caused by red blood cell destruction
exchange transfusion	simultaneous blood extraction and replacement in an individual
autologous (aw-TOL-uh-gus) **transfusion**	donation of blood for later use by that same person
sickle cell anemia (uh-NEE-mee-uh)	inherited form of anemia in which the red blood cells are abnormally shaped
thalassemia (thal-uh-SEE-mee-uh)	inherited form of anemia characterized by an inability to produce adequate amounts of hemoglobin
jaundice (JAWN-dis)	yellowish skin due to accumulated bilirubin
nutritional anemia (uh-NEE-mee-uh)	anemia caused by dietary deficiency of nutrients that are essential to red blood cell formation
pernicious anemia (pur-NISH-us uh-NEE-mee-uh)	anemia caused by vitamin B_{12} deficiency usually resulting from a lack of intrinsic factor
Schilling (SHIL-ing) **test**	diagnostic tool to determine whether the body absorbs vitamin B_{12} by determining the amount of radioactive vitamin B_{12} excreted in the urine

KEY TERM PRACTICE: *Anemia*

1. Identify two hereditary forms of anemia. _____

2. The form of anemia that results from a vitamin B_{12} deficiency is _____.

3. The _____ is a diagnostic tool used to determine whether the body absorbs vitamin B_{12} by determining the amount of radioactive vitamin B_{12} that is excreted in the urine.

4. A donation of blood for later use by that same person is termed an _____ and is derived from the word part _____, which refers to "self."

5. _____ is a general term for a blood disorder.

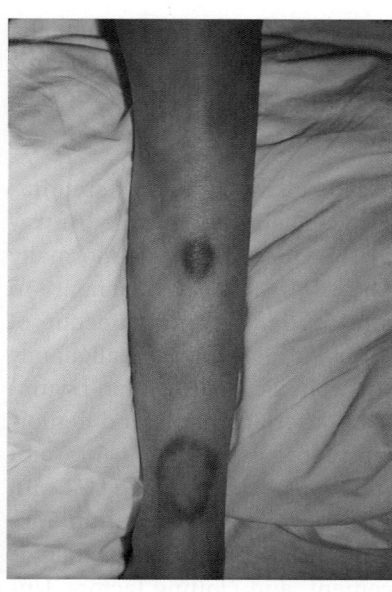

Figure 10-12 Ecchymoses in a patient with hemophilia.

Bleeding, Coagulation, and Platelet Disorders

hemophilia

Hemophilia is a hereditary blood disorder, found almost exclusively in males, caused by a clotting factor deficiency in which the blood clots much more slowly than normally, resulting in extensive bleeding from even minor injuries. Hemarthrosis, hematoma, ecchymosis, and gastrointestinal bleeding characterize it. **Hemarthrosis** is bleeding in the joints. A **hematoma** is a semisolid mass of clotted blood in the tissues, and **ecchymosis** (bruise) refers to bleeding into surrounding tissues (**Figure 10-12**).

The clinical picture, bleeding time, prolonged partial thromboplastin time test, and plasma prothrombin time test lead to the diagnosis. **Bleeding time** is the average time it takes for bleeding to stop after the skin (earlobe or fingertip) has been superficially lanced. **Partial thromboplastin time (PTT)** and **plasma prothrombin time (PT; protime)** are tests used to determine clotting time. Normal PTT is 35 to 50 seconds. Hemophiliacs and patients on heparin, warfarin, or aspirin may have a prolonged time. This test is usually done every 1 to 3 months to monitor heparin or other anticoagulant therapies. Normal PT is 9 to 17 seconds. Prolonged times are seen with hemophilia, infection, heart attack, disseminated intravascular coagulation (described below), and anticoagulant therapy. Treatment involves antihemophilic factor transfusions and limiting activities that have the risk of injury. **Antihemophilic factor (AHF)** is clotting factor VIII, which is administered to individuals with hemophilia to assist with blood coagulation.

purpura

Purpura is a condition in which bleeding under the skin causes purplish blotches to appear on the skin. Two types are allergic (caused by sensitization to food, drugs, or insect bites) and fibrinolytic (characterized by bleeding and rapid clot fibrinolysis). Typical skin lesions of petechiae (tiny, purplish skin spots), ecchymoses, and vibices (lines of bleeding) vary with the type of purpura. An ecchymosis differs from petechiae only in size. The lesions first appear red, gradually darkening to purple, fading to brown and yellow, and eventually disappearing. The usual duration is 2 to 3 weeks. No treatment is necessary.

disseminated intravascular coagulation (DIC)

A disorder of the clotting cascade characterized by simultaneous bleeding and clottingis is called **disseminated intravascular coagulation (DIC)**. In DIC, fibrin is abnormally generated in the circulating blood. It is usually secondary to another condition such as **septicemia** (bacterial infection of the blood; formerly known as blood poisoning), malignancy (cancer), trauma, or an obstetric complication. Signs and symptoms include venous thrombosis, arterial emboli, and hemorrhage (**Figure 10-13**). Laboratory studies, patient history, and the clinical picture confirm the diagnosis. Prolonged PT and PTT are evident. Immediate treatment involves antibiotics (when bacterial infection is present), heparin (unless there is head injury), platelet replacement, and clotting factors. Untreated DIC can be life threatening because hypotension (low blood pressure) develops and the vascular volume is depleted.

A thrombosis is treated with **thrombolytic** drugs, such as aspirin, streptokinase, and TPA, that break up or dissolve thrombi. Aspirin is considered a thrombolytic agent because it inhibits vasoconstriction and platelet aggregation by blocking the synthesis of thromboxane (a substance formed in platelets). **Streptokinase** and tissue plasminogen activator help to dissolve clots.

thrombocytopenia

A clotting disorder caused by a decreased platelet count is termed **thrombocytopenia**. It is characterized by bleeding from small vessels throughout the body. It may be caused by platelet production failure or increased platelet destruction. Signs and symptoms include petechiae and mucosal bleeding. There is generally no bleeding into tissues, as is commonly seen in coagulation disorders. It is diagnosed by history, ruling out any drugs that interfere with platelet formation, blood tests, hemoglobin count, and bone marrow aspiration biopsy.

A **bone marrow aspiration biopsy** involves inserting a needle directly into the bone marrow to remove cells for later examination (**Figure 10-14**). This diagnostic procedure is useful for identifying the shapes and sizes of red blood cells and white blood cells. Platelet transfusions are used to treat thrombocytopenia.

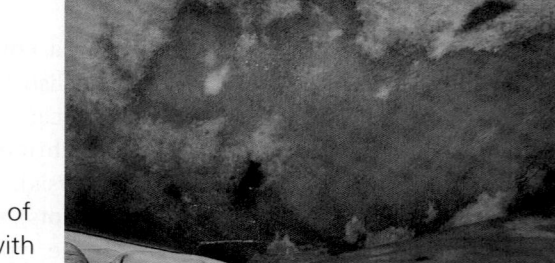

Figure 10-13 Patchy hemorrhages of the skin on the thigh of a patient with DIC associated with cancer.

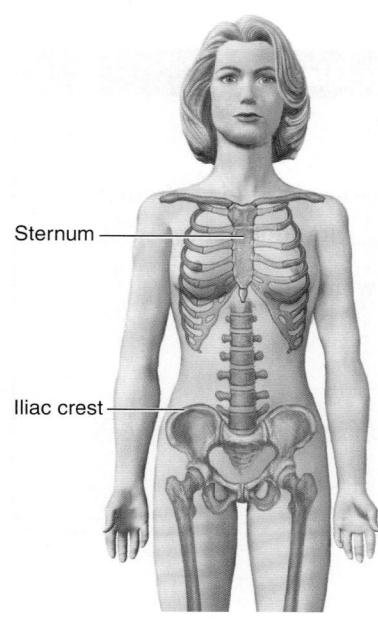

Sternum

Iliac crest

Figure 10-14 Usual sites for a bone marrow aspiration biopsy are the sternum and iliac crest.

KEY TERM	Definition
hemophilia (hee-moh-FIL-ee-uh)	inherited blood clotting disorder
hemarthrosis (hee-mahr-THROH-sis)	bleeding into a joint
hematoma (hee-muh-TOH-muh)	semisolid mass of clotted blood in the tissues
ecchymosis (eck-i-MOH-sis)	bleeding into surrounding tissue; also called a bruise
bleeding time	average time it takes bleeding to stop after the skin (earlobe or fingertip) has been superficially lanced
partial thromboplastin (throm-oh-PLAS-tin) **time (PTT)**	test of time it takes for blood to clot
plasma prothrombin (proh-THROM-bin) **time (PT; protime)**	test of time it takes for blood to clot
antihemophilic (an-tee-hee-moh-FIL-ick) **factor (AHF)**	clotting factor VIII used to treat hemophilia
purpura (PURE-pew-ruh)	condition characterized by hemorrhage into the skin
disseminated intravascular coagulation (DIC) (di-SEM-i-nay-tid in-truh-VAS-kew-lur koh-ag-yoo-LAY-shun)	disorder of the clotting cascade characterized by simultaneous bleeding and clotting
septicemia (sep-ti-SEE-mee-uh)	bacterial infection of the blood; formerly known as blood poisoning
thrombolytic (throm-boh-LIT-ick)	agent that dissolves a thrombus (clot)
streptokinase (strep-toh-KIGH-nace)	enzyme that dissolves blood clots
thrombocytopenia (throm-boh-sigh-toh-PEE-nee-uh)	clotting disorder caused by a decreased number of platelets
bone marrow aspiration biopsy (as-pi-RAY-shun BYE-op-see)	removal of bone marrow for clinical examination

continued

continued from page 477

> **K E Y   T E R M   P R A C T I C E :** *Bleeding, Coagulation, and Platelet Disorders*
>
> **1.** Identify an inherited bleeding disorder that primarily affects males. _____
>
> **2.** _____ is the clotting disorder caused by a decreased platelet count; the term is derived from the word part _____, which means "blood clot," and _____ for "deficiency."
>
> **3.** A _____ is an agent that destroys a blood clot and is formed from the word part _____ for "blood clot."
>
> **4.** The medical term for a semisolid mass of clotted blood in the tissues is _____.
>
> **5.** _____ is the average time it takes bleeding to stop after the skin (earlobe or fingertip) has been superficially lanced.

Other Blood Disorders

Because of its very nature, blood is susceptible to an extensive list of disorders.

leukopenia   An abnormally low total white blood cell count (below 5,000 cells/ mm^3 of blood) is referred to as **leukopenia**. The leukopenias are diagnosed through blood studies.

neutropenia   **Neutropenia** is a type of leukopenia characterized by a decreased number of neutrophils, which leads to an increased susceptibility to infection. The condition is usually caused by drug toxicity (side effect of some cancer treatments) or drug allergy. Weakness, fatigue, fever, and mucous membrane ulcers are common signs and symptoms.

hemochromatosis   **Hemochromatosis** is a genetic disorder in which iron is deposited in the tissues. The excessive accumulation of iron in the body leads to liver damage, diabetes mellitus (due to iron presence in the pancreas), and bronze discoloration of the skin. The accumulation of hemosiderin, a golden yellow-brown protein, causes the skin bronzing. The condition is diagnosed by the clinical picture, physical examination, and evidence of elevated serum iron (Fe) levels. It is treated by phlebotomy until serum Fe levels are restored to normal. **Phlebotomy** or **venipuncture** is a puncture made by a needle inserted into the vein to draw blood (**Figure 10-15**). Phlebotomy to treat hemochromatosis is bloodletting for therapeutic purposes to reduce the amount of blood in the body.

leukocytosis   **Leukocytosis** is a condition resulting from an abnormally high leukocyte (white blood cell) count that exceeds 10,000 cells/mm^3 of blood. It indicates acute infection but may follow vigorous exercise or excessive loss of body fluids.

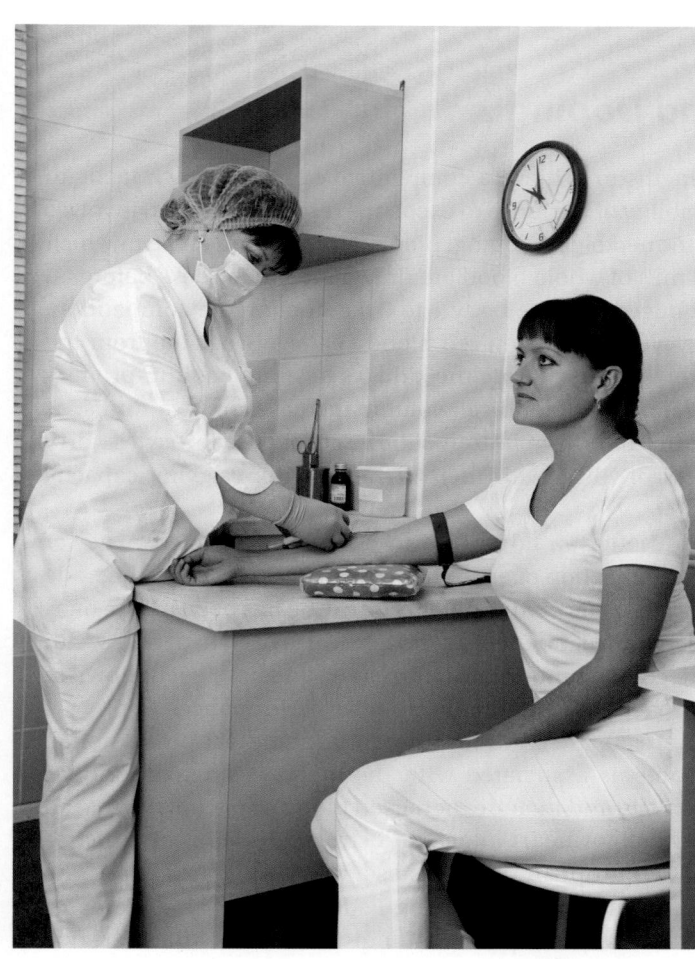

Figure 10-15 Practitioner drawing a blood sample from the arm vein of a patient using a needle and syringe.

infectious mononucleosis (IM)	Commonly referred to as the "kissing disease" because it is frequently spread through saliva. **Infectious mononucleosis (IM)** is a contagious disease caused by the Epstein-Barr virus (EBV). The virus affects lymphatic tissue and is characterized by leukocytosis accompanied by pharyngitis (inflamed throat), fever, lymphadenopathy (enlarged lymph nodes), and splenomegaly. Blood tests and the clinical picture confirm the diagnosis. Most cases involve children and young adults. Antiviral medications and supportive therapy are the only treatment options. Most patients recover, but relapses can occur.
polycythemia	**Polycythemia** is a disorder marked by an abnormally high number of red blood cells in the circulating blood. It results from chronic obstructive pulmonary disease (COPD), which is caused by decreased oxygen levels (including those at high altitudes), cardiac disease, and other conditions in which the body compensates for low levels of oxygen in the tissues and blood. **Cyanosis**, bluish skin discoloration because there is not enough oxygen in the blood, is a common sign.

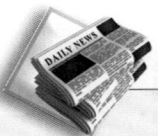

IN THE NEWS: Blood Doping

Serious athletes go to great lengths to achieve a competitive edge. One such tactic to increase aerobic capacity (the ability of the lungs to exchange respiratory gases) involves autologous transfusion and is termed blood doping. Blood doping is a practice in which one to four units (450 to 1,800 mL) of whole blood are drawn off 3 to 8 weeks before an athletic event and then reintroduced into the body 1 to 7 days before the competition. Physiologically, it induces polycythemia. When red blood cell levels decline from the draining process, erythropoietin is released from the kidneys to stimulate RBC production in the bone marrow. Therefore, red blood cell volume increases on two fronts: as a result of increased production and via reintroduction. Because erythrocytes carry oxygen, the increased numbers of RBCs with their higher oxygen-carrying capacity should enhance performance.

The practice does appear to offer an advantage to endurance athletes. A newer form of blood doping involves the injection of epoetin. Epoetin, also known by the trade names of Procrit and Epogen, is synthetic erythropoietin. The drug has been on the market since 1988 and is beneficial in the treatment of anemia. It is also used in patients with kidney dysfunction. Epoetin injections stimulate RBC formation and have been shown to significantly improve aerobic capacity and endurance exercise performance.

As with any drug whose effects are not monitored by a medical professional, its use has inherent risks. Problems associated with the increased hematocrit are related to the higher blood viscosity and include increased blood pressure, decreased cardiac output, and increased risk for heart attack and stroke. Epoetin administration has caused the deaths of 18 European bicyclists as a result of heart attack. The International Cycling Union and International Skiing Federation monitor hematocrit and hemoglobin concentrations in competing athletes in an effort to thwart this practice. Moreover, blood doping and/or ancillary epoetin injections are considered a form of cheating and are banned from Olympic games.

Blood doping is not always linked to athletic performance. In October 2010, Canadian authorities reported a new problem concerning blood doping: patients using blood doping to gain admittance into cancer clinical trials. In three cases, patients who did not meet eligibility requirements because of low albumin, platelet, or hemoglobin levels received transfusions, which then raised their levels sufficiently to participate in the trials. Scientists conducting research and designing studies must take this practice into consideration when determining eligibility requirements.

Polycythemia vera is a chronic form of polycythemia with an unknown cause. It is characterized by bone marrow hyperplasia, leading to erythrocytosis, increased blood volume, and skin redness. Phlebotomy is used to treat the condition (**Figure 10-16**).

An abnormal hematocrit or RBC count diagnoses both polycythemia conditions. There may also be accompanying splenomegaly.

multiple myeloma　　**Multiple myeloma** is a condition in which tumors composed of bone marrow–derived cells occur. It is an uncommon disease affecting more men than women. It is characterized by anemia, hemorrhage, recurrent infections, and weakness. Signs include accumulations of abnormal or malignant plasma cells in the bone marrow, especially

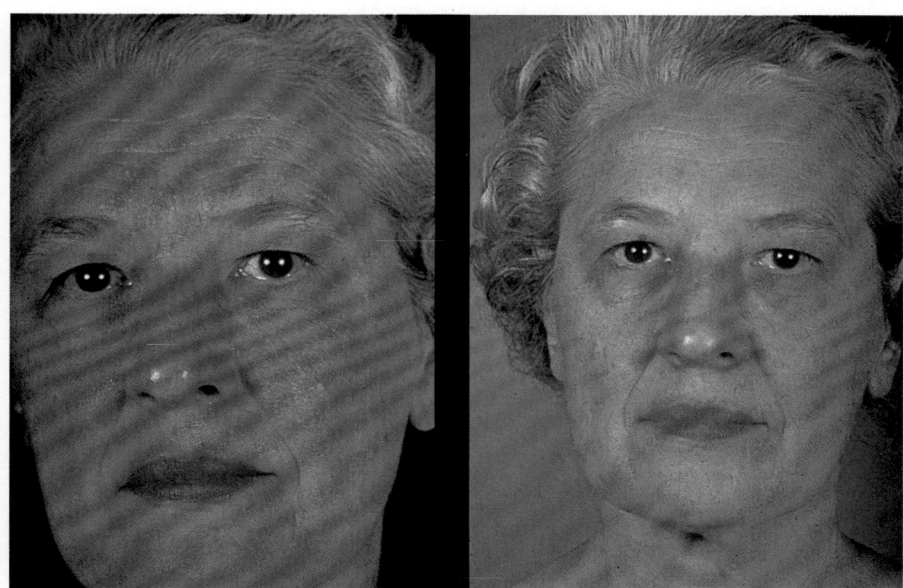

Figure 10-16 Adult woman with polycythemia vera showing reduction in facial redness after phlebotomy.

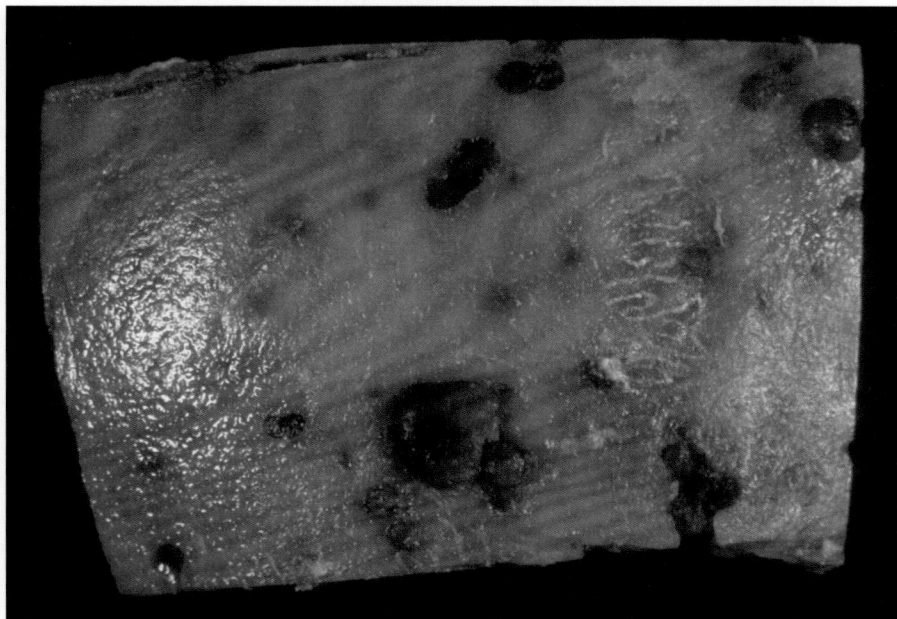

Figure 10-17 A segment of the skull from a patient with multiple myeloma showing numerous punched-out lesions.

in the skull, causing palpable bone swellings (**Figure 10-17**). X-rays, bone biopsy, and evidence of abnormal proteins known as *Bence Jones proteins* in the serum and urine make the diagnosis.

Treatment includes chemotherapy, bone marrow transplant, and plasmapheresis. **Plasmapheresis** is a process in which blood is taken from the patient, separated into plasma and cells, and then the cells are transfused back into the patient's bloodstream. The plasma of the patient is depleted, but the cellular components remain. The median survival of individuals with multiple myeloma is 3 years.

KEY TERM	Definition
leukopenia (lew-koh-PEE-nee-uh)	abnormally low white blood cell (leukocyte) count
neutropenia (new-troh-PEE-nee-uh)	decreased neutrophil levels
hemochromatosis (hee-moh-kroh-muh-TOH-sis)	chronic genetic disease characterized by iron deposits in the body
phlebotomy (fle-BOT-uh-mee)	puncture made in a vein to withdraw blood; also called venipuncture
venipuncture (veen-i-PUNK-chur)	puncture made in a vein to withdraw blood; also called phlebotomy
leukocytosis (lew-koh-sigh-TOH-sis)	abnormally high leukocyte count
infectious mononucleosis (IM) (mon-oh-new-klee-OH-sis)	Epstein-Barr virus (EBV) infection that affects lymphatic tissue and is characterized by leukocytosis
polycythemia (pol-ee-sigh-THEEM-ee-uh)	disorder marked by an abnormally high number of red blood cells in the circulating blood
cyanosis (sigh-uh-NOH-sis)	bluish skin discoloration due to lack of oxygen
polycythemia vera (pol-ee-sigh-THEEM-ee-uh VEER-uh)	a chronic form of polycythemia with an unknown cause
multiple myeloma (migh-eh-LOH-muh)	tumors composed of cells derived from bone marrow that cause palpable swellings on bones
plasmapheresis (plaz-muh-fe-REE-sis)	process in which blood is taken from the patient, separated into plasma and cells, and then the cells are transfused back into the patient's bloodstream

KEY TERM PRACTICE: *Other Blood Disorders*

1. An abnormally low white blood cell count is termed _____ and is derived from the word part _____ for "white blood cell" and _____ for "deficiency."

2. _____ is a procedure that involves withdrawing blood from a patient, removing the plasma, and then reintroducing the blood cells back into the patient.

3. _____ is a bluish skin discoloration due to a lack of oxygen.

4. _____ is caused by the Epstein-Barr virus (EBV), which affects lymphatic tissues and is characterized by leukocytosis.

5. A disorder marked by an abnormally high number of red blood cells in the circulating blood and is found in people with COPD is called _____ .

Hemolytic Disease of the Newborn (HDN) or Erythroblastosis Fetalis

hemolytic disease of the newborn (HDN) or erythroblastosis fetalis

Hemolytic disease of the newborn (HDN) is an RBC-related disorder caused by a cross-reaction between fetal and maternal blood types and it involves the Rh factor. It occurs only when the mother is Rh$^-$ and the fetus is Rh$^+$. With this serious blood disease of fetuses and newborn babies, antibodies produced by an Rh$^-$ mother destroy the red blood cells of an Rh$^+$ fetus. During the first pregnancy, this combination causes no problems, but a subsequent pregnancy is at risk because some Rh$^+$ cells from the first

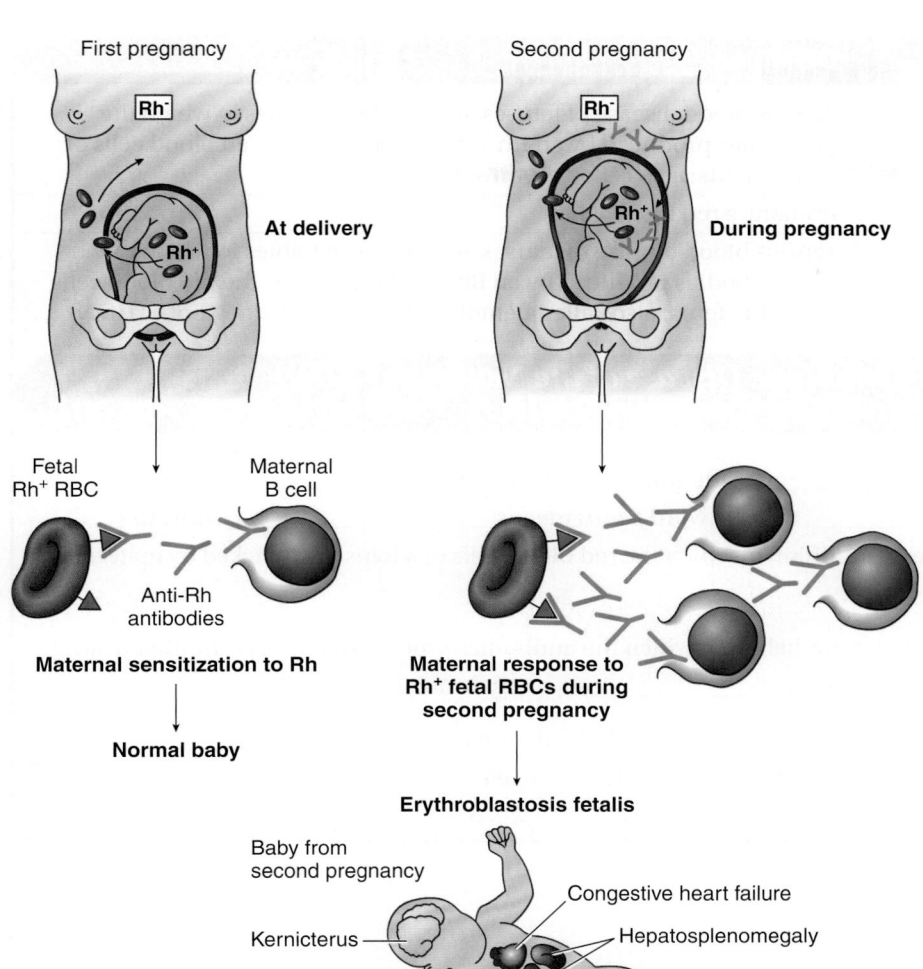

First pregnancy

Rh⁻

At delivery

Rh⁺

Second pregnancy

Rh⁻

Rh⁺

During pregnancy

Fetal
Rh⁺ RBC

Maternal
B cell

Anti-Rh
antibodies

Maternal sensitization to Rh

Normal baby

**Maternal response to
Rh⁺ fetal RBCs during
second pregnancy**

Erythroblastosis fetalis

Baby from
second pregnancy

Kernicterus

Jaundice

Hemolytic anemia

Congestive heart failure

Hepatosplenomegaly

Edema

Figure 10-18 Erythroblastosis fetalis is due to maternal fetal Rh incompatibility. Sensitization of the Rh⁻ mother with Rh⁺ RBCs in the first pregnancy leads to the formation of anti-Rh antibodies. These antibodies cross the placenta and damage the Rh⁺ fetus in subsequent pregnancies

child may have entered the maternal circulation through damaged placental tissues. When this occurs, the mother produces antibodies against the Rh⁺ blood cells. If a second Rh⁺ child is conceived, that child is at risk because the anti-Rh antibodies from the maternal circulation can pass through the placenta, enter the fetal blood, and attack the fetal blood cells. The fetus develops HDN when the maternal antibodies react with the fetal Rh antigens, destroying fetal RBCs and producing anemia (**Figure 10-18**). As the fetal demand for blood increases, RBCs begin leaving the bone marrow and enter the bloodstream before completing their development. These immature red blood cells are called **erythroblasts**, and the Latin term for fetus is fetalis, so HDN is also known as **erythroblastosis fetalis**.

A commercial protein preparation, RhoGAM, is now administered to Rh⁻ mothers, regardless of the number of pregnancies. This product protects the Rh⁺ fetus from antibodies produced by its Rh⁻ mother.

KEY TERM	Definition
hemolytic (hee-moh-LIT-ick) **disease of the newborn (HDN)**	serious blood disease of fetuses and newborn babies in which the antibodies produced by an Rh$^-$ mother destroy the red blood cells of an Rh$^+$ fetus; also called erythroblastosis fetalis
erythroblasts (e-RITH-roh-blasts)	immature red blood cells
erythroblastosis fetalis (e-rith-roh-blas-TOH-sis fee-TAY-lis)	serious blood disease of fetuses and newborn babies in which the antibodies produced by an Rh$^-$ mother destroy the red blood cells of an Rh$^+$ fetus; also called hemolytic disease of the newborn (HDN)

KEY TERM PRACTICE: *Hemolytic Disease of the Newborn (HDN) or Erythroblastosis Fetalis*

1. The word part *erythro-* means _____; the word part *-blast* means _____; the word part *-osis* refers to _____; and the word *fetalis* means _____. Thus the word _____ describes a condition in which the red blood cells of a fetus are attacked by maternal antibodies.

2. A serious blood disease of fetuses and newborn babies in which the antibodies produced by an Rh$^-$ mother destroy the red blood cells of an Rh$^+$ fetus is known as _____ or erythroblastosis fetalis.

3. Immature red blood cells are known as _____, derived from the word part _____ for "red blood cell" and _____ for "immature precursor cell."

Leukemia

leukemia

Leukemia is a type of cancer characterized by production of increased numbers of immature or abnormal leukocytes (white blood cells). The increased WBC production suppresses the production of normal blood cells, leading to anemia. Leukemias were formerly classified as acute or chronic, based on life expectancy, but they are now categorized as acute or chronic according to cellular maturity. The Leukemia & Lymphoma Society identifies the four most common types of leukemia as acute lymphoblastic leukemia (ALL), chronic lymphocytic leukemia (CLL), acute myeloid leukemia (AML), and chronic myeloid leukemia (CML). Because the leukocytes of individuals with leukemia are either immature or incapable of fighting infection, a mild infection may be fatal. The disease is further classified on the basis of cell count, cell type, degree of differentiation, and rapidity of onset. Signs and symptoms of all leukemias include joint and bone pain, liver enlargement, spleen enlargement, and enlarged lymph nodes. Leukemia has an unknown cause but may be precipitated by viral infection, chemical exposure, or genetic disposition.

Chemotherapy is the use of chemical agents to treat disease, especially cancer. Agents that prevent the development, maturation, or spread of cancer cells are termed **antineoplastic drugs**.

Bone marrow transplant (BMT) and **stem cell transplant** are treatment options for blood diseases. They involve the transfer of bone marrow or stem cells from one person to another. Both procedures require donor tissue. Bone marrow transplants are used as a last resort when other therapeutic measures fail. It is an extremely dangerous procedure because the recipient's immune response must be suppressed and all malignant cells destroyed by aggressive treatment before the donor's marrow is intravenously infused. The new marrow then repopulates the marrow cavity and begins producing healthy cells. Stem cell transplants involve the transfer of stem cells from one person to another. The aim is to have normal cell proliferation.

acute lymphoblastic leukemia (ALL)

Acute lymphoblastic leukemia (ALL) is a disease characterized by increased formation of immature lymphocytes (lymphoblasts) that are unable to fight infection. It is also called acute lymphocytic leukemia and acute lymphoid leukemia. It is marked by a rapid onset (acute) with severe anemia, hemorrhage, and increased susceptibility to infection. Although the cause is unknown, the condition can occur after radiation or chemical exposure or viral infection. It is treated by aggressive chemotherapy, antibiotics, bone marrow transplant, or stem cell transplant. ALL is the most common type of cancer in children aged 1 to 7, and the prognosis is good for children under age 5. The adult form of ALL is treatable, but the prognosis is not as optimistic.

chronic lymphocytic leukemia (CLL)

Chronic lymphocytic leukemia (CLL) is a cancer in which the bone marrow makes too many mature, but still abnormal, lymphocytes. It is the most common type of leukemia in adults. CLL is slow-growing in some people, but faster-growing in others. Diagnosis is made by blood and bone marrow studies. Chemotherapy and radiation are treatment options.

acute myeloid leukemia (AML)

Acute myeloid leukemia (AML) is a fast-growing cancer of the blood and bone marrow, causing the marrow to produce abnormal lymphoblasts that are incapable of fighting infections. It has several alternate names including acute myelogenous leukemia, acute myelocytic leukemia, acute myeloblastic leukemia, and acute granulocytic leukemia. The cause is unknown but radiation exposure and viral infections have been implicated. Signs and symptoms include fever, headache, joint and bone pain, bruising, and enlarged lymphatic organs. The clinical picture, along with blood and bone marrow studies, confirms the diagnosis. It is treated with chemotherapy and bone marrow transplant or stem cell transplant.

chronic myeloid leukemia (CML)

Chronic myeloid leukemia (CML) is a slowly progressing disease in which too many immature white blood cells, which are incapable of fighting infection, are made in the bone marrow. It is also known as chronic myelogenous leukemia, chronic granulocytic leukemia, and chronic myelocytic leukemia. Weight loss, fatigue, hepatomegaly, splenomegaly, leukocytosis, thrombocytosis, bleeding, and bruising are common. Exposure to ionizing radiation increases the risk of disease. Diagnosis is made by blood and bone marrow studies. Chronic myelocytic leukemia is treated with antineoplastic drugs and chemotherapy.

KEY TERM	Definition
leukemia (lew-KEE-mee-uh)	a type of cancer characterized by the production of increased numbers of immature or abnormal leukocytes (white blood cells)
chemotherapy (kee-moh-THERR-uh-pee)	the use of chemical agents to treat disease, especially cancer
antineoplastic (an-tee-nee-oh-PLAS-tick) drugs	agents that prevent the development, maturation, or spread of cancer cells
bone marrow transplant	transfer of bone marrow from one person to another
stem cell transplant	transfer of stem cells from one person to another
acute lymphoblastic leukemia (ALL) (uh-KEWT lim-foh-BLAST-ick lew-KEE-mee-uh)	disease characterized by increased formation of immature lymphocytes (lymphoblasts) that are unable to fight infection
chronic lymphocytic leukemia (CLL) (KRON-ick lim-foh-SIT-ick lew-KEE-mee-uh)	cancer in which the bone marrow makes too many mature, but still abnormal, lymphocytes
acute myeloid leukemia (AML) (uh-KEWT MIGH-eh-loid lew-KEE-mee-uh)	fast-growing cancer of the blood and bone marrow, causing the marrow to produce abnormal lymphoblasts that are incapable of fighting infections
chronic myeloid leukemia (CML) (KRON-ick MIGH-eh-loid lew-KEE-mee-uh)	slowly progressing disease in which too many immature white blood cells, which are incapable of fighting infection, are made in the bone marrow

KEY TERM PRACTICE: *Leukemia*

1. _____ is a type of cancer characterized by the production of increased numbers of immature or abnormal leukocytes (white blood cells).

2. The transfer of bone marrow from one person to another is called a _____.

3. _____ is a fast-growing cancer of the blood and bone marrow, causing the marrow to produce abnormal blast cells that are incapable of fighting infections.

4. _____ is a slowly progressing disease in which too many immature white blood cells, which are incapable of fighting infection, are made in the bone marrow.

5. Agents that prevent the development, maturation, or spread of cancer cells are termed _____.

LIFE SPAN

Blood cells develop from the mesoderm germ layer, one of the primary layers formed early in embryonic life. While in utero, the mesoderm gives rise to other tissues and blood, which then forms from several sites, including the liver and spleen. By the seventh gestational month, the bone marrow takes over the role of hemopoiesis.

Fetal hemoglobin (HbF) is the form found in the body while still in the womb. It is different from infant and adult hemoglobin (HbA). HbF has a greater affinity for oxygen than does HbA, the form produced after birth and throughout life. After birth, HbF is destroyed by the infant's liver and replaced by newly formed HbA.

Blood disorders that occur early in life, such as hemophilia and von Willebrand disease, a coagulation disorder, are usually genetically determined. Childhood and adolescence are unremarkable relative to blood transformation.

Age-related blood changes include decreased hematocrit and blood pooling in the legs that results from ineffective vein valve function. Many disorders are usually secondary to cardiovascular disease. Late-life leukemias may result from declining immune function.

COMMON Abbreviations

Abbreviation	Term
Ab	antibody
Ag	antigen
AHF	antihemophilic factor; factor VIII
ALL	acute lymphoblastic leukemia
ALT	alanine aminotransferase
AML	acute myeloid leukemia
AST	aspartate aminotransferase
BMT	bone marrow transplant
CBC	complete blood count
chol	cholesterol
CLL	chronic lymphocytic leukemia
CML	chronic myeloid leukemia
DIC	disseminated intravascular coagulation
EBV	Epstein-Barr virus
EPO	erythropoietin
Fe	iron
HbF	fetal hemoglobin
HbO_2	oxyhemoglobin
HbS	sickle cell hemoglobin
Hct	hematocrit
HDL	high-density lipoprotein
HDN	hemolytic disease of the newborn
Hgb	hemoglobin
IM	infectious mononucleosis
LDL	low-density lipoprotein
O_2	oxygen
PCV	packed cell volume
PHSC	pluripotential hemopoietic stem cell
protime	plasma prothrombin time
PT	plasma prothrombin time
PTA	prothrombin tissue activator
PTT	partial thromboplastin time
RBC	red blood cell
Rh	Rhesus
SGOT	serum glutamic-oxaloacetic transaminase

continued

continued from page 487

Abbreviation	Term
SGPT	serum glutamic-pyruvic transaminase
TPA; tPA	tissue plasminogen activator
WBC	white blood cell

COMMON ABBREVIATIONS EXERCISES

1. The abbreviation HbF refers to _____.

2. When referring to the blood, PCV is the abbreviation for _____.

3. _____ is the abbreviation for erythropoietin.

4. Give the two abbreviations for tissue plasminogen activator. _____

5. LDL is the abbreviation for _____.

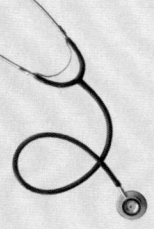

Case Study

Mr. Sanderson, 55 years old, has been sent to the outpatient laboratory where John is the attending phlebotomist. Mr. Sanderson has a history of deep vein thrombosis and neuropathy (nerve disease) secondary to diabetes mellitus. As a monitoring process to evaluate the effectiveness of his medications and assess liver function, Mr. Sanderson has had blood studies done on a regular basis.

Anthropomorphic data noted that Mr. Sanderson is 6 feet 2 inches tall and weighs 230 lb. The physician ordered a complete blood chemistry, immunological studies, and diagnostic panels. The patient fasted for 12 hours but took his medications the morning of the draw. His medications consisted of a 20-mg tablet of atorvastatin (Lipitor) once per day, a 2-mg tablet of warfarin (Coumadin) once per day, and an 81-mg tablet of aspirin three times per week. Atorvastatin is used in the treatment of hyperlipidemia, and warfarin is an oral anticoagulant.

The blood was drawn and sent for analysis. Immediate results were obtained for PTT, bleeding time, and PT.

Case Study Questions

Select the best answer to each of the following questions.

1. **PTT is the abbreviation for**

   _____.

   a. partial thromboplastin time
   b. plasma prothrombin time
   c. plasma timed test
   d. partial thrombocyte test

2. **Atorvastatin is used in the treatment of hyperlipidemia. It acts to** _____.

   a. increase blood lipid levels
   b. decrease blood lipid levels

   c. keep blood lipid levels constant
   d. coagulate blood

3. **Warfarin is a drug that**

   _____.

   a. promotes clotting
   b. inhibits thrombosis
   c. promotes lipid formation
   d. is used to treat hemophilia

continued

continued from page 488

4. **Mr. Sanderson's PTT time was 80 sec; the normal range is 35 to 50 sec. The prolonged time could be caused by _____.**

   a. warfarin therapy
   b. Coumadin therapy
   c. aspirin therapy
   d. all of these

5. **Mr. Sanderson's PT was 18 sec; normal PT time is within 2 sec of the control, which is 11 to 15 sec. The prolonged time may be the result of _____.**

   a. fasting
   b. vitamin K therapy
   c. Coumadin therapy
   d. none of these

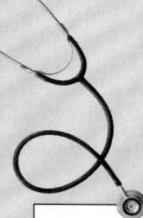

Real World Report

CENTRAL HOSPITAL LABORATORY: LAB ONE

Run Date:	September 29, 2011
Patient Name:	Max Sanderson
Sex:	Male
DOB:	March 3, 1956
Date/Time Last Meal:	09/28/2011 @ 7:30 P.M.
Date/Time Collected:	09/29/2011 @ 8:30 A.M.
Date Recd.: 09/29/2011	Date Rptd: 09/29/2011

TEST RESULTS

- Serum: normal

BLOOD CHEMISTRY AND IMMUNOLOGY

Determination	Results	Reference Range	Low	Normal	High
Glucose	85.0 mg/dL	70–125 mg/dL		X	
Fructosamine	1.6 mmol/L	1.2–2.1 mmol/L		X	
BUN	14.0 mg/dL	5–25 mg/dL		X	
Creatinine	1.0 mg/dL	0.5–1.5 mg/dL		X	
Alkaline phosphatase	68.0 Units/L	30–115 Units/L		X	
Total bilirubin	0.5 mg/dL	0.1–1.2 mg/dL		X	

continued

continued from page 489

Determination	Results	Reference Range	Low	Normal	High
AST (SGOT)	22.0 Units/L	0–41 Units/L		X	
ALT (SGPT)	27.0 Units/L	0–45 Units/L		X	
Total protein	6.9 g/dL	6.0–8.5 g/dL		X	
Albumin	4.4 g/dL	3.0–5.5 g/dL		X	
Globulin	2.5 g/dL	1.0–4.5 g/dL		X	
Cholesterol	251.0 mg/dL	75–260 mg/dL		X	
Triglycerides	209.0 mg/dL	10–190 mg/dL			X
HDL cholesterol	33.0 mg/dL	31–56 mg/dL		X	
Chol/HDL ratio	7.6	0–4.9			X
LDL cholesterol	176.0 mg/dL	60–160 mg/dL			X
LDL/HDL ratio	5.34	1.82–6.06		X	
PSA	0.2	0.4	X		
HIV	nonreactive	nonreactive			

Real World Report Questions

The following exercises review the medical terms in the preceding medical report. The central laboratory where John works receives the reports, which are then forwarded to the physician's office. Abnormal values are indicated in some areas.

1. **The report indicates that Mr. Sanderson's "Chol/HDL ratio" is high.**

   a. Chol is the abbreviation for _____.

   b. HDL is the abbreviation for _____.

2. **Mr. Sanderson's LDL cholesterol is also high. LDL is the abbreviation for _____.**

3. **According to the laboratory report, the patient's AST (SGOT) is within normal limits.**

   a. AST is the abbreviation for _____.

   b. SGOT is the abbreviation for _____.

   c. AST and SGOT are synonymous terms. True or False? _____

4. **Mr. Sanderson's total bilirubin is within normal limits. Bilirubin is _____.**

   a. a bile pigment

   b. a form of PSA

   c. another term for cholesterol

   d. a form of albumin

Review and Application

Multiple-Choice Questions

Select the best answer to each of the following questions.

1. The blood has a role in _____.
   a. nutrient transport b. gas exchange c. temperature regulation d. all of these

2. The word part *-poiesis* means _____.
   a. production, producing b. blood c. condition of blood d. green colored

3. The word part *leuko-* means _____.
   a. cell b. white c. red d. thrombopenia

4. Thrombus refers to _____.
   a. oxygen b. hemoglobin c. a blood clot in a vessel d. bilirubin

5. Hemoglobin with oxygen is called _____.
   a. oxyhemoglobin b. deoxyhemoglobin c. hemosiderin d. a hemocyte

6. A _____ is an immature erythrocyte.
   a. reticulocyte b. leukocyte c. neutrophil d. monocyte

7. Granular leukocytes include _____.
   a. monocytes b. lymphocytes c. basophils d. erythrocytes

8. *Pernicious* means _____.
   a. increased leukocyte levels b. decreased leukocyte levels c. excessive nutrients d. highly destructive and potentially fatal

9. A hematoma is _____.
   a. pain within the blood system b. an alternate term for erythrocytes c. a semisolid mass of clotted blood d. an abnormally low erythrocyte count

10. Cells that assist clot formation are _____.
    a. platelets b. eosinophils c. agglutinogens d. antibodies

11. The fluid portion of blood is called _____.
    a. the hematocrit b. plasma c. fibrin d. thrombin

12. For health reasons, it is better to have a greater circulating level of _____ than _____.
    a. LDL; HDL b. cholesterol; HDL c. fat; cholesterol d. HDL; LDL

13. The medical term for stoppage of uncontrolled bleeding is _____.
    a. thrombostasis b. hemostasis c. coagustasis d. embolism

14. A person with antigens A and B on her erythrocytes is said to have Type _____ blood.
    a. A b. B c. AB d. O

15. A person with B antibodies has Type _____ blood.
    a. A b. B c. AB d. O

16. The universal donor has Type _____ blood.

    a. A   b. B   c. AB   d. O

17. Bluish skin discoloration is termed _____.

    a. jaundice   b. cyanosis   c. bilirubin   d. sepsis

18. The average time it takes for bleeding to stop after the skin has been superficially lanced is known as the _____ time.

    a. bleeding   b. pro   c. clotting   d. TPA

19. _____ refers to the use of chemical agents to treat disease.

    a. Chemotherapy   b. Nutritional therapy   c. Pharmacology   d. Antineoplasia

20. Administering synthetic erythropoietin stimulates erythrocyte production. This is known medically as _____.

    a. erythroeisis   b. cytopenia   c. proerythroblasts   d. erythropoiesis

21. Fibrinogen is _____.

| a. soluble and dissolves easily | b. insoluble and dissolves easily | c. soluble and does not dissolve | d. insoluble and does not dissolve |

Word Parts Exercises

Using the following word parts, form a medical term for each definition. Each word part is used only once.

-cyte
erythro-
hemo-
-philia
phlebo-
-tomy

22. vein incision _____

23. inherited clotting disorder _____

24. red blood cell _____

Matching Exercises

Match the disorder with its description.

_____ 25. disseminated intravascular coagulation

_____ 26. infectious mononucleosis

_____ 27. chronic lymphocytic leukemia

_____ 28. hemochromatosis

_____ 29. nutritional anemia

a. viral infection of lymphatic tissue
b. chronic disease with iron deposits in tissues
c. cancer characterized by mature, abnormal lymphocytes
d. anemia caused by dietary deficiency
e. simultaneous bleeding and clotting

Match the anemia with its description.

_____ 30. aplastic anemia

_____ 31. hemolytic anemia

_____ 32. hemorrhagic anemia

_____ 33. sickle cell anemia

a. anemia with hemoglobin S
b. anemia caused by excessive blood loss
c. anemia caused by bone marrow failure
d. anemia caused by RBC destruction

Definitions

Define the following terms.

34. lipoprotein _____

35. prothrombin _____

36. phlebotomy _____

37. agglutination _____

38. osmotic pressure _____

39. packed cell volume _____

40. white blood cells _____

41. hemoglobin count _____

Provide a medical term for the following definitions

42. large eater _____

43. affinity for neutral dye _____

44. formation of leukocytes _____

45. blood stoppage _____

46. against clotting _____

47. toxic blood _____

Alternate Terms

Give an alternate term for each of the following terms.

48. agglutinin _____

49. antigen _____

50. bruise _____

51. red blood cell _____

52. white blood cell _____

Spelling

Identify the correctly spelled term in each set.

53. _____
   a. erythrocyte
   b. errythrocyte
   c. erithrocyte
   d. erythracyte

54. _____
   a. aglutinin
   b. egglutinin
   c. agglutinin
   d. agglutinnin

55. _____
   a. hemaglobin
   b. hemeglobin
   c. hemoglobun
   d. hemoglobin

56. _____
   a. pluripotential
   b. pleuripotentshul
   c. plurepotentcial
   d. pluripotintial

57. _____
   a. albumen
   b. albumin
   c. allbumen
   d. albumine

58. _____
   a. proethrombin
   b. prothrombin
   c. protrombin
   d. prothrumbin

Unscramble

Unscramble the letters to form a medical term.

59. poailymecyht _____

60. matameho _____

61. slumboe _____

62. nistfransuo _____

63. teauc _____

Abbreviations

Provide the term for the abbreviations and then define the terms.

64. Hct _____

65. EPO _____

66. PCV _____

67. CBC _____

Analogies

Provide a medical term to complete a meaningful analogy.

68. Leukocytosis is to leukopenia as _____ is to erythropenia.

69. Blue is to cyanosis as _____ is to jaundice.

70. RBC is to erythrocyte as _____ is to leukocyte.

Short Answer

Answer the following questions.

71. John Doe has Type O blood. What type blood can he successfully receive in a blood transfusion?

_____

72. In what two circumstances might a person simultaneously have a decreased red blood cell count and an increased reticulocyte count?

_____

Labeling

Label the structures in the following diagram.

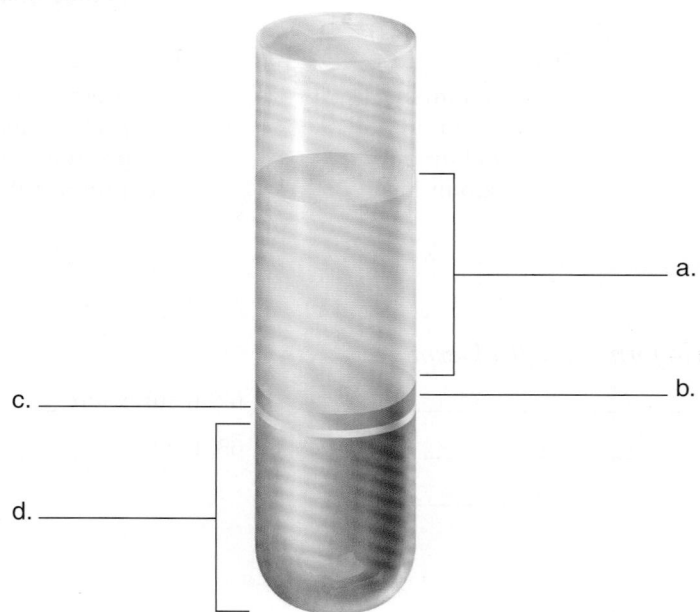

a.

b.

c. _____

d. _____

Word Search

Find the medical terms hidden in the puzzle.

U	C	K	E	G	I	C	Y	P	O	C	E	W	J	X	S
B	O	G	S	R	C	E	L	E	N	T	Q	W	N	T	N
A	A	M	I	J	Y	A	P	I	C	K	O	E	S	I	U
S	G	J	K	N	S	T	M	I	R	W	O	A	B	Y	N
O	U	B	C	M	L	U	H	N	S	S	L	O	W	D	I
P	L	O	A	J	B	X	M	R	I	B	L	I	H	O	N
H	A	G	G	L	U	T	I	N	O	G	E	N	M	B	I
I	T	T	A	O	W	L	O	R	O	C	E	S	G	I	T
L	I	S	D	T	Q	P	H	M	N	H	Y	T	M	T	U
S	O	U	G	A	H	T	E	P	U	I	O	T	X	N	L
F	N	G	W	I	Y	H	M	U	R	E	S	L	E	A	G
I	X	J	L	R	N	I	B	U	R	I	L	I	B	S	G
B	M	S	E	S	L	I	H	P	O	R	T	U	E	N	A
R	W	A	J	V	F	I	B	R	I	N	O	G	E	N	Z
I	L	A	N	T	I	G	E	N	F	K	K	D	M	R	S
N	E	Q	M	I	D	N	V	O	X	Y	N	Y	U	S	M

agglutinin
agglutinogen
albumin
antibody
antigen
basophils
bilirubin
coagulation
eosinophils
erythroblasts
erythrocytes
fibrin
fibrinogen
hemoglobin
neutrophils
plasma
serum

Vocabulary Review

Review the key terms from this chapter, study the spelling and pronunciation of each term, and write its definition in the space provided. Listen to the audio available for most terms at http://thepoint.lww.com/nath2e and pronounce each term for yourself. Then check the box when you feel confident that you know the definition and can pronounce the term correctly.

Key Term	Pronunciation	Definition
❏ **acute lymphoblastic leukemia (ALL)**	(uh-KEWT lim-foh-BLAST-ick lew-KEE-mee-uh)	_____
❏ **acute myeloid leukemia (AML)**	(uh-KEWT MIGH-eh-loid lew-KEE-mee-uh)	_____
❏ **agglutination**	(uh-gloo-ti-NAY-shun)	_____
❏ **agglutinin**	(uh-GLOO-ti-nin)	_____
❏ **agglutinogen**	(uh-GLOO-tin-oh-jen)	_____
❏ **albumin**	(al-BEW-min)	_____
❏ **anemia**	(uh-NEE-mee-uh)	_____
❏ **antibody (Ab)**	(AN-tee-bod-ee)	_____
❏ **anticoagulant**	(an-tee-koh-AG-yoo-lunt)	_____

Key Term	Pronunciation	Definition
❏ antigen (Ag)	(AN-ti-jen)	_____
❏ antihemophilic factor (AHF)	(an-tee-hee-moh-FIL-ick)	_____
❏ antineoplastic drugs	(an-tee-nee-oh-PLAS-tick)	_____
❏ aplastic anemia	(ay-PLAS-tick uh-NEE-mee-uh)	_____
❏ autologous transfusion	(aw-TOL-uh-gus)	_____
❏ basophils	(BAY-soh-fils)	_____
❏ bilirubin	(bil-i-ROO-bin)	_____
❏ bleeding time		_____
❏ bone marrow aspiration biopsy	(as-pi-RAY-shun BYE-op-see)	_____
❏ bone marrow transplant		_____
❏ chemotherapy	(kee-moh-THERR-uh-pee)	_____
❏ chronic lymphocytic leukemia (CLL)	(KRON-ick lim-foh-SIT-ick lew-KEE-mee-uh)	_____
❏ chronic myeloid leukemia (CML)	(KRON-ick MIGH-eh-loid lew-KEE-mee-uh)	_____
❏ coagulation	(koh-ag-yoo-LAY-shun)	_____
❏ complete blood count (CBC)		_____
❏ cyanosis	(sigh-uh-NOH-sis)	_____
❏ differential white blood count	(dif-ur-EN-shul)	_____
❏ disseminated intravascular coagulation (DIC)	(di-SEM-i-nay-tid in-truh-VAS kew-lur koh-ag-yoo-LAY-shun)	_____
❏ dyscrasia	(dis-KRAY-zee-uh)	_____
❏ ecchymosis	(eck-i-MOH-sis)	_____
❏ embolism	(EM-boh-liz-um)	_____
❏ embolus	(EM-boh-lus)	_____
❏ eosinophils	(ee-oh-SIN-uh-fils)	_____
❏ erythroblastosis fetalis	(e-rith-roh-blas-TOH-sis-fee-TAY-lis)	_____
❏ erythroblasts	(e-RITH-roh-blasts)	_____
❏ erythrocytes	(e-RITH-roh-sites)	_____
❏ erythrocytosis	(e-rith-roh-sigh-TOH-sis)	_____
❏ erythropenia	(e-rith-roh-PEE-nee-uh)	_____
❏ erythropoiesis	(e-rith-roh-poy-EE-sis)	_____
❏ erythropoietin (EPO)	(e-rith-roh-POY-e-tin)	_____
❏ exchange transfusion		_____
❏ fibrin	(FIGH-brin)	_____
❏ fibrinogen	(figh-BRIN-oh-jen)	_____
❏ globulin	(GLOB-yoo-lin)	_____
❏ hemarthrosis	(hee-mahr-THROH-sis)	_____

Key Term	Pronunciation	Definition
❏ **hematocrit (Hct)**	(hee-MAT-oh-krit)	_____
❏ **hematology**	(he-muh-TOL-oh-jee)	_____
❏ **hematoma**	(hee-muh-TOH-muh)	_____
❏ **hematopoiesis**	(hee-mat-oh-poy-EE-sis)	_____
❏ **hemochromatosis**	(hee-moh-kroh-muh-TOH-sis)	_____
❏ **hemoglobin (Hg, Hgb)**	(HEE-muh-gloh-bin)	_____
❏ **hemoglobin count**	(HEE-muh-GLOH-bin)	_____
❏ **hemolytic anemia**	(hee-moh-LIT-ick uh-NEE-mee-uh)	_____
❏ **hemolytic disease of the newborn (HDN)**	(hee-moh-LIT-ick)	_____
❏ **hemophilia**	(hee-moh-FIL-ee-uh)	_____
❏ **hemopoiesis**	(hee-moh-poy-EE-sis)	_____
❏ **hemorrhage**	(HEM-ur-rij)	_____
❏ **hemorrhagic anemia**	(hem-uh-RAJ-ick uh-NEE-mee-uh)	_____
❏ **hemostasis**	(hee-moh-STAY-sis)	_____
❏ **heparin**	(HEP-uh-rin)	_____
❏ **high-density lipoprotein (HDL)**	(lip-oh-PROH-teen)	_____
❏ **histamine**	(HIS-tuh-meen)	_____
❏ **immunity**	(i-MEW-ni-tee)	_____
❏ **infectious mononucleosis (IM)**	(mon-oh-new-klee-OH-sis)	_____
❏ **jaundice**	(JAWN-dis)	_____
❏ **leukemia**	(lew-KEE-mee-uh)	_____
❏ **leukocytes**	(LEW-koh-sites)	_____
❏ **leukocytosis**	(lew-koh-sigh-TOH-sis)	_____
❏ **leukopenia**	(lew-koh-PEE-nee-uh)	_____
❏ **leukopoiesis**	(lew-koh-poy-EE-sis)	_____
❏ **lipoprotein**	(lip-oh-PROH-teen)	_____
❏ **low-density lipoprotein (LDL)**	(lip-oh-PROH-teen)	_____
❏ **lymphocytes**	(LIM-foh-sites)	_____
❏ **macrophage**	(MACK-roh-faij)	_____
❏ **monocytes**	(MON-oh-sites)	_____
❏ **multiple myeloma**	(migh-eh-LOH-muh)	_____
❏ **neutropenia**	(new-troh-PEE-nee-uh)	_____
❏ **neutrophils**	(NEW-truh-filz)	_____
❏ **nutritional anemia**	(uh-NEE-mee-uh)	_____
❏ **osmotic pressure**	(oz-MOT-ick)	_____

Key Term	Pronunciation	Definition
❏ oxyhemoglobin (HbO$_2$)	(ock-se-HEE-muh-gloh-bin)	_____
❏ packed cell volume (PCV)		_____
❏ partial thromboplastin time (PTT)	(throm-boh-PLAS-tin)	_____
❏ pernicious anemia	(pur-NISH-us uh-NEE-mee-uh)	_____
❏ phlebotomy	(fle-BOT-uh-mee)	_____
❏ plasma	(PLAZ-muh)	_____
❏ plasma prothrombin time (PT; protime)	(proh-THROM-bin)	_____
❏ plasmapheresis	(plaz-muh-fe-REE-sis)	_____
❏ platelets	(PLAIT-lits)	_____
❏ pluripotential hemopoietic stem cell (PHSC)	(ploo-ree-POH-ten-shul hee-moh-poy-ET-ick STEM SELL)	_____
❏ polycythemia	(pol-ee-sigh-THEEM-ee-uh)	_____
❏ polycythemia vera	(pol-ee-sigh-THEEM-ee-uh VEER-uh)	_____
❏ prothrombin	(proh-THROM-bin)	_____
❏ purpura	(PURE-pew-ruh)	_____
❏ red blood cell count		_____
❏ red blood cells (RBCs)		_____
❏ reticulocyte	(re-TICK-yoo-loh-site)	_____
❏ Rh factor		_____
❏ Schilling test	(SHIL-ing)	_____
❏ septicemia	(sep-ti-SEE-mee-uh)	_____
❏ serotonin	(seer-oh-TOH-nin)	_____
❏ serum	(SEER-um)	_____
❏ sickle cell anemia	(uh-NEE-mee-uh)	_____
❏ stem cell transplant		_____
❏ streptokinase	(strep-toh-KIGH-nace)	_____
❏ thalassemia	(thal-uh-SEE-mee-uh)	_____
❏ thrombin	(THROM-bin)	_____
❏ thrombocytes	(THROM-boh-sites)	_____
❏ thrombocytopenia	(throm-boh-sigh-toh-PEE-nee-uh)	_____
❏ thrombolytic	(throm-boh-LIT-ick)	_____
❏ thrombus	(THROM-bus)	_____
❏ tissue plasminogen activator (TPA, tPA)	(plaz-MIN-oh-jen)	_____
❏ transfusion	(trans-FYOO-zhun)	_____
❏ venipuncture	(veen-i-PUNK-chur)	_____
❏ white blood cells (WBCs)		_____

Answers

Word Grouping Exercises

Definition	Word Part	Definition	Word Part
base, basis	basi-, basio-, baso-	fiber	fibr-, fibro-
affinity for, craving for	phil-, -phile, -philia, -philic	fibrin	fibrino-
bile	bili-	granular	granulo-
blood	A. hem-, hema- B. hemat-, hemato-, hemo-	iron	sidero-
blood clot, coagulation, thrombin	thromb-, thrombo-	lymph (tissue fluid in a lymphatic vessel)	lymph-, lympho-
blue	cyan-, cyano-	neutral	neutr-, neutro-
bone marrow	myel-, myelo-	nucleus	nucle-, nucleo-
causing lysis (destruction)	-lytic	plasma (liquid part of blood)	plasma-, plasmat-, plasmato-, plasmo-
cell	-cyte	presence of oxygen	oxy-
color	chrom-, chromat-, chromato-, chromo-	production, producing	-poiesis
condition of blood	-emia	red, red blood cell	erythr-, erythro-
deficiency	-penia	sepsis, septic (blood infection)	septic-, septico-
denoting appearance	phen-, pheno-	serum, serous	sero-
eating, devouring	A. -phage, -phagia, -phagy B. phago-	several	pluri-
excessive discharge, hemorrhage	-rrhagia	vein	phleb-, phlebo-
		white, white blood cell	leuk-, leuko-

Word Building Exercises

Word Part	Meaning	Common or Known Word	Example Medical Term
leuk-, leuko-	white, white blood cell	leukemia	leukocyte
cyan-, cyano-	blue	cyanide	cyanosis
-emia	condition of blood	anemia	anemia
fibr-, fibro-	fiber	fiber	fibrosis
hem-, hema-	blood	hemorrhoids	hemostasis
hemat-, hemato-, hemo-	blood	hematoma	hematopoiesis
neutr-, neutro-	neutral	neutral	neutrophil
oxy-	presence of oxygen	oxygen	oxygen
phleb-, phlebo-	vein	phlebotomist	phlebotomy

Word Part	Meaning	Common or Known Word	Example Medical Term
phil-, -phile, -philia, -philic	affinity for, craving for	pedophilia	hemophilia
pluri-	several	plural	pluripotent
septic-, septico-	sepsis, septic (blood infection)	septic system	septicemia
sero-	serum, serous	serum	serum
thromb-, thrombo-	blood clot, coagulation, thrombin	thrombus	thrombocyte

Key Terms Practice

Blood Preview

1. hemopoiesis; hematopoiesis; *hem-* and *hemato-*; *-poiesis*
2. serum
3. albumin, globulin, and fibrinogen
4. pluripotential hemopoietic stem cell (PHSC); *pluri-*; *hemo-*; *-poiesis*
5. Plasma

Red Blood Cells (RBCs) or Erythrocytes

1. erythropoiesis; *erythro-*; *-poiesis*
2. oxyhemoglobin (HbO_2)
3. Bilirubin
4. reticulocyte
5. Hemoglobin (Hg, Hgb)

White Blood Cells (WBCs) or Leukocytes

1. neutrophil
2. monocytes and lymphocytes
3. Immunity
4. leukopoiesis; *leuko-*; *-poiesis*
5. differential white blood count

Platelets or Thrombocytes

1. platelets; thrombocytes
2. *thrombo-*; *-cyte*

Lipoproteins

1. lipoprotein
2. high-density lipoprotein (HDL)
3. low-density lipoprotein (LDL)

Blood Clotting

1. thrombus
2. tissue plasminogen activator (TPA)
3. hemostasis
4. coagulation
5. hemorrhage

Blood Types

1. agglutination
2. agglutinogen; antigen (Ag)
3. transfusion
4. agglutinin; antibody (Ab)
5. Rh factor

Anemia

1. sickle cell anemia and thalassemia
2. pernicious anemia
3. Schilling test
4. autologous transfusion; *auto-*
5. Dyscrasia

Bleeding, Coagulation, and Platelet Disorders

1. hemophilia
2. Thrombocytopenia; *thrombo-*; *-penia*
3. thrombolytic; *thrombo-*
4. hematoma
5. Bleeding time

Other Blood Disorders

1. leukopenia; *leuko-*; *-penia*
2. Plasmapheresis
3. Cyanosis
4. Infectious mononucleosis (IM)
5. polycythemia

Hemolytic Disease of the Newborn (HDN) or Erythroblastosis Fetalis

1. red; immature precursor cell; condition of; fetus; erythroblastosis fetalis
2. hemolytic disease of the newborn (HDN)
3. erythroblasts; *erythro-*; *-blast*

Leukemia

1. Leukemia
2. bone marrow transplant
3. Acute myeloid leukemia (AML)
4. Chronic myeloid leukemia (CML)
5. antineoplastic drugs

Common Abbreviations Exercises

1. HbF = fetal hemoglobin
2. PCV = packed cell volume
3. EPO = erythropoietin
4. tissue plasminogen activator = TPA and tPA
5. LDL = low-density lipoprotein

Case Study

1. a is the correct answer.
   - b is incorrect because the abbreviation for plasma prothrombin time is PT.
   - c and d are incorrect because these are made-up tests.
2. b is the correct answer.
   - a and c are incorrect because atorvastatin decreases blood lipid levels.
   - d is incorrect because atorvastatin does not act as a clotting agent.
3. b is the correct answer.
   - a is incorrect because clotting agents enhance clotting.
   - c is incorrect because warfarin is an anticoagulant; drugs typically do not promote fat formation.
   - d is incorrect because hemophilia would be treated with a clotting agent.
4. d is the correct answer.
   - All answers are correct because all these agents act as anticoagulants.
5. c is the correct answer.
   - a is incorrect because fasting does not affect clotting time.
   - b is incorrect because vitamin K therapy acts as a clotting agent and thus would decrease the PT time.
   - d is incorrect because c is the correct answer.

Real World Report

1. a. cholesterol; b. high-density lipoprotein
2. low-density lipoprotein
3. a. aspartate aminotransferase; b. serum glutamic-oxaloacetic transaminase; c. True
4. a

Review and Application

1. d	4. c	7. c	10. a
2. a	5. a	8. d	11. b
3. b	6. a	9. c	12. d

13. b	18. a	23. hemophilia	28. b
14. c	19. a	24. erythrocyte	29. d
15. a	20. d	25. e	30. c
16. d	21. a	26. a	31. d
17. b	22. phlebotomy	27. c	32. b

33. a

34. lipoprotein = blood plasma complex that contains both lipid (fat) and soluble proteins

35. prothrombin = plasma protein that converts to thrombin during blood clotting

36. phlebotomy = puncture made in a vein to withdraw blood

37. agglutination = clumping of blood cells

38. osmotic pressure = fluid pressure in the blood vessels

39. packed cell volume = fraction of whole blood that is made up of red blood cells; also called the hematocrit (Hct)

40. white blood cells = granular and agranular cells of whole blood that play a role in immunity; also called leukocytes

41. hemoglobin count = test used to measure hemoglobin content in a blood sample

42. macrophage

43. neutrophil

44. leukopoiesis

45. hemostasis

46. anticoagulant

47. septicemia

48. agglutinin = antibody

49. antigen = agglutinogen

50. bruise = ecchymosis

51. red blood cell = erythrocyte

52. white blood cell = leukocyte

53. a

54. c

55. d

56. a

57. b

58. b

59. polycythemia

60. hematoma

61. embolus

62. transfusion

63. acute

64. Hct = hematocrit; fraction of whole blood that is made up of red blood cells; also called the packed cell volume (PCV)

65. EPO = erythropoietin; hormone released from kidneys that promotes red blood cell production

66. PCV = packed cell volume; fraction of whole blood that is made up of red blood cells; also called the hematocrit (Hct)

67. CBC = complete blood count; diagnostic test that measures blood cell types and levels in a sample of blood

68. erythrocytosis

69. yellow

70. WBC

71. John can receive only blood Type O.

72. The individual may have severe hemorrhage or low blood oxygen levels.

Labeling

a. Plasma   **b.** Platelets

c. White blood cells   **d.** Red blood cells

Word Search

U	C	K	E	G	I	C	Y	P	O	C	E	W	J	X	S
B	O	G	S	R	C	E	L	E	N	T	Q	W	N	T	N
A	A	M	I	J	Y	A	P	I	C	K	O	E	S	I	U
S	G	J	K	N	S	T	M	I	R	W	O	A	B	Y	N
O	U	B	C	M	L	U	H	N	S	S	L	O	W	D	I
P	L	O	A	J	B	X	M	R	I	B	L	I	H	O	N
H	A	G	G	L	U	T	I	N	O	G	E	N	M	B	I
I	T	T	A	O	W	L	O	R	O	C	E	S	G	I	T
L	I	S	D	T	Q	P	H	M	N	H	Y	T	M	T	U
S	O	U	G	A	H	T	E	P	U	I	O	T	X	N	L
F	N	G	W	I	Y	H	M	U	R	E	S	L	E	A	G
I	X	J	L	R	N	I	B	U	R	I	L	I	B	S	G
B	M	S	E	S	L	I	H	P	O	R	T	U	E	N	A
R	W	A	J	V	F	I	B	R	I	N	O	G	E	N	Z
I	L	A	N	T	I	G	E	N	F	K	K	D	M	R	S
N	E	Q	M	I	D	N	V	O	X	Y	N	Y	U	S	M

agglutinin
agglutinogen
albumin
antibody
antigen
basophils
bilirubin
coagulation
eosinophils
erythroblasts
erythrocytes
fibrin
fibrinogen
hemoglobin
neutrophils
plasma
serum

Vocabulary Review

Key Term	Definition	Key Term	Definition
acute lymphoblastic leukemia (ALL)	disease characterized by increased formation of immature lymphocytes (lymphoblasts) that are unable to fight infection	**agglutinogen**	protein (antigen) on the surface of the red blood cell that determines the blood type; an antigen
acute myeloid leukemia (AML)	fast-growing cancer of the blood and bone marrow, causing the marrow to produce abnormal lymphoblasts that are incapable of fighting infections	**albumin**	white-colored protein found in plasma that gives blood its viscosity
		anemia	condition characterized by red blood cell deficiency or hemoglobin deficiency
agglutination	clumping of blood cells	**antibody (Ab)**	substance in blood plasma that causes clumping when it reacts with a specific antigen; an agglutinin
agglutinin	substance in blood plasma that causes clumping when it reacts with a foreign antigen; an antibody		
		anticoagulant	substance that prevents blood clotting

Key Term	Definition
antigen (Ag)	protein on the surface of the red blood cell that determines the blood type; an agglutinogen
antihemophilic factor (AHF)	clotting factor VIII used to treat hemophilia
antineoplastic drugs	agents that prevent the development, maturation, or spread of cancer cells
aplastic anemia	anemia caused by failure of the red bone marrow to produce enough red blood cells
autologous transfusion	donation of blood for later use by that same person
basophils	type of granular white blood cell that releases heparin, histamine, and serotonin
bilirubin	orange-yellow bile pigment formed from the breakdown of hemoglobin
bleeding time	average time it takes bleeding to stop after the skin (earlobe or fingertip) has been superficially lanced
bone marrow aspiration biopsy	removal of bone marrow for clinical examination
bone marrow transplant	transfer of bone marrow from one person to another
chemotherapy	the use of chemical agents to treat disease, especially cancer
chronic lymphocytic leukemia (CLL)	cancer in which the bone marrow makes too many mature, but still abnormal, lymphocytes
chronic myeloid leukemia (CML)	slowly progressing disease in which too many immature white blood cells, which are incapable of fighting infection, are made in the bone marrow
coagulation	thickening of blood to form a clot
complete blood count (CBC)	diagnostic test that measures blood cell types and levels in a sample of blood
cyanosis	bluish skin discoloration due to lack of oxygen
differential white blood count	test that determines the number of each type of white blood cell in a blood sample
disseminated intravascular coagulation (DIC)	disorder of the clotting cascade characterized by simultaneous bleeding and clotting

Key Term	Definition
dyscrasia	general term for a blood disorder
ecchymosis	bleeding into surrounding tissue; also called a bruise
embolism	blood vessel obstruction caused by an embolus
embolus	thrombus that migrates and lodges in the bloodstream
eosinophils	type of granular white blood cell that increases in number during parasitic infections and allergic reactions
erythroblastosis fetalis	serious blood disease of fetuses and newborn babies in which the antibodies produced by an Rh^- mother destroy the red blood cells of an Rh^+ fetus; also called hemolytic disease of the newborn (HDN)
erythroblasts	immature red blood cells
erythrocytes	mature cells shaped like biconcave discs without a nucleus that contain hemoglobin for the transport of oxygen and carbon dioxide; also called red blood cells
erythrocytosis	abnormally high number of red blood cells; also called polycythemia
erythropenia	deficiency in the number of red blood cells
erythropoiesis	formation of red blood cells that begins in the red bone marrow and ends with the release of mature cells
erythropoietin (EPO)	hormone released from kidneys that promotes red blood cell production
exchange transfusion	simultaneous blood extraction and replacement in an individual
fibrin	insoluble protein formed from fibrinogen during the clotting process
fibrinogen	protein found in plasma that plays an essential role in blood clotting
globulin	protein group found in the plasma that has an immune function
hemarthrosis	bleeding into a joint
hematocrit (Hct)	fraction of whole blood that is made up of red blood cells; also called the packed cell volume (PCV)

Key Term	Definition	Key Term	Definition
hematology	branch of medicine devoted to the study of blood and diseases of the blood	leukemia	a type of cancer characterized by the production of increased numbers of immature or abnormal leukocytes (white blood cells)
hematoma	semisolid mass of clotted blood in the tissues	leukocytes	granular and agranular cells of whole blood that play a role in immunity; also called white blood cells
hematopoiesis	production of red blood cells, white blood cells, and platelets, which occurs in the red bone marrow; also called hemopoiesis	leukocytosis	abnormally high leukocyte count
		leukopenia	abnormally low white blood cell (leukocyte) count
hemochromatosis	chronic genetic disease characterized by iron deposits in the body	leukopoiesis	formation of white blood cells
hemoglobin (Hg, Hgb)	protein found in red blood cells that reversibly binds and transports oxygen and carbon dioxide	lipoprotein	blood plasma complex that contains both lipid (fat) and soluble proteins
hemoglobin count	test used to measure hemoglobin content in a blood sample	low-density lipoprotein (LDL)	lipoprotein that transports cholesterol to the cells and tissues; also referred to as LDL cholesterol or "bad cholesterol"
hemolytic anemia	anemia caused by red blood cell destruction		
hemolytic disease of the newborn (HDN)	serious blood disease of fetuses and newborn babies in which the antibodies produced by an Rh$^-$ mother destroy the red blood cells of an Rh$^+$ fetus; also called erythroblastosis fetalis	lymphocytes	agranular white blood cells that are active in the immune response
		macrophage	phagocytic cell derived from a monocyte
		monocytes	agranular white blood cells that consume foreign particles and cellular debris
hemophilia	inherited blood clotting disorder	multiple myeloma	tumors composed of cells derived from bone marrow that cause palpable swellings on bones
hemopoiesis	production of red blood cells, white blood cells, and platelets, which occurs in the red bone marrow; also called hematopoiesis		
		neutropenia	decreased neutrophil levels
hemorrhage	uncontrolled, profuse bleeding	neutrophils	most common type of granular white blood cell that contains antibiotic-like proteins
hemorrhagic anemia	anemia caused by excessive bleeding		
hemostasis	stoppage of uncontrolled bleeding	nutritional anemia	anemia caused by dietary deficiency of nutrients that are essential to red blood cell formation
heparin	an anticoagulant or antiplatelet factor		
high-density lipoprotein (HDL)	lipoprotein that transports cholesterol to the liver for excretion in bile; also referred to as HDL cholesterol or "good cholesterol"	osmotic pressure	fluid pressure in the blood vessels
		oxyhemoglobin (HbO$_2$)	bright red compound formed when oxygen combines with hemoglobin
histamine	chemical that stimulates blood vessel dilation (expansion)	packed cell volume (PCV)	fraction of whole blood that is made up of red blood cells; also called the hematocrit (Hct)
immunity	protection against disease		
infectious mononucleosis (IM)	Epstein-Barr virus (EBV) infection that affects lymphatic tissue and is characterized by leukocytosis	partial thromboplastin time (PTT)	test of time it takes for blood to clot
jaundice	yellowish skin due to accumulated bilirubin	pernicious anemia	anemia caused by vitamin B$_{12}$ deficiency usually resulting from a lack of intrinsic factor

Key Term	Definition	Key Term	Definition
phlebotomy	puncture made in a vein to withdraw blood; also called venipuncture	septicemia	bacterial infection of the blood; formerly known as blood poisoning
plasma	liquid, noncellular portion of whole blood	serotonin	chemical that stimulates blood vessel constriction (narrowing)
plasma prothrombin time (PT; protime)	test of time it takes for blood to clot	serum	blood plasma without the clotting protein fibrinogen
plasmapheresis	process in which blood is taken from the patient, separated into plasma and cells, and then the cells are transfused back into the patient's bloodstream	sickle cell anemia	inherited form of anemia in which the red blood cells are abnormally shaped
platelets	cellular fragments found in whole blood that play a role in controlling blood loss and in blood clotting; also called thrombocytes	stem cell transplant	transfer of stem cells from one person to another
		streptokinase	enzyme that dissolves blood clots
pluripotential hemopoietic stem cell (PHSC)	stem cell found in the red bone marrow that forms all other blood cells	thalassemia	inherited form of anemia characterized by an inability to produce adequate amounts of hemoglobin
polycythemia	disorder marked by an abnormally high number of red blood cells in the circulating blood	thrombin	protein that induces the conversion of fibrinogen to fibrin to form a clot
polycythemia vera	a chronic form of polycythemia with an unknown cause	thrombocytes	cellular fragments found in whole blood that play a role in controlling blood loss and in blood clotting; also called platelets
prothrombin	plasma protein that converts to thrombin during blood clotting		
purpura	condition characterized by hemorrhage into the skin	thrombocytopenia	clotting disorder caused by a decreased number of platelets
red blood cell count	measurement of the number of red blood cells per microliter (mcL) of whole blood	thrombolytic	an agent that dissolves a thrombus (clot)
red blood cells (RBCs)	mature cells shaped like biconcave discs without a nucleus that contain hemoglobin for the transport of oxygen and carbon dioxide; also called erythrocytes	thrombus	abnormal blood clot that remains at the site of formation
		tissue plasminogen activator (TPA, tPA)	naturally produced and genetically engineered anticlotting enzyme
reticulocyte	immature red blood cell	transfusion	transfer of blood from one person to another
Rh factor	a specific antigen found on the surface of red blood cells; those with the Rh factor are Rh^+ and those without it are Rh^-	venipuncture	puncture made in a vein to withdraw blood; also called phlebotomy
Schilling test	diagnostic tool to determine whether the body absorbs vitamin B_{12} by determining the amount of radioactive vitamin B_{12} excreted in the urine	white blood cells (WBCs)	granular and agranular cells of whole blood that play a role in immunity; also called leukocytes

C H A P T E R

11

Cardiovascular System

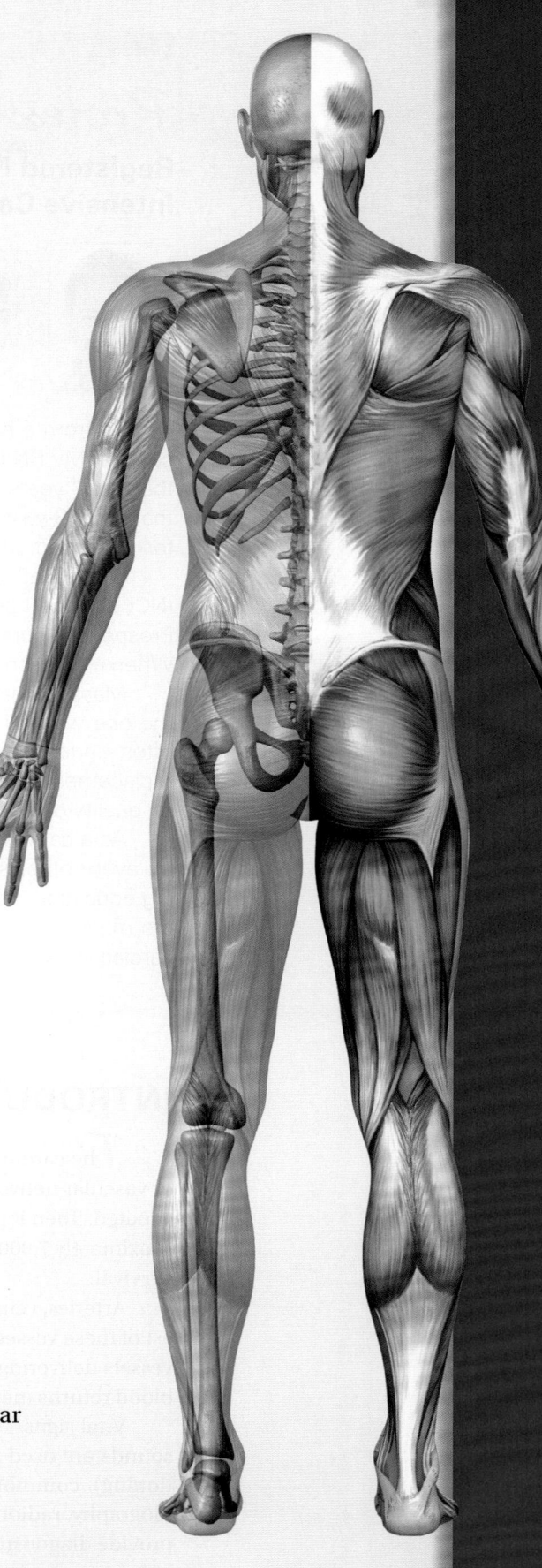

OBJECTIVES

After completing this chapter, you should be able to:

1. State the meaning of word parts related to the cardiovascular system.

2. Identify and label anatomical features of the heart and trace the pathway of blood through the heart.

3. Identify common arteries and veins.

4. Explain how blood pressure is measured.

5. Define common signs, symptoms, and treatments of various cardiovascular system diseases.

6. Define clinical tests and diagnostic procedures related to the cardiovascular system.

7. Describe anatomical and physiological alterations throughout the life span.

8. Define common abbreviations related to the cardiovascular system.

9. Define terms used in medical reports involving the cardiovascular system.

10. Define, spell, and pronounce the chapter's medical terms correctly.

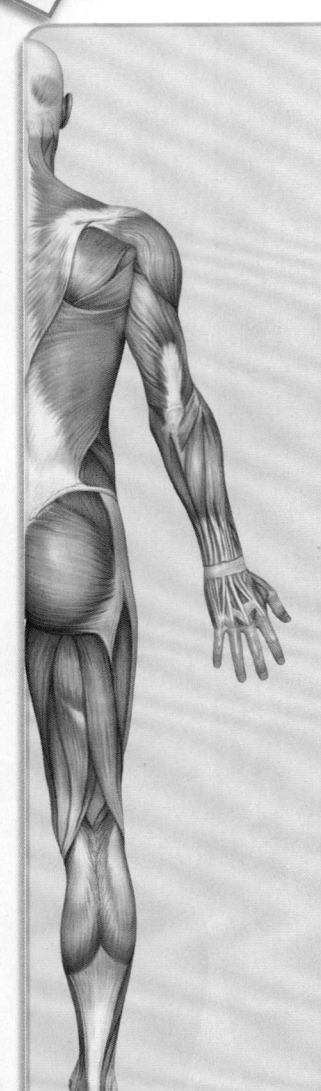

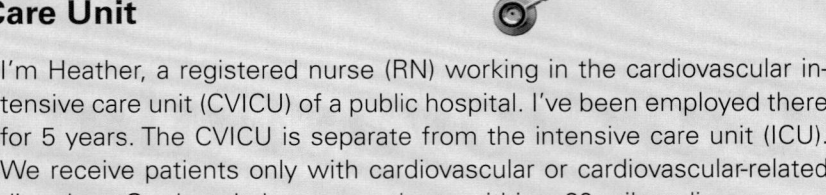

Professional Profile

Registered Nurse in a Cardiovascular Intensive Care Unit

I'm Heather, a registered nurse (RN) working in the cardiovascular intensive care unit (CVICU) of a public hospital. I've been employed there for 5 years. The CVICU is separate from the intensive care unit (ICU). We receive patients only with cardiovascular or cardiovascular-related disorders. Our hospital serves patients within a 60-mile radius.

I received my RN diploma and associate of arts (AA) in natural science degree from a hospital-based school of nursing, which has an affiliation with a local college. My RN program was a "3 + 1" program, which means that after completing the first 3 years of the program, I graduated with a diploma and an AA degree. After that initial 3-year course of study, as a graduate of the program I was able to continue for 1 year more to earn a bachelor of science in nursing (BSN) degree.

One month after graduating, I passed the National Council Licensure Examination (NCLEX) and began my full-time nursing career, working on the rehabilitation floor. Prospective nurses are required to pass the NCLEX to be licensed in the nursing field. When a position in the CVICU opened up, I applied and was transferred.

Many cardiac patients are in serious condition when they arrive at a CVICU like the one where I work. The acuity level ranges from moderate to high. Patients have often undergone major medical procedures, such as coronary artery bypass, valve replacement, and vascular and thoracic surgery. Regardless of the situation, we focus on quality care for patients and their families.

As a cardiovascular nurse, I realize that the cardiovascular system has an impact on every other system in the human body. For this reason I appreciate the continuing education, update programs and conferences, and advanced training courses that are mandatory. As a cardiovascular nurse, I must also regularly update my advanced cardiac life support (ACLS) certification.

INTRODUCTION

*T*he cardiovascular (CV) system is composed of the heart and the body's blood vessels, or vascular network. The heart pumps blood that is low in oxygen to the lungs, where it is oxygenated. Then it pumps oxygen-rich blood to the entire body. Each day, the heart pumps approximately 7,000 L (1,855 gallons) of blood throughout the body. The heart's work ensures our survival.

Arteries, veins, and capillaries make up the body's blood vessels. Capillaries are the smallest of these vessels. They are the sites of nutrient and gas exchange. Blood flows through blood vessels delivering electrolytes, hormones, nutrients, and oxygen to tissues. At the same time blood returns metabolic waste products to proper organs for removal.

Vital signs—such as blood pressure, pulse, respiratory rate, and temperature—and heart sounds are used to assess the cardiac patient. In addition to normal physiology (body functioning), common disorders of the cardiovascular system are described in this chapter. Radiography, radionuclide imaging, catheterization, electrocardiography, and echocardiograms provide diagnostic evidence of cardiac or vascular pathology.

MEDICAL TERM PARTS

Word Parts

Medical term prefixes, suffixes, and combining forms related to the cardiovascular system are introduced in this section.

Word Part	Meaning
angi-, angio-	vessel, vascular
arteri-, arterio-	artery, arterial
athero-	fatty, pasty materials
atrio-	atrium
brady-	slow
cardi-, cardio-	heart
chord-	cord
eury-	broad, wide
parieto-	wall of the body
phleb-, phlebo-	vein
-pnea	breath, respiration
pulmo-, pulmon-, pulmono-	lungs
sphygm-, sphygmo-	pulse
steth-, stetho-	chest or breast
tachy-	rapid, quick, accelerated
vas-, vasculo-, vaso-	blood vessel
veni-, veno-	veins
ventriculo-	ventricle

Word Grouping Exercises

Using the *Medical Term Parts* table, identify the prefix, suffix, or combining forms for each of the following definitions. The first one has been done as an example.

Definition	Word Part
heart	*cardi-, cardio-*
artery, arterial	
atrium	
blood vessel	
breath, respiration	
broad, wide	
chest or breast	

continued

continued from page 509

Definition	Word Part
cord	
fatty, pasty materials	
lungs	
pulse	
rapid, quick, accelerated	
slow	
vein	
veins, ventricle	
vessel, vascular	
wall of the body	

Word Building Exercises

Word parts introduced in the *Medical Term Parts* section are listed in the following table. For this exercise, first supply the meaning of each word part, then use the word part to build a word you already know. The word you list under *Common or Known Word* does not have to be a medical term; a commonly used word is fine. Be sure, however, that the word correctly reflects the intended meaning. The first one has been done as an example. Check your answers in a dictionary.

Word Part	Meaning	Common or Known Word	Example Medical Term
angi-, angio-	*vessel, vascular*	*angina*	angiogram
arteri-, arterio-			artery
athero-			atherosclerosis
cardi, cardio-			cardiac
phleb-, phlebo-			thrombophlebitis
pulmo-, pulmon-, pulmono-			pulmonary artery
steth-, stetho-			stethoscope
tachy-			tachycardia
vas-, vasculo-, vaso-			vascular

ANATOMY AND PHYSIOLOGY

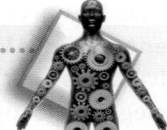

The Heart

The **heart** is a four-chambered, pumping organ located in the thoracic cavity. It receives its own oxygen and nutrition from the coronary circulation (the heart's blood supply). It delivers oxygen and nutrients to all parts of the body by pumping blood through the blood vessels. Most of the blood swooshing through the heart's chambers gets sent to other body regions.

The heart lies within the mediastinum of the thorax. Its general structure is that of a hollow, funnel-shaped muscular pump. The heart is in a tilted position with the inferior **apex** (point) of the left lower chamber resting on the diaphragm. You can find the **apical heartbeat** by listening between the fifth and sixth ribs, the location of the heart's apex. The bulk of the heart lies left of the sternum (**Figure 11-1**).

Your heart is about the size of your own clenched fist. The average heart is approximately 13 cm (5.2 in.) long and 8 cm (3.2 in.) wide. Heart size, however, depends on the individual and his or her usual level of exercise. Because it is a muscle, aerobic exercise can cause the heart to hypertrophy (increase in size), which enables the heart to pump more efficiently. This improved function brings about improved blood circulation.

A fibroserous membrane called the **pericardium** (*peri-* = around; *cardi-* = heart) surrounds and protects the heart. The pericardium has two layers: an inner visceral layer (epicardium) and an outer parietal layer. The **visceral pericardium (epicardium)** adheres to the heart's surface. The parietal layer forms a loose-fitting sac that shields the heart from friction. The thick middle **myocardium** (*my-* = muscle) consists mostly of cardiac muscle tissue. The inner lining is the **endocardium**. This inner layer is continuous with the inner lining of blood vessels (**Figure 11-2**).

Within the heart are four chambers and four valves. The two upper chambers, called **atria** (singular = atrium), receive blood from veins and have thin walls. They are called atria because in earlier times, the atrium was the first room that guests entered in a house. Accordingly, the atrium is the chamber that blood first enters in the heart.

The two lower chambers, called **ventricles**, force blood out of the heart into arteries. The term *ventricle* is derived from Latin and refers to small body cavities, in this case, the two lower heart chambers. The left ventricle has a thicker wall than the right ventricle because its stronger muscle pushes blood throughout the whole body. The right ventricle pumps blood a shorter distance to the lungs.

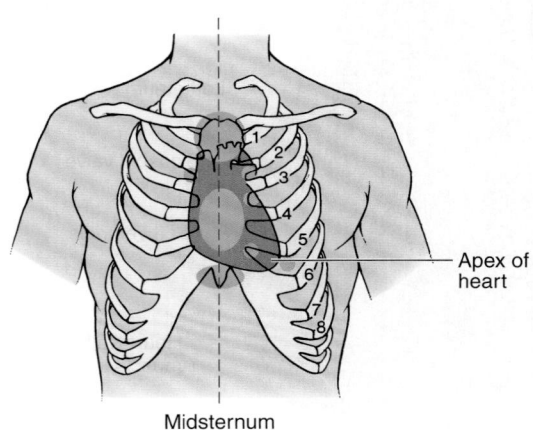

Figure 11-1 The position of the heart.

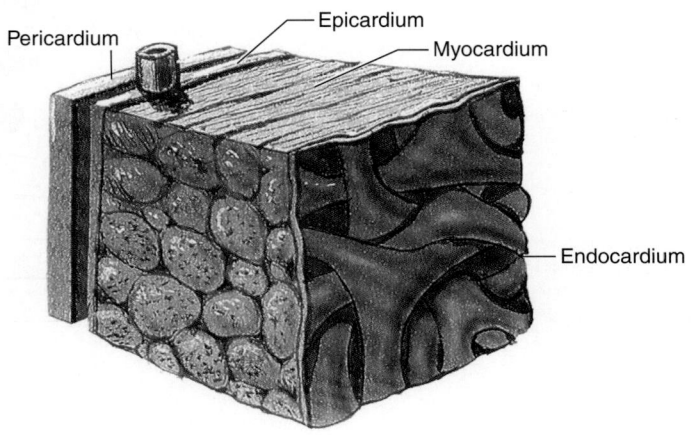

Figure 11-2 The cardiac wall is composed of three layers: epicardium, myocardium, and endocardium.

Valves prevent the backflow of blood during heart contraction or relaxation. The heart has four valves: two **atrioventricular (AV) valves** and two **semilunar (SL) valves** (**Figure 11-3**). The atrioventricular valves are so named because they are located between the atria and the ventricles. There they safeguard the openings between the upper and lower chambers, ensuring that blood flows in one direction only. The semilunar valves are composed of a set of three semilunar cusps and are located between the heart and the aorta and the heart and the pulmonary trunk.

The valves are identified according to the number of flaps, called cusps, they contain. The **tricuspid valve**, or **right atrioventricular (AV) valve**, has three cusps and is located between the right atrium and right ventricle. (To remember this side, think "*try* to be right" for *tri*cuspid.) It prevents backflow of blood from the right ventricle into the right atrium. Likewise, the **bicuspid valve**, or **left atrioventricular (AV) valve**, has two cusps and is found between the left atrium and left ventricle (**Figure 11-3**). The left AV valve is also called the **mitral valve** because it is shaped like a miter, the hat traditionally worn by bishops.

Chordae tendineae are fibrous cords that look like strings. The chordae tendineae attach the papillary muscles to the cusps of the AV valves. Chordae tendineae keep the flaps pointing in the correct direction. **Papillary muscles** are bulges in the heart wall. These muscles "tug on the heartstrings."

The two semilunar valves of the heart are so named because they are shaped like a half moon. The **pulmonary valve** (or pulmonary semilunar valve) is located at the entrance to the pulmonary trunk, the blood vessel that branches into the pulmonary arteries leading to the lungs. The pulmonary valve prevents blood from moving from the pulmonary trunk back into the right ventricle. The **aortic valve** (or aortic semilunar valve) is located at the entrance to the **aorta**, a large artery arising from the left ventricle. The aorta branches into several other arteries. This valve prevents blood from flowing from the aorta back into the left ventricle (**Figure 11-4**).

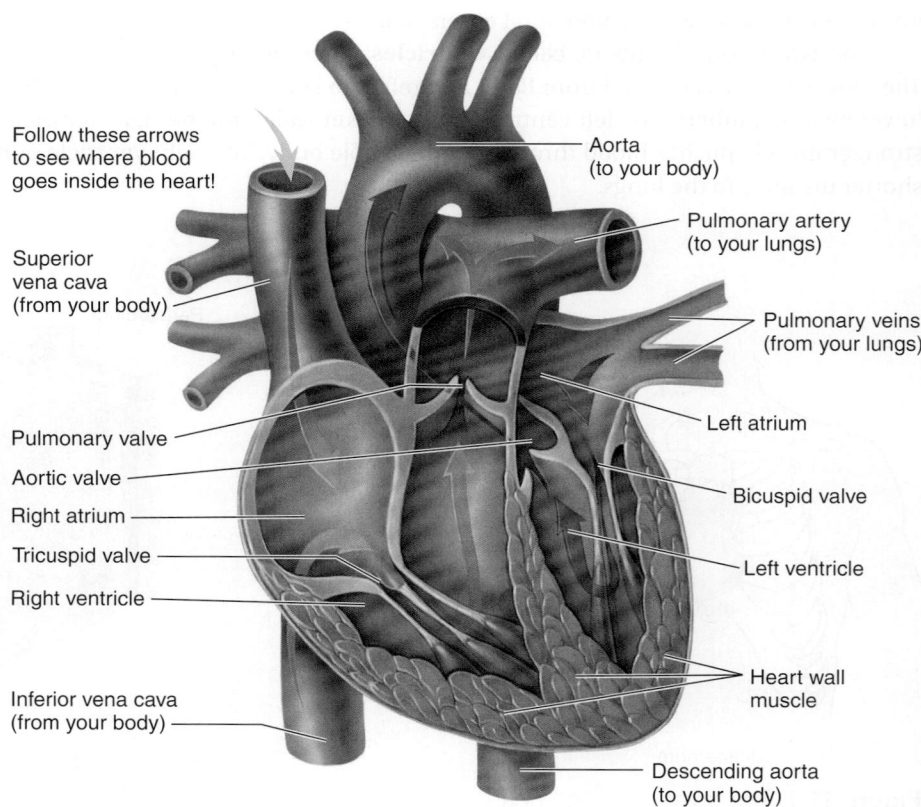

Figure 11-3 The chambers and valves of the heart.

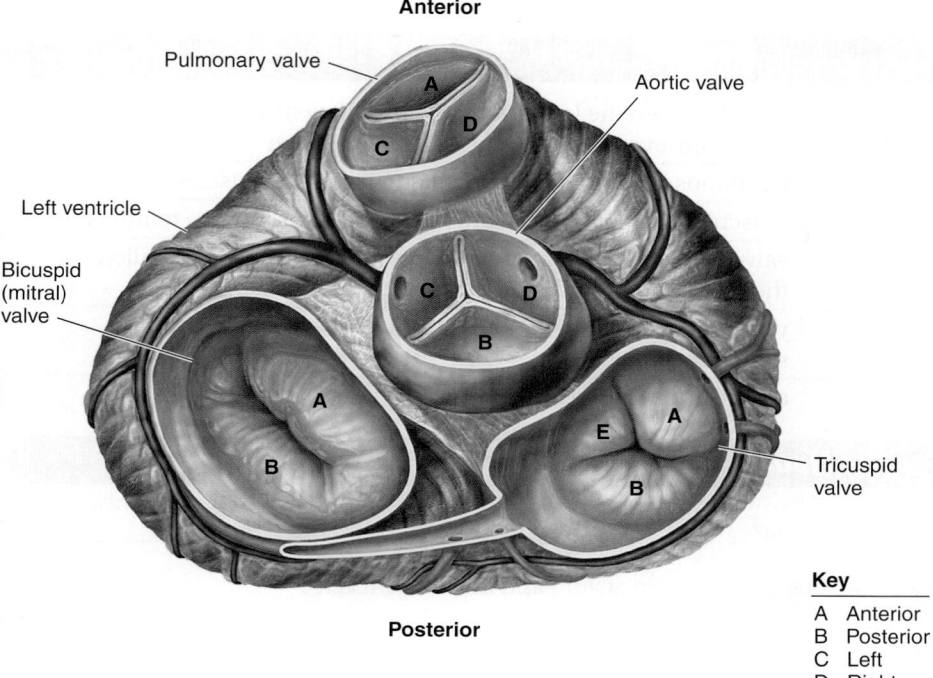

Anterior

Pulmonary valve

Aortic valve

Left ventricle

Bicuspid
(mitral)
valve

Tricuspid
valve

Posterior

Key
A Anterior
B Posterior
C Left
D Right
E Septal

Figure 11-4 The valves of the heart.

KEY TERM	Definition
heart	organ that pumps blood
apex	lowest, left-most heart point
apical (AY-pi-kul) **heartbeat**	heartbeat heard at the apex of the heart
pericardium (perr-i-KAHR-dee-um)	membrane that encircles the heart
visceral pericardium (VIS-ur-ul perr-i-KAHR-dee-um)	membrane directly on the heart; also called the epicardium
epicardium (ep-i-KAHR-dee-um)	membrane directly on the heart; also called the visceral pericardium
myocardium (migh-oh-KAHR-dee-um)	middle layer made of heart muscle
endocardium (en-doh-KAHR-dee-um)	membrane lining the inner heart
atria (AY-tree-uh)	the two upper heart chambers
ventricles (VEN-tri-kulz)	the two lower heart chambers
atrioventricular (ay-tree-oh-ven-TRICK-yoo-lur) **(AV) valves**	valves between the atria and the ventricles; the bicuspid and tricuspid valves
semilunar (sem-ee-LOO-nur) **(SL) valves**	valve between the heart and the aorta and the valve between the heart and the pulmonary trunk
tricuspid (trye-KUS-pid) **valve**	valve between the right atrium and the right ventricle; also called the right atrioventricular valve
right atrioventricular (ay-tree-oh-ven-TRICK-yoo-lur) **(AV) valve**	valve between the right atrium and the right ventricle; also called the tricuspid valve
left atrioventricular (ay-tree-oh-ven-TRICK-yoo-lur) **(AV) valve**	valve between the left atrium and the left ventricle; also called the bicuspid valve or mitral valve
bicuspid (bye-KUS-pid) **valve**	valve between the left atrium and the left ventricle; also called the left atrioventricular valve or mitral valve

continued

continued from page 513

KEY TERM	Definition
mitral (MIGH-trul) **valve**	valve between the left atrium and the left ventricle; also called the left atrioventricular valve or bicuspid valve
chordae tendineae (KOR-dee TEN-di-nee-ee)	tendinous cords in heart attached to papillary muscles
papillary (PAP-i-lerr-ee) **muscles**	muscular projections that are attached to the chordae tendineae
pulmonary (PUL-muh-nerr-ee) **valve**	valve between the heart and the pulmonary trunk; also called the pulmonary semilunar valve
aortic (ay-OR-tick) **valve**	valve between the heart and the aorta; also called the aortic semilunar valve
aorta (ay-OR-tuh)	a large artery in the body that arises from the left ventricle

KEY TERM PRACTICE: *The Heart*

1. What is the medical term that means heart muscle? _____

2. What are the terms for the heart valve located between the left atrium and the left ventricle?

 a. _____

 b. _____

 c. _____

3. Give the term for the lowest, left-most point of the heart. _____

4. Give the alternate term for the visceral pericardium. _____

5. Name the blood vessel arising from the left ventricle. _____

Blood Vessels

The heart and the network of blood vessels make up the cardiovascular system, or CV system. The word parts *cardi-* and *cardio-* mean "heart." They are derived from the Latin word for heart, *cardium,* which is based on the Greek term *kardia.* Note the *c* and *k* variation—some terms pertaining to the CV system use the letters interchangeably; for example, both ECG and EKG are acceptable abbreviations for the word *electrocardiogram.* There is a minor difference between the cardiovascular system and the circulatory system. The CV system includes the heart and affiliated blood vessels, but the circulatory system includes the entire cardiovascular system plus the lymphatic vessels, which are outside the CV system (see Chapter 13).

The cardiovascular system includes the body's blood vessels (derived from the word part *vas-,* meaning "vessel"). The body has a closed, continuous circuit of blood vessels. **Arteries** carry blood away from the heart (**Figure 11-5A**). As a tip, associate the *a* in *a*rtery with the *a* in *a*way. **Veins** return blood to the heart. Unlike arteries, veins have valves to prevent backflow of blood (**Figure 11-5B**). Veins are less elastic and have less smooth muscle tissue than arteries. Arteries and veins both have three layers—tunica intima, tunica media, and tunica externa— and are lined with endothelium. At any one time, more than 60% of the body's blood is located in our network of veins.

Capillaries are tiny blood vessels that provide a bridge between the smallest branches of arteries, called **arterioles**, and the smallest branches of veins, called **venules**. The capillary network allows microscopic molecules (gases, nutrients, and wastes) to be exchanged quickly between blood and tissue fluid nearly everywhere throughout the body (**Figure 11-6**). If you strung together all of your blood vessels, they would circle the Earth 2.5 times. **Figures 11-7** and **11-8** show the body's major arteries and veins, respectively, and **Tables 11-1** and **11-2** give their pronunciations.

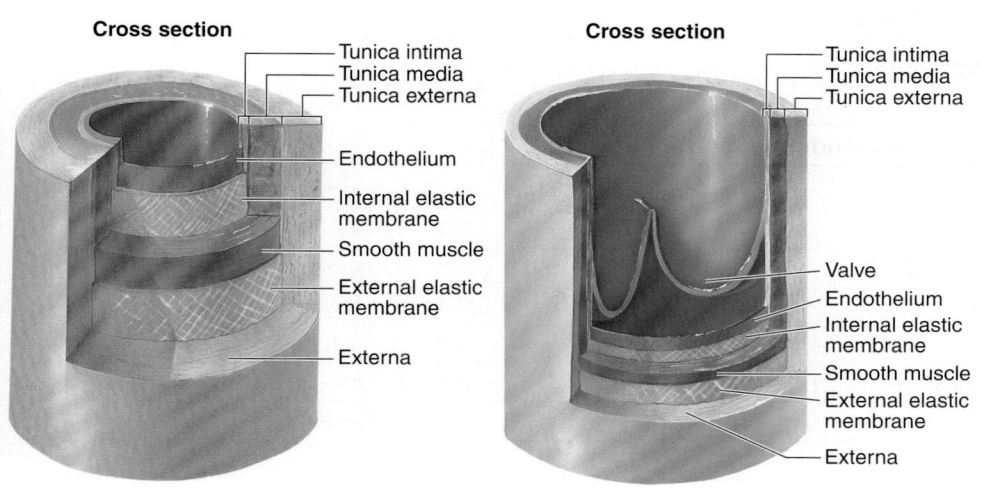

Figure 11-5 (A) The artery wall in cross section. **(B)** The vein wall and valve in cross section.

Cross section
- Tunica intima
- Tunica media
- Tunica externa
- Endothelium
- Internal elastic membrane
- Smooth muscle
- External elastic membrane
- Externa

Cross section
- Tunica intima
- Tunica media
- Tunica externa
- Valve
- Endothelium
- Internal elastic membrane
- Smooth muscle
- External elastic membrane
- Externa

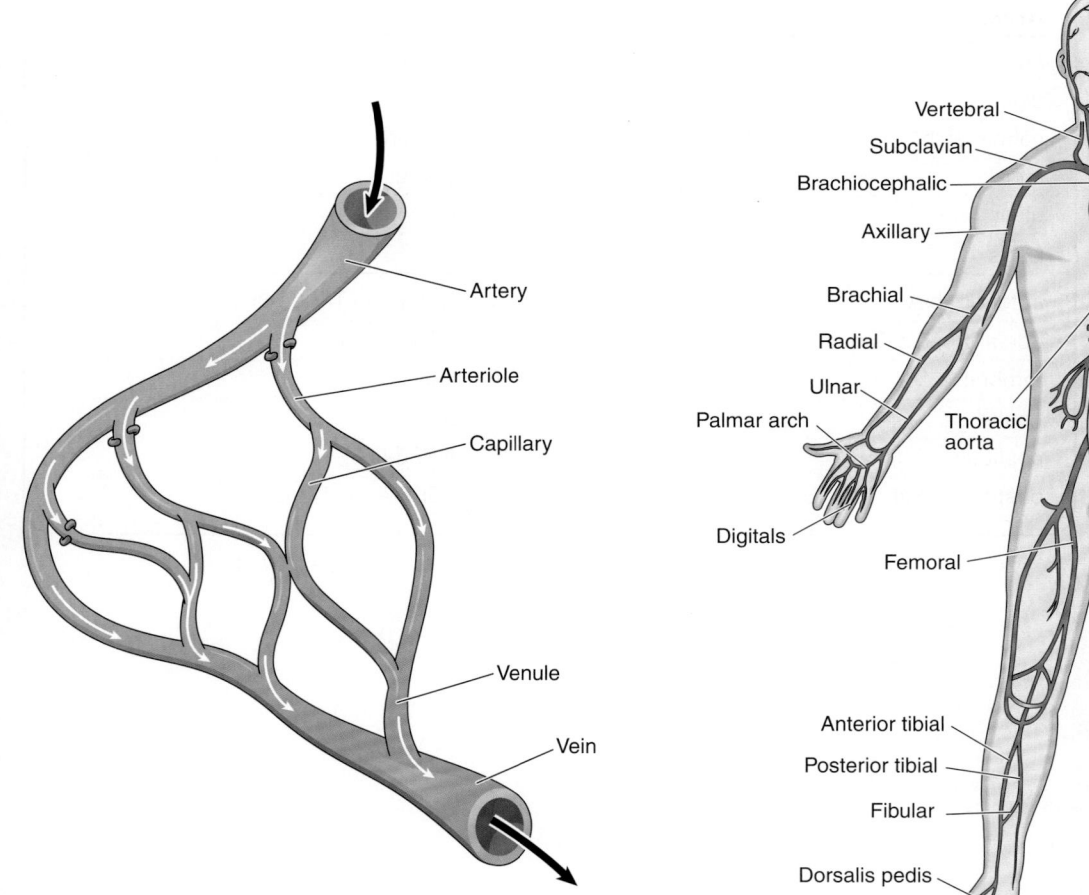

- Artery
- Arteriole
- Capillary
- Venule
- Vein

Figure 11-6 The capillary network allows for the exchange of molecules between the blood and the surrounding tissue fluid.

- Vertebral
- Subclavian
- Brachiocephalic
- Axillary
- Brachial
- Radial
- Ulnar
- Palmar arch
- Digitals
- Thoracic aorta
- Femoral
- Anterior tibial
- Posterior tibial
- Fibular
- Dorsalis pedis
- Common carotid
- Aortic arch
- Intercostals
- Renal
- Common iliac
- Internal iliac
- External iliac
- Popliteal

Figure 11-7 Common arteries.

T A B L E **11-1**

COMMON SYSTEMIC ARTERIES

Common Arteries	Pronunciation
Cervical Region	
common carotid	KOM-mun ka-ROT-id
vertebral	VUR-te-brul
Thoracic and Abdominopelvic Regions	
aortic arch	ay-OR-tick arch
axillary	ACK-si-lerr-ee
brachiocephalic	bray-kee-oh-se-FAL-ick
common iliac	KOM-mun IL-ee-ack
external iliac	ECKS-tur-nul IL-ee-ack
intercostals	in-tur-KOS-tuls
internal iliac	IN-tur-nul IL-ee-ack
renal	REE-nul
subclavian	sub-KLAY-vee-un
thoracic aorta	thor-AS-ick ay-OR-tuh
Arms	
brachial	BRAY-kee-ul
digitals	DIJ-ih-tuls
palmar arch	PAL-mur arch
radial	RAY-dee-ul
ulnar	UL-nur
Legs	
anterior tibial	an-TEER-ee-or TIB-ee-ul
dorsalis pedis (top of foot)	dor-SAY-lis PE-dis
femoral	FEM-uh-rul
fibular	FIB-yoo-lur
popliteal	pop-li-TEE-ul
posterior tibial	pos-TEER-ee-or TIB-ee-ul

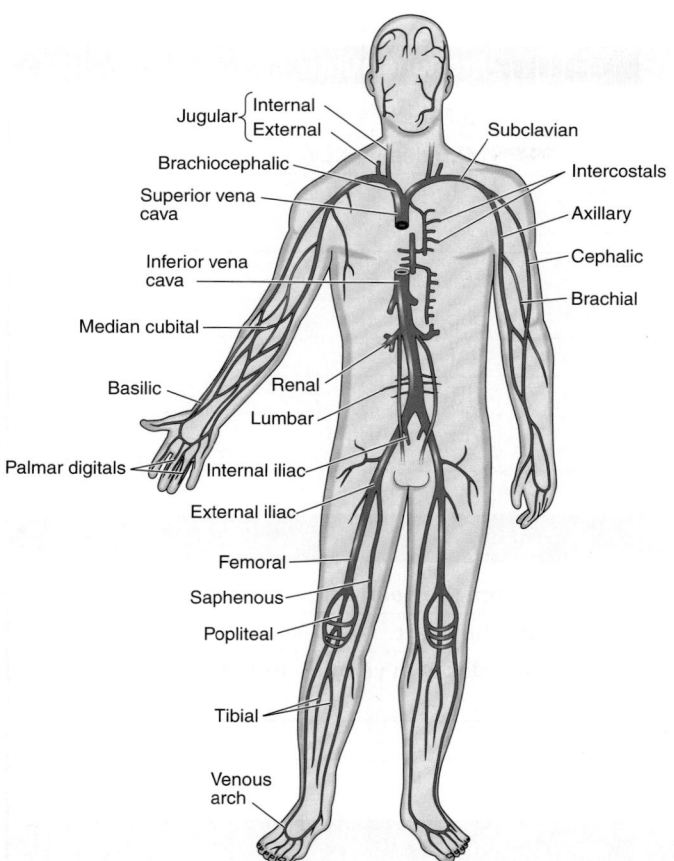

Jugular {Internal / External}
Subclavian
Brachiocephalic
Intercostals
Superior vena cava
Axillary
Inferior vena cava
Cephalic
Brachial
Median cubital
Basilic
Renal
Lumbar
Palmar digitals
Internal iliac
External iliac
Femoral
Saphenous
Popliteal
Tibial
Venous arch

Figure 11-8 Common veins.

T A B L E 11-2	COMMON SYSTEMIC VEINS
Common Veins	**Pronunciation**
Cervical Region	
external jugular	ECKS-tur-nul JUG-yoo-lur
internal jugular	IN-tur-nul JUG-yoo-lur
Thoracic and Abdominopelvic Regions	
axillary	ACK-si-lerr-ee
brachiocephalic	bray-kee-oh-se-FAL-ick
external iliac	ECKS-tur-nul IL-ee-ack
inferior vena cava	VEE-nuh KAY-vuh
intercostals	in-tur-KOS-tulz
internal iliac	IN-tur-nul IL-ee-ack
lumbar	LUM-bahr
renal	REE-nul
subclavian	sub-KLAY-vee-un
superior vena cava	VEE-nuh KAY-vuh
Arms	
basilic	ba-SIL-ick
brachial	BRAY-kee-ul

continued

continued from page 517

Common Veins	Pronunciation
cephalic	se-FAL-ick
median cubital	MEE-dee-un KEW-bi-tul
palmar digitas	PAL-mur DIJ-i-tuls
Legs	
femoral	FEM-uh-rul
popliteal	pop-li-TEE-ul
saphenous	SAF-e-nus
tibial	TIB-ee-ul
venous arch (top of foot)	VEE-nus ARCH

KEY TERM	Definition
arteries (AHR-tur-eez)	blood vessels that carry blood away from the heart
veins	blood vessels that carry blood toward the heart
capillaries (KAP-i-lair-eez)	small blood vessels that connect arterioles with venules and the sites of gas, nutrient, and waste exchange
arterioles (ahr-TEER-ee-ohlz)	smallest branches of arteries
venules (VEN-yoolz)	smallest branches of veins

KEY TERM PRACTICE: *Blood Vessels*

1. What is the plural form for each of the following terms?

a. artery = _____

b. vein = _____

c. capillary = _____

2. A _____ carries blood toward the heart; an _____ carries blood away from the heart.

3. The smallest arteries are termed _____.

4. The smallest veins are termed _____.

Cardiac Blood Flow

The heart lies between the lungs where it is near the sites of gas exchange in the lungs. Blood traveling throughout the blood vessels in the body releases its oxygen supply along the route. An average blood cell travels about 9 miles per day throughout the body's blood vessels!

Circulatory routes or circuits are pathways through which blood flows to and from the heart and various organs. The **systemic circuit** takes oxygenated blood from the left ventricle to the aorta, which then divides into branches that distribute the blood to the rest of the body (**Figure 11-9**). This blood returns to the heart through large veins called the **superior vena cava** and **inferior vena cava** (plural = venae cavae). This low-oxygen, high–carbon dioxide blood then enters the right atrium of the heart. Blood flows through this systemic circuit as follows:

heart → aorta → arteries → arterioles → capillaries →
venules → veins → superior and inferior venae cavae → heart

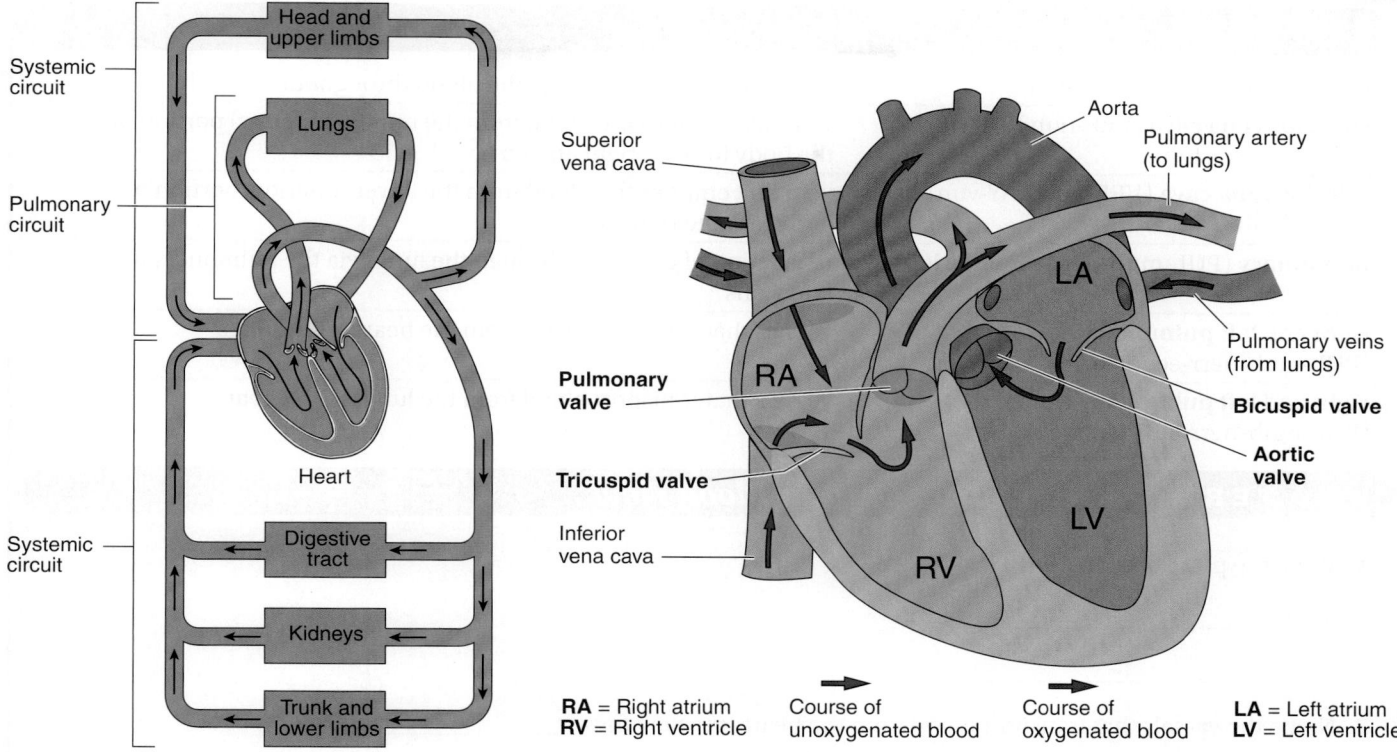

Figure 11-9 The systemic and pulmonary circuits.

Figure 11-10 The unidirectional passage of blood through the heart is maintained by heart valves.

In the **pulmonary circuit**, the heart pumps deoxygenated blood from its right ventricle to the lungs, where the blood picks up oxygen and then is returned to the left atrium of the heart (**Figure 11-9**). The blood is first pumped into the **right** and **left pulmonary arteries**, which transport blood to the right and left lungs. In the lungs, the supply of oxygen is replenished, and the accumulated carbon dioxide is exhaled. The newly oxygenated blood then returns to the left atrium via the **right** and **left pulmonary veins**.

When you think about the heart muscle, remember that the left myocardium is thicker because it pumps oxygenated blood to all parts of the body through the systemic circulation. Greater muscle mass is needed for this work. The myocardium on the right side is thinner because the right side of the heart pumps deoxygenated blood just a short distance to the lungs through the pulmonary circulation. Most veins carry deoxygenated blood, and most arteries transport oxygenated blood in the body. However, notice that the pulmonary circulation is different: The pulmonary veins carry oxygenated blood, and the pulmonary arteries carry deoxygenated blood. If you consider the pathway of blood to and from the heart, this makes sense because blood enters the lungs through the pulmonary arteries to become oxygen rich and then exits through the pulmonary veins. Keep in mind that arteries carry blood away from the heart, while veins carry blood to the heart. Therefore, the pulmonary arteries leave the heart, and the pulmonary veins enter the heart.

The action of the valves maintains the one-way passage of blood through the heart (**Figure 11-10**). The path is as follows:

inferior vena cava and superior vena cava → right atrium → tricuspid valve
→ right ventricle → pulmonary valve → right and left pulmonary arteries
→ right and left lungs → right and left pulmonary veins → left atrium → bicuspid valve
→ left ventricle → aortic valve → aorta → systemic circulation → back to
superior vena cava and inferior vena cava

KEY TERM	Definition
systemic (sis-TEM-ick) **circuit**	general circulatory route of the blood throughout the body
superior vena cava (VEE-nuh KAY-vuh)	vein that empties the blood from the upper (superior) portion of the body into the right atrium
inferior vena cava (VEE-nuh KAY-vuh)	vein that empties the blood from the lower (inferior) portion of the body into the right atrium
pulmonary (PUL-muh-nerr-ee) **circuit**	circulation of the blood through the lungs via the pulmonary arteries and veins
right and **left pulmonary** (PUL-muh-nerr-ee) **arteries**	vessels that transport blood from the heart to the lungs
right and **left pulmonary** (PUL-muh-nerr-ee) **veins**	vessels that transport blood from the lungs to the heart

KEY TERM PRACTICE: *Cardiac Blood Flow*

1. Write the plural forms of each given term.

   a. vena = _____

   b. cava = _____

2. Name the vessels that transport blood from the heart *into* the lungs. _____

3. Name the vessels that transport blood *out* of the lungs to the heart. _____

4. The _____ circuit transports blood throughout the body, while the _____ circuit transports blood throughout the lungs.

Coronary Circulation

The **coronary circulation** involves those arteries and veins that supply and drain the heart itself with blood (**Figure 11-11A**). The word *corona* means "crown," and the coronary arteries encircle the heart exterior like a crown, supplying the myocardium with blood for nourishment. The **right coronary artery** and **left coronary artery**, which are the first two branches off the aorta, supply the heart. The **circumflex artery** supplies blood to the walls of the left atrium and left ventricle. Then the deoxygenated blood is returned to the right atrium through the great cardiac vein and coronary sinus (**Figure 11-11B**). If blood flow to the heart is interrupted, new circulatory routes can develop over time. This formation of new blood vessels is termed **angiogenesis**.

KEY TERM	Definition
coronary (KOR-uh-nerr-ee) **circulation**	blood supply to the heart tissue
right coronary (KOR-uh-nerr-ee) **artery**	artery supplying blood to the heart tissue
left coronary (KOR-uh-nerr-ee) **artery**	artery supplying blood to the heart tissue
circumflex (SUR-kum-flecks) **artery**	vessel that supplies blood to the left atrium and left ventricle
angiogenesis (an-jee-oh-JEN-e-sis)	formation of new blood vessels

continued

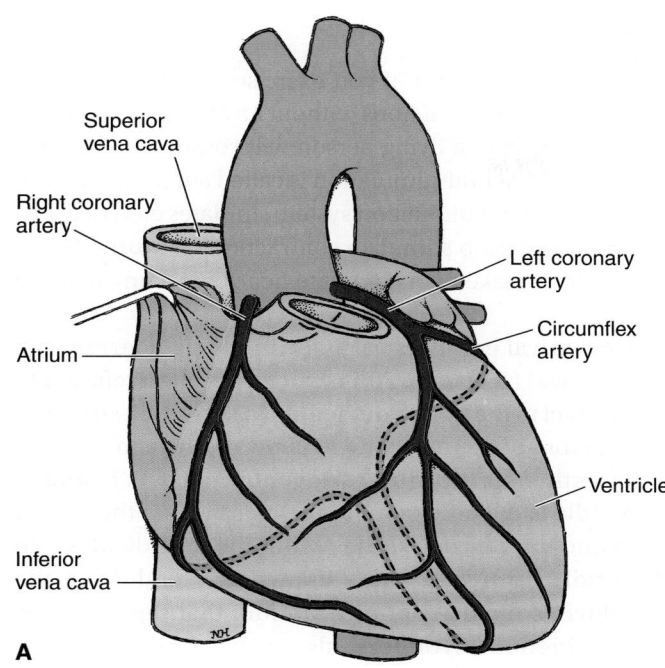

Superior
vena cava

Right coronary
artery

Left coronary
artery

Circumflex
artery

Atrium

Ventricle

Inferior
vena cava

A

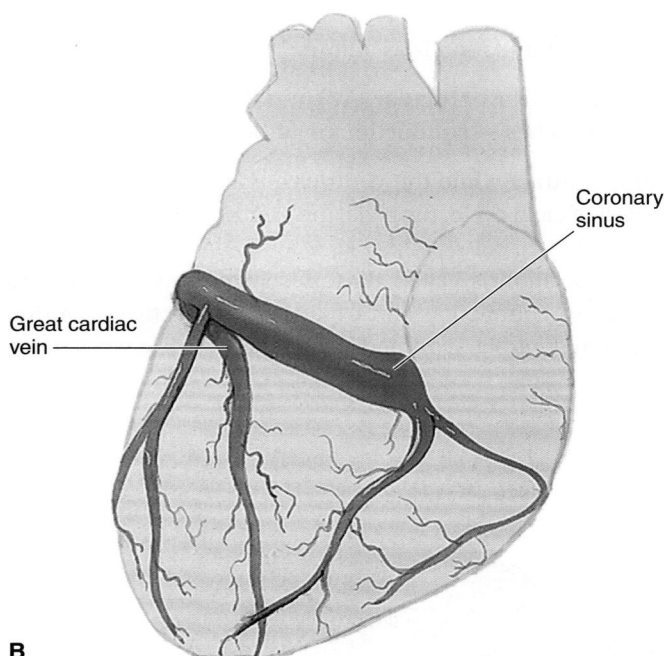

Coronary
sinus

Great cardiac
vein

B

Figure 11-11 (A) The right and left coronary arteries and circumflex artery supply blood to the heart muscle; anterior view. **(B)** The cardiac veins and coronary sinus return blood to the heart; posterior view.

continued from page 520

KEY TERM PRACTICE: *Coronary Circulation*

1. Heart tissue is supplied with oxygen-rich blood via the _____ circulation.

2. The formation of new blood vessels is termed _____.

3. Name three important arteries making up the coronary circulation that supply the heart muscle with nourishing blood. _____

Cardiac Conducting System

The average heart beats 36 million times per year—more if you exercise. The heart has the ability to generate electrical impulses to stimulate contractions without any input from nerves or hormones. For this reason, a heart removed from a living person will continue to beat for nearly 2 minutes. This ability to contract without neural stimulation is called automaticity. The **cardiac conducting system** (also called the cardiac conduction system) initiates electrical impulses and conducts them through the entire heart to stimulate contractions (**Figure 11-12**). The resulting series of myocardial contractions make up a complete heartbeat, known as the **cardiac cycle**.

In the cardiac conducting system, electrical impulses originate in the right atrium at a mass of conduction tissue called the **sinoatrial (SA) node**. This structure is often referred to as the heart's pacemaker. Impulses then travel to the **atrioventricular (AV) node**, a structure in the right atrium. There they are delayed for about 0.1 second to allow the atria to contract before the ventricles contract. The impulses then spread to the **atrioventricular (AV) bundle**, also called the bundle of His. The AV bundle is the only point in the heart where there is an electrical connection between the atria and the ventricles. The AV bundle then divides into two branches, called **right** and **left bundle branches**. These branches extend down the sides of the interventricular septum, which is the mass of myocardium that separates the ventricles. The branches end in the **conduction myofibers**, also called **Purkinje fibers** (named after a Czech physiologist), which are heart cells that stimulate the heart ventricles to contract.

In summary, the pathway for electrical stimulation is as follows:

SA node → AV node → atrioventricular (AV) bundle →
right and left bundle branches → conduction myofibers

During the cardiac cycle, the atria contract while the ventricles relax; then as the ventricles contract, the atria relax. At the end of each cycle, the atria and ventricles both relax for a moment, and then a new cycle begins.

Contraction is called **systole**, and relaxation is called **diastole**. *Systole* and *diastole* are derived from the Greek language and mean contraction and expansion, respectively. During systole, the ventricle walls come together to contract. During diastole, the ventricle walls move apart and relax.

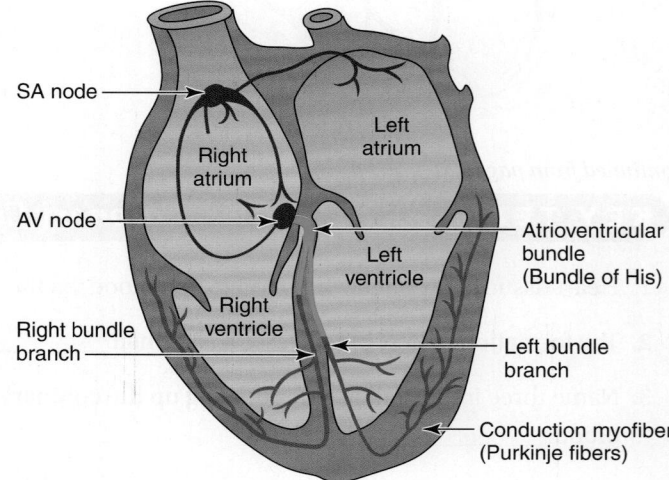

Figure 11-12 The heart initiates electrical impulses and conducts them through the heart walls to stimulate contraction.

KEY TERM	Definition
cardiac (KAHR-dee-ack) **conducting system**	electrical impulses that guide the heart to contract; also called the cardiac conduction system
cardiac cycle (KAHR-dee-ack SIGH-kul)	a complete round of heart contraction and relaxation; a complete heartbeat
sinoatrial (sigh-noh-AY-tree-ul) **(SA) node**	conduction tissue in the right atrium, where the heart's electrical impulses originate
atrioventricular (ay-tree-oh-ven-TRICK-yoo-lur) **(AV) node**	conduction tissue that delays the heart's electrical impulses slightly
atrioventricular (ay-tree-oh-ven-TRICK-yoo-lur) **(AV) bundle**	arises from the atrioventricular node and transmits impulses to the ventricle muscle fibers; also called bundle of His
right and **left bundle branches**	conduction fibers that originate at the atrioventricular bundle and separate along the interventricular septum
conduction myofibers (migh-oh-FIGH-burz)	heart cells that stimulate heart ventricles to contract; also called Purkinje fibers
Purkinje (PUR-kin-jee) **fibers**	heart cells that stimulate heart ventricles to contract; also called conduction myofibers
systole (SIS-toh-lee)	contraction of the heart
diastole (dye-AS-toh-lee)	relaxation of the heart

KEY TERM PRACTICE: *Cardiac Conducting System*

1. What is the medical term for each given eponym?

   a. bundle of His _____

   b. Purkinje fibers _____

2. A complete round of heart contraction and heart relaxation is termed _____.

3. The medical term for contraction is _____.

4. Relaxation of the heart is termed _____.

5. Trace the pathway of electrical stimulation in the heart. _____

Blood Pressure and Other Vital Signs

Blood pressure (BP) is the force that blood exerts against the arterial walls. The device used to measure blood pressure is a **sphygmomanometer**. This instrument has an inflatable cuff, bulb, and gauge that measure pressure in millimeters of mercury, abbreviated mmHg. The word part *sphygmo-* means "pulse"; so, this "blood pressure cuff" is an instrument that measures pulsating blood. The measurement indicates the pressure on the arterial wall at the highest and lowest pressures: when the ventricle undergoes systole (contraction) and diastole (relaxation). It is written as a fraction with the systolic pressure over the diastolic pressure, for example, 120/80 mmHg. **Systolic blood pressure** (the top number) represents contraction pressure, and **diastolic blood pressure** (the bottom number) represents relaxation or recoil pressure. Associate the *d* in *d*own with the *d* in *d*iastolic to remember that diastolic pressure is the number on bottom. A typical blood pressure is 120/80 mmHg. Optimal blood pressure to reduce the risk of heart disease is lower than 120/80 mmHg.

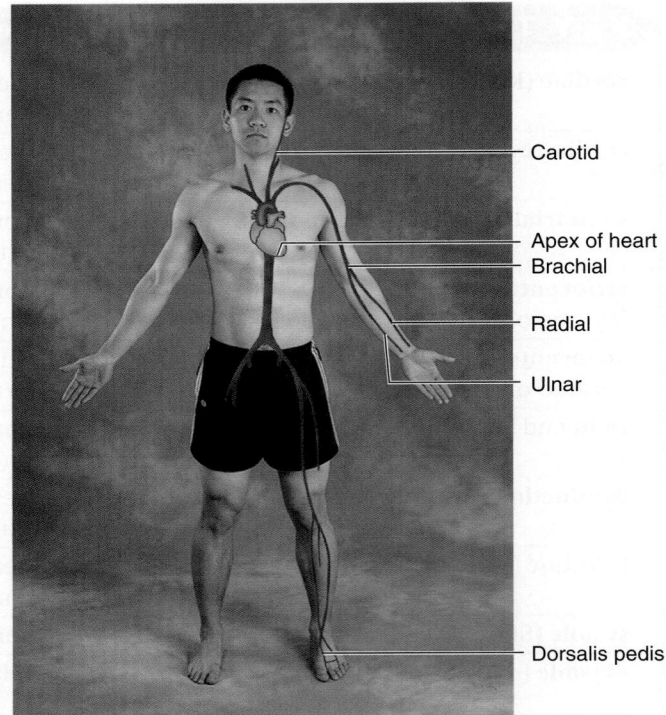

Carotid

Apex of heart
Brachial

Radial

Ulnar

Dorsalis pedis

Figure 11-13 Pulse points. Shown here are anatomical locations where an artery crosses bone or firm tissue and can be palpated for a pulse.

The expansion of an artery with each heartbeat is termed **pulse**. It can be detected by palpating the superficial arteries. Commonly used pulse points are the carotid artery in the neck, the brachial artery in the arm, the radial artery and ulnar artery in the wrist, and the dorsalis pedis artery in the foot (**Figure 11-13**).

Many factors affect blood pressure. They include chemicals, temperature, emotions, age, gender, and signals from the nervous system. Pulse and blood pressure, along with temperature and breathing rate, are **vital signs** directly related to the cardiovascular system. *Vital* refers to life, and these are clinical measurements of key body functions.

Listening to sounds made by internal organs, especially the heart and lungs, is called auscultation. The instrument used to listen is a **stethoscope**. The word comes from the Greek *stethos* meaning "chest" and *skopein* meaning "to examine."

Each cardiac cycle generates four sounds, but in a normal, healthy adult, only the first two are regularly heard. The first typical sound, *lubb,* is produced by the contraction (systole) of ventricles. The second softer sound, *dupp,* is marked by the beginning of ventricular relaxation (diastole). Both sounds represent the closing of heart valves.

KEY TERM	Definition
blood pressure (BP)	pressure exerted by the circulating blood on the arterial walls
sphygmomanometer (sfig-moh-muh-NOM-e-tur)	instrument used to measure blood pressure
systolic (sis-TOL-ick) **blood pressure**	arterial blood pressure during ventricular contraction
diastolic (dye-us-TOL-ick) **blood pressure**	arterial blood pressure during ventricular relaxation
pulse	palpable throbbing of an artery with each heartbeat
vital signs	objective measurements of key body functions, such as temperature, breathing rate, pulse, and blood pressure
stethoscope (STETH-uh-skope)	instrument used to hear sounds within the body

continued

continued from page 524

KEY TERM PRACTICE: *Blood Pressure and Other Vital Signs*

1. What is the medical term for the instrument that measures blood pressure using a pressure cuff? _____

2. The throbbing of an artery that can be felt is known as your _____.

3. The medical instrument placed on the chest and used to listen to the heart is called a _____.

4. The pressure applied to the arterial walls by circulating blood is the _____.

5. The opposite of systolic blood pressure, or ventricular contraction, is _____, or ventricular relaxation.

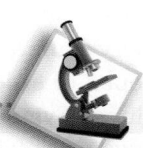

THE CLINICAL DIMENSION

Pathology of the cardiovascular system falls into several broad categories. Many diseases are partly due to an individual's genes or are the result of lifestyle factors. Viral and bacterial infections are implicated in several CV disorders. Congenital diseases are those that are present at birth. Fortunately, a number of treatments are available for the numerous pathological conditions.

Congenital Heart Defects

Congenital heart defects are conditions present at birth. Congenital vascular disorders affect the blood vessels but are not as common as heart defects.

aortic coarctation
Congenital narrowing of the aorta is termed **aortic coarctation** (**Figure 11-14**). It results in upper extremity hypertension (high blood pressure), excessive left ventricular workload, and diminished blood supply to the abdominal organs and lower extremities.

The newborn will present with symptoms of congestive heart failure (described later in this chapter) and hypotension (low blood

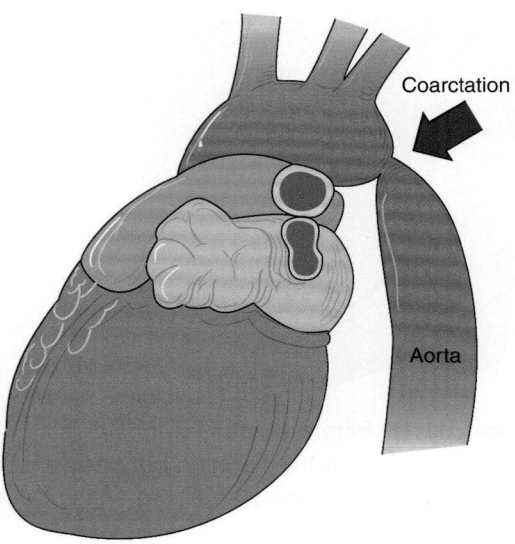

Figure 11-14 Coarctation of the aorta showing the deformed descending aorta.

pressure). Older children exhibit upper extremity hypertension. Aortic coarctation is diagnosed by chest x-ray, echocardiogram, and magnetic resonance imaging (MRI) if the previous two are inconclusive.

An **echocardiogram** is a pictorial representation of the heart using ultrasound. Infants younger than 1 year are treated by **aortoplasty** (surgical repair of the aorta).

atrial septal defect

Atrial septal defect is an opening in the septum between the atria, causing blood to shunt from the left atrium to the right atrium (**Figure 11-15**). (The pressure in the left atrium is slightly greater than pressure in the right, so blood flows from high to low.) The right side of the heart becomes overloaded and hypertrophies in response to the greater blood volume.

patent ductus arteriosus (PDA)

In the condition **patent ductus arteriosus (PDA)**, the ductus arteriosus (an opening between the aorta and the pulmonary artery in the fetus) persists after birth (**Figure 11-16**). Patent means open or exposed. Thus, oxygenated blood is pushed back to the lungs. Symptoms include thrill on palpation and signs of congestive heart failure. A **thrill** is a palpable vibration caused by turbulent blood flow. The alternate term for thrill is **fremitus**. These vibrations feel like the throat of a purring cat. If the PDA is small, the individual may be asymptomatic (without symptoms). Chest x-ray, abnormal electrocardiogram, and echocardiogram are used to make the diagnosis.

The **electrocardiogram (ECG, EKG)** is an electrical recording of the heart's electrical activity, traced as a graph. It detects and records electrical activity during contraction. (As noted earlier in this chapter, sometimes electrocardiogram is abbreviated as EKG, which stems from the Greek word *kardia* for heart.) The letters P, QRS, and T, are used to represent parts of the record of

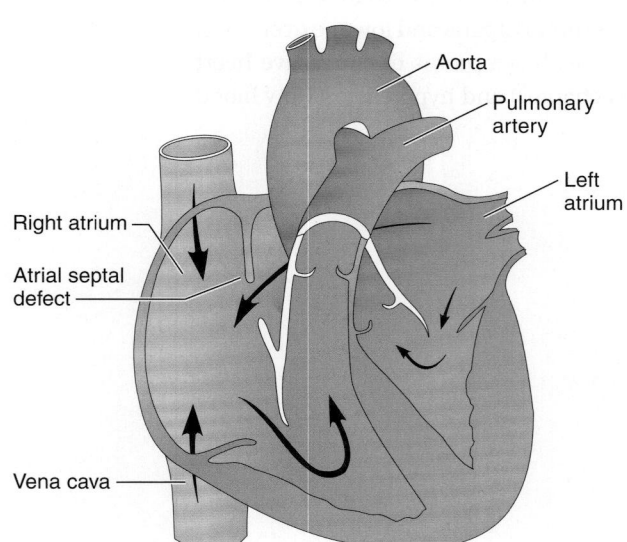

Figure 11-15 An atrial septal defect is an opening in the septum between the atria, causing blood to shunt from the left atrium to the right atrium.

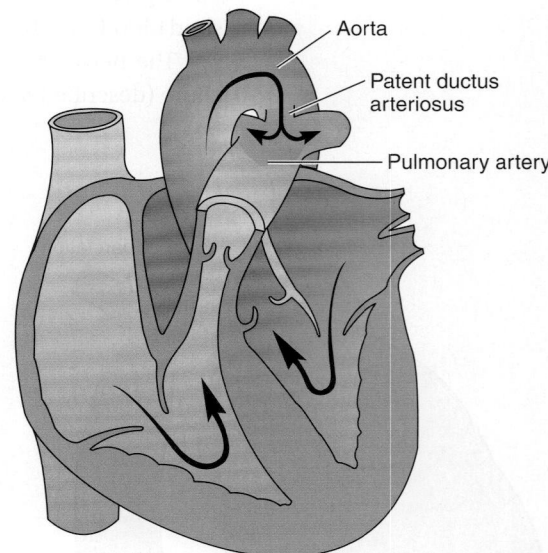

Figure 11-16 Patent ductus arteriosus is a condition in which the opening between the aorta and the pulmonary artery persists after birth.

heart activity. Graphical representation resembles peaks, valleys, dips, and humps (**Figure 11-17**). The **P wave** represents the electrical impulse that stimulates atrial contraction. The **QRS complex** demonstrates the electrical impulse during ventricular contraction. Atrial relaxation takes place at the same time as ventricular contraction, but it cannot be seen on the ECG because the QRS complex is a bigger event that masks it. The **T wave** shows the electrical activity during ventricular relaxation.

tetralogy of Fallot

As its name suggests, the congenital condition called **tetralogy of Fallot** (*tetra-* = four) is a complex of four heart defects (**Figure 11-18**). These are pulmonary stenosis (narrowing of the pulmonary artery), an opening in the interventricular septum

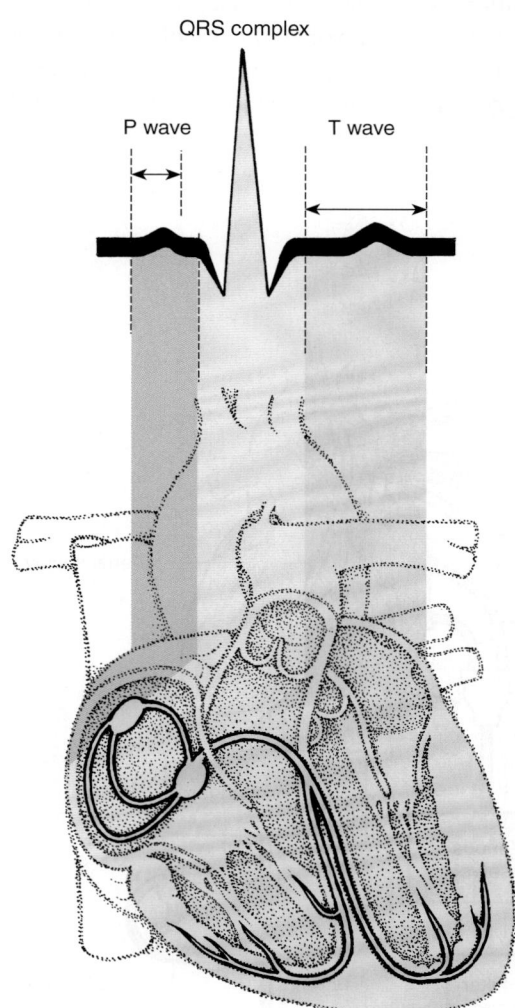

Figure 11-17 Correlation of the ECG and the contractions of the heart. Impulse spreads across atria, triggering atrial contractions, known as the P wave and shown in green. The ventricles then contract, indicated by the QRS complex in yellow. The T wave, in pink, shows ventricular relaxation.

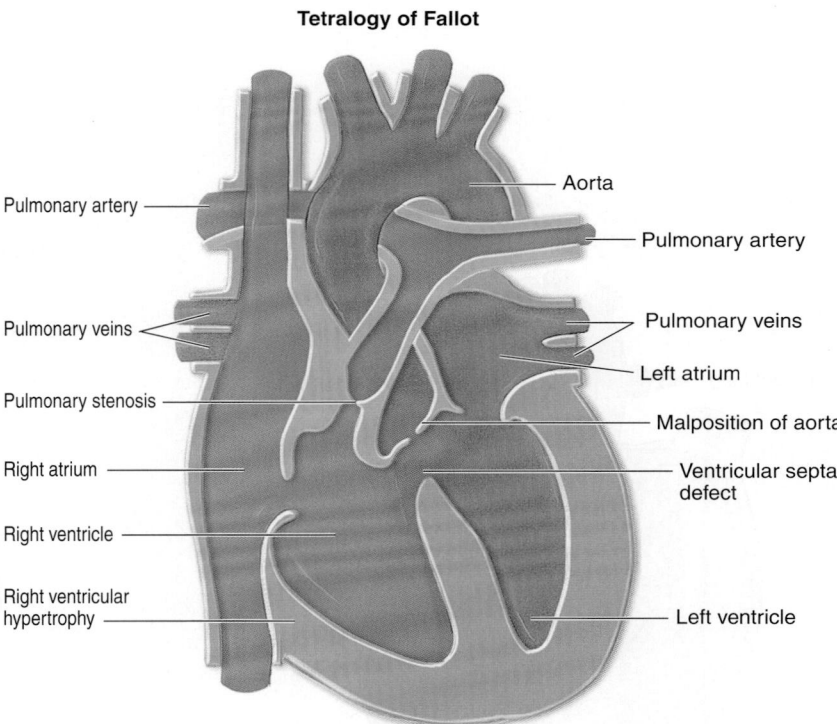

Figure 11-18 Tetralogy of Fallot consists of four congenital heart defects: ventricular septal defect, pulmonary stenosis, malposition of aorta, and right ventricular hypertrophy.

(ventricular septal defect), abnormal position of the aorta over both ventricles (malposition of aorta), and right ventricular hypertrophy. Signs and symptoms are **dyspnea** (difficulty breathing or shortness of breath), cyanosis (bluish discoloration due to lack of oxygen), and restlessness. Chest x-rays reveal the abnormality, and an ECG indicates right ventricular hypertrophy. Treatment involves a patch closure of the septal defect and a resection (removal) at the stenosis.

ventricular septal defect   A **ventricular septal defect** occurs when there is an opening between the two ventricles that allows blood to shuttle back and forth (**Figure 11-19**). If the hole does not close, there is risk of right heart failure or left heart failure. A chest x-ray or ECG is used for diagnosis. Treatment includes a patch closure using synthetic material, and cardiopulmonary bypass is necessary during this procedure. Cardiopulmonary bypass involves the use of a **heart–lung machine**. During some types of surgery, this device serves as a pump and blood oxygenator, replacing the jobs of the heart and lungs (**Figure 11-20**).

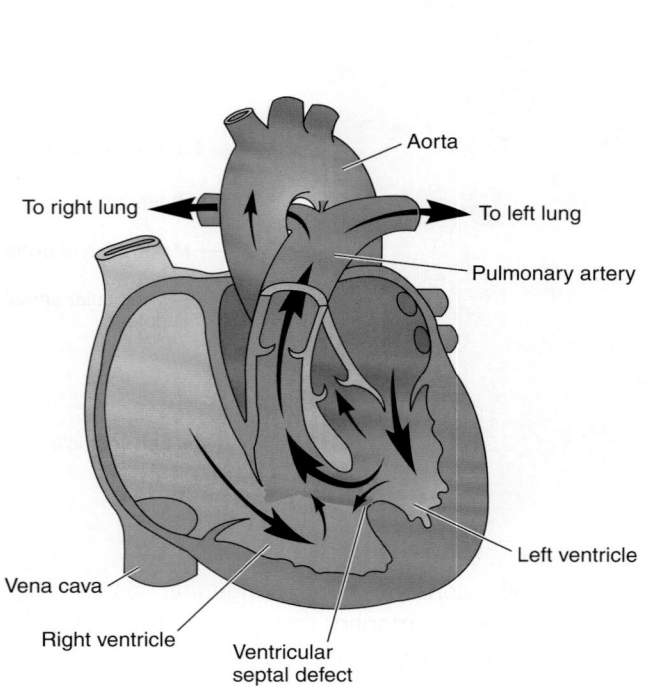

Figure 11-19 Ventricular septal defect. Oxygenated blood is allowed to travel from the left ventricle to the right ventricle and into the pulmonary trunk.

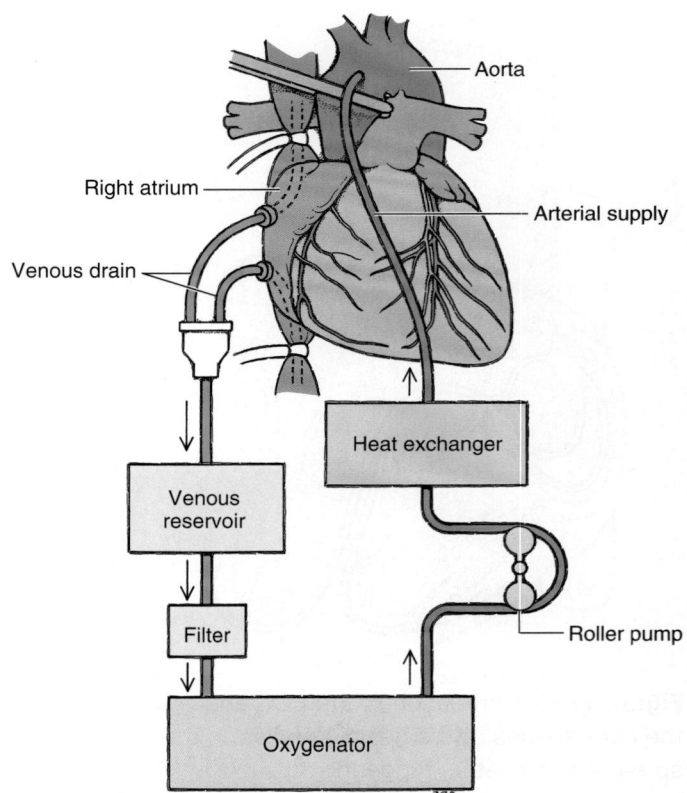

Figure 11-20 A heart–lung machine uses a pump that serves both as the heart and as the lungs to provide circulation outside the body during cardiac surgery.

KEY TERM	Definition
aortic coarctation (AY-or-tick koh-ark-TAY-shun)	congenital narrowing of the aorta
echocardiogram (eck-oh-KAHR-dee-oh-gram)	image of the heart produced by ultrasound
aortoplasty (ay-or-toh-PLAS-tee)	surgical repair of the aorta
atrial septal (AY-tree-ul SEP-tul) **defect**	abnormal opening between the atria that allows blood to shunt back and forth
patent ductus arteriosus (PDA) (PAT-unt DUCK-tus ahr-teer-ee-OH-sus)	condition in which the ductus arteriosus remains open after birth, allowing oxygenated blood back into the lungs
thrill	palpable vibration caused by turbulent blood flow; also called a fremitus
fremitus (FREM-i-tus)	palpable vibration caused by turbulent blood flow; also called a thrill
electrocardiogram (ECG, EKG) (ee-leck-troh-KAHR-dee-oh-gram)	record of the electrical activity of the heart
P wave	section of the ECG showing atrial contraction
QRS complex	section of the ECG showing ventricular contraction
T wave	section of the ECG showing ventricular relaxation
tetralogy (te-TRAL-oh-jee) **of Fallot** (fahl-OH)	four congenital heart defects appearing together
dyspnea (disp-NEE-uh)	difficulty breathing or shortness of breath
ventricular septal (ven-TRICK-yoo-lur SEP-tul) **defect**	abnormal opening between the ventricles that allows blood to shunt back and forth
heart–lung machine	device that serves as artificial heart and lungs during some cardiac procedures

KEY TERM PRACTICE: *Congenital Heart Defects*

1. Four congenital heart defects—pulmonary stenosis, ventricular septal defect, abnormal aorta positioning, and ventricular hypertrophy—are characteristics of this condition. _____

2. An opening between the two atria that allows blood to shunt back and forth is termed _____; and a similar opening between the ventricles is called _____.

3. A record of the electrical activity in the heart is called an _____, and is abbreviated as _____ or _____.

4. An _____ is a surgical repair of the aorta.

5. Turbulent blood flow creates a palpable vibration known as a _____ or _____.

Coronary Artery Disease

coronary artery disease (CAD)

Coronary artery disease (CAD) is a condition in which the myocardium receives inadequate blood supply. It may result from problems with the coronary arteries, such as atherosclerosis, coronary artery spasm, or blood clots. It is usually caused by **plaque** (lipid deposits) in the arterial **lumen**, the space inside the vessel. This hardening of the arteries causing loss of elasticity is termed **arteriosclerosis**, and atherosclerosis represents a major type. **Atherosclerosis** is arteriosclerosis characterized by lipid deposits on the lining of large-sized and medium-sized arteries that lead to lumen narrowing

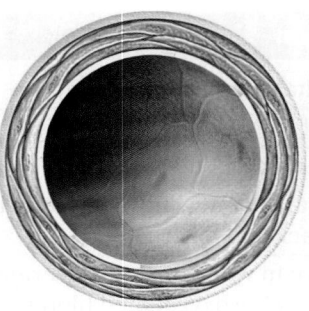
Normal vessel

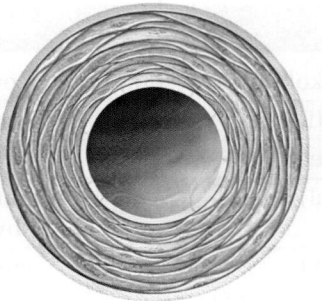
Arteriosclerosis

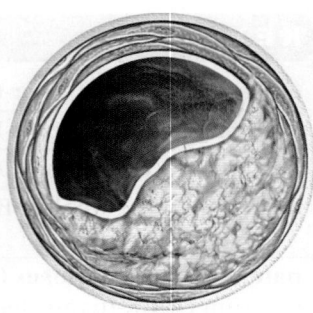
Atherosclerosis

Figure 11-21 Arterio-sclerosis and athero-sclerosis. Coronary artery disease is usually caused by plaque on the arterial lumen.

(Figure 11-21). The word part *athero-* means "fatty" or "lipid" deposit. Treatments of many forms of CAD involve atherectomy or endarterectomy. An **atherectomy** is the surgical removal of plaque from an artery, and an **endarterectomy** is the surgical removal of the fatty deposits along the endothelium, which is the inner lining of the artery. The removal results in a smooth lining.

Tests assessing coronary artery function are the exercise stress test and cardiac catheterization. The **exercise stress test** monitors heart rate, blood pressure, and ECG while the patient exercises. Abnormal results indicate coronary artery blockage. During a **cardiac catheterization**, a long, flexible tube is inserted into cardiac vessels via a peripheral artery or vein, such as a vessel in the thigh. Images produced from the procedure can show vessel blockage.

CAD has a gradual onset. Early signs and symptoms include blockage of a vessel, nausea, and weakness. Advanced signs such as **angina pectoris**—pain in the chest that radiates to the left shoulder—may not even occur until there is 75% occlusion (blockage) in a vessel. Angina pectoris is caused by localized **ischemia**, inadequate blood and oxygen supply to heart tissue. Risk factors for CAD include elevated levels of low-density lipoproteins (LDLs), which are fat and protein molecules that transport cholesterol to cells and tissues, and decreased levels of high-density lipoproteins (HDLs), which are fat and protein molecules that carry cholesterol away from arteries. As a memory tool, think of HDLs as *h*ealthy and *h*elpful and LDLs are *l*ousy and *l*ethal. Other risk factors are sedentary lifestyle and genetic predisposition (hereditary factors that make a person more susceptible to a disease).

A stress test, thallium scan, cardiac catheterization, ECG, Holter monitor ECG, or angiogram helps make the diagnosis. The **thallium scan** diagnoses coronary artery disease through the use of a radioactive isotope of thallium. Thallium is given via an intravenous drip, and the patient undergoes a physical stress test. The isotope collects in areas of poor circulation and can be seen as an image on the scanner. An **angiogram** is an x-ray of blood vessels after injecting a radiopaque dye into the bloodstream. The dye enables the vessels to be "mapped."

A **Holter monitor** is a small, portable ECG device that the patient wears continuously for 24 hours to record heart activity over an extended time period. During this time, the patient records symptoms and activities in a diary. The resulting graph reflects heart activity under a variety of situations in which the patient normally engages.

CAD can be treated with drugs or surgery. Drug therapy includes administration of **vasodilators**, drugs that cause blood vessel dilation

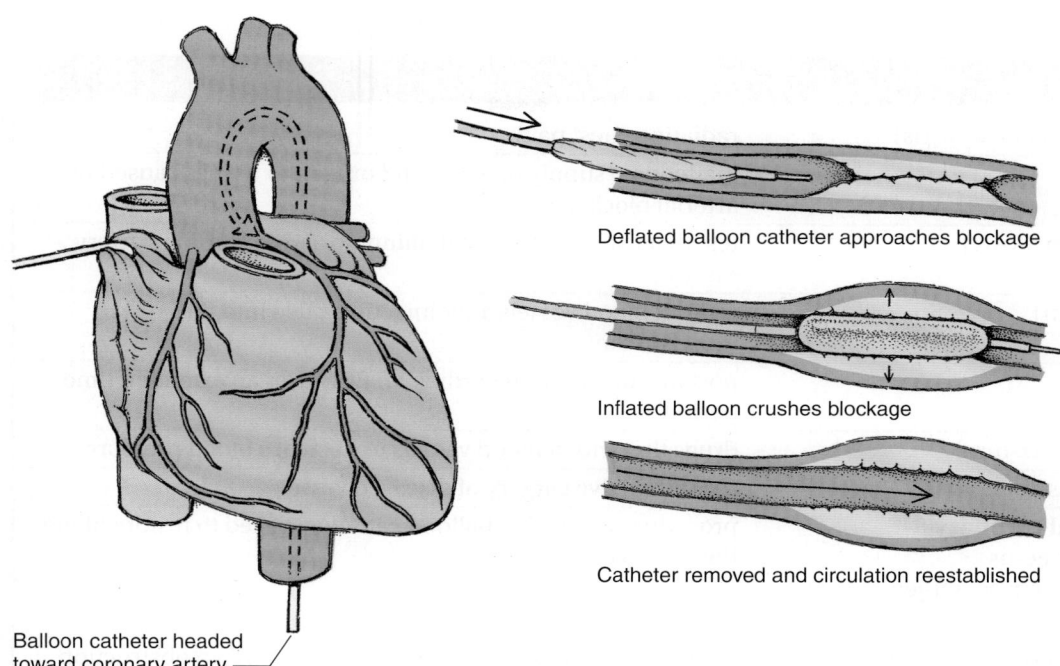

Deflated balloon catheter approaches blockage

Inflated balloon crushes blockage

Catheter removed and circulation reestablished

Balloon catheter headed toward coronary artery

Figure 11-22 Percutaneous transluminal coronary angioplasty

(expansion) and relaxation. Angioplasty, percutaneous transluminal coronary angioplasty, and coronary artery bypass graft surgery are invasive options. **Angioplasty** is the reconstructive surgery of diseased vessels. **Percutaneous transluminal coronary angioplasty (PTCA)** is a procedure in which a catheter is guided into the coronary arteries. Once the catheter is inserted, a balloon catheter is threaded through it and positioned at the occlusion. The balloon is then inflated, expanding the artery and restoring blood flow (**Figure 11-22**). **Coronary artery bypass graft (CABG) surgery** is an operation that creates a detour around obstructions in the coronary vessels. A heart-healthy diet, consisting of low fat and low salt intake, and physical exercise are therapeutic.

KEY TERM	Definition
coronary (KOR-uh-nerr-ee) **artery disease (CAD)**	condition in which the myocardium receives inadequate blood supply
plaque (PLACK)	lipid deposits on the arterial wall
lumen (LEW-min)	space inside the tubular artery
arteriosclerosis (ahr-teer-ee-oh-skle-ROH-sis)	hardening of the arteries
atherosclerosis (ath-ur-oh-skle-ROH-sis)	plaque formation on the inner arterial wall
atherectomy (ath-eh-RECK-toh-mee)	surgical removal of a plaque deposit from an artery
endarterectomy (en-do-ahr-terr-ECK-toh-mee)	atherectomy that includes removal of diseased portions of the arterial linings, leaving a smooth lining
exercise stress test	test that measures heart rate, blood pressure, and ECG while a patient exercises
cardiac catheterization (KAHR-dee-ack kath-e-tur-i-ZAY-shun)	procedure in which a flexible tube is inserted into the coronary vessels via a peripheral artery or vein for imaging purposes

continued

continued from page 531

KEY TERM	Definition
angina pectoris (an-JYE-nuh PECK-to-ris)	radiating chest pain
ischemia (is-KEE-mee-uh)	inadequate supply of blood and oxygen to tissues caused by arterial blockage
thallium scan (THAL-ee-um SKAN)	test that uses radioactive thallium to assess coronary artery disease
angiogram (AN-jee-oh-gram)	x-ray of blood vessels after injecting a dye into the bloodstream
Holter monitor	portable device for recording an ECG over an extended time period
vasodilators (vay-zoh-dye-LAY-turz)	drugs that widen blood vessels to decrease blood pressure
angioplasty (AN-jee-oh-plas-tee)	reconstructive surgery of diseased vessels
percutaneous transluminal coronary angioplasty (pur-kew-TAY-nee-us trans-LEW-mi-nul KOR-uh-nerr-ee AN-jee-oh-plas-tee) **(PTCA)**	procedure in which a balloon catheter is used to restore blood flow in a blocked vessel
coronary artery (KOR-uh-nerr-ee AHR-tur-ee) **bypass graft (CABG) surgery**	surgery to create an arterial diversion around an obstruction in the coronary vessels

KEY TERM PRACTICE: *Coronary Artery Disease*

1. Narrowing of the arterial lumen, called _____, can lead to arterial wall inelasticity known as

   _____.

2. The medical term for lipid deposits on the arterial lumen is _____.

3. This surgery, abbreviated CABG, is used to create arterial diversions around obstructions in coronary vessels.

   _____

4. An x-ray of blood vessels after injecting a radiopaque dye into the bloodstream is termed an _____.

5. _____ are drugs used to decreased blood pressure because they widen blood vessels.

Heart Disorders

cardiac arrest

The cessation of normal, effective heart action is termed **cardiac arrest**. Underlying coronary blood vessel disease that leads to ventricular tachycardia and/or ventricular fibrillation usually causes it. **Tachycardia** is a rapid heart rate (more than 90 beats per minute). **Fibrillation** is irregular, uncoordinated, fast contractions. It is usually described as quivering because there are no full contractions. A quivering heart looks like worms squirming in a small bag. **Palpitation**, fluttering heart, is often associated with irregular rhythm or tachycardia. In some cases, **bradycardia** (heart rate below 50 beats per minute) leads to cardiac arrest. The diagnosis is based on the absence of a palpable pulse, no respirations, bluish lips and pale skin, and an abnormal ECG.

Cardiopulmonary resuscitation combined with cardiac defibrillation must be administered within minutes of cardiac arrest to prevent death. **Cardiopulmonary resuscitation (CPR)** is a lifesaving procedure that consists of chest compressions that push the heart to stimulate blood flow, alternated with breaths to keep the lungs oxygenated. The American Heart Association also encourages hands-only CPR as a lifesaving action. Hands-only CPR involves pushing hard and fast on the center of the chest and can be used on adults. **Defibrillation** is stopping an asynchronous (uncoordinated) heart contraction by applying an electrical current via a defibrillator. When defibrillation is provided within 5 to 7 minutes of cardiac arrest, the survival rate is approximately 49%. Cardiac drugs are also administered.

heart block

The condition called **heart block** occurs when the nerve impulses are abnormal, which results in uncoordinated contractions of atria and ventricles. This conduction disturbance may be caused by drugs or by a disturbance of the heart's ability to conduct electrical impulses from the atria to the ventricles via the AV node. An artificial pacemaker may correct this problem. An **artificial pacemaker** is a permanent, battery-operated device that is surgically implanted into the chest wall. The artificial pacemaker assumes the role of the SA node, which is no longer properly regulating heart rate activity (**Figure 11-23**).

cardiac tamponade

Cardiac tamponade is heart compression as the result of fluid accumulation in the pericardial sac. Causes include blood vessel breakage. It results in decreased return of blood to the heart, and restricted heart filling. Signs and symptoms are rapidly falling blood pressure, dyspnea, a weak and thready (lacking fullness) pulse, and decreased consciousness. The sac requires immediate drainage via pericardiocentesis.

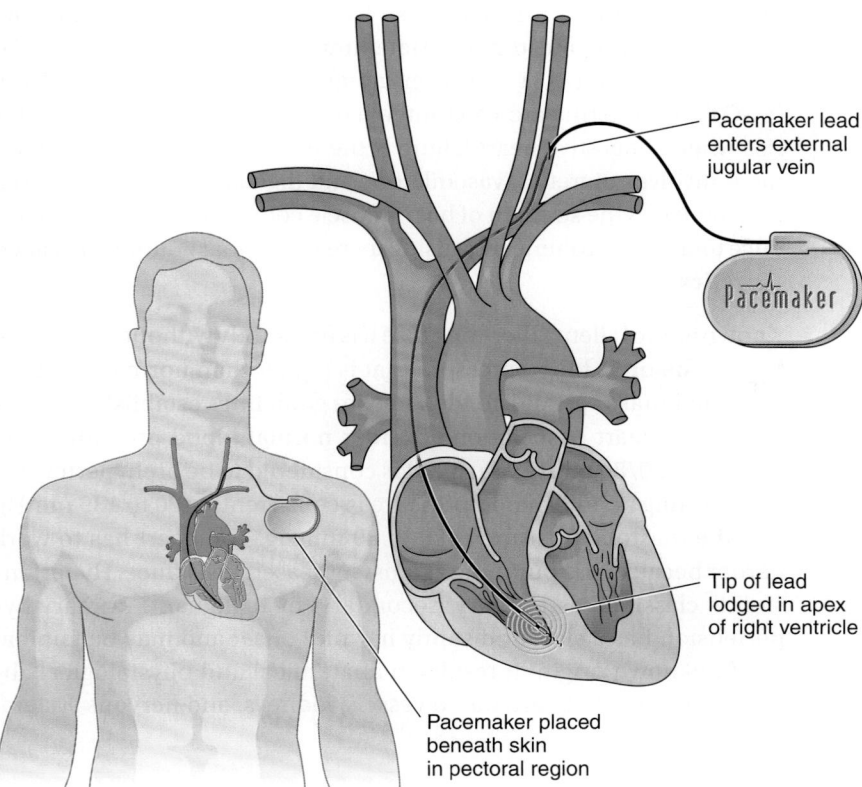

Pacemaker lead enters external jugular vein

Tip of lead lodged in apex of right ventricle

Pacemaker placed beneath skin in pectoral region

Figure 11-23 Placement of an artificial pacemaker. The lead is placed in an atrium or ventricle, usually on the right side.

Pericardiocentesis is an invasive procedure in which fluid is removed from the pericardial sac using a needle or catheter. The procedure can also serve as a diagnostic tool because the fluid can be chemically analyzed for microbes. Surgery may be required to repair the breakage.

cardiomyopathy

Disease of the myocardium (heart muscle) is called **cardiomyopathy**. Cardiomyopathy is characterized by ventricular dysfunction and myocardium enlargement. Cardiomyopathy is diagnosed by the history and physical examination. Cardiomegaly (heart enlargement) is apparent on an echocardiogram, radionuclide scan, or transesophageal echocardiogram, and the ECG is abnormal. A **radionuclide scan** involves the injection of radioactive substances into the bloodstream. Computerized scanning isolates the radioisotope and forms images of the heart. In **transesophageal echocardiography**, a combination endoscope/ultrasound probe is inserted into the esophagus to examine the nearby heart. Pulsating waves from the ultrasound probe create the picture. Treatment involves the use of drugs to reduce the heart's workload, bed rest, and heart transplant.

congestive heart failure (CHF)

Congestive heart failure (CHF) results when the heart cannot pump enough blood to meet the oxygen demands of the body. Blood remains in the heart because the muscle cannot pump it out fast enough, thereby causing an abnormal amount of blood in the veins. Causes include hypertension, CAD, chronic obstructive pulmonary disease (COPD; a progressive lung disease characterized by difficulty breathing), and cardiomyopathy. Common signs and symptoms include increased respiration rate to compensate for inadequate oxygen delivery, distended veins in the neck, and edema (swelling) in the extremities, notably the ankles and feet. It is diagnosed by history, physical examination, echocardiogram, and the aspartate aminotransferase (AST) test. An alternate term for AST is serum glutamic:oxaloacetic transaminase (SGOT). Both terms are used interchangeably. AST (or SGOT) levels rise when congestive heart failure is the result of liver damage. Treatment involves diuretics, vasodilators, and digitalis. **Digitalis** is a drug that increases the strength of heart muscle contractions. Drugs that reduce total blood volume by causing increased urinary output are called **diuretics**.

hypertension

Known as the "silent killer" because it is frequently without symptoms, **hypertension** is blood pressure that is higher than normal range for the individual's age and gender. Recent guidelines established by the American Heart Association consider normal blood pressure to be less than 120/80 mmHg. An adult is considered to be prehypertensive if the resting systolic blood pressure is consistently 120 to 139 mmHg and the diastolic pressure is 80 to 89 mmHg. The heart has to work harder because it is pumping against increased resistance. Hypertension is classified as primary, secondary, or malignant. Primary hypertension has a slow and subtly harmful onset and may be familial or of unknown origin. It results in anatomical and physiological abnormalities in the heart, blood vessels, kidneys, and nervous system.

This form of hypertension is poorly understood. Secondary hypertension is the result of having another known disease, stress, or from some drugs used to treat other conditions. Signs for both may include epistaxis (nose bleed) or **syncope** (loss of consciousness or fainting due to lack of oxygen to the brain). The diagnosis is based on blood pressure readings greater than 140/90 to 159/99 mmHg over a period of time.

An arsenal of drug therapies to target a variety of physiological signs and symptoms of hypertension is available. Common drug treatments include diuretics to reduce total blood volume and beta-adrenergic blockers, angiotensin-converting enzyme (ACE) inhibitors, and calcium channel blockers. **Angiotensin-converting enzyme (ACE) inhibitors** act on the kidney. ACE inhibitors produce vasodilation to lower blood pressure. Drugs that slow the heart rate and dilate vessels belong to the class of drugs called **beta-adrenergic blockers. Calcium channel blockers** slow the heart rate, dilate blood vessels, and reduce nervous conduction and excitability. A healthy diet and exercise are also recommended.

Malignant hypertension is rapidly progressive, severe hypertension of unknown cause. Signs and symptoms include headache, blurred vision, dyspnea, and blood pressure greater than 200/120 mmHg. The person is at risk for a **cerebrovascular accident (CVA)**, or stroke, and irreversible kidney damage. It is treated aggressively with intravenous vasodilators and drug therapy for life.

myocardial infarction (MI)

Heart attack is the common term for **myocardial infarction (MI)**, localized heart tissue death (ischemia). The term *infarct* refers to an area of dead tissue. With an MI, heart tissue dies when one of the coronary arteries becomes blocked. Signs and symptoms are crushing chest pain radiating to the left arm, back, and jaw; irregular heartbeat; dyspnea; and **diaphoresis** (profuse-sweating). History and physical examination, ECG, radiographic studies, and laboratory tests make the initial diagnosis. Elevated cardiac enzyme and abnormal isoenzyme levels confirm the diagnosis. Cardiac enzyme tests are blood tests that determine if cardiac tissue damage is present. Two important enzyme tests are the creatine kinase (CK) test and the lactic dehydrogenase (LDH) test. Levels of creatine kinase, an important substance in muscle tissue, rise 6 to 24 hours after an MI. LDH levels are elevated in patients with congestive heart failure and also peak 48 hours after an MI. There is a 6-hour window of opportunity to halt the progression of the cardiac event before permanent damage results. However nearly 65% of MI deaths occur within the first hour.

Immediate treatment includes ingestion of 325 mg of aspirin and defibrillation if necessary. Other treatments include oxygen therapy, thrombolytic (clot breaking) drugs, and nitroglycerin. **Nitroglycerin** is a fast-acting coronary vasodilator. It is administered sublingually (under the tongue) or through an intravenous drip. Bypass surgery and angioplasty are invasive treatment options. **Bypass surgery** is an operation in which blood flow is restored by the creation of a diversionary channel (**Figure 11-24**).

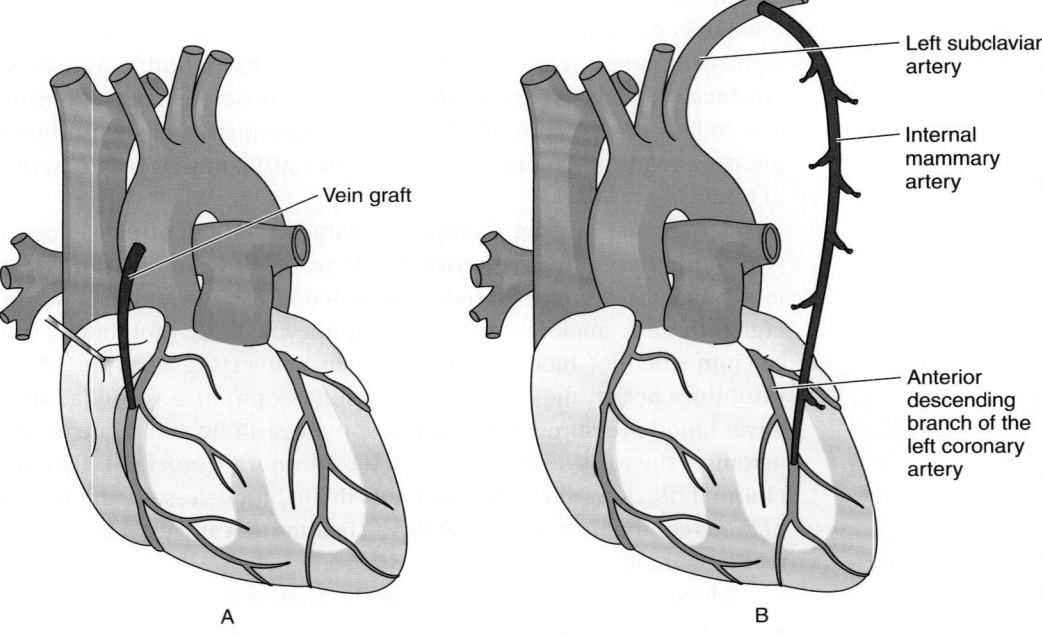

Figure 11-24 Bypass surgery. **(A)** A segment of the saphenous vein carries blood from the aorta to a part of the right coronary artery that is distal to a blockage. **(B)** The mammary artery is used to bypass an obstruction in the left anterior descending coronary artery.

KEY TERM	Definition
cardiac (KAHR-dee-ack) **arrest**	sudden stoppage of the heart
tachycardia (tack-i-KAHR-dee-uh)	rapid heart rate, above 90 beats per minute
fibrillation (fib-ri-LAY-shun)	irregular, uncoordinated heart contractions
palpitation (pal-pi-TAY-shun)	fluttering heart
bradycardia (brad-ee-KAHR-dee-uh)	slow heart rate, below 50 beats per minute
cardiopulmonary resuscitation (CPR) (kahr-dee-oh-PUL-muh-nerr-ee)	emergency technique to restore the heartbeat and breathing by alternating chest compressions with artificial respiration
defibrillation (dee-fib-ri-LAY-shun)	shocking the heart with a defibrillator to restore the regular heartbeat
heart block	condition caused by an impairment of the conducting system
artificial pacemaker	electrical device that restores normal heart rhythm
cardiac tamponade (KAHR-dee-ack tam-puh-NADE)	heart compression caused by fluid accumulation in the pericardial sac
pericardiocentesis (perr-i-kahr-dee-oh-sen-TEE-sis)	drainage of the pericardial sac by a needle or catheter
cardiomyopathy (kahr-dee-oh-migh-OP-uh-thee)	disease of the myocardium (heart muscle)
radionuclide scan (ray-dee-oh-NEW-klide SKAN)	computer-generated images made using radionuclides injected into the bloodstream
transesophageal echocardiography (trans-ee-sof-uh-JEE-ul eck-oh-kahr-dee-OG-ruh-fee)	ultrasound examination of the heart via an endoscope through the esophagus
congestive heart failure (CHF)	disease in which the heart muscle cannot keep pace to provide the body with oxygenated blood
digitalis (dij-i-TAL-is)	drug that increases the strength of heart muscle contraction
diuretics (dye-yoo-RET-icks)	drugs that increase urination

continued

continued from page 536

KEY TERM	Definition
hypertension (high-pur-TEN-shun)	chronic abnormally high blood pressure
syncope (SING-kuh-pee)	loss of consciousness as a result of lack of oxygen to the brain; fainting
angiotensin- (an-jee-oh-TEN-sin) **converting enzyme (ACE) inhibitors**	drugs that act on the kidneys to decrease blood pressure
beta-adrenergic (ad-re-NUR-jick) **blocker**	drug that slows the heart rate
calcium channel blocker	drug used to induce muscle relaxation and slow the heart rate
cerebrovascular (se-ree-broh-VAS-kyu-lur) **accident (CVA)**	stroke
myocardial infarction (MI) (migh-oh-KAHR-dee-ul in-FARK-shun)	heart tissue ischemia; also called a heart attack
diaphoresis (dye-uh-foh-REE-sis)	heavy sweating
cardiac (KAHR-dee-ack) **enzyme test**	examines heart muscle enzymes to assess cardiac tissue damage
nitroglycerin (nigh-troh-GLIS-ur-in)	fast-acting vasodilator drug
bypass (BYE-pass) **surgery**	operation in which blood flow is restored through the creation of a diversionary channel

KEY TERM PRACTICE: *Heart Disorders*

1. Abnormally high blood pressure is termed _____.

2. _____ describes heart muscle disease.

3. The term for heavy sweating is _____.

4. A _____ is another term for a stroke.

5. _____ is the term for a fluttering heart; _____ refers to irregular, uncoordinated heart contractions.

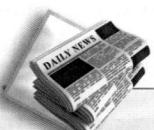

IN THE NEWS: Aspirin

The phrase is familiar: "Aspirin, the wonder drug." Is it really? Or is this marketing hype? The pharmaceutical name for aspirin is acetylsalicylic acid (ASA), and it is a common nonsteroidal anti-inflammatory drug (NSAID). Its properties are numerous, ranging from anti-inflammatory effects to acting as an analgesic, antipyretic (fever reducer), and thrombolytic.

Studies indicate that prophylactic aspirin therapy is beneficial for secondary prevention of vascular events in individuals with a history of CV disease. The U.S. Food and Drug Administration (FDA) has approved aspirin use at 325 mg/day for primary myocardial infarction prevention. Aspirin used clinically at a dosage level of 81 mg/day (baby aspirin) demonstrated antiplatelet effects that last 8 to 10 days, the life span of a platelet.

Other research demonstrated that aspirin administration of 325 mg/day decreased the incidence of transient ischemic attacks (TIAs; also known as mini-strokes, which

continued

continued from page 537

IN THE NEWS: Aspirin

resolve within 24 hours), unstable angina, coronary artery thrombosis with MI, and thrombosis after CABG surgery. Aspirin administration of 325 mg every other day decreased MI incidence 40% in another study population.

The findings appear promising in terms of disease prevention. Yet, aspirin ingestion of 500 mg/day greatly increases the incidence of gastrointestinal bleeding and may increase the occurrence of stomach ulcers. Therefore, aspirin should be used cautiously and only under the guidance of a health care professional.

Heart Disorders Associated with the Lungs

cor pulmonale

Cor pulmonale is characterized by acute right heart strain or chronic right ventricular hypertrophy resulting from lung disease (**Figure 11-25**). *Cor* means "heart" and *pulmon-* means "lung." The impaired blood flow to the lungs causes the right ventricle to work harder. Common signs and symptoms include dyspnea, distended neck veins, and hepatomegaly (enlarged liver). The diagnosis is made through the history, physical examination, x-ray studies, and an echocardiogram that shows heart enlargement. Medical care involves treating the underlying pulmonary condition along with digitalis.

pulmonary edema

Fluid effusion (oozing of liquid) into lung air sacs is termed **pulmonary edema**. It is caused by left heart failure that results from chronic hypertension, cardiomyopathy, or myocardial infarction. Signs and symptoms are dyspnea, **orthopnea** (difficulty breathing except when standing erect or sitting upright), increased heart and respiration rates, and hemoptysis. **Hemoptysis** is the coughing up of blood or mucus containing blood. The word *hemoptysis* is formed from the word part *hemo-* for "blood" and the word part *-ptysis*, the Greek term for "spitting." The history, physical examination, clinical picture, x-rays, and echocardiogram that show an enlarged heart are used to confirm the diagnosis. Treatments include oxygen therapy; use of the **Fowler position** (semireclining in bed); and drug treatment with diuretics, digitalis, and beta-adrenergics.

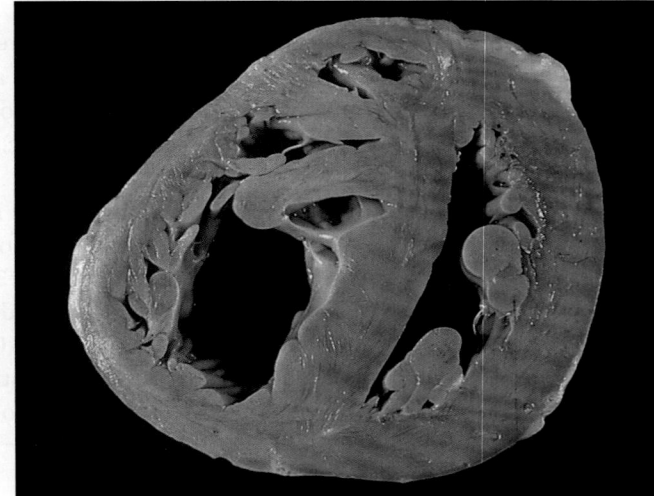

Figure 11-25 Cor pulmonale. A heart section showing a greatly hypertrophied right ventricle, which has the same wall thickness as that of the left ventricle.

KEY TERM	Definition
cor pulmonale (KOR pul-mo-NAY-lee)	disease characterized by right ventricular hypertrophy (enlargement) caused by lung disease
pulmonary edema (PUL-muh-nerr-ee e-DEE-muh)	fluid leakage into the lung air sacs caused by left heart failure
orthopnea (or-THOP-nee-uh)	difficulty breathing except when sitting or standing straight
hemoptysis (hee-MOP-ti-sis)	coughing up blood
Fowler position	semireclining in bed

KEY TERM PRACTICE: *Heart Disorders Associated with the Lungs*

1. Fluid filling the lung air sacs is called _____.

2. The disease characterized by right ventricular hypertrophy resulting from lung disease is termed _____.

3. Coughing up blood is termed _____.

4. _____ is difficulty breathing except when sitting or standing.

5. This term describes a position in which the person is semireclining in bed. _____

Inflammation Disorders

endocarditis   **Endocarditis** is inflammation of the endocardium. It is usually secondary to bacterial or fungal infection elsewhere in the body. Individuals with a history of rheumatic disease are at greater risk for endocarditis than the general population. Endocardial inflammation is characterized by growth on the heart valves that causes improper closure, which can be heard as a murmur (**Figure 11-26**). A **murmur** is the soft blowing or fluttering sound heard with a stethoscope placed on the chest. Signs and symptoms include fever, chills, fatigue, and generalized weakness. Diagnosis is made through complete blood cell count (CBC); elevated erythrocyte sedimentation rate (ESR); blood cultures to identify the causative microorganism; and detection of **arrhythmia**, an irregular

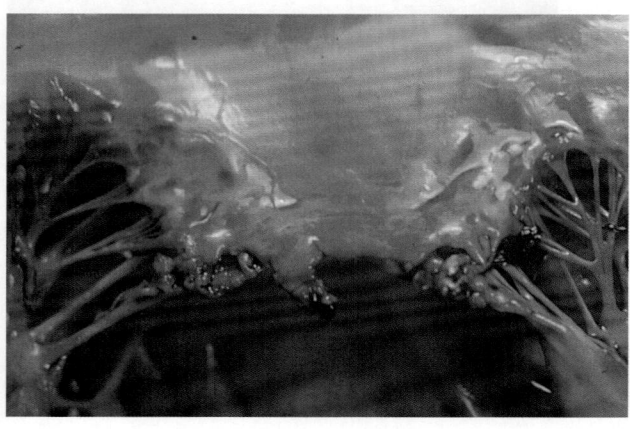

Figure 11-26 Bacterial endocarditis. The mitral valve shows destructive growths, which have eroded through the valve.

heartbeat that can result in flutter, fibrillation, or dysrhythmia. **Dysrhythmia** is an irregularity in an otherwise normal heart rhythm. Treating the underlying cause with antibiotics is the first step. After recovery, prophylactic (preventing or helping prevent disease) antibiotics are prescribed to individuals undergoing procedures with risk of bacterial infection. For example, patients with a history of endocarditis take antibiotics before having dental work done.

myocarditis Inflammation of the myocardium is called **myocarditis**. Its causes are varied and include infection, toxin exposure, and chronic cocaine use. Fatigue, dyspnea, and arrhythmia are common signs and symptoms. Increased cardiac enzyme levels, increased white blood cell count, abnormal ECG, and heart enlargement confirm the diagnosis. In some cases, a heart tissue biopsy is necessary. Treatment is aimed at managing the underlying cause and providing rest.

pericarditis **Pericarditis** is an acute or chronic inflammation of the pericardium (**Figure 11-27**). It has varied causes, including bacterial or viral infection, trauma, and cancer. It may occur secondary to myocardial infarction. Fever, malaise (general ill feeling), chest pain, and friction rub (sound resulting from rubbing of two serous surfaces) heard with a stethoscope are common signs and symptoms. Pericarditis is diagnosed through blood studies, ECG, and echocardiography. Bacterial cases are treated with antibiotics once the microbe has been identified, analgesics to control pain, and nonsteroidal anti-inflammatory drugs (NSAIDs) for inflammation.

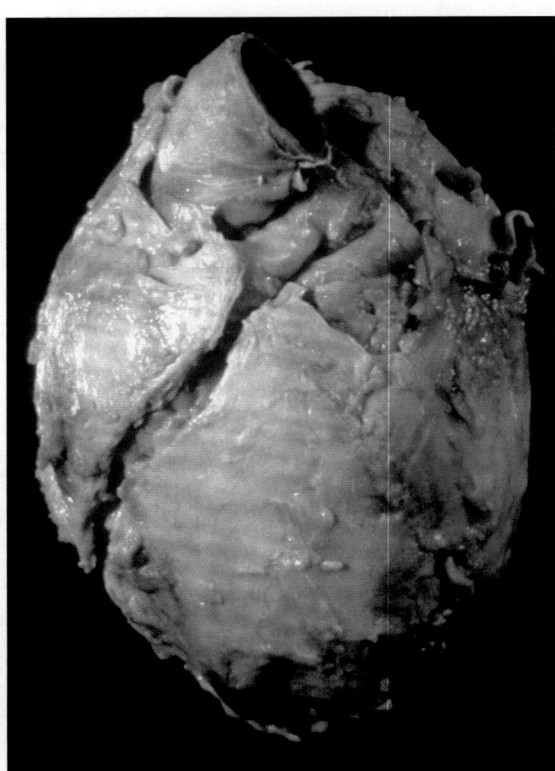

Figure 11-27 Pericarditis. The heart is encased in a fibrotic, thickened pericardium.

KEY TERM	Definition
endocarditis (en-doh-kahr-DYE-tis)	inflammation of the endocardium
murmur	soft blowing or fluttering heart sound
arrhythmia (uh-RITH-mee-uh)	irregular heartbeat
dysrhythmia (dis-RITH-mee-uh)	an irregularity in the normal heart rhythm
myocarditis (migh-oh-kahr-DYE-tis)	inflammation of the myocardium
pericarditis (perr-i-kahr-DYE-tis)	inflammation of the pericardium

KEY TERM PRACTICE: *Inflammation Disorders*

1. Define the following word parts.

a. *endo-* _____

b. *myo-* _____

c. *peri-* _____

d. *cardi-* _____

e. *-itis* _____

2. An inflammation of the myocardium is termed _____.

3. An inflammation of the pericardium is termed _____.

4. A _____ is a soft blowing or fluttering heart sound.

5. An inflammation of the heart's inner lining is called _____.

Shock

shock   **Shock** results when blood flow to and perfusion of tissues is inadequate. Less blood returns to the heart causing collapse (failure) of the cardiovascular system. Main types of shock include hypovolemic, cardiogenic, and septic. Hypovolemic shock results from inadequate blood volume. Inadequate cardiac function results in cardiogenic shock. Septic shock is associated with infection that causes low blood pressure (hypotension). Signs and symptoms include hypotension, weak pulse, tachycardia, decreased urinary output, coldness, sweating, and irregular respirations. It is diagnosed by the clinical picture and must be treated immediately because it is life threatening. The form determines the treatment options, but in all cases measures are taken to restore blood pressure and stimulate the heart to contract more forcefully.

KEY TERM	Definition
shock	condition resulting from inadequate blood flow through the body to nourish tissues

KEY TERM PRACTICE: *Shock*

1. The condition resulting from inadequate blood flow through the body to nourish tissues is termed _____.

Heart Valve Diseases

Valvular heart diseases are acquired or congenital and cause improper functioning of heart valves.

rheumatic heart disease (RHD)

Rheumatic heart disease (RHD) is a delayed **sequela** (disorder caused by a previous disease) of rheumatic fever. That is, RHD results from rheumatic fever, an acute disease caused by group A streptococcal infection. Signs and symptoms of rheumatic fever include fever, sore throat, joint swelling, and heart valve damage (**Figure 11-28**). RHD can be successfully treated with antibiotics. Valvular disturbances and inflammatory lesions in the heart, blood vessels, and joints characterize rheumatic heart disease. Carditis, arthritis, and skin rash may also be present. Rheumatic heart disease is diagnosed through a history of rheumatic fever and elevated levels of cardiac enzymes. Surgical repair of damaged heart valves may be necessary.

valvular regurgitation (valvular insufficiency)

Valvular regurgitation (valvular insufficiency) is characterized by a leaky state of one or more of the cardiac valves. With this condition, the valve does not close tightly during contraction, allowing blood to reenter the atrium. A scarred valve that results from rheumatic fever often causes it. Signs and symptoms are fatigue, dyspnea, and heart murmur. Valvular insufficiency is diagnosed through the history, presence of a murmur, ECG, x-ray, or cardiac catheterization. It is treated with bed rest, oxygen therapy, antibiotics, and diuretics.

mitral valve prolapse (MVP)

A mild condition in which the left bicuspid (mitral) flaps do not close properly is termed **mitral valve prolapse (MVP)** (**Figure 11-29**). Most often it is a congenital disorder. The prolapse (slippage of the valves from their usual position) causes blood regurgitation (backflow). There are usually no signs or symptoms because the

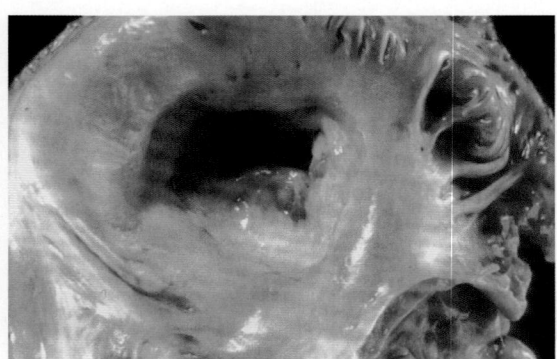

Figure 11-28 Rheumatic heart disease. A view of the mitral valve from the left atrium shows rigid, thickened, and fused leaflets with a narrow orifice, creating the characteristic "fish mouth" appearance of rheumatic mitral stenosis.

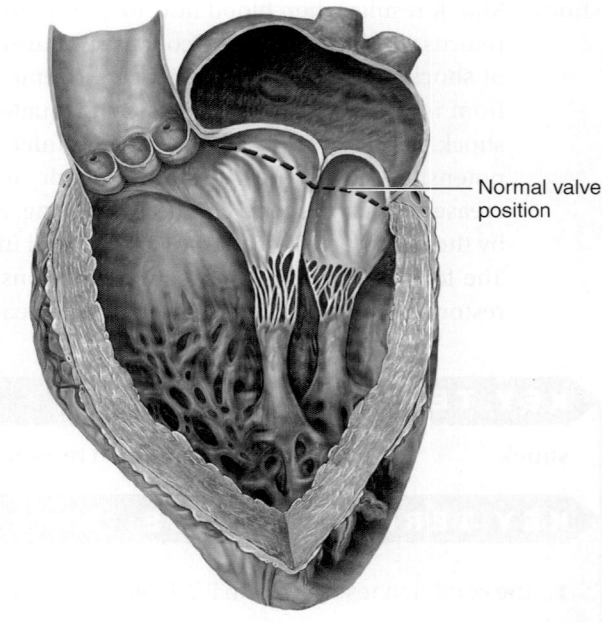

Normal valve position

Figure 11-29 Mitral valve prolapse.

volume of blood flowing in the opposite direction through the defective valve is not significant. Mitral valve prolapse is generally discovered during a routine stethoscope auscultation. It can be detected at any age. The diagnosis is confirmed by the presence of a heart murmur or by echocardiogram evidence. Treatment is normally not required but may include avoidance of stimulants such as caffeine, nicotine, and decongestants, and administration of beta-blockers.

mitral stenosis

Mitral stenosis is narrowing of the opening of the mitral valve (see **Figure 11-28**). The primary cause is rheumatic heart disease. It appears that this is an autoimmune disorder because the antibodies formed after rheumatic fever continue to attack the heart tissue. Primary signs and symptoms are cough, dyspnea, and hemoptysis. The diagnosis is confirmed through the presence of a heart murmur and constriction shown by echocardiogram. Treatments include drugs to reduce the heart workload, anticoagulants, **commissurotomy** (surgical opening of a narrowed valve), and valve replacement.

KEY TERM	Definition
rheumatic (roo-MAT-ick) **heart disease**	valvular disease of the heart as a result of rheumatic fever
sequela (se-KWEL-uh)	disorder caused by a previous disease
valvular regurgitation (VAL-vyoo-lur ree-gur-jih-TAY-shun)	disorder characterized by a leaky state of one or more of the cardiac valves that allows for backward flow of blood; also called valvular insufficiency
valvular insufficiency (VAL-vyoo-lur in-suh-FISH-en-see)	disorder characterized by a leaky state of one or more of the cardiac valves that allows for backward flow of blood; also called valvular regurgitation
mitral (MIGH-trul) **valve prolapse (MVP)**	improper closure of the mitral (bicuspid) valve
mitral stenosis (MIGH-trul ste-NOH-sis)	narrowed mitral valve opening that impedes blood flow
commissurotomy (com-i-shur-OT-oh-mee)	surgical opening of a narrowed heart valve

KEY TERM PRACTICE: *Heart Valve Diseases*

1. Which heart disease may result from rheumatic fever? _____

2. The disorder characterized by a leaky state of one or more of the cardiac valves that allows for backward flow of blood is known by these two terms. _____

3. _____ is a narrowing of the mitral valve.

4. A disorder that is caused by a previous disease in the same individual is termed _____.

5. The surgical opening of a narrowed valve is called a _____.

Vein and Artery Disorders

peripheral vascular disease (PVD)

Peripheral vascular disease (PVD) describes progressive occlusions (blockages) of small arteries and arterioles that supply the extremities. It is a common secondary condition in diabetes mellitus, and atherosclerosis is a primary risk factor.

vascular murmur

A **vascular murmur** is a finding that originates in blood vessels as a result of turbulent flow. Vascular murmurs create thrills and are common to an **arteriovenous fistula**, a surgically created connection directly between an artery and a vein (**Figure 11-30**). Vascular surgeons perform this procedure on dialysis patients (those whose kidneys are not functioning) to provide easy access to a vessel for treatment. Naturally formed arteriovenous fistulas do occur, but they are abnormal conditions.

aneurysm

An **aneurysm** is a thin, weakened section of an arterial wall that bulges outward, forming a sac. Remember, the word part *eury-* means broad or wide. The localized, abnormal bulge usually progresses in size and causes a **bruit**, which is a swishing sound that results from turbulent blood flow. Medical professionals are taught the phrase "palpate a thrill and auscultate a bruit." The signs and symptoms of aneurysms may include pain, pressure at the site, and hemorrhage. Atherosclerotic plaque buildup causes them. Common sites are along the abdominal aorta.

There are three classifications of aneurysms: saccular, fusiform, and dissecting. As its name suggests, a **saccular aneurysm** is a sac-like bulge on one side of an artery. A **fusiform aneurysm** is an elongated, spindle-shaped dilation of the arterial wall. A **dissecting aneurysm** is a splitting of the arterial wall (usually the inner lining) layers, creating a bulge between the layers (**Figure 11-31**). Dissecting aneurysms are created by blood

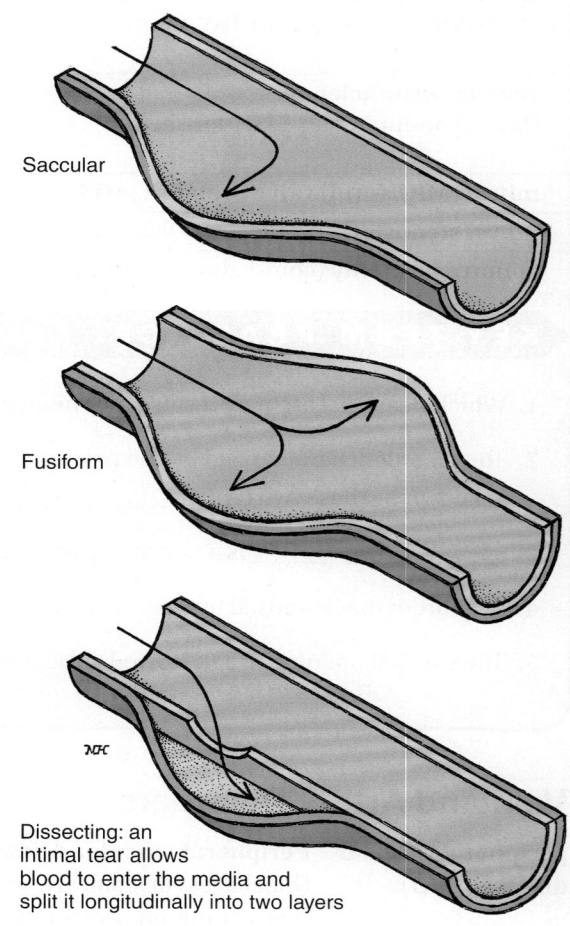

Saccular

Fusiform

Dissecting: an intimal tear allows blood to enter the media and split it longitudinally into two layers

Figure 11-31 Aneurysm.

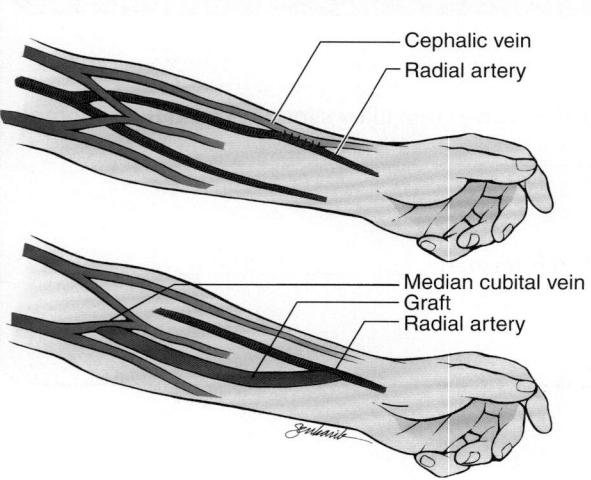

Cephalic vein
Radial artery

Median cubital vein
Graft
Radial artery

Figure 11-30 An arteriovenous fistula (top) is created by a side-to-side connection between the artery and the vein. A graft (bottom) can be established between the artery and the vein.

forcing its way through a tear in the intima between the arterial layers. A **false aneurysm**, or pseudoaneurysm, mimics an aneurysm and is composed of fibrous tissue. A rupture of all arterial layers that causes a swelling in an artery creates a pseudoaneurysm. Hematomas are commonly the underlying cause of aneurysms, which are diagnosed by bruit presence and palpation. Radiographic, CT, and MRI studies reveal their presence. Surgical repair is the primary treatment.

phlebitis

Phlebitis is the term for vein inflammation. Its cause is unknown, and it typically affects lower leg regions. Injury, surgery, and obesity have been implicated as possible causative factors. Other instances include travelers who sit for prolonged periods without changing position, pregnant women, women who have just delivered babies, and smokers who take birth control pills. Pain and edema are frequent signs and symptoms. Phlebitis is diagnosed through the history, physical examination, and visual inspection.

Most cases of phlebitis are acute and resolve, using only analgesics to control pain. Massage is not recommended because it may stimulate either clot formation or emboli release. In elderly, overweight people, who have skin changes from chronic phlebitis, it is difficult to get the underlying inflamed veins to heal. In some cases, treatment should include elevation of the limbs for improved drainage, antibiotics for underlying skin infection, and blood thinners.

thrombophlebitis

Thrombophlebitis is vein inflammation associated with a thrombus. It is caused by blood pooling or injury affecting the inner lining of the vein. A **deep vein thrombosis (DVT)** refers to a blood clot in a deep vein. Signs and symptoms include pain, edema, and warmth in the affected area; however, sometimes the phlebitis is silent and the first clinical indication is swelling from the thrombosed veins. It is diagnosed by the clinical picture, physical examination, venography, or Doppler ultrasonography. **Venography** is an x-ray of the veins after injecting a contrast dye that shows up on x-rays; it provides a pictorial venogram or phlebogram. **Doppler ultrasonography** is a noninvasive procedure for assessing blood flow velocity, direction, and occlusions. It uses high-frequency sound waves reflecting off internal body parts to create images.

The goal of therapy is to dissolve the clot. Anticlotting agents, such as heparin, are used to dissolve underlying clots, and coumarin is used to prevent further clotting. Because the clot could break loose, travel, and block a major vessel, immobilization of the affected part, along with heparin, is prescribed. Surgical intervention may be necessary.

varicose veins

A vein that has become abnormally swollen and knotted (**tortuous**) as a result of defective valves is called a **varicose vein** (**Figure 11-32**). The causes include standing or sitting for prolonged periods, which allows blood to pool, and pregnancy, which creates pressure on veins, thereby affecting blood flow. Leg cramps, pain, and edema are signs and symptoms. Visual inspection and patient history lead to the diagnosis.

Treatment options are varied. Exercises, changing position while standing, vein ligation, stripping, and sclerosing solutions are possible medical therapies. **Vein ligation** is the surgical tying off of a vein to close an area's blood supply. **Vein stripping** refers to surgical removal of a vein after ligation. **Vein sclerosing** involves injecting a solution that

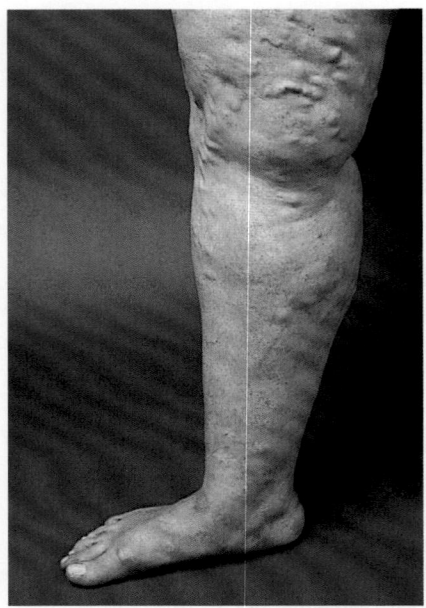

Figure 11-32 Varicose veins.

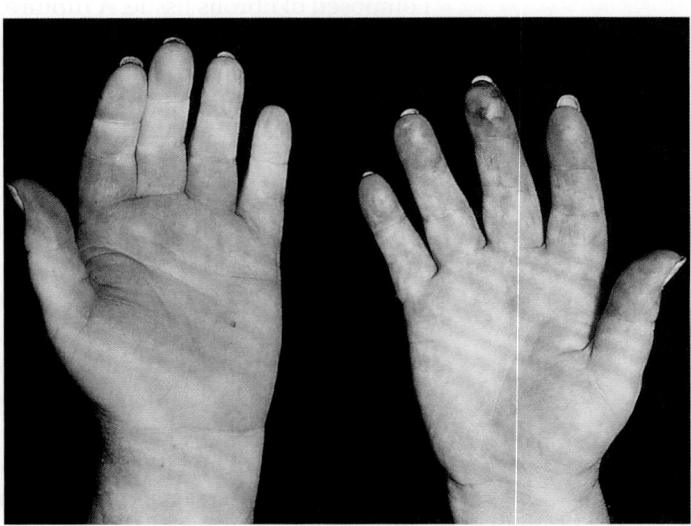

Figure 11-33 Raynaud phenomenon is characterized by color changes on the hands.

causes the vein to harden and eventually atrophy. After a ligation or sclerosing procedure, new blood vessels develop.

Raynaud phenomenon

Raynaud phenomenon is characterized by intermittent episodes of pallor (pale appearance), cyanosis, or rubor (redness) of fingers and/or toes that is induced by cold or emotions (**Figure 11-33**). It is often secondary to or concomitant (existing along) with an autoimmune disease and is more common in women than men. Pain, numbness, and discoloration often occur with this disorder. The effects are the result of arteries and arterioles that undergo spasm and constriction. A Raynaud phenomenon episode resolves after application of warmth. Smoking aggravates the condition. Diagnosis is made by the clinical picture and visual inspection. Treatment involves use of warm compresses, smoking cessation, and avoidance of cold temperatures. Vasodilators may be prescribed.

KEY TERM	Definition
peripheral vascular (pe-RIF-e-rul VAS-kew-lur) **disease (PVD)**	progressive disorder caused by occlusions of the small arteries and arterioles that supply the extremities
vascular (VAS-kew-lur) **murmur**	condition that originates in the blood vessels as a result of turbulent blood flow
arteriovenous fistula (ahr-teer-ee-oh-VEE-nus FIS-tew-luh)	direct connection between an artery and a vein
aneurysm (AN-yoo-riz-um)	abnormal outward bulge in an artery
bruit (broo-EE)	abnormal swishing sound, caused by turbulent blood flow, heard through a stethoscope
saccular aneurysm (SACK-yoo-lur AN-yoo-riz-um)	sac-shaped outward bulge on an artery

continued

continued from page 546

KEY TERM	Definition
fusiform aneurysm (FEW-zi-form AN-yoo-riz-um)	spindle-shaped outpouching on an artery
dissecting aneurysm (AN-yoo-riz-um)	abnormal bulge between the layers of an arterial wall
false aneurysm (AN-yoo-riz-um)	rupture of the arterial walls, causing swelling
phlebitis (fle-BYE-tis)	vein inflammation
thrombophlebitis (throm-boh-fle-BYE-tis)	vein inflammation with thrombus
deep vein thrombosis (throm-BOH-sis) **(DVT)**	blood clot in a deep vein
venography (vee-NOG-ruh-fee)	x-ray examination of the veins after injecting a dye that absorbs the x-rays
Doppler (DOP-lur) **ultrasonography**	a noninvasive procedure that uses high-frequency sound waves reflecting off internal body parts to create images and assess blood flow velocity, direction, and occlusions
tortuous (TOR-choo-us)	swollen and knotted
varicose (VAR-i-koce) **veins**	knotted, swollen veins
vein ligation (lye-GAY-shun)	surgical tying of a vein
vein stripping	surgical removal of a vein
vein sclerosing (skle-ROCE-ing)	surgical hardening of a vein
Raynaud (reh-NOH) **phenomenon**	artery and arteriole spasms in the fingers and toes causing cold, numb, and painful digits

KEY TERM PRACTICE: *Vein and Artery Disorders*

1. _____ is the medical term for vein inflammation.

2. _____ is the word used to describe vein inflammation with clot formation.

3. The surgical removal of a vein is termed _____.

4. A direct connection between an artery and a vein is called an _____.

5. A _____ is an abnormal swishing sound caused by turbulent blood flow.

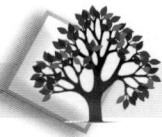

LIFE SPAN

Beginning on the 15th day of development in the uterus, blood vessels begin to form. The fetal heart begins to beat around week 4. Important fetal structures, such as the foramen ovale, ductus arteriosus, and ductus venosus, function until birth. While the fetus is in the uterus, the foramen ovale and ductus arteriosus allow blood to bypass the nonfunctioning lungs, and the ductus venosus permits blood to bypass the fetal liver. At birth, the umbilical vein and two umbilical arteries, which enable nutrient and waste exchange between mother and fetus, stop functioning.

As the infant develops, blood vessels enlarge and the heart tissue grows. Blood pressure also undergoes considerable change. The average BP for a baby is 90/55 mm Hg. During childhood, there is a gradual increase in both systolic and diastolic pressures. As we age, blood pressure increases because the arteries become stiffer.

Atherosclerosis is the most common cardiovascular age-related disorder in Western populations, but little is known of its relationship to aging. It is known that cholesterol deposition is a normal part of aging and begins as fatty streaks (superficial fatty patches on the arterial wall) while an individual is still very young. Research has demonstrated that the earliest stage of atherosclerosis is that fatty streak, which lays the foundation for deposition later in life; but the streak appears not to be clinically significant. The only human tissue in which fatty streaks are not evident is fetal tissue. Fatty streaks form fibrous plaques that result in the formation of a connective tissue matrix around age 18 years. At age 24, about 30% of coronary vessels show evidence of a fatty streak, and at age 40, there is nearly 80% involvement. Fibrous plaques can lead to complicated lesions, which are calcifications of the inner lining of the blood vessel and may be associated with a clinical event.

The role of cholesterol in aging vessels is still under investigation. To date, there is no strong predictability factor in the elderly population regarding cholesterol levels and heart attack risks. Geriatric research indicates that high cholesterol may serve a protective function in old age because cholesterol in the elderly population may detoxify bacteria.

Cardiac changes with age include an increased incidence of angina, myocardial infarction, and cardiac arrest. There is thickening of the endocardium while myocardial tissue mass may decline. Women lag slightly behind men in incidence of cardiovascular disease until menopause, when the protective effects of the female hormone, estrogen, diminish. At age 65 years, the risks of disease are equal for males and females.

Diet modification, aerobic exercise, and cigarette smoking cessation all help lower cardiovascular disease risk and are beneficial for decreasing disease occurrence. Diet modification can assist in controlling hypertension, and smoking cessation does much for diminishing microvascular (very small blood vessel) disease.

COMMON Abbreviations

Abbreviation	Term
AA	associate of arts
ACE inhibitors	angiotensin-converting enzyme inhibitors
ACLS	advanced cardiac life support
ASA	acetylsalicylic acid
AST	aspartate aminotransferase
AV	atrioventricular; arteriovenous
BP	blood pressure
BSN	bachelor of science in nursing
CABG	coronary artery bypass graft
CAD	coronary artery disease
CBC	complete blood (cell) count
CHF	congestive heart failure
CK	creatine kinase
CK-MB	creatine phosphokinase muscle and brain
COPD	chronic obstructive pulmonary disease
CPR	cardiopulmonary resuscitation
CV	cardiovascular
CVA	cerebrovascular accident
CVICU	cardiovascular intensive care unit

continued

continued from page 548

Abbreviation	Term
DVT	deep vein thrombosis
ECG	electrocardiogram
EKG	electrocardiogram
ESR	erythrocyte sedimentation rate
FDA	Food and Drug Administration
HDL	high-density lipoprotein
ICU	intensive care unit
LDH	lactic dehydrogenase
LDL	low-density lipoprotein
MI	myocardial infarction
mmHg	millimeters of mercury
MRI	magnetic resonance imaging
MVP	mitral valve prolapse
NCLEX	National Council Licensure Examination
NSAIDs	nonsteroidal anti-inflammatory drugs
PDA	patent ductus arteriosus
PTCA	percutaneous transluminal coronary angioplasty
PVD	peripheral vascular disease
RHD	rheumatic heart disease
RN	registered nurse
SA	sinoatrial
SGOT	serum glutamic:oxaloacetic transaminase; AST
SL	semilunar
TIA	transient ischemic attack
2D	two dimensional

COMMON ABBREVIATIONS EXERCISES

1. TIA is the abbreviation for _____

2. Write the abbreviation for millimeters of mercury. _____

3. CV is the abbreviation for _____

4. MVP is the abbreviation for _____

5. PDA stands for _____

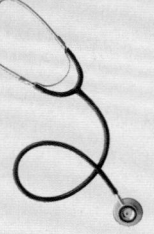

Case Study

Mr. Jay Tigress, age 67 years, was brought to the emergency department by ambulance. Before arrival at the hospital, he had been suffering alternating bouts of diarrhea and vomiting. He had flu-like symptoms and was unable to walk due to intense weakness. Mr. Tigress stated that he had been unable to keep any food down for several days and last remembered eating some oatmeal and applesauce 2 days earlier. He was extremely confused, but stated he was a diabetic and had not taken his insulin injection in nearly 2 days. Initial examination and blood chemistry profile revealed the following data.

Measure	Value	Measure	Value (Normal Value)
Weight	247 lb	Blood glucose	60 mg/dL (70–100)
BP	90/60 mmHg	Serum potassium	10 mEq/L (3.8–5.0)
Pulse	50	Serum phosphorus	4.1 mEq/L (1.8–2.6)
Respirations	40	Plasma/serum creatinine	3.2 mEq/L (0.6–1.2)
Temperature	35°C	Serum sodium	100 mEq/L (135–145)
Skin color	pale	CK-MB	65% of total isoenzyme (0–6)

A Foley urinary catheter was inserted; chest x-rays, ECG, and Doppler ultrasonography were ordered. Mr. Tigress was admitted to the CVICU, where Heather was the charge nurse that night.

Case Study Questions

Select the best answer to each of the following questions.

1. **Mr. Tigress has a BP of 90/60. BP is an abbreviation for _____.**
   a. bicuspid pressure
   b. blood pressure
   c. bradycardia pressure
   d. beating pressure

2. **A BP of 90/60 means _____.**
   a. the systolic pressure is 90 and the diastolic pressure is 60
   b. the diastolic pressure is 90 and the systolic pressure is 60
   c. the pulse pressure is 30
   d. a and c

3. **An ECG was ordered to evaluate _____.**
   a. brain function
   b. cardiac function
   c. liver function
   d. kidney function

4. **An elevated CK-MB is an indication of _____.**
   a. renal failure
   b. liver failure
   c. damaged cardiac tissue
   d. hypertension

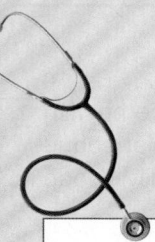

Real World Report

Mr. Tigress was admitted to Heather's floor, the CVICU, because he was experiencing multiple organ failure secondary to renal failure. His heart was fragile. The following is the cardiologist's report.

CENTRAL HOSPITAL: ECHOCARDIOGRAM REPORT

NAME: Jay Tigress   DOB: 01/02/1944
ATTENDING: J. L. Manjunata, MD   AGE: 67 years
ORDERING: M. M. Isaac, MD   DATE: 04/05/2011

REASON FOR STUDY

- Heart failure

PROCEDURE

The patient underwent M-Mode, 2D, continuous-wave, and pulse-wave Doppler.

RESULTS

- The left ventricle demonstrates mild increase in cavity size with severe systolic dysfunction. Ejection fraction is estimated to be no more than 25%. Hypokinesis is global.
- The right ventricle is normal in size and function.
- Normal size atria and aortic root.
- The mitral valve is mildly thickened. Trivial degree of mitral regurgitation is present.
- The aortic valve was not very well visualized but appears to have normal flow characteristics.
- Tricuspid valve was not very well visualized, but there is no significant (trivial) regurgitation present.
- Pulmonic valve was not visualized.
- Small to moderate size circumferential pericardial effusion that does not seem to be hemodynamically significant.
- No intracardiac mass or thrombi.

CONCLUSION

This is an abnormal study that demonstrates evidence of a mildly dilated left ventricle with severe systolic dysfunction. Ejection fraction is 25%. Mild to moderate circumferential pericardial effusion is present without hemodynamics of significance. No significant valvular abnormalities are seen.

continued

continued from page 551

Real World Report Questions

The following exercises review the medical terms in the preceding medical report. Two terms may be new to you: M-Mode and 2D Doppler. M-Mode Doppler ultrasound is a diagnostic procedure that uses Doppler sound waves so that the echoes displayed correlate to time (T) and motion (M). It is often referred to as TM-Mode Doppler ultrasound. 2D Doppler ultrasound returns a two-dimensional image.

1. **The left ventricle demonstrates severe systolic dysfunction. Define *systolic dysfunction* and explain its effects.**

   _____

   _____

   _____

2. **The report notes that hypokinesis is global.**

   a. The word part *hypo-* means _____.

   b. The word part *-kinesis* means _____.

   c. Thus, the word *hypokinesis* means _____.

3. **The mitral valve is mildly thickened and a trivial degree of regurgitation is present.**

   a. Another term for mitral valve is _____.

   b. What is another way of stating "trivial degree of mitral valve regurgitation"?

   _____

   _____

   _____

4. **Pericardial effusion is present.**

   a. The word part *peri-* means _____.

   b. The word part *-cardi* refers to _____.

   c. Thus, the term *pericardial effusion* refers to _____.

5. **No significant valvular abnormalities are seen. What valves were evaluated?**

   _____

   _____

   _____

Review and Application

Multiple-Choice Questions

Select the best answer to each of the following questions.

1. Components of the cardiovascular system include _____.
   a. the heart   b. arteries   c. veins   d. all of these

2. Which structure is *not* a layer of cardiac tissue? _____
   a. atrium   b. endocardium   c. myocardium   d. pericardium

3. The two upper chambers of the heart are the _____.
   a. ventricles   b. atria   c. semilunar valves   d. atrioventricular valves

4. The two lower chambers of the heart are the _____.
   a. ventricles   b. atria   c. semilunar valves   d. atrioventricular valves

5. The two semilunar valves are the _____.
   a. aortic and bicuspid   b. pulmonary and bicuspid   c. aortic and pulmonary   d. tricuspid and mitral

6. The term _____ means vein.
   a. arteriole   b. vena   c. cava   d. aorta

7. Pulmonary _____ carry blood to the _____.
   a. veins; lungs   b. venules; lungs   c. arteries; lungs   d. arteries; heart

8. A _____ monitor is a portable _____ machine.
   a. Fowler; sonogram   b. Holter; sonogram   c. Fowler; ECG   d. Holter; ECG

9. The heart's pacemaker is the _____.
   a. sinoatrial node   b. atrioventricular node   c. cardiac conducting cycle   d. atrioventricular bundle

10. The word part *cardio-* refers to _____; the word part *myo-* means _____; and the word part *-pathy* refers to _____.
    a. heart; heart; disease   b. head; muscle; occupation   c. heart; muscle; disease   d. coronary; disease; course of treatment

11. The procedure in which fluid is aspirated from the sac surrounding the heart is termed _____.
    a. myocardiocentesis   b. pericardiocentesis   c. endocardiocentesis   d. cardiac effusion

12. Systolic blood pressure measures arterial blood pressure during ventricular _____.
    a. relaxation   b. repolarization   c. fibrillation   d. contraction

13. The general blood circulatory route through the body is termed the _____ circuit.
    a. pulmonary   b. systemic   c. circulatory   d. coronary

14. These two structures empty blood into the right atrium. _____
    a. superior vena cava and inferior vena cava   b. bicuspid and tricuspid valve   c. right and left ventricle   d. aorta and aortic semilunar valve

15. The *lubb-dupp* sound the heart makes is caused by _____.
   a. contraction of ventricles, followed by relaxation of ventricles
   b. systole, followed by diastole
   c. the closing of heart valves
   d. all of these

16. Heart defects that are present at birth are called _____.
   a. genital
   b. progenital
   c. congenital
   d. congenial

17. A heartbeat that is irregular and uncoordinated with fast contractions is called _____.
   a. tachycardia
   b. fibrillation
   c. bradycardia
   d. defibrillation

18. _____ is a noninvasive procedure for assessing blood flow velocity, direction, and occlusions.
   a. Venography
   b. Thallium scanning
   c. Doppler ultrasonography
   d. Electrocardiogram

19. _____ is the surgical tying off of a vein to close an area's blood supply, while _____ involves injecting a solution that causes the vein to harden and eventually atrophy.
   a. Sclerosing; ligation
   b. Stripping; sclerosing
   c. Ligation; stripping
   d. Ligation; sclerosing

Word Parts

Using the following word parts, form a medical term for each definition. Each word part is used only once.

cardi-   -itis   phleb-
cardi-   -itis   thrombo-
cardi-   -itis   -um
endo-   myo-   -um
endo-   phleb-

20. vein inflammation with clot formation _____

21. inner heart lining _____

22. heart muscle _____

23. inflammation of the heart inner lining _____

24. vein inflammation _____

Matching Exercises

Match the disorder with its description.

_____ 25. congestive heart failure

_____ 26. congenital heart defect

_____ 27. aneurysm

_____ 28. varicose veins

_____ 29. cardiac arrest

a. stretching of vessel; especially near a valve
b. heart stoppage
c. heart cannot keep up with body's oxygen demands
d. bulging of arterial wall
e. patent ductus arteriosus

Match the sign or symptom with its description.

_____ 30. ischemia

_____ 31. angina

_____ 32. bradycardia

_____ 33. tachycardia

_____ 34. bruit

a. abnormally slow heart rate
b. pain
c. sound heard in a vessel as a result of turbulent flow
d. interruption of blood flow caused by an obstruction
e. abnormally rapid heart rate

Match the clinical test or diagnostic procedure with its description.

_____ 35. venography

_____ 36. angiogram

_____ 37. pericardiocentesis

_____ 38. echocardiogram

_____ 39. exercise

a. radiograph of blood vessels
b. phlebography
c. ultrasound of heart
d. monitor of heart rate, BP, and ECG, while on a tread mill
e. procedure for stress test extracting fluid from pericardial sac

Match the treatment with its description.

_____ 40. defibrillation

_____ 41. angioplasty

_____ 42. nitroglycerin

_____ 43. digitalis

_____ 44. vasodilator

a. vessel-dilating agent
b. sublingual vasodilator
c. surgery of diseased vessels
d. shocking the heart with a defibrillator to restore the regular heartbeat
e. drug that increases heart contractions

Definitions

Define the following terms.

45. hypertension _____

46. cardiology _____

47. angiogenesis _____

Alternate Terms

Give an alternate term for each of the following terms.

48. cerebrovascular accident _____

49. fremitus _____

50. left atrioventricular valve _____

51. myocardial infarction _____

52. right atrioventricular valve _____

Spelling

Identify the correctly spelled term in each set.

53. _____
    a. infarktion
    b. infarction
    c. infarckion
    d. infarcktion

54. _____
    a. cor pulmonale
    b. kor pulmonale
    c. cor pulmonole
    d. kor pulmunale

55. _____
    a. cardiac tampanade
    b. kardiac tampanade
    c. cardiac tamponade
    d. cardiack temponade

56. _____
    a. anurism
    b. aneurizm
    c. aneurism
    d. aneurysm

57. _____
    a. Raynawd
    b. Raynoe
    c. Raynaud
    d. Reynaud

58. _____
    a. angeeogenesis
    b. angiogenesis
    c. angiogeneses
    d. anjeogenesis

Unscramble

Unscramble the letters to form a medical term.

59. marthahyir _____

60. rumrum _____

61. sleup _____

62. roonyacr _____

Abbreviations

Provide the terms for the abbreviations and then define the terms.

63. RHD _____

64. CAD _____

65. ASA _____

66. DVT _____

67. CPR _____

68. PTCA _____

Analogies

Provide a medical term to complete a meaningful analogy.

69. Veins are to venules as _____ are to arterioles.

70. Aortic or pulmonary is to semilunar as bicuspid or tricuspid is to _____.

Short Answer

Answer the following questions.

71. Explain why there is a difference in muscle wall thickness between the left and the right ventricles. _____

72. What is the purpose of the flaps, or cusps, in the left and right atrioventricular valves? _____

73. A patient is diagnosed with tetralogy of Fallot, which is composed of four defects. List the defects and briefly describe what each means. _____

74. Identify which vein carries oxygenated blood and why it makes sense to refer to this as vein. _____

Arrange the medical terms so they describe the correct blood flow pattern in the body.

75. arteries   aorta   veins
    venules   capillaries   arterioles

heart → _____ → _____ → _____ → _____ → _____ → _____

76. left ventricle   left atrium
    bicuspid valve   lungs
    pulmonary arteries   pulmonary veins
    right ventricle   tricuspid valve

right atrium → _____ → _____ → _____ → _____ → _____ → _____ → _____ → _____
→ _____

77. AV bundle   AV node
    conduction myofibers   bundle branches

SA node → _____ → _____ → _____ → _____

Labeling

Label the structures in the following diagram.

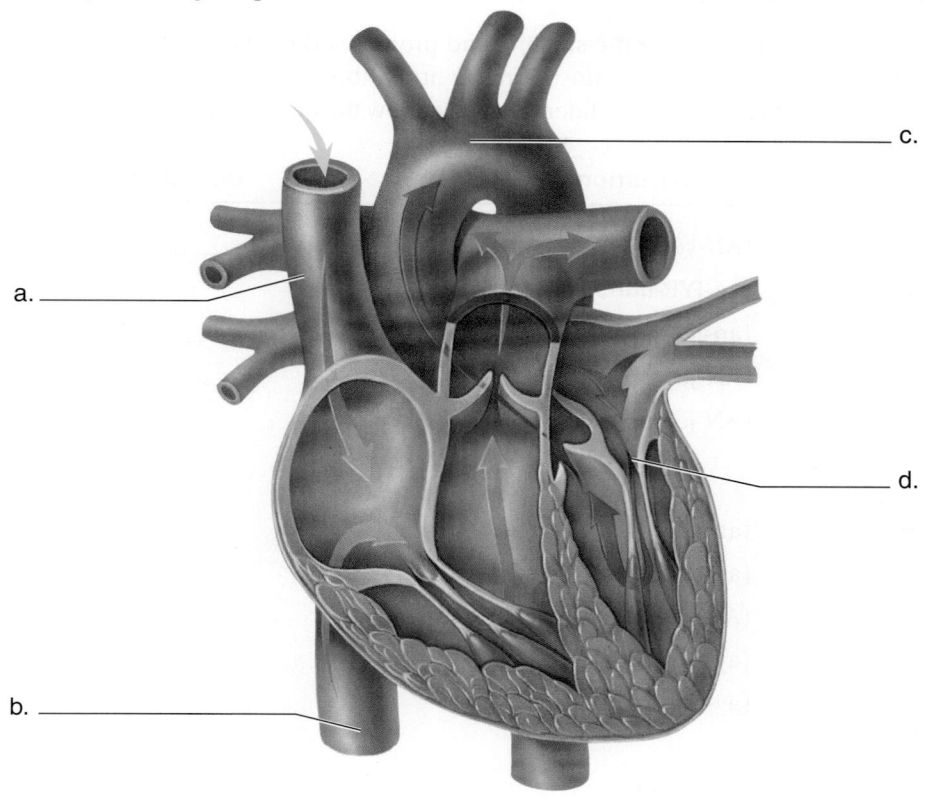

a.

b.

c.

d.

Word Search

Find the medical terms hidden in the puzzle.

D	Q	F	N	A	Y	V	H	U	H	D	A
T	T	E	H	R	S	H	T	E	S	Y	E
I	S	C	H	E	M	I	A	U	C	S	N
F	K	K	I	V	U	P	T	Q	B	P	P
B	X	E	H	R	S	I	C	A	C	N	O
B	X	D	B	K	M	E	W	L	O	E	H
L	E	N	Y	E	S	R	Q	P	E	A	T
A	I	D	R	A	C	Y	H	C	A	T	R
J	T	F	E	P	O	C	N	Y	S	J	O
D	I	A	P	H	O	R	E	S	I	S	H

bruit
diaphoresis
dyspnea
fremitus
ischemia
orthopnea
plaque
syncope
tachycardia

Vocabulary Review

Review the key terms from this chapter, study the spelling and pronunciation of each term, and write its definition in the space provided. Listen to the audio available for most terms at http://thepoint.lww.com/nath2e and pronounce each term for yourself. Then check the box when you feel confident that you know the definition and can pronounce the term correctly.

Key Term	Pronunciation	Definition
❏ aneurysm	(AN-yoo-riz-um)	_____
❏ angina pectoris	(an-JYE-nuh PECK-to-ris)	_____
❏ angiogenesis	(an-jee-oh-JEN-e-sis)	_____
❏ angiogram	(AN-jee-oh-gram)	_____
❏ angioplasty	(AN-jee-oh-plas-tee)	_____
❏ angiotensin-converting enzyme (ACE) inhibitors	(an-jee-oh-TEN-sin)	_____
❏ aorta	(ay-OR-tuh)	_____
❏ aortic coarctation	(AY-or-tick koh-ark-TAY-shun)	_____
❏ aortic valve	(ay-OR-tick)	_____
❏ aortoplasty	(ay-or-toh-PLAS-tee)	_____
❏ apex		_____
❏ apical heartbeat	(AY-pi-kul)	_____
❏ arrhythmia	(uh-RITH-mee-uh)	_____
❏ arteries	(AHR-tur-eez)	_____
❏ arterioles	(ahr-TEER-ee-ohlz)	_____
❏ arteriosclerosis	(ahr-teer-ee-oh-skle-ROH-sis)	_____
❏ arteriovenous fistula	(ahr-teer-ee-oh-VEE-nus FIS-tew-luh)	_____
❏ artificial pacemaker		_____
❏ atherectomy	(ath-eh-RECK-toh-mee)	_____
❏ atherosclerosis	(ath-ur-oh-skle-ROH-sis)	_____
❏ atria	(AY-tree-uh)	_____
❏ atrial septal defect	(AY-tree-ul SEP-tul)	_____
❏ atrioventricular (AV) bundle	(ay-tree-oh-ven-TRICK-yoo-lur)	_____
❏ atrioventricular (AV) node	(ay-tree-oh-ven-TRICK-yoo-lur)	_____
❏ atrioventricular (AV) valves	(ay-tree-oh-ven-TRICK-yoo-lur)	_____
❏ beta-adrenergic blocker	(ad-re-NUR-jick)	_____
❏ bicuspid valve	(bye-KUS-pid)	_____
❏ blood pressure (BP)		_____

Key Term	Pronunciation	Definition
❏ bradycardia	(brad-ee-KAHR-dee-uh)	
❏ bruit	(broo-EE)	
❏ bypass surgery	(BYE-pass)	
❏ calcium channel blocker		
❏ capillaries	(KAP-i-lair-eez)	
❏ cardiac arrest	(KAHR-dee-ack)	
❏ cardiac catheterization	(KAHR-dee-ack kath-e-tur-i-ZAY-shun)	
❏ cardiac conducting system	(KAHR-dee-ack)	
❏ cardiac cycle	(KAHR-dee-ack SIGH-kul)	
❏ cardiac enzyme test	(KAHR-dee-ack)	
❏ cardiac tamponade	(KAHR-dee-ack tam-puh-NADE)	
❏ cardiomyopathy	(kahr-dee-oh-migh-OP-uh-thee)	
❏ cardiopulmonary resuscitation (CPR)	(kahr-dee-oh-PUL-muh-nerr-ee)	
❏ cerebrovascular accident (CVA)	(se-ree-broh-VAS-kyu-lur)	
❏ chordae tendineae	(KOR-dee TEN-di-nee-ee)	
❏ circumflex-artery	(SUR-kum-flecks)	
❏ commissurotomy	(com-i-shur-OT-oh-mee)	
❏ conduction myofibers	(migh-oh-FIGH-burz)	
❏ congestive heart failure (CHF)		
❏ cor pulmonale	(KOR pul-mo-NAY-lee)	
❏ coronary artery bypass graft (CABG) surgery	(KOR-uh-nerr-ee AHR-tur-ee)	
❏ coronary artery disease (CAD)	(KOR-uh-nerr-ee)	
❏ coronary circulation	(KOR-uh-nerr-ee)	
❏ deep vein thrombosis (DVT)	(throm-BOH-sis)	
❏ defibrillation	(dee-fib-ri-LAY-shun)	
❏ diaphoresis	(dye-uh-foh-REE-sis)	
❏ diastole	(dye-AS-toh-lee)	
❏ diastolic blood pressure	(dye-us-TOL-ick)	
❏ digitalis	(dij-i-TAL-is)	
❏ dissecting aneurysm	(AN-yoo-riz-um)	
❏ diuretics	(dye-yoo-RET-icks)	
❏ Doppler ultrasonography	(DOP-lur)	
❏ dyspnea	(disp-NEE-uh)	

Key Term	Pronunciation	Definition
❑ dysrhythmia	(dis-RITH-mee-uh)	_____
❑ echocardiogram	(eck-oh-KAHR-dee-oh-gram)	_____
❑ electrocardiogram (ECG, EKG)	(ee-leck-troh-KAHR-dee-oh-gram)	_____
❑ endarterectomy	(en-doh-ahr-terr-ECK-toh-mee)	_____
❑ endocarditis	(en-doh-kahr-DYE-tis)	_____
❑ endocardium	(en-doh-KAHR-dee-um)	_____
❑ epicardium	(ep-i-KAHR-dee-um)	_____
❑ exercise stress test		_____
❑ false aneurysm	(AN-yoo-riz-um)	_____
❑ fibrillation	(fib-ri-LAY-shun)	_____
❑ Fowler position		_____
❑ fremitus	(FREM-i-tus)	_____
❑ fusiform aneurysm	(FEW-zi-form AN-yoo-riz-um)	_____
❑ heart		_____
❑ heart block		_____
❑ heart–lung machine		_____
❑ hemoptysis	(hee-MOP-ti-sis)	_____
❑ Holter monitor		_____
❑ hypertension	(high-pur-TEN-shun)	_____
❑ inferior vena cava	(VEE-nuh KAY-vuh)	_____
❑ ischemia	(is-KEE-mee-uh)	_____
❑ left atrioventricular valve	(ay-tree-oh-ven-TRICK-yoo-lur)	_____
❑ left coronary artery	(KOR-uh-nerr-ee)	_____
❑ lumen	(LEW-min)	_____
❑ mitral insufficiency	(MIGH-trul)	_____
❑ mitral stenosis	(MIGH-trul ste-NOH-sis)	_____
❑ mitral valve	(MIGH-trul)	_____
❑ mitral valve prolapse (MVP)	(MIGH-trul)	_____
❑ murmur		_____
❑ myocardial infarction (MI)	(migh-oh-KAHR-dee-ul in-FARK-shun)	_____
❑ myocarditis	(migh-oh-kahr-DYE-tis)	_____
❑ myocardium	(migh-oh-KAHR-dee-um)	_____
❑ nitroglycerin	(nigh-troh-GLIS-ur-in)	_____
❑ orthopnea	(or-THOP-nee-uh)	_____
❑ P wave		_____
❑ palpitation	(pal-pi-TAY-shun)	_____

Key Term	Pronunciation	Definition
❏ papillary muscles	(PAP-i-lerr-ee)	_____
❏ patent ductus arteriosus (PDA)	(PAT-unt DUCK-tus ahr-teer-ee-OH-sus)	_____
❏ percutaneous transluminal coronary angioplasty (PTCA)	(pur-kew-TAY-nee-us trans-LEW-mi-nul KOR-uh-nerr-ee AN-jee-oh-plas-tee)	_____
❏ pericardiocentesis	(perr-i-kahr-dee-oh-sen-TEE-sis)	_____
❏ pericarditis	(perr-i-kahr-DYE-tis)	_____
❏ pericardium	(perr-i-KAHR-dee-um)	_____
❏ peripheral vascular disease (PVD)	(pe-RIF-e-rul VAS-kew-lur)	_____
❏ phlebitis	(fle-BYE-tis)	_____
❏ plaque	(PLACK)	_____
❏ pulmonary circuit	(PUL-muh-nerr-ee)	_____
❏ pulmonary edema	(PUL-muh-nerr-ee e-DEE-muh)	_____
❏ pulmonary valve	(PUL-muh-nerr-ee)	_____
❏ pulse		_____
❏ Purkinje fibers	(PUR-kin-jee)	_____
❏ QRS complex		_____
❏ radionuclide scan	(ray-dee-oh-NEW-klide SKAN)	_____
❏ Raynaud phenomenon	(reh-NOH)	_____
❏ rheumatic heart disease	(roo-MAT-ick)	_____
❏ right and left bundle branches		_____
❏ right and left pulmonary arteries	(PUL-muh-nerr-ee)	_____
❏ right and left pulmonary veins	(PUL-muh-nerr-ee)	_____
❏ right atrioventricular valve	(ay-tree-oh-ven-TRICK-yoo-lur)	_____
❏ right coronary artery	(KOR-uh-nerr-ee)	_____
❏ saccular aneurysm	(SACK-yoo-lur AN-yoo-riz-um)	_____
❏ semilunar (SL) valves	(sem-ee-LOO-nur)	_____
❏ sequela	(se-KWEL-uh)	_____
❏ shock		_____
❏ sinoatrial node (SA)	(sigh-noh-AY-tree-ul)	_____
❏ sphygmomanometer	(sfig-moh-muh-NOM-e-tur)	_____
❏ stethoscope	(STETH-uh-skope)	_____
❏ superior vena cava	(VEE-nuh KAY-vuh)	_____
❏ syncope	(SING-kuh-pee)	_____
❏ systemic circuit	(sis-TEM-ick)	_____
❏ systole	(SIS-toh-lee)	_____

Key Term	Pronunciation	Definition
❏ systolic blood pressure	(sis-TOL-ick)	_____
❏ T wave		_____
❏ tachycardia	(tack-i-KAHR-dee-uh)	_____
❏ tetralogy of Fallot	(te-TRAL-oh-jee of fahl-OH)	_____
❏ thallium scan	(THAL-ee-um SKAN)	_____
❏ thrill		_____
❏ thrombophlebitis	(throm-boh-fle-BYE-tis)	_____
❏ tortuous	(TOR-choo-us)	_____
❏ transesophageal echocardiography	(trans-ee-sof-uh-JEE-ul eck-oh-kahr-dee-OG-ruh-fee)	_____
❏ tricuspid valve	(trye-KUS-pid)	_____
❏ valvular insufficiency	(VAL-vyoo-lur in-suh-FISH-en-see)	_____
❏ valvular regurgitation	(VAL-vyoo-lur ree-gur-jih-TAY-shun)	_____
❏ varicose veins	(VAR-i-koce)	_____
❏ vascular murmur	(VAS-kew-lur)	_____
❏ vasodilators	(vay-zoh-dye-LAY-turz)	_____
❏ vein ligation	(lye-GAY-shun)	_____
❏ vein sclerosing	(skle-ROCE-ing)	_____
❏ vein stripping		_____
❏ veins		_____
❏ venography	(vee-NOG-ruh-fee)	_____
❏ ventricles	(VEN-tri-kulz)	_____
❏ ventricular septal defect	(ven-TRICK-yoo-lur SEP-tul)	_____
❏ venules	(VEN-yoolz)	_____
❏ visceral pericardium	(VIS-ur-ul perr-i-KAHR-dee-um)	_____
❏ vital signs		_____

Answers

Word Grouping Exercises

Definition	Word Part	Definition	Word Part
heart	cardi-, cardio-	chest or breast	steth-, stetho-
artery, arterial	arteri-, arterio-	cord	chord-
atrium	atrio-	fatty, pasty materials	athero-
blood vessel	vas-, vasculo-, vaso-	lungs	pulmo-, pulmon-, pulmono-
breath, respiration	-pnea	pulse	sphygm-, sphygmo-
broad, wide	eury-	rapid, quick, accelerated	tachy-

Definition	Word Part	Definition	Word Part
slow	brady-	ventricle	ventriculo-
vein	phleb-, phlebo-	vessel, vascular	angi-, angio-
veins	veni-, veno-	wall of the body	parieto-

Word Building Exercises

Word Part	Meaning	Common or Known Word	Example Medical Term
angi-, angio-	vessel, vascular	angina	angiogram
arteri-, arterio-	artery, arterial	arteriosclerosis	artery
athero-	fatty, pasty materials	atherosclerosis	atherosclerosis
cardi, cardio-	heart	cardiac	cardiac
phleb-, phlebo-	vein	phlebotomy	thrombophlebitis
pulmo-, pulmon-, pulmono-	lung, pulmonary	pulmonologist	pulmonary artery
steth-, stetho-	chest or breast	stethoscope	stethoscope
tachy-	rapid, quick, accelerated	tachymeter	tachycardia
vas-, vasculo-, vaso-	small vessel, vascular	vascular	vascular

Key Term Practice

The Heart

1. myocardium
2. a. bicuspid valve; b. mitral valve; c. left atrioventricular valve
3. apex
4. epicardium
5. aorta

Blood Vessels

1. a. arteries; b. veins; c. capillaries
2. vein; artery
3. arterioles
4. venules

Cardiac Blood Flow

1. a. venae; b. cavae
2. pulmonary arteries
3. pulmonary veins
4. systemic; pulmonary

Coronary Circulation

1. coronary
2. angiogenesis
3. right coronary artery, left coronary artery, circumflex artery

Cardiac Conducting System

1. a. atrioventricular (AV) bundle; b. conduction myofibers
2. cardiac cycle
3. systole
4. diastole
5. SA node → AV node → atrioventricular (AV) bundle → right and left bundle branches → conduction myofibers

Blood Pressure and Other Vital Signs

1. sphygmomanometer
2. pulse
3. stethoscope
4. blood pressure
5. diastolic blood pressure

Congenital Heart Defects

1. tetralogy of Fallot
2. atrial septal defect; ventricular septal defect
3. electrocardiogram; ECG; EKG
4. aortoplasty
5. thrill; fremitus

Coronary Artery Disease

1. atherosclerosis; arteriosclerosis
2. plaque
3. coronary artery bypass graft surgery
4. angiogram
5. Vasodilators

Heart Disorders

1. hypertension
2. Cardiomyopathy
3. diaphoresis
4. cardiovascular accident (CVA)
5. Palpitation; fibrillation

Heart Disorders Associated with the Lungs

1. pulmonary edema
2. cor pulmonale
3. hemoptysis
4. Orthopnea
5. Fowler position

Inflammation Disorders

1. a. inner; b. muscle; c. around; d. heart; e. inflammation of
2. myocarditis
3. pericarditis
4. murmur
5. endocarditis

Shock

1. shock

Heart Valve Diseases

1. rheumatic heart disease (RHD)
2. valvular regurgitation and valvular insufficiency
3. mitral stenosis
4. sequela
5. commissurotomy

Vein and Artery Disorders

1. Phlebitis
2. Thrombophlebitis
3. vein stripping
4. arteriovenous fistula
5. bruit

Common Abbreviations Exercises

1. TIA = transient ischemic attack
2. millimeters of mercury = mmHg
3. CV = cardiovascular
4. MVP = mitral valve prolapse
5. PDA = patent ductus arteriosus

Case Study

1. b is the correct answer.
   - a, c, and d are incorrect because they are fictitious.
2. d is the correct answer.
   - b is incorrect because 90 is the systolic reading and 60 is the diastolic reading.
3. b is the correct answer.
   - a is incorrect because an ECG does not assess brain function.
   - c is incorrect because an ECG does not assess liver function.
   - d is incorrect because an ECG does not assess kidney function.

4. c is the correct answer.
   - a is incorrect because CK-MB is a measurement of the creatine kinase in muscle and brain, not the kidneys.
   - b is incorrect because CK-MB is a measurement of the creatine kinase in muscle and brain, not the liver.
   - d is incorrect because Mr. Tigress is experiencing hypotension.

Real World Report

1. Systolic dysfunction means that the contraction of the heart ventricles is not performing optimally. When systolic dysfunction occurs, the force of contraction that enables pumping of the blood through the systemic and pulmonary circuits is diminished.
2. a. diminished, slow, or below; b. motion or movement; c. diminished or slow motion or movement
3. a. bicuspid valve or left atrioventricular valve; b. There is little backflow of blood from the left ventricle into the left atrium, or the mitral valve prolapse is not significant.
4. a. around; b. heart; c. the presence of fluid and/or blood in the area surrounding the heart or in the pericardial space.
5. mitral valve, aortic valve, and tricuspid valve

Review and Application

1. d
2. a
3. b
4. a
5. c
6. b
7. c
8. d
9. a
10. c
11. b
12. d
13. b
14. a
15. d
16. c
17. b
18. c
19. d
20. thrombophlebitis
21. endocardium
22. myocardium
23. endocarditis
24. phlebitis
25. c
26. e
27. d
28. a
29. b
30. d
31. b
32. a
33. e
34. c
35. b
36. a
37. e
38. c
39. d
40. d
41. c
42. b
43. e
44. a
45. abnormally high blood pressure
46. study of the heart
47. formation of new blood vessels
48. stroke
49. thrill
50. bicuspid valve or mitral valve
51. heart attack
52. tricuspid valve
53. b
54. a
55. c
56. d
57. c
58. b
59. arrhythmia
60. murmur
61. pulse
62. coronary
63. RHD = rheumatic heart disease; valvular disease of the heart as a result of rheumatic fever
64. CAD = coronary artery disease; condition in which the myocardium receives inadequate blood supply
65. ASA = acetylsalicylic acid; another term for aspirin, a common drug taken to prevent heart attacks.
66. DVT = deep vein thrombosis; blood clot in a deep vein
67. CPR = cardiopulmonary resuscitation; emergency technique to restore the heartbeat and breathing by alternating chest compressions with artificial respiration
68. PTCA = percutaneous transluminal coronary angioplasty; procedure in which a balloon catheter is used to restore blood flow in a blocked vessel
69. arteries
70. atrioventricular
71. The left ventricle wall is thicker than the right because this part of the heart is responsible for pumping blood systemically (throughout the body), whereas the right ventricle merely has to push the blood to the nearby lungs.
72. The cusps prevent backflow of blood from the ventricle into the atrium.

73. (1) Pulmonary stenosis: narrowing of the pulmonary artery; (2) ventricular septal defect: an opening in the interventricular septum; (3) abnormal aorta positioning: abnormal position of the aorta over both ventricles; (4) right ventricular hypertrophy: enlargement of the right ventricle.

74. The pulmonary vein carries oxygenated blood. Veins carry blood to the heart, and the pulmonary veins carry the recently oxygenated blood from the lungs to the heart. This blood will then be sent to the rest of the body.

75. heart → aorta → arteries → arterioles → capillaries → venules → veins

76. right atrium → tricuspid valve → right ventricle → pulmonary arteries → lungs → pulmonary veins → left atrium → bicuspid valve → left ventricle

77. SA node → AV node → AV bundle → bundle branches → conduction myofibrils

   A = superior vena

   B = inferior vena cava

   C = aorta

   D = bicuspid valve

Word Search

```
+  +  +  +  +  +  +  +  +  +  D  A
+  +  +  +  +  +  +  T  E  S  Y  E
I  S  C  H  E  M  I  A  U  +  S  N
+  +  +  +  +  U  +  T  Q  +  P  P
+  +  +  +  R  +  I  +  A  +  N  O
+  +  +  B  +  M  +  +  L  +  E  H
+  +  +  +  E  +  +  +  P  +  A  T
A  I  D  R  A  C  Y  H  C  A  T  R
+  +  F  E  P  O  C  N  Y  S  +  O
D  I  A  P  H  O  R  E  S  I  S  +
```

bruit
diaphoresis
dyspnea
fremitus
ischemia
orthopnea
plaque
syncope
tachycardia

Vocabulary Review

Key Term	Definition
aneurysm	abnormal outward bulge in an artery
angina pectoris	radiating chest pain
angiogenesis	formation of new blood vessels
angiogram	x-ray of blood vessels after injecting a dye into the bloodstream
angioplasty	reconstructive surgery of diseased vessels
angiotensin-converting enzyme (ACE) inhibitors	drugs that act on the kidneys to decrease blood pressure
aorta	largest artery in the body that arises from the left ventricle
aortic coarctation	congenital narrowing of the aorta
aortic valve	valve between the heart and the aorta; also called the aortic semilunar valve

Key Term	Definition
aortoplasty	surgical repair of the aorta
apex	lowest, left-most heart point
apical	heartbeat heard at the apex of the heart
arrhythmia	irregular heartbeat
arteries	blood vessels that carry blood away from the heart
arterioles	smallest branches of arteries
arteriosclerosis	hardening of the arteries
arteriovenous fistula	direct connection between an artery and a vein
artificial pacemaker	electrical device that restores normal heart rhythm
atherectomy	surgical removal of a plaque deposit from an artery

Key Term	Definition	Key Term	Definition
atherosclerosis	plaque formation on the inner arterial wall	chordae tendineae	tendinous cords in heart attached to papillary muscles
atria	the two upper heart chambers	circumflex artery	vessel that supplies blood to the left atrium and left ventricle
atrial septal defect	abnormal opening between the atria that allows blood to shunt back and forth	commissurotomy	surgical opening of a narrowed heart valve
atrioventricular (AV) bundle	arises from the atrioventricular node and transmits impulses to the ventricle muscle fibers; also called bundle of His	conduction myofibers	heart cells that stimulate heart ventricles to contract; also called Purkinje fibers
atrioventricular (AV) node	conduction tissue that delays the heart's electrical impulses slightly	congestive heart failure (CHF)	disease in which the heart muscle cannot keep pace to provide the body with oxygenated blood
atrioventricular (AV) valves	valves between the atria and the ventricles; the bicuspid and the tricuspid valves	cor pulmonale	disease characterized by right ventricular hypertrophy (enlargement) caused by lung disease
beta-adrenergic blocker	drug that slows the heart rate	coronary artery bypass graft (CABG) surgery	surgery to create an arterial diversion around an obstruction in the coronary vessels
bicuspid valve	valve between the left atrium and the left ventricle; also called the left atrioventricular valve or mitral valve	coronary artery disease (CAD)	condition in which the myocardium receives inadequate blood supply
blood pressure (BP)	pressure exerted by the circulating blood on the arterial walls	coronary circulation	blood supply to the heart tissue
bradycardia	slow heart rate, below 50 beats per minute	deep vein thrombosis (DVT)	blood clot in a deep vein
bruit	abnormal swishing sound, caused by turbulent blood flow, heard through a stethoscope	defibrillation	shocking the heart with a defibrillator to restore the regular heartbeat
bypass surgery	operation in which blood flow is restored through the creation of a diversionary channel	diaphoresis	heavy sweating
calcium channel blocker	drug used to induce muscle relaxation and slow the heart rate	diastole	relaxation of the heart
		diastolic blood pressure	arterial blood pressure during ventricular relaxation
capillaries	small blood vessels that connect arterioles with venules and the sites of gas, nutrient, and waste exchange	digitalis	drug that increases the strength of heart muscle contraction
cardiac arrest	sudden stoppage of the heart	dissecting aneurysm	abnormal bulge between the layers of an arterial wall
cardiac catheterization	procedure in which a flexible tube is inserted into the coronary vessels via a peripheral artery or vein for imaging purposes	diuretics	drugs that increase urination
cardiac conducting system	electrical impulses that guide the heart to contract; also called the cardiac conduction system	Doppler ultrasonography	a noninvasive procedure that uses high-frequency sound waves reflecting off internal body parts to create images and assess blood flow velocity, direction, and occlusions
cardiac cycle	a complete round of heart contraction and relaxation; a complete heartbeat	dyspnea	difficulty breathing or shortness of breath
cardiac enzyme test	examines heart muscle enzymes to assess cardiac tissue damage	dysrhythmia	an irregularity in the normal heart rhythm
cardiac tamponade	heart compression caused by fluid accumulation in the pericardial sac	echocardiogram	image of the heart produced by ultrasound
cardiomyopathy	disease of the myocardium (heart muscle)	electrocardiogram (ECG, EKG)	record of the electrical activity of the heart
cardiopulmonary resuscitation (CPR)	emergency technique to restore the heartbeat and breathing by alternating chest compressions with artificial respiration	endarterectomy	atherectomy that includes removal of diseased portions of the arterial linings, leaving a smooth lining
cerebrovascular accident (CVA)	stroke	endocarditis	inflammation of the endocardium
		endocardium	membrane lining the inner heart

Key Term	Definition	Key Term	Definition
epicardium	membrane directly on the heart; also called the visceral pericardium	patent ductus arteriosus (PDA)	condition in which the ductus arteriosus remains open after birth, allowing oxygenated blood back into the lungs
exercise stress test	test that measures heart rate, blood pressure, and ECG while a patient exercises	percutaneous transluminal coronary angioplasty (PTCA)	procedure in which a balloon catheter is used to restore blood flow in a blocked vessel
false aneurysm	rupture of the arterial walls, causing swelling		
fibrillation	irregular, uncoordinated heart contractions	pericardiocentesis	drainage of the pericardial sac by a needle or catheter
Fowler position	semireclining in bed	pericarditis	inflammation of the pericardium
fremitus	palpable vibration caused by turbulent blood flow; also called a thrill	pericardium	membrane that encircles the heart
fusiform aneurysm	spindle-shaped outpouching on an artery	peripheral vascular disease (PVD)	progressive disorder caused by occlusions of the small arteries and arterioles that supply the extremities
heart	organ that pumps blood		
heart block	condition caused by an impairment of the conducting system	phlebitis	vein inflammation
		plaque	lipid deposits on the arterial wall
heart–lung machine	device that serves as artificial heart and lungs during some cardiac procedures	pulmonary circuit	circulation of the blood through the lungs via the pulmonary arteries and veins
hemoptysis	coughing up blood	pulmonary edema	fluid leakage into the lung air sacs caused by left heart failure
Holter monitor	portable device for recording an ECG over an extended time period	pulmonary valve	valve between the heart and the pulmonary trunk; also called the pulmonary semilunar valve
hypertension	chronic abnormally high blood pressure		
inferior vena cava	vein that empties the blood from the lower (inferior) portion of the body into the right atrium		
		pulse	palpable throbbing of an artery with each heartbeat
ischemia	inadequate supply of blood and oxygen to tissues caused by arterial blockage	Purkinje fibers	heart cells that stimulate heart ventricles to contract; also called conduction myofibers
left atrioventricular valve	valve between the left atrium and the left ventricle; also called the bicuspid valve or mitral valve	QRS complex	section of the ECG showing ventricular contraction
left coronary artery	artery supplying blood to the heart tissue	radionuclide scan	computer-generated images made using radionuclides injected into the bloodstream
lumen	space inside the tubular artery		
mitral stenosis	narrowed mitral valve opening that impedes blood flow	Raynaud phenomenon	artery and arteriole spasms in the fingers and toes causing cold, numb, and painful digits
mitral valve	valve between the left atrium and the left ventricle; also called the left atrioventricular valve or bicuspid valve		
		rheumatic heart disease	valvular disease of the heart as a result of rheumatic fever
mitral valve prolapse (MVP)	improper closure of the mitral (bicuspid) valve	right and left bundle branches	conduction fibers that originate at the atrioventricular bundle and separate along the interventricular septum
murmur	soft blowing or fluttering heart sound		
myocardial infarction (MI)	heart tissue ischemia; also called a heart attack	right and left pulmonary arteries	vessels that transport blood from the heart to the lungs
myocarditis	inflammation of the myocardium		
myocardium	middle layer made of heart muscle	right and left pulmonary veins	vessels that transport blood from the lungs to the heart
nitroglycerin	fast-acting vasodilator drug		
orthopnea	difficulty breathing except when sitting or standing straight	right atrioventricular valve	valve between the right atrium and the right ventricle; also called the tricuspid valve
P wave	section of the ECG showing atrial contraction		
		right coronary artery	artery supplying blood to the heart tissue
palpitation	fluttering heart		
papillary muscles	muscular projections that are attached to the chordae tendineae	saccular aneurysm	sac-shaped outward bulge on an artery

Key Term	Definition	Key Term	Definition
semilunar (SL) valves	valve between the heart and the aorta and the valve between the heart and the pulmonary trunk	**transesopha- geal echocar- diography**	ultrasound examination of the heart via an endoscope through the esophagus
sequela	disorder caused by a previous disease	**tricuspid valve**	valve between the right atrium and the right ventricle; also called the right atrio- ventricular valve
shock	condition resulting from inadequate blood flow through the body to nourish tissues	**valvular insufficiency**	disorder characterized by a leaky state of one or more of the cardiac valves that allows for backward flow of blood; also called valvular regurgitation
sinoatrial (SA) node	conduction tissue in the right atrium, where the heart's electrical impulses originate	**valvular regurgitation**	disorder characterized by a leaky state of one or more of the cardiac valves that allows for backward flow of blood; also called valvular insufficiency
sphygmoma- nometer	instrument used to measure blood pressure	**varicose veins**	knotted, swollen veins
stethoscope	instrument used to hear sounds within the body	**vascular murmur**	condition that originates in the blood vessels as a result of turbulent blood flow
superior vena cava	vein that empties the blood from the up- per (superior) portion of the body into the right atrium	**vasodilators**	drugs that widen blood vessels to de- crease blood pressure
syncope	loss of consciousness as a result of lack of oxygen to the brain; fainting	**vein ligation**	surgical tying of a vein
systemic circuit	general circulatory route of the blood throughout the body	**vein sclerosing**	surgical hardening of a vein
systole	contraction of the heart	**vein stripping**	surgical removal of a vein
systolic blood pressure	arterial blood pressure during ventricular contraction	**veins**	blood vessels that carry blood toward the heart
T wave	section of the ECG showing ventricular relaxation	**venography**	x-ray examination of the veins after injecting a dye that absorbs the x-rays
tachycardia	rapid heart rate, above 90 beats per minute	**ventricles**	the two lower heart chambers
tetralogy of Fallot	four congenital heart defects appearing together	**ventricular septal defect**	abnormal opening between the ventricles that allows blood to shunt back and forth
thallium scan	test that uses radioactive thallium to assess coronary artery disease	**venules**	smallest branches of veins
thrill	palpable vibration caused by turbulent blood flow; also called a fremitus	**visceral pericardium**	membrane directly on the heart; also called the epicardium
thrombophle- bitis	vein inflammation with thrombus	**vital signs**	objective measurements of key body func- tions, such as temperature, breathing rate, pulse, and blood pressure
tortuous	swollen and knotted		

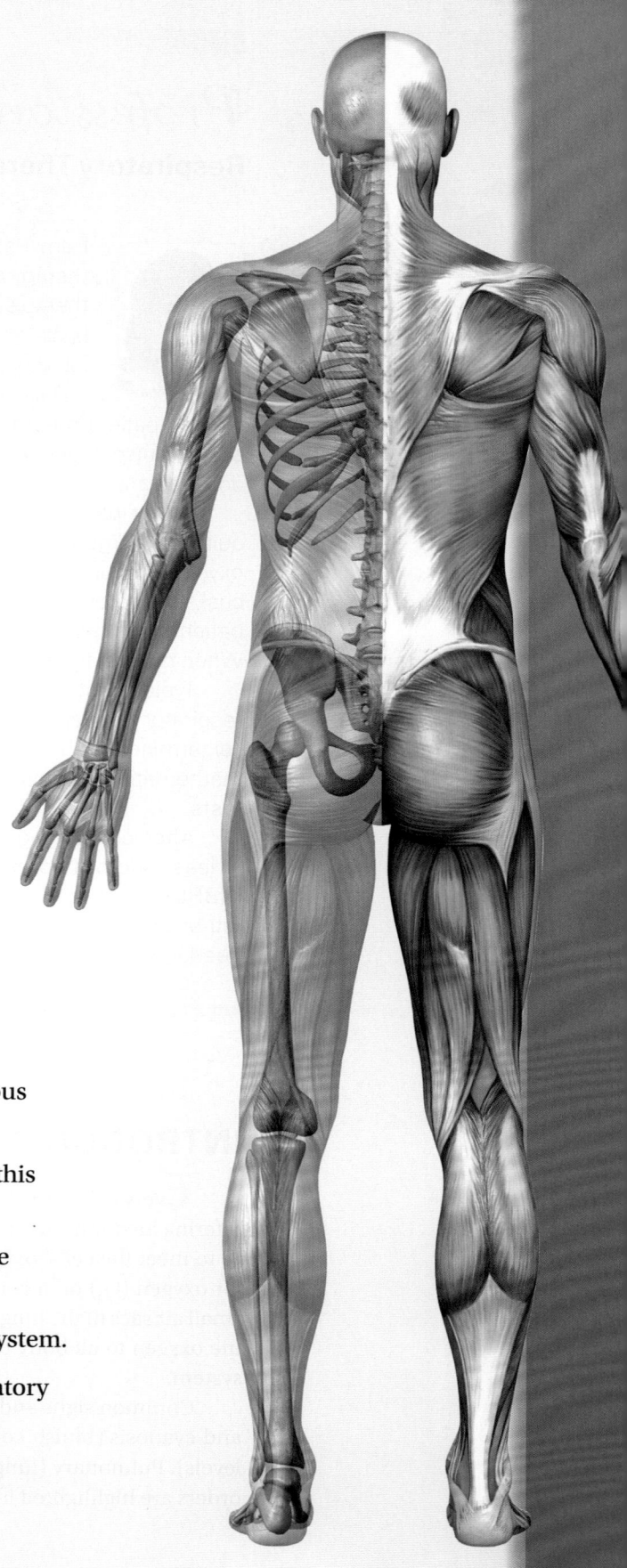

CHAPTER 12

Respiratory System

OBJECTIVES

After completing this chapter, you should be able to:

1. State the meanings of word parts related to the respiratory system.

2. Identify and label key structures of the respiratory system.

3. Explain functions of the respiratory system.

4. Describe how inhalation and exhalation occur.

5. Define terms for signs, symptoms, and treatments of various respiratory system diseases.

6. Define clinical tests and diagnostic procedures related to this system.

7. Describe changes in the respiratory system throughout the life span.

8. Define common abbreviations related to the respiratory system.

9. Define terms used in medical reports involving the respiratory system.

10. Define, spell, and pronounce the chapter's medical terms correctly.

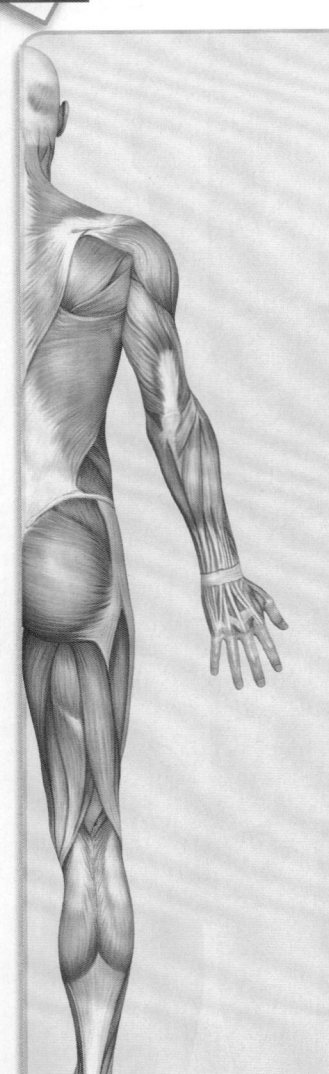

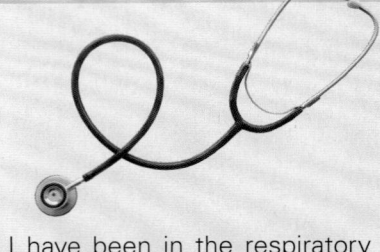

Professional Profile

Respiratory Therapist

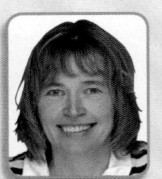

I am Pat, a respiratory therapist (RT). I have been in the respiratory therapy department of the hospital for 20 years. In addition to work as a therapist, my role has expanded over the past 2 decades from providing basic respiratory care to being in a supervisory position. Moreover, my job description has evolved to include cardiopulmonary and infant care.

Daily activities of work in a hospital include pulmonary function testing and patient breathing treatments. Spirometry and blood gas concentration analyses are also routinely performed. I use math skills daily for computing medication dosages and gas concentrations.

I treat patients of all ages with various types of disorders, including those requiring emergency care. Patients who need respiratory care are treated with oxygen, oxygen mixtures, chest physiotherapy ("poundings" or percussion to dislodge mucus), and aerosol medications. As an RT, I place Venturi masks and nasal cannulas on patients and monitor patients who are on ventilators that deliver pressurized oxygen. When making treatment decisions, physicians rely on the records kept by me as an RT.

Typical respiratory therapy programs take 2 years to complete. Along with focal respiratory therapy courses, other areas of study within the curriculum include medical terminology, human anatomy and physiology, chemistry, physics, microbiology, and mathematics. Respiratory therapy courses cover procedures, equipment, and clinical tests.

After completing the formalized education, as a prospective RT I had to pass at least one of two examinations offered by the National Board for Respiratory Care (NBRC): certified respiratory therapist (CRT) and registered respiratory therapist (RRT). Either one is the standard for licensure in many states, but the RRT certification is needed if the therapist is to become a supervisor.

INTRODUCTION

*E*very cell in the body requires oxygen. The main purposes of the respiratory system are filtering incoming air, transporting air from the environment to the lungs, and exchanging gases to meet the cells' oxygen requirement. The respiratory system trades carbon dioxide (CO_2) for oxygen (O_2) on a continuous basis (**Figure 12-1**). The capillary network that lies close to small air sacs in the lungs called alveoli takes up the oxygen. The red blood cells then distribute the oxygen to all body parts. Oxygen delivery is critical for normal functioning of every body system.

Common signs and symptoms of respiratory disorders are coughing, shortness of breath, and cyanosis (bluish coloration in the mucous membranes resulting from low blood oxygen levels). Pulmonary (lung) function tests and diagnostic procedures related to respiratory disorders are highlighted in this chapter.

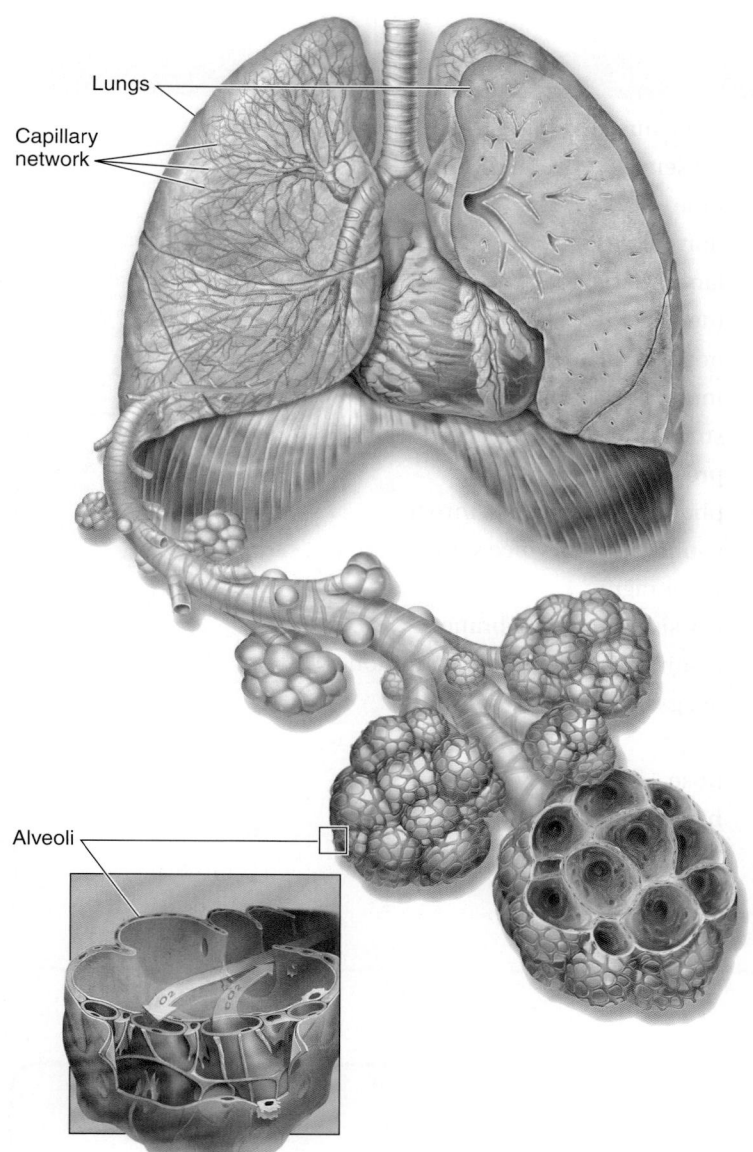

Figure 12-1 The respiratory system exchanges carbon dioxide (CO_2) for oxygen (O_2) on a continuous basis.

MEDICAL TERM PARTS

Word Parts

Medical term prefixes, suffixes, and combining forms related to the respiratory system are introduced in this section.

Word Part	Meaning
alveolo-	alveolus (air cell), alveolar
anthraco-	coal, charcoal, carbon
atel-, atelo-	imperfect, incomplete
brady-	slow

continued

continued from page 573

Word Part	Meaning
bronch-, bronchi-, broncho-	bronchus, windpipe
-capnia	presence of carbon dioxide
chron-, chrono-	time
eu-	normal, true
laryng-, laryngo-	larynx, laryngeal
muc-, muci-, muco-	mucus
nas-, naso-	nose, nasal
oro-	mouth, oral
orth-, ortho-	straight
oxy-	presence of oxygen
pharyng-, pharyngo-	pharynx, pharyngeal, throat
phon-, phono-	sound, speech, voice sounds
phren-, phreno-	diaphragm
pleur-, pleura-, pleuro-	rib, side, lung membrane
-pnea	respiration, respiratory condition
pneum-, pneumo-, pneumon-, pneumono-	air, gas, lung, breathing
pulmo-, pulmon-, pulmono-	lungs
rhin-, rhino-	nose
spir-, spiro-	breathing
tachy-	rapid, quick
thorac-, thoracico-, thoraco-	chest
trache-, tracheo-	trachea, tracheal

Word Grouping Exercises

Using the *Medical Term Parts* table, identify the prefix, suffix, or combining form for each of the following definitions. The first one has been done as an example.

Definition	Word Part
imperfect, incomplete	*atel-, atelo-*
air, gas, lung, breathing	
alveolus (air cell), alveolar	
breathing	
bronchus, windpipe	
chest	
coal, charcoal, carbon	
diaphragm	
larynx, laryngeal	
lungs	

continued

continued from page 574

Definition	Word Part
mouth, oral	
mucus	
normal, true	
nose	
nose, nasal	
pharynx, pharyngeal, throat	
presence of carbon dioxide	
presence of oxygen	
rapid, quick	
respiration, respiratory condition	
rib, side, lung membrane	
slow	
sound, speech, voice sounds	
straight	
time	
trachea, tracheal	

Word Building Exercises

Word parts introduced in the *Medical Term Parts* section are listed in the following table. For this exercise, first supply the meaning of each word part, then use the word part to build a word you already know. The word you list under *Common or Known Word* does not have to be a medical term; a commonly used word is fine. Be sure, however, that the word correctly reflects the intended meaning. The first one has been done as an example. Check your answers in a dictionary.

Word Part	Meaning	Common or Known Word	Example Medical Term
orth-, ortho-	*straight*	*orthodontics*	orthopnea
anthraco-			anthracosis
bronch-, bronchi, broncho-			bronchoscopy
chron-, chrono-			chronic
laryng-, laryngo-			laryngospasm
muc-, muci-, muco-			mucus

continued

continued from page 575

Word Part	Meaning	Common or Known Word	Example Medical Term
nas-, naso-			nasal cavity
oro-			oral cavity
phon-, phono-			aphonia
-pnea			apnea
pneum-, pneumo-, pneumon-, pneumono-			pneumonia
pulmo-, pulmon-, pulmono-			pulmonary
tachy-			tachypnea
thorac-, thoraci-, thoraco-			thoracentesis
trache-, tracheo-			tracheostomy

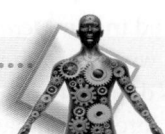

ANATOMY AND PHYSIOLOGY

Respiratory System Preview

The respiratory system has two portions: the upper respiratory tract and the lower respiratory tract (**Figure 12-2**). The upper structures are the nose, nasal cavity, paranasal sinuses, and pharynx. Lower respiratory structures include the larynx (voice box), trachea (windpipe), bronchial tree, and lungs. Consider the *L* as a memory aid: *l*ower structures begin with the *l*arynx and end with the *l*ungs. The mouth and nose are structures through which air is breathed. The **nasal cavity** is the space on either side of the nasal septum. The septum divided the cavity into halves. Four pairs of sinuses, air-filled cavities in the face and skull bones that open into the nasal passages, lessen the weight of the skull. The region between the mouth and the esophagus (tube for food, leading to the stomach) is the **pharynx**, commonly called the throat. *Pharynx* and *larynx* have tricky pronunciations. They are pronounced "FAIR-inks" and "LAIR-inks," respectively.

The **larynx** or voice box is the most superior structure of the lower respiratory system. The tube that conducts air from the larynx to the bronchial tree is the **trachea** or

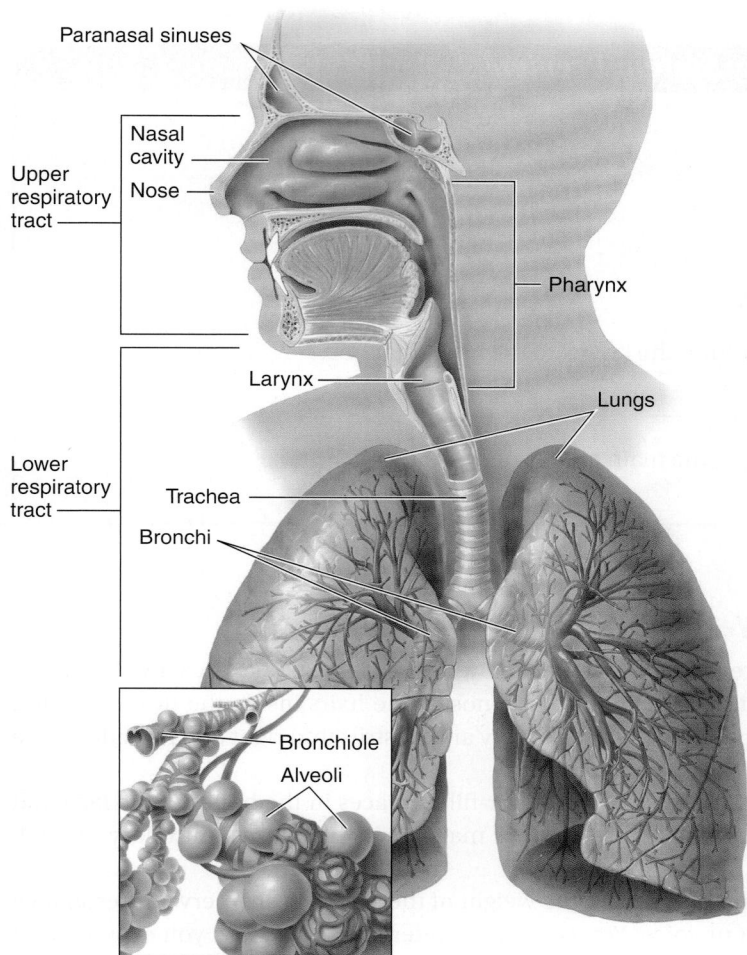

Paranasal sinuses

Nasal cavity

Nose

Upper respiratory tract

Pharynx

Larynx

Lungs

Lower respiratory tract

Trachea

Bronchi

Bronchiole

Alveoli

Figure 12-2 The structures of the upper and lower respiratory system.

windpipe. The **bronchial tree** consists of air-passage tubes leading from the trachea to the lungs. It begins with the left bronchus and right bronchus, which branch into smaller and smaller bronchioles in each lung. The right and left **lungs**, located in the rib cage, are the respiratory organs involved in breathing. Deeper in the lungs are the alveoli, where the oxygen you inhale diffuses into your blood, and carbon dioxide is removed from your blood.

KEY TERM	Definition
nasal cavity (NAY-zul KAV-i-tee)	the space on either side of the nasal septum
pharynx (FAIR-inks)	region between the mouth and the esophagus; also called the throat
larynx (LAIR-inks)	voice box
trachea (TRAY-kee-uh)	tube that conducts air from the larynx to the bronchial tree; also called the windpipe
bronchial (BRONK-ee-ul) **tree**	branches of the bronchi
lungs	organs of breathing

continued

continued from page 577

KEY TERM PRACTICE: *Respiratory System Preview*

1. What is the plural form for each given term?

  a. pharynx = _____

  b. larynx = _____

2. The word part *bronch-* means _____.

3. The _____ is a tube that conducts air from the larynx to the bronchial tree.

4. The space on either side of the nasal septum is the _____.

5. Gas exchange takes place in the _____, the main organs of breathing.

Nose, Nasal Cavity, and Paranasal Sinuses

The skull and facial bones are structures associated with the nose and nasal cavity. The **nares** (singular = *naris*) are nostrils opening out of the nose. Fine hairs inside the nose filter and screen particles. The wall separating the nasal cavity and nostrils into right and left sides is the **nasal septum**.

Paranasal sinuses, or **sinuses**, are hollow, air-filled spaces in the bones of the face that are lined with mucous membrane. There are four major pairs of sinuses: maxillary, frontal, ethmoidal, and sphenoidal (**Figure 12-3**).

The paranasal sinuses not only lessen the weight of the skull but also serve as resonance chambers for the sound of your voice. You can easily understand this when you experience a common head cold: When your sinuses are "plugged," your voice sounds different because the sound waves are not being conducted across clear air space. Instead, they travel through the fluid-filled cavities, creating a muffled sound.

The sinuses also drain mucus into the nose. If this drainage is blocked because of an infection or allergic reaction, the membranes become inflamed and swollen. Fluids build up and increase pressure in the sinuses, resulting in a sinus headache.

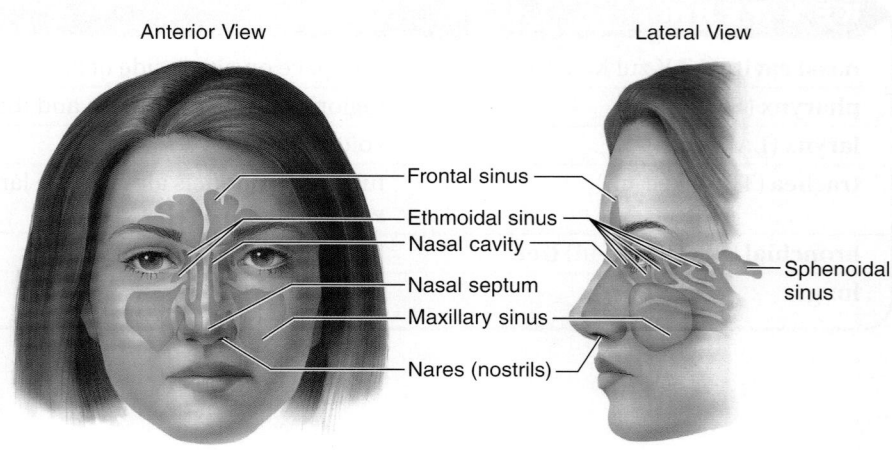

Figure 12-3 The nasal cavity and paranasal sinuses.

KEY TERM	Definition
nares (NAY-res)	nostrils
nasal septum (SEP-tum)	wall dividing the nasal cavity into right and left sides
paranasal sinuses (pair-uh-NAY-zul SIGH-nus-ez)	hollow, air-filled spaces in the bones of the face that are lined with mucous membrane; also called sinuses
sinuses (SIGH-nus-ez)	hollow, air-filled spaces in the bones of the face that are lined with mucous membrane; also called paranasal sinuses

KEY TERM PRACTICE: *Nose, Nasal Cavity, and Paranasal Sinuses*

1. What is the singular form for each given term?

   a. nares = _____

   b. sinuses = _____

2. This structure separates the nasal cavity into left and right sides. _____

3. Air-filled spaces within the skull and facial bones make up the _____, also simply referred to as _____.

Pharynx

The pharynx, commonly called the throat, connects the oral (mouth) and nasal cavities to the esophagus (tube that leads from the mouth to the stomach) and trachea. The pharynx is located behind the oral cavity and is the passageway for air to reach the trachea. Also part of the digestive system, it is a pathway for food from the oral cavity to the esophagus. The pharynx also aids in speech by forming vowel sounds.

From superior to inferior, there are three regions of the pharynx: nasopharynx, oropharynx, and laryngopharynx. The **nasopharynx** is the upper portion, and the auditory tubes open into this part. This explains why ear infections commonly spread to the throat and vice versa. The **pharyngeal tonsil**, also called the **adenoid**, is found on the posterior wall of the nasopharynx. The middle segment, located posterior to the mouth, is the **oropharynx**. It contains the **palatine tonsils**, often simply known as the tonsils. The lingual tonsil is at the base of the tongue. The tonsils are made of lymphatic tissue and play a role in immunity. The oropharynx functions in both digestion and respiration because it carries both food and air. The most inferior section of the pharynx is the **laryngopharynx** (**Figure 12-4**).

KEY TERM	Definition
nasopharynx (nay-zoh-FAIR-inks)	region of the pharynx behind the nasal cavity
pharyngeal tonsil (fuh-RIN-jee-ul TON-sil)	lymphatic tissue on the posterior wall of the nasopharynx; also called the adenoid
adenoid (AD-e-noid)	lymphatic tissue on the posterior wall of the nasopharynx; also called the pharyngeal tonsil
oropharynx (or-oh-FAIR-inks)	region of the pharynx located near the back of the mouth
palatine tonsils (PAL-uh-tine TON-sils)	lymphatic tissue embedded in wall of oropharynx; commonly referred to as the tonsils
laryngopharynx (la-ring-oh-FAIR-inks)	lower-most region of the pharynx located near the larynx

continued

continued from page 579

KEY TERM PRACTICE: *Pharynx*

1. The word part *naso-* refers to _____; so the region of the pharynx near the nasal passage is termed the _____.

2. The word part _____ refers to "the mouth," so the region of the pharynx extending from the oral cavity is the _____.

3. The word part _____ means "larynx;" therefore, the _____ is the region of the pharynx posterior to the larynx.

4. Provide the alternate term for adenoid. _____

5. Which tonsils are located in the wall of the oropharynx and commonly referred to simply as "tonsils"?

   _____

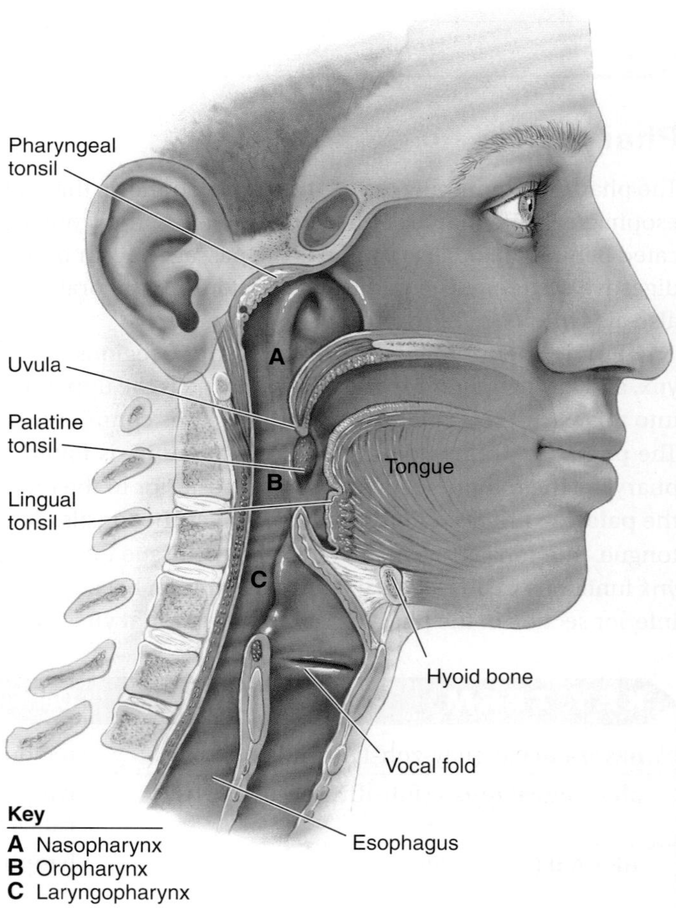

Figure 12-4 The pharynx, commonly called the throat, connects the nasal and oral cavities to the esophagus and trachea.

Key
A Nasopharynx
B Oropharynx
C Laryngopharynx

Larynx

The larynx, or voice box, is an enlargement in the airway between the pharynx and the top of the trachea. Associate the *l* in *l*ower with the *l* in *l*arynx to remember that the larynx is lower than (inferior to) the pharynx. It is often called the voice box because it contains the vocal

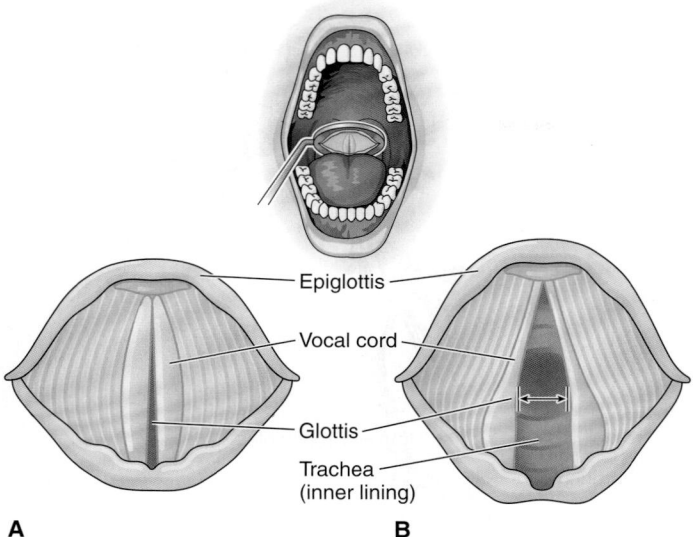

Figure 12-5 The vocal cords with **(A)** glottis closed and **(B)** glottis open.

cords. The **uvula** is a fleshy flap at the back of the oral cavity that hangs above the throat. Air enters the larynx through a slit-like opening called the **glottis**. A flap of cartilage known as the **epiglottis** protects the glottis. The epiglottis covers the glottis during swallowing to prevent food or liquids from entering the respiratory tract and the uvula helps prevent food from entering the pharynx too soon. It is interesting to note that it is physically impossible to swallow and inhale at the same time! The **vocal cords** vibrate to produce sound. There are two types of vocal cords: false and true. False vocal cords do not produce sound. True vocal cords vibrate to produce sound (**Figure 12-5**).

KEY TERM	Definition
uvula (YOO-vyoo-luh)	fleshy flap at the back of the oral cavity that hangs above the throat
glottis (GLOT-is)	a slit-like opening where air enters the larynx
epiglottis (ep-i-GLOT-is)	flap of cartilage that guards the glottis during swallowing
vocal cords	structures that vibrate in the larynx to produce sound

KEY TERM PRACTICE: *Larynx*

1. The slit-like opening where air enters the larynx is termed the _____, and the _____ is a flap of cartilage that protects this structure.

2. The structures capable of producing sound are termed _____.

3. The _____ is a fleshy extension that hangs at the back of the oral cavity above the throat.

Trachea and Bronchial Tree

The trachea, or windpipe, is a flexible tube extending from the larynx into the thorax, where it divides into the right and left primary **bronchi** (singular = *bronchus*). The trachea has approximately 20 C-shaped open rings of cartilage arranged one above the other to prevent collapse. The cartilage does not form a complete circle because the smooth esophagus (food tube) is

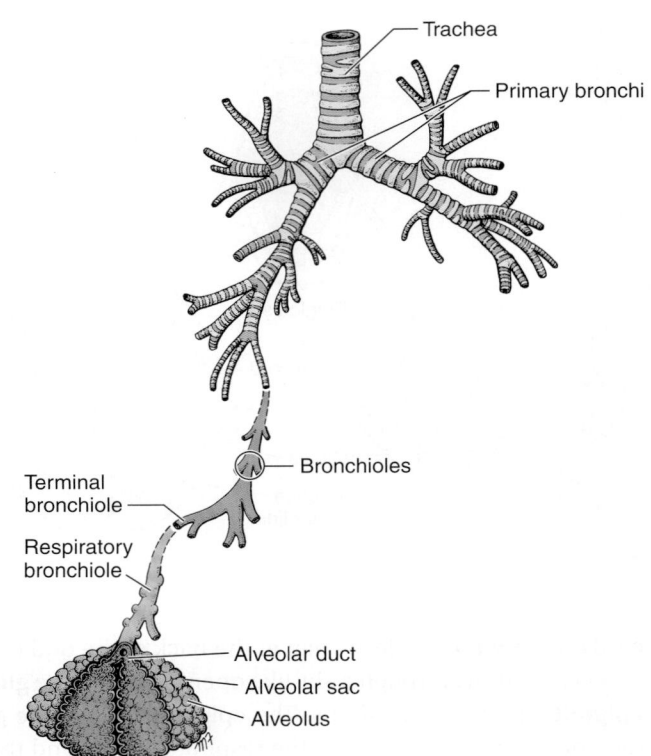

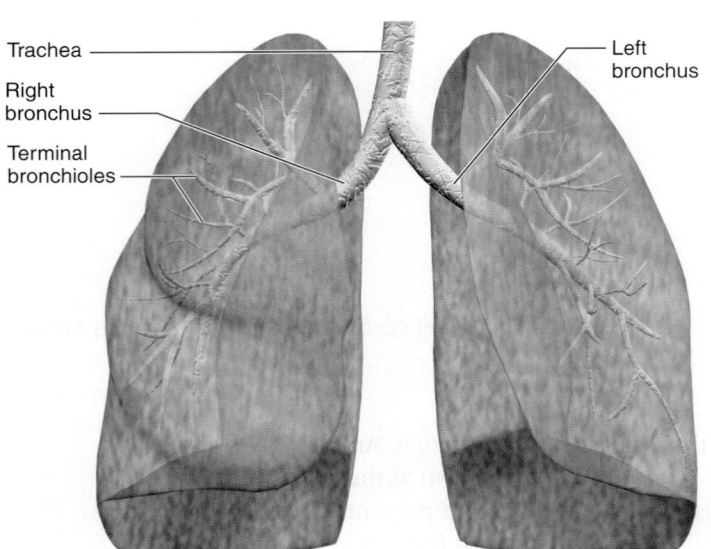

Figure 12-6 The structures of the trachea and bronchial tree.

Figure 12-7 The conducting airways are the primary bronchi, bronchioles, and terminal bronchioles. The respiratory airways include millions of alveoli.

nestled against it. Functions of the trachea include transporting air between the larynx and the bronchi and protecting the bronchial tree from inhaled particles.

The bronchial tree is the branched airway leading from the trachea to the alveoli (air sacs) in the lungs (**Figure 12-6**). The right and left bronchi are the main segments that branch into the smaller and smaller bronchi. The right bronchus is larger in diameter and slightly more vertical than the left. For this reason, an accidentally inhaled object is more likely to become lodged in the right lung than in the left lung. Bronchi eventually branch to form small **bronchioles**, which further subdivide into **terminal bronchioles**. The nasal cavity, pharynx, larynx, trachea, bronchi, and terminal bronchioles make up the **conducting airway**, or the parts of the respiratory tract that distribute air.

As the branching tubes become finer and finer, the amount of cartilage in them decreases and finally disappears in the small bronchioles to permit diffusion of oxygen and carbon dioxide gas across their surfaces. The terminal bronchioles connect with respiratory bronchioles, which mark the beginning of the **respiratory airway**. The respiratory airway ends in tiny air sacs, called **alveoli**, the sites of gas exchange between alveolar air and blood. Each lung has approximately 150 million alveoli. **Figure 12-7** shows the pathway of air through the lungs.

KEY TERM	Definition
bronchi (BRONK-eye)	the two main branches (left and right) off the trachea
bronchioles (BRONK-ee-ohlz)	small subdivisions of bronchi
terminal bronchioles (BRONK-ee-ohlz)	subdivision of the bronchioles

continued

continued from page 582

KEY TERM	Definition
conducting airway	respiratory structures involved with air distribution
respiratory (RES-pi-ruh-tor-ee) **airway**	respiratory structures involved with gas exchange
alveoli (al-VEE-oh-lye)	tiny air sacs in lungs where gases are exchanged between alveolar air and blood

KEY TERM PRACTICE: *Trachea and Bronchial Tree*

1. The first branches of the respiratory tree off the trachea are the left and right _____.

2. The _____ are the sites of gas exchange between the alveolar air and blood.

3. The _____ is the segment of the respiratory tract involved with air distribution, while the _____ is the segment involved with gas exchange.

4. _____ are respiratory branches coming between smaller bronchi and terminal bronchioles.

5. The _____ are located between bronchioles and alveoli.

Lungs

The lungs are paired, spongy organs of breathing located in the thoracic (chest) cavity. They are separated by the mediastinum. The lungs of an average male hold 6 L (6.4 qt) of air. The average female lungs can hold 4.2 L (4.5 qt) of air.

Two separate serous membranes, the visceral pleura and parietal pleura, enclose the lungs. The **visceral pleura** is an inner layer of serous membrane attached to the outside surface of each lung. The outer **parietal pleura** is a serous membrane that lines the inner wall of the thoracic cavity. These pleural surfaces are lubricated by serous fluid to reduce friction, and the interaction between these membranes is important to physical lung action.

Each lung is shaped somewhat like a cone, with the upper **apex** pointing to the first rib and the lower **base** resting on the diaphragm (breathing muscle). On the mediastinal surface of each lung is the **hilum**, a wedge-shaped depression. The right and left lungs are anatomically different because the heart occupies a portion of the left side of the body. The right lung has three lobes. The left lung is composed of only two lobes, and it also contains the cardiac notch, occupied by the heart (**Figure 12-8**). Alveoli are the basic functional units of the lungs because they are the sites of gas exchange. Alveoli are lined with epithelium that allows for the oxygen–carbon dioxide swap. In these tiny, thin-walled structures, oxygen leaves the lungs and enters the bloodstream, while carbon dioxide leaves the blood to be blown off when we exhale.

Surfactant is a normal lung secretion that prevents the alveolar walls from sticking together. In this way it helps to keep the alveoli from collapsing. Surfactant also makes it easier for the lungs to expand and contract.

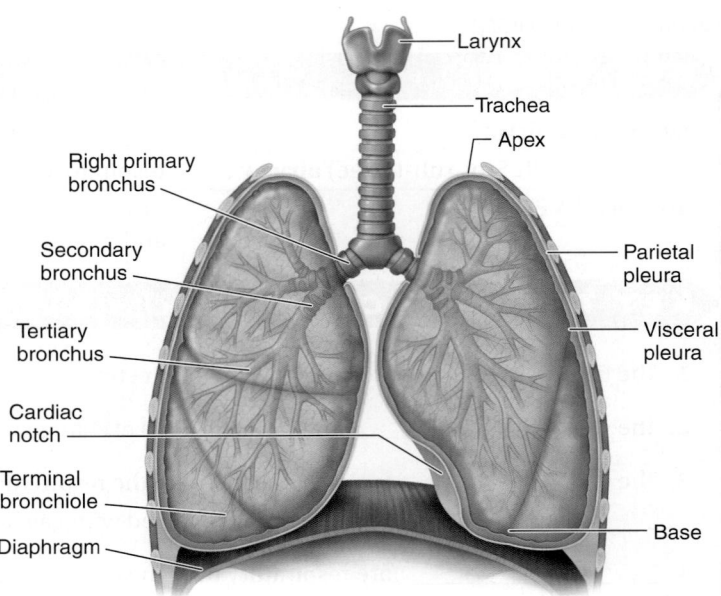

Figure 12-8 The lungs are paired, spongy organs of breathing located in the thoracic cavity.

KEY TERM	Definition
visceral pleura (VIS-ur-ul PLOOR-uh)	serous membrane on the lung surface
parietal pleura (puh-RYE-e-tul PLOOR-uh)	serous membrane lining the thoracic cavity
apex (AY-pex)	rounded top portion of lung pointing toward the first rib
base	lower part of lung that rests on the diaphragm
hilum (HIGH-lum)	wedge-shaped depression on the mediastinal surface of each lung
surfactant (sur-FACK-tunt)	substance that helps to prevent the alveoli from collapsing

KEY TERM PRACTICE: *Lungs*

1. The _____ pleura is the membrane directly on the lung surface, and the _____ pleura lines the thoracic cavity around the lung.

2. This part of each lung rests on the diaphragm. _____

3. _____ is a normal lung secretion that prevents the alveoli from sticking together and collapsing.

4. The _____ is a wedge-shaped depression on the mediastinal surface of the lung.

5. The rounded portion of the lung that points toward the first rib is called the _____.

Functions of the Respiratory System

The respiratory system delivers oxygen to cells via the bloodstream, while at the same time it removes the metabolic waste product, carbon dioxide. The respiratory system also maintains blood pH and acid–base balance. The pH is a measure of blood acidity or alkalinity, a critical factor for blood. Other functions are warming, moistening, and filtering incoming air. As part of filtering, particles are either expelled through coughing or sneezing or are swallowed.

Normal functioning requires inhalation and exhalation. You take about 24,000 breaths per day. Air intake through the mouth or nose for delivery to the lungs is termed **inhalation**, or *inspiration*. Breathing out is termed **exhalation**, or *expiration*. Exhaled air contains the waste products of cellular metabolism, mostly carbon dioxide.

The entire process of gas exchange between the external atmosphere and body cells is termed **respiration**. This process depends on **pulmonary ventilation**, the act of breathing using the lungs, which provides the necessary oxygen for respiration. From a strict biological perspective, respiration takes place at the cellular level and depends on ventilation, but the term *respiration* is often used synonymously with *breathing* (inhalation and exhalation).

Inhalation and exhalation result from changes in the size of the thoracic cavity. The **diaphragm** is a curved muscle that separates the thoracic cavity and abdominal cavity and is the main muscle of breathing. (When pronouncing the word, notice the silent *g*.)

During inhalation (breathing in), pressure inside the lungs and alveoli is reduced as the diaphragm moves downward, expanding the thoracic cage. Because the outside air has a greater pressure, the lungs expand.

During exhalation (breathing out), the diaphragm relaxes, making the chest cavity smaller and causing a decrease in lung volume. A relaxed diaphragm appears dome shaped, causing air to be pushed up and out.

Modified respiratory movements, also called nonrespiratory air movements, are actions that involve the respiratory system, but are not directly involved with breathing. Such movements include coughing, crying, hiccupping, laughing, sighing, sneezing, talking, and yawning. A cough, or **tussis**, is a rapid rush of air to remove the substance that triggered the cough. Sneezing clears the upper respiratory passages. (Particles from a sneeze fly at a rate of 103 miles per hour.) Hiccupping is the result of a spasm in the larynx that occurs from an abrupt, involuntary contraction of the diaphragm, which causes an intake of breath and closes the vocal cords. Yawning is thought to aid respiration by providing an occasional deep breath. During **eupnea**, or normal quiet breathing, not all alveoli are ventilated and some blood may pass through without being well oxygenated. This low blood oxygen concentration somehow triggers the yawn reflex.

KEY TERM	Definition
inhalation (in-huh-LAY-shun)	process of inhaling or inspiring
exhalation (ecks-huh-LAY-shun)	process of exhaling or expiring
respiration (res-pi-RAY-shun)	chemical processes occurring in tissues for gas exchange; commonly called breathing
pulmonary (PUL-moh-nerr-ee) **ventilation**	breathing, respiration
diaphragm (DYE-uh-fram)	curved muscle that separates the thoracic cavity and abdominal cavity
tussis (TUS-is)	cough
eupnea (yoop-NEE-uh)	normal breathing

KEY TERM PRACTICE: *Functions of the Respiratory System*

1. _____ is breathing in, and _____ is breathing out.

2. The medical term for breathing is _____, which is derived from the word part _____, which means "lungs."

3. The term for normal, quiet breathing is _____, derived from the word part _____, meaning "normal, true," and _____, which means "respiration."

4. _____ is the medical term for a cough.

5. The base of the lung sits on this main muscle of breathing known as the _____.

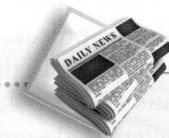

IN THE NEWS: Hypothermia and the Diving Reflex

It's a miracle! A young boy has an underwater accident while sledding on a cold winter day. After being submerged in icy, frigid lake water for over a half hour, he is rushed to the hospital, where he later recovers with no long-lasting damage. His is not an isolated incident; such cases have been reported for many years. What is preventing death in these near-drowning victims?

A person can survive immersion in cold water because of two factors: hypothermia and the diving reflex. Hypothermia sets in when the body loses heat faster than it can generate it. Hypothermia occurs in water 25 times faster than in air of the same temperature.

The diving reflex enables air-breathing, water-dwelling mammals—such as whales—to remain submerged for extended periods without surfacing for oxygen. In humans, the diving reflex is initiated when the body suddenly comes in contact with cold water. Immediately, blood flow is shunted to the vital areas of the heart, lungs, and brain and is shut off from the extremities and gut. Peripheral arteries constrict, the heart rate becomes bradycardic, and the oxygen supply to the heart and brain is enhanced. Laryngospasm protects against water inhalation. The cold water reduces the need for oxygen in body tissues. In warm water, hypoxia (inadequate tissue oxygenation) would lead to irreversible brain damage within 5 minutes; but in cold water, victims have survived hypoxia lasting 2 hours.

Investigations of near-drowning survival are based on documentation from available case studies, so data are limited. Although the relationship between hypothermia and the diving reflex remains unclear, it is known that an accident victim should not be considered dead until he or she is "warm and dead" because this phenomenon demonstrates that a cold body could be very much alive.

Pulmonary Function Tests

Tests can be performed to assess and evaluate respiratory function. The instrument used is a **spirometer** (Figure 12-9). The **pulmonary function test (PFT)** is a series of tests using diagnostic spirometry that determines lung volumes and capacities. These tests involve the person

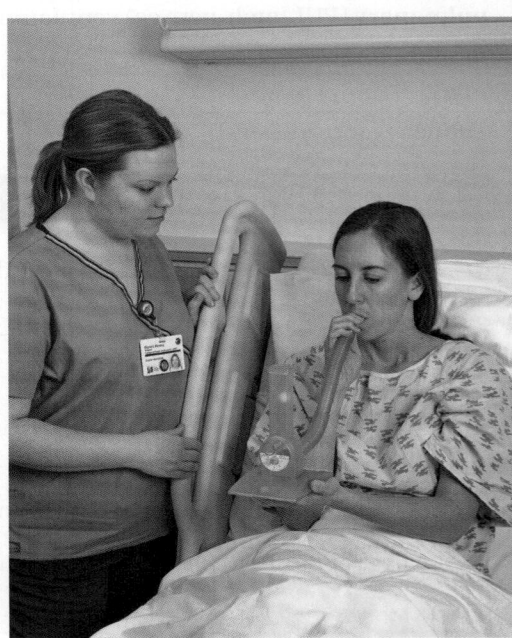

Figure 12-9 An incentive spirometer is a medical device used to help patients improve lung function.

directly and require active breathing. They are useful in diagnosing and determining the extent of pulmonary disease. They are also called ventilation tests.

Tidal volume (TV) is the volume of air that is inhaled or exhaled in a single breath. The volume of air that can be inhaled with forced breathing in addition to tidal volume is termed the **inspiratory reserve volume (IRV)**. The **expiratory reserve volume (ERV)** is the volume of air that can be exhaled during forced breathing in addition to tidal volume. **Vital capacity (VC)** is the maximum amount of air a person can exhale after taking the deepest breath possible. **Residual volume (RV)** is the volume of air that remains in the lungs after complete exhalation. **Total lung capacity (TLC)** is the total volume of air that the lungs can hold. Important values are identified in **Table 12-1**.

TABLE 12-1

PULMONARY VOLUMES AND CAPACITIES

Volume	Description	Average Value
Tidal volume (TV)	volume of air entering or exiting the lungs during normal breathing	500 mL
Inspiratory reserve (IRV)	volume of air entering the lungs plus the tidal volume during forced inhalation	3000 mL volume
Expiratory reserve volume (ERV)	volume of air exiting the lungs plus the tidal volume during forced exhalation	1000 mL
Vital capacity (VC) (VC = TV + IRV + ERV)	maximum volume of air that can be exhaled after taking the deepest possible breath	4500 mL
Residual volume (RV)	volume of air in the lungs at all times	1500 mL
Total lung capacity (TLC) (TLC = VC + RV)	volume of air that the lungs can hold	6000 mL

KEY TERM	Definition
spirometer (spye-ROM-e-tur)	device that measures inhaled and exhaled air volumes
pulmonary (PUL-moh-nerr-ee) **function test (PFT)**	evaluates and assesses lung function by measuring lung volumes and capacities
tidal volume (TV)	amount of air inhaled or exhaled in a single breath
inspiratory (in-SPYE-ruh-tor-ee) **reserve volume (IRV)**	amount of air that can be forcefully breathed in after normal inhalation
expiratory (eck-SPYE-ruh-tor-ee) **reserve volume (ERV)**	amount of air that can be forcefully expired after normal exhalation
vital capacity (VC)	amount of air that can be exhaled after the deepest possible inhalation
residual volume (RV)	amount of air remaining in the lungs after complete exhalation
total lung capacity (TLC)	total volume of air the lungs can hold

continued

continued from page 587

KEY TERM PRACTICE: *Pulmonary Function Tests*

1. The instrument used to measure pulmonary volumes and capacities is termed a _____.

2. _____ describes the amount of air moved in a single breath.

3. The maximum amount of air that a person can exhale after taking the deepest possible breath is termed _____.

4. _____ is the total volume of air that the lungs can hold.

5. The _____ is a series of tests that provide pulmonary volumes and capacities.

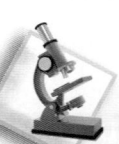

THE CLINICAL DIMENSION

Signs and symptoms of respiratory disorders are generally marked by abnormal breathing patterns, sounds, and mucus production; visible physical manifestations; and physiological alterations. **Auscultation** (listening to sounds made by the respiratory structures with a stethoscope) and **percussion** (tapping on the chest or back during auscultation to determine the presence of normal air content in the lungs) are commonly the first steps in diagnosing lung conditions (**Figure 12-10**). Treatment of respiratory disorders is aimed at increasing lung function and enhancing oxygen delivery or use. Common indications, tests, and treatments of respiratory system disorders are reviewed in this section.

Altered Breathing

Recall that normal, quiet breathing is called eupnea. The normal resting breathing rate for an adult is 12 to 20 respirations per minute. **Dyspnea** is shortness of breath, labored breathing, or difficulty breathing. **Bradypnea** is an abnormally slow breath rate, usually less than 12 breaths per minute. **Hyperpnea** is an involuntary, compensatory increased breathing rate to meet an increased oxygen demand. This deep, fast breathing is common after physical exercise. An abnormally rapid breathing rate is **tachypnea**. It is usually greater than 20 breaths per minute.

Figure 12-10 Locations for **(A)** percussion and **(B)** auscultation.

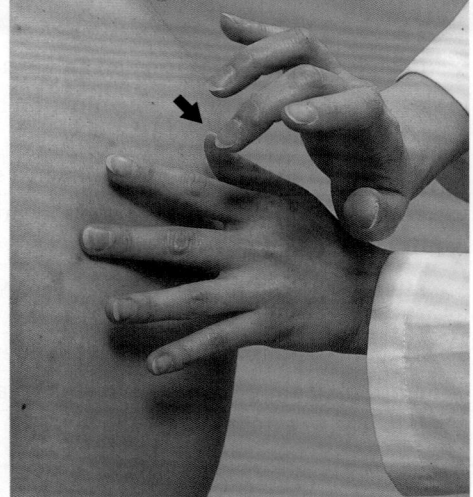
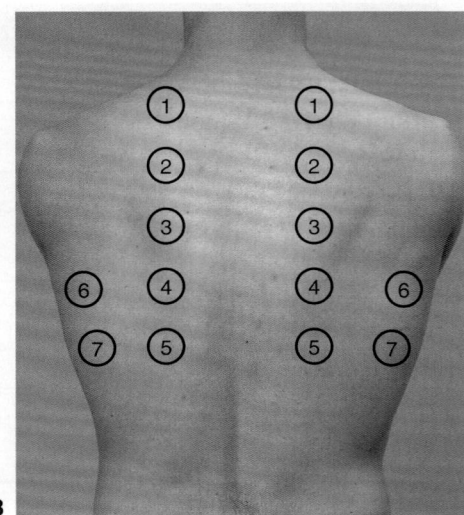

A   B

There are other terms associated with altered breathing resulting from abnormal gas levels. **Asphyxia** is impaired or absent exchange of oxygen (O_2) and carbon dioxide (CO_2) during breathing that results in suffocation. **Hyperventilation** is excessive inhalation and exhalation that leads to decreased CO_2 levels. **Hypoventilation** is decreased breathing rate that often results in increased levels of CO_2.

apnea	**Apnea** refers to the temporary absence of breathing, and several forms exist. For example, **reflex apnea** is the temporary loss of breath due to a sudden painful or cold stimulation to the skin. This is why an infant gasps after receiving an injection or a person gasps in response to the chill of a cold shower. **Sleep apnea** occurs during sleep and is associated with frequent awakening and daytime sleepiness.
Biot respirations	**Biot respirations** are an irregular breathing pattern represented by alternating periods of apnea with four or five breaths having the same depth. Biot respirations result from lesions in the respiratory centers in the brainstem.
Cheyne–Stokes respiration	An alternating pattern of apnea and deep, rapid breathing is termed **Cheyne-Stokes respiration**, after Scottish doctor John Cheyne and Irish doctor William Stokes. Cheyne–Stokes breathing is characterized by a cyclical pattern of breathing that completely stops and then returns to normal. It is commonly observed in comatose patients and often indicates impending death.
Kussmaul respirations	**Kussmaul respirations** are described as "air hunger" because the respirations are rapid and deep without pauses. They are characteristic of acidosis.

KEY TERM	Definition
auscultation (aws-kul-TAY-shun)	listening to body sounds using a stethoscope
percussion	tapping on the chest or back during auscultation to determine the presence of normal air content in the lungs
dyspnea (disp-NEE-uh)	difficulty breathing
bradypnea (brad-ip-NEE-uh)	abnormally slow breathing rate
hyperpnea (high-pur-NEE-uh)	increased rate and depth of breathing
tachypnea (tack-ip-NEE-uh)	rapid breathing rate
asphyxia (as-FICK-see-uh)	impaired or absent exchange of oxygen (O_2) and carbon dioxide (CO_2) during breathing that results in suffocation
hyperventilation (high-pur-ven-ti-LAY-shun)	excessive inhalation and exhalation that leads to decreased CO_2 levels
hypoventilation (high-poh-ven-ti-LAY-shun)	decreased breathing rate that often results in increased levels of CO_2
apnea (AP-nee-uh)	temporary absence of breathing
reflex apnea (AP-nee-uh)	sudden, temporary loss of breath; a gasp
sleep apnea (AP-nee-uh)	cessation of breathing during sleep that causes one to awaken and is associated with daytime sleepiness

continued

continued from page 589

KEY TERM	Definition
Biot respirations (bee-OH res-pi-RAY-shunz)	alternating periods of apnea with breaths of the same depth
Cheyne–Stokes respiration (CHAIN-STOKES res-pi-RAY-shun)	alternating pattern of apnea and deep, rapid breathing
Kussmaul respirations (KOOS-mawl res-pi-RAY-shuns)	rapid and deep respirations; referred to as air hunger

KEY TERM PRACTICE: *Altered Breathing*

1. The word part _____ refers to "slow," and the word part _____ refers to "respiration"; so, the term _____ describes a slow breathing rate.

2. The word part *tachy-* means _____, and the word part *-pnea* means _____; so, the term _____ describes a rapid breathing rate.

3. _____ is an abnormally slow and shallow breathing that leads to a buildup of carbon dioxide in the blood.

4. _____ is rapid breathing that leads to a loss of carbon dioxide from the blood.

5. The temporary absence of breathing is termed _____.

Cardiovascular Disorders Affecting Lungs

pulmonary embolism

A **pulmonary embolism** is a blood clot or mass that lodges in a pulmonary artery, obstructing blood flow. An embolism often originates in a deep vein and travels to the lungs (**Figure 12-11**). A common pathway is as follows:

leg vein → inferior vena cava → right atrium → right ventricle → pulmonary artery

Signs and symptoms include dyspnea, tachypnea, and chest pain. If the embolism is large, **cyanosis** (bluish coloration of skin and mucous membranes because of low oxygen levels), shock, or sudden death is likely. The clinical picture, rales (abnormal hissing), magnetic resonance imaging (MRI) studies, x-ray, or pulmonary angiogram diagnoses an embolism. It is important to prevent emboli in patients, especially those with thrombophlebitis or individuals who are immobile for long periods of time.

Rales are abnormal hissing, whistling, or rattling lung or airway sounds heard on auscultation. Although rales are subjectively characterized, they fall into categories such as coarse, medium, fine, moist (gurgling), and dry. Rales are the result of turbulent airflow. Oxygen therapy, mucolytics (mucus-thinning agents), anticoagulants, and thrombolytics (blood clot dissolvers) are prescribed.

Oxygen therapy involves oxygen being delivered by nasal cannula, Venturi mask, or an oxygen tent. A flexible tube inserted into the nostrils to deliver oxygen through the nasal passages is called a **nasal cannula**. A **Venturi mask** is a facial mask worn by the patient that delivers a precise, continuous high-flow oxygen mixture.

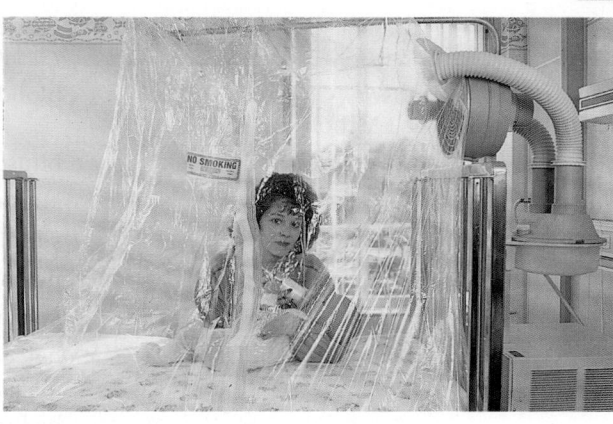

Figure 12-12 Infant in an oxygen tent.

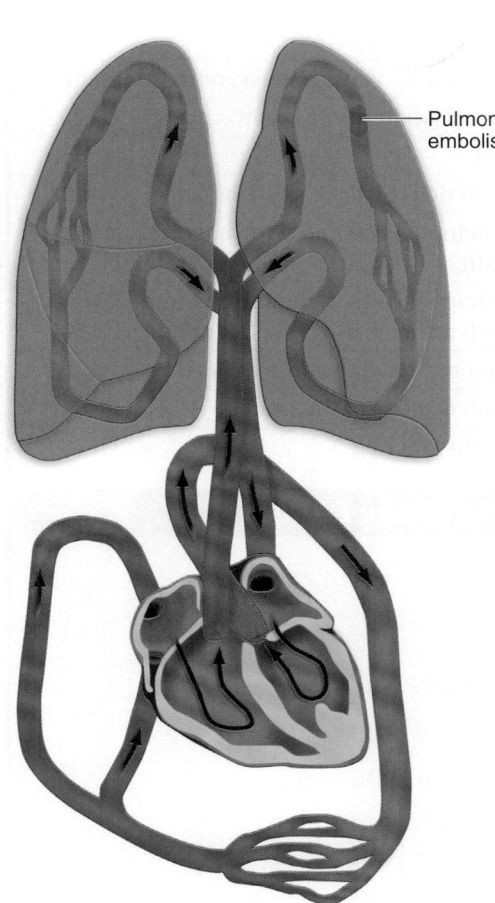

Figure 12-11 Pulmonary embolism. A common pathway for a blood clot to travel to the lungs.

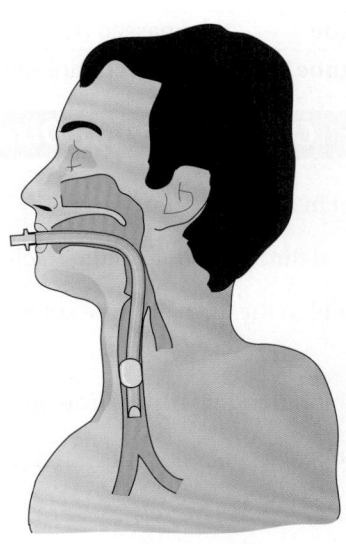

Figure 12-13 Endotracheal tube in place.

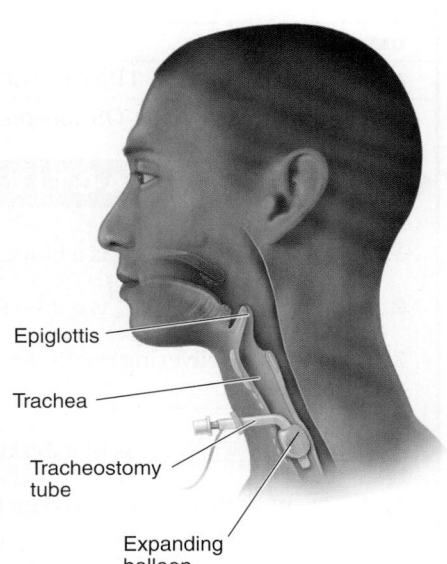

Figure 12-14 A tracheostomy tube is a flexible tube inserted into the trachea to deliver oxygen to the lungs.

A **resuscitation bag** is an inflatable, balloon-like device that can be attached to an oxygen face mask, endotracheal tube (see below), or tracheostomy tube (see below) to pump oxygen or air into the lungs. The bag allows for manual ventilation. A **nebulizer** is a device that delivers a fine mist or spray for inhalation drug delivery. It is also known as an **atomizer. Oxygen tents** are transparent, plastic tent-like structures that enclose a patient in bed while pumping oxygen into the enclosure to assist with breathing (**Figure 12-12**).

An **endotracheal tube** is a flexible tube inserted into the mouth or nose and passed through the glottis to deliver positive-pressure oxygen to the lungs (**Figure 12-13**). Trache tubes, as they are commonly called, are used to facilitate breathing during surgery or when respiratory assistance is needed.

A flexible tube inserted into a tracheal opening to deliver oxygen to the lungs is termed a **tracheostomy tube**. The tube is inserted inferior to an obstruction to effectively provide oxygen (**Figure 12-14**).

KEY TERM	Definition
pulmonary embolism (PUL-moh-nerr-ee EM-boh-liz-um)	blood clot lodged in a pulmonary artery
cyanosis (sigh-uh-NOH-sis)	bluish colored tissue due to a lack of oxygen in the blood
rales (RAHLZ)	abnormal hissing or whistling respiratory sounds
oxygen therapy	supplying oxygen via a nasal cannula, Venturi mask, or oxygen tent
nasal cannula (KAN-yoo-luh)	flexible tube placed in the nostrils to deliver oxygen
Venturi (ven-TUE-ree) **mask**	face mask that delivers oxygen
resuscitation (ree-sus-i-TAY-shun) **bag**	bag that is manually pumped to deliver air or oxygen
nebulizer (NEB-yoo-lye-zur)	device for administering medicinal liquid in the form of a spray to be breathed through the mouth or nose; also called an atomizer
atomizer (AT-uh-migh-zur)	device for administering medicinal liquid in the form of a spray to be breathed through the mouth or nose; also called a nebulizer
oxygen tent	structure that surrounds a patient in bed to supply oxygen
endotracheal (en-doh-TRAY-kee-ul) **tube**	tube passed through the mouth or nose to the trachea
tracheostomy (tray-kee-OS-toh-mee) **tube**	tube placed through a hole in the trachea

KEY TERM PRACTICE: *Cardiovascular Disorders Affecting Lungs*

1. A _____ is a blood clot in the pulmonary artery.

2. A _____ is a tube placed through a hole in the trachea.

3. A device for delivering medicinal liquid in the form of a fine spray that is inhaled is called a _____ or _____.

4. _____ is bluish skin coloration that results from inadequate oxygen in the tissues.

5. A face mask that delivers oxygen is known as a _____,

Cystic Fibrosis

cystic fibrosis   Cystic fibrosis (CF) is an inherited disorder of various glands resulting in the production of excessive, thick mucus, which ultimately obstructs the gastrointestinal tract and lungs causing infections. Pulmonary failure is the primary cause of death. The disease begins in infancy and childhood. Children are taught to pronounce this difficult term by calling it "65 roses."

Characteristics of the disease include pancreatic enzyme deficiency, progressive infectious pulmonary disease, malabsorption of nutrients, and elevated salt (sodium chloride) concentrations in the sweat. Chronic cough with purulent sputum (mucus that contains pus) is a primary sign. **Sputum** is thick mucus from the respiratory tract. It often contains a mixture of saliva, pus, microbes, and inhaled particles, which is **expectorated** (coughed up and spit out). Sputum is also commonly called **phlegm**. Labored breathing as a result of airway obstruction results in **hypoxia** (inadequate oxygen in the tissues), clubbing of fingers, and cyanosis. **Clubbing of fingers** is overly rounded fingertips resulting from long-term decreased oxygen supply to the extremities (**Figure 12-15**).

Diagnosis is confirmed by physical examination, family history, pulmonary function tests, tests measuring oxygen levels, chest x-rays, and sweat tests. The **peak expiratory flow (PEF) test** uses a peak expiratory flow meter

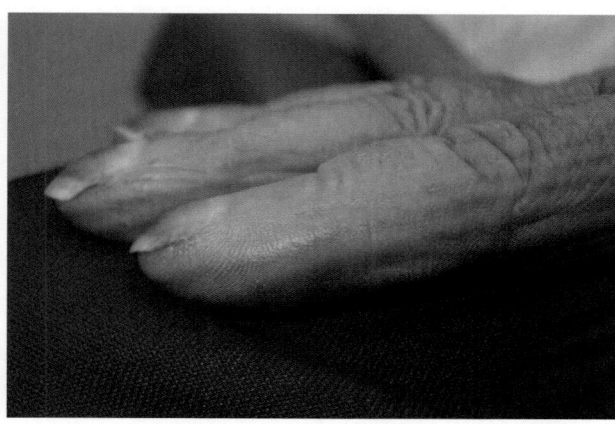

Figure 12-15 Clubbing of fingers results from a long-term decreased oxygen supply to the extremities.

to measure the volume of air after forced expiration. It is also used to monitor asthma and drug therapy in lung diseases. **Pulse oximetry** measures the oxygen in the blood using a photoelectric instrument called a **pulse oximeter**. The pulse oximeter is clipped to a fingertip or earlobe and is usually left in place on hospital patients so that oxygen levels can be continuously monitored.

Advances in research and an intense effort by the scientific community in developing new therapies have greatly increased the life expectancy of patients with CF. The management plan includes careful use of antibiotics to control pulmonary infection, aggressive chemotherapeutic pulmonary measures to thin mucous secretions, postural drainage to evacuate excess mucus (see below), a flutter device to loosen mucous secretions in the lungs, oxygen infusion to inflate the lungs, and—as a last resort—lung transplantation.

Noninvasive measures can assist with breathing. **Postural drainage (PD)** involves positioning the body in various poses to allow gravity to move secretions out of the lungs to be coughed out (**Figure 12-16**). Percussion often accompanies postural drainage poses. This form of percussion involves cupping the hands and striking the chest and back over the lung fields to loosen mucus so it can be expectorated. Percussions are commonly called "poundings." A recent innovation, the therapy vest, increases the efficacy of displacing the mucus from more areas of the lung fields.

KEY TERM	Definition
cystic fibrosis (SIS-tick figh-BROH-sis)	inherited disorder characterized by thick mucous secretions that block the internal passages, including the lungs
sputum (SPEW-tum)	fluid or semifluid mucus mixture; also called phlegm
expectorated (eck-speck-toh-RATE-ed)	coughed up and spit out
phlegm (FLEM)	fluid or semifluid mucus mixture; also called sputum
hypoxia (high-POCK-see-uh)	inadequate oxygen in the tissues
clubbing of fingers	fingertips that are rounded like a club as a result of chronic inadequate oxygen delivery to the tissues
peak expiratory (eck-SPYE-ruh-tor-ee) **flow (PEF) test**	uses a PEF meter to measure the volume of air after forced expiration
pulse oximetry (ock-SIM-e-tree)	measurement of oxygen in the blood
pulse oximeter (ock-SIM-e-tur)	small instrument that measures the amount of oxygen in blood
postural (POS-chur-ul) **drainage (PD)**	positioning the body to allow gravity to drain mucus from areas of the lungs

continued

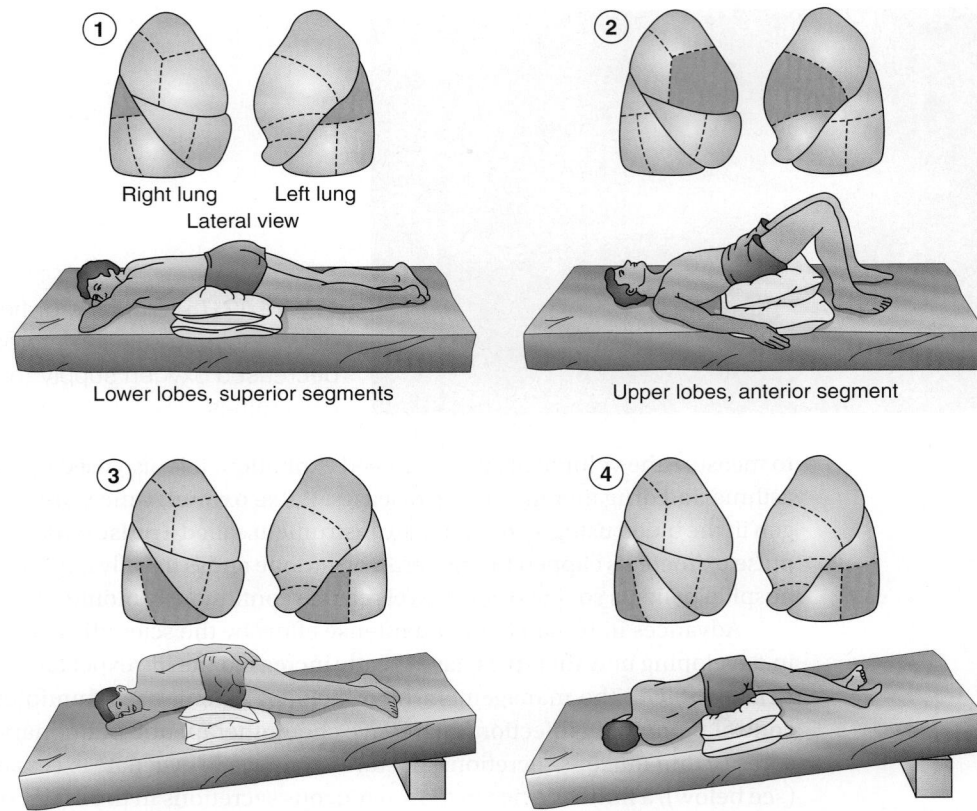

Figure 12-16 Postural drainage positions and the areas of lung drained by each position.

Right lung Left lung
Lateral view

Lower lobes, superior segments

Upper lobes, anterior segment

Lower lobes, anterior basal segment

Upper lobes, lateral basal segment

continued from page 593

KEY TERM PRACTICE: *Cystic Fibrosis*

1. The word part _____ means "below normal"; and inadequate oxygen in the tissues is termed _____.

2. An inherited disorder characterized by abnormal mucus production that clogs airways is termed _____.

3. _____ is a measurement of oxygen in the blood using a device clamped on the patient's finger.

4. To _____ is to cough something up from the airways and spit it out.

5. A fluid or semifluid mixture coughed up from the lungs is called _____ or _____.

Chronic Obstructive Pulmonary Disease

chronic obstructive pulmonary disease (COPD)

Chronic obstructive pulmonary disease (COPD) is a general term describing various lung diseases with permanent or temporary narrowing of the small bronchi, including bronchiectasis, bronchitis, emphysema, and asthma (discussed in the next section). In all cases, gas exchange is inadequate due to the inability to freely ventilate the lungs. COPDs tend to be progressive and irreversible.

bronchiectasis   Bronchiectasis is chronic dilation of the respiratory passages, causing tussis and excessive mucus production. It is characterized by sac-shaped or tubular dilation of the bronchus or bronchi resulting from obstruction and infection. It takes several years to develop and is caused by smoking, obstruction, or corrosive gas inhalation. Other signs include mucopurulent (mucus with pus) sputum, hemoptysis (coughing up blood or bloody mucus), and recurrent pneumonia. The history and physical examination, x-rays, computerized tomography (CT) scans, bronchoscopy, sputum culture, and pulmonary function tests diagnose bronchiectasis.

Bronchoscopy uses a thin, lighted instrument called a **bronchoscope**, which is inserted into the mouth and down the trachea to the bronchi, enabling the clinician to visually inspect the structures (**Figure 12-17**). If necessary, lung tissue can be removed (**lung biopsy**) or other foreign matter can be extracted for evaluation. Lung biopsies are used to test for pathology. Bronchodilators, postural drainage, and avoidance of irritants are treatment options. **Bronchodilators** are drugs that ease breathing by relaxing the air passages.

bronchitis   **Bronchitis** is inflammation of the bronchial mucous membranes, causing breathing problems and coughing episodes. Two forms exist: acute and chronic. **Acute bronchitis** is characterized by a sharp, rapid onset with a short duration. Infectious agents in the lower respiratory tract cause it. Signs and symptoms include cough, variable sputum production, fever, soreness beneath the sternum, and rales. The symptoms subside within 1 week, but the cough persists for 2 to 3 weeks.

Chronic bronchitis is long lasting and is typified by excessive mucus secretion with chronic, productive (sputum-producing) cough (**Figure 12-18**). It can lead to asthma and often occurs with emphysema,

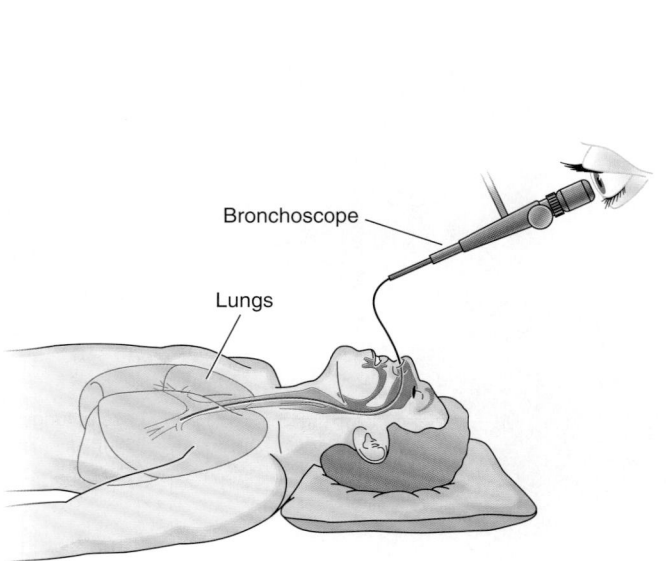

Figure 12-17 Bronchoscopy allows for visualization of respiratory structures.

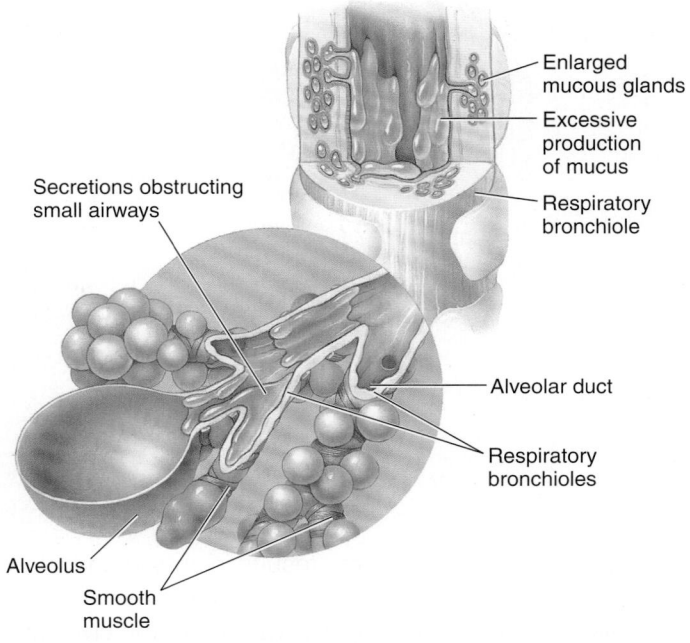

Figure 12-18 Mucus buildup in bronchitis.

tuberculosis, and heart failure. Signs and symptoms of all forms include dyspnea, wheezing (breathing with a whistling sound), fever, and cough. Bronchitis is diagnosed by the clinical picture, x-ray studies of the lungs, pulmonary function tests, and blood/sputum analyses. Treatment options include increasing fluid intake, humidifying rooms, using bronchodilators, and smoking cessation.

emphysema

Emphysema involves an anatomical alteration of the lungs characterized by enlarged air sacs and destructive changes to the alveolar walls (**Figure 12-19**). The deterioration of the alveoli leads to loss of elasticity, which is the loss of their ability to spring back to their original shape. Breathing and gas exchange are hindered. Signs and symptoms include gradual breathing difficulty, dyspnea, tachypnea, wheezing, persistent cough, reduced ability to exhale air, rhonchi (coarse rales), and inflated lungs at the end of exhalation. Progression of the disease is marked by a **barrel chest** (increased chest size, resembling a barrel shape), cyanosis surrounding the mouth, and right ventricular heart failure.

Long-term cigarette smoking, repeated respiratory infections, exposure to environmental hazards, or α_1-antitrypsin (α_1-antiprotease) deficiency are causes. Diagnosis is made by clinical history and physical examination, pulmonary function tests (PFTs), and x-rays. Radiographic studies show translucent-appearing lungs, flattened diaphragm, and cardiomegaly (enlarged heart). Treatments include smoking cessation, increased protein intake, vitamin supplements, oxygen therapy, bronchodilators, and possible prophylactic (preventive) antibiotics. Emphysema is a frequent cause of death in smokers.

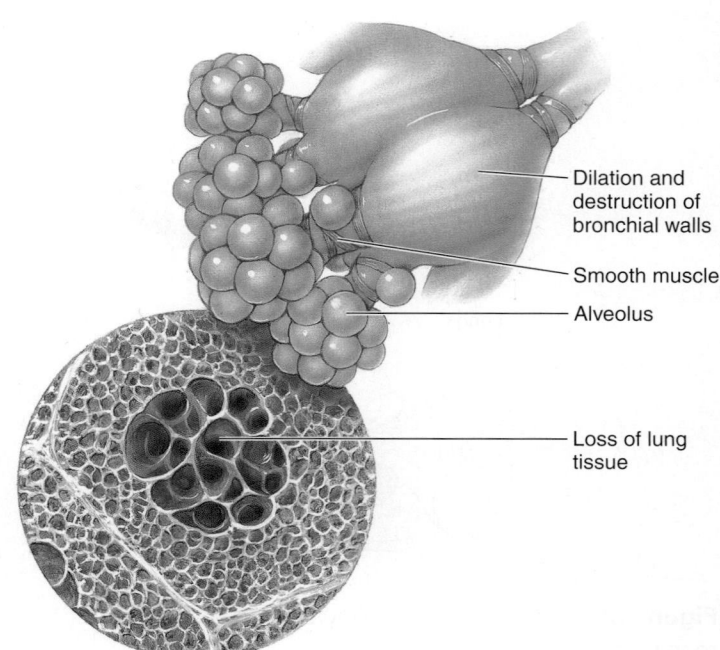

Dilation and destruction of bronchial walls

Smooth muscle

Alveolus

Loss of lung tissue

Figure 12-19 Emphysema results in an anatomical alteration of the lungs, characterized by air sac enlargement and destructive changes to the alveolar walls, leading to loss of elasticity.

KEY TERM	Definition
chronic obstructive pulmonary (PUL-moh-nerr-ee) **disease (COPD)**	general term describing lung disease affecting the bronchial tree
bronchiectasis (bronk-ee-ECK-tuh-sis)	chronic dilation of the airways
mucopurulent (mew-koh-PEW-roo-lunt)	pertaining to mucus with pus
hemoptysis (hee-MOP-ti-sis)	coughing up blood or bloody mucus
bronchoscopy (brong-KOS-kuh-pee)	procedure for viewing the inside of the respiratory structures using a bronchoscope
bronchoscope (BRONK-oh-skope)	thin, lighted instrument used to view respiratory structures during a bronchoscopy
lung biopsy (BYE-op-see)	removal of lung tissue for diagnostic evaluation
bronchodilators (bronk-oh-DYE-lay-turz)	drugs that ease breathing by relaxing the air passages
bronchitis (bron-KIGH-tis)	inflammation of the bronchial tubes
acute bronchitis (bron-KIGH-tis)	sudden and short-lasting inflammation of the bronchial tubes
chronic bronchitis (bron-KIGH-tis)	long-lasting inflammation of the bronchial tubes
emphysema (em-fi-SEE-muh)	chronic lung disorder characterized by enlarged air sacs
barrel chest	abnormal rounded chest cavity

KEY TERM PRACTICE: *Chronic Obstructive Pulmonary Disease*

1. The word part _____ refers to "the bronchus," and _____ is the suffix for "inflammation"; therefore, the term _____ describes *inflammation of the bronchial passages*.

2. Short-term bronchial inflammation is termed _____, and long-term bronchial inflammation is known as _____.

3. The coughing up of blood or mucus containing blood is termed _____.

4. A _____ is the removal of lung tissue for diagnostic evaluation.

5. _____ is a chronic disorder characterized by enlarged air sacs that results in breathing impairment.

Asthma

Asthma **Asthma** is a disease of the respiratory system caused by an allergic reaction or other form of hypersensitivity in the airways. The condition is characterized by the narrowing and constriction of the air passages (**Figure 12-20**). Signs and symptoms include coughing, chest tightness, dyspnea, shallow respirations, rhonchi, wheezing, bronchospasms, and mucus production. A harsh rattling sound caused by a partially obstructed airway is referred to as a **rhonchus** (plural = *rhonchi*). A **wheeze** is a whistling or sighing noise that indicates mucus buildup. Some wheezes can be heard without a stethoscope. A **bronchospasm** is contraction of smooth muscle in the walls of the bronchi and bronchioles, causing narrowing of the bronchial tubes. Individuals with asthma have greater difficulty exhaling than inhaling.

Asthma may have a hereditary component. Asthma is diagnosed by pulmonary function tests, peak airflow measurements, history, and physical examination. **Bronchial asthma** is characterized by attacks of dyspnea and bronchial tube spasms. It is frequently caused by an allergic reaction and results in partial

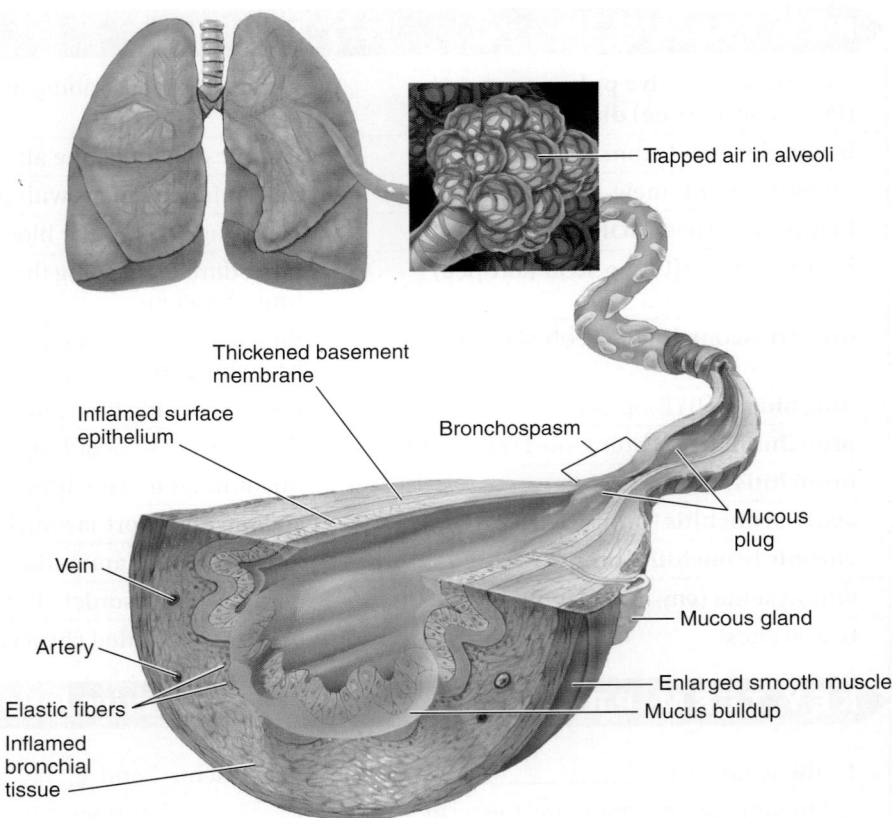

Trapped air in alveoli

Thickened basement membrane

Inflamed surface epithelium

Bronchospasm

Mucous plug

Vein

Mucous gland

Artery

Enlarged smooth muscle

Elastic fibers

Mucus buildup

Inflamed bronchial tissue

Figure 12-20 Asthma results in restricted airways.

closure of the air passages, inflammation, inflated alveoli, and excess mucus production. Treatments include avoidance of allergy-causing substances, bronchodilators (drugs that increase the diameter of the pulmonary air passages), and anti-inflammatories.

Exercise-induced asthma is constriction of the bronchial tubes caused by exercise. Exercise normally results in relaxation of the bronchial tree smooth muscle, but, in people with asthma, bronchospasm and mucus secretion follow the initial bronchodilation. The episode normally occurs within 5 to 15 minutes after exercise. It is diagnosed by the clinical picture and spirometriy. Treatment is usually not necessary because recovery is spontaneous, occurring 30 to 90 minutes after exercise.

KEY TERM	Definition
asthma (AZ-muh)	breathing disorder characterized by chest tightness and airway constriction
rhonchus (RONK-us)	harsh rattling sound
wheeze	audible whistling breath sound
bronchospasm (BRONK-oh-spaz-um)	contraction of smooth muscle in the walls of the bronchi and bronchioles, causing narrowing of the bronchial tubes
bronchial asthma (BRONK-ee-ul AZ-muh)	form of asthma with attacks of dyspnea and bronchial spasms
exercise-induced asthma (AZ-muh)	form of asthma with bronchoconstriction caused by exercise

continued

continued from page 598

KEY TERM PRACTICE: *Asthma*

1. The medical term for a harsh rattling sound is _____.

2. A _____ describes the contraction of the bronchial smooth muscle causing narrowing of the bronchial tubes.

3. This type of asthma occurs within 5 to 15 minutes after exercising. _____

4. An audible whistling breath sound is termed a _____.

5. _____ is a breathing disorder characterized by chest tightness and airway constriction in which individuals have a more difficult time exhaling than inhaling.

Inhalation Disorders

pneumoconiosis   Any lung disease caused by dust inhalation, especially metallic dust or mineral dusts that produce fibrosis (scarring) of pulmonary tissue, is termed **pneumoconiosis**. The term coniosis means "disease or morbid condition caused by dust inhalation." Pneumoconiosis is frequently job related and may develop after 2 to 30 years of daily exposure. The average time for disease development appears to be 10 years. It is characterized by progressive, chronic lung inflammation. Dyspnea, dry cough that becomes productive, tachypnea, malaise (generalized tiredness), and recurrent infections are hallmarks of advanced disease. Numerous forms exist, including anthracosis, asbestosis, berylliosis, and silicosis.

  Anthracosis, also called black lung disease, results from inhalation of smoke or coal dust and is common in coal miners. **Asbestosis** is caused by prolonged exposure to asbestos dust. **Berylliosis** is caused by exposure to beryllium. **Silicosis** occurs in quarry workers and stone masons who inhale silica dust (**Figure 12-21**). Treatment is symptomatic and supportive because there is no cure. Bronchodilators, oxygen therapy, physical therapy, and corticosteroids may be helpful.

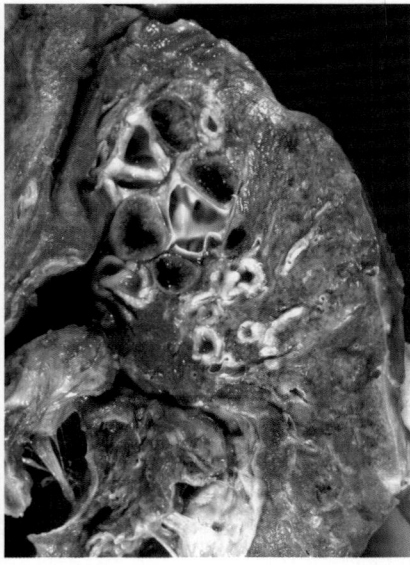

Figure 12-21 Lung with silicosis.

KEY TERM	Definition
pneumoconiosis (new-moh-koh-nee-OH-sis)	disease caused by inhaling mineral or metallic dust over a long period of time
anthracosis (an-thruh-KOH-sis)	pneumoconiosis caused by inhalation of coal dust
asbestosis (as-bes-TOH-sis)	pneumoconiosis caused by inhalation of asbestos fibers
berylliosis (be-ril-ee-OH-sis)	pneumoconiosis caused by inhalation of beryllium
silicosis (sil-i-KOH-sis)	pneumoconiosis caused by inhalation of silica dust

KEY TERM PRACTICE: *Inhalation Disorders*

1. The general term used to describe lung diseases caused by mineral dust inhalation is _____, which is derived from the word part _____, meaning "lung," and the word *coniosis*, which refers to a "condition caused by dust inhalation."

2. The word part _____ means "coal," and *-osis* is a suffix meaning _____; so _____ is a lung condition caused by inhaling coal dust.

3. _____ is pneumoconiosis that is caused by inhalation of asbestos.

4. Pneumoconiosis caused by inhalation of beryllium is termed _____.

5. Inhalation of silica dust can lead to a type of pneumoconiosis called _____.

Upper Respiratory Disorders

upper respiratory infection (URI)

An **upper respiratory infection (URI)** is an acute infection causing inflammation that affects the upper respiratory structures. Signs and symptoms vary with the particular strain of microbe and can include nasal congestion, sneezing, watery eyes, sore throat, voice hoarseness, and coughing. Headache, fever, chills, and malaise may also occur.

About half of all adult cases of URI are caused by **rhinoviruses**, which are RNA viruses that infect the upper respiratory system. The diagnosis is made by assessing the common signs and symptoms and, if necessary, sputum or nasal cultures. There is no cure. Treatment consists of rest, drinking plenty of fluids, nutrition therapy, and use of decongestants. **Decongestants** reduce or relieve nasal congestion.

nasal polyps

Nasal polyps are small, round-shaped growths projecting from the mucous membranes of the nose into the nasal cavity (**Figure 12-22**). They usually are not harmful, but large ones may interfere with nose breathing. Polyps are caused by overproduction of mucus, usually resulting from **allergic rhinitis**, inflammation of the nasal mucous membranes as a result of allergen reaction. They are identified using a **nasal speculum**, an instrument for looking into the nasal cavity. Polyps can be surgically removed or treated with a steroid injection directly into the growth.

acute rhinitis

Acute rhinitis, also called **nasal catarrh**, is an inflammation of the nasal mucous membranes. It is characterized by sneezing, **lacrimation** (production of tears), and **coryza** (secretion of watery mucus discharged from the nose, commonly called a runny nose). Also known as the common

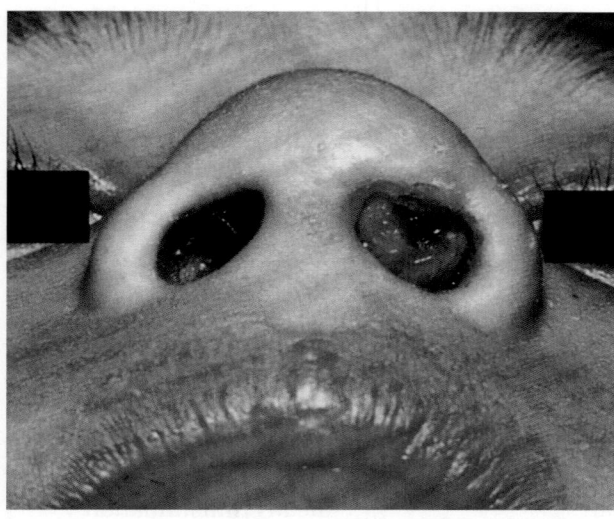

Figure 12-22 Nasal polyp.

head cold, this viral infection differs from other viral-based illness such as influenza in that it is not accompanied by fever. Rhinitis is treated symptomatically.

sinusitis   Inflammation of mucous membranes of any of the sinuses is **sinusitis**. It is characterized by pain, headache, and pressure. Nasal discharge is usually yellow-green, indicating the infection is bacterial in origin. The patient history is generally enough to confirm the diagnosis. X-ray scans, if necessary, may reveal fluid-filled cavities that appear white; normal air-filled cavities appear dark on x-ray films. Sinusitis is treated with antibiotics if the causative agent is bacterial. Decongestants, antihistamines, and analgesics may also provide relief.

pharyngitis   **Pharyngitis**, commonly known as a sore throat, is an inflammation of the pharynx. Dry, painful throat; chills; fever; **dysphonia** (hoarseness); **dysphagia** (difficulty swallowing); and a red, swollen pharynx typify the condition. It is caused by a viral or bacterial infection or by chemical or smoke inhalation. Physical examination and patient history confirm the diagnosis. Antibiotics are prescribed for a bacterial infection. Otherwise, the treatment involves soothing throat lozenges, getting plenty of rest and fluids, and using over-the-counter medications to treat symptoms.

KEY TERM	Definition
upper respiratory (RES-pi-ruh-tor-ee) **infection (URI)**	acute infection causing inflammation that affects the upper respiratory structures
rhinoviruses (rye-noh-VYE-rus-ez)	any of many RNA viruses that cause upper respiratory tract infections
decongestant	drug that reduces nasal congestion
nasal polyp (POL-ip)	benign growth on the nasal mucous membranes
allergic rhinitis (rye-NIGH-tis)	nasal inflammation resulting from an allergy
nasal speculum (SPECK-yoo-lum)	instrument for viewing the nasal cavity
acute rhinitis (rye-NIGH-tis)	inflammation of the nasal cavity caused by infection; also called nasal catarrh
nasal catarrh (kuh-TAHR)	inflammation of the nasal cavity caused by infection; also called acute rhinitis

continued

continued from page 601

KEY TERM	Definition
lacrimation (lack-ri-MAY-shun)	tear production
coryza (koh-RYE-zuh)	runny nose
sinusitis (sigh-nuh-SIGH-tis)	inflammation of the sinuses
pharyngitis (fair-in-JYE-tis)	inflammation of the pharynx; also called a sore throat
dysphonia (dis-FOH-nee-uh)	hoarseness
dysphagia (dis-FAY-jee-uh)	difficulty swallowing

KEY TERM PRACTICE: *Upper Respiratory Disorders*

1. Difficulty swallowing is called _____.

2. The word part *rhin-* means _____, and the word part _____ means "inflammation"; therefore, an inflammation of the nasal cavity is termed _____.

3. _____ is the medical term for a runny nose.

4. The word part _____ refers to "the pharynx," and the suffix _____ means "inflammation"; therefore, _____ is an inflammation of the pharynx.

5. A _____ is a drug used to reduce nasal congestion.

Lower Respiratory Disorders

laryngitis

Inflammation of the larynx is termed **laryngitis**, which is usually accompanied by hoarseness, **aphonia** (loss of voice), and coughing. Depending on the causative agent, sore throat, fever, and malaise may also occur. It can be viral or bacterial in origin and frequently occurs along with other conditions such as syphilis and tuberculosis. Tonsillitis, sinusitis, smoke or chemical inhalation, and excessive voice use are also common causes of laryngitis. The diagnosis is made by the patient history and physical examination, although laryngoscopy may be performed for confirmation purposes.

Examination of the larynx with a **laryngoscope** (an instrument with a light and telescope for viewing the larynx) is termed **laryngoscopy**. In addition to diagnostic purposes, laryngoscopy may also be used to facilitate the passage of a breathing tube through the larynx. Treatment involves voice rest, humidity therapy to thin the mucous secretions, increased fluid intake, and throat lozenges.

histoplasmosis

Histoplasmosis is a mild respiratory infection caused by the fungus *Histoplasma capsulatum*, which can progress to other body systems. It is initially asymptomatic. Then dyspnea, malaise, fever, splenomegaly (enlarged spleen), and hepatomegaly (enlarged liver) occur. Infection results from inhaling contaminated dust or bird feces particles. Histoplasmosis is diagnosed by skin test, blood studies, and sputum or tissue samples confirming the presence of the fungus. Antifungal drugs are used to treat the condition.

pneumonia

Lung inflammation with **exudate** (seeping mass of cells and fluid) is termed **pneumonia**. The condition is caused by viral or bacterial infection or, less commonly, a chemical or physical irritant. Common pneumonia-causing microorganisms are *Klebsiella pneumoniae*, *Streptococcus pneumoniae*, and *Mycoplasma pneumoniae*. In addition to viral and bacterial types, **aspiration pneumonia** is a form that results from the inhalation of foreign material, such as food or vomit, into the bronchi. It can also develop secondary to the presence of fluid, blood, saliva, or gastric contents in the airways. When the pneumonia occurs in patchy areas within a lung field, it is termed bronchopneumonia. When the pneumonia affects one or more lobes, or part of a lobe, it is termed **lobar pneumonia** (Figure 12-23).

Cough, fever, and dyspnea are major signs and symptoms. Chest pain depends on the area of lung field affected. Pneumonia is diagnosed by the history and physical examination, x-ray evaluations, sputum studies, and blood culture. **Sputum studies** are tests that look for the presence of abnormal cells in sputum. Sputum is also often obtained for **culture and sensitivity (C&S) studies**, whereby the sample is grown on nutritive media, and infectious microbes (causative agents) are identified and tested for antibiotic sensitivity. Once the organism is known, appropriate antimicrobial therapy can begin. Management involves treating the underlying cause, bed rest, fluids, and postural drainage. Fluid aspiration from the lung may also be required.

An infection and inflammation of lungs relatively common in young children and the elderly is **respiratory syncytial virus (RSV) pneumonia**. It produces cold-like symptoms, nasal congestion, otitis media (middle ear infection), coughing, fever, malaise, and lethargy. The greatest number of cases occurs between December and March. It is a viral infection spread by contact with secretions of infected individuals. RSV pneumonia is diagnosed by the patient's history, physical examination, and sputum culture. It is treated with antiviral medications, rest, and fluid intake.

Legionnaires' disease or **legionellosis**

Legionnaires' disease, also called **legionellosis**, is a form of pneumonia caused by the *Legionella pneumophila* bacterium. The microbe causes acute lobar pneumonia and affects other body systems. It was first recognized in an outbreak in July 1976, at an American Legion conference in Philadelphia. It is spread mainly by water droplets in air conditioning systems; warm, moist environments such as spas and hot tubs; and grocery

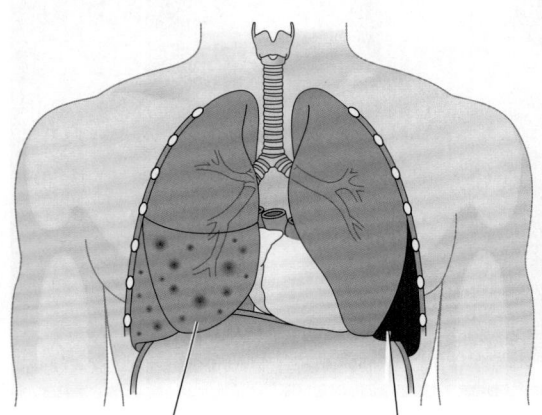

Bronchopneumonia   Lobar pneumonia

Figure 12-23 The red areas indicate bronchopneumonia and lobar pneumonia.

store vegetable misting systems. *L. pneumophila* infection is not contagious. Signs and symptoms include malaise, headache, cough, chills, fever, chest pain, dyspnea, and myalgia. The diagnosis is based on the history and physical examination, x-rays, and blood sputum studies. Presence of the bacterium in the sputum or urine confirms the diagnosis. Antibiotic therapy is necessary, and prevention measures are used to avoid outbreaks.

influenza

Influenza, commonly called the flu, is an acute respiratory infection caused by a specific virus. Because there is usually an epidemic every 1 to 4 years, annual preventive vaccination programs start in early fall. Sudden onset, cough, headache, runny nose, fever, chills, and myalgia (muscle pain) characterize influenza. Complications include bronchitis, sinusitis, and otitis media (ear infection). Three general types—designated A, B, and C—have been identified, but mutant strains are prevalent.

Influenza is quickly transmitted among people because of the short incubation period of 1 to 3 days. It tends to be more serious in young, elderly, and immunocompromised people. It is spread through inhalation of the virus, and the signs and symptoms are often indistinguishable from those of the common cold. Definitive diagnosis is made by isolating the virus from a throat culture. There is no cure, so the condition is treated symptomatically. Rest and increased fluid intake are generally prescribed. Vaccines are administered before an outbreak, and individuals typically require 2 to 4 weeks to develop active immunity.

tuberculosis (TB)

Tuberculosis (TB) is an infectious disease caused by *Mycobacterium tuberculosis* in which rounded swellings, called tubercles, form on the mucous membranes, especially in the lungs (**Figure 12-24**). Although it infects lung tissue primarily, it can attack most body organs. It is characterized by fever, weight loss, tussis, chest pain, and hemoptysis. It is transmitted when a person inhales droplets containing the microbe after

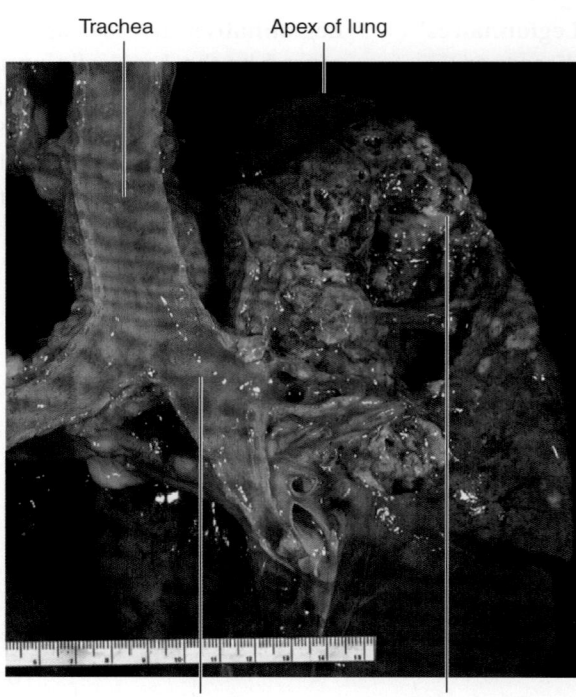

Trachea   Apex of lung

Bronchus   Tubercles in apical region

Figure 12-24 Tuberculosis is an infections disease in which rounded swellings called tubercles occur in the apical regions of the lungs.

an infected person coughs or sneezes. It is diagnosed by a positive tuberculin test followed by chest x-rays that reveal walled-off tubercles in the lungs. The **tuberculin test**, or **Mantoux test**, is a skin test used to diagnose infection by *Mycobacterium tuberculosis*. The acid-fast bacilli (AFB) staining procedure is useful for detecting acid-fast bacilli, such as *M. tuberculosis*. Sputum cultures identifying the AFB also provide confirmation. Tuberculosis is treated aggressively with isoniazid (INH) and rifampin.

KEY TERM	Definition
laryngitis (lair-in-JYE-tis)	larynx inflammation
aphonia (ay-FOH-nee-uh)	loss of the voice
laryngoscope (la-RING-goh-skope)	lighted instrument with a short metal or plastic tube used for examining the larynx
laryngoscopy (lair-ing-GOS-kuh-pee)	visual examination of the larynx using a lighted instrument called a laryngoscope
histoplasmosis (his-toh-plaz-MOH-sis)	fungal infection of the lungs
exudate (ECKS-yoo-date)	seeping mass of cells and fluid
pneumonia (new-MOH-nee-uh)	inflammation of the lungs
aspiration pneumonia (as-pi-RAY-shun new-MOH-nee-uh)	inflammation of the lungs that results from inhaling a substance into the lung field
lobar pneumonia (LOH-bar new-MOH-nee-uh)	inflammation of the lungs affecting one or more lobes or parts of a lobe
sputum (SPEW-tum) **studies**	tests to evaluate substances found in sputum
culture and sensitivity (C&S) studies	tests to identify microbes and the effectiveness of various antibiotics
respiratory syncytial (RES-pi-ruh-tor-ee sin-SISH-ul) **virus (RSV) pneumonia** (new-MOH-nee-uh)	lung inflammation caused by RSV
Legionnaires' (lee-juh-NAIRZ) **disease**	pneumonia caused by *Legionella pneumophila;* also called legionellosis
legionellosis (lee-juh-nell-OH-sis)	pneumonia caused by *Legionella pneumophila;* also called Legionnaires' disease
influenza (in-floo-EN-zuh)	viral infection producing fever, sore throat, cough, and muscle pain; flu
tuberculosis (tew-bur-kew-LOH-sis) **(TB)**	infectious disease affecting the lungs caused by *Mycobacterium tuberculosis*
tuberculin (TOO-berk-yoo-lun) **test**	intradermal test used to establish past or present tuberculosis infection; also called the Mantoux test
Mantoux (MAN-too) **test**	intradermal test used to establish past or present tuberculosis infection; also called the tuberculin test

KEY TERM PRACTICE: *Lower Respiratory Disorders*

1. Inflammation of the lungs is termed _____.

2. An infectious disease affecting the lungs that is caused by *Mycobacterium tuberculosis* is called _____.

3. Provide the two names for the lung disease caused by *Legionella pneumophila*. _____

4. Give the two names for the skin test used to provide a diagnosis for tuberculosis. _____

5. The type of pneumonia that results from inhaling a substance into the lung field is termed _____.

Lung Cancer

lung cancer   Malignant tumors of the lung tissue are termed **lung cancer** (**Figure 12-25**). Lung cancer is the leading cause of cancer deaths in the United States. Early stages are asymptomatic, but later the affected individual experiences cough, wheezing, and hemoptysis. Common sites of metastasis (tumor spread) are the brain, liver, bone, and skin. Cigarette smoking or passive exposure to cigarette smoke causes 85% to 90% of all lung cancer. Lung cancer is initially diagnosed by chest x-rays and sputum studies. Tissue biopsy indicating the presence of cancerous cells confirms the diagnosis. It is treated aggressively by surgery, radiation, and chemotherapy.

mesothelioma   **Mesothelioma** is a cancer derived from the lining cells of the pleura or peritoneum that grows as a thick sheet covering the organs. A chronic inflammatory state is thought to contribute to the disease. An association between asbestos exposure and disease development has been established. The cancer is usually asymptomatic in the early stages but progresses to include signs and symptoms of dyspnea and pleuritic pain. Chest x-rays identify the cancer. Treatment includes radiation, chemotherapy, and partial or complete **lobectomy** (surgical removal of all or part of a lung).

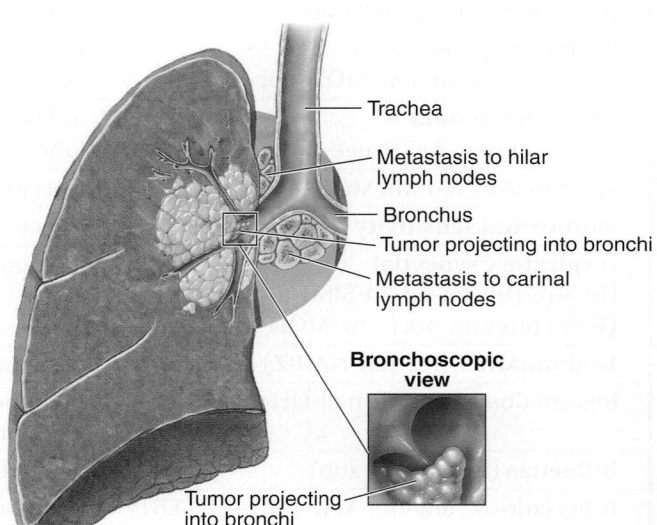

Trachea
Metastasis to hilar lymph nodes
Bronchus
Tumor projecting into bronchi
Metastasis to carinal lymph nodes

Bronchoscopic view

Tumor projecting into bronchi

Figure 12-25 Cancer of the right lung, anterior view.

KEY TERM	Definition
lung cancer	malignant tumors of the lung tissue
mesothelioma (mez-oh-thee-lee-OH-muh)	cancer derived from the lining cells of the pleura and peritoneum, associated with asbestos exposure
lobectomy (loh-BECK-toh-mee)	surgical removal of all or part of a lung

KEY TERM PRACTICE: *Lung Cancer*

1. Cancer of the lung tissue is termed _____.

2. Surgical removal of all or part of a lung is termed _____.

3. _____ is a cancer derived from the lining cells of the pleura or peritoneum.

Pneumothorax and Hemothorax

pneumothorax   The abnormal presence of air or gas in the pleural cavity between the lungs and chest wall, which causes pain and difficulty breathing, is a **pneumothorax** (**Figure 12-26**). Pneumothoraces result in collapse or partial collapse of the lung. They are characterized by severe dyspnea; sudden chest pain; and rapid, weak pulse. Causes of a pneumothorax include alveoli erosion from tumor or disease, spontaneous tear, improper artificial ventilation, or traumatic injury.

Diagnosis is made by the history and physical examination and confirmed through chest x-rays and the presence of diminished breath sounds. Treatment involves placing the person in the Fowler or semi-Fowler position (sitting position or semireclining position in bed respectively), oxygen therapy, and thoracentesis. **Thoracentesis** is a needle aspiration of the pleural cavity through the chest wall for fluid or air withdrawal. Removed fluid can then be analyzed for infection or pathology.

hemothorax   Blood in the pleural cavity is termed **hemothorax**. It is caused by trauma or a tear in a pulmonary vessel. Signs and symptoms are similar to those of pneumothorax. Hemothorax is diagnosed by diminished or absent breath sounds, chest x-rays indicating that blood is present in the pleural cavity, and patient distress. Medical intervention involves treating the underlying cause, thoracentesis, and blood replacement if necessary.

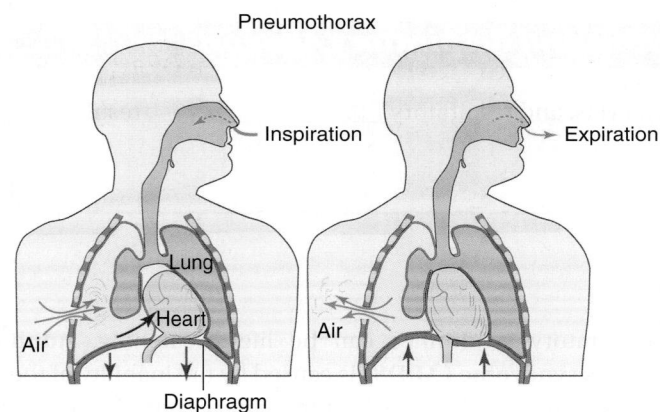

Figure 12-26 Pneumothorax. Left illustration shows how the heart and lungs are affected during inspiration in a person with a pneumothorax. Right illustration shows how the heart and lungs are affected during expiration in a person with a pneumothorax.

KEY TERM	Definition
pneumothorax (new-moh-THOR-acks)	abnormal presence of air or gas in the pleural cavity
thoracentesis (thoh-ruh-sen-TEE-sis)	needle aspiration of the pleural cavity through the chest wall for fluid or air withdrawal
hemothorax (hee-moh-THOR-acks)	blood in the pleural cavity

KEY TERM PRACTICE: *Pneumothorax and Hemothorax*

1. _____ is the general term for air or gas in the pleural cavity; _____ is the medical term for blood in the pleural cavity.

2. A needle aspiration of the pleural cavity through the chest wall for fluid or air withdrawal is termed a _____.

Respiratory Acidosis and Respiratory Alkalosis

respiratory acidosis The lungs play a role in regulating the pH (the acidity or alkalinity) of blood. **Respiratory acidosis** is a condition in which hypoventilation (decreased breathing) causes increased blood carbon dioxide and decreased blood pH (acidosis). If the lungs cannot "blow off" excess carbon dioxide, it accumulates, causing the blood pH to drop. A sign of respiratory acidosis is decreased respiratory rate. Underlying causes may be COPD, pulmonary embolus, or neuromuscular disease.

respiratory alkalosis **Respiratory alkalosis** is a condition in which increased breathing (hyperventilation) increases blood pH. The increased breathing causes the elimination of too much carbon dioxide, leading to alkalosis. Underlying causes contributing to the disorder include exercise, anxiety, and blood poisoning with gram-negative (G–) bacteria. Treatment of both respiratory alkalosis and respiratory acidosis involves restoring normal breathing patterns.

KEY TERM	Definition
respiratory acidosis (RES-pi-ruh-tor-ee as-i-DOH-sis)	low blood pH caused by carbon dioxide retention
respiratory alkalosis (RES-pi-ruh-tor-ee al-kuh-LOH-sis)	increased blood pH due to elimination of too much carbon dioxide

KEY TERM PRACTICE: *Respiratory Acidosis and Respiratory Alkalosis*

1. Respiratory _____ results in elevated blood pH levels, and respiratory _____ results in below normal blood pH levels.

Respiratory Syndromes

adult respiratory distress syndrome (ARDS) As a group, respiratory syndromes can be life-threatening. **Adult respiratory distress syndrome (ARDS)** is caused by the inability of the lungs to take in oxygen. It is characterized by **hypercapnia** (excessive amount of carbon dioxide in the blood), **acidemia** (acidic blood from decreased pH levels), and severe **hypoxemia** (inadequate amount of oxygen in the blood). ARDS is typified by severe dyspnea, rapid and shallow respirations, cyanosis, rales, rhonchi, and wheezing. The cause is pulmonary edema (lung swelling) and respiratory failure when the alveoli fill with exudate.

pulmonary edema **Pulmonary edema** occurs when fluid accumulates in the lungs producing severe dyspnea. Pulmonary edema is commonly caused by left heart failure. The syndrome results in pulmonary hypertension and hypoxemia. Radiologic studies confirm the clinical picture. Treatment entails oxygen therapy and air administered under positive pressure during expiration (exhalation) to keep the alveoli expanded. This air delivery is termed **positive end-expiratory pressure (PEEP)**.

altitude sickness **Altitude sickness**, also called **mountain sickness**, is a syndrome caused by exposure to the low partial pressure of oxygen at high altitude. It is characterized by nausea, headache, dyspnea, malaise, and insomnia. It can lead to pulmonary edema and adult respiratory distress syndrome.

infant respiratory distress syndrome (IRDS)

Infant respiratory distress syndrome (IRDS) is a disease of unknown cause that affects premature infants and newborns during the first few days after birth. It is also known as **neonatal respiratory distress syndrome (NRDS)** and **hyaline membrane disease (HMD)**. Respiratory distress, nasal flaring, cyanosis, and alveolar collapse are characteristics. The disorder is diagnosed by arterial blood gases that show inadequate gas exchange and chest x-rays that reveal the presence of a hyaline membrane. **Arterial blood gas (ABG)** is a test used to measure blood pH, the partial pressures of carbon dioxide and oxygen, and the bicarbonate ion (HCO_3^-) concentration.

Treatments include mechanical ventilation and CPAP. A **mechanical ventilator**, often referred to as a respirator, supplies negative or positive pressure to the lungs to support breathing. **Continuous positive airway pressure (CPAP)** supplies positive pressure throughout the entire respiratory cycle (**Figure 12-27**).

sudden infant death syndrome (SIDS)

Sudden infant death syndrome (SIDS) is the sudden, unexpected, unexplained death of an apparently healthy infant. Other names include cot death, crib death, and sleep apnea syndrome. It occurs most commonly in infants between 1 and 4 months old during sleep. Autopsies reveal no conclusive evidence to support a cause of this syndrome. The incidence is greater in homes in which the infant is exposed to cigarette smoking before and after birth. Other risk factors include inadequate prenatal care, low birth weight, young maternal age, and maternal hard drug use. Since 1992, the American Academy of Pediatrics has recommended that infants be placed on their backs while sleeping. Although back sleeping is no guarantee against SIDS, research has shown this is a safer sleeping position for infants.

respiratory failure

Respiratory failure takes place when the respiratory system cannot keep pace with the body's demand for oxygen. Insufficient carbon dioxide is eliminated. The buildup of carbon dioxide results in hypercapnia. If the situation does not resolve, coma follows. Treatment of respiratory failure requires mechanical ventilation.

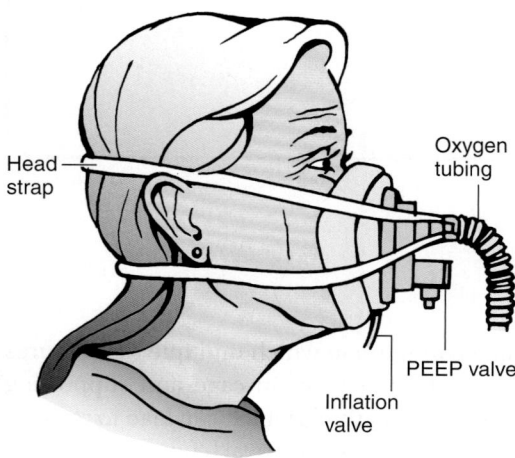

Head strap

Oxygen tubing

PEEP valve

Inflation valve

Figure 12-27 Administering oxygen by face mask with continuous positive airway pressure (CPAP).

KEY TERM	Definition
adult respiratory (RES-pi-ruh-tor-ee) **distress syndrome (ARDS)**	disorder marked by hypercapnia, acidemia, and severe hypoxemia resulting in cyanosis
hypercapnia (high-pur-KAP-nee-uh)	too much carbon dioxide in the blood
acidemia (as-i-DEE-mee-uh)	abnormally low blood pH
hypoxemia (high-pock-SEE-mee-uh)	inadequate oxygen in the blood
pulmonary edema (PUL-moh-nerr-ee e-DEE-muh)	fluid accumulation in the lungs causing breathing difficulty
positive end-expiratory (eck-SPYE-ruh-tor-ee) **pressure (PEEP)**	positive-pressure air delivered during expiration (exhalation)
altitude sickness	illness caused by the ascent to a high altitude and the resulting shortage of oxygen; also called mountain sickness
mountain sickness	illness caused by the ascent to a high altitude and the resulting shortage of oxygen; also called altitude sickness
infant respiratory (RES-pi-ruh-tor-ee) **distress syndrome (IRDS)**	disorder marked by breathing difficulty and cyanosis in the infant or newborn; also called NRDS and HMD
neonatal respiratory (RES-pi-ruh-tor-ee) **distress syndrome (NRDS)**	disorder marked by breathing difficulty and cyanosis in the infant or newborn; also called IRDS and HMD
hyaline (HIGH-uh-lin) **membrane disease (HMD)**	disorder marked by breathing difficulty and cyanosis in the infant or newborn; also called IRDS and NRDS
arterial (ahr-TEER-ee-ul) **blood gas (ABG)**	evaluation of blood pH, CO_2, O_2, and HCO_3^- concentrations
mechanical ventilator	machine for moving air into and out of a person's lungs; also called a respirator
continuous positive airway pressure (CPAP)	positive-pressure air delivered throughout the respiratory cycle
sudden infant death syndrome (SIDS)	sudden, unexpected, unexplained death of a sleeping infant
respiratory (RES-pi-ruh-tor-ee) **failure**	respiratory system is unable to meet the oxygen demands of the body, and carbon dioxide levels increase

KEY TERM PRACTICE: *Respiratory Syndromes*

1. What condition results when the respiratory system cannot keep pace with the body's oxygen demands and the carbon dioxide levels rise? _____

2. The unexplained death of an otherwise healthy infant that occurs during sleep is known as _____.

3. _____ is fluid accumulation in the lungs causing breathing difficulty.

4. Inadequate oxygen in the blood is termed _____ for the word part _____, meaning "below," and the word part _____, meaning "condition of the blood."

5. Abnormally low blood pH is termed _____.

Trauma and Poisoning

flail chest

Flail chest is a life-threatening condition in which multiple rib fractures cause thoracic cage instability. The unstable rib cage and supporting muscles cannot function to support breathing, which can lead to respiratory failure. The hindered action is called paradoxical (contrary to usual).

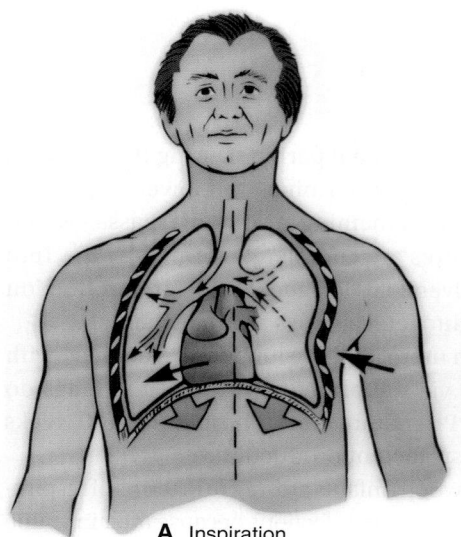 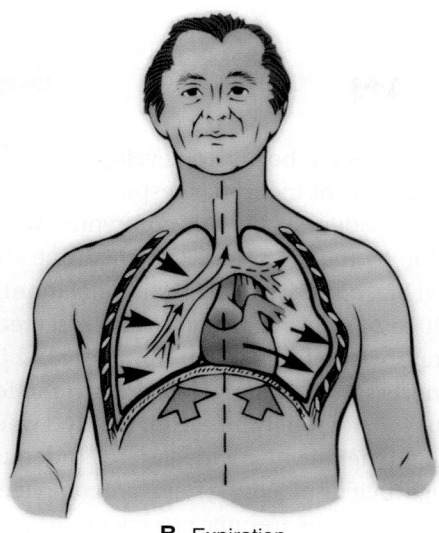

A Inspiration   **B** Expiration

Figure 12-28 Flail chest is a condition of paradoxical chest wall movement, resulting from trauma to the rib cage and muscles.

In **paradoxical respiration**, the lung deflates during inhalation, and inflates during exhalation (**Figure 12-28**). The physical examination, clinical picture, and chest x-ray confirm the diagnosis. Treatment consists of healing the rib fractures, possible mechanical ventilation, or oxygen administration.

carbon monoxide poisoning   Carbon monoxide (CO) is a colorless, odorless gas that forms from the burning of carbon-containing fuels with insufficient air turnover. **Carbon monoxide poisoning** occurs when CO instead of oxygen combines with hemoglobin (Hb) molecules, which normally carry oxygen in the blood. This results in hypoxia. The skin appears a cherry red color, even though tissues are really anoxic, or deprived of oxygen. Symptoms and signs of CO poisoning are shallow breathing and ruddy complexion. Hemoglobin does not easily release carbon monoxide, so individuals suffering from CO poisoning must be treated in hyperbaric oxygen chambers, which are pressurized containers that force oxygen into the blood.

KEY TERM	Definition
flail chest	fracture of the rib cage that causes paradoxical chest wall movement
paradoxical respiration (pair-uh-DOCK-si-kul res-pi-RAY-shun)	breathing that is contrary to usual movements in that the lung deflates during inhalation, and inflates during exhalation
carbon monoxide poisoning	disorder resulting from hemoglobin combining with CO instead of hemoglobin combining with oxygen

KEY TERM PRACTICE: *Trauma and Poisoning*

1. A rib cage fracture causing paradoxical breathing describes _____.

2. _____ occurs when carbon monoxide instead of oxygen is attached to hemoglobin.

3. The term _____ is used to describe breathing that is contrary to usual movements in that the lung deflates during inhalation, and inflates during exhalation.

LIFE SPAN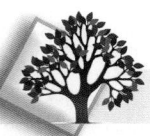

The respiratory system begins to develop early in the gestational period. During the 4th week of embryonic growth, the upper respiratory structures begin forming, and lower respiratory structures are evident at the 5th embryonic week. The remaining respiratory passages and lungs develop by the 8th week. Bronchial tree structures are completely formed by the 16th week of fetal life, and by the 6th gestational month, alveoli are formed. Surfactant production begins by 20 to 24 weeks of gestation and is secreted into fetal airways around week 30.

Respiratory structures are nonfunctional while in utero, and the lungs are even filled with fluid. The necessary oxygen is delivered to the fetus via the placenta. At birth, the lungs do function but will not totally inflate for nearly 3 weeks. Premature infants born at 28 to 30 weeks can breathe on their own provided there is adequate surfactant production.

Although their respiratory systems are complete, newborn infants are fragile in terms of respiratory function. Newborns are quite susceptible to upper respiratory infections because their immune system is immature. In addition, their tonsils and epiglottis are rather large, so infants up to 3 months of age must breathe through the nose. Mouth breathing would not supply enough oxygen for adequate lung inflation. For this reason, nasal congestion in young infants can be a serious problem.

Newborns and children have fewer alveoli than adults, but the number of alveoli increases until approximately age 8. Children have a faster metabolic rate than do adults, and accordingly, they consume more oxygen per body weight. If children grow up in a home where cigarette smoke is prevalent, they may never attain optimal respiratory capacity and their organ reserve will be diminished.

With aging, lung tissue becomes less elastic and more rigid. Arthritic changes in the rib cage alter pulmonary function, and there is a decline in blood oxygen levels and lung capacity. The vital capacity, or the maximum amount of air a person can exhale after taking the deepest breath possible, can diminish up to 35% by age 70 years. Respiratory muscle strength and endurance decrease up to 20%, but these values can be enhanced with physical exercise. Blood pH and the amount of carbon dioxide carried in the blood remain relatively constant with advancing age.

COPD is not a normal change of aging. Older adults are more susceptible to respiratory infections and pulmonary disorders such as pneumonia, influenza, and bronchitis. As of 2010, pneumonia was the fifth leading cause of death in people older than 65 years, especially during the winter months of flu season. It is critical to administer pneumococcal and flu vaccines to this group.

COMMON Abbreviations

Abbreviation	Term
ABG	arterial blood gas
AFB	acid-fast bacilli
ARDS	adult respiratory distress syndrome
CF	cystic fibrosis
CO	carbon monoxide
CO$_2$	carbon dioxide
COPD	chronic obstructive pulmonary disease
CPAP	continuous positive airway pressure

continued

continued from page 612

Abbreviation	Term
CRT	certified respiratory therapist
C&S	culture and sensitivity
CT	computerized tomography
ERV	expiratory reserve volume
FEV_1	forced expiratory volume at 1 second
FVC	forced vital capacity
G−	gram-negative
HCO_3^-	bicarbonate ion
HMD	hyaline membrane disease
INH	isoniazid; isonicotinic acid hydrazide
IRDS	infant respiratory distress syndrome
IRV	inspiratory reserve volume
MRI	magnetic resonance imaging
NBRC	National Board for Respiratory Care
NRDS	neonatal respiratory distress syndrome
O_2	oxygen
P	partial pressure
PCO_2	partial pressure of carbon dioxide
PD	postural drainage
PEEP	positive end-expiratory pressure
PEF	peak expiratory flow
PFT	pulmonary function test
RRT	registered respiratory therapist
RSV	respiratory syncytial virus
RT	respiratory therapist
RV	residual volume
SIDS	sudden infant death syndrome
TB	tuberculosis
TLC	total lung capacity
TV	tidal volume
URI	upper respiratory infection
VC	vital capacity

COMMON ABBREVIATIONS EXERCISES

1. Give the abbreviation for oxygen. _____

2. CO is the abbreviation for _____.

3. ABG is the abbreviation for _____.

4. Give the abbreviation for gram-negative. _____

5. PFT is the abbreviation for _____.

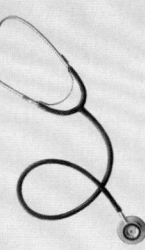

Case Study

Mrs. June Sawyer, age 55 years, has a history of COPD with severe pulmonary fibrosis. She presented in her physician's office with dyspnea, vomiting, headache, and dizziness as her chief complaints. The physical examination revealed nothing remarkable. Partial CT scans of the sinuses were ordered. Soft tissue and bone windows were used for the examination. The following results were obtained:

- Clear sinuses
- Clear nasal airway
- Normal nasal conchae
- No soft tissue masses
- No bone destructive changes
- No nasal cavity soft tissue displacement
- Normal orbital contents

The physician ordered pulmonary function tests.

Case Study Questions

Select the best answer to each of the following questions.

1. **Mrs. Sawyer presented with dyspnea. Dyspnea means _____.**
   a. being off balance
   b. thirsty
   c. difficulty swallowing
   d. breathing difficulty

2. **The report indicates that there are no soft tissue masses. An example of a soft tissue mass would be _____.**
   a. paranasal sinuses
   b. the septum
   c. nasal polyps
   d. the nasal cavity

3. **The nasal cavity soft tissue refers to the _____.**
   a. external nares
   b. septum
   c. lungs
   d. sinuses

4. **Given the clinical picture and the results of this CT study, Mrs. Sawyer _____.**
   a. probably has a sinus infection
   b. is suffering from TB
   c. does not have a sinus infection
   d. is healthy and requires no further treatment

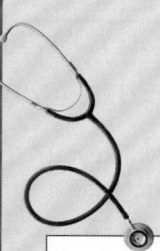

Real World Report

Mrs. June Sawyer's family physician sent her to the respiratory therapy department for a complete pulmonary function test. The examination revealed the following results.

CENTRAL HOSPITAL: PULMONARY CARE UNIT

NAME: June Sawyer

SEX: Female

ORDERPHYS: R. L. Keefer, MD

DOB: February 9, 1956

AGE: 55

EXAM DATE: November 1, 2011

INDICATION FOR STUDY

Pulmonary function studies were done on this patient, who has a history of chronic obstructive pulmonary disease and severe pulmonary fibrosis.

SPIROMETRY

Spirometry showed severe reduction in forced vital capacity, profound reduction in forced expiratory volume at 1 s (FEV_1), with severe reduction in the FEV_1 to forced vital capacity (FVC) ratio (FEV_1/FVC). Midexpiratory flow rates were profoundly reduced. Borderline improvement was noted in forced vital capacity after bronchodilator treatment. Maximum voluntary ventilation was severely reduced.

LUNG VOLUMES

Lung volumes measured by body plethysmography showed increased total lung capacity with marked increase in residual volume.

AIRWAY MECHANICS

Airway resistance was markedly increased and airway conductance was reduced.

DIFFUSION

Diffusion capacity was severely reduced.

OVERALL IMPRESSION

Overall, this study shows evidence of profound obstructive ventilatory impairment associated with severe overinflation and severe diffusion abnormalities consistent with severe chronic obstructive pulmonary disease and emphysema.

Dictated by: M. E. Chabath, MD

continued

continued from page 615

Real World Report Questions

The following exercises review the medical terms used in the preceding medical report. A term with which you may not be familiar is *plethysmography* (pleth-iz-MOG-ruh-fee). *Plethysmos* is the Greek term for "increase"; thus plethysmography is a technique to measure increased lung volume or other changes.

1. The pulmonary function tests are done to
   _____.

2. The tests involved spirometry.

   a. Spirometry measures _____.

   b. Vital capacity is _____.

   c. Bronchodilator treatment is used to
      _____.

3. Lung volumes were measured. Define the following terms.

   a. TLC = _____

   b. residual volume = _____

4. The report indicated that there was reduced conductance. What structures are involved in the conducting airway?

   _____

   _____

   _____

5. What type of COPD does Mrs. Sawyer have?

   _____

Review and Application

Multiple-Choice Questions

Select the best answer to each of the following questions.

1. Cavities within skull bones that lighten the weight of the cranium are called _____.
   - a. bases
   - b. sinuses
   - c. polyps
   - d. passages

2. _____ is oxygen use occurring at the cellular level.
   - a. Respiration
   - b. Pulmonation
   - c. Ventilation
   - d. Inhalation

3. The _____ is a cartilaginous partition separating the nasal cavity into left and right sections.
   - a. bronchioles
   - b. alveoli
   - c. septum
   - d. vestibule

4. The medical term for a cough is _____.
   - a. tussis
   - b. expectorate
   - c. phlegm
   - d. sputum

5. The anatomical structure that covers the trachea during swallowing is the _____.
   - a. glottis
   - b. epiglottis
   - c. cricoid cartilage
   - d. upper vestibular fold

6. The slit-like opening where air enters the larynx is the _____.
   - a. epiglottis
   - b. vocal cords
   - c. apex
   - d. glottis

7. Identify the form of lung cancer in which fibrous tissue derived from the pleura forms and grows in sheets over the organs. _____
   - a. tussis
   - b. pertussis
   - c. mesothelioma
   - d. emphysema

8. Structures of the conducting airway of the respiratory system include _____.
   - a. larynx, pharynx, and alveoli
   - b. trachea, bronchi, and alveoli
   - c. bronchi, bronchioles, and alveoli
   - d. larynx, bronchi, and bronchioles

9. Structures of the respiratory airway include _____.
   - a. bronchioles and alveoli
   - b. trachea and alveoli
   - c. trachea and bronchioles
   - d. bronchi and trachea

10. _____ therapy is a treatment in which oxygen is supplied via a nasal cannula, Venturi mask, or oxygen tent.
   - a. Breathing
   - b. Oxygen
   - c. Nitrogen
   - d. Ventilation

11. The substance that decreases surface tension is _____.
   - a. antitrypsin
   - b. antiprotease
   - c. alpha$_1$
   - d. surfactant

12. _____ is a test used to evaluate blood pH, CO_2, O_2, and HCO_3^- concentrations in order to diagnose IRDS.
   - a. Oxygen therapy
   - b. Continuous-positive airway pressure
   - c. Arterial blood gas
   - d. Positive end-expiratory pressure

13. Cessation of breathing is known as _____.
   - a. eupnea
   - b. dyspnea
   - c. bradypnea
   - d. apnea

14. Pulmonary function tests use a device called a _____.
   - a. ventilator
   - b. respirator
   - c. spirometer
   - d. nasal cannula

15. Chronic dilation of the respiratory passages causing tussis is termed _____.
   - a. bradypnea
   - b. hyperventilation
   - c. bronchiectasis
   - d. hyperpnea

16. An abnormally rapid breathing rate is _____.
    a. tachypnea   b. Biot respirations   c. hypoventilation   d. bradypnea

17. _____ is an abnormal hissing or whistling lung sound.
    a. Sputum   b. Rale   c. Phlegm   d. Dysphonia

18. A flexible tube inserted into the mouth or nose to deliver oxygen to the lungs is a/an _____.
    a. bronchoscopy   b. thoracotomy   c. endotracheal tube   d. auscultation

19. Identify the instrument that measures the amount of oxygen in blood. _____
    a. lung scan   b. MRI machine   c. spirometer   d. pulse oximeter

20. Inflammation of the lungs that affects one or more lobes or parts of a lobe is called _____.
    a. nasal polyp   b. lung cancer   c. nasal catarrh   d. lobar pneumonia

21. As the bronchial tree branches into smaller structures, the amount of cartilage _____.
    a. increases   b. decreases

Word Parts Exercises

Using the following word parts, form a medical term for each definition. Each word part is used only once.

broncho-   -itis
bronchiole   laryngo-
-centesis   spasm
-ectomy   thorac-

22. surgical puncture of thorax to remove fluid _____

23. surgical removal of larynx _____

24. involuntary contraction of bronchus _____

25. inflammation of bronchiole _____

Matching Exercises

Match the disorder with its description.

_____ 26. cystic fibrosis

_____ 27. emphysema

_____ 28. bronchiectasis

_____ 29. anthracosis

_____ 30. silicosis

a. COPD with enlarged air sacs
b. genetic disorder with abnormally thick mucous secretion
c. pneumoconiosis caused by silica inhalation
d. chronic dilation of airways
e. pneumoconiosis caused by coal dust

Match the sign or symptom with its description.

_____ 31. dyspnea

_____ 32. exudate

_____ 33. mucopurulent

_____ 34. stridor

_____ 35. tactile fremitus

a. seeping of mass of cells and fluid
b. vibration felt by the hand on chest while a person talks
c. harsh sound heard on inhalation that is caused by air passing through a constricted passageway
d. labored breathing
e. pertaining to mucus with pus

Match the clinical test or diagnostic procedure with its description.

_____ 36. bronchoscope

_____ 37. nasal speculum

_____ 38. sputum studies

_____ 39. laryngoscope

_____ 40. laryngoscopy

a. evaluation of substances found in the sputum
b. instrument for viewing the nasal cavity
c. lighted instrument with a short metal or plastic tube used for examining the larynx
d. thin, lighted instrument used to view respiratory structures during a bronchoscopy
e. visual examination of the larynx

Match the breathing type with its description.

_____ 41. Kussmaul respirations

_____ 42. hyperpnea

_____ 43. Biot respirations

_____ 44. bradypnea

_____ 45. Cheyne–Stokes respirations

a. alternating apnea with breathing of same depth
b. alternating pattern of apnea and deep, rapid breathing
c. air hunger
d. increased rate and depth of breathing
e. abnormally slow breathing rate

Match the medical term with its description.

_____ 46. aphonia

_____ 47. dysphonia

_____ 48. tussis

_____ 49. phlegm

_____ 50. rhonchus

a. thick mucus that is abnormally produced
b. loss of voice
c. impaired voice
d. coarse rale produced by air passage through a partially obstructed bronchus
e. cough

Match the medical term with its description.

_____ 51. spirometer

_____ 52. expiratory reserve volume (ERV)

_____ 53. tidal volume (TV)

_____ 54. eupnea

_____ 55. residual volume (RV)

a. amount of air inhaled or exhaled in a single breath
b. amount of air forcefully exhaled after normal expiration
c. device that measures inhaled and exhaled air volumes
d. amount of air in the lungs at all times
e. normal breathing

Match the medical term with its description.

_____ 56. total lung capacity

_____ 57. asphyxia

_____ 58. inspiratory reserve volume (IRV)

_____ 59. vital capacity (VC)

_____ 60. anatomical dead space

a. space containing air that does not reach alveoli
b. amount of air forcefully breathed in
c. amount of air expired after deepest possible breath
d. volume of air the lungs can hold
e. impaired oxygen and carbon dioxide exchange resulting in suffocation

Match the drug therapy with its description.

_____ 61. isoniazid

_____ 62. bronchodilator

_____ 63. expectorant

_____ 64. decongestant

a. drug that reduces congestion
b. drug used to treat TB
c. drug that relaxes bronchial smooth muscles
d. drug that stimulates phlegm secretion to be coughed out

Definitions

Define the following terms.

65. pulmonology _____

66. pneumonitis _____

67. hypercapnia _____

68. tracheotomy _____

Provide a medical term for the following definitions.

69. coughing up blood or bloody sputum _____

70. audible whistling breath sound that can be heard without using a stethoscope _____

71. difficulty swallowing _____

72. too much carbon dioxide in the blood _____

73. inadequate oxygen in the blood _____

Alternate Terms

Give an alternate term for each of the following terms.

74. acute rhinitis _____

75. adenoid _____

76. atomizer _____

77. hyaline membrane disease (HMD) _____

78. mechanical ventilator _____

79. mountain sickness _____

Spelling

Identify the correctly spelled term in each set.

80. _____
a. resusitation
b. resuscitation
c. resusutation
d. rescuscitation

81. _____
a. paradoxical
b. paridoxical
c. pearadoxical
d. paradocsical

82. _____
a. legionelosis
b. legionellosis
c. legunellosis
d. legunullosis

83. _____
a. neumonia
b. pnumonia
c. pneumonia
d. pneumonuh

84. _____
a. tuburculosis
b. tubercolosis
c. terberculosis
d. tuberculosis

85. _____
a. rinitis
b. rhinitis
c. rhynitis
d. rhinitus

Unscramble

Unscramble the letters to form a medical term.

86. yegnxo _____

87. nalnacu _____

88. tyorrerispa _____

89. finezanlu _____

90. mustpu _____

Abbreviations

Provide the terms for the abbreviation and then define the terms.

91. RSV = _____

92. SIDS = _____

93. COPD = _____

94. PEEP = _____

95. C&S = _____

96. URI = _____

Analogies

Provide a medical term to complete a meaningful analogy.

97. Inspiration is to expiration as hypoventilation is to _____

98. Inhalation is to exhalation as _____ is to alkalosis.

99. _____ is to slow respiration rate as tachypnea is to abnormally high respiration rate.

Short Answer

Answer the following questions.

100. Joey was sucking on a throat lozenge when he accidentally choked. The lozenge became wedged in his right bronchus. Provide a plausible explanation for it to be in the right bronchus instead of the left bronchus.

_____

101. If an individual loses the gag reflex, a protective mechanism to prevent choking, food particles can be accidentally inhaled. What type of lung disorder is likely to develop? _____

102. What is the difference between sleep apnea and reflex apnea? _____

Labeling

Label the structures in the following diagram.

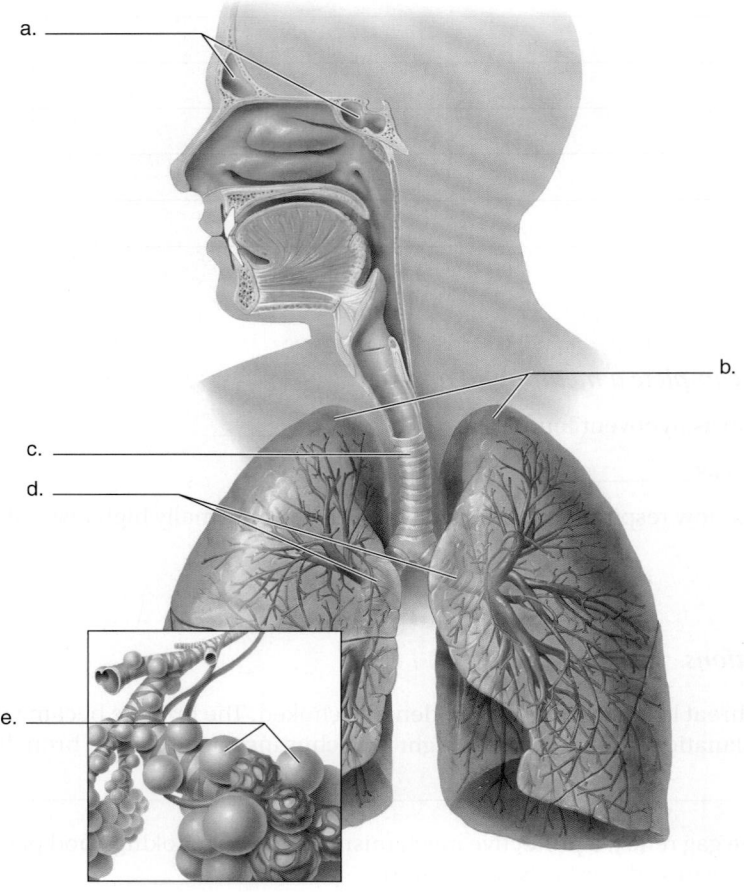

Word Search

Find the medical terms hidden in the puzzle.

F	W	N	B	E	K	D	U	P	P	D	E	A
C	P	Y	S	I	N	U	S	I	T	I	S	L
K	T	Y	Q	R	I	K	R	D	I	O	M	L
L	A	C	W	I	O	G	P	S	W	N	E	E
K	C	T	V	A	R	X	Y	E	Z	E	C	R
P	E	R	C	U	S	S	I	O	N	D	H	G
S	I	T	I	G	N	Y	R	A	L	A	L	I
R	H	I	N	O	V	I	R	U	S	E	S	C
E	E	R	T	L	A	I	H	C	N	O	R	B
P	Y	L	O	P	L	A	S	A	N	T	I	E
S	I	T	I	N	I	H	R	O	J	X	K	Z

adenoid
allergic rhinitis
bronchial tree
laryngitis
nasal polyp
percussion
rhinoviruses
sinusitis

Vocabulary Review

Review the key terms from this chapter, study the spelling and pronunciation of each term, and write its definition in the space provided. Listen to the audio available for most terms at http://thepoint.lww.com/nath2e and pronounce each term for yourself. Then check the box when you feel confident that you know the definition and can pronounce the term correctly.

Key Term	Pronunciation	Definition
❏ acidemia	(as-i-DEE-mee-uh)	_____
❏ acute bronchitis	(bron-KIGH-tis)	_____
❏ acute rhinitis	(rye-NIGH-tis)	_____
❏ adenoid	(AD-e-noid)	_____
❏ adult respiratory distress syndrome (ARDS)	(RES-pi-ruh-tor-ee)	_____
❏ allergic rhinitis	(rye-NIGH-tis)	_____
❏ altitude sickness		_____
❏ alveoli	(al-VEE-oh-lye)	_____
❏ anthracosis	(an-thruh-KOH-sis)	_____
❏ apex	(AY-pex)	_____
❏ aphonia	(ay-FOH-nee-uh)	_____
❏ apnea	(AP-nee-uh)	_____
❏ arterial blood gas (ABG)	(ahr-TEER-ee-ul)	_____
❏ asbestosis	(as-bes-TOH-sis)	_____
❏ asphyxia	(as-FICK-see-uh)	_____
❏ aspiration pneumonia	(as-pi-RAY-shun new-MOH-nee-uh)	_____
❏ asthma	(AZ-muh)	_____
❏ atomizer	(AT-uh-migh-zur)	_____
❏ auscultation	(aws-kul-TAY-shun)	_____
❏ barrel chest		_____
❏ base		_____
❏ berylliosis	(be-ril-ee-OH-sis)	_____
❏ Biot respirations	(bee-OH res-pi-RAY-shunz)	_____
❏ bradypnea	(brad-ip-NEE-uh)	_____
❏ bronchi	(BRONK-eye)	_____
❏ bronchial asthma	(BRONK-ee-ul AZ-muh)	_____
❏ bronchial tree	(BRONK-ee-ul)	_____
❏ bronchiectasis	(bronk-ee-ECK-tuh-sis)	_____
❏ bronchioles	(BRONK-ee-ohlz)	_____
❏ bronchitis	(bron-KIGH-tis)	_____
❏ bronchodilators	(bronk-oh-DYE-lay-turz)	_____

Key Term	Pronunciation	Definition
❏ bronchoscope	(BRONK-oh-skope)	_____
❏ bronchoscopy	(brong-KOS-kuh-pee)	_____
❏ bronchospasm	(BRONK-oh-spaz-um)	_____
❏ carbon monoxide poisoning		_____
❏ Cheyne–Stokes respiration	(CHAIN-STOKES res-pi-RAY-shun)	_____
❏ chronic bronchitis	(bron-KIGH-tis)	_____
❏ chronic obstructive pulmonary disease (COPD)	(PUL-moh-nerr-ee)	_____
❏ clubbing of fingers		_____
❏ conducting airway		_____
❏ continuous positive airway pressure (CPAP)		_____
❏ coryza	(koh-RYE-zuh)	_____
❏ culture and sensitivity (C&S) studies		_____
❏ cyanosis	(sigh-uh-NOH-sis)	_____
❏ cystic fibrosis	(SIS-tick figh-BROH-sis)	_____
❏ decongestant		_____
❏ diaphragm	(DYE-uh-fram)	_____
❏ dysphagia	(dis-FAY-jee-uh)	_____
❏ dysphonia	(dis-FOH-nee-uh)	_____
❏ dyspnea	(disp-NEE-uh)	_____
❏ emphysema	(em-fi-SEE-muh)	_____
❏ endotracheal tube	(en-doh-TRAY-kee-ul)	_____
❏ epiglottis	(ep-i-GLOT-is)	_____
❏ eupnea	(yoop-NEE-uh)	_____
❏ exercise-induced asthma	(AZ-muh)	_____
❏ exhalation	(ecks-huh-LAY-shun)	_____
❏ expectorated	(eck-speck-toh-RATE-ed)	_____
❏ expiratory reserve volume (ERV)	(eck-SPYE-ruh-tor-ee)	_____
❏ exudate	(ECKS-yoo-date)	_____
❏ flail chest		_____
❏ glottis	(GLOT-is)	_____
❏ hemoptysis	(hee-MOP-ti-sis)	_____
❏ hemothorax	(hee-moh-THOR-acks)	_____
❏ hilum	(HIGH-lum)	_____
❏ histoplasmosis	(his-toh-plaz-MOH-sis)	_____
❏ hyaline membrane disease (HMD)	(HIGH-uh-lin)	_____

Key Term	Pronunciation	Definition
❏ hypercapnia	(high-pur-KAP-nee-uh)	
❏ hyperpnea	(high-pur-NEE-uh)	
❏ hyperventilation	(high-pur-ven-ti-LAY-shun)	
❏ hypoventilation	(high-poh-ven-ti-LAY-shun)	
❏ hypoxemia	(high-pock-SEE-mee-uh)	
❏ hypoxia	(high-POCK-see-uh)	
❏ infant respiratory distress syndrome (IRDS)	(RES-pi-ruh-tor-ee)	
❏ influenza	(in-floo-EN-zuh)	
❏ inhalation	(in-huh-LAY-shun)	
❏ inspiratory reserve volume (IRV)	(in-SPYE-ruh-tor-ee)	
❏ Kussmaul respirations	(KOOS-mawl res-pi-RAY-shuns)	
❏ lacrimation	(lack-ri-MAY-shun)	
❏ laryngitis	(lair-in-JYE-tis)	
❏ laryngopharynx	(la-ring-oh-FAIR-inks)	
❏ laryngoscope	(la-RING-goh-skope)	
❏ laryngoscopy	(lair-ing-GOS-kuh-pee)	
❏ larynx	(LAIR-inks)	
❏ legionellosis	(lee-juh-nell-OH-sis)	
❏ Legionnaires' disease	(lee-juh-NAIRZ)	
❏ lobar pneumonia	(LOH-bar new-MOH-nee-uh)	
❏ lobectomy	(loh-BECK-toh-mee)	
❏ lung biopsy	(BYE-op-see)	
❏ lung cancer		
❏ lungs		
❏ Mantoux test	(MAN-too)	
❏ mechanical ventilator		
❏ mesothelioma	(mez-oh-thee-lee-OH-muh)	
❏ mountain sickness		
❏ mucopurulent	(mew-koh-PEW-roo-lunt)	
❏ nares	(NAY-res)	
❏ nasal cannula	(KAN-yoo-luh)	
❏ nasal catarrh	(kuh-TAHR)	
❏ nasal cavity	(NAY-zul KAV-i-tee)	
❏ nasal polyp	(POL-ip)	
❏ nasal septum	(SEP-tum)	
❏ nasal speculum	(SPECK-yoo-lum)	
❏ nasopharynx	(nay-zoh-FAIR-inks)	

Key Term	Pronunciation	Definition
❏ nebulizer	(NEB-yoo-lye-zur)	_____
❏ neonatal respiratory distress syndrome (NRDS)	(RES-pi-ruh-tor-ee)	_____
❏ oropharynx	(or-oh-FAIR-inks)	_____
❏ oxygen tent		_____
❏ oxygen therapy		_____
❏ palatine tonsils	(PAL-uh-tine TON-sils)	_____
❏ paradoxical respiration	(pair-uh-DOCK-si-kul res-pi-RAY-shun)	_____
❏ paranasal sinuses	(pair-uh-NAY-zul-SIGH-nus-ez)	_____
❏ parietal pleura	(puh-RYE-e-tul-PLOOR-uh)	_____
❏ peak expiratory flow (PEF) test	(eck-SPYE-ruh-tor-ee)	_____
❏ percussion		_____
❏ pharyngeal tonsil	(fuh-RIN-jee-ul TON-sil)	_____
❏ pharyngitis	(fair-in-JYE-tis)	_____
❏ pharynx	(FAIR-inks)	_____
❏ phlegm	(FLEM)	_____
❏ pneumoconiosis	(new-moh-koh-nee-OH-sis)	_____
❏ pneumonia	(new-MOH-nee-uh)	_____
❏ pneumothorax	(new-moh-THOR-acks)	_____
❏ positive end-expiratory pressure (PEEP)	(eck-SPYE-ruh-tor-ee)	_____
❏ postural drainage (PD)	(POS-chur-ul)	_____
❏ pulmonary edema	(PUL-moh-nerr-ee e-DEE-muh)	_____
❏ pulmonary embolism	(PUL-moh-nerr-ee EM-boh-liz-um)	_____
❏ pulmonary function test (PFT)	(PUL-moh-nerr-ee)	_____
❏ pulmonary ventilation	(PUL-moh-nerr-ee)	_____
❏ pulse oximeter	(ock-SIM-e-tur)	_____
❏ pulse oximetry	(ock-SIM-e-tree)	_____
❏ rales	(RAHLZ)	_____
❏ reflex apnea	(AP-nee-uh)	_____
❏ residual volume (RV)		_____
❏ respiration	(res-pi-RAY-shun)	_____
❏ respiratory acidosis	(RES-pi-ruh-tor-ee as-i-DOH-sis)	_____
❏ respiratory airway	(RES-pi-ruh-tor-ee)	_____
❏ respiratory alkalosis	(RES-pi-ruh-tor-ee al-kuh-LOH-sis)	_____

Key Term	Pronunciation	Definition
❏ respiratory failure	(RES-pi-ruh-tor-ee)	_____
❏ respiratory syncytial virus (RSV) pneumonia	(RES-pi-ruh-tor-ee sin-SISH-ul) (new-MOH-nee-uh)	_____ _____
❏ resuscitation bag	(ree-sus-i-TAY-shun)	_____
❏ rhinoviruses	(rye-noh-VYE-rus-ez)	_____
❏ rhonchus	(RONK-us)	_____
❏ silicosis	(sil-i-KOH-sis)	_____
❏ sinuses	(SIGH-nus-ez)	_____
❏ sinusitis	(sigh-nuh-SIGH-tis)	_____
❏ sleep apnea	(AP-nee-uh)	_____
❏ spirometer	(spye-ROM-e-tur)	_____
❏ sputum	(SPEW-tum)	_____
❏ sputum studies	(SPEW-tum)	_____
❏ sudden infant death syndrome (SIDS)		_____
❏ surfactant	(sur-FACK-tunt)	_____
❏ tachypnea	(tack-ip-NEE-uh)	_____
❏ terminal bronchioles	(BRONK-ee-ohlz)	_____
❏ thoracentesis	(thoh-ruh-sen-TEE-sis)	_____
❏ tidal volume (TV)		_____
❏ total lung capacity (TLC)		_____
❏ trachea	(TRAY-kee-uh)	_____
❏ tracheostomy tube	(tray-kee-OS-toh-mee)	_____
❏ tuberculin test	(TOO-berk-yoo-lun)	_____
❏ tuberculosis (TB)	(tew-bur-kew-LOH-sis)	_____
❏ tussis	(TUS-is)	_____
❏ upper respiratory infection (URI)	(RES-pi-ruh-tor-ee)	_____
❏ uvula	(YOO-vyoo-luh)	_____
❏ Venturi mask	(ven-TUE-ree)	_____
❏ visceral pleura	(VIS-ur-ul-PLOOR-uh)	_____
❏ vital capacity (VC)		_____
❏ vocal cords		_____
❏ wheeze		_____

Answers

Word Grouping Exercises

Definition	Word Part	Definition	Word Part
imperfect, incomplete	atel-, atelo-	nose	rhin-, rhino-
air, gas, lung, breathing	pneum-, pneumo-, pneumon-, pneumono-	nose, nasal	nas-, naso-
alveolus (air cell), alveolar	alveolo-	pharynx, pharyngeal, throat	pharyng-, pharyngo-
breathing	spir-, spiro-	presence of carbon dioxide	-capnia
bronchus, windpipe	bronch-, bronchi-, broncho-	presence of oxygen	oxy-
chest	thorac-, thoracico-, thoraco-	rapid, quick	tachy-
coal, charcoal, carbon	anthraco-	respiration, respiratory condition	-pnea
diaphragm	phren-, phreno-	rib, side, lung membrane	pleur-, pleura-, pleuro-
larynx, laryngeal	laryng-, laryngo-	slow	brady-
lungs	pulmo-, pulmon-, pulmono-	sound, speech, voice sounds	phon-, phono-
mouth, oral	oro-	straight	orth-, ortho-
mucus	muc-, muci-, muco-	time	chron-, chrono-
normal, true	eu-	trachea, tracheal	trache-, tracheo-

Word Building Exercises

Word Part	Meaning	Common or Known Word	Example Medical Term
orth-, ortho-	straight	orthodontics	orthopnea
anthraco-	coal, charcoal, carbon	anthrax	anthracosis
bronch-, bronchi, broncho-	bronchus, windpipe	bronchitis	bronchoscopy
chron-, chrono-	time	chronometer	chronic
laryng-, laryngo-	larynx, laryngeal	laryngitis	laryngospasm
muc-, muci-, muco-	mucus	mucous membrane	mucus
nas-, naso-	nose, nasal	nasogastric	nasal cavity
oro-	mouth, oral	orator	oral cavity
phon-, phono-	sound, speech, voice	phonetics	aphonia
-pnea	respiration, respiratory condition	sleep apnea	apnea
pneum-, pneumo-, pneumon-, pneumono-	air, gas, lung, breathing	pneumonia	pneumonia
pulmo-, pulmon-, pulmono-	lungs	pulmonologist	pulmonary
tachy-	rapid, quick	tachymeter	tachypnea
thorac-, thoracico-, thoraco-	chest	thoracic	thoracentesis
trache-, tracheo-	trachea, tracheal	tracheitis	tracheostomy

Key Term Practice

Respiratory System Preview

1. a. pharynges; b. larynges
2. bronchus, windpipe
3. trachea
4. nasal cavity
5. lungs

Nose, Nasal Cavity, and Paranasal Sinuses

1. a. naris; b. sinus
2. septum
3. paranasal sinuses; sinuses

Pharynx

1. nose, nasal; nasopharynx
2. *Oro-*; oropharynx
3. *laryng-, laryngo-*; laryngopharynx
4. pharyngeal tonsil
5. palatine tonsils

Larynx

1. glottis; epiglottis
2. true vocal cords
3. uvula

Trachea and Bronchial Tree

1. bronchi
2. alveoli
3. conducting airway; respiratory airway
4. Bronchioles
5. terminal bronchioles

Lungs

1. visceral; parietal
2. base
3. Surfactant
4. hilum
5. apex

Functions of the Respiratory System

1. Inhalation; exhalation
2. pulmonary ventilation; *pulmo-, pulmon-, pulmono-*
3. eupnea; *eu-; -pnea*
4. Tussis
5. diaphragm

Pulmonary Function Tests

1. spirometer
2. Tidal volume
3. vital capacity
4. Total lung capacity
5. pulmonary function test (PFT)

Altered Breathing

1. *brady-; -pnea*; bradypnea
2. rapid, quick; respiration, respiratory condition; tachypnea
3. Hypoventilation
4. Hyperventilation
5. apnea

Cardiovascular Disorders Affecting Lungs

1. pulmonary embolism
2. tracheostomy tube
3. nebulizer or atomizer
4. Cyanosis
5. Venturi mask

Cystic Fibrosis

1. *hypo-*; hypoxia
2. cystic fibrosis
3. Pulse oximetry
4. expectorate
5. sputum; phlegm

Chronic Obstructive Pulmonary Disease

1. *bronch-, bronchi-, broncho-; -itis*; bronchitis
2. acute bronchitis; chronic bronchitis
3. hemoptysis
4. lung biopsy
5. Emphysema

Asthma

1. rhonchus
2. bronchospasm
3. exercise-induced asthma
4. wheeze
5. Asthma

Inhalation Disorders

1. pneumoconiosis; *pneumo-*
2. *anthrac-*; condition of; anthracosis
3. Asbestosis
4. berylliosis
5. silicosis

Upper Respiratory Disorders

1. dysphagia
2. nose, nasal; *-itis*; rhinitis
3. Coryza
4. *pharyng-, pharyngo-; -itis*; pharyngitis
5. decongestant

Lower Respiratory Disorders

1. pneumonia
2. tuberculosis
3. Legionnaires' disease and legionellosis
4. tuberculin test and Mantoux test
5. aspiration pneumonia

Lung Cancer

1. lung cancer
2. lobectomy
3. Mesothelioma

Pneumothorax and Hemothorax

1. Pneumothorax; hemothorax
2. thoracentesis

Respiratory Acidosis and Respiratory Alkalosis

1. alkalosis; acidosis

Respiratory Syndromes

1. respiratory failure
2. sudden infant death syndrome (SIDS)
3. Pulmonary edema
4. hypoxemia; *hypo-; -emia*
5. acidemia

Trauma and Poisoning

1. flail chest
2. Carbon monoxide poisoning
3. paradoxical respiration

Common Abbreviations Exercises

1. oxygen = O_2
2. CO = carbon monoxide
3. ABG = arterial blood gas
4. gram-negative = G–
5. PFT = pulmonary function test

Case Study

1. d is the correct answer.
   - a is incorrect because being off balance describes vertigo.
   - b is incorrect because thirsty describes dipsia.
   - c is incorrect because difficulty swallowing describes dysphagia.
2. c is the correct answer.
   - a is incorrect because paranasal sinuses are hollow, air-filled spaces in the bones of the face that are lined with mucous membrane.
   - b is incorrect because the septum is a cartilaginous partition dividing the nasal cavity into right and left sides.
   - d is incorrect because the nasal cavity is the space between the nostrils.

3. b is the correct answer.
   - a is incorrect because the external nares are nostrils.
   - c is incorrect because the lungs are not found in the nasal cavity.
   - d is incorrect because the sinuses are not soft tissue but rather are spaces located within the skull bones.
4. c is the correct answer.
   - a is incorrect because the report indicated clear sinuses; thus she does not have an infection.
   - b is incorrect because a CT scan of the skull would not indicate TB, which is a lung infection; a lung x-ray would be needed.
   - d is incorrect because she is experiencing dyspnea, vomiting, and dizziness, which are all abnormal signs and symptoms; thus further study is warranted.

Real World Report

1. evaluate and assess lung function and performance
2. a. lung capacities and volumes; b. the amount of air that can be exhaled from the lungs after the deepest possible breath; c. expand and relax the breathing passages, especially those of the bronchial tree.
3. a. total lung capacity, which is the total volume of air the lungs can hold; b. the amount of air that is constantly present in the lungs
4. nasal cavity, pharynx, larynx, trachea, bronchi, and terminal bronchioles
5. emphysema

Review and Application

1. b	23. laryngectomy	45. b	66. inflammation of lung
2. a	24. bronchospasm	46. b	67. excessive carbon dioxide in blood
3. c	25. bronchiolitis	47. c	68. surgical opening in trachea
4. a	26. b	48. e	69. hemoptysis
5. b	27. a	49. a	70. wheeze
6. d	28. d	50. d	71. dysphagia
7. c	29. e	51. c	72. hypercapnia
8. d	30. c	52. b	73. hypoxemia
9. a	31. d	53. a	74. nasal catarrh
10. b	32. a	54. e	75. pharyngeal tonsil
11. d	33. e	55. d	76. nebulizer
12. c	34. c	56. d	77. infant respiratory distress syndrome (IRDS)
13. d	35. b	57. e	and neonatal respiratory distress syndrome
14. c	36. d	58. b	(NRDS)
15. c	37. b	59. c	78. respirator
16. a	38. a	60. a	79. altitude sickness
17. b	39. c	61. b	80. b
18. c	40. e	62. c	81. a
19. d	41. c	63. d	82. b
20. d	42. d	64. a	83. c
21. b	43. a	65. study of the	84. d
22. thoracentesis	44. e	lungs	85. b

86. oxygen
87. cannula
88. respiratory
89. influenza
90. sputum
91. RSV = respiratory syncytial virus; virus that causes lung inflammation and RSV pneumonia
92. SIDS = sudden infant death syndrome; sudden, unexpected, unexplained death of a sleeping infant
93. COPD = chronic obstructive pulmonary disease; general term describing lung disease affecting the bronchial tree
94. PEEP = positive end-expiratory pressure; positive-pressure air delivered during expiration
95. C&S = culture and sensitivity; tests to identify microbes and the effectiveness of various antibiotics
96. URI = upper respiratory infection; acute infection causing inflammation that affects the upper respiratory structures

97. hyperventilation
98. acidosis
99. Bradypnea
100. Inhaled particles are more likely to be lodged in the right bronchus than the left bronchus because the right bronchus is slightly larger in diameter and positioned in a more vertical direction than the left bronchus.
101. Aspiration pneumonia is the type of pneumonia likely to result from food particles inhaled into the lower airways.
102. Sleep apnea is the cessation of breathing during sleep that causes one to awaken and is associated with daytime sleepiness. Reflex apnea is a sudden, temporary loss of breath and is a sign, not a disease.

Labeling

a. paranasal sinuses   **b.** lungs   **c.** trachea

d. bronchi   **e.** alveoli

Word Search

+	+	+	+	+	+	+	+	+	+	D	+	A
+	+	+	S	I	N	U	S	I	T	I	S	L
+	+	+	+	+	+	+	+	+	+	O	+	L
+	+	+	+	+	+	+	+	+	+	N	+	E
+	+	+	+	+	+	+	+	+	+	E	+	R
P	E	R	C	U	S	S	I	O	N	D	+	G
S	I	T	I	G	N	Y	R	A	L	A	+	I
R	H	I	N	O	V	I	R	U	S	E	S	C
E	E	R	T	L	A	I	H	C	N	O	R	B
P	Y	L	O	P	L	A	S	A	N	+	+	+
S	I	T	I	N	I	H	R	+	+	+	+	+

adenoid
allergic rhinitis
bronchial tree
laryngitis
nasal polyp
percussion
rhinoviruses
sinusitis

Vocabulary Review

Key Term	Definition	Key Term	Definition
acidemia	abnormally low blood pH	bronchi	the two main branches (left and right) off the trachea
acute bronchitis	sudden and short-lasting inflammation of the bronchial tubes	bronchial asthma	form of asthma with attacks of dyspnea and bronchial spasms
acute rhinitis	inflammation of the nasal cavity caused by infection; also called nasal catarrh	bronchial tree	branches of the bronchi
		bronchiectasis	chronic dilation of the airways
adenoid	lymphatic tissue on the posterior wall of the nasopharynx; also called the pharyngeal tonsil	bronchioles	small subdivisions of bronchi
		bronchitis	inflammation of the bronchial tubes
		bronchodilators	drugs that ease breathing by relaxing the air passages
adult respiratory distress syndrome (ARDS)	disorder marked by hypercapnia, acidemia, and severe hypoxemia resulting in cyanosis	bronchoscope	thin, lighted instrument used to view respiratory structures during a bronchoscopy
allergic rhinitis	nasal inflammation resulting from an allergy	bronchoscopy	procedure for viewing the inside of the respiratory structures using a bronchoscope
altitude sickness	illness caused by the ascent to a high altitude and the resulting shortage of oxygen; also called mountain sickness	bronchospasm	contraction of smooth muscle in the walls of the bronchi and bronchioles, causing narrowing of the bronchial tubes
alveoli	tiny air sacs in lungs where gases are exchanged between alveolar air and blood		
anthracosis	pneumoconiosis caused by inhalation of coal dust	carbon monoxide poisoning	disorder resulting from hemoglobin combining with CO instead of hemoglobin combining with oxygen
apex	rounded top portion of lung pointing toward the first rib	Cheyne–Stokes respiration	alternating pattern of apnea and deep, rapid breathing
aphonia	loss of the voice	chronic bronchitis	long-lasting inflammation of the bronchial tubes
apnea	temporary absence of breathing		
arterial blood gas (ABG)	evaluation of blood pH, CO_2, O_2, and HCO_3^- concentrations	chronic obstructive pulmonary disease (COPD)	general term describing lung disease affecting the bronchial tree
asbestosis	pneumoconiosis caused by inhalation of asbestos fibers		
asphyxia	impaired or absent exchange of oxygen (O_2) and carbon dioxide (CO_2) during breathing that results in suffocation	clubbing of fingers	fingertips that are rounded like a club as a result of chronic inadequate oxygen delivery to the tissues
aspiration pneumonia	inflammation of the lungs that results from inhaling a substance into the lung field	conducting airway	respiratory structures involved with air distribution
asthma	breathing disorder characterized by chest tightness and airway constriction	continuous positive airway pressure (CPAP)	positive-pressure air delivered throughout the respiratory cycle
atomizer	device for administering medicinal liquid in the form of a spray to be breathed through the mouth or nose; also called a nebulizer	coryza	runny nose
		culture and sensitivity (C&S) studies	tests to identify microbes and the effectiveness of various antibiotics
auscultation	listening to body sounds using a stethoscope	cyanosis	bluish colored tissue due to a lack of oxygen in the blood
barrel chest	abnormal rounded chest cavity		
base	lower part of lung that rests on the diaphragm	cystic fibrosis	inherited disorder characterized by thick mucous secretions that block the internal passages, including the lungs
berylliosis	pneumoconiosis caused by inhalation of beryllium	decongestant	drug that reduces nasal congestion
Biot respirations	alternating periods of apnea with breaths of the same depth	diaphragm	curved muscle that separates the thoracic cavity and abdominal cavity
bradypnea	abnormally slow breathing rate	dysphagia	difficulty swallowing

Key Term	Definition	Key Term	Definition
dysphonia	hoarseness	laryngoscope	lighted instrument with a short metal or plastic tube used for examining the larynx
dyspnea	difficulty breathing	laryngoscopy	visual examination of the larynx using a lighted instrument called a laryngoscope
emphysema	chronic lung disorder characterized by enlarged air sacs	larynx	voice box
endotracheal tube	tube passed through the mouth or nose to the trachea	legionellosis	pneumonia caused by *Legionella pneumophila*; also called Legionnaires' disease
epiglottis	flap of cartilage that guards the glottis during swallowing	Legionnaires' disease	pneumonia caused by *Legionella pneumophila*; also called legionellosis
eupnea	normal breathing	lobar pneumonia	inflammation of the lungs affecting one or more lobes or parts of a lobe
exercise-induced asthma	form of asthma with bronchoconstriction caused by exercise	lobectomy	surgical removal of all or part of a lung
exhalation	process of exhaling or expiring	lung biopsy	removal of lung tissue for diagnostic evaluation
expectorated	coughed up and spit out	lung cancer	malignant tumors of the lung tissue
expiratory reserve volume (ERV)	amount of air that can be forcefully expired after normal exhalation	lungs	organs of breathing
exudate	seeping mass of cells and fluid	Mantoux test	intradermal test used to establish past or present tuberculosis infection; also called the tuberculin test
flail chest	fracture of the rib cage that causes paradoxical chest wall movement	mechanical ventilator	machine for moving air into and out of a person's lungs; also called a respirator
glottis	a slit-like opening where air enters the larynx	mesothelioma	cancer derived from the lining cells of the pleura and peritoneum, associated with asbestos exposure
hemoptysis	coughing up blood or bloody mucus	mountain sickness	illness caused by the ascent to a high altitude and the resulting shortage of oxygen; also called altitude sickness
hemothorax	blood in the pleural cavity	mucopurulent	pertaining to mucus with pus
hilum	wedge-shaped depression on the mediastinal surface of each lung	nares	nostrils
histoplasmosis	fungal infection of the lungs	nasal cannula	flexible tube placed in the nostrils to deliver oxygen
hyaline membrane disease	disorder marked by breathing difficulty and cyanosis in the infant or newborn; also called IRDS and NRDS	nasal catarrh	inflammation of the nasal cavity caused by infection; also called acute rhinitis
hypercapnia	too much carbon dioxide in the blood	nasal cavity	the space on either side of the nasal septum
hyperpnea	increased rate and depth of breathing	nasal polyp	benign growth on the nasal mucous membranes
hyperventilation	excessive inhalation and exhalation that leads to decreased CO_2 levels	nasal septum	wall dividing the nasal cavity into right and left sides
hypoventilation	decreased breathing rate that often results in increased levels of CO_2	nasal speculum	instrument for viewing the nasal cavity
hypoxemia	inadequate oxygen in the blood	nasopharynx	region of the pharynx behind the nasal cavity
hypoxia	inadequate oxygen in the tissues	nebulizer	device for administering medicinal liquid in the form of a spray to be breathed through the mouth or nose; also called an atomizer
infant respiratory distress syndrome (IRDS)	disorder marked by breathing difficulty and cyanosis in the infant or newborn; also called NRDS and HMD		
influenza	viral infection producing fever, sore throat, cough, and muscle pain; flu	neonatal respiratory distress syndrome (NRDS)	disorder marked by breathing difficulty and cyanosis in the infant or newborn; also called IRDS and HMD
inhalation	process of inhaling or inspiring		
inspiratory reserve volume (IRV)	amount of air that can be forcefully breathed in after normal inhalation		
Kussmaul respirations	rapid and deep respirations; referred to as air hunger		
lacrimation	tear production		
laryngitis	larynx inflammation		
laryngopharynx	lower-most region of the pharynx located near the larynx		

Key Term	Definition	Key Term	Definition
oropharynx	region of the pharynx located near the back of the mouth	rales	abnormal hissing or whistling respiratory sounds
oxygen tent	structure that surrounds a patient in bed to supply oxygen	reflex apnea	sudden, temporary loss of breath; a gasp
oxygen therapy	supplying oxygen via a nasal cannula, Venturi mask, or oxygen tent	residual volume (RV)	amount of air remaining in the lungs after complete exhalation
palatine tonsils	lymphatic tissue embedded in wall of oropharynx; commonly referred to as the tonsils	respiration	chemical processes occurring in tissues for gas exchange; commonly called breathing
paradoxical respiration	breathing that is contrary to usual movements in that the lung deflates during inhalation and inflates during exhalation	respiratory acidosis	low blood pH caused by carbon dioxide retention
		respiratory airway	respiratory structures involved with gas exchange
paranasal sinuses	hollow, air-filled spaces in the bones of the face that are lined with mucous membrane; also called sinuses	respiratory alkalosis	increased blood pH due to elimination of too much carbon dioxide
parietal pleura	serous membrane lining the thoracic cavity	respiratory failure	respiratory system is unable to meet the oxygen demands of the body, and carbon dioxide levels increase
peak expiratory flow (PEF) test	uses a PEF meter to measure the volume of air after forced expiration	respiratory syncytial virus (RSV) pneumonia	lung inflammation caused by RSV
percussion	tapping on the chest or back during auscultation to determine the presence of normal air content in the lungs	resuscitation bag	bag that is manually pumped to deliver air or oxygen
pharyngeal tonsil	lymphatic tissue on the posterior wall of the nasopharynx; also called the adenoid	rhinoviruses	any of many RNA viruses that cause upper respiratory tract infections
pharyngitis	inflammation of the pharynx; also called a sore throat	rhonchus	harsh rattling sound
		silicosis	pneumoconiosis caused by inhalation of silica dust
pharynx	region between the mouth and the esophagus; also called the throat	sinuses	hollow, air-filled spaces in the bones of the face that are lined with mucous membrane; also called paranasal sinuses
phlegm	fluid or semifluid mucus mixture; also called sputum		
pneumoconiosis	disease caused by inhaling mineral or metallic dust over a long period of time	sinusitis	inflammation of the sinuses
pneumonia	inflammation of the lungs	sleep apnea	cessation of breathing during sleep that causes one to awaken and is associated with daytime sleepiness
pneumothorax	abnormal presence of air or gas in the pleural cavity		
positive end-expiratory pressure (PEEP)	positive-pressure air delivered during expiration (exhalation)	spirometer	device that measures inhaled and exhaled air volumes
		sputum	fluid or semifluid mucus mixture; also called phlegm
postural drainage (PD)	positioning the body to allow gravity to drain mucus from areas of the lungs	sputum studies	tests to evaluate substances found in sputum
pulmonary edema	fluid accumulation in the lungs causing breathing difficulty	sudden infant death syndrome (SIDS)	sudden, unexpected, unexplained death of a sleeping infant
pulmonary embolism	blood clot lodged in a pulmonary artery	surfactant	substance that helps to prevent the alveoli from collapsing
pulmonary function test (PFT)	evaluates and assesses lung function by measuring lung volumes and capacities	tachypnea	rapid breathing rate
		terminal bronchioles	subdivision of the bronchioles
pulmonary ventilation	breathing, respiration	thoracentesis	needle aspiration of the pleural cavity through the chest wall for fluid or air withdrawal
pulse oximeter	small instrument that measures the amount of oxygen in blood		
pulse oximetry	measurement of oxygen in the blood	tidal volume (TV)	amount of air inhaled or exhaled in a single breath

Key Term	Definition	Key Term	Definition
total lung capacity (TLC)	total volume of air the lungs can hold	upper respiratory infection (URI)	acute infection causing inflammation that affects the upper respiratory structures
trachea	tube that conducts air from the larynx to the bronchial tree	uvula	fleshy flap at the back of the oral cavity that hangs above the throat
tracheostomy tube	tube placed through a hole in the trachea	Venturi mask	face mask that delivers oxygen
tuberculin test	intradermal test used to establish past or present tuberculosis infection; also called the Mantoux test	visceral pleura	serous membrane on the lung surface
		vital capacity (VC)	amount of air that can be exhaled after the deepest possible inhalation
tuberculosis (TB)	infectious disease affecting the lungs caused by *Mycobacterium tuberculosis*	vocal cords	structures that vibrate in the larynx to produce sound
tussis	cough	wheeze	audible whistling breath sound

CHAPTER 13

Lymphatic System and Immunity

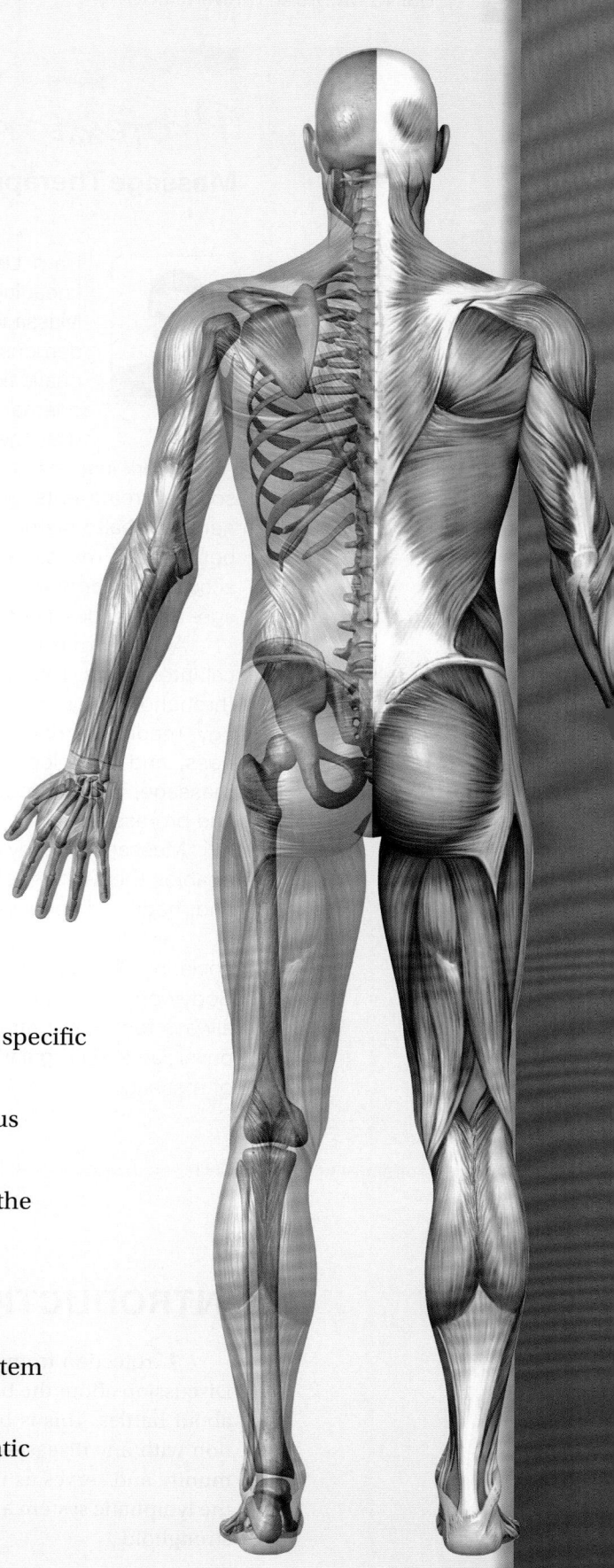

OBJECTIVES

After completing this chapter, you should be able to:

1. State the meanings of word parts related to the lymphatic system and immunity.

2. List key functions of the lymphatic system.

3. Describe lymphatic vessels, their locations, and how lymph circulates throughout the body.

4. Explain the difference between nonspecific immunity and specific immunity and their function to overall body functioning.

5. Define common signs, symptoms, and treatments of various lymphatic system and immunity diseases.

6. Explain clinical tests and diagnostic procedures related to the lymphatic system and immunity.

7. Describe anatomical and physiological alterations of the lymphatic system and immunity throughout the life span.

8. Define common abbreviations related to the lymphatic system and immunity.

9. Define terms used in medical reports involving the lymphatic system and immunity.

10. Define, spell, and pronounce the chapter's medical terms correctly.

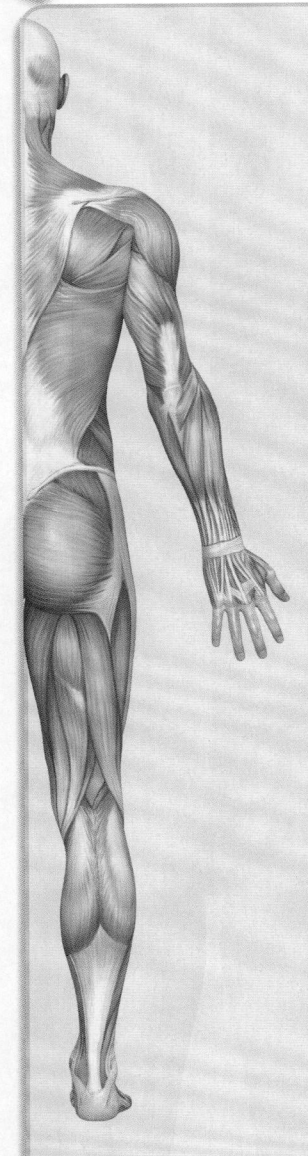

Professional Profile

Massage Therapist

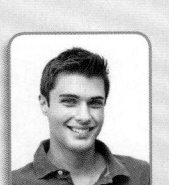

I am Lee, a massage therapist (MT). I provide treatment by rubbing, kneading, and manipulating the muscles for medical and healing purposes. Massage therapy is beneficial to good health and well-being. Research is demonstrating its therapeutic merit, especially in immune function, lymphatic flow, and stress reduction. Massage therapy is used to treat lymphedema by stimulating undamaged lymph nodes and encouraging fluid drainage from swollen areas through the application of pressure and motion.

I work in a spa environment, but there is a physician on staff who performs other sorts of treatments, primarily for patients with cancer. For each new client, a comprehensive health history is obtained, and for established clients, the history is updated before each massage session. As with any allied health profession, I must maintain accurate records, document treatments, ensure confidentiality, and be sensitive to age- and gender-related issues.

A typical massage therapy program consists of 720 hours of coursework and clinical internships. The hands-on approach enables students to practice in-class material throughout their educational program. Courses include anatomy, physiology, kinesiology, medical terminology, first aid, cardiopulmonary resuscitation (CPR), HIV awareness, and herbology, along with Swedish massage, sports massage, seated chair massage, prenatal massage, and lymphatic massage. Students also study business and professionalism.

Massage therapy is a discipline in which practice enhances technique. Experience enables the MT to feel for fine nuances in the physical body, observe client reactions, and modify as necessary with greater confidence.

I am licensed by the state medical board, the American Massage Therapy Association (AMTA), and the National Certification Board for Therapeutic Massage and Bodywork (NCBTMB). Job satisfaction is high, primarily because the clients almost always feel better after a treatment. The profession is results oriented, and the staff physician and I regularly provide informative community presentations on the benefits of massage.

INTRODUCTION

*P*rotection from disease enables us to live in a world ripe with microscopic adversity. Discussion about the body's lymphatic system and immune response often sounds like a talk about battles. This is because the body is constantly engaged in a "me versus them" situation with any disease-causing agent. The lymphatic system provides the foundation for immunity and serves as the relentless warrior and constant guard. The coordinated actions of the lymphatic system and immunity prevent millions of infinitesimal organisms from taking a stronghold.

Distinguishing "self" from "nonself" is key to protection. Anything that is nonself, such as a virus, bacterium, or toxin, is eliminated by two specialized mechanisms: nonspecific (innate) immunity and specific (adaptive) immunity. Neither type operates in isolation. They are complementary operations that require the coordination of the total immune response.

A common characteristic of all immune disorders is increased susceptibility (likelihood of being affected) to infection. Immunodeficiency diseases result from defective operations of the immune system. Pathology of the lymphatic system and subsequent acute, chronic, or recurrent disease is the topic of *The Clinical Dimension* section of this chapter.

MEDICAL TERM PARTS

Word Parts

Medical term prefixes, suffixes, and combining forms related to the lymphatic system and immunity are introduced in this section.

Word Part	Meaning
allo-	other, different
aut-, auto-	self, same
chyl-, chylo-	chyle, fat droplets in lymph
-gen,	substance that produces something
heter-, hetero-	other, different
immuno-	immune, immunity, protected
iso-	like
lact-, lacti-, lacto-	milk
lymph-, lympho-	lymph
lymphaden-, lymphadeno-	lymph nodes
lymphangi-, lymphangio-	lymphatic vessels
path-, patho-, -pathy	disease
phago-	eating, devouring
rhin-, rhino-	nose
splen-, spleno-	spleen
thym-, thymi-, thymo-	thymus
tonsillo-	tonsil
tox-, toxi-, toxico-, toxo-	poison, toxin
xeno-	strange, foreign

Word Grouping Exercises

Using the *Medical Term Parts* table, identify the prefix, suffix, or combining form for each of the following definitions. The first one has been done as an example.

Definition	Word Part
chyle, fat droplets in lymph	*chyl-, chylo-*
disease	
eating, devouring	
immune, immunity, protected	
like	
lymph	
lymph nodes	
lymphatic vessels	
milk	
nose	
other, different	A. B.
poison, toxin	
self, same	
spleen	
strange, foreign	
substance that produces something	
thymus	
tonsil	

Word Building Exercises

Word parts introduced in the *Medical Term Parts* section are listed in the following table. For this exercise, first supply the meaning of each word part, then use the word part to build a word you already know. The word you list under *Common or Known Word* does not have to be a medical term; a commonly used word is fine. Be sure, however, that the word correctly reflects the intended meaning. The first one has been done as an example. Check your answers in a dictionary.

Word Part	Meaning	Common or Known Word	Example Medical Term
xeno-	*strange, foreign*	*xenolith*	xenograft
allo-			allogeneic
aut-, auto-			autoimmune

continued

continued from page 640

Word Part	Meaning	Common or Known Word	Example Medical Term
-gen			antigen
heter-, hetero-			heterograft
immuno-			immunologic response
iso-			isograft
lact-, lacti-, lacto-			lacteal
lymph-, lympho-			lymph node
path-, patho-, -pathy			pathogen
phago-			phagocyte
rhin-, rhino-			rhinitis
thym-, thymi-, thymo-			thymus gland
tonsillo-			tonsillitis
tox-, toxi-, toxico-, toxo-			lymphotoxin

ANATOMY AND PHYSIOLOGY

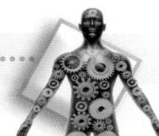

Lymphatic System and Immunity Preview

The lymphatic system and immunity are considered together because each supports the other, and both are important for a healthy immune response. Structures of the lymphatic system include lymph nodes, lymphatic vessels, and various lymphatic organs. Major roles of the lymphatic system include returning tissue fluid to the bloodstream, providing defense against **pathogens** (disease-causing agents), and removing proteins from tissue spaces. **Lymph** is a fluid drained from tissue spaces that has entered the lymphatic system. Lymph contains white blood cells, mostly **lymphocytes**, which are cells that protect against infection. Lymphocytes are grouped into three categories: T cells, B cells, and NK cells. T cells are responsible for cell-mediated immunity—destroying invaders by direct contact. T cells (also known as T lymphocytes) are so named because they mature in the thymus. B cells (also known as B lymphocytes) are formed in the bone marrow, and these cells create antibodies in response to specific antigens. NK cells (also known as natural killer lymphocytes) respond to foreign cells without being previously sensitized to their antigens. Lymphatic vessels, simply called **lymphatics**, transport lymph in a system separate from the blood vessels. The lymphatic vessels serve as the conduit between the lymphatic system and the blood vessels. The exchange occurs at lymphatic capillaries, which are more porous than blood capillaries. Because they are porous, lymphatic capillaries can collect interstitial fluid formed from blood plasma that has escaped the blood vessels. Lymph is then transported to collecting ducts and then into the right and left subclavian veins that empty into the bloodstream (**Figure 13-1**).

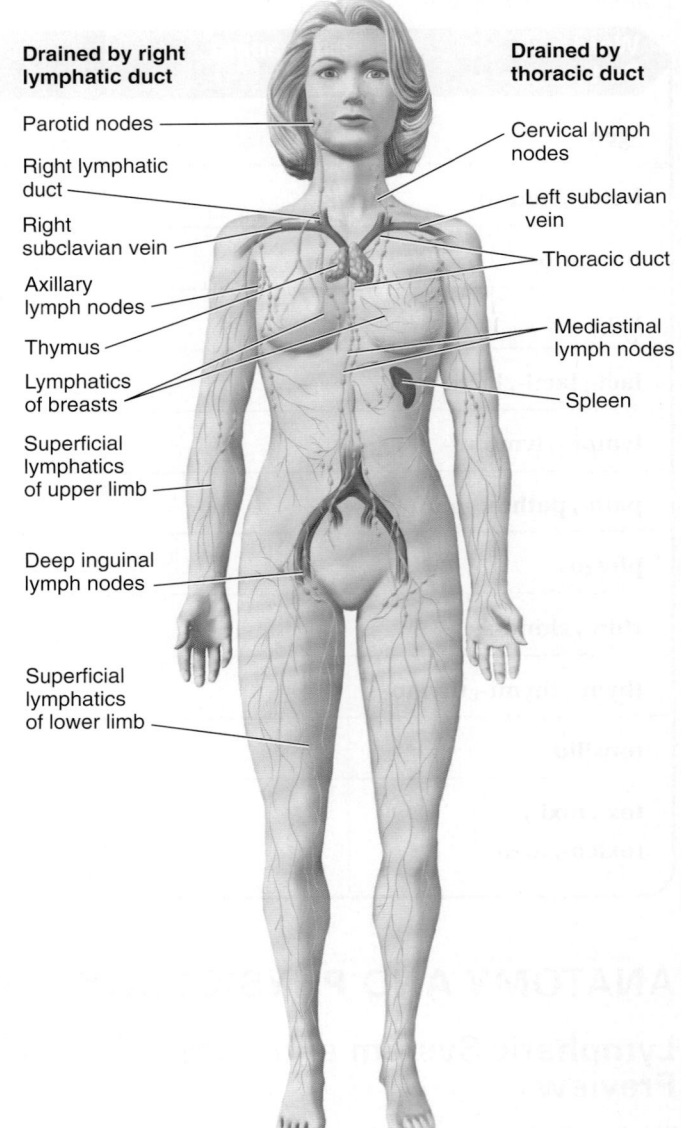

Drained by right lymphatic duct

Parotid nodes

Right lymphatic duct

Right subclavian vein

Axillary lymph nodes

Thymus

Lymphatics of breasts

Superficial lymphatics of upper limb

Deep inguinal lymph nodes

Superficial lymphatics of lower limb

Drained by thoracic duct

Cervical lymph nodes

Left subclavian vein

Thoracic duct

Mediastinal lymph nodes

Spleen

Figure 13-1 An overview of the lymphatic system.

Unlike the cardiovascular system, which has the heart to pump blood through the vessels, lymph flows through lymphatics by lymphokinetic factors. These factors include compression of muscles, breathing, and moving. That is, lymph flow is dependent on a body moving. If you sit for long periods of time without moving, you experience lymph pooling in your legs. The moving lymph is filtered through **lymph nodes**, bean-shaped structures distributed along lymphatics much like beads on a necklace.

Lymphatic organs are populated with lymphocytes. Major lymphatic organs are the tonsils, thymus, and spleen. Your **tonsils** are masses of lymphatic tissue in walls of the pharynx. The **thymus** is a pyramid-shaped organ consisting of two lobes located in the mediastinum, directly posterior to the sternum. It functions in immunity by promoting the development of T cells. The **spleen**, a large mass of lymphatic tissue located in the left hypochondriac region, is the largest lymphatic organ. It is a nonvital organ involved with lymphocyte production.

Another function of the lymphatic system is the transport of lipids from the intestinal tract to the circulatory system. Special lymphatic structures in the intestinal wall called **lacteals** carry recently digested fats in the form of chyle from the small intestine to the thoracic duct, which empties into the left subclavian vein. The word part *lact-* refers to "milk," and the fluid from lacteals is milky in color.

Immunity is the ability of the body to resist disease. It is provided by nonspecific and specific defenses. **Nonspecific immunity** (or *innate immunity*) is generalized immunity that protects the body through various defenses and does not discriminate one threat from another. These defenses include physical barriers, phagocytes, NK cells, inflammation, and fever. On the other hand, **specific immunity** (or *adaptive immunity*) is aimed directly at particular antigens. Specific immunity involves T cells and B cells. Both kinds of immunity work simultaneously on a continuous basis.

Basic terms associated with the immune response are antibody, antigen, and immunoglobulin. An **antigen (Ag)** is a foreign protein or nonself substance that triggers an immune response by causing the formation of antibodies. An **antibody (Ab)** is a protein that responds to the presence of an antigen and works to eliminate that particular antigen. Likewise, immunoglobulins (Ig) are body glycoproteins that act like antibodies. For example, bacteria and viruses contain antigens that stimulate antibody or immunoglobulin formation.

KEY TERM	Definition
pathogens (PATH-oh-jenz)	disease-causing agents
lymph (LIMF)	tissue fluid that has entered the lymphatic system
lymphocytes (LIM-foh-sites)	white blood cells found in lymph
lymphatics (lim-FAT-icks)	collecting vessels that transport lymph
lymph (LIMF) **nodes**	bean-shaped masses of lymphatic tissue distributed along lymphatics that filter lymph
tonsils	masses of lymphatic tissue in the pharynx
thymus (THY-mus)	lymphatic organ, located in the mediastinum, where T cells mature
spleen	largest lymphatic organ located in the left hypochondriac region and is a site for lymphocyte production
lacteals (LACK-tee-ulz)	lymphatics in the intestinal wall that transport recently digested fats to the bloodstream
immunity	the body's ability to resist disease
nonspecific immunity	generalized resistance to disease; also called innate immunity
specific immunity	resistance against particular antigens; also called adaptive immunity
antigen (AN-ti-jen) **(Ag)**	protein that provokes an immune response
antibody (AN-tee-bod-ee) **(Ab)**	protein produced in response to a particular antigen that works to eliminate that specific antigen

KEY TERM PRACTICE: *Lymphatic System and Immunity Preview*

1. The word part _____ refers to *lymph*, and the word part _____ means *cell*. So a _____ is a *white blood cell in lymphatic tissue*.

2. Identify two types of immunity. _____

3. Collecting vessels that transport lymph are known as _____.

4. _____ are bean-shaped masses of lymphatic tissue distributed along lymphatics that filter lymph.

5. _____ is the body's ability to resist disease.

Lymph Nodes, Lymphocytes, and Lymphatics

Bean-shaped structures located along lymphatics are lymph nodes. Their size varies, ranging from 1 to 20 mm. Lymph nodes occur in groups throughout the body. Lymph node clusters are found in the axillary, cervical, and inguinal regions. They contain phagocytes, which digest foreign substances, and germinal centers, which produce lymphocytes. Lymph is filtered through lymph nodes to sift out pathogens, such as viruses and bacteria. The lymph enters an afferent lymphatic, sifts through the lymph node, and exits an efferent lymphatic.

Lymph nodes have several distinct regions. The capsule is the dense layer that encloses a lymph node, the cortex is the outer region, and the medulla is the inner region. T cells can be found in the cortex and B cells are in the medulla. **Lymph nodes** are areas of dense masses of lymphocytes within lymph nodes. Areas of rapidly dividing lymphocytes within the lymph nodules are termed **germinal centers** (**Figure 13-2**). When an infection is present, the germinal centers form and release lymphocytes for combat.

Lymphatics begin where lymphatic capillaries interlace with the capillary beds of the cardiovascular system, forming vast networks (**Figure 13-3**). Lymphatic vessels run alongside blood vessels. Lymphatics merge to form greater vessels called lymphatic trunks, which eventually empty into two large collecting ducts. These two collecting ducts, called the thoracic duct and right lymphatic duct, drain into the left and right subclavian veins. The **thoracic duct** collects lymph from all but the upper right body quadrant. The thoracic duct empties into the left subclavian vein. The **right lymphatic duct** is smaller than the thoracic duct and collects lymph from the upper right body quadrant, superior to the diaphragm, including the right arm and right regions of the chest, neck, and head. The right lymphatic duct empties into the right subclavian vein (**Figure 13-4**). The pathway of lymph is as follows:

interstitial fluid → lymph capillaries → lymphatics → lymphatic trunks → thoracic duct or right lymphatic duct → left or right subclavian vein

Lymphatics are often associated with blood vessels, but are not part of the cardiovascular system. Like veins, lymphatics contain valves that prevent the backflow of lymph. Because pressures within lymphatics are low, the valves are important to maintaining normal lymph flow toward the chest.

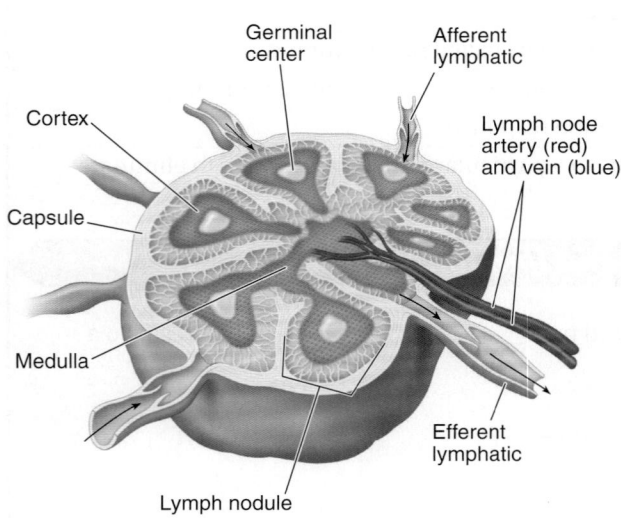

Figure 13-2 A typical lymph node showing lymph flow through several distinct areas.

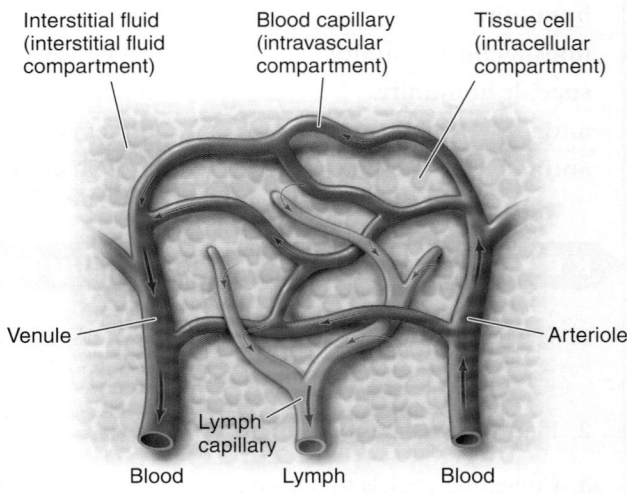

Figure 13-3 The structural relationship between the capillary bed in the vascular system and the lymph capillaries in the lymphatic system.

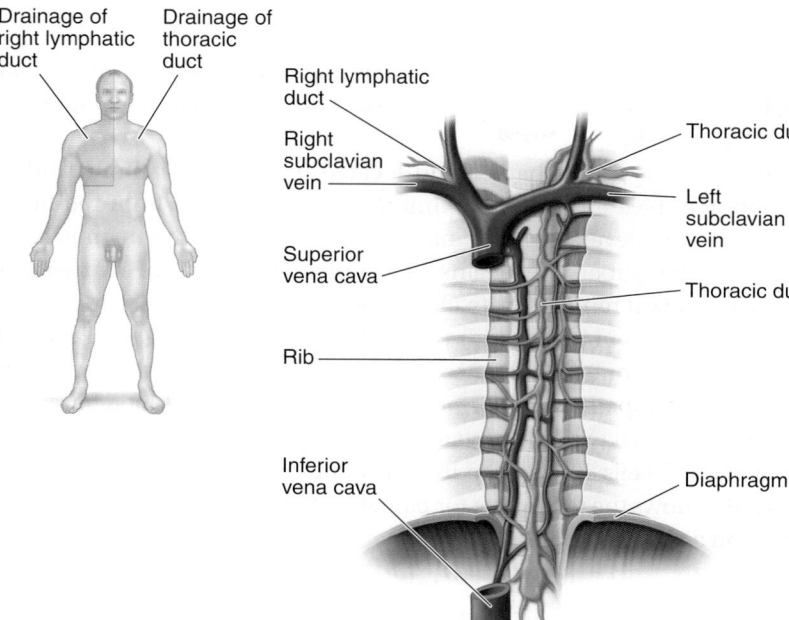

Figure 13-4 The drainage of the thoracic duct and the right lymphatic duct.

KEY TERM	Definition
lymph nodules (LIMF NOD-yoolz)	areas of dense masses of lymphocytes within lymph nodes
germinal (JUR-mi-nul) **centers**	areas of rapidly dividing lymphocytes within lymph nodules
thoracic (thoh-RAS-ick) **duct**	large lymphatic duct that drains lymph from all but the right upper quadrant of the body and returns it to the bloodstream via the left subclavian vein
right lymphatic (lim-FAT-ick) **duct**	smaller lymphatic duct that drains lymph from the upper right body quadrant superior to the diaphragm and returns it to the bloodstream via the right subclavian vein

KEY TERM PRACTICE: *Lymph Nodes, Lymphocytes, and Lymphatics*

1. The _____ is a lymphatic duct that drains lymph from the upper right body quadrant superior to the diaphragm.

2. The _____ is a large lymphatic duct that drains lymph from all but the upper right quadrant of the body and returns it to the bloodstream via the left subclavian vein.

3. _____ are areas of rapidly dividing lymphocytes within lymph nodules.

4. Areas of dense masses of lymphocytes within lymph nodes are termed _____.

Tonsils, Thymus, and Spleen

Tonsils are oval masses of lymphatic tissue. Five tonsils are found in the oral region: left and right lingual, left and right palatine, and a single pharyngeal tonsil. The pharyngeal tonsil is also called the **adenoid** (Figure 13-5).

As noted earlier, the thymus is a lymphatic gland located in the mediastinum and is important in T cell development (see Figure 13-1). Immature T cells travel from red bone marrow to the thymus, where they develop into mature T cells. In a child, the thymus is an important site of immunity. After puberty, it begins to atrophy, and much of its tissue is replaced by fat so that only a remnant remains in an elderly person.

The spleen is about 12 cm (5 in.) in length with two distinct regions: white pulp and red pulp. The white pulp is active in the immune response and the red pulp is a blood reservoir. In addition to its roles related to hematopoiesis (blood formation), blood storage, blood filtration, and antibody production, it is involved with the **phagocytosis** (the engulfing and ingesting) of particles, such as bacteria and old cells. The spleen hypertrophies during infection and atrophies in old age. Figure 13-6A shows the technique for palpating the spleen and Figure 13-6B depicts an enlarged spleen on a cadaver.

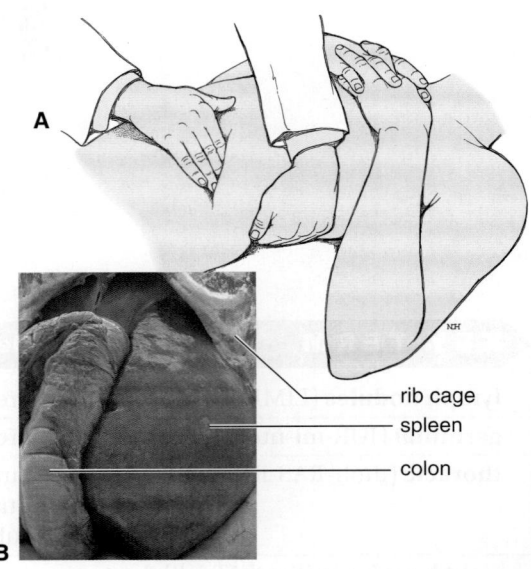

A

rib cage
spleen
colon

B

Figure 13-6 (A) Palpation technique used in diagnosis. (B) Enlarged spleen seen at autopsy.

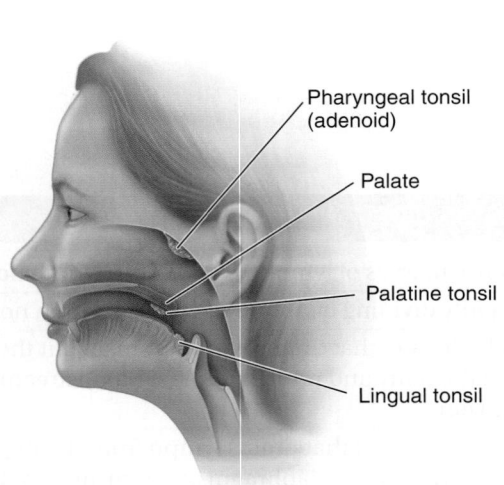

Pharyngeal tonsil (adenoid)

Palate

Palatine tonsil

Lingual tonsil

Figure 13-5 The locations of the tonsils.

KEY TERM	Definition
adenoid (AD-eh-noid)	another term for the pharyngeal tonsil
phagocytosis (fag-oh-sigh-TOH-sis)	ingestion of particles, such as bacteria and worn-out cells

KEY TERM PRACTICE: *Tonsils, Thymus, and Spleen*

1. What is the alternate term for the pharyngeal tonsil? _____

2. _____ is the ingestion of particles, such as bacteria and worn-out cells.

Nonspecific Defenses and Specific Defenses

Nonspecific and specific defenses interact to provide protection every day without us being aware of their actions. Both types of defenses work together to prevent **infection**, the growth of pathogens in the body. Two terms are important to note when dealing with the immune system: resistance and susceptibility. The ability to ward off or not to succumb to disease is termed **resistance**. Lack of resistance and the likelihood of developing a disease is called **susceptibility**. The body uses several lines of nonspecific defenses (also called innate defenses) to prevent illness. These defenses prevent pathogens from gaining access to the body and destroy them without distinguishing one type of offender from another. The major types of nonspecific defenses are as follows:

- *Physical barriers*. Physical barriers include the skin and mucous membranes. As the first line of defense, they keep pathogens and harmful substances from entering your body.
- *Phagocytes*. **Phagocytes** are scavenger cells in the bloodstream that ingest bacteria, foreign particles, and other cells.
- *Immune surveillance*. With immune surveillance, the immune system recognizes and destroys abnormal cells in peripheral tissues.
- *Interferons*. **Interferons (IFNs)** are proteins produced by various cells in response to viral infections. These proteins then inhibit virus replication.
- *Complement system*. The complement system consists of circulating proteins that cause the destruction of abnormal cells.
- *Inflammation*. Inflammation is a response to abnormal changes in tissues and it limits the spread of injury or infection. The so-called cardinal signs of inflammation are rubor (redness), calor (heat or warmth), tumor (swelling), and dolor (pain).
- *Fever*. Fever is a rise in the core body temperature, which activates immune responses.

Specific defenses (also known as adaptive defenses) target individual threats by activating and coordinating T cells and B cells. Direct attack on a pathogen by T cells is called **cell-mediated immunity** (*cellular immunity*). Cell-mediated immunity defends against pathogens *inside* cells. B cells provide **antibody-mediated immunity**. Antibody-mediated immunity is also called *humoral* (fluid) *immunity* because this type of immunity defends against pathogens in body fluids.

Immunity, like defenses, is classified as either nonspecific (innate) or specific (adaptive). **Innate immunity** is genetically determined; that is, a person is born with it. It is commonly called *natural immunity*. **Adaptive immunity** is not present at birth. A person acquires this type of resistance only after being exposed to a particular antigen. Within the adaptive immunity category, there are two types: active and passive. **Active immunity** is resistance that results from previous exposure to a particular antigen, whether that antigen was in the environment (*naturally acquired active immunity*) or was introduced by a vaccine (*artificially induced active immunity*). **Passive immunity** is resistance that results from the actual transfer of antibodies to a person. For example, *naturally acquired passive immunity* occurs when a baby receives antibodies from the mother either during gestation when antibodies crossed the placenta or through breast milk while feeding. *Artificially induced passive immunity* occurs when a person receives antibodies directly through an injection (**Figure 13-7**).

The likelihood of being sick varies among individuals, but stress is a major risk factor for disease. Stress is known to affect the entire body, and may diminish the immune response. Current research demonstrates a link between the mind and the body's resistance or susceptibility to disease and physiological decline. **Psychoneuroimmunology (PNI)** is an area of science that focuses on the association between emotions and other psychological states and their effects on the immune system.

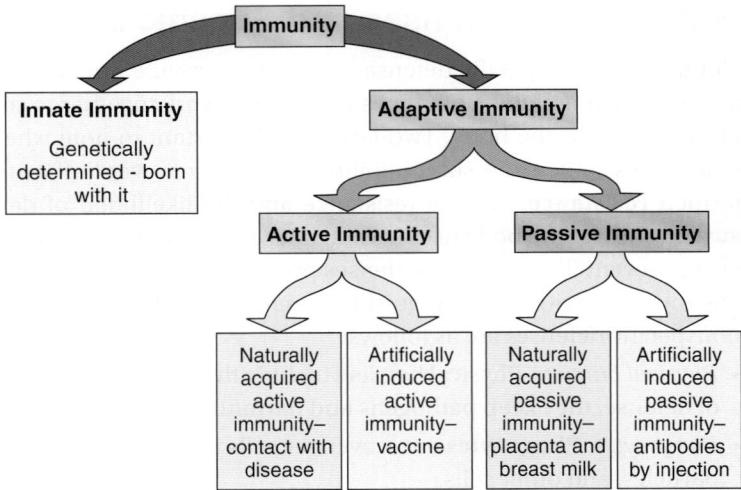

Figure 13-7 Types of immunity.

KEY TERM	Definition
infection	growth of pathogens in the body
resistance	ability to ward off infection
susceptibility	likelihood of developing a disease
phagocytes (FAG-oh-sites)	scavenger cells in the blood that ingest bacteria, foreign particles, and other cells
interferons (in-tur-FEER-onz) **(IFNs)**	proteins produced by various cells in response to viral infections
cell-mediated immunity	direct attack on a pathogen by T cells; also called cellular immunity
antibody-mediated immunity	resistance that results from antibodies directed at specific antigens; also called humoral immunity
innate immunity	genetically determined resistance that a person is born with; also called natural immunity
adaptive immunity	type of resistance acquired only after being exposed to a particular antigen
active immunity	resistance that results from previous exposure to a particular antigen
passive immunity	resistance that results from the actual transfer of antibodies to a person
psychoneuroimmunology (PNI) (sigh-koh-new-roh-im-yoo-NOL-uh-jee)	field of science that deals with the association between emotions and other psychological states and their effects on the immune system

KEY TERM PRACTICE: *Nonspecific Defenses and Specific Defenses*

1. _____ is growth of pathogens in the body.

2. _____ is an area of science that focuses on the association between emotions and other psychological states and their effects on the immune system.

3. Resistance that results from previous exposure to a particular antigen is termed _____.

4. Resistance that results from the actual transfer of antibodies to a person is called _____.

5. _____ are scavenger cells in the blood that ingest bacteria, foreign particles, and other cells; the term is derived from the word part _____ for *eating* and the word part _____ for *cell*.

Major Types of T Cells and B Cells

T cells, also called T lymphocytes, are formed in the red bone marrow and then migrate to the thymus where they mature and become fully functional in immunity. The *T* indicates it is from the *t*hymus. T cells have long life spans (months to years) and are further categorized by function. There are four major types of T cells:

- **Cytotoxic T (T_c) cells**, directly attack other cells both physically and chemically. T_c cells engage in cell-to-cell combat by secreting toxins that puncture and destroy other cells.

- **Helper T (T_H) cells** cooperate with B cells, which are important in specific immunity, to amplify antibody production. Helper T cells are aptly named for they also assist in recruiting other T cell populations.

- **Memory T cells** are long-lived lymphocytes that respond to subsequent invasion by the same antigen. These cells lie in wait for the reappearance of a specific antigen.

- **Suppressor T (T_s) cells** inhibit other T cells and B cells. They help to prevent the destruction of uninfected self cells and to wind down the immune reaction after the initial response.

   B cells are also called B lymphocytes, and they are not dependent on the thymus to mature. *B* cells get their name because they are derived from the red *b*one marrow. B cells circulate freely in blood and lymph, searching for foreign antigens. **Memory B cells** have a role in antibody-mediated immunity and function, the same as memory T cells do in cell-mediated immunity. When stimulated by an antigen, these B cells differentiate into large numbers of **plasma cells** that eventually make specific antibodies in response to the antigen. Antibodies are made only if an antigen is detected. The antibody is a specific protein produced in response to the presence of a particular antigen. The antibodies circulate and bind to the antigens that stimulated their production. **Figure 13-8** summarizes the events of the immune response.

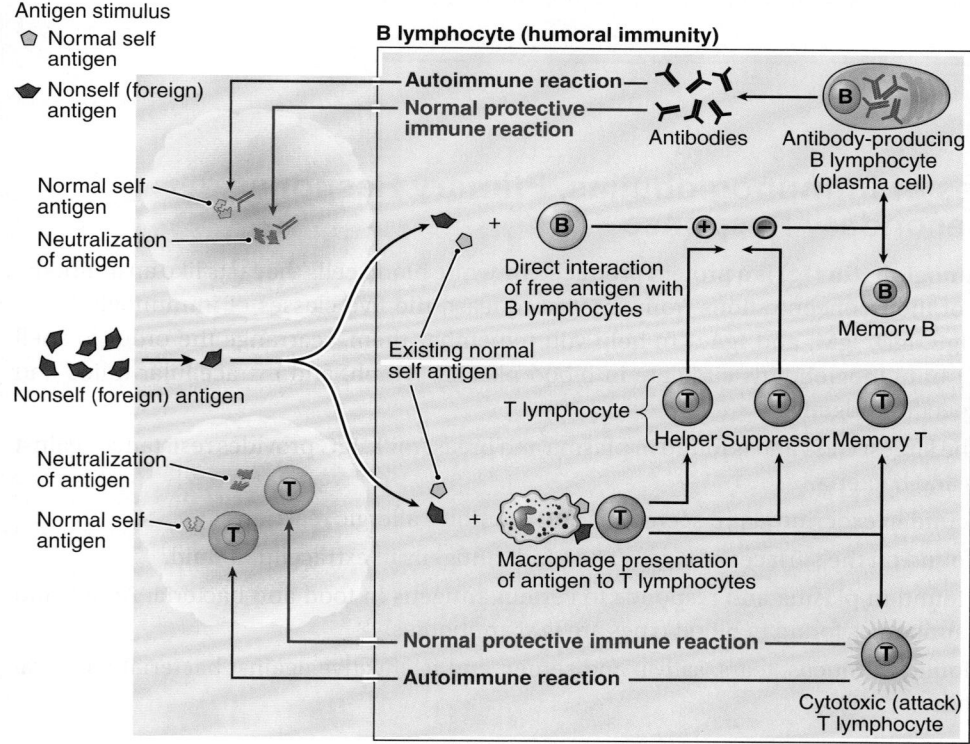

Figure 13-8 Sequence of immune reactions. In normal protective immune reactions, a foreign antigen stimulates T and B cells, which react to neutralize it. In autoimmune reactions (discussed later), self antigens stimulate T cell and B cell reactions against the body for reasons that are unknown.

KEY TERM	Definition
T cells	lymphocytes derived from the thymus; also called T lymphocytes
cytotoxic (sigh-toh-TOCK-sick) T (T_C) cells	lymphocytes that directly attack other cells both physically and chemically
helper T (T_H) cells	lymphocytes that cooperate with B cells to amplify antibody production
memory T cells	long-lived lymphocytes that can respond to subsequent encounters by the same antigen
suppressor T (T_S) cells	lymphocytes that inhibit other T cells and B cells
B cells	lymphocytes that can differentiate into plasma cells when stimulated by an antigen
memory B cells	B lymphocytes that mediate immunologic memory
plasma (PLAZ-muh) cells	antibody-producing cells that are derived from B cells

KEY TERM PRACTICE: *Major Types of T Cells and B Cells*

1. _____ are antibody-producing cells that are derived from B cells.

2. Lymphocytes derived from the thymus are called _____.

3. Long-lived lymphocytes that can respond to subsequent encounters by the same antigen are termed _____.

4. _____ are lymphocytes that can differentiate into plasma cells when stimulated by an antigen.

5. Lymphocytes that cooperate with B cells to amplify antibody production are known as _____.

Classes of Immunoglobulins, Primary Response, and Secondary Response

An **immunoglobulin (Ig)** is a protein produced by white blood cells that acts like an antibody. In order of their concentrations from greatest to least, the five classes of immunoglobulins are IgG, IgE, IgD, IgM, and IgA. (To help you remember them, rearrange the order to spell *MADGE.*) Immunoglobulins circulate in blood plasma, lymph, and extracellular fluids and bind to specific antigens.

- IgG is the largest class and is found in plasma and breast milk. IgG provides resistance against viruses and bacteria.
- IgE is found in exocrine gland secretions and promotes allergic reactions.
- IgD is found on the surfaces of B cells and binds antigens in extracellular fluid.
- IgM is found in plasma and responds to certain antigens in food and bacteria. Anti-A and anti-B antibodies found in blood types are IgM antibodies.
- IgA is found in mucus, tears, saliva, and semen and is effective against bacterial and viral infections.

Immune activation involves exposure to an antigen. The initial response to antigen exposure is called the **primary response**. When the antigen reappears, the repeat encounter is termed the **secondary response**. The primary response takes time to develop, because B cells must be activated. These B cells must then differentiate into plasma cells, which will then make the appropriate antibody. If the body encounters that particular antigen again, the memory B cells "remember" the first exposure, recognize the antigen, and take action by releasing the specific antibody. Essentially, it is memory recall. The secondary response produces more quantities of antibodies, is quicker to respond, and is longer in duration than the primary response (**Figure 13-9**). That is why we usually have each childhood disease, such as chickenpox, only once in our lifetime. This is also the basic principle behind immunizations (vaccines).

A **vaccine** is a preparation that stimulates the production of antibodies and provides immunity against disease. Each vaccine is prepared from the causative agent of a disease, its products, or a synthetic substitute, treated to act as an antigen without inducing the disease. Vaccines provide immunity because the antigen stimulates antibody production. Four basic types of vaccines are used today:

- *Killed vaccines*. These preparations contain killed, but previously harmful microbes that have been destroyed by heat or chemicals. Examples of killed vaccines are influenza, hepatitis A, polio, and rabies.

- *Attenuated vaccines*. These preparations contain live virus particles that grow in the person who is vaccinated, but they do not cause disease because the vaccine virus has been altered to a nonpathogenic form. These are the preferred type for healthy adults. Examples of attenuated vaccines are measles, rubella, and mumps.

- *Sub-unit vaccines*. These preparations contain purified fragments of the virus's antigen. The hepatitis B virus vaccine is an example.

- *Toxoid vaccines*. These preparations are made from inactivated toxins, rather than from the microbes. Examples of toxoid vaccines include tetanus and diphtheria.

Vaccines are basically harmless when given as an injection, oral preparation, or inhalant. The body recognizes the antigen as foreign, mounts an immune response, and produces memory cells, so that any future encounter with the pathogen will be swiftly eliminated.

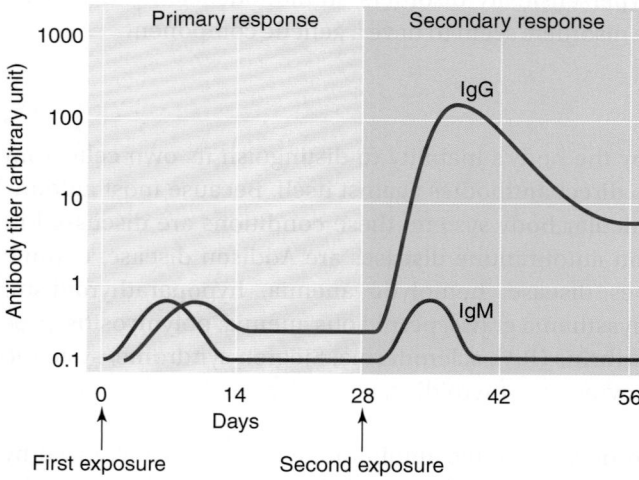

Figure 13-9 The level of antibodies in the primary and secondary responses to a specific antigen.

KEY TERM	Definition
immunoglobulin (Ig) (im-yoo-noh-GLOB-yoo-lin)	protein produced by white blood cells that acts like an antibody; the classes are IgG, IgE, IgD, IgM, and IgA
primary response	initial immune reaction to the first encounter with a foreign antigen
secondary response	immune reaction to a second (or later) encounter with a known antigen, due to memory cells
vaccine (vack-SEEN)	preparation that stimulates the production of antibodies and provides immunity against disease

KEY TERM PRACTICE: *Classes of Immunoglobulins, Primary Response, and Secondary Response*

1. A preparation that stimulates the production of antibodies and provides immunity against disease is termed a

    _____.

2. An _____ is a protein produced by white blood cells that acts like an antibody; the classes are IgG, IgE, IgD, IgM, and IgA.

3. The initial immune reaction to the first encounter with a foreign antigen is the _____.

4. The _____ is an immune reaction to a second (or later) encounter with a known antigen, due to memory cells.

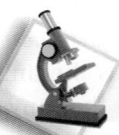

THE CLINICAL DIMENSION

Pathology related to the lymphatic system and immunity can be grouped into five basic categories: autoimmune diseases, hypersensitivity disorders, immunodeficiency disorders, infections, and tumors. Many of these disorders seem to have a genetic component.

Autoimmune Diseases

Autoimmune diseases are caused by the body's inability to distinguish its own cells from foreign material, causing the body to direct antibodies against itself. Because most autoimmune diseases have effects in a particular body system, these conditions are discussed in each relevant chapter. Some common autoimmune diseases are Addison disease, chronic hepatitis, glomerulonephritis, Graves disease, hemolytic anemia, hypoparathyroidism, Type 1 diabetes, multiple sclerosis, myasthenia gravis, pernicious anemia, polymyositis, psoriasis, rheumatic fever, rheumatoid arthritis (RA), scleroderma, Sjögren syndrome, systemic lupus erythematosus (SLE), thrombocytopenia, thyroiditis, ulcerative colitis, and vitiligo.

Sjögren syndrome   **Sjögren syndrome** is a chronic autoimmune disease characterized by degeneration of the salivary and lacrimal glands, causing dryness of the mouth and eyes. It is seen in menopausal women and is often associated with rheumatoid arthritis. It is named for Henrik Sjögren, the Swedish ophthalmologist who first described the condition.

KEY TERM	Definition
autoimmune (aw-toh-i-MEWN) **diseases**	disorders in which the immune response is directed against the body's own tissues
Sjögren (SHOE-greyn) **syndrome**	autoimmune disease marked by degeneration of the salivary and lacrimal glands causing dryness of the mouth and eyes

KEY TERM PRACTICE: *Autoimmune Diseases*

1. A disease in which the immune response is directed at the body's own tissues is termed an _____.

2. _____ is an autoimmune disease marked by degeneration of the salivary and lacrimal glands, causing dryness of the mouth and eyes.

Hypersensitivity Disorders

A reaction in which specific antibodies develop in response to an antigen is termed **sensitization**. Sensitization can be induced by immunization.

hypersensitivity   **Hypersensitivity** refers to an abnormal, overreaction to an allergen (antigen). Hypersensitivity disorders are characterized by an exaggerated reaction to a stimulus. Examples of disproportionate responses include allergies, asthma, and anaphylaxis (discussed below). Foods such as shellfish and peanuts trigger hypersensitivity reactions in susceptible persons. The effects of hypersensitivity disorders range from mild to severe.

One treatment for hypersensitivity is desensitization, but it is not effective for the majority of the population. **Desensitization** is a treatment for allergies that makes the individual insensitive to an antigen through antigen administration. Small amounts of the antigen (usually a protein) are injected over a period of time, initiating antibody production so that eventually the person will no longer mount a hypersensitivity reaction. This treatment is also called **hyposensitization**.

allergy   An extreme sensitivity reaction to a normally harmless substance that is touched, breathed in, or ingested is termed **allergy**. Common examples are allergic rhinitis and latex allergy. **Allergic rhinitis** is an allergic reaction to an inhaled particle. Runny nose, itchy eyes, and congestion characterize it. If it occurs seasonally in response to particles such as pollen from trees, grasses, weeds, or flowers, it is called **hay fever**. Year-round occurrence is termed **perennial allergic rhinitis**. Both are treated with decongestants and antihistamines. **Decongestants** are drugs that reduce or relieve nasal congestion, which often accompanies allergies. Drugs that prevent or diminish histamine effects are **antihistamines**. Histamine is a potent capillary dilator, which is evident in the face during an allergic reaction as nasal swelling, itchy eyes, and swollen cheeks. As the name suggests, antihistamines counter the effects of histamine to reduce the signs and symptoms.

An emerging allergy, particularly in the health care field where workers wear latex gloves, is the hypersensitivity to latex, called **latex allergy**.

Latex is a sap derived from the rubber tree that can cause localized irritation on the skin or systemic effects that are life threatening.

Various skin tests are diagnostic tools for determining sensitivity or immunity to specific antigens that are applied to or injected into the skin. Common skin tests include the intradermal test, patch test, and prick test. The **intradermal test** involves the injection of a small amount of antigen into the skin. Positive intradermal tests are indicated by a raised reddened area called a **wheal** that appears on the skin. A test for allergens in which a patch is saturated with allergens and then applied to the skin for a period of time is the **patch test** (Figure 13-10A and B). The **prick test** is one in which a small amount of antigen is poked into the skin. Positive tests are indicated by erythema (patches of redness on the skin), a round hard swelling, or itching.

asthma

A reactive airway disorder characterized by bronchospasm and mucus secretion is called **asthma**. Asthma is often caused by allergies. Other signs and symptoms include coughing, difficulty breathing, and a feeling of tightness in the chest.

Several types of asthma exist. **Acute asthma** has a sudden onset. It is severe and marked by coughing and difficulty breathing. **Extrinsic asthma** is caused by sensitivity to inhalants, drugs, foods, pollen, mold, animal dander, or environmental allergen. When the cause cannot be determined, and extrinsic asthma has been ruled out, the condition is called **intrinsic asthma**. **Status asthmaticus** is severe, prolonged asthma that can lead to respiratory distress and failure. Treatment for all forms involves bronchodilator use. **Bronchodilators** are drugs that widen and relax pulmonary passages, thereby making breathing easier. In some cases, preventive maintenance drugs are used.

anaphylaxis

An extreme hypersensitivity reaction is termed **anaphylaxis**. At times, the term anaphylaxis is used for anaphylactic shock. The reaction may be fatal if asphyxiation or cardiovascular collapse occurs.

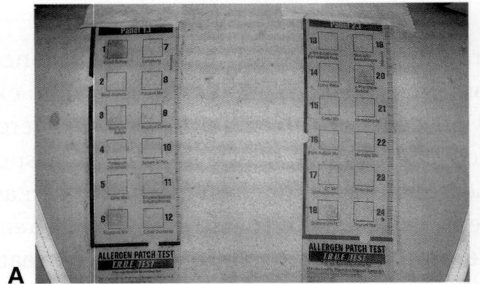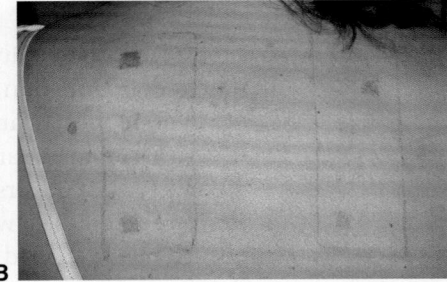

Figure 13-10 Test patches. **(A)** These test patches will be removed after 48 hours. **(B)** The final reading at 96 hours shows positive reactions to various allergens.

KEY TERM	Definition
sensitization (sen-si-ti-ZAY-shun)	a reaction in which specific antibodies develop in response to an antigen
hypersensitivity (high-pur-sen-si-TIV-i-tee)	abnormal overreaction to an allergen
desensitization (dee-sen-si-ti-ZAY-shun)	treatment for making a person insensitive to an antigen; also called hyposensitization
hyposensitization (high-poh-sen-sih-tih-ZAY-shun)	treatment for making a person insensitive to an antigen; also called desensitization
allergy	extreme sensitivity reaction to a normally harmless substance
allergic rhinitis (rye-NIGH-tis)	inflammation of the nasal mucous membranes caused by allergen inhalation
hay fever	allergy to seasonal plant allergens such as pollen
perennial allergic rhinitis (rye-NIGH-tis)	year-round allergy to environmental allergens
decongestants	drugs that relieve nasal congestion
antihistamines	drugs that inhibit the physiological effects of histamine
latex (LAY-tecks) **allergy**	allergic reaction to natural rubber latex
intradermal (in-truh-DUR-mul) **test**	detects sensitivity to an antigen after it is injected into the skin
wheal	raised, reddened area caused by a sensitivity reaction
patch test	determines sensitivity to an antigen after a patch saturated with antigens is placed on the skin
prick test	detects a reaction to an antigen after it is poked into the skin
asthma (AZ-muh)	reactive airway disorder characterized by bronchospasm and mucus secretion
acute asthma (AZ-muh)	sudden, severe asthma that causes coughing and difficulty breathing
extrinsic asthma (ecks-TRIN-sick AZ-muh)	asthma caused by sensitivity to inhalants, drugs, foods, pollen, mold, animal dander, or environmental allergen
intrinsic asthma (in-TRIN-sick AZ-muh)	asthma of unknown cause
status asthmaticus (STAT-us az-MAT-i-kus)	severe, prolonged asthma that can lead to respiratory distress and failure
bronchodilators (bronk-oh-dye-LAY-turz)	drugs that widen and relax pulmonary passages, thereby making breathing easier
anaphylaxis (an-uh-fi-LACK-sis)	an extreme hypersensitivity reaction that can be fatal; the term may be used for anaphylactic shock

KEY TERM PRACTICE: *Hypersensitivity Disorders*

1. Seasonal allergies are called _____, and allergies that last throughout the entire year are referred to as _____.

2. Inflammation of the nasal mucous membranes resulting from allergies is known as _____; it is derived from the word part _____, which means *nose*.

3. _____ is an extreme hypersensitivity reaction that can be fatal.

4. Drugs that widen and relax pulmonary passages, thereby making breathing easier, are termed _____.

5. The treatment for making a person insensitive to an allergen is called _____ or _____.

Immunodeficiency Disorders

Immunodeficiency disorders are characterized by the inability to mount an adequate immune response to disease. These disorders are either innate or acquired.

acquired immunodeficiency syndrome (AIDS)

Acquired immunodeficiency syndrome (AIDS) is the disease caused by infection with the retrovirus **human immunodeficiency virus (HIV)**, which destroys certain white blood cells. A retrovirus is a type of virus whose genetic information is found in its RNA rather than its DNA. This virus cannot survive outside living cells and is transmitted though body fluids, blood, and contaminated needles. The HIV binds to receptors on helper T (T_H) cells. HIV attacks T_H cells and renders them incapable of mounting an immune response. In this way it hinders the very system that normally protects the body. AIDS lowers the body's immunity by decreasing the number of helper T cells, reversing the ratio of helper T cells to suppressor T cells, and allowing malignancy of lymphoid tissue to develop.

Signs and symptoms of the disease may not appear for several years after infection, as the virus remains latent (dormant). Despite its latency, disease transmission is possible throughout the course of disease development, beginning with the initial infection when it may not be apparent. Manifestations of AIDS in patients who have not yet developed major deficient immune function, characterized by fever with generalized **lymphadenopathy** (disease affecting lymph nodes), diarrhea, weight loss, and opportunistic infections, is known as the **AIDS-related complex**. An **opportunistic infection** is an infection that occurs because of a weakened immune response; the infection would not normally occur in a healthy person. In AIDS patients, a relatively minor disease becomes life threatening as a result of impaired immune function. Common infections in the AIDS patient are *Candida* (type of yeast infection), tuberculosis, herpes simplex, herpes zoster, *Pneumocystis jiroveci* pneumonia, and Kaposi sarcoma, among others (**Figure 13-11**). *Pneumocystis jiroveci* was formerly known as *Pneumocystis carinii*. End stages are marked by neurological involvement. Diagnosis of HIV is made by blood or saliva tests.

There is no cure for AIDS. Treatment is aimed at improving the patient's immune status and preventing infections. Pharmacological therapy consists of antiviral, reverse transcriptase (RT), and protease inhibitor drugs given in combinations often called "cocktails." When other treatments fail, **immunotherapy** (serotherapy), therapy that strengthens the immune system function—for example, with monoclonal antibodies—is used to treat AIDS. A **monoclonal antibody (MAB or MoAb)** is an antibody produced by a single (mono) cell line and consists of identical antibody molecules (clones). In AIDS patients, HIV-specific antibodies are cloned to combat HIV infection. Each year about 5 million people contract AIDS worldwide, and 3 million die of it. It is estimated that 40 to 50 million people are living with the disease. The incidence of AIDS is approximately equal between males and females.

1 Chorioretinitis
  • *Cytomegalovirus*

2 Encephalitis
  • *Cytomegalovirus*
  • *Toxoplasma*

3 Meningitis
  • *Cryptococcus*

4 Stomatitis
  • *Candida*

5 Esophagitis
  • *Candida*
  • *Cytomegalovirus*

6 Bone marrow infections
  • *Mycobacterium avium*

7 Pneumonia
  • *Pneumocystis jiroveci*
  • *Mycobacterium avium*

8 Gastritis, enteritis, colitis
  • *Candida*
  • *Cytomegalovirus*
  • *Mycobacterium avium*

9 Proctitis
  • *Candida*

10 Vaginitis
  • *Candida*

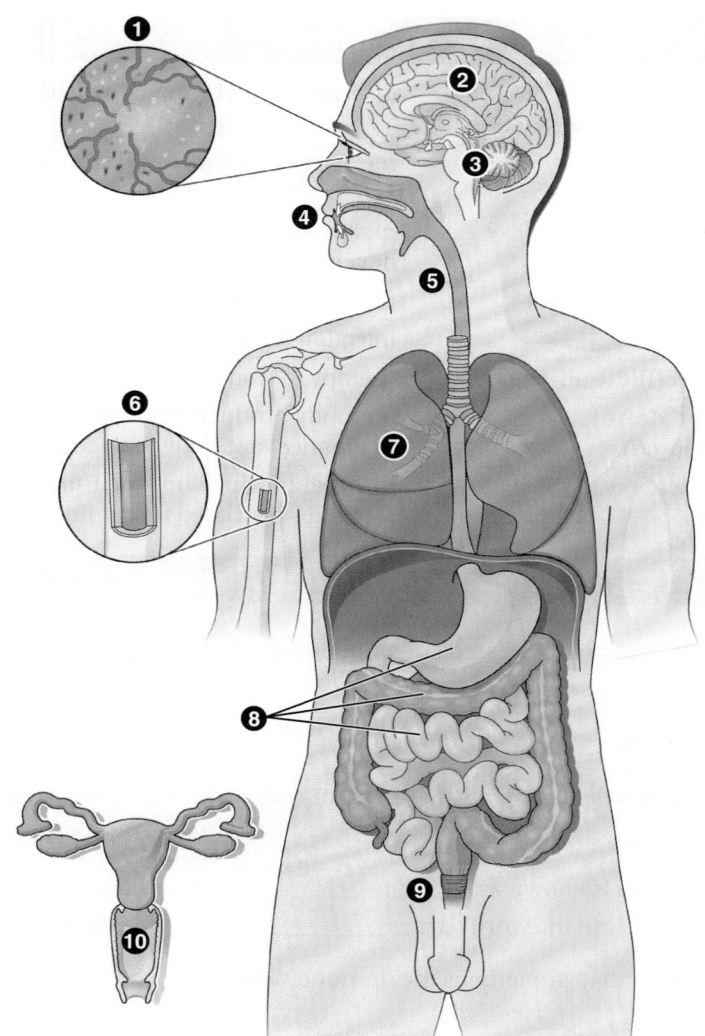

Figure 13-11 Opportunistic and AIDS-related infections.

severe combined immunodeficiency (SCID)

Severe combined immunodeficiency (SCID) is an inherited disorder characterized by the impairment of both cell-mediated and antibody-mediated immunity. The first sign is chronic infections early in infancy once immunity transferred from the mother has waned. Initial diagnosis is made by clinical history of low-grade fever and recurring infections. It is confirmed by lymph node biopsy that demonstrates absent lymph follicles and blood tests that indicate low B cell and T cell counts.

Individuals with SCID are placed in a completely sterile environment to prevent infections. Currently, the only other treatment option remains a bone marrow transplant to restore immune function. Gene therapies are also in clinical trials. The much publicized case of David Vetter, the boy who lived in a plastic bubble, illustrated this often-fatal infirmity.

KEY TERM	Definition
acquired immunodeficiency (im-yoo-noh-de-FISH-un-see) **syndrome (AIDS)**	disease caused by infection with HIV
human immunodeficiency (im-yoo-noh-de-FISH-un-see) **virus (HIV)**	retrovirus that causes AIDS
AIDS-related complex	manifestations of AIDS in patients who have not yet developed major deficient immune function
lymphadenopathy (lim-fad-e-NOP-uh-thee)	disease affecting the lymph nodes
opportunistic infection	infection that occurs because of a weakened immune response
immunotherapy (im-yoo-noh-THERR-uh-pee)	therapy that strengthens the immune system
monoclonal antibody (MAB or MoAb) (mon-oh-KLOH-nul AN-tee-bod-ee)	antibody produced by a single (mono) cell line and consists of identical antibody molecules (clones)
severe combined immunodeficiency (SCID) (im-yoo-noh-de-FISH-un-see)	disorder in which both cell-mediated immunity and antibody-mediated immunity are impaired

KEY TERM PRACTICE: *Immunodeficiency Disorders*

1. Identify the disorder in which both cell-mediated and antibody-mediated immunity are impaired.
   _____

2. Identify the virus that causes AIDS. _____

3. An _____ occurs when generally harmless microbes cause pathology when the host's immune response is impaired.

4. Disease affecting the lymph nodes is known as _____, and is derived from the word part _____ for *lymph*, and the word part _____ for *disease*.

5. _____ is therapy that strengthens the immune system.

Infections

Infections and **lymphangitis** (inflammation of the lymphatics) are common to lymphatic organs because these structures are involved in eradicating pathogens.

elephantiasis

Elephantiasis is a chronic disease in which parasitic worms obstruct lymphatics, causing swelling of parts of the body, such as the legs and scrotum, and hardening of the surrounding skin. The swelling of lymphatics in the extremities is termed **lymphedema** (**Figure 13-12**). Elephantiasis is caused by the filaria (parasitic roundworm) *Wuchereria bancrofti*, which infects lymphatic tissues. The disease is common in tropical and subtropical regions and is diagnosed by the presence of microfilariae in blood smears. It is treated with the drugs diethylcarbamazine and metronidazole.

infectious mononucleosis (IM)

An acute disorder caused by the Epstein-Barr virus (EBV) is **infectious mononucleosis (IM)**, also known as "mono" or the "kissing disease." Signs and symptoms are fever, fatigue, generalized malaise, lymph node enlargement, and sore throat. The virus infects B cells, and latent infections are common. Once afflicted, the individual carries the virus for life. The clinical

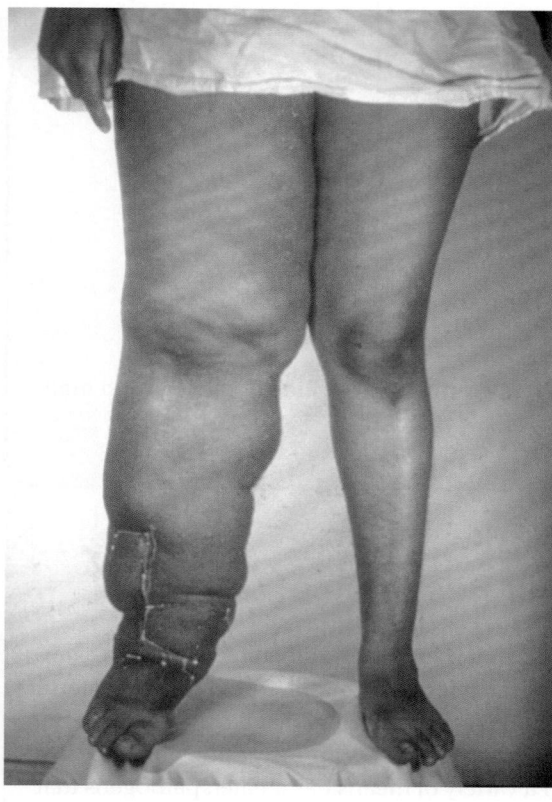

Figure 13-12 Lymphedema of the right lower extremity in a patient with elephantiasis.

and physical exam provide the initial diagnosis, and blood tests indicating elevated lymphocytes confirm the findings. Treatment options are antiviral medication administration and rest.

tonsillitis   **Tonsillitis** is inflammation of the tonsils. It is generally caused by a bacterial or viral infection and is characterized by swelling and pain, sore throat, and fever. It is diagnosed by the clinical picture and identification of the culprit organism by a throat swab. When tonsillitis is bacterial in origin, antibiotics are prescribed. **Tonsillectomy** (removal of the tonsils) is performed only as a last resort, because the tonsils play a key role in fighting infection.

KEY TERM	Definition
lymphangitis (lim-fan-JYE-tis)	inflammation of the lymphatics
elephantiasis (el-eh-fan-TYE-uh-sis)	lymphatic disease caused by filaria (parasitic roundworm) that is characterized by swelling of the legs and male scrotum
lymphedema (lim-feh-DEE-muh)	swelling of lymphatics in the extremities
infectious mononucleosis (IM) (mon-oh-new-klee-OH-sis)	disease caused by the Epstein-Barr virus (EBV) that infects B cells
tonsillitis (ton-si-LYE-tis)	inflammation of the tonsils usually due to bacterial or viral infection
tonsillectomy (ton-sil-LECK-toh-mee)	surgical removal of the tonsils

continued

continued from page 659

KEY TERM PRACTICE: *Infections*

1. _____ refers to inflammation of the tonsils.

2. Surgical removal of the tonsils is termed _____.

3. The disease caused by the Epstein-Barr virus (EBV) that infects B cells is termed _____.

4. Inflammation of the lymphatics is called _____, and is derived from the word part _____ for *lymphatic vessels* and the word part _____ for *inflammation*.

5. The lymphatic disease caused by filaria (parasitic roundworm) that is characterized by swelling of the legs and male scrotum is known as _____.

IN THE NEWS: Antimicrobial Resistance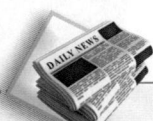

Have you heard of a "superinfection"? It is one that is extremely difficult to treat with available antimicrobics because of resistant strains of bacteria. An antimicrobic is a general term for a drug that destroys microbes, and an antibiotic is a drug aimed at destroying bacteria, a specific type of microbe. Antimicrobial resistance (AMR) is an increasing public health problem. The overuse of antibiotics through a variety of means has created pathogens that are remarkably resilient to drugs meant to kill them. A common example is methicillin-resistant *Staphylococcus aureus* (MRSA) infection. This strain of bacteria has become resistant to the antibiotic, methicillin, used to treat ordinary staphylococcal infections. It is spread by skin-to-skin contact. Most MRSA infections occur in health care settings, but they also occur in the wider community. For example, high school wrestlers, child care workers, and people living in crowded conditions are at greater risk of infection. Another example is multidrug-resistant tuberculosis (MDR-TB), which leads to 150,000 annual deaths worldwide.

According to the Centers for Disease Control and Prevention (CDC), bacterial infections worldwide are becoming resistant to drugs that once were effective. Bacteria develop resistance to drugs through a few mechanisms. For example, bacteria destroy the effect of the drug, they mutate to avoid the sensitive step that the drug is designed to affect, or they evolve in ways that do not allow the drug to enter.

The problem—namely, unneeded, intensive overuse of antibiotics—stems from several causes. Millions of prescriptions for antimicrobics in the United States are unnecessary. For example, too many antibiotics are prescribed for viral infections, for which they offer no benefit, and taking an antibiotic for a virus-based infection increases the risk of a future drug-resistant infection. Compounding the problem is the fact that antibiotics are not always taken as prescribed. Patients cut short the course of treatment because symptoms have disappeared. Failing to adhere to prescription instructions may not kill all the bacteria, allowing the remaining microbes to become drug resilient. Antimicrobial agents are also being added to soaps, detergents, lotions, and countless other household products, and there is no proven benefit of these products to public health. This adds to the predicament. Simple soap with good hand washing will suffice. Antibacterial products should be reserved for the health care setting and for individuals with compromised immune systems.

New drug development cannot keep pace with the rate of microbial resistance. In 2011, the World Health Organization (WHO) called on key stakeholders, including policy makers and planners, the public and patients, practitioners and prescribers, pharmacists and dispensers, and the pharmaceutical industry to act responsibly to halt the spread of antimicrobial resistance worldwide.

Tumors

Tumors are abnormal, uncontrolled growths that may occur in lymphatic vessels, tissues, and organs. Tumors have no physiological function and are classified as either benign (having a mild or harmless effect) or malignant (capable of spreading and causing harm). Cancer of the lymphatic system is termed **lymphoma**. Monoclonal antibody treatments are effective for treating lymphomas when they are tagged with a radionuclide to deliver radiation to the cancerous tissue.

Hodgkin disease (HD) | **Hodgkin disease (HD)** is a malignant lymphoma characterized by lymphadenopathy and sometimes **splenomegaly** (enlarged spleen) and hepatomegaly (enlarged liver), but there is no pain. The presence of Reed-Sternberg (or Sternberg-Reed) cells, giant lymphocytes with one or two large nuclei, indicates HD. Approximately 40% of lymphomas are Hodgkin type, and they generally affect individuals who are either between 15 and 35 years old or over age 50. It may be precipitated by a viral infection. The clinical picture and scintigraphy or lymphangiography confirm the diagnosis.

Scintigraphy is a diagnostic procedure for examining lymphatics after injection of a radioactive tracer using a scintillation (gamma) camera. After lymphatic absorption of the radioactive substance, the scanner detects the radioactive tracer and makes a two-dimensional image called a **scintigram** or **scintiscan.** Scintigraphic studies are useful for measuring lymphatic metastases (tumors that have spread).

Lymphangiography involves the injection of dye into lymphatic vessels (lymphatics). The nodes absorb the dye and x-ray images reveal nodal conditions. It is used to stage the disease (determine the level of disease progression), locate the source of the lymphedema, and evaluate the treatment.

Total nodal radiation, immunosuppressive drugs (such as azathioprine), corticosteroids, and chemotherapy are used in treating the disease. With **radiation therapy**, or **radiotherapy**, x-rays are aimed at the tumor to kill cancerous cells. **Azathioprine (AZT)** is a drug that suppresses the body's immune response. **Corticosteroids** are drugs that are similar to or identical to the natural corticosteroids secreted by the adrenal gland. Corticosteroids have both anti-inflammatory and immunosuppressive actions.

Toxic immunosuppressive drugs for the treatment of Hodgkin disease and tumors of the lymphatic system are cyclosporine and cyclophosphamide. **Cyclosporine** is an immunosuppressant drug derived from soil fungi that selectively depresses T_H cells, and **cyclophosphamide** suppresses B cells and antibody formation. **Cytotoxic drugs** are nonselective drugs that prevent cell division in replicating cells. A common four-drug chemotherapy regimen for the treatment of Hodgkin disease is mechlorethamine, Oncovin (vincristine), prednisone, and procarbazine (MOPP).

non-Hodgkin lymphoma (NHL) | **Non-Hodgkin lymphoma (NHL)** is the general term used to describe the diverse group of other lymphomas. Some evidence suggests that these lymphomas have a genetic predisposition. Treatment of NHL may be unnecessary until later stages, in which radiation,

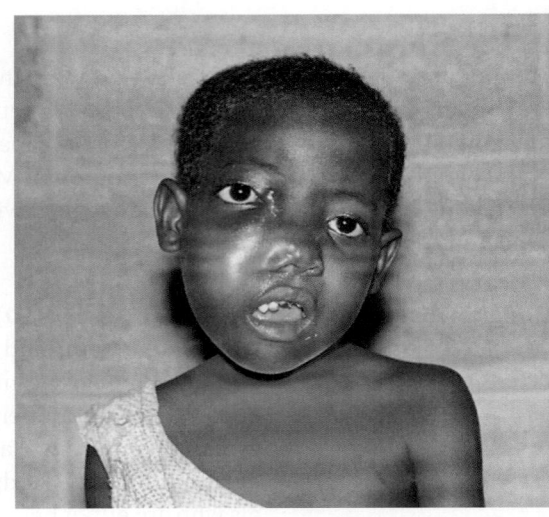

Figure 13-13 Burkitt lymphoma. A tumor of the jaw distorts the child's face.

chemotherapy, and bone marrow transplants (discussed later in this chapter) may be used.

Burkitt lymphoma

Burkitt lymphoma, a malignant tumor affecting B cells, is an example of an NHL. This cancer, occurring primarily in children in Central Africa, frequently affects the jaw and abdominal lymph nodes (**Figure 13-13**). Viral infections, including EBV, have been implicated in the disease. A clinical history of fever and night sweats provides the initial diagnosis. Advanced disease is marked by hepatomegaly and splenomegaly, and tissue biopsy is used to confirm the diagnosis.

Kaposi sarcoma (KS)

Kaposi sarcoma (KS) is cancer of the skin and lymph nodes. It is marked by purplish-red skin patches and occurs mainly in people with depressed immune systems, such as patients with AIDS (see **Figure 20-7**). Treatment is primarily supportive.

KEY TERM	Definition
lymphoma (lim-FOH-muh)	cancer of the lymphatic system
Hodgkin (HOJ-kin) **disease (HD)**	malignant lymphoma characterized by lymphadenopathy and sometimes splenomegaly and hepatomegaly
splenomegaly (splee-noh-MEG-uh-lee)	enlarged spleen
scintigraphy (sin-TIG-ruh-fee)	procedure using a scintillation (gamma) camera in which lymphatic absorption of a radioactive substance leads to a computer-created image
scintigram (SIN-ti-gram)	two-dimensional image of the distribution of a radioactive tracer in a body organ that is obtained using a special scanner; also called a scintiscan
scintiscan (SIN-ti-skan)	two-dimensional image of the distribution of a radioactive tracer in a body organ that is obtained using a special scanner; also called a scintigram

continued

continued from page 662

KEY TERM	Definition
lymphangiography (lim-fan-jee-OG-ruh-fee)	imaging of the lymphatic vessels (lymphatics) using an injected dye
radiation therapy	treating a disease by using targeted x-rays to kill cancerous cells; another term for radiotherapy
radiotherapy	treating a disease by using targeted x-rays to kill cancerous cells; another term for radiation therapy
azathioprine (ay-zuh-THIGH-oh-preen) **(AZT)**	immunosuppressive drug
corticosteroids (kor-ti-koh-STEER-oidz)	anti-inflammatory, immunosuppressive drugs that are similar to or identical to naturally secreted corticosteroids from the adrenal gland
cyclosporine (sigh-kloh-SPOR-een)	immunosuppressive drug that suppresses T_H cells
cyclophosphamide (sigh-kloh-FOS-fuh-mide)	immunosuppressive drug that suppresses B cells and antibody formation
cytotoxic (sigh-toh-TOCK-sick) **drugs**	chemical agents that prevent cell division in replicating cells, often used in cancer treatment
non-Hodgkin (HOJ-kin) **lymphoma (NHL)**	general term used to describe the diverse group of lymphomas that are not Hodgkin lymphoma
Burkitt (BUR-kit) **lymphoma**	a non-Hodgkin lymphoma of B cells that frequently affects the jaw and abdominal lymph nodes
Kaposi sarcoma (KS) (KA-poh-zee sahr-KOH-muh)	cancer of the skin and lymph nodes that is characterized by purplish-red skin patches and occurs primarily in people with depressed immune systems

KEY TERM PRACTICE: *Tumors*

1. Cancer of the lymphatic system is termed _____, and is derived from the word part _____ for *lymph* and the word part _____ that means *tumor*.

2. Cancer of the skin and lymph nodes that is characterized by purplish-red skin patches is _____.

3. _____ are chemical agents that prevent cell division in replicating cells and are often used to treat cancer. The term is derived from the word part _____ that means *cell* and the word part _____ that means *poison*.

4. The general term used to describe the diverse group of lymphomas that are not Hodgkin lymphoma is _____.

5. The medical term for an enlarged spleen is _____, from the word part _____ for *spleen* and the word part _____ for *large*.

Transplants

A **transplant** involves transferring an organ or tissue between a compatible donor and a recipient. The immune system is of great concern when dealing with tissue or organ transplants because the body recognizes the imported tissue as foreign. Medical transplants are performed out of necessity. Compatibility—the degree of similarity that exists between the donor tissue and recipient tissue—is a major factor. In order for a T cell to recognize an antigen, that antigen must be bound to glycoproteins in the cell membrane. The structure of these glycoproteins is genetically determined and found in a region of chromosome 6 known as the *major histocompatibility complex* (MHC). These glycoproteins are also called MHC proteins or *human leukocyte antigens* (HLAs). MHC proteins must be considered when performing a transplant. To reduce the risk of tissue rejection in transplant surgery, the tissue that is transplanted must be as much like the recipient's as possible. Cyclosporine drugs that dampen the immune response are used primarily to prevent organ and tissue rejection in transplant surgery. If the immune response is impeded, the body will not mount a full-blown attack on the implanted tissue. As a result, however, the patient's generalized risk of infection also increases.

Grafts are any living tissues or organs used for transplants. Typically, portions are transplanted to another body part to replace nonfunctional or absent tissue.

Bone marrow transplants involve extracting cells from functioning red bone marrow and transferring them to an immunosuppressed patient. Several types of transplants exist:

- *Allograft.* An **allograft** is a tissue graft from one member of a species to a genetically different member of the same species. An example would be a tissue transplant between siblings.
- *Autograft.* An **autograft** tissue graft is obtained from the patient's own body. In autografts, tissue is collected and used immediately or frozen for later use.
- *Syngraft.* A **syngraft** is a tissue graft taken from an individual genetically identical to the recipient of the graft. For example, a syngraft occurs between identical twins.
- *Xenograft.* A **xenograft** is a tissue transplant from an animal of one species to one of another species. An example is using valves from a pig heart to replace human heart valves.

graft versus host disease (GVHD)	**Graft versus host disease (GVHD)** is an immune reaction in transplant recipients. It occurs most frequently with red bone marrow transplants in which the donor's immune cells attack the recipient's tissues. The situation is complicated by the fact that the red bone marrow recipient is already immunosuppressed to receive the transplant. The newly transplanted donor's cells react against the recipient's (host's) antigens, creating systemic effects. Signs and symptoms include rash, diarrhea, gastrointestinal distress, and hepatosplenomegaly. Treatment depends on the individual patient. If the condition is not resolved, it could lead to death.

Immunosuppressive drugs are used to overcome tissue rejection. Some are selective in their actions, and others target the entire immune response. **Tissue rejection** involves antibody production against the proteins (antigens) in a transplanted organ. Drugs that affect T cell activity by depleting their numbers are used to hamper T cell–mediated immunity and are beneficial in the prevention of tissue and organ rejection.

KEY TERM	Definition
transplant	tissue transfer between a compatible donor and a recipient
grafts	living tissues or organs used for transplants
bone marrow transplants	red bone marrow cells collected and transferred from one individual to another
allograft (AL-oh-graft)	transplant between compatible donor and recipient of the same species
autograft (AW-toh-graft)	transplant tissue sample taken from the patient's own body
syngraft (SIN-graft)	transplant between identical twins
xenograft (ZEE-noh-graft)	transplant between two different species
graft versus host disease (GVHD)	immunologic reaction involving the attack of host cells by donor immune cells
tissue rejection	destruction of transplanted tissue by the immune response

continued

continued from page 664

KEY TERM PRACTICE: *Transplants*

1. The medical term for an immunologic reaction involving the attack of host cells by donor immune cells is _____.

2. Give the term for each of the following definitions.

   a. transplant tissue between identical twins _____

   b. transplant tissue sample taken from the patient's own body _____

   c. transplant tissue between two different species _____

   d. transplant between compatible donor and recipient _____

3. Destruction of transplanted tissue by the immune response is termed _____.

4. _____ is a tissue transfer between a compatible donor and a recipient.

5. _____ are living tissues or organs used for transplants.

LIFE SPAN

Lymphatic system development begins early in embryonic life. By the fifth gestational week, lymphatics and lymph nodes are apparent. Except for the thymus gland, which is derived from the endoderm, lymphatics and organs are derived from the mesoderm. The lymphatic vessels originate from lymph sacs that developed from veins. Lymphocytes are derived from hematopoietic (blood) tissue.

The thymus gland is of particular importance regarding immune function. At birth, the thymus is relatively large and continues to grow until puberty and early adolescence, when it reaches its maximum size. Thereafter, it gradually diminishes in size and function. As the thymus gland continues to atrophy, T cells decline in number, and the remaining T cells fail to function as well as their predecessors. In this sense, the thymus loses a portion of its ability to protect against the invasion of bacteria and viruses. It may also fail to protect against abnormal cell growth, as in cancers.

The human immune system becomes less efficient throughout the aging process, but the relationship between decreased immune response and aging is not well understood. Decreased function may be the result of diminished organ reserve, which is the ability to function beyond the usual needs. Along with the functional decline, autoantibodies within the blood tend to rise, thereby increasing the risk of developing autoimmune diseases. The B cells also function less well, so their capacity to proliferate and release specific antibodies is diminished in elderly immune systems.

Other age-related changes in immunity are decreased lymphocyte response to antigens, decreased antibody titer (blood test used to determine the concentration of an antibody) after vaccination, slower antibody response, increased susceptibility to infections, and prolonged infectious episodes. Conversely, some elderly persons have no immunologic changes and have immune systems that are as vigorous as when they were young.

COMMON Abbreviations

Abbreviation	Term
Ab	antibody
Ag	antigen
AIDS	acquired immunodeficiency syndrome
AMR	antimicrobial resistance
AMTA	American Massage Therapy Association
AZT	azathioprine
CDC	Centers for Disease Control and Prevention
CPR	cardiopulmonary resuscitation
EBV	Epstein-Barr virus
GVHD	graft versus host disease
HIV	human immunodeficiency virus
HD	Hodgkin disease
HLA	human leukocyte antigen
IFN	interferon
Ig	immunoglobulin
IM	infectious mononucleosis
KS	Kaposi sarcoma
MAB	monoclonal antibody
MHC	major histocompatibility complex
MoAb	monoclonal antibody
MRSA	methicillin-resistant *Staphylococcus aureus*
MT	massage therapist
NCBTMB	National Certification Board for Therapeutic Massage and Bodywork
NHL	non-Hodgkin lymphoma
NK cells	natural killer cells
NSAID	nonsteroidal anti-inflammatory drug
PNI	psychoneuroimmunology
RA	rheumatoid arthritis
RT	reverse transcriptase
SCID	severe combined immunodeficiency
SLE	systemic lupus erythematosus
T_C cell	cytotoxic T cell
T_H cell	helper T cell
T_S cell	suppressor T cell

continued

continued from page 666

COMMON ABBREVIATIONS EXERCISES

1. PNI is the abbreviation for _____.

2. GVHD is the abbreviation for _____.

3. Give the abbreviation for helper T cell. _____

4. Give the abbreviation for nonsteroidal anti-inflammatory drug. _____

5. MRSA is the abbreviation for _____.

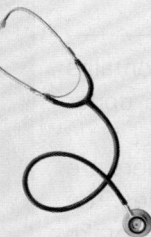

Case Study

Mrs. Eleanor Chime is 67 years old and has a history of melanoma (cancer derived from skin melanocytes) on her back. The melanoma metastasized to regional lymph nodes with concomitant splenomegaly and hepatomegaly. Her lungs and brain are not affected.

She is not very ambulatory because of arthritis and suffers from lymphedema, notably in her legs. Analgesics and nonsteroidal anti-inflammatory drugs (NSAIDs) provide some relief. Mrs. Chime's oncologist recommended massage therapy for lymphedema relief.

Case Study Questions

Select the best answer to each of the following questions.

1. Splenomegaly is best described as _____.

   a. enlargement of the spleen
   b. a papule on the epidermis
   c. cancer of the spleen
   d. non-Hodgkin lymphoma

2. Lymphedema is best described as _____.

   a. enlargement of the lymph nodes
   b. swelling of lymphatic tissue
   c. an autoimmune disease
   d. all of these

3. Lymphedema could result from _____.

   a. obstructed lymphatics
   b. immobility
   c. decreased fluid intake
   d. a and b

4. Why might Mrs. Chime experience relief after having massage therapy? _____

   a. The oils used increase lymph flow.
   b. Manual manipulation and compression enhance lymph flow.
   c. Reclining while receiving a massage increases lymph flow.
   d. Massage therapy is counterintuitive, and the benefit she proclaims is merely perceived and not actual.

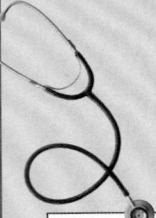

Real World Report

Mrs. Chime brought her medical report to the spa so that the physician on staff and Lee could review it. Her oncologist believes that massage therapy will assist with her persistent lymphedema.

CENTRAL NUCLEAR MEDICINE IMAGING

NAME: Eleanor Chime

AGE: 67

DATEORD: May 2, 2011

DOB: January 23, 1944

EXAM DATE: May 3, 2011

ORDPHYS: R. J. Meter, DO

CLINICAL INFORMATION:

Melanoma in the back; persistent lymphedema

LYMPHOSCINTIGRAPHY

After four separate intradermal injections of technetium-99m sulfur colloid (each injection contains approximately 90 mCi) surrounding the previous excisional biopsy at the posterior aspect of the upper lumbar region, scintigraphic evaluation was obtained.

Lymphatic drainage was noted toward the right axilla soon after the injection was completed. There are two separate areas of prominent radionuclide concentration within the right-side axillary lymph nodes. The lateral projection also shows two additional areas of mildly to moderately increased lymph nodal uptake adjacent to the above-described prominent lymph nodal uptake. There was no lymphatic drainage noted in the groin region.

At the end of the scintigraphic study, the two prominent uptakes in the right axillary lymph nodes were localized using a small amount of radioisotopic marker and the corresponding areas were marked on the skin. The patient tolerated the procedure well and left the department for sentinel node sampling.

DICTATED BY: E. Matters, MD

This document has been reviewed and electronically approved.

Real World Report Questions

The following exercise reviews the medical terms used in the preceding medical report. Two terms may be unfamiliar: Technetium-99m is used as a radiopharmaceutical for scanning purposes. The abbreviation mCi stands for millicurie, which is a unit of radioactivity equal to 3.7×10^7 disintegrations per second.

1. **Mrs. Chime was sent for sentinel node sampling. A sentinel node is the most important node that draws from the area of the tumor. Nodes adjacent to the tumor that receive drainage from the tumor site are sentinel nodes. If the sentinel node does not show cancerous cells during microscopic examination, it may not be necessary to remove any more lymph nodes. Define the following medical terms or phrases.**

a. scintigraphic study _____

b. biopsy _____

c. posterior aspect _____

d. upper lumbar region _____

e. right-side axillary lymph nodes _____

f. increased nodal uptake refers to _____

g. lymphedema _____

Review and Application

Multiple-Choice Questions

Select the best answer to each of the following questions.

1. Tissue fluid that has entered the lymphatic system is termed _____.
   a. plasma   b. blood   c. lymph   d. serum

2. The lymphatic organ located in the mediastinum deep to the sternum is the _____.
   a. thymus   b. thyroid   c. parathyroid   d. spleen

3. _____ is the medical term for a lymphatic in the intestinal wall that transports recently digested fats to the bloodstream.
   a. Lacteal   b. Allergy   c. Lymph   d. Antibody

4. The _____ duct drains lymph from the entire body except the upper right quadrant.
   a. right lymphatic   b. lymphatic   c. thoracic   d. plasma

5. Resistance that results from previous exposure to a particular antigen is known as _____.
   a. active immunity   b. adaptive immunity   c. cell-mediated immunity   d. antibody-mediated immunity

6. Cancer of the lymphatic system is termed a _____.
   a. capsule   b. lymphocyte   c. lymphoma   d. lymph node

7. Disease resistance as a result of antibodies is called _____ defense.
   a. nonspecific   b. specific   c. physical   d. symbiotic

8. Inflammation of the tonsils is termed _____.
   a. tonsillopharyngitis   b. tonsillectomy   c. pharyngitis   d. tonsillitis

9. Proteins produced by various cells in response to viral infections are termed _____.
   a. interferons   b. antigens   c. macrophages   d. phagocytes

10. The lymphatic organ that decreases in size as we age is the _____.
    a. spleen   b. lymph node   c. lung   d. thymus

11. _____ is the ability to ward off infection.
    a. Susceptibility   b. Resistance   c. Fever   d. Complement

12. Cell-mediated immunity involves _____.
    a. T cells   b. antibodies   c. memory cells   d. plasma cells

13. Lymphocytes that directly attack other cells both physically and chemically are called _____.
    a. cytotoxic T cells   b. B cells   c. helper T cells   d. suppressor T cells

14. Immune reaction to a first encounter is called the _____ response.
    a. plasma   b. primary   c. secondary   d. HLA

15. T cells mature in the _____.
    a. thyroid   b. tonsils   c. T lymphocytes   d. thymus

16. An alternative term for adenoid is _____.
    a. pharyngeal tonsil   b. antigen   c. immunoglobulin   d. antibody

17. The type of immunity present after recovering from an infection is _____ immunity.
    a. naturally acquired active   b. naturally acquired passive   c. artificially induced   d. innate

18. The immunity conferred to an infant through breast milk is called _____ immunity.
    a. naturally acquired active   b. naturally acquired passive   c. innate   d. artificially induced

19. _____ are preparations that stimulate the production of antibodies and provide immunity against disease.
    a. Cytotoxic drugs   b. Antibiotics   c. Vaccines   d. Immunosuppressants

20. Which of the following are lymphokinetic factors? _____
    a. skeletal muscle contractions   b. arterial pulses   c. postural changes   d. all of the above

21. Which pathway correctly identifies lymph flow through the body? _____
    a. interstitial fluid → lymphatic trunks → lymph capillaries → thoracic duct or right lymphatic duct
    b. thoracic duct or right lymphatic duct → lymphatic trunks → lymphatic capillaries → tissue fluid
    c. lymph capillaries → lymphatics → lymphatic trunks → thoracic duct or right lymphatic duct
    d. lymphatics → lymph capillaries → lymphatic trunks → tissue fluid

22. Lymph vessels (lymphatics) are most similar to _____.
    a. arteries with valves   b. veins with valves   c. arterioles with capillaries   d. venules with capillaries

23. Lymph flow would be the greatest _____.
    a. during sleep   b. during flight in an aircraft   c. while bathing   d. while exercising

24. Lymphatic obstruction resulting from infection in the thumb might cause enlarged lymph nodes in the _____ region.
    a. cervical   b. axillary   c. pelvic   d. inguinal

25. HIV is transmitted to people by _____.
    a. body fluids and blood   b. skin touching   c. contaminated needle sharing   d. a and c

Word Parts Exercises

Using the following word parts, form a medical term for each definition. Each word part is used only once.

-angiogram   -ectomy   lymph-
lymphadeno-   -pathy   splen-

26. removal of the spleen _____

27. enlarged lymph nodes _____

28. x-ray of lymphatic tissue after dye injection _____

Matching Exercises

Match the T cell type with its description.

_____ 29. helper T cell

_____ 30. suppressor T cell

_____ 31. cytotoxic T cell

_____ 32. memory T cell

a. inhibits other T cells and B cells
b. long-lived cell that responds to future encounters with a known antigen
c. assists other cells in their actions
d. directly attacks foreign antigens

Match the drug with its classification or mode of action.

_____ 33. antihistamine

_____ 34. corticosteroid

_____ 35. cyclosporine

_____ 36. cytotoxic drugs

a. anti-inflammatory, immunosuppressant
b. targets replicating cells
c. inhibits effects of histamine
d. immunosuppressant, T_H depressor

Match the graft type with its definition.

_____ 37. allograft

_____ 38. autograft

_____ 39. syngraft

_____ 40. xenograft

a. tissue from same species
b. tissue from different species
c. tissue from self
d. tissue from identical twin

Match the disorder with its description.

_____ 41. severe combined immunodeficiency syndrome (SCID)

_____ 42. anaphylaxis

_____ 43. acquired immunodeficiency syndrome (AIDS)

_____ 44. asthma

_____ 45. perennial allergic rhinitis

a. disease caused by HIV
b. extreme hypersensitivity to antigen, protein, or drug
c. absence of both cell-mediated and antibody-mediated immunity
d. year-round allergy to environmental allergens
e. reactive airway disorder characterized by bronchospasm and mucus secretion

Match the test with its description.

_____ 46. HLA test

_____ 47. biopsy

_____ 48. prick test

_____ 49. intradermal test

_____ 50. lymphangiography

a. detects reaction to antigen after it is poked into the skin
b. detects sensitivity to an antigen after it is injected into the skin
c. test used to determine compatibility in transplant procedures between donor and patients through antigen detection
d. dye injected into lymphatics for x-ray imaging
e. extraction of tissue sample for examination

Definitions

Define the following terms.

51. splenomegaly _____

52. lymphoma _____

53. lymphadenectomy _____

54. T cells _____

55. lymph nodes _____

Provide a medical term for the following definitions.

56. A two-dimensional image of an organ obtained using a scintiscanner is termed a _____ or _____.

57. immune reaction to a second (or later) encounter with a known antigen due to memory cells _____

58. resistance against particular antigens; also called adaptive immunity _____

59. genetically determined resistance that a person is born with _____

60. resistance that results from the actual transfer of antibodies to a person _____

Alternate Terms

Give an alternate term for each of the following terms.

61. anaphylactic shock _____

62. humoral immunity _____

63. cellular immunity _____

64. hyposensitization _____

65. T lymphocytes _____

66. B lymphocytes _____

67. innate immunity _____

68. adaptive immunity _____

Spelling

Identify the correctly spelled term in each set.

69. _____

   a. lymphangitis
   b. lymphoangitis
   c. limfangitis
   d. lymphengitis

70. _____

   a. anephylaxis
   b. enaphylaxis
   c. anaphylaxes
   d. anaphylaxis

71. _____

   a. imunodeficiency
   b. immunodeficiency
   c. imunnodeficiency
   d. imminudeficiency

72. _____

   a. humoral
   b. hummoral
   c. humorel
   d. humorol

73. _____

   a. elefantiasis
   b. elephantiasisl
   c. elefanntiasis
   d. elephantasis

Unscramble

Unscramble the letters to form a medical term.

74. fragtonex _____

75. mylph _____

76. mathas _____

77. shinriit _____

78. minutyim _____

Abbreviations

Provide the term for the abbreviations and then define the terms.

79. AZT = _____

80. HD = _____

81. Ag = _____

82. AIDS = _____

83. Ab = _____

84. GVHD = _____

85. Ig = _____

Analogies

Provide a medical term to complete a meaningful analogy.

86. Hepatomegaly is to enlarged liver as _____ is to enlarged spleen.

87. HIV is to AIDS as filaria is to _____.

Short Answer

Answer the following questions.

88. Heinz has been feeling a bit under the weather, but he does not have the flu. Upon physical examination, it was discovered that his lymph nodes in the cervical region were slightly enlarged and palpable. Provide a plausible explanation.

   _____

89. Carla is a third-year nursing student. A blood test showed she had antibodies to EBV but she denies being sick with EBV. Explain why she has antibodies to EBV.

   _____

Labeling

Label the structures in the following diagram.

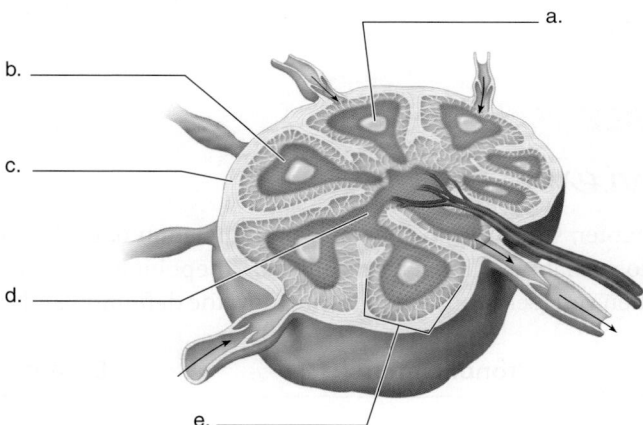

Word Search

Find the medical terms hidden in the puzzle.

```
L N L J S P A A U Y Q P G S Y Y
Y I L Y R N P N T T H S P H T V
M L F D M P E I T A A L K I O S
P U S P F P N G G I E T L G N D
H B H M N U H O O E G I H D S J
A O U W M O C O N H B E E T I J
T L E M V Y F U C I T O N Y L I
I G I K T D F Q T Y B A R M S T
C O Q E X M X P Q K T N P I Y I
S N S W T C E V G G Y E N P D X
X U X X C S U M Y H T S J O J
F M E H S N O I T C E F N I B N
A M H U P H A G O C Y T O S I S
V I S Q W M Z F K D P E J B T T
X X S F Q M W F J N I J Q R N E
L A C T E A L S C U E V B N A L
```

antibody
antigen
immunity
immunoglobulin
infection
lacteals
lymphatics
lymphocytes
pathogens
phagocytes
phagocytosis
spleen
susceptibility
thymus
tonsils

Vocabulary Review

Review the key terms from this chapter, study the spelling and pronunciation of each term, and write its definition in the space provided. Listen to the audio available for most terms at http://thepoint.lww.com/nath2e and pronounce each term for yourself. Then check the box when you feel confident that you know the definition and can pronounce the term correctly.

Key Term	Pronunciation	Definition
❑ acquired immunodeficiency syndrome (AIDS)	(im-yoo-noh-de-FISH-un-see)	_____
❑ active immunity		_____
❑ acute asthma	(AZ-muh)	_____
❑ adaptive immunity		_____
❑ adenoid	(AD-eh-noid)	_____
❑ AIDS-related complex		_____
❑ allergic rhinitis	(rye-NIGH-tis)	_____
❑ allergy		_____
❑ allograft	(AL-oh-graft)	_____

Key Term	Pronunciation	Definition
❏ anaphylaxis	(an-uh-fi-LACK-sis)	
❏ antibody (Ab)	(AN-tee-bod-ee)	
❏ antibody-mediated immunity		
❏ antigen (Ag)	(AN-ti-jen)	
❏ antihistamines		
❏ asthma	(AZ-muh)	
❏ autograft	(AW-toh-graft)	
❏ autoimmune diseases	(aw-toh-i-MEWN)	
❏ azathioprine (AZT)	(ay-zuh-THIGH-oh-preen)	
❏ B cells		
❏ bone marrow transplant		
❏ bronchodilators	(bronk-oh-dye-LAY-turz)	
❏ Burkitt lymphoma	(BUR-kit)	
❏ cell-mediated immunity		
❏ corticosteroids	(kor-ti-koh-STEER-oidz)	
❏ cyclophosphamide	(sigh-kloh-FOS-fuh-mide)	
❏ cyclosporine	(sigh-kloh-SPOR-een)	
❏ cytotoxic drugs	(sigh-toh-TOCK-sick)	
❏ cytotoxic T (T_C) cells	(sigh-toh-TOCK-sick)	
❏ decongestant		
❏ desensitization	(dee-sen-si-ti-ZAY-shun)	
❏ elephantiasis	(el-eh-fan-TYE-uh-sis)	
❏ extrinsic asthma	(ecks-TRIN-sick AZ-muh)	
❏ germinal centers	(JUR-mi-nul)	
❏ graft versus host disease (GVHD)		
❏ grafts		
❏ hay fever		
❏ helper T (T_H) cells		
❏ Hodgkin disease (HD)	(HOJ-kin)	
❏ human immunodeficiency virus (HIV)	(im-yoo-noh-de-FISH-un-see)	
❏ hypersensitivity	(high-pur-sen-si-TIV-i-tee)	
❏ hyposensitization	(high-poh-sen-sih-tih-ZAY-shun)	
❏ immunity		
❏ immunoglobulin (Ig)	(im-yoo-noh-GLOB-yoo-lin)	
❏ immunotherapy	(im-yoo-noh-THERR-uh-pee)	
❏ infection		
❏ infectious mononucleosis (IM)	(mon-oh-new-klee-OH-sis)	

Key Term	Pronunciation	Definition
❑ innate immunity		
❑ interferons (IFNs)	(in-tur-FEER-onz)	
❑ intradermal test	(in-truh-DUR-mul)	
❑ intrinsic asthma	(in-TRIN-sick AZ-muh)	
❑ Kaposi sarcoma (KS)	(KA-poh-zee sahr-KOH-muh)	
❑ lacteals	(LACK-tee-ulz)	
❑ latex allergy	(LAY-tecks)	
❑ lymph	(LIMF)	
❑ lymph nodes	(LIMF)	
❑ lymph nodules	(LIMF NOD-yoolz)	
❑ lymphadenopathy	(lim-fad-e-NOP-uh-thee)	
❑ lymphangiography	(lim-fan-jee-OG-ruh-fee)	
❑ lymphangitis	(lim-fan-JYE-tis)	
❑ lymphatics	(lim-FAT-icks)	
❑ lymphedema	(lim-feh-DEE-muh)	
❑ lymphocytes	(LIM-foh-sites)	
❑ lymphoma	(lim-FOH-muh)	
❑ memory B cells		
❑ memory T cells		
❑ monoclonal antibody (MAB or MoAb)	(mon-oh-KLOH-nul AN-tee-bod-ee)	
❑ non-Hodgkin lymphoma (NHL)	(HOJ-kin)	
❑ nonspecific immunity		
❑ opportunistic infection		
❑ passive immunity		
❑ patch test		
❑ pathogens	(PATH-oh-jenz)	
❑ perennial allergic rhinitis	(rye-NIGH-tis)	
❑ phagocytes	(FAG-oh-sites)	
❑ phagocytosis	(fag-oh-sigh-TOH-sis)	
❑ plasma cells	(PLAZ-muh)	
❑ prick test		
❑ primary response		
❑ psychoneuroimmunology (PNI)	(sigh-koh-new-roh-im-yoo-NOL-uh-jee)	
❑ radiation therapy		
❑ radiotherapy		
❑ resistance		
❑ right lymphatic duct	(lim-FAT-ick)	

Key Term	Pronunciation	Definition
❏ scintigram	(SIN-ti-gram)	
❏ scintigraphy	(sin-TIG-ruh-fee)	
❏ scintiscan	(SIN-ti-skan)	
❏ secondary response		
❏ sensitization	(sen-si-ti-ZAY-shun)	
❏ severe combined immunodeficiency syndrome (SCID)	(im-yoo-noh-de-FISH-un-see)	
❏ Sjögren syndrome	(SHOE-greyn)	
❏ specific immunity		
❏ spleen		
❏ splenomegaly	(splee-noh-MEG-uh-lee)	
❏ status asthmaticus	(STAT-us az-MAT-i-kus)	
❏ suppressor T (T_s) cells		
❏ susceptibility		
❏ syngraft	(SIN-graft)	
❏ T cells		
❏ thoracic duct	(thoh-RAS-ick)	
❏ thymus	(THY-mus)	
❏ tissue rejection		
❏ tonsillectomy	(ton-sil-LECK-toh-mee)	
❏ tonsillitis	(ton-si-LYE-tis)	
❏ tonsils		
❏ transplant		
❏ vaccine	(vack-SEEN)	
❏ wheal		
❏ xenograft	(ZEE-noh-graft)	

Answers

Word Grouping Exercises

Definition	Word Part	Definition	Word Part
chyle, fat droplets in lymph	chyl-, chylo-	lymph	lymph-, lympho-
disease	patho, patho-, -pathy	lymph nodes	lymphaden-, lymphadeno-
eating, devouring	phago-	lymphatic vessels	lymphangi-, lymphangio-
immune, immunity, protected	immuno-	milk	lact-, lacti-, lacto-
like	iso-	nose	rhin-, rhino-

Definition	Word Part	Definition	Word Part
other, different	A. allo- B. heter-, hetero-	strange, foreign	xeno-
poison, toxin	tox-, toxi-, toxico-, toxo-	substance that produces something	-gen
self, same	aut-, auto-	thymus	thym-, thymi-, thymo-
spleen	splen-, spleno-	tonsil	tonsillo-

Word Building Exercises

Word Part	Meaning	Common or Known Word	Example Medical Term
xeno-	strange, foreign	xenolith	xenograft
allo-	other, different	allograft	allogeneic
aut-, auto-	self, one's own	autonomous	autoimmune
-gen	substance that produces something	antigen	antigen
heter-, hetero-	other, different	heterosexual	heterograft
immuno-	immune, immunity, protected	immunology	immunologic response
iso-	like	isolate	isograft
lact-, lacti-, lacto-	milk	lactate	lacteal
lymph-, lympho-	lymph	lymphoma	lymph node
path-, patho-, -pathy	disease	pathophysiology	pathogen
phago-	eating, devouring	phagocytosis	phagocyte
rhin-, rhino-	nose	rhinoceros	rhinitis
thym-, thymi-, thymo-	thymus	thyme	thymus gland
tonsillo-	tonsil	tonsillectomy	tonsillitis
tox-, toxi-, toxico-, toxo-	toxic, poisonous	toxic	lymphotoxin

Key Term Practice

Lymphatic System and Immunity Preview

1. *lympho-*; *-cyte*; lymphocyte
2. nonspecific immunity; specific immunity
3. lymphatics
4. Lymph nodes
5. Immunity

Lymph Nodes, Lymphocytes, and Lymphatics

1. right lymphatic duct
2. thoracic duct
3. Germinal centers
4. lymph nodules

Tonsils, Thymus, and Spleen

1. adenoid
2. Phagocytosis

Nonspecific Defenses and Specific Defenses

1. Infection
2. Psychoneuroimmunology (PNI)
3. active immunity
4. passive immunity
5. Phagocytes; *phago-*; *-cyte*

Major Types of T Cells and B Cells

1. Plasma cells
2. T cells
3. memory T cells
4. B cells
5. helper T (T$_H$) cells

Classes of Immunoglobulins, Primary Response, and Secondary Response

1. vaccine
2. immunoglobulin (Ig)
3. primary response
4. secondary response

Autoimmune Diseases

1. autoimmune disease
2. Sjögren syndrome

Hypersensitivity Disorders

1. hay fever; perennial allergic rhinitis
2. allergic rhinitis; *rhin-*
3. Anaphylaxis
4. bronchodilators
5. desensitization; hyposensitization

Immunodeficiency Disorders

1. severe combined immunodeficiency disease
2. human immunodeficiency virus (HIV)
3. opportunistic infection
4. lymphadenopathy; *lymphadeno-; -pathy*
5. Immunotherapy

Infections

1. Tonsillitis
2. tonsillectomy
3. infectious mononucleosis (IM)
4. lymphangitis; *lymphang-; -itis*
5. elephantiasis

Tumors

1. lymphoma; *lymph-; -oma*
2. Kaposi sarcoma (KS)
3. Cytotoxic drugs; *cyto-; -toxic*
4. non-Hodgkin lymphoma (NHL)
5. splenomegaly; *spleno-; -megaly*

Transplants

1. graft versus host disease (GVHD)
2. a. syngraft; b. autograft; c. xenograft; d. allograft
3. tissue rejection
4. Transplant
5. Grafts

Common Abbreviations Exercises

1. PSI = psychoneuroimmunology
2. GVHD = graft versus host disease
3. helper T cell = T$_H$ cell
4. nonsteroidal anti-inflammatory drug = NSAID
5. MRSA = methicillin-resistant *Staphylococcus aureus*

Case Study

1. a is the correct answer.
   - b is incorrect because a papule is a small hard bump on the skin.
   - c is incorrect because the word part *-megaly* refers to *enlarged.*
   - d is incorrect because splenomegaly refers to an enlargement of the spleen.

2. b is the correct answer.
   - a is incorrect because the word part *-edema* refers to *swelling* not *enlargement*.
   - c is incorrect because an autoimmune disease is characterized by the body attacking itself because it can no longer recognize self from nonself tissue.
   - d is incorrect because answers a and c are incorrect.
3. d is the correct answer.
   - c is incorrect because a decreased fluid intake does not cause lymphedema; in fact, fluid restriction often lessens the severity of the swelling.
4. b is the correct answer.
   - a is incorrect because the oils have nothing to do with moving lymphatic fluid.
   - c is incorrect because movement, not reclining, contributes to lymph movement; in fact, elevating a body part will move lymph as a result of gravity.
   - d is incorrect because massage therapy is beneficial for enhancing fluid movement, especially when the body part does not get much exercise. Furthermore, perceived benefits are also beneficial because there is a strong link between psychological and physiological well-being.

Real World Report

1. a. an evaluation of lymph nodes via a two-dimensional image produced by radioactive tracer distribution
   b. surgical extraction of tissue for examination purposes
   c. the back side of the body
   d. the small of the back
   e. those located in the armpit region on the anatomical right side of the body
   f. an area in which the radioactive material (technetium-99m) was dense
   g. swelling in the extremities as a result of lymph accumulation

Review and Application

1. c	18. b	35. d
2. a	19. c	36. b
3. a	20. d	37. a
4. c	21. c	38. c
5. a	22. b	39. d
6. c	23. d	40. b
7. b	24. b	41. c
8. d	25. d	42. b
9. a	26. splenectomy	43. a
10. d	27. lymphadenopathy	44. e
11. b	28. lymphangiogram	45. d
12. a	29. c	46. c
13. a	30. a	47. e
14. b	31. d	48. a
15. d	32. b	49. b
16. a	33. c	50. d
17. a	34. a	51. splenomegaly = enlarged spleen

52. lymphoma = tumor of lymph tissue
53. lymphadenectomy = removal of lymph node
54. T cells = lymphocytes derived from the thymus; also called T lymphocytes
55. lymph nodes = bean-shaped masses of lymphatic tissue distributed along lymphatics that filter lymph
56. scintigram; scintiscan
57. secondary response
58. specific immunity
59. innate immunity
60. passive immunity
61. anaphylaxis
62. antibody-mediated immunity
63. cell-mediated immunity
64. desensitization
65. T cells
66. B cells
67. nonspecific immunity
68. specific immunity
69. a
70. d
71. b
72. a
73. b
74. xenograft
75. lymph
76. asthma
77. rhinitis

78. immunity
79. AZT = azathioprine; immunosuppressive drug
80. HD = Hodgkin disease; malignant lymphoma characterized by lymphadenopathy and sometimes splenomegaly and hepatomegaly
81. Ag = antigen; protein that provokes an immune response
82. AIDS = acquired immunodeficiency syndrome; disease caused by infection with HIV
83. Ab = antibody; protein produced in response to a particular antigen that works to eliminate that specific antigen
84. GVHD = graft verus host disease; immunologic reaction involving the attack of host cells by donor immune cells
85. Ig = immunoglobulin; protein produced by white blood cells that acts like an antibody; the classes are IgG, IgE, IgD, IgM, and IgA
86. splenomegaly
87. elephantiasis
88. Heinz probably has an infection because enlarged lymph nodes are an indication that the body is mounting an immune response.
89. The Epstein-Barr virus causes infectious mononucleosis. Once infected with the virus, the virus will always remain in the body, although there may be no outward signs or symptoms after recovery. However, circulating antibodies indicate either previous infection or exposure.

Labeling

a. germinal center
b. cortex
c. capsule
d. medulla
e. lymph nodule
f. efferent lymphatic
g. afferent lymphatic

Word Search

```
L  N  L  J  S  P  A  A  U  Y  Q  P  G  S  Y  Y
Y  I  L  Y  R  N  P  N  T  T  H  S  P  H  T  V
M  L  F  D  M  P  E  I  T  A  A  L  K  I  O  S
P  U  S  P  F  P  N  G  G  I  E  T  L  G  N  D
H  B  H  M  N  U  H  O  O  E  G  I  H  D  S  J
A  O  U  W  M  O  C  O  N  H  B  E  E  T  I  J
T  L  E  M  V  Y  F  U  C  I  T  O  N  Y  L  I
I  G  I  K  T  D  F  Q  T  Y  B  A  R  M  S  T
C  O  Q  E  X  M  X  P  Q  K  T  N  P  I  Y  I
S  N  S  W  T  C  E  V  G  G  Y  E  N  P  D  X
X  U  X  X  X  C  S  U  M  Y  H  T  S  J  O  J
F  M  E  H  S  N  O  I  T  C  E  F  N  I  B  N
A  M  H  U  P  H  A  G  O  C  Y  T  O  S  I  S
V  I  S  Q  W  M  Z  F  K  D  P  E  J  B  T  T
X  X  S  F  Q  M  W  F  J  N  I  J  Q  R  N  E
L  A  C  T  E  A  L  S  C  U  E  V  B  N  A  L
```

antibody
antigen
immunity
immunoglobulin
infection
lacteals
lymphatics
lymphocytes
pathogens
phagocytes
phagocytosis
spleen
susceptibility
thymus
tonsils

Vocabulary Review

Key Term	Definition	Key Term	Definition
active immunity	resistance that results from previous exposure to a particular antigen	**anaphylaxis**	an extreme hypersensitivity reaction that can be fatal; the term may be used for anaphylactic shock
acquired immunodeficiency syndrome (AIDS)	disease caused by infection with HIV	**antibody (Ab)**	protein produced in response to a particular antigen that works to eliminate that specific antigen
acute asthma	sudden, severe asthma that causes coughing and difficulty breathing	**antibody-mediated immunity**	resistance that results from antibodies directed at specific antigens; also called humoral immunity
adaptive immunity	type of resistance acquired only after being exposed to a particular antigen	**antigen (Ag)**	protein that provokes an immune response
adenoid	another term for the pharyngeal tonsil	**antihistamines**	drugs that inhibit the physiological effects of histamine
AIDS-related complex	manifestations of AIDS in patients who have not yet developed major deficient immune function	**asthma**	reactive airway disorder characterized by bronchospasm and mucus secretion
allergic rhinitis	inflammation of the nasal mucous membranes caused by allergen inhalation	**autograft**	transplant tissue sample taken from the patient's own body
allergy	extreme sensitivity reaction to a normally harmless substance	**autoimmune diseases**	disorders in which the immune response is directed against the body's own tissues
allograft	transplant between compatible donor and recipient of the same species	**azathioprine (AZT)**	immunosuppressive drug

Key Term	Definition
B cells	lymphocytes that can differentiate into plasma cells when stimulated by an antigen
bone marrow transplants	red bone marrow cells collected and transferred from one individual to another
bronchodilators	drugs that widen and relax pulmonary passages, thereby making breathing easier
Burkitt lymphoma	a non-Hodgkin lymphoma of B cells that frequently affects the jaw and abdominal lymph nodes
cell-mediated immunity	direct attack on a pathogen by T cells; also called cellular immunity
corticosteroids	anti-inflammatory, immunosuppressive drugs that are similar to or identical to naturally secreted corticosteroids from the adrenal gland
cyclophosphamide	immunosuppressive drug that suppresses B cells and antibody formation
cyclosporine	immunosuppressive drug that suppresses T_H cells
cytotoxic drugs	chemical agents that prevent cell division in replicating cells, often used in cancer treatment
cytotoxic T (T_C) cells	lymphocytes that directly attack other cells both physically and chemically
decongestants	drugs that relieve nasal congestion
desensitization	treatment for making a person insensitive to an antigen; also called hyposensitization
elephantiasis	lymphatic disease caused by filaria (parasitic roundworm) that is characterized by swelling of the legs and male scrotum
extrinsic asthma	asthma caused by sensitivity to inhalants, drugs, foods, pollen, mold, animal dander, or environmental allergen
germinal centers	areas of rapidly dividing lymphocytes within lymph nodules
graft versus host disease (GVHD)	immunologic reaction involving the attack of host cells by donor immune cells
grafts	living tissues or organs used for transplants
hay fever	allergy to seasonal plant allergens such as pollen
helper T (T_H) cells	lymphocytes that cooperate with B cells to amplify antibody production
Hodgkin disease (HD)	malignant lymphoma characterized by lymphadenopathy and sometimes splenomegaly and hepatomegaly

Key Term	Definition
human immunodeficiency virus (HIV)	retrovirus that causes AIDS
hypersensitivity	abnormal overreaction to an allergen
hyposensitization	treatment for making a person insensitive to an antigen; also called desensitization
immunity	the body's ability to resist disease
immunoglobulin (Ig)	protein produced by white blood cells that acts like an antibody; the classes are IgG, IgE, IgD, IgM, and IgA
immunotherapy	therapy that strengthens the immune system
infection	growth of pathogens in the body
infectious mononucleosis (IM)	disease caused by the Epstein-Barr virus (EBV) that infects B cells
innate immunity	genetically determined resistance that a person is born with; also called natural immunity
interferons (IFNs)	proteins produced by various cells in response to viral infections
intradermal test	detects sensitivity to an antigen after it is injected into the skin
intrinsic asthma	asthma of unknown cause
Kaposi sarcoma (KS)	cancer of the skin and lymph nodes that is characterized by purplish-red skin patches and occurs primarily in people with depressed immune systems
lacteals	lymphatics in the intestinal wall that transport recently digested fats to the bloodstream
latex allergy	allergic reaction to natural rubber latex
lymph	tissue fluid that has entered the lymphatic system
lymph nodes	bean-shaped masses of lymphatic tissue distributed along lymphatics that filter lymph
lymph nodules	areas of dense masses of lymphocytes within lymph nodes
lymphadenopathy	disease affecting the lymph nodes
lymphangiography	imaging of the lymphatic vessels (lymphatics) using an injected dye
lymphangitis	inflammation of the lymphatics
lymphatics	collecting vessels that transport lymph
lymphedema	swelling of lymphatics in the extremities
lymphocytes	white blood cells found in lymph
lymphoma	cancer of the lymphatic system
memory B cells	B lymphocytes that mediate immunologic memory
memory T cells	long-lived lymphocytes that can respond to subsequent encounters by the same antigen

Key Term	Definition
monoclonal antibody (MAB or MoAb)	antibody produced by a single (mono) cell line and consists of identical antibody molecules (clones)
non-Hodgkin lymphoma (NHL)	general term used to describe the diverse group of lymphomas that are not Hodgkin lymphoma
nonspecific immunity	generalized resistance to disease; also called innate immunity
opportunistic infection	infection that occurs because of a weakened immune response
passive immunity	resistance that results from the actual transfer of antibodies to a person
patch test	determines sensitivity to an antigen after a patch saturated with antigens is placed on the skin
pathogens	disease-causing agents
perennial allergic rhinitis	year-round allergy to environmental allergens
phagocytes	scavenger cells in the blood that ingest bacteria, foreign particles, and other cells
phagocytosis	ingestion of particles, such as bacteria and worn-out cells
plasma cells	antibody-producing cells that are derived from B cells
prick test	detects a reaction to an antigen after it is poked into the skin
primary response	initial immune reaction to the first encounter with a foreign antigen
psychoneuroimmu-nology (PNI)	field of science that deals with the association between emotions and other psychological states and their effects on the immune system
radiation therapy	treating a disease by using targeted x-rays to kill cancerous cells; another term for radiotherapy
radiotherapy	treating a disease by using targeted x-rays to kill cancerous cells; another term for radiation therapy
resistance	ability to ward off infection
right lymphatic duct	smaller lymphatic duct that drains lymph from the upper right body quadrant superior to the diaphragm and returns it to the bloodstream via the right subclavian vein
scintigram	two-dimensional image of the distribution of a radioactive tracer in a body organ that is obtained using a special scanner; also called a scintiscan
scintigraphy	procedure using a scintillation (gamma) camera in which lymphatic absorption of a radioactive substance leads to a computer-created image

Key Term	Definition
scintiscan	two-dimensional image of the distribution of a radioactive tracer in a body organ that is obtained using a special scanner; also called a scintigram
secondary response	immune reaction to a second (or later) encounter with a known antigen, due to memory cells
sensitization	a reaction in which specific antibodies develop in response to an antigen
severe combined immunodeficiency syndrome (SCID)	disorder in which both cell-mediated immunity and antibody-mediated immunity are impaired
Sjögren syndrome	autoimmune disease marked by degeneration of the salivary and lacrimal glands, causing dryness of the mouth and eyes
specific immunity	resistance against particular antigens; also called adaptive immunity
spleen	largest lymphatic organ located in the left hypochondriac region and is a site for lymphocyte production
splenomegaly	enlarged spleen
status asthmaticus	severe, prolonged asthma that can lead to respiratory distress and failure
suppressor T (T_s) cells	lymphocytes that inhibit other T cells and B cells
susceptibility	likelihood of developing a disease
syngraft	transplant between identical twins
T cells	lymphocytes derived from the thymus; also called T lymphocytes
thoracic duct	large lymphatic duct that drains lymph from all but the right upper quadrant of the body and returns it to the bloodstream via the left subclavian vein
thymus	lymphatic organ, located in the mediastinum, where T cells mature
tissue rejection	destruction of transplanted tissue by the immune response
tonsillectomy	surgical removal of the tonsils
tonsillitis	inflammation of the tonsils usually due to bacterial or viral infection
tonsils	masses of lymphatic tissue in the pharynx
transplant	tissue transfer between a compatible donor and a recipient
vaccine	preparation that stimulates the production of antibodies and provides immunity against disease
wheal	raised, reddened area caused by a sensitivity reaction
xenograft	transplant between two different species

CHAPTER

14

Digestive System

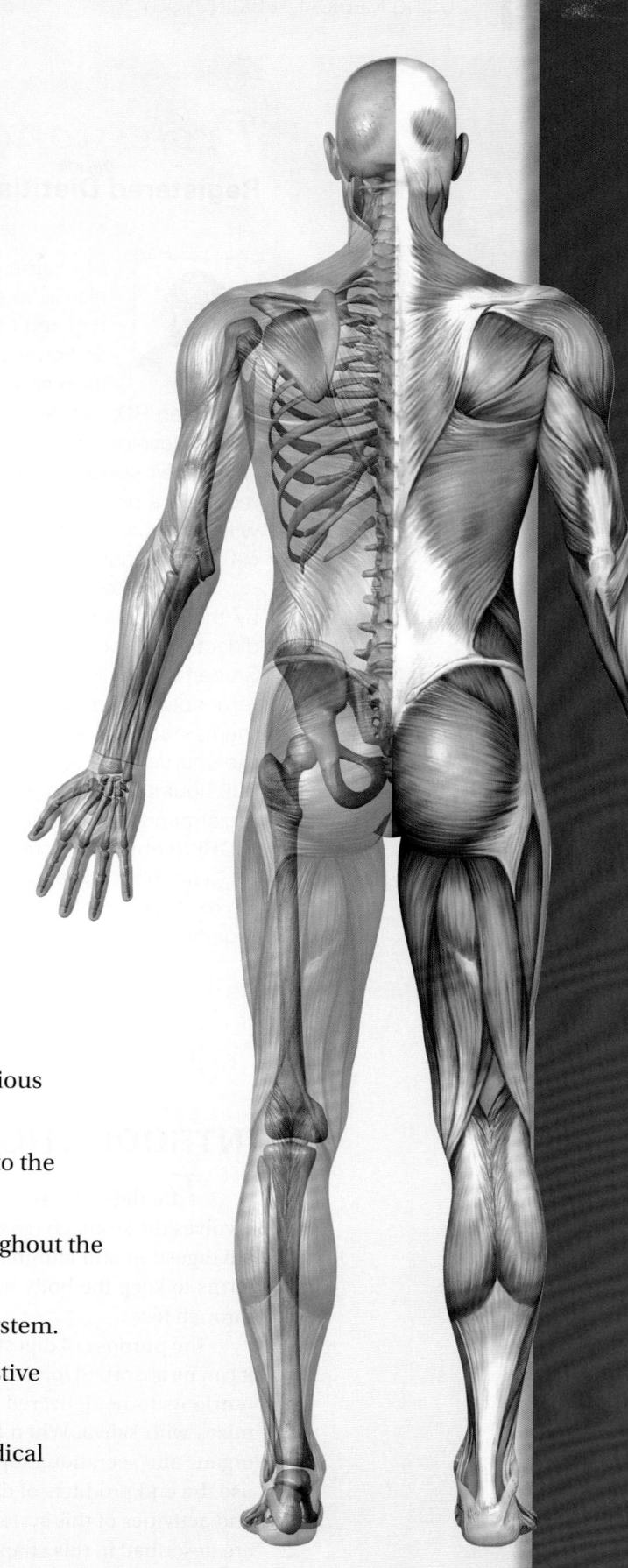

OBJECTIVES

After completing this chapter, you should be able to:

1. State the meanings of word parts related to the digestive system.

2. Identify and locate organs of the digestive system.

3. Outline the pathway of food ingestion through the gastrointestinal tract.

4. List the nutrients necessary for life.

5. Define common signs, symptoms, and treatments of various digestive system diseases.

6. Explain clinical tests and diagnostic procedures related to the digestive system.

7. Describe anatomical and physiological alterations throughout the lifespan.

8. Define common abbreviations related to the digestive system.

9. Define terms used in medical reports involving the digestive system.

10. Correctly define, spell, and pronounce the chapter's medical terms.

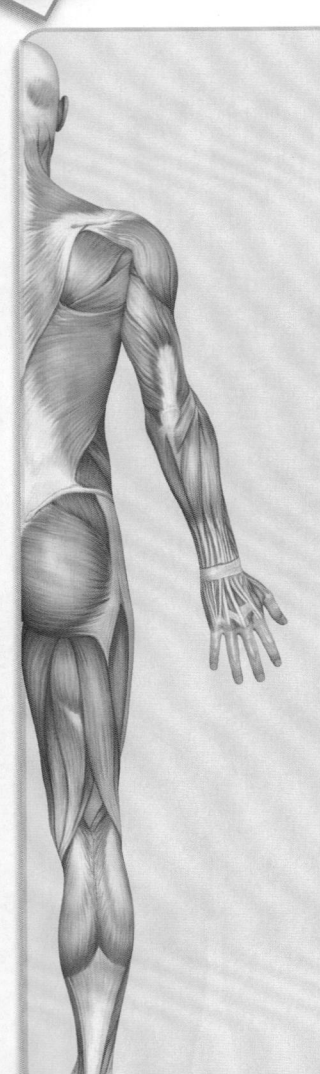

Professional Profile

Registered Dietitian

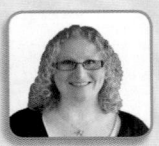

My name is Jane, and I'm a registered dietitian (RD). (Note that *dietician* is an accepted spelling variation of *dietitian*.) I work in a clinical setting and I specialize in renal and diabetic care. I plan nutrition programs and provide nutritional services to patients with diabetes. Many already have renal failure and require hemodialysis (artificial blood filtering).

As an RD, I assess the nutritional needs of patients on an individual basis. I focus on the development and implementation of dietary programs while I educate people about their specific food requirements and restrictions. In the dialysis unit, nutritional reports are generated monthly for evaluation. Much of my time is spent in conference with physicians and other members of the patient's health care team so that the medical and nutritional needs can be coordinated.

I completed a Bachelor of Science degree in dietetics from a program accredited by the American Dietetic Association (ADA). There are two parts to the curriculum: didactic and practice. The academic component is referred to as the didactic part. Students take a variety of courses, including biology, anatomy, physiology, medical terminology, food and nutrition science, chemistry, biochemistry, accounting, management, statistics, sociology, microbiology, business, and communication. After finishing the coursework, students must complete a dietetic internship (practice). Mine was a 900-hour supervised practicum. Finally, as a prospective RD, I had to pass the national registration examination administered by the Commission on Dietetic Registration (CDR) to obtain the credentials to practice.

I am both a licensed dietitian (LD), and an RD with the ADA. I took advanced training to obtain certification in both renal nutrition and diabetes education. To maintain my registrations, I must participate in continuing professional education.

INTRODUCTION

The digestive system is also referred to as the gastrointestinal (GI) system because it involves the stomach (*gastro-*) and intestines (*intestinal*). The primary functions of the system are digestion and elimination. Digestion involves the breakdown of food into smaller, usable forms to keep the body healthy, and elimination is the expulsion of digestive waste products through feces.

The purpose of digestion is to alter the physical and chemical composition of food so that it can be absorbed for cellular use. One digestive system action is to supply the blood with vital nutrients to be delivered to the body's cells. Digestion begins in the mouth as soon as food mixes with saliva. When food particles progress through the intestinal tracts, movements of organs and secretions supplied by accessory structures continue the process. The body's cells use the end products of digestion, and waste substances become excrement. Other functions and activities of this system and its parts, along with congenital and structural abnormalities, are described in this chapter.

Nutrition is a key aspect of total body health and must be considered with digestive processes. The field is expanding as the connection between nutrition and health becomes further defined. Nutrition is one area in which intervention strategies can be immediately implemented and positive outcomes easily achieved.

MEDICAL TERM PARTS

Word Parts

Medical term prefixes, suffixes, and combining forms related to the digestive system are introduced in this section.

Word Part	Meaning
amino-	compound containing —NH$_2$
amyl-, amylo-	starch
appendico-	appendix
-ase	enzyme
bili-	bile
bucco-	cheek
cec-, ceco-	cecum
celio-, celo-	abdomen, belly
cephal-, cephalo-	head
chol-, chole-, cholo-	bile
chyl-, chylo-	chyle (milky fluid taken up by intestines)
colo-	colon
dent-, denti-, dento-	teeth, dental
duoden-, duodeno-	duodenum
enter-, entero-	intestine
galact-, galacto-	milk
gastr-, gastro-	stomach
gloss-, glosso-	tongue
gluco-, glyco-	glucose, sugar
hepat-, hepato-	liver
hernio-	hernia
ileo-	ileum
jejun-, jejuno-	jejunum
linguo-	tongue
lip-, lipo-	lipid, fat
lith-, litho-	stone, calculus
oro-	mouth
palato-	palate
pancreat-, pancreatico-, pancreato-, pancreo-	pancreas
peritoneo-	peritoneum (abdominopelvic cavity lining)

continued

continued from page 687

Word Part	Meaning
-phagia	eating, devouring
pharyng-, pharyngo-	pharynx
proct-, procto-	anus, rectum
ptyal-, ptyalo-	salivary glands, saliva
pylor-, pyloro-	pylorus, muscular opening
rect-, recto-	rectum
sacchar-, sacchari-, saccharo-	sugar
sial-, sialo-	saliva, salivary glands
sigmoid-, sigmoido-	sigmoid, S-shaped
stom-, stomat-, stomato-	mouth
uvul-, uvulo-	uvula
vermi-	worm, worm-like

Word Grouping Exercises

Using the *Medical Term Parts* table, identify the prefix, suffix, or combining form for each of the following definitions. The first one has been done as an example.

Definition	Word Part
appendix	*appendico-*
abdomen, belly	
anus, rectum	
bile	A. B.
cecum	
cheek	
chyle (milky fluid taken up by intestines)	
colon	
compound containing —NH$_2$	
duodenum	
eating, devouring	
enzyme	
glucose, sugar	
head	
hernia	
ileum	
intestine	
jejunum	
lipid, fat	

continued

by a mucous membrane. **Papillae** (*papilla* = singular) are small, conical projections on the tongue surface, some of which contain taste buds.

The entire process of taking in food and swallowing it is termed **ingestion**. The act of swallowing is called **deglutition**.

The pharynx (throat) receives the bolus and automatically continues deglutition to the esophagus. The **uvula**, a fleshy V-shaped extension hanging from the soft palate above the tongue, closes and seals the entrance to the throat. The bolus is then transported through the esophagus to the stomach by peristalsis. It takes approximately 10 seconds for food to reach the stomach after swallowing.

KEY TERM	Definition
salivary (SAL-i-verr-ee) **glands**	exocrine structures that secrete saliva
parotid (puh-ROT-id) **glands**	salivary glands in front of and below the external ears
submandibular (sub-man-DIB-yoo-lur) **glands**	salivary glands below the mandible (lower jaw)
sublingual (sub-LING-gwul) **glands**	salivary glands beneath the tongue
mastication (mas-ti-KAY-shun)	chewing
bolus (BOH-lus)	ball of chewed food
papillae (pa-PIL-ee)	small projections on the tongue
ingestion (in-JES-chun)	taking food into the body; eating
deglutition (dee-gloo-TISH-un)	swallowing
uvula (YOO-vew-luh)	fleshy appendage hanging from the soft palate at the entrance to the throat

KEY TERM PRACTICE: *Oral Cavity*

1. Give the singular and plural forms of the term meaning small projections on the tongue _____

2. The _____ is the fleshy structure hanging from the soft palate.

3. The word part *sub-* means _____, and the word part *linguo-* means _____, so the salivary gland beneath the tongue is the _____ gland.

4. Another term for swallowing is _____.

5. A _____ is a ball of chewed food.

Teeth

Teeth are important structures for the digestive system as a whole. Children have 20 **deciduous** (primary) **teeth** (**Figure 14-3A**), which are shed and replaced by the permanent teeth. *Deciduous* means "shed after a stage of development," as in deciduous trees, whose leaves fall off during the autumn. The 32 **permanent** (secondary) **teeth** are the final adult teeth (**Figure 14-3B**).

Different kinds of teeth are adapted to handle foods in various ways, such as biting, grasping, and grinding. The eight **incisors** are adapted for biting, the four **cuspids** (canines) grasp and tear food, and the eight **bicuspids** (premolars) and 12 **molars** do the job of grinding. The *buccal corridor* is the alignment of our teeth within the jaw.

The **gingiva** is the mucous membrane surrounding the teeth and is more commonly known as the *gum*. The typical tooth consists of a crown, neck, and root, and teeth are composed of cementum, enamel, dentin, pulp, nerves, and blood vessels. The exposed part of the tooth,

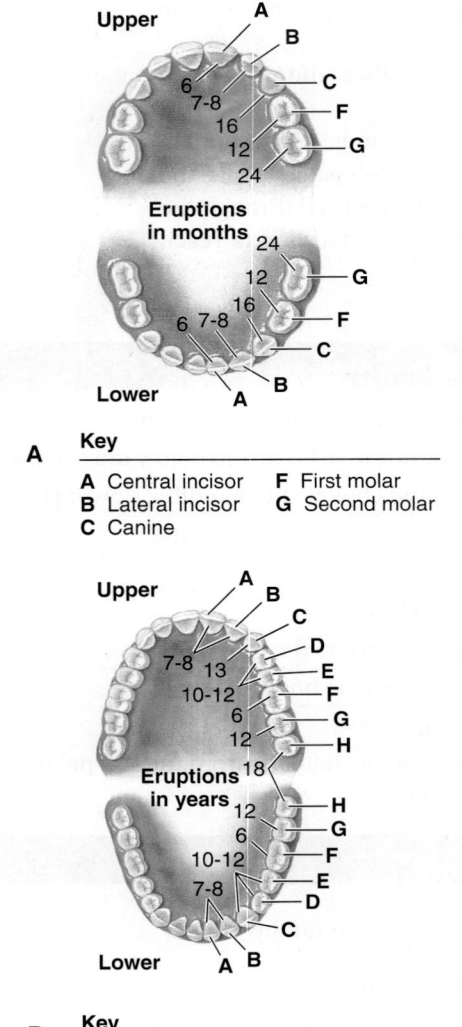

A

Key

A Central incisor	**F** First molar
B Lateral incisor	**G** Second molar
C Canine	

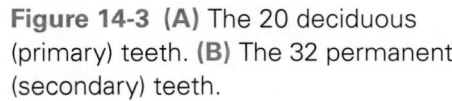

B

Key

A Central incisor	**E** Second premolar
B Lateral incisor	**F** First molar
C Canine	**G** Second molar
D First premolar	**H** Third molar

Figure 14-3 **(A)** The 20 deciduous (primary) teeth. **(B)** The 32 permanent (secondary) teeth.

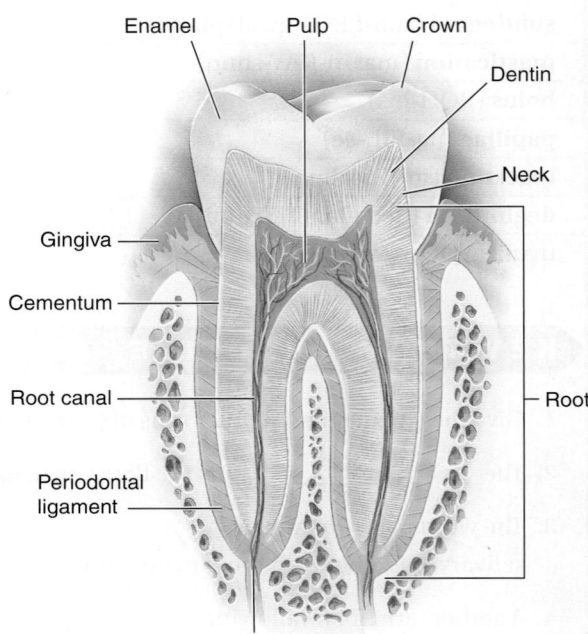

Figure 14-4 This longitudinal section shows normal tooth anatomy.

called the **crown,** extends beyond the gingiva (gum) line. The **neck** is the portion at the gingiva between the root and the crown. **Roots** anchor teeth to bone. The **root canal** is the tooth cavity containing pulp, nerves, and blood vessels.

Enamel, the hardest substance in the human body, covers the crown and consists of calcium salts in a crystalline form. **Dentin** forms the bulk of a tooth underneath the enamel. It is similar to bone, but harder. The pulp cavity is surrounded by dentin and contains blood vessels, nerves, and connective tissue called pulp. **Pulp** is the soft, internal portion of the tooth. **Cementum** is the thin layer of bony tissue that covers the dentin of the roots and neck of teeth. The *periodontal ligament* helps anchor the tooth in the bone (**Figure 14-4**).

KEY TERM	Definition
deciduous (de-SID-yoo-us) **teeth**	the 20 early teeth that are shed and replaced by permanent teeth; also called primary teeth
permanent teeth	the 32 adult teeth; also called secondary teeth
incisors (in-SIGH-zurz)	front cutting teeth (four in upper jaw, four in lower jaw)
cuspids (KUS-pidz)	teeth with only one point; also called canines
bicuspids (bye-KUS-pidz)	teeth with two points; also called premolars
molars (MOH-lurz)	teeth that grind and pulverize food
gingiva (JIN-ji-vuh)	mucous membrane surrounding the teeth; also called the gum
crown	exposed part of a tooth
neck	area between the crown and the root of a tooth
roots	parts of teeth embedded in tissue that anchor teeth to bone
root canal	tooth cavity in the root containing pulp, nerves, and blood vessels
enamel	calcified substance covering the tooth's crown
dentin (DEN-tin)	calcified substance underneath the tooth enamel
pulp	soft interior of the tooth
cementum (se-MEN-tum)	thin layer of bony tissue covering the dentin of the roots and neck of a tooth

KEY TERM PRACTICE: *Teeth*

1. Name the four types of adult teeth. _____

2. _____ is the thin layer of bony tissue covering the dentin of the roots and neck of a tooth.

3. The mucous membrane surrounding the teeth is called the _____ or the gum.

4. _____ is the calcified substance covering the tooth's crown.

5. The exposed part of the tooth is known as the _____.

Esophagus

The digestive system is often divided into two parts: upper and lower gastrointestinal tracts. The upper gastrointestinal (UGI) tract includes the esophagus, stomach, and duodenum (first segment of the small intestine). The lower gastrointestinal tract includes structures distal to the small intestine. The **esophagus** is the collapsible, muscular tube extending from the pharynx to the stomach. It is about 25 cm (10 in.) long and 2 cm (0.80 in.) wide (**Figure 14-5**).

The lining of the esophagus is made of tissue that resists abrasion. The opening where the esophagus passes through the diaphragm (the muscle of breathing that separates the thorax and the abdomen) is termed the **esophageal hiatus**. *Hiatus* means an opening in an organ. A circular band of muscle at the distal end of the esophagus forms the **lower esophageal sphincter (LES)** (**Figure 14-6**). The LES prevents the backflow of food from the stomach into the esophagus.

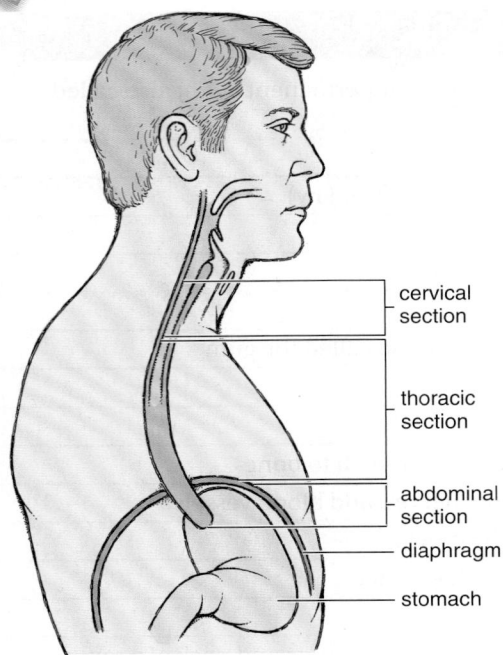

Figure 14-5 Sections of the esophagus.

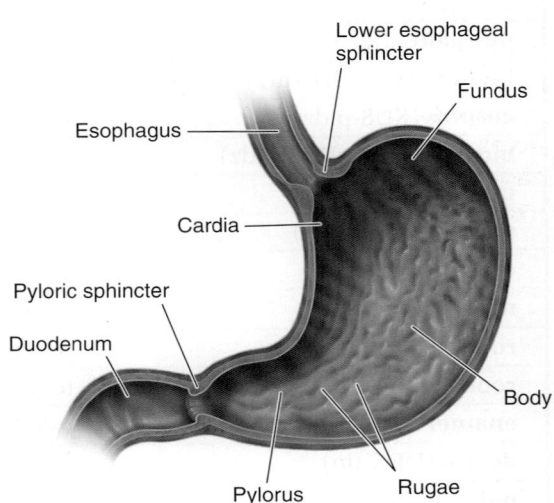

Figure 14-6 The stomach has four main anatomical regions.

KEY TERM	Definition
esophagus (ee-SOF-uh-gus)	muscular tube connecting the pharynx to the stomach
esophageal hiatus (ee-sof-uh-JEE-ul high-AY-tus)	opening in the diaphragm for the esophagus to pass through
lower esophageal sphincter (ee-sof-uh-JEE-ul SFINK-tur)	circular band of muscle between the stomach and the esophagus that prevents backflow of stomach contents into the esophagus

KEY TERM PRACTICE: *Esophagus*

1. The _____ is a muscular tube that connects the pharynx to the stomach.

2. The opening in the diaphragm through which the esophagus passes is termed the _____.

3. The _____ is a circular band of muscle between the stomach and the esophagus that prevents the backflow of stomach contents into the esophagus.

Stomach

The abdominopelvic cavity has a smooth, transparent membrane lining called the **peritoneum**. This membrane doubles back over the surfaces of abdominal and pelvic organs, surrounding them and forming a continuous sac.

The **stomach** is a J-shaped organ that lies mostly left of the midline, inferior to the diaphragm. It receives and briefly stores food from the esophagus and aids in mechanical (by muscular mixing) and chemical (by digestive enzymes) digestion. Food can remain in the stomach for 3 to 4 hours.

The stomach has four main anatomical regions: cardia, fundus, body, and pylorus. The **cardia** is nearest the esophageal opening and is the smallest part. Located above the cardia is a dome-shaped temporary storage area called the **fundus**. Swallowed air often fills this area. **Eructation** refers to the belching or burping of stomach air through the mouth. The largest region of the stomach is referred to as the **body**. Gastric glands in the body secrete acids and enzymes. Last, the **pylorus** narrows and connects to the duodenum at the **pyloric sphincter**, a muscular band that prevents backflow.

Digestion begins once food has entered the mouth, and the volume of the stomach changes, depending on how much you eat. **Rugae**, natural folds in the stomach, distend (stretch) to accommodate these changes (**Figure 14-6**). *Gastric* means "pertaining to the stomach," and gastric secretions are regulated by nervous responses. As the stomach fills, its muscular wall stretches and the internal pressure remains constant. When partially digested food mixes with gastric secretions, it leaves the stomach and enters the small intestine as a thick, pasty mass termed **chyme**. *Chymos* is the Greek term for *juice*. Chyme is moved by peristalsis to the pyloric region of the stomach. The pyloric region then pumps chyme into the small intestine.

Vomiting, or **emesis**, occurs in response to gastric irritation. The actual act is the result of a complex nervous reflex triggered by the irritation. Sensory impulses travel from the site of gastric irritation to the vomiting center in the medulla oblongata. The diaphragm moves downward over the stomach and squeezes it on all sides. Motor responses then cause the contents to be dispelled. These involuntary muscle spasms cause the discharge of stomach contents through the mouth.

Chemical digestion within the digestive tract involves a series of enzymatically controlled catabolic (breakdown) reactions. Enzymes, proteins synthesized by the body, promote these reactions by acting as catalysts. **Catalysts** accelerate the rate of chemical reactions without being changed or used up in the process. Enzymes need specific pH levels for optimal functioning and can be activated or inactivated by agents that physically or chemically alter their molecular structures. Enzyme names generally end in the suffix *-ase* and their word parts are useful in identifying the types of food they metabolize. For example, **lipase** (*lip-* = lipid) breaks down lipids, and **amylase** (*amyl-* = starch) breaks down starches.

Specialized cells called mucous cells secrete mucus, which coats the lining of the stomach and prevents it from digesting itself. Other cells secrete hydrochloric acid (HCl) and **pepsin**, a protein-digesting enzyme that is most active in acidic (low-pH) environments. Still other cells secrete **intrinsic factor**, a protein that the body needs in order to absorb vitamin B_{12} in the small intestine.

After digestion, absorption takes place. **Absorption** is the passage of nutrients from the digestive tract into the blood or lymph for distribution to body cells. Absorption of nutrients does not occur in the stomach because the gastric wall is impermeable to most matter. Most absorption occurs along the length of the small intestine.

KEY TERM	Definition
peritoneum (perr-i-toh-NEE-um)	membrane that lines the abdominopelvic cavity and covers the internal organs contained within the cavity
stomach	organ in which food is stored after swallowing and that aids in mechanical and chemical digestion
cardia (KAHR-dee-uh)	smallest stomach area adjacent to the esophagus
fundus (FUN-dus)	dome-shaped stomach region
eructation (ee-ruck-TAY-shun)	belching, burping
body	largest region of stomach between the fundus and the pylorus
pylorus (pye-LOR-us)	region of the stomach opening into the small intestine

continued

continued from page 697

KEY TERM	Definition
pyloric sphincter (pye-LOH-rick SFINK-tur)	circular muscle enclosing pylorus between the stomach and the small intestine
rugae (ROO-gee)	stomach folds that allow the stomach to distend
chyme (KIME)	semisolid paste formed in the stomach that is a mixture of gastric juice and food
emesis (EM-eh-sis)	vomiting
catalysts (KAT-uh-lists)	chemicals that speed up chemical reactions without being changed or used up in the process
lipase (LIP-ace)	fat-breaking enzyme
amylase (AM-il-ace)	starch-breaking enzyme
pepsin (PEP-sin)	a protein-digesting enzyme
intrinsic factor	substance secreted by stomach cells that promotes the absorption of vitamin B_{12} in the small intestine
absorption	passage of nutrients from the digestive tract into the blood or lymph for distribution to body cells

KEY TERM PRACTICE: *Stomach*

1. Name the four regions of the stomach. _____

2. _____ is a protein secreted by stomach cells that is necessary for the absorption of vitamin B_{12} in the small intestine.

3. _____ are stomach folds that enable the stomach to distend.

4. _____ is a protein-digesting enzyme.

5. The medical term for burping is _____.

Small Intestine

The **small intestine** is the segment of the GI tract between the stomach and the large intestine. The term *small* used to describe the small intestine is deceptive. *Small* indicates the narrow diameter of this portion of the intestine, but the small intestine is quite lengthy, approximately 6.4 m (21 ft) long, considerably longer than the large intestine. Most food digestion and nutrient absorption occur in the small intestine.

The small intestine has three major sections: duodenum, jejunum, and ileum. The **duodenum**, which is about 30 cm (12 in.) long, is the first section of the small intestine. It receives a mixture of partly digested food and digestive secretions from the stomach, bile from the gallbladder, and pancreatic juice from the pancreas. The **jejunum**, approximately 2.4 m (8 ft) long, makes up the next section of the intestine. This section is where most chemical digestion and nutrient absorption take place. The **ileum** is the remaining section, about 3.7 m (12 ft) long. It leads to the large intestine. Note the spelling of this term so you do not to confuse it with the large coxal bone, the il*i*um. To help you remember the order, from proximal to distal, think,"***D***on't ***j***ump ***i***n" for ***d***uodenum, ***j***ejunum, and ***i***leum (**Figure 14-7**).

The interior intestinal wall has finger-like projections called **villi** and hair-like extensions called **microvilli**, which increase the absorptive surface area of the lining. The villi and

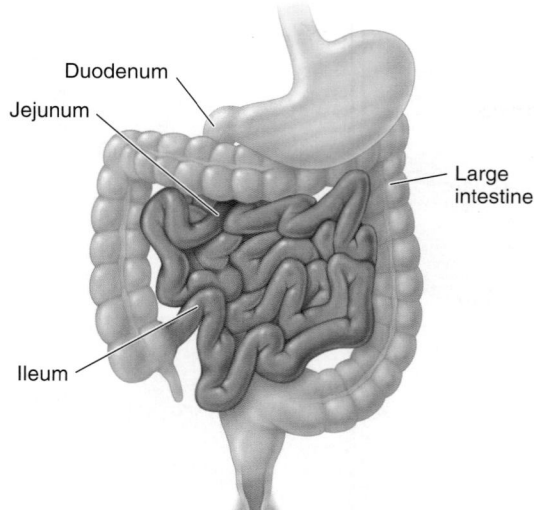

Duodenum
Jejunum
Large intestine
Ileum

Figure 14-7 The three segments of the small intestine are the duodenum, jejunum, and ileum.

microvilli resemble a fine carpet of velvet on the inside of the small intestine. These structures absorb nutrients.

Movement of intestinal contents is under nervous control. Major mixing movements are called segmentation, and other movements are a result of peristalsis. The growling stomach and intestinal sounds often heard are called **borborygmi** and result from gas and/or fluid moving through the GI tract.

KEY TERM	Definition
small intestine (in-TES-tin)	segment of gastrointestinal tract between stomach and large intestine involved with nutrient absorption
duodenum (dew-oh-DEE-num)	first section of small intestine beginning at the stomach
jejunum (je-JOO-num)	middle section of small intestine; location of most chemical digestion and nutrient absorption
ileum (IL-ee-um)	last section of small intestine, leading to the large intestine
villi (VIL-eye)	finger-like projections from the interior intestinal wall
microvilli (migh-kroh-VIL-eye)	hair-like projections that increase the absorptive surface area of intestines
borborygmi (bor-boh-RIG-migh)	rumbling or gurgling noises produced by movement of gas and/or fluid in the GI tract

KEY TERM PRACTICE: *Small Intestine*

1. Name the three sections of the small intestine. _____

2. Provide the singular and plural forms for hair-like projections in the intestine that increase the absorptive surface area. _____

3. Provide the singular and plural forms for finger-like projections from the interior intestinal wall. _____

4. The _____ is the segment of the gastrointestinal tract between the stomach and large intestine.

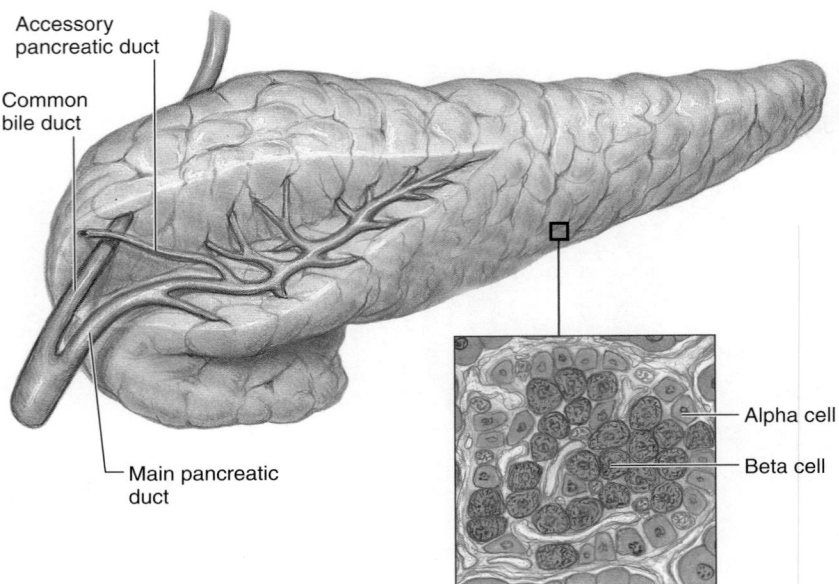

Figure 14-8 The general anatomy of the pancreas.

Pancreas

The **pancreas** is an elongated, somewhat flattened organ located posterior to the stomach. It is about 15 cm (6 in.) in length and is conveniently located for secreting digestive pancreatic juices directly into the small intestine. The pancreas is an endocrine gland when secreting insulin (from beta cells) and glucagon (from alpha cells) and an exocrine gland when secreting **pancreatic juice**, an alkaline mixture of digestive enzymes. Alkaline pancreatic juice enzymes break down different types of nutrients. The pancreas plays an important role in the digestion process when acting as an exocrine gland.

Extending the length of the pancreas is a tube called the **pancreatic duct**. This duct connects to the duodenum (first segment of the small intestine) at the common bile duct (CBD), the same place where the bile duct from the liver and gallbladder joins the duodenum (**Figure 14-8**).

KEY TERM	Definition
pancreas (PAN-kree-us)	gland with endocrine and exocrine functions sandwiched between the stomach and the small intestine
pancreatic (pan-kree-AT-ick) **juice**	alkaline secretion from the pancreas that contains digestive enzymes
pancreatic (pan-kree-AT-ick) **duct**	pancreas excretory tube emptying into the duodenum

KEY TERM PRACTICE: *Pancreas*

1. What is the gland that has both endocrine and exocrine functions and is involved with digestion? _____

2. The pancreas produces _____, which is a secretion that contains digestive enzymes.

3. The _____ is a tube leading from the pancreas into the duodenum.

Liver and Gallbladder

The **liver** is a vascular, glandular organ that secretes bile, and plays a role in many metabolic functions. It is the largest visceral organ in the body, weighing about 1.5 kg (3.3 lb), and is located in the upper right and central portions of the abdominal cavity, just inferior to the diaphragm. Structurally, it is divided into lobes with smaller subdivisions called lobules. The falciform ligament separates the right and left lobes and attaches the liver to the anterior abdominal wall. The four lobes of the liver are the left, right, caudate, and quadrate lobes.

Lobules are the functional units of the liver that contain hepatocytes. Liver cells, or **hepatocytes**, secrete bile that is transported to the gallbladder for storage. Because hepatocytes can regenerate, liver tissue can regrow.

Bile is a yellowish-green alkaline fluid that emulsifies (disperses and suspends) fats in water-soluble salts to make them more water soluble. Bile has digestive functions. In addition to emulsification, the bile aids in the absorption of fatty acids, cholesterol, and certain vitamins. The bile pigment bilirubin is a product of red blood cell breakdown.

Bile flows from the liver to the small intestine (duodenum) through a series of ducts. The left and right hepatic ducts unite to form the **common hepatic duct**. Bile from the common hepatic duct takes one of two courses: It may flow into the CBD, which empties into the duodenum, or it may enter the **cystic duct**, which enters the gallbladder. The cystic duct from the gallbladder and the common hepatic ducts from the liver each carry bile and merge to form the **common bile duct (CBD)** (**Figure 14-9**). The **hepatic portal vein** transports blood from the intestinal capillaries to the liver, where some absorbed nutrients can be processed and foreign substances and damaged red blood cells can be removed.

Metabolism refers to the sum of the chemical and physical changes occurring in the body. It consists of anabolism (building processes) and catabolism (breakdown processes). Anabolism is the body's ability to convert small molecules into larger ones, and catabolism refers to converting large molecules into smaller particles. The liver functions in carbohydrate metabolism by forming glycogen from glucose (blood sugar), breaking down glycogen to glucose, or producing glucose from sources other than sugar. **Glycogenesis** is the formation of glycogen from glucose, **glycogenolysis** is the breakdown of glycogen to glucose, and **gluconeogenesis** is the formation of glucose from noncarbohydrates, such as proteins or fats. Remember that the word part *glyco-* refers to "glucose", the word part *-genesis* means "formation of something," and the word *lysis* describes "breaking apart."

The greenish colored **gallbladder** is another complementary digestive gland. It is a small, muscular sac located on the right underside of the liver (**Figure 14-9**). The word *gall* means

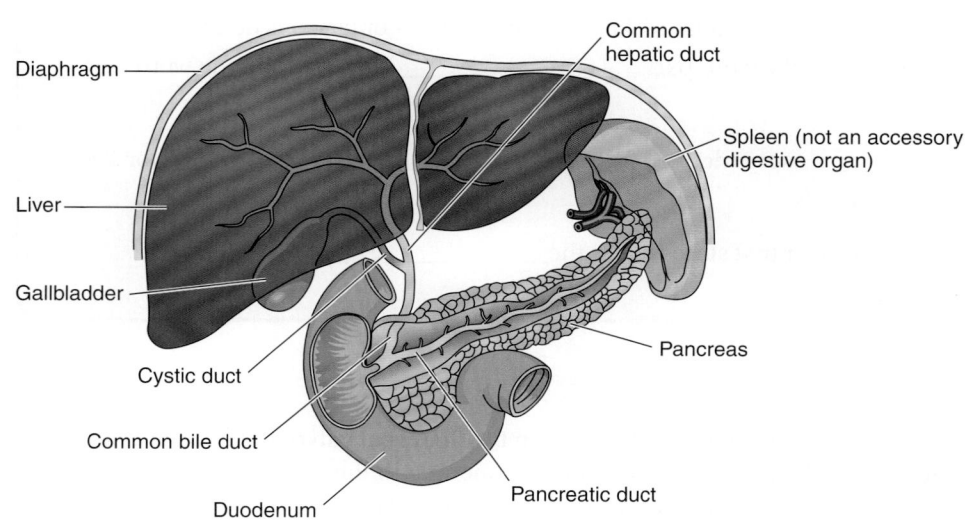

Figure 14-9 The accessory organs of digestion.

"bile," and this organ stores bile until it is needed for digestive processes in the small intestine. The gallbladder releases between 600 and 1,000 mL (20 and 33.8 oz) of bile per day, and 40 to 70 mL (1.4 to 2.4 oz) of bile is stored per day. Bile is ejected into the CBD under the influence of the intestinal hormone, cholecystokinin (CCK). The fat-soluble vitamins (A, D, E, and K) depend on bile for their absorption. The liver reabsorbs much of the bile secreted.

KEY TERM	Definition
liver	largest visceral organ, that secretes bile and plays a role in many metabolic functions
lobules (LOB-yoolz)	functional units of liver that contain hepatocytes
hepatocytes (HEP-a-toh-sites)	liver cells
bile	yellowish-green alkaline fluid secreted by the liver and passed into the duodenum
common hepatic (he-PAT-ick) duct	duct formed by the union of the left hepatic duct and right hepatic duct
cystic duct	duct of the gallbladder
CBD	duct formed by the union of the cystic duct and the hepatic duct
hepatic (he-PAT-ick) portal vein	vessel that delivers blood from the digestive system to the liver
metabolism (muh-TAB-oh-liz-um)	all chemical and physical activity in the body, consisting of anabolism (building processes) and catabolism (breakdown processes)
glycogenesis (glye-koh-JEN-e-sis)	glycogen formation from glucose
glycogenolysis (glye-koh-jen-OL-i-sis)	breaking down glycogen into glucose
gluconeogenesis (gloo-koh-nee-oh-JEN-e-sis)	glucose formation from noncarbohydrates, such as proteins and fats
gallbladder	sac-like organ on the undersurface of the liver that stores bile

KEY TERM PRACTICE: *Liver and Gallbladder*

1. Identify the duct formed by the union of the cystic duct and the hepatic duct. _____

2. The medical term for breaking down glycogen into glucose is _____, and it is derived from the word part _____ for *glucose* and _____ for *breaking down*.

3. _____ is the medical term for the formation of glucose from proteins or fats; it is derived from the word part _____ for *glucose*, the word part _____ for *new*, and the word part _____ for *formation of*.

4. Liver cells are known as _____, a term derived from the word part _____ for *liver* and the word part _____ for *cells*.

5. The sac-like organ on the undersurface of the liver that stores bile is the _____.

Large Intestine

The **large intestine**, or large bowel, extends from the **ileocecal valve** (the circular muscle between the ileum and the cecum) to the anus, an opening to the outside. The large intestine is approximately 1.5 m (5 ft) long. It forms, stores, and expels waste matter. The last stage of chemical digestion takes place in the large intestine through the actions of bacteria rather than by intestinal enzymes. The large intestine also receives undigested wastes from the small intestine; secretes mucus; reabsorbs water and electrolytes; and absorbs vitamins K, B$_{12}$, thiamin, and riboflavin synthesized by intestinal bacteria. **Electrolytes** are minerals such as sodium, potassium, phosphorus, and calcium that are dissolved as ions. Most water is reabsorbed in the large intestine, and diarrhea results when excess fluid and electrolytes are not absorbed back into the body through the intestinal wall. This is usually the result of a bacterial infection.

The large intestine is anatomically divided into the cecum, colon, rectum, and anal canal. The **cecum** is the beginning, pouch-like portion of the large intestine to which the small intestine is connected. Attached to the cecum is a worm-like lymphatic structure known as the vermiform (*vermis* = worm) appendix or **appendix**. Although its size and shape vary considerably among individuals, it averages 9 cm (3.5 in.) in length. In addition to having some immune function, recent studies propose that the appendix harbors and protects bacteria that are beneficial to the colon. For example, if a person has a bout of diarrhea, resident bacteria are flushed out. Afterward, the appendix may repopulate the colon. The **colon**, or main portion of the large intestine, has four subdivisions—ascending, transverse, descending, and sigmoid.

The **ascending colon** is the region from the cecum to the right colic (hepatic) flexure, the bend at the liver border that creates a right angle between portions of the colon. The **transverse colon** is the horizontal section between the right colic (hepatic) **flexure** (bend) and the left colic (splenic) flexure, the bend closest to the spleen. The transverse colon then turns inferiorly to become the **descending colon**. The last part is the **sigmoid colon**, so named because its shape resembles the Greek letter sigma (σ), which looks like a truncated *S*. It continues to the **rectum**, the last part of the digestive tract.

The last portion of the rectum is the **anal canal**, which ends at the **anus**, the opening to the outside. Two circular bands of muscle, the internal and external anal sphincters, control the passage of materials to the outside (**Figure 14-10**). **Defecation** is the medical term for

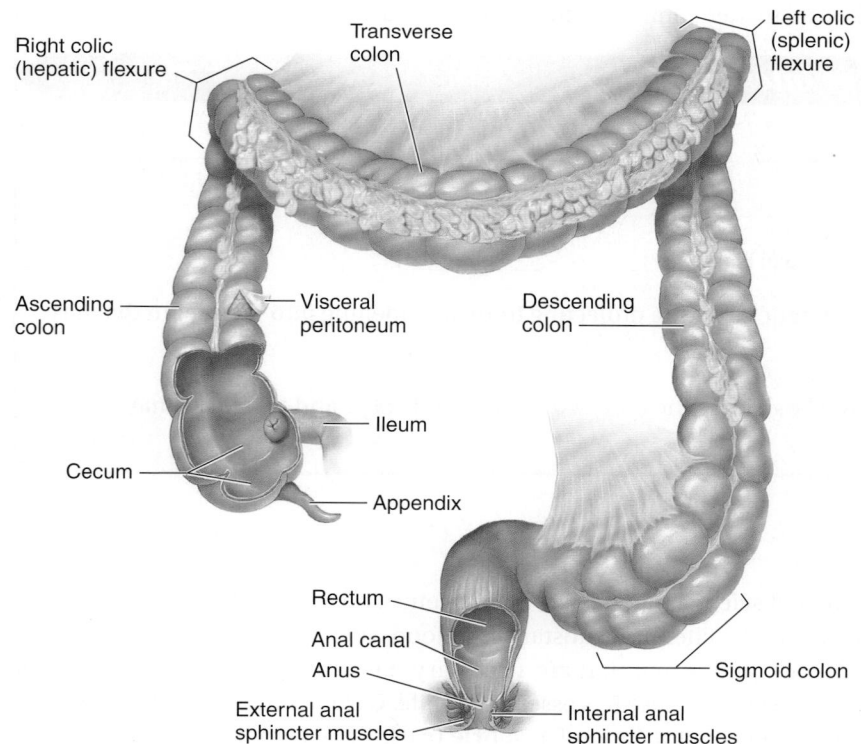

Figure 14-10 The large intestine is anatomically divided into the cecum, colon, rectum, and anal canal.

expelling **feces**, or solid waste, from the bowel. Defecation is more commonly known as a bowel movement (BM). The composition of feces includes undigested food, bacteria, water, and bile pigments. During defecation, internal abdominal pressure increases and forces the feces into the rectum. Peristaltic waves are triggered, and the internal and external anal sphincters relax. Feces are then forced to the outside.

KEY TERM	Definition
large intestine (in-TES-tin)	portion of the intestine between the small intestine and the anus that forms, stores, and expels waste matter
ileocecal (il-ee-oh-SEE-kul) **valve**	circular muscle (sphincter) between the ileum and the cecum
electrolytes (ee-LECK-troh-lites)	minerals (ions) dissolved in solution and circulating in body fluids
cecum (SEE-kum)	pouch where the large intestine begins
appendix	small worm-like lymphatic structure projecting from and opening into the cecum
colon (KOH-lun)	main part of large intestine, beginning at the cecum and ending at the rectum
ascending colon (KOH-lun)	section of the large intestine from the cecum to the right colic (hepatic) flexure
transverse colon (KOH-lun)	section of the large intestine between the right colic (hepatic) flexure and the left colic (splenic) flexure
flexure (FLECK-shur)	bend
descending colon (KOH-lun)	section of the large intestine between the left colic (splenic) flexure and the sigmoid colon
sigmoid colon (SIG-moid KOH-lun)	section of the large intestine between the descending colon and the rectum
rectum (RECK-tum)	section of the large intestine between the sigmoid colon and the anal canal
anal canal	portion of the large intestine between the rectum and the anus
anus (AY-nus)	opening to the exterior through which feces exit the body
defecation (def-e-KAY-shun)	bowel movement
feces (FEE-seez)	solid waste matter eliminated from the bowel during defecation

KEY TERM PRACTICE: *Large Intestine*

1. Name the four regions of the colon. _____

2. The medical term for bowel movement is _____.

3. Solid waste matter that is eliminated from the bowel is called _____.

4. The _____ is a worm-like lymphatic structure projecting from and opening into the cecum that has an immune function.

5. The _____ is the section of the large intestine between the sigmoid colon and the anal canal.

Nutrition

Nutrition is the branch of science that deals with nutrients and the role food plays in health and disease. **Nutrients** are the chemical substances in food, such as carbohydrates, proteins, lipids, vitamins, minerals, and water, that are necessary for normal body functions. Water (H_2O) is considered a nutrient because it is essential for life. Carbohydrates, proteins, and lipids provide energy to the body in the form of a **calorie (cal)**: 1 g of carbohydrate equals 4 cal,

1 g of protein equals 4 cal, and 1 g of fat equals 9 cal. Calories are important in maintaining body function, and a measure of metabolism is known as the basal metabolic rate. The **basal metabolic rate (BMR)** is the average caloric expenditure of a person under basal (basic, fundamental) conditions. Breathing, keeping warm, and other vital functions are examples of basal conditions.

A **carbohydrate (CHO)** is an organic compound that contains carbon (C), hydrogen (H), and oxygen (O). Carbohydrates are important sources of food energy and include sugar, starch, and cellulose (plant fiber).

Proteins are dietary compounds made up of chains of **amino acids**. There are two types of amino acids: essential and nonessential. Essential amino acids must be obtained from food because the body either does not make them at all or does not make them in sufficient supply to meet its demands. The body manufactures nonessential amino acids, and for this reason, they are not essential in the diet.

Lipids are organic nutrients consisting of fats and oils. They are important energy reserves and are composed mostly of triglycerides.

Vitamins are essential organic (carbon-containing) nutrients that occur naturally in food. They are required for normal growth and maintenance. (The word *vitamin* is derived from the Latin word *vitalis*, meaning *life*.) Vitamins must be obtained through food because the body does not manufacture them. However, intestinal bacteria do synthesize vitamin K and some B vitamins. Because vitamins are calorie free, they provide no energy source, yet they are essential for metabolic pathways and energy transformation. Vitamins are classified as fat-soluble or water-soluble. The fat-soluble vitamins are A, D, E, and K. All others are water-soluble. Fat-soluble vitamins are absorbed with fats and can be stored in the body; bile salts promote their absorption.

Minerals are inorganic ions functioning as electrolytes. Minerals play important roles in physiological systems, such as muscle contraction, nerve impulse transmission, and electrolyte balance. Minerals in the body are identified as bulk or trace, depending on the amount necessary. Common bulk body minerals are calcium, potassium, chlorine, sodium, phosphorus, and magnesium. Trace minerals are needed in very small amounts and include chromium, cobalt, copper, iodine, iron, manganese, selenium, sulfur, and zinc. **Figure 14-11** shows some common vitamins and minerals, along with their sources, benefits, results of deficiency, and recommended dietary allowance.

KEY TERM	Definition
nutrition	branch of science that deals with nutrients in health and disease
nutrients	chemical substances in food that include carbohydrates, proteins, lipids, vitamins, minerals, and water
calorie (KAL-oh-ree) **(cal)**	the energy value in food
basal metabolic (met-uh-BOL-ick) **rate (BMR)**	quantity of energy the body expends performing basic physiological tasks
carbohydrate	organic compound containing carbon, hydrogen, and oxygen and includes sugar, starch, and cellulose
protein	a dietary compound made of amino acids
amino (uh-MEE-noh) **acids**	the building blocks of proteins
lipids (LIP-ids)	organic nutrients consisting of fats and oils
vitamins	essential organic nutrients necessary for normal metabolism
minerals	inorganic ions functioning as electrolytes

continued

continued from page 705

KEY TERM PRACTICE: *Nutrition*

1. The building blocks of protein are called _____.

2. List the six nutrients necessary for life. _____

3. _____ is the branch of science that deals with nutrients in health and disease.

4. The _____ is the quantity of energy the body expends performing basic physiological tasks.

5. A _____ is the energy value in food.

Vitamins & minerals	Sources	Benefits	Deficiency	Recommended dietary allowance (RDA)
vitamin A*	sweet potatoes, carrots, milk	improved skin resistance to infection; good eyesight	night blindness, xerophthalmia	1000 mcg retinol equivalents (5000 IU)
vitamin D*	sunlight, dairy products	strengthens bone development	rickets	5–10 mcg (1000–1200 IU)
vitamin E*	green leafy vegetables, nuts, whole grains, wheat germ	oxidative protection of red blood cells	anemia	8–10 mg (30 IU)
vitamin K*	green leafy vegetables, tomatoes	blood clotting cascade	bleeding diathesis	70–140 mcg
vitamin B_1† (thiamine)	whole grains, vegetables, nuts, wheat germ	carbohydrate metabolism	beriberi	1–1.5 mg
vitamin B_2† (riboflavin)	animal products, mushrooms, broccoli	protein metabolism, skin and eye protectant	angular stomatitis/ blepharitis	1.2–1.5 mg
vitamin B_6† (pyridoxine)	brewer's yeast, whole grains, nuts, meat	helps regulate central nervous system	peripheral neuropathy, seizures	1.7–2 mg
vitamin B_{12}†	animal products, fish, soybeans	red blood cell formation	mental status changes	3 mcg
folic acid	green leafy vegetables, liver, yeast	protect against birth defects, red blood cell production	anemia	0.4 mg (or 400 mcg)
vitamin C†	broccoli, tomatoes, Brussels sprouts, citrus fruits	resistance to stress; oral hygiene; wound healing	scurvy	60 mg
niacin†	nuts, poultry, fish	cholesterol-lowering agent, coenzyme in oxidations, reductions	pellagra	13–16 mg
calcium	dairy products	bone growth; nerve, muscle function	rickets, osteomalacia, osteoporosis	800 mg
potassium	tomatoes, citrus fruits	cellular function	Ileus, muscle weakness	1.8–6 g
sodium	most foods	cellular function	weakness, confusion	1–3.3 g
phosphorus	cereals, dairy products	cellular function	mental status changes, osteomalacia	800 mg
iron	green leafy vegetables, dried fruits, meat, wheat germ	red blood cell formation	anemia	10–18 mg
iodine	some dairy products, seafood, iodized salt	normal thyroid function, topical antiseptic	goiter	150 mcg

* fat soluble
† water soluble

Figure 14-11 Common vitamins and minerals.

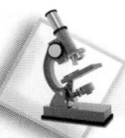

THE CLINICAL DIMENSION

Diagnosing and treating digestive system disorders require a comprehensive, balanced approach. Evaluation tools are numerous and must be used in conjunction with the detailed history and physical examination. This section describes the medical management of common gastrointestinal pathologies.

Oral Cavity Disorders

Dentistry is the medical science concerned with the prevention and treatment of tooth and gum diseases. Dentists graduate from dental school and pass appropriate licensing exams to practice in the field. Oral cavity disorders are the focus of this section.

Missing teeth may result from decay, accident, or congenital disorders. Impacted teeth occur because of the lack of jaw space to accommodate the teeth. This is a common occurrence with third molars (wisdom teeth) when adjacent teeth block their eruption. A dentist diagnoses teeth abnormalities with x-rays. Implants and bridges may be used to replace absent teeth.

Orthodontics is the branch of dentistry concerned with the prevention and correction of teeth irregularities. It uses braces to move the teeth or other measures to adjust the underlying bone.

Discolored teeth that are not characteristically white have several underlying causes. With age, teeth become darker and more yellow, and smoking and food stains can also cause tooth discoloration. Tetracycline (an antibiotic) taken during pregnancy can affect the tooth color of the developing child, and when taken by children, the drug can affect the color of the permanent teeth. Oral examination provides the diagnosis. Treatment options include teeth cleaning with a rotary polisher, bleaches, synthetic veneers, caps, and crowns. Veneers, caps, and crowns create artificial tooth surfaces.

malocclusion	**Malocclusion**, or misaligned teeth, is the abnormal positioning of the teeth when the jaw is closed. Treatment involves extraction or orthodontics.
periodontal disease	**Periodontal disease** refers to pathology of the tissues that surround the neck and root of a tooth, including the underlying bone. It is marked by **gingivitis**, inflammation of the gingivae (gums) around the roots of the teeth (**Figure 14-12**).
dental caries	**Dental caries**, commonly called cavities or tooth decay, results when bacteria in plaque destroy tooth tissue. In dentistry, **plaque** refers to an abnormal hardened buildup of saliva, mucus, bacteria, and food

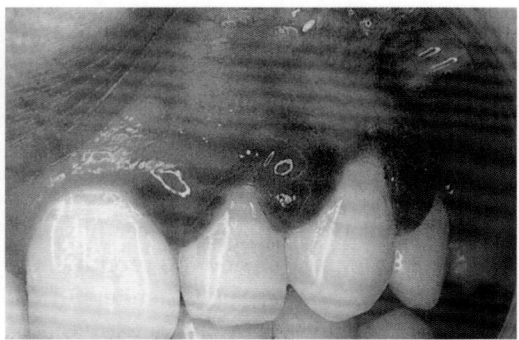

Figure 14-12 The gingival margins are reddened and swollen in this case of gingivitis.

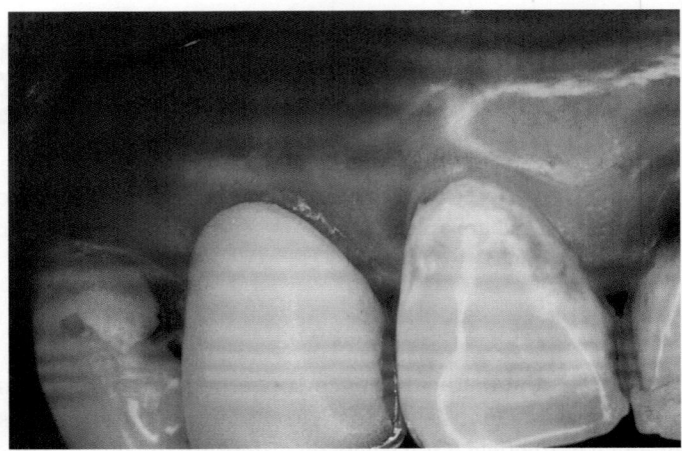

Figure 14-13 Plaque buildup on the surfaces of teeth.

residue on the tooth surface that causes tooth or gingival disease (**Figure 14-13**). In the process of breaking down sugars, the bacteria form enamel-eroding acids.

Periodontal disease and dental caries often have overlapping signs and symptoms. Signs and symptoms of caries include temperature and sweet sensitivity, **halitosis** (bad-smelling breath), pain, or an **abscess** (pus-filled sac around root). X-rays confirm the diagnosis. Treatment involves removing the diseased portion, filling in the space or performing a root canal (removal of the infected pulp, filling the canal with an impervious material, and sealing the canal in the roots to prevent subsequent infection); sometimes treatment involves tooth extraction. Good oral hygiene, which includes brushing, flossing, and regular professional cleaning, is a preventive measure.

bruxism	**Bruxism** is the unconscious habit of clenching and grinding the teeth that occurs during sleep or in stressful situations. It can lead to excessive wear on the teeth.
temporomandibular joint (TMJ) syndrome	**Temporomandibular joint (TMJ) syndrome** is an inflammation or disease of the temporal bone and mandible (lower jaw) articulation characterized by limited jaw movement and pain. Clicking sounds while chewing are common. It can be caused by malocclusion, arthritis, or degenerative joint disease. The oral examination and x-rays diagnose it. The treatment depends on the underlying cause. Options include cortisone injection, grinding of the teeth surfaces, or wearing of specially created mouth appliances to correct the bite.
aphtha	A painful oral ulcer of unknown cause is known as an **aphtha**. The common term is *canker sore*. Its appearance is correlated with stress or illness. It is diagnosed by oral examination and usually heals spontaneously within 1 to 2 weeks. Antiseptic or steroid mouthwashes may be used to treat it.
cold sores	Herpes simplex virus 1 (HSV-1) causes **cold sores** (fever blisters), small painful blisters on or near the lips or inside the mouth. They often recur at irregular intervals. The term *fever blister* refers to the fact that the eruptions often reappear during an illness with a fever

(febrile illness). The virus enters the body through interruptions in the mucous membranes or skin. Tingling and numbness in the area may precede their onset. Visual examination is enough for a clear diagnosis. Topical creams and ice application are treatments.

thrush

White spots on the tongue and buccal (cheek) mucous membrane characterize **thrush**, caused by the fungus *Candida albicans* (**Figure 14-14**). It occurs most commonly in infants and young children. The organism is part of the normal mouth flora, but antibiotic use, impaired immunity, or lowered resistance disrupts the natural balance, thereby creating the condition. Oral examination or lesion analysis confirms the diagnosis. It is treated with antifungal medications. Eating yogurt containing active yeast cultures while taking antibiotics is a preventive measure for thwarting thrush onset. (The microbes in yogurt assist in maintaining stability by restoring microbial life that was killed by the antibiotics.)

necrotizing ulcerative gingivitis

A noncontagious ulcerative infection of the oral membranes and gingivae is termed **necrotizing ulcerative gingivitis**. Microorganisms that are normally present in the mouth cause the condition when they overpopulate as a result of poor hygiene, vitamin B deficiency, or immune disorder. Painful, swollen gums, metallic taste, and halitosis are characteristic signs and symptoms. Contributing factors include stress, cigarette smoking, and infection. The infection is diagnosed by dental examination. Treatments are antibiotics, hydrogen peroxide mouthwash, and professional teeth cleaning.

oral leukoplakia

Oral leukoplakia is an abnormal thickening and whitening of mucous membranes in the mouth. It may be a precancerous condition. The tongue and mouth are white and rough, and the hardened surface is sensitive to heat (**Figure 14-15**). It is diagnosed by oral examination. A tissue biopsy is warranted if the condition does not resolve within 2 to 3 weeks. Treatment involves identifying the source of irritation (such as ill-fitting dentures) and eliminating it.

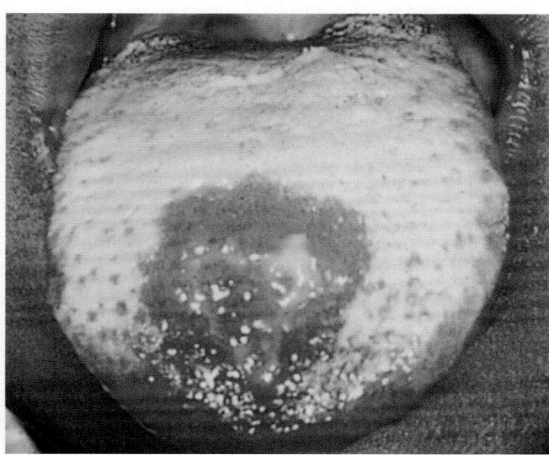

Figure 14-14 *Candida albicans* infection (thrush).

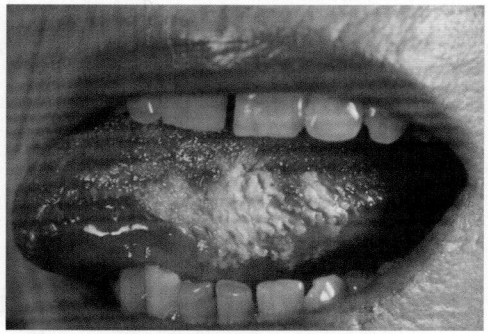

Figure 14-15 Leukoplakia. White plaques resembling corrugated cardboard are fixed to the mucous membrane.

KEY TERM	Definition
orthodontics (or-thoh-DON-ticks)	dentistry concerned with the prevention and correction of teeth irregularities
malocclusion (mal-oh-KLOO-zhun)	abnormal positioning of the upper and lower teeth when closing the jaw
periodontal (perr-ee-oh-DON-tul) **disease**	pathology of the tissues that surround the neck and root of a tooth, including the underlying bone
gingivitis (jin-ji-VYE-tis)	inflammation of the gingivae (gums) around the roots of the teeth
dental caries (KAIR-eez)	cavities or tooth decay
plaque (PLACK)	hardened film of saliva, mucus, bacteria, and food residue on the tooth surface
halitosis (hal-i-TOH-sis)	bad-smelling breath
abscess (AB-ses)	pus-filled cavity created by bacterial infection and inflammation
bruxism (BRUK-sizm)	unconscious habit of clenching the teeth that occurs during sleep or in stressful situations and leads to excessive wear on the teeth
temporomandibular (tem-puh-roh-man-DIB-yoo-lur) **joint (TMJ) syndrome**	inflammation of the temporal bone and mandible articulation characterized by limited jaw movement and pain
aphtha (AF-thuh)	white oral ulcer of unknown cause; also called a canker sore
cold sores	small painful blisters in the mouth or on the surrounding lips caused by herpes simplex virus 1 (HSV-1); also called a fever blister
thrush	*Candida albicans* fungal infection of the mouth characterized by white patches
necrotizing ulcerative gingivitis (NECK-roh-tize-ing UL-sur-uh-tiv jin-ji-VYE-tis)	painful ulcerative condition of the mouth caused by normal mouth microorganisms
oral leukoplakia (lew-koh-PLAY-kee-uh)	abnormal thickening and whitening of mucous membranes in the mouth

KEY TERM PRACTICE: *Oral Cavity Disorders*

1. *Candida albicans* is the causative agent for which oral cavity disorder? _____

2. An abnormal thickening and whitening of mucous membranes in the mouth is termed _____; it is derived from the word _____, which means *mouth*, and the word part _____, which means *white*.

3. _____ is the medical term for a canker sore.

4. An abnormal positioning of the upper and lower teeth when closing the jaw is termed _____.

5. _____ is the medical term for bad-smelling breath.

Ulcers

ulcer   An **ulcer** is a slow-healing sore on the surface of an organ or tissue resulting from loss of tissue. It is often accompanied by inflammation.

peptic ulcers   **Peptic ulcers** are sores (lesions) in the digestive tract, typically in the stomach or duodenum, caused by stomach acid and the digestive action of pepsin. The type depends on its location:

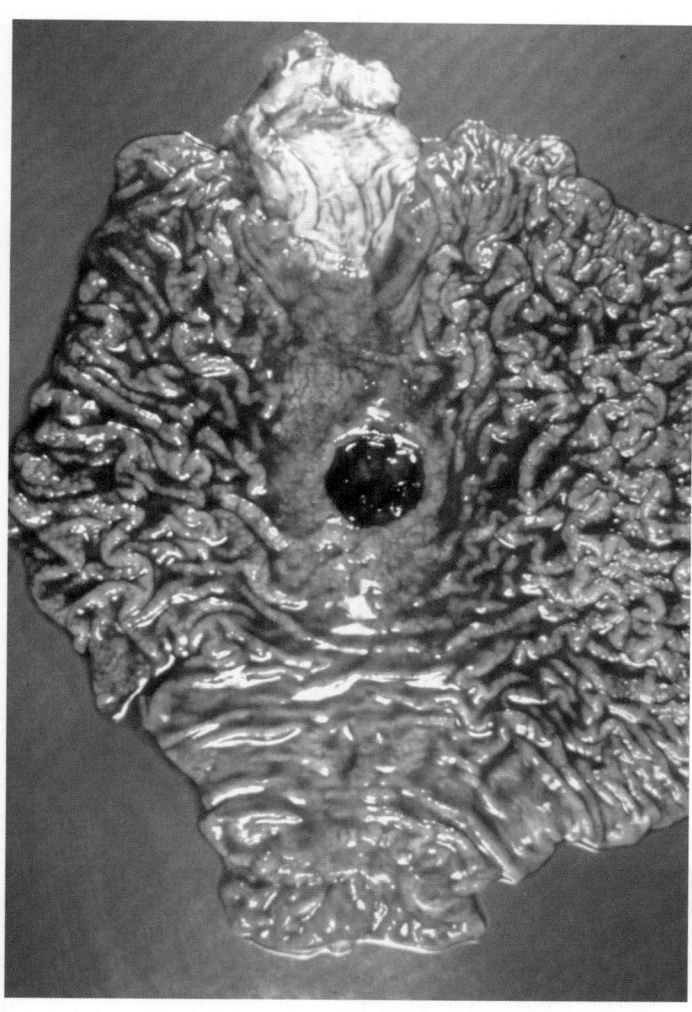

Figure 14-16 The stomach has been opened to reveal a sharply demarcated, deep gastric ulcer.

- A **gastric ulcer** is a sore in the stomach with inflammation (**Figure 14-16**).
- A **duodenal ulcer** is a sore in the first section of the small intestine. Ninety percent of duodenal ulcers are caused by *Helicobacter pylori* infection.

Signs and symptoms of ulcers affecting the digestive system include epigastric pain, heartburn, pain that occurs 2 hours after eating, occult blood (hidden blood in the stool), and bloody stools. **Heartburn** is named for its burning or warm sensation felt beneath the sternum. An alternate term for heartburn is **pyrosis**, derived from the word part *pyr-,* which means *fire* or *heat.* Heartburn (pyrosis) is caused by esophageal **regurgitation**, backflow of gastric juice into the esophagus. Ulcers can also be caused by nonsteroidal anti-inflammatory drug (NSAID) use, alcohol and aspirin overuse, smoking, and psychological stress.

Diagnosis of peptic ulcers is made by the history and physical examination, serum gastrin test, barium studies, endoscopy, diagnostic studies indicating the presence of *H. pylori* infection, stool samples, and biopsy to rule out (R/O) or confirm cancer. Normally, the acidity of the stomach creates an inhospitable environment for microbial growth, but the bacterium *H. pylori* thrives in the low pH of gastric secretions. *H. pylori* is so named because it was originally identified in the pyloric region of the stomach. The **serum gastrin test** evaluates levels of the hormone gastrin in blood serum. Elevated gastrin levels may be a sign of gastric ulcers, pernicious anemia, or pancreatic tumor.

Treatment choices consist of diet and lifestyle modifications, increased exercise, and use of antacids, antibiotics, or other drugs. Agents, such as calcium carbonate, that reduce or neutralize acidity, especially in the stomach, are termed **antacids. Antibiotics** are medicines that inhibit bacterial growth or kill bacteria. They are used to treat ulcers caused by *H. pylori*. Other drugs that block or inhibit acid secretion include H_2 receptor antagonists (cimetidine or Tagamet) and proton pump inhibitors (omeprazole or Prilosec, lansoprazole or Prevacid, and esomeprazole or Nexium).

KEY TERM	Definition
ulcer (UL-sur)	slow-healing sore on the surface of an organ or tissue resulting from loss of tissue
peptic ulcers (PEP-tick UL-surs)	sores in the digestive tract caused by excessive secretion of acid and the digestive action of pepsin
gastric ulcer (GAS-trick UL-sur)	sore on the stomach lining with inflammation
duodenal ulcer (dew-oh-DEE-nul UL-sur)	sore on the duodenum lining
heartburn	burning or warm sensation felt just below the sternum that results from regurgitation of gastric juice into the esophagus; another term for pyrosis
pyrosis (pye-ROH-sis)	burning or warm sensation felt just below the sternum that results from regurgitation of gastric juice into the esophagus; another term for heartburn
regurgitation (ree-gur-ji-TAY-shun)	backflow of digestive juice into the esophagus
serum gastrin (SEER-um GAS-trin) **test**	test for levels of the gastric and intestinal hormone, gastrin, in blood serum
antacid	agent that neutralizes acid
antibiotic	medicine that inhibits bacterial growth or kills bacteria

KEY TERM PRACTICE: *Ulcers*

1. A _____ is a slow-healing sore on the surface of an organ or tissue.

2. A sore on the membrane lining the stomach is termed a _____ ulcer, derived from the word part _____, which refers to *stomach*.

3. An _____ is an agent that neutralizes acids.

4. A burning or warm sensation felt just below the sternum that results from regurgitation of gastric juice into the esophagus is termed _____ or _____.

5. _____ is the backflow of digestive juice into the esophagus.

Appendicitis

appendicitis A serious medical condition in which the appendix becomes inflamed is called **appendicitis**. Signs and symptoms are pain in the right lower quadrant, nausea, vomiting, constipation, or diarrhea. The medical term for an unsettled feeling in the stomach with an urge to vomit is **nausea**. Difficulty emptying the bowels or infrequent bowel movements is called **constipation**. Feces are generally hard and dry with constipation. The opposite of constipation is increased frequency of watery feces, termed **diarrhea**. Diarrhea, constipation, and **fecal incontinence** (inability to control defecation) may have accompanying excessive gas in the GI tract known as **flatulence**.

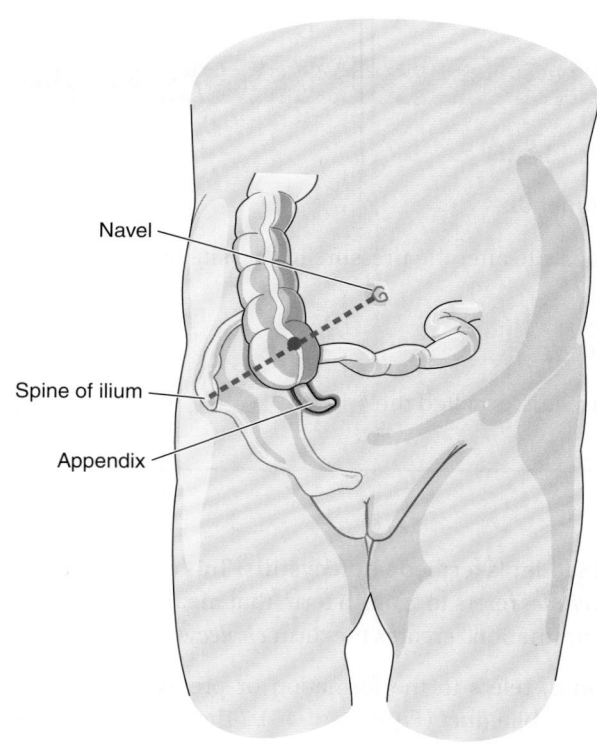

Navel

Spine of ilium

Appendix

Figure 14-17 Location of appendicitis on female child. McBurney point is indicated as dot on center of dashed line drawn between the anterior spine of ilium and the navel.

The cause of appendicitis is poorly understood, but the condition results in an obstructed structure in which bacteria multiply, compromise circulation, and create infection. It most commonly occurs between the ages of 20 and 40. The patient's history and physical examination, McBurney point tenderness, and rebound pain are used for diagnosis. The **McBurney point** is a 5.08-cm (2-in.) spot located over the appendix base where extreme sensitivity indicates appendicitis (**Figure 14-17**). The Aaron sign refers to pain when pressure is applied over the McBurney point. **Rebound pain**, also called the Blumberg sign is soreness that is greater at a sensitive site after releasing palpating pressure. It assists in distinguishing between appendicitis pain (great rebound pain) and gas pain. Another test for appendicitis is the Rovsing sign, pain in the right lower quadrant when pressure is applied to the left lower quadrant. Appendicitis is treated by appendectomy and broad-spectrum antibiotic therapy. Untreated appendicitis is lethal because a ruptured appendix leads to peritonitis and shock.

KEY TERM	Definition
appendicitis (a-pen-di-SIGH-tis)	inflammation of the appendix with severe pain
nausea (NAW-zee-uh)	unsettled feeling in the stomach with the urge to vomit
constipation	difficulty emptying the bowels or infrequent bowel movements
diarrhea (dye-uh-REE-uh)	increased frequency of watery feces
fecal incontinence (FEE-kul in-KON-ti-nence)	inability to control defecation
flatulence (FLAT-yoo-lents)	excessive amount of gas in the GI tract
McBurney point	site of extreme tenderness over the appendix, indicating appendicitis
rebound pain	soreness that is greater at a site after the pressure to that site has been removed

continued

continued from page 713

KEY TERM PRACTICE: *Appendicitis*

1. Increased frequency of watery feces is termed _____.

2. _____ is the term describing inflammation of the appendix.

3. _____ is best described as soreness that is greater at a site after the pressure to that site has been removed.

4. An unsettled feeling in the stomach with the urge to vomit is termed _____.

5. The site of extreme tenderness over the appendix, indicating appendicitis, is called the _____.

Gallbladder Disorders

cholecystitis Inflammation of the gallbladder is termed **cholecystitis**. This condition is so called because the prefix *chole-* refers to "gall," a term that means "bile." Adding the suffix *-itis* for "inflammation" creates the term *cholecystitis*.

cholelithiasis or gallstones **Cholelithiasis**, or **gallstones**, refers to the formation or presence of calculi (stones) in the gallbladder or bile duct (**Figure 14-18**). (The word part *litho-* means "stone" or "calculus.") Gallstones develop by several processes. For example, if the bile is too concentrated, liver cells create too much cholesterol, which comes out of solution and forms crystals, or if the gallbladder is inflamed, gallstones may form. Although the stones are formed from cholesterol, their course of development is not known. The person may be asymptomatic unless there is an obstruction.

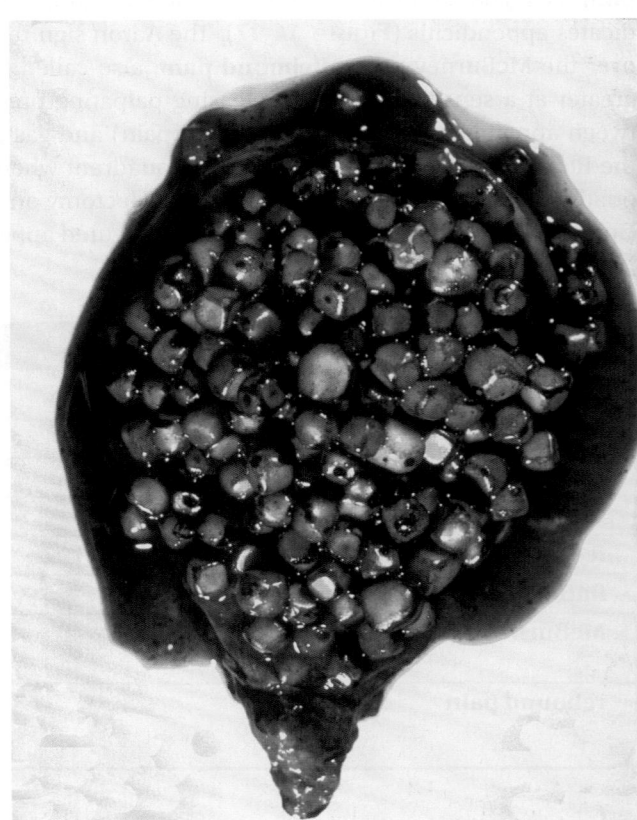

Figure 14-18 The gallbladder has been opened to reveal numerous yellow cholesterol gallstones.

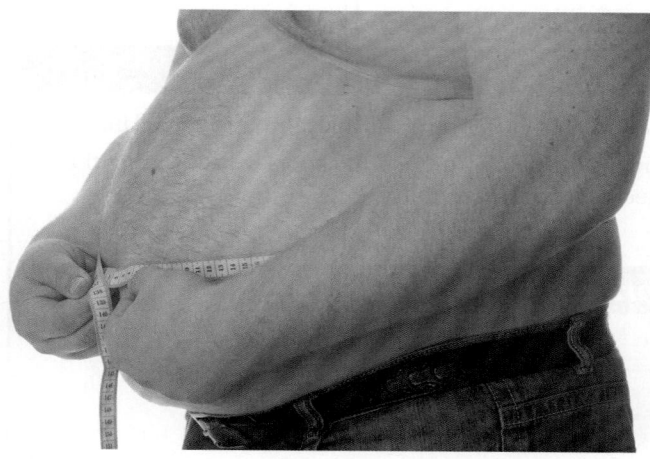

Figure 14-19 Photograph showing obesity.

Signs and symptoms may include colicky pain (pain in the colon), epigastric or right upper quadrant pain radiating to the scapular region, and jaundice. **Colic** is acute abdominal pain that increases in severity, reaches a peak, and then slowly subsides. It is usually the result of spasmodic smooth muscle contractions in the colon.

Cholelithiasis is often associated with a high-calorie/high-cholesterol diet and obesity. **Obesity** is an excessive accumulation of fat beyond physical requirements. It is characterized by body weight that is 20% or more in excess of ideal weight for a person's sex and height (**Figure 14-19**). In the United States, obesity is the leading nutrition disorder and is responsible for more than 280,000 deaths per year. Cholelithiasis is diagnosed through the history and physical examination, ultrasonography, radioisotope scan, oral cholecystogram, and intravenous cholangiogram. A **cholecystogram** is a radiograph of the gallbladder taken after the patient has swallowed a contrast dye that shows up in an x-ray image. The **cholangiogram** is an x-ray image of the bile ducts after dye introduction.

Conservative treatment options include diet therapy to decrease fat intake. Laparoscopic cholecystectomy or extracorporeal shock wave lithotripsy (ESWL) may also be used. The excision of the gallbladder and cystic duct is termed **cholecystectomy**. The surgical procedure can be performed using a **laparoscope**, a tube-shaped instrument that is inserted through the abdominal wall for viewing the internal organs. **Extracorporeal shock wave lithotripsy (ESWL)** involves directing high-energy sound waves to the site of the gallstone or other stone concentration to destroy it. The pieces are then small enough to pass normally through the gallbladder and bile ducts.

KEY TERM	Definition
cholecystitis (koh-lee-sis-TIGH-tis)	inflammation of the gallbladder
cholelithiasis (koh-lee-li-THIGH-uh-sis)	presence of calculi in the gallbladder or bile ducts; also called gallstones
gallstones	presence of calculi in the gallbladder or bile ducts; also called cholelithiasis
colic (KOL-ick)	attack of abdominal pain caused by colonic spasms
obesity	body weight 20% or more in excess of ideal weight for a person's sex and height
cholecystogram (kohl-ee-SIS-toh-gram)	x-ray of the gallbladder
cholangiogram (kohl-AN-jee-oh-gram)	x-ray of the bile ducts after introduction of a contrast dye
cholecystectomy (koh-lee-sis-TECK-toh-mee)	surgical removal of the gallbladder

continued

continued from page 715

KEY TERM	Definition
laparoscope (LAP-uh-roh-skope)	instrument used to view the inside of the body through a small incision
extracorporeal shock wave lithotripsy (ecks-truh-kor-POH-ree-ul SHOCK WAVE lith-oh-TRIP-see) **(ESWL)**	fragmentation of stones using ultrasound shock waves so that the pulverized pieces can pass naturally

KEY TERM PRACTICE: *Gallbladder Disorders*

1. The formation or presence of gallbladder calculi is termed _____.

2. _____ is an x-ray image of the bile ducts after dye injection.

3. An attack of abdominal pain caused by colonic spasms is termed _____.

4. Inflammation of the gallbladder is called _____ and is derived from the word part _____ for "bile (gall)" and the word part _____ for "inflammation of."

5. A _____ is the surgical removal of the gallbladder and is derived from the word part _____ for *bile (gall)* and the word part _____ for *surgical removal of.*

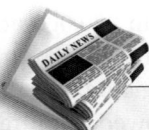

IN THE NEWS: Obesity in America

Is there really an obesity problem in the United States? Government agencies and scientific health organizations now use data collected by the National Center for Health Statistics (NCHS) and the Centers for Disease Control and Prevention (CDC) from cross-sectional surveys to establish statistically significant information relative to obesity. These continuous surveys have been the standard since 1999; and since 1991, obesity has increased by nearly 60% in American adults. Obesity is now considered an epidemic.

According to the most recent National Health and Nutrition Examination Survey (NHANES), nearly 64.5% of Americans older than 20 years are considered overweight, and of these overweight Americans, nearly one-third are obese. Overweight and obesity are known risk factors for several disorders, including diabetes mellitus; cardiovascular disease; gallbladder disease; respiratory disorders; and cancers of the breast, colon, gallbladder, kidney, rectum, and uterus.

Findings from the studies indicate that in the United States, approximately 280,000 deaths annually can be attributed to unhealthy dietary habits, lack of physical activity, and sedentary behavior. Despite the known and publicized risks associated with being overweight, the prevalence has steadily increased between both genders and across all ages, ethnic groups, and educational levels. Although there is no accepted definition distinguishing overweight from obesity in the 6- to 19-year-old age group, 15.3% of children ages 6 to 11 years and 15.5% of adolescents ages 12 to 19 years are overweight.

Another striking discovery is that among individuals with Type 1 diabetes, 67% have a body mass index (BMI) greater than 27 and 46% have a BMI greater than 30. The BMI is an indicator of the appropriateness of a person's weight for his or her height and provides a fairly accurate estimate of body fat content. Underweight is a BMI of less than 18.5, normal is between 18.5 and 25, overweight is between 25 and 30, and obese is 30 or higher.

continued

continued from page 716

IN THE NEWS: Obesity in America

The figures are nearly as staggering for the prevalence of high blood cholesterol, cancer, and mortality. An average annual total of 10.2 million people reported treatment for diabetes during 1997–1998 compared to 18.2 million persons in 2006–2007. According to the American Diabetes Association (ADA), the economic cost of diabetes in the United States in 2007 (the latest year for which there are figures) was estimated at $174 billion.

Americans appear to be quite concerned about their weight problem. In fact, nearly $42 billion is spent annually on weight-loss products and services. However, less than one-third (31.8%) of the adult population engages in physical activity, which is known to help reduce obesity and disease risk.

Pancreas Disorders

pancreatitis

Chronic or acute inflammation of the pancreas is known as **pancreatitis**. Signs and symptoms are edema, inflammation, pain radiating to the back, nausea, vomiting, diaphoresis (profuse sweating), tachycardia (rapid heart rate), and tender abdomen. Advanced cases lead to malabsorption and diabetes mellitus. Causes of pancreatitis are varied and include autodigestion from digestive juices secreted, alcoholism, biliary tract disease, infection, trauma, drugs, hyperlipidemia, and gallstones. The history and physical examination, x-rays, sonograms, CT scan, hyperglycemia (increased blood glucose), and increased serum amylase and lipase levels within the first 3 days of the attack confirm the diagnosis. Elevated serum amylase occurs with pancreatic disease and pancreatic duct obstruction. Increased serum lipase levels result from acute pancreatitis. Urine amylase amounts increase 7 to 10 days after the onset of pancreatic disease. Treatment includes intravenous electrolyte replacement, nothing ingested by mouth, feeding by a nasogastric tube, antibiotics if an infection is present, and pain medications. At times it is necessary to bypass the oral cavity to deliver nutrients, dyes, or medications directly into the stomach. This is accomplished by means of a **nasogastric (NG) tube**, a flexible structure inserted through the nose that ends in the stomach (**Figure 14-20**).

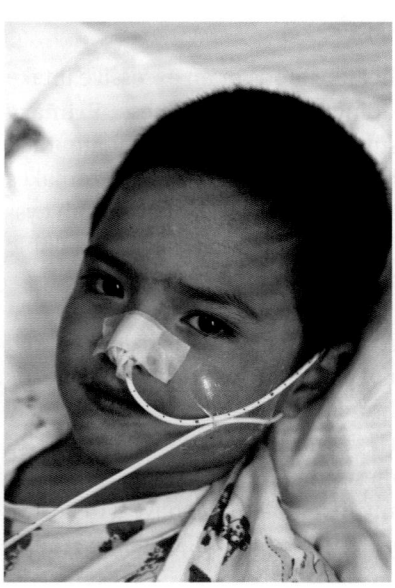

Figure 14-20 A nasogastric tube inserted into a child. The nasogastric tube can be secured by gently placing the tubing behind the child's ear and taping the tubing to the child's cheek.

cystic fibrosis (CF)   A genetic disease starting in infancy that affects various exocrine glands in addition to respiratory structures is **cystic fibrosis (CF)**. Secretion of thick mucus that blocks internal passages, absence of pancreatic enzymes, and inadequate absorption of fat-soluble vitamins characterize the disease. Signs and symptoms include frequent respiratory infections, **anorexia** (appetite loss), and failure to gain weight. It is diagnosed by the history and physical examination and a sweat test revealing elevated sodium and chloride levels. Treatment aimed at the digestive malfunction includes vitamin and mineral supplementation, diet therapy, and ingestion of pancreatic enzymes to assist with food metabolism.

KEY TERM	Definition
pancreatitis (pan-kree-uh-TYE-tis)	pancreas inflammation
nasogastric (nay-zoh-GAS-trick) **(NG) tube**	small tube inserted through the nose to the stomach for feeding purposes
cystic fibrosis (SIS-tick figh-BROH-sis) **(CF)**	hereditary disease associated with dysfunction of the exocrine glands and respiratory structures
anorexia (an-oh-RECK-see-uh)	loss of appetite

KEY TERM PRACTICE: *Pancreas Disorders*

1. The word part _____ means *pancreas* and the word part *-itis* means _____; thus inflammation of the pancreas is termed _____.

2. The medical term for loss of appetite is _____.

3. A hereditary disease associated with dysfunction of the exocrine glands and respiratory structures is called _____.

4. A small tube inserted through the nose to the stomach for feeding purposes is termed a _____.

Eating, Nutritional, and Metabolic Disorders

primary malnutrition   Malnutrition results from a lack of healthy foods or an excessive intake of unhealthy foods in the diet leading to physical illness. **Primary malnutrition** is a condition resulting from an inadequate diet. **Secondary malnutrition** results when an individual's pathology makes a normally adequate diet insufficient. For example, a person with cystic fibrosis may eat a balanced, nutrient-rich diet, but many fat-soluble vitamins will not be adequately absorbed as a result of the disease.

anorexia nervosa (AN)   **Anorexia nervosa (AN)** is a psychological eating disorder marked by profound food aversion and fear of becoming overweight that leads to emaciation and malnutrition. **Emaciation** describes an extremely lean body caused by starvation that leads to muscle atrophy and depletion of fat reserves. The person denies hunger pains and self-imposes starvation. It occurs more commonly in females who have a distorted body image, are excessive exercisers, strive for high achievement, and have a compulsive personality. In addition to severe weight and appetite loss, other signs are hypotension (low blood pressure), bradycardia (slow heart rate), and hypothermia (abnormally low body temperature). Serious ill health and death can result without intervention. Treatment includes psychiatric counseling, hospitalization to monitor food intake and electrolytes, and diet therapy.

bulimia

Bulimia (bulimia nervosa) is a condition characterized by bouts of overeating followed by undereating, laxative use, or self-induced vomiting. The individual engages in binge eating to overcome an insatiable appetite but then attempts to purge the body of the recently eaten food. For this reason it is commonly called the binge–purge syndrome. Bulimia is associated with depression and anxiety about weight gain and obesity. Common signs are laxative and diuretic abuse, along with tooth decay from erosion caused by vomited acidic gastric secretions. Other signs and symptoms mimic those of anorexia nervosa. The person often vomits in secret and denies it when questioned. The cause is unknown. The history and physical examination provide the diagnosis. Treatment for this life-threatening disease requires a multidimensional approach that includes diet therapy and counseling.

kwashiorkor

Two types of protein-energy malnutrition (PEM) are kwashiorkor and marasmus. **Kwashiorkor** is a type of malnutrition in children characterized by deficiency of calories in general and of protein in particular. A Ghanaian term, *kwashiorkor* means "the evil spirit that infects the first child when the second child is born." It is a common disorder in African children weaned from protein-rich breast milk to a traditional cornmeal diet that is deficient in protein. Signs and symptoms include extreme weight loss, edema, ascites (fluid-filled abdomen), lethargy, failure to grow, skin and hair changes, fatty liver, and weakness (**Figure 14-21**). Sometimes mental retardation results due to the lack of proteins needed for neuron development. Treatment involves a nutritious diet with added protein.

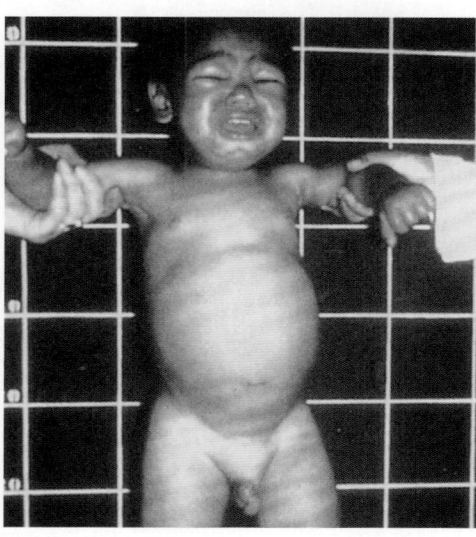

Figure 14-21 A child with kwashiorkor and the characteristic ascites (fluid-filled abdomen).

marasmus

Occurring in infants and young children, **marasmus** is chronic, severe wasting of body tissues caused by prolonged nutritional deficiency. It is referred to as the disease of starvation. Marasmus is characterized by loss of subcutaneous fat, wrinkled skin, loss of muscle tissue and strength, failure to grow, and lethargy. It is difficult to distinguish between marasmus and kwashiorkor, and recent research suggests that they are stages of the same disease, because marasmus (deficiency of all nutrients) can progress to kwashiorkor. Diagnosis is made by the history and physical examination. Treatment involves nutrition therapy that includes a nutrient-rich diet.

phenylketonuria (PKU)

Phenylketonuria (PKU) is a genetic disorder characterized by an inability to convert the essential amino acid, phenylalanine, to the nonessential amino acid, tyrosine. The genetic mutation causes the body to be deficient in the enzyme phenylalanine hydroxylase, which is necessary for the conversion. Signs and symptoms include excessive amounts of phenylalanine in the blood, eczema, fair hair, seizures, and neuronal function impairment. If not treated, it can result in mental retardation. It is diagnosed shortly after birth by elevated plasma concentration of phenylalanine after milk or formula ingestion. Treatment involves controlling the amount of phenylalanine in the diet, especially during childhood when the nervous system is developing. Adults with PKU can relax their dietary restrictions, but pregnant women must adhere to the strict phenylalanine-restricted diet to protect the fetus. Diet sodas carry a warning label for people with PKU that states the drink contains phenylalanine (**Figure 14-22**).

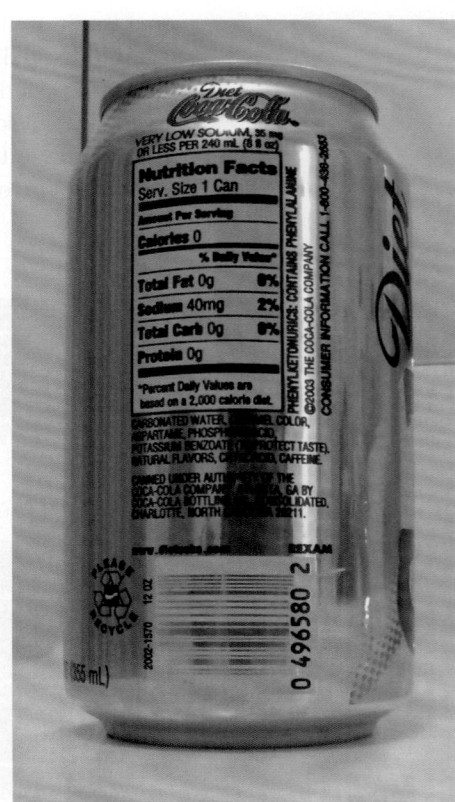

Figure 14-22 Diet soda with the mandatory phenylalanine warning.

KEY TERM	Definition
primary malnutrition	poor health resulting from an inadequate diet
secondary malnutrition	poor health resulting from a disease process that makes a normally healthy diet inadequate
anorexia nervosa (AN) (an-oh-RECK-see-uh nur-VOH-suh)	psychological disorder characterized by not eating because of morbid fear of weight gain
emaciation (ee-may-see-AY-shun)	excessive leanness caused by muscle wasting
bulimia (bew-LIM-ee-uh)	psychological disorder characterized by binge eating and self-induced purging; also called bulimia nervosa
kwashiorkor (kwah-shee-OR-kor)	malnutrition in children characterized by ascites and caused by deficiency of calories in general and of protein in particular
marasmus (muh-RAZ-mus)	malnutrition in infants and young children characterized by loss of subcutaneous fat and wrinkled skin and caused by prolonged nutritional deficiency
phenylketonuria (PKU) (fen-il-kee-toh-NEW-ree-uh)	hereditary metabolic disorder characterized by a deficiency of phenylalanine hydroxylase

KEY TERM PRACTICE: *Eating, Nutritional, and Metabolic Disorders*

1. _____ is the eating disorder marked by self-induced vomiting after eating.

2. This type of malnutrition results from an inadequate diet. _____

3. This type of malnutrition results from a disease process that makes a normally healthy diet inadequate. _____

4. _____ is excessive leanness caused by muscle wasting.

5. _____ is a psychological disorder characterized by not eating because of morbid fear of weight gain.

Gastroesophageal Disorders

gastroesophageal reflux disease (GERD)

Gastroesophageal reflux disease (GERD) is characterized by regurgitation (reflux) of acidic gastric juice into the esophagus (**Figure 14-23**). It often results in belching with vomitus in the mouth. Coughing and wheezing resulting from throat irritation are common. GERD leads to dysphagia, esophageal ulcers, and esophageal hemorrhage. **Dysphagia**—from the word part *-phagia,* which refers to a "condition involving eating or swallowing"—means difficulty swallowing. (Be sure not to confuse this term with *dysphasia,* whose word part *-phasia* means "speech disorder or difficulty speaking." Think *g* for *gastric,* as in dysphagia, and *s* for *speech,* as in dysphasia.) Tooth enamel erosion occurs from the acidic chyme in the mouth. Causes include overeating and pregnancy, which increase abdominal pressure; hiatal hernia (protrusion of the stomach through the esophageal hiatus); some medications; coffee; and alcohol.

The clinical picture and history, barium swallow, endoscopy, or biopsy confirms the diagnosis. Barium is a radiographic contrast medium used for GI studies. Barium sulfate ($BaSO_4$) is a whitish,

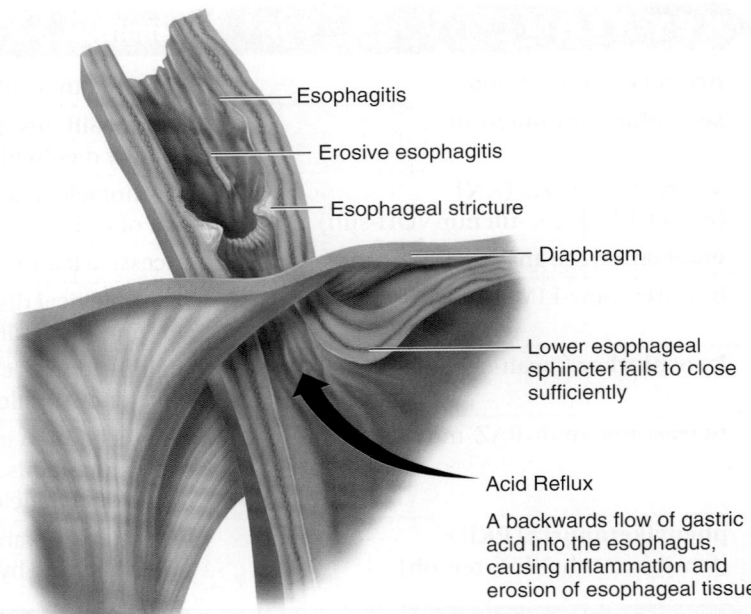

Esophagitis

Erosive esophagitis

Esophageal stricture

Diaphragm

Lower esophageal
sphincter fails to close
sufficiently

Acid Reflux

A backwards flow of gastric
acid into the esophagus,
causing inflammation and
erosion of esophageal tissue

Figure 14-23 Gastroesophageal reflux disease (GERD).

yellowish, odorless powder that is used in medical tests because x-rays cannot penetrate it, so it serves as a contrast medium that is easily viewed. The **barium swallow** examination is a series of x-rays taken after swallowing barium sulfate. This test determines pharyngeal and esophageal abnormalities, identifies tumors, and demonstrates the presence of a hiatal hernia. A series of contrast x-rays taken of the esophagus, stomach, and duodenum after swallowing barium sulfate is termed an **upper gastrointestinal series (UGIS)**.

A fiberoptic instrument called an **endoscope** that allows for visual examination of the organ interior may be used to examine the esophagus, stomach, and duodenum. The endoscope is also used for biopsy, which is tissue removal for diagnostic study.

Mild cases of GERD are treated by elevating the head and chest after eating, ingesting small meals to prevent overstretching the stomach, eating the last meal at least 4 hours before sleeping, losing weight if overweight, limiting alcohol consumption, and eliminating smoking. Severe cases can be treated pharmacologically with drugs that reduce acid output.

esophageal varices   Twisted, swollen esophageal veins are termed **esophageal varices** (*varix* = dilated vein). The swollen, twisted veins could rupture (**Figure 14-24**). Esophageal varices are common complications with liver cirrhosis (fibrous liver). The varices are caused by portal hypertension—pressure that develops from poor venous return to the liver. Diagnosis is made by physical examination, clinical picture, history of cirrhosis, and endoscopy. Treatment is aimed at controlling bleeding.

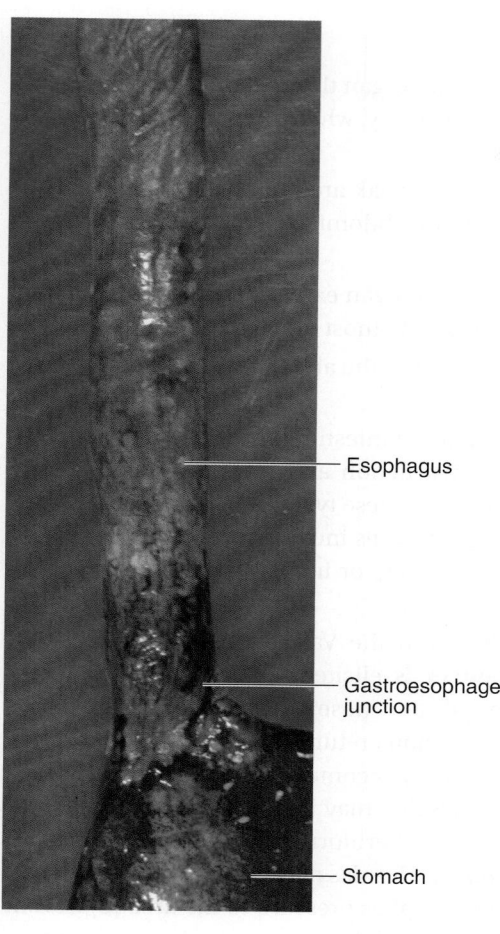

Esophagus

Gastroesophageal junction

Stomach

Figure 14-24 Esophageal varices. Numerous prominent blue venous channels are seen beneath the mucous membrane of the everted esophagus, particularly above the gastroesophageal junction.

KEY TERM	Definition
gastroesophageal (gas-troh-ee-sof-uh-JEE-ul) **reflex disease (GERD)**	regurgitation of acidic gastric juice into the esophagus
dysphagia (dis-FAY-jee-uh)	difficulty swallowing
barium (BAIR-ee-um) **swallow**	radiographic study of the pharynx and esophagus after swallowing barium sulfate
upper gastrointestinal series (UGIS)	x-rays of the esophagus, stomach, and duodenum after swallowing barium sulfate
endoscope (EN-doh-skope)	fiberoptic scope used for viewing inside the body
esophageal varices (ee-sof-uh-JEE-ul VAIR-i-seez)	twisted, swollen veins in the esophagus

KEY TERM PRACTICE: *Gastroesophageal Disorders*

1. GERD is the abbreviation for _____.

2. Twisted and swollen veins in the esophagus are termed _____.

3. X-rays of the esophagus, stomach, and duodenum after swallowing barium sulfate are used for an _____.

4. Difficulty swallowing is called _____.

5. An _____ is a fiberoptic scope used for viewing the inside of the body.

Hernias

hernia

A **hernia** is an abnormal protrusion of an organ through the wall of its cavity. Hernias usually occur in the abdominal cavity, where the intestine abnormally projects through the wall.

- An **abdominal hernia** results when a weak area of muscle allows an abdominal organ to protrude through the abdominal wall. The umbilicus is a common site (see **Figure 6-9**).
- An **inguinal hernia** is one in which an organ extends through the inguinal canal in the groin region. This type occurs most often in males.
- If the organ can be manipulated back into the abdominal cavity, it is said to be a **reducible hernia**.
- A **strangulated hernia** results when the intestine is not reducible and the blood flow is interrupted. Fecal obstruction and intestinal gangrene are complications of a strangulated hernia. These types of hernia are characterized by pain radiating from the site. Causes include trauma, excessive abdominal pressure caused by heavy lifting, or increased pressure resulting from pregnancy.

Palpation, radiographic studies, and the Valsalva maneuver are used for diagnosis. The **Valsalva maneuver** is elicited when the patient forcefully exhales while closing the mouth and nose. This movement increases intrathoracic pressure and impedes venous return (return of blood through the veins) to the heart, causing a hernia to become more pronounced.

Treatment depends on the type. Some may be reduced by manual manipulation, whereas others may require a herniorrhaphy or truss. Surgical repair of a hernia is called **herniorrhaphy**. Hernias may be treated using a **truss**, which is a pad attached to a belt that applies pressure to the area to prevent recurrence of a reduced hernia or to prevent the increase in size of a hernia.

hiatal hernia

Protrusion of the stomach through the esophageal hiatus is termed **hiatal hernia** (**Figure 14-25**). It is associated with esophageal regurgitation and

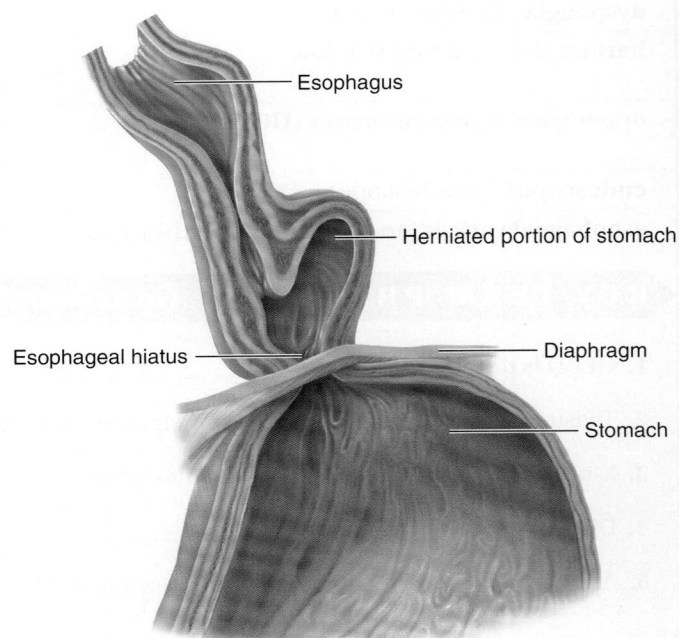

Esophagus

Herniated portion of stomach

Esophageal hiatus — Diaphragm

Stomach

Figure 14-25 Hiatal hernia.

GERD. It can have an unknown cause; be a congenital defect; or result from obesity, old age, or trauma. The initial diagnosis is made by x-ray evaluation and confirmed through barium radiographic studies and/or endoscopy. Conservative treatments, such as eating smaller portions and remaining upright after meals to allow gravity to assist in keeping the food down, are applied first. Specific drugs, such as cholinergics, may be used to strengthen the sphincter muscles. Surgical repair is a last resort.

KEY TERM	Definition
hernia (HUR-nee-uh)	abnormal protrusion of an organ through the wall of its cavity
abdominal hernia (ab-DOM-i-nul HUR-nee-uh)	abnormal protrusion of an organ through the abdominal wall
inguinal hernia (ING-gwi-nul HUR-nee-uh)	abnormal protrusion of an organ through the inguinal canal in the groin region
reducible hernia (re-DEW-si-bul HUR-nee-uh)	abnormal protrusion of an organ through the wall of its cavity that can be physically manipulated back into normal position
strangulated hernia (HUR-nee-uh)	interruption of blood flow in an abnormal protrusion of the intestine, possibly leading to fecal obstruction and gangrene
Valsalva (vahl-SAHL-vuh) **maneuver**	action of exhaling when the mouth and nostrils are closed, increasing internal pressure and causing a hernia to become more pronounced
herniorrhaphy (hur-nee-OR-uh-fee)	surgical repair of a hernia
truss	pad attached to a belt that applies pressure to a reduced hernia to prevent recurrence or to prevent the increase in size of a hernia
hiatal hernia (high-AY-tul HUR-nee-uh)	protrusion of the stomach through the esophageal hiatus (opening in diaphragm)

KEY TERM PRACTICE: *Hernias*

1. Which type of hernia results from a protrusion of the stomach through the diaphragm? _____

2. The surgical repair of a hernia is termed _____ and is derived from the word part *hernio-* for

   _____.

3. A pad attached to a belt that applies pressure to a reduced hernia to prevent recurrence or to prevent the increase in size of a hernia is called a _____.

4. An _____ is an abnormal protrusion of an organ through the inguinal canal in the groin region.

5. A _____ is an abnormal protrusion of an organ through the wall of its cavity that can be physically manipulated back into normal position.

Small Intestine Disorders

gastroenteritis or **traveler's diarrhea**   Commonly known as "traveler's diarrhea," **gastroenteritis** is inflammation of the mucous membrane of both the stomach and intestine. The acidity of the stomach generally protects the GI tract from bacterial invasion, but in some instances the microbes are able to survive and cause infection. Bacteria, toxins produced by bacteria, and parasites cause gastroenteritis. A person contracts the illness by ingesting

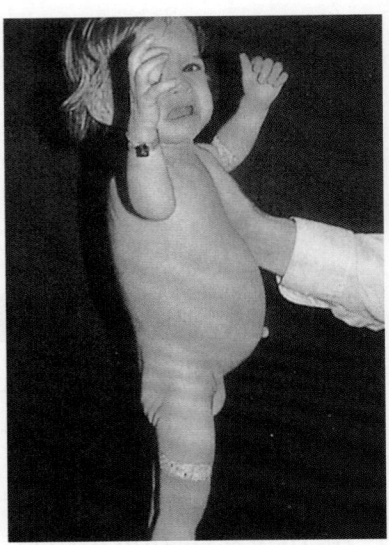

Figure 14-26 A child with celiac disease. Notice the protruding abdomen and wasted buttocks.

contaminated food or water. Stress is also a culprit. Signs and symptoms are diarrhea, cramps, and mucus and blood in the stool. The history and physical examination, along with a stool sample to identify the causative agent, are used for diagnosis. Treatment depends on the cause, but the condition is usually self-limiting and resolves with simple hydration therapy.

celiac disease   *Celiac* means "involving the abdomen." **Celiac disease** (celiac sprue) is a disorder caused by gluten sensitivity or intolerance that hinders the digestive system's ability to metabolize fat. Gluten is a protein in wheat. It is characterized by chronic inflammation and atrophy of the mucosa of the upper small intestine. Manifestations include diarrhea, malabsorption, steatorrhea, nutritional and vitamin deficiencies, and failure to thrive (**Figure 14-26**). Greasy, fatty feces is termed **steatorrhea**. The feces have a high fat content as a result of the reduced absorption of fat by the intestine. Celiac disease is diagnosed by tests indicating abnormal-appearing villi and a positive response to a gluten-free diet. The disease may have a genetic component and is thought to be an immune reaction to gluten.

Celiac disease is treated by strict adherence to a gluten-free diet and corticosteroid drugs aimed at diminishing the immune response. This disease is associated with the development of abdominal lymphoma.

KEY TERM	Definition
gastroenteritis (gas-troh-en-tur-EYE-tis)	inflammation of the mucous membrane of both the stomach and intestine; also called traveler's diarrhea
celiac (SEE-lee-ack) **disease**	malabsorption disorder caused by gluten sensitivity that hinders the digestive system's ability to metabolize fat; also called celiac sprue
steatorrhea (stee-uh-toh-REE-uh)	greasy, fatty feces

continued

continued from page 726

KEY TERM PRACTICE: *Small Intestine Disorders*

1. Inflammation of the stomach and intestines is termed _____, which is derived from the word part _____, meaning *stomach*; the word part _____, meaning *intestines*; and the suffix _____, meaning *inflammation*.

2. The medical term for greasy, fatty feces is _____.

3. _____ is a malabsorption disorder caused by gluten sensitivity that hinders the digestive system's ability to metabolize fat.

Large Intestine Disorders

ileus

Obstruction of the intestines causing failure to pass feces is termed **ileus**. (The failure to pass feces can also be caused by inadequate peristalsis in intestinal smooth muscles.) **Adhesions** (intestinal bands of scar tissue), calculi (stones), surgical or traumatic injury, infection, or tumors may be the cause of the obstruction. Following a surgery that requires general anesthesia, patients may experience ileus until their intestines "recover" from the inhibitory effects of the anesthesia. Signs and symptoms include extreme pain, abdominal distention, and vomiting. Treatment involves removing the source of obstruction or restoring muscle activity.

inflammatory bowel disease (IBD)

Inflammatory bowel disease (IBD) is a general term for bowel disorders that cause irritation, swelling, and tenderness. Two types of inflammatory bowel disease are Crohn disease and ulcerative colitis (covered in a later section).

Crohn disease or regional enteritis

Crohn disease, also known as **regional enteritis**, is a chronic inflammatory disorder of the intestines, usually affecting the terminal ileum, but possibly affecting other parts of the gastrointestinal tract. It is characterized by cramps, abdominal pain, diarrhea, fever, anorexia, and weight loss. The cause is unknown, but it may have a genetic component, and autoimmunity has been implicated.

Crohn disease is diagnosed by barium enema radiographic studies revealing diseased segments that are separated by normal bowel. Colonoscopy may also have diagnostic value. There is no cure, so the disease is treated symptomatically using anticholinergics and immunosuppressants. **Anticholinergics** are drugs that block or neutralize the effects of the neurotransmitter acetylcholine (Ach). A drug that inhibits the immune response is called an **immunosuppressant**.

diverticulosis

Similar sounding conditions are diverticulosis and diverticulitis. An abnormal pouch or sac opening from the intestine is termed a **diverticulum** (*diverticula* = plural). The presence of diverticula is called **diverticulosis** (**Figure 14-27**). Diverticulosis is common in middle

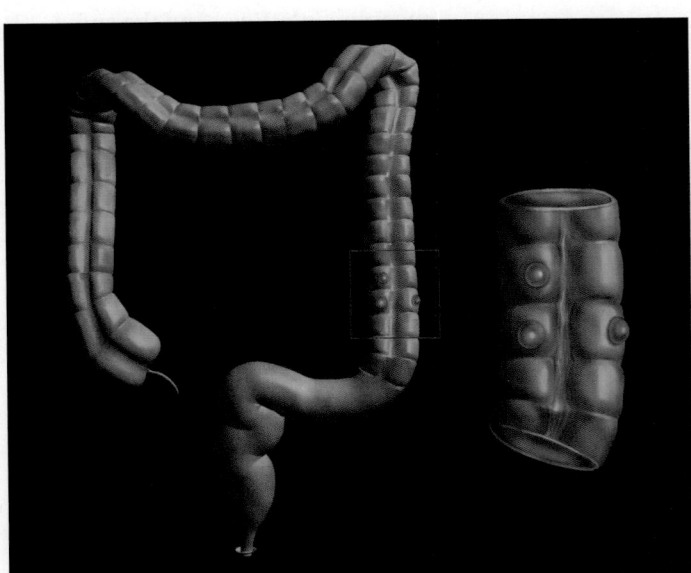

Figure 14-27 Diverticulosis is seen in a segment of the descending colon.

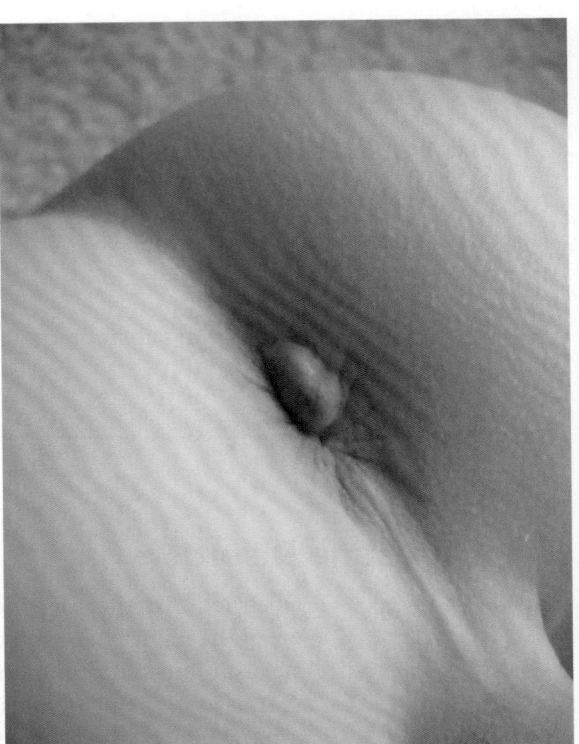

Figure 14-28 External hemorrhoid in a 2-year-old male with recurrent straining because of chronic constipation.

age and is usually asymptomatic with no inflammation. If signs and symptoms are present, they tend to be occasional pain, flatulence, and constipation. The cause of diverticulosis is inadequate fiber intake that prevents the bowel lumen from fully expanding, thereby creating diverticula pouches. It is more common after age 35 years. Treatment consists of increasing fluids and fiber in the diet, decreasing stress, and exercising. Anticholinergic drugs may be prescribed.

diverticulitis

Diverticulitis is inflammation of a diverticulum and results when fecal matter is trapped in a diverticulum. (A patient has to have diverticulosis to be afflicted with diverticulitis.) Signs and symptoms of diverticulitis include severe abdominal pain, fever, and bloody stools. If the wall is perforated, **peritonitis** (inflammation of the peritoneum) can result. Chronic forms of diverticulitis create adhesions, abscesses (localized pus collections), and fistulas (abnormal passages between two hollow organs). The cause is a low-fiber diet that is often accompanied by inadequate fluid intake. The clinical picture, sigmoidoscopy, colonoscopy, and barium enema study (if the intestine is not perforated) provide the diagnosis. Treatments are increased fluid and fiber intake and a regimen of exercise. Surgery may be necessary to remove any diseased intestinal portions.

hemorrhoids

Varicose veins in the lower rectum or anal wall are called **hemorrhoids**, commonly known as piles (**Figure 14-28**). Internal (toward the interior) hemorrhoids are located within the rectal wall, and external (toward the outside) hemorrhoids are found in the anal wall. Pain, pruritus (itching), protrusion through the anus, hematochezia, and bleeding (especially after defecation) are common signs and symptoms. **Hematochezia** is the passage of bloody stools. The term is used to distinguish this type of blood passage from the passage of dark, sticky feces containing partly digested blood called **melena**. Causes include constipation, straining while defecating, and pregnancy. Visual examination is generally all that is necessary to confirm the diagnosis.

Treatments include relieving constipation, increasing dietary fiber, anti-inflammatory drugs, and topical anti-itch creams. Ligation, cryosurgery, or hemorrhoidectomy may be necessary. An operation that ties a bleeding vessel with a knotted surgical ligature is called **ligation**. **Cryosurgery** involves a localized freezing of the bleeding hemorrhoid site. Surgical removal of hemorrhoids is termed **hemorrhoidectomy**.

KEY TERM	Definition
ileus (IL-ee-us)	obstruction of the intestines (or inactive peristalsis) causing failure to pass feces
adhesions (ad-HEE-zhunz)	intestinal bands of scar tissue
inflammatory bowel disease (IBD)	general term for bowel disorders that cause irritation, swelling, and tenderness
Crohn (KROHN) **disease**	chronic inflammatory disorder of the intestines, usually affecting the terminal ileum, but possibly affecting other parts of the gastrointestinal tract; also called regional enteritis
regional enteritis (en-tur-EYE-tis)	chronic inflammatory disorder of the intestines, usually affecting the terminal ileum, but possibly affecting other parts of the gastrointestinal tract; also called Crohn disease
anticholinergics (an-tee-koh-lin-UR-jicks)	drugs that block or neutralize the effects of the neurotransmitter acetylcholine (Ach)
immunosuppressant (im-yoo-noh-suh-PRES-unt)	drug that inhibits the immune response
diverticulum (dye-vur-TICK-yoo-lum)	abnormal pouch or sac opening from the intestine
diverticulosis (dye-vur-tick-yoo-LOH-sis)	presence of diverticula (abnormal pouches in the bowel)
diverticulitis (dye-vur-tick-yoo-LYE-tis)	inflammation of the diverticula
peritonitis (perr-i-toh-NIGH-tis)	inflammation of the peritoneum
hemorrhoids (HEM-uh-roidz)	painful varicose veins in the lower rectum or anal wall
hematochezia (hee-muh-toh-KEE-zee-uh)	passage of bloody stools
melena (me-LEE-nuh)	passage of dark, sticky feces containing partly digested blood
ligation (lye-GAY-shun)	tying a bleeding vessel with a knotted surgical ligature
cryosurgery (krye-oh-SUR-juh-ree)	surgery in which extremely cold temperature is applied to destroy tissue or stop bleeding
hemorrhoidectomy (hem-oh-roid-ECK-tuh-mee)	surgical removal of hemorrhoids

continued

continued from page 729

KEY TERM PRACTICE: *Large Intestine Disorders*

1. The word part _____ refers to the *peritoneum* and the word part _____ means *inflammation*; so inflammation of the peritoneum is termed _____.

2. What is the surgical procedure in which extremely cold temperature is used to destroy tissue or stop bleeding? _____

3. Give the singular and plural forms for the medical terms describing an abnormal pouch or sac opening from the intestine. _____

4. _____ are intestinal bands of scar tissue.

5. The surgical removal of hemorrhoids is termed _____.

Colon Disorders

colitis

Colitis is a general term for colon inflammation. Signs and symptoms include diarrhea, abdominal cramps, or constipation.

irritable bowel syndrome (IBS)

Irritable bowel syndrome (IBS) is a condition characterized by recurrent pain with constipation or diarrhea or alternating attacks of these. In most cases, no underlying pathology is found. IBS is associated with uncoordinated and inefficient contractions of the large intestine. **Spastic colon** is a nonspecific term used to describe symptoms such as abdominal pain, flatulence, and alternating diarrhea with constipation. Spastic colon is thought to occur as a result of increased muscular function of the colon. Colonic disorders are diagnosed by the history and physical examination. Treatment involves ingesting bulking agents or fiber and possibly taking anticholinergic drugs.

ulcerative colitis

Ulcerative colitis is a chronic disease of unknown cause characterized by ulceration of the colon and rectum with rectal bleeding, inflammation, abdominal pain, and diarrhea (**Figure 14-29**). The history and physical

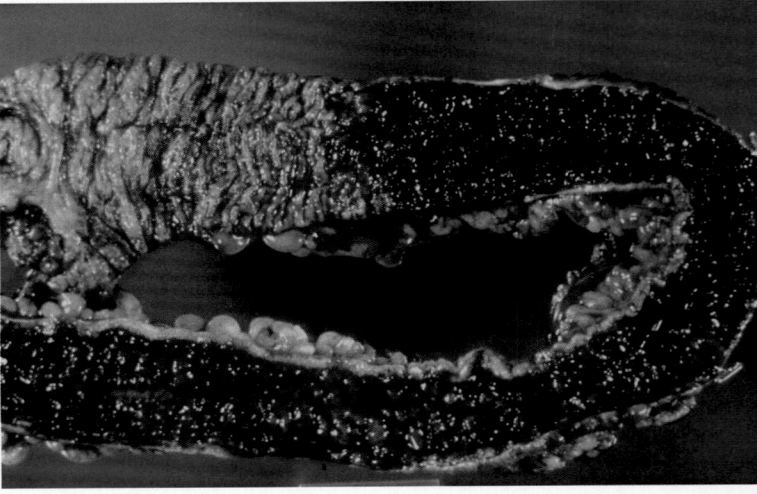

Figure 14-29 Ulcerative colitis beginning in the ascending colon and most severe in the rectosigmoid area.

examination, barium enema studies, colonoscopy, and biopsy are used for diagnosis. Treatment involves eating a well-balanced diet. Anticholinergic drugs and corticosteroids may be prescribed. Surgical removal of a severely diseased portion of the colon may be necessary because ulcerative colitis is associated with the development of colon cancer.

colorectal cancer   **Colorectal cancer** is the term used to describe several forms of cancer within the colon and/or rectum. Signs and symptoms are anemia, occult blood, diarrhea, constipation, **dyspepsia** (indigestion), and pain, or it may be totally asymptomatic. The term **occult** means the blood is not obvious and can only be detected by chemical or microscopic evaluation. The **fecal occult blood test** is the analysis of feces to determine the abnormal presence of blood in the stool. The cause of colorectal cancer is unknown, but there are several predisposing factors, including diets high in red meat, fat, and refined foods and low in fiber. Crohn disease and polyps (growths on the intestinal wall) are also associated with the development of cancer (**Figure 14-30**).

After the initial history and physical examination, fecal occult blood test, barium enema, sigmoidoscopy, colonoscopy, CT scan, or magnetic resonance imaging (MRI) studies confirm the diagnosis. The lower GI studies generally evaluate the status of the colon. The infusion of barium sulfate into the rectum and colon for diagnostic x-ray evaluation of the lower intestinal tract is termed **barium enema (BE)**.

Colonoscopy and sigmoidoscopy are performed with an endoscope that is inserted into the anus and through the rectum for viewing the interior of the large intestine. **Colonoscopy** is visual examination of the entire large intestine to the cecum using a colonoscope, whereas **sigmoidoscopy** examines the interior of the sigmoid colon and rectum using a sigmoidoscope. Biopsies can be obtained through the endoscope. These tests are performed to detect tumors, ulcers, or polyps.

Treatments include surgery, colostomy, chemotherapy, and radiation therapy. A **colostomy** is the surgical construction of an artificial connection between the colon and the skin (**Figure 14-31**). The operation is performed to bypass a damaged part of the colon and create an opening, other than the anus, to the exterior.

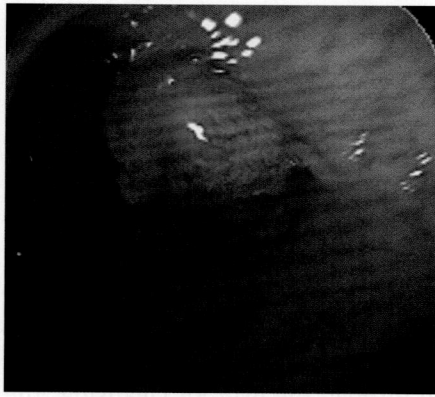

Figure 14-30 Endoscopic ultrasound for rectal cancer staging showing a rectal polyp.

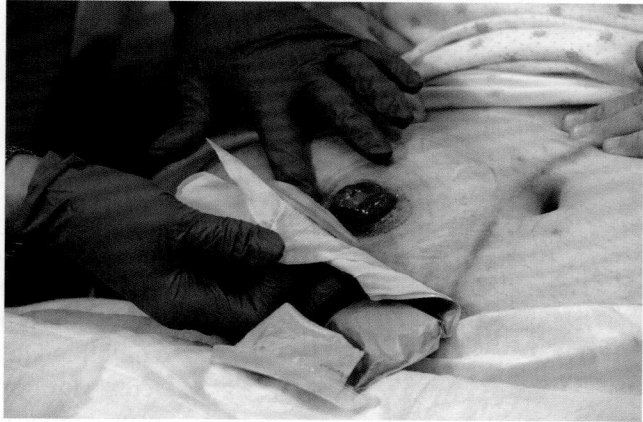

Figure 14-31 Changing a colostomy pouch on a patient.

KEY TERM	Definition
colitis (koh-LYE-tis)	inflammation of the colon
irritable bowel syndrome (IBS)	condition characterized by recurrent pain with constipation or diarrhea or alternating attacks of constipation and diarrhea
spastic colon (SPAS-tick KOH-lun)	nonspecific term used to describe symptoms such as abdominal pain, flatulence, and alternating diarrhea with constipation thought to occur as a result of increased muscular function of the colon
ulcerative colitis (UL-sur-uh-tiv koh-LYE-tis)	chronic disease of unknown cause characterized by ulceration of the colon and rectum with rectal bleeding, inflammation, abdominal pain, and diarrhea
colorectal cancer	general term for various cancers within the colon and/or rectum
dyspepsia (dis-PEP-see-uh)	indigestion
occult	hidden and only detectable by chemical or microscopic evaluation
fecal (FEE-kul) **occult blood test**	analysis of feces to determine the abnormal presence of blood in the stool
barium enema (BAIR-ee-um EN-e-muh) **(BE)**	the infusion of barium sulfate into the rectum and colon for diagnostic x-ray evaluation of the lower intestinal tract
colonoscopy (KOH-lun-OS-kuh-pee)	visual examination of the colon using a colonoscope
sigmoidoscopy (sig-moy-DOS-koh-pee)	visual examination of the sigmoid colon and rectum using a sigmoidoscope
colostomy (koh-LOS-tuh-mee)	surgical construction of an artificial opening between the colon and the exterior

KEY TERM PRACTICE: *Colon Disorders*

1. Inflammation of the colon is termed _____, which is derived from the word part _____, meaning *colon*, and the suffix _____, meaning *inflammation*.

2. A _____ describes a visual examination of the colon using a colonoscope

3. The medical term for indigestion is _____.

4. Introduction of barium sulfate into the rectum and colon for diagnostic x-ray evaluation of the lower intestinal tract describes a _____.

5. _____ is a condition characterized by recurrent pain with constipation or diarrhea or alternating attacks of constipation and diarrhea.

Liver Disorders

cirrhosis   **Cirrhosis** is a chronic, progressive liver disease marked by inflammation, degeneration, and regeneration with widespread fibrous tissue. The disease is characterized by the replacement of healthy hepatocytes with scar tissue, creating a nodular condition known as hobnail liver (**Figure 14-32**). The resultant scar tissue interferes with normal trickling of venous blood through the liver for cleansing. The causes range from idiopathic (no known origin) and exposure to toxic chemicals to chronic alcoholism, hepatitis, and parasites. Signs and symptoms include weight loss, decreased appetite, nausea, vomiting, indigestion, abnormal abdominal

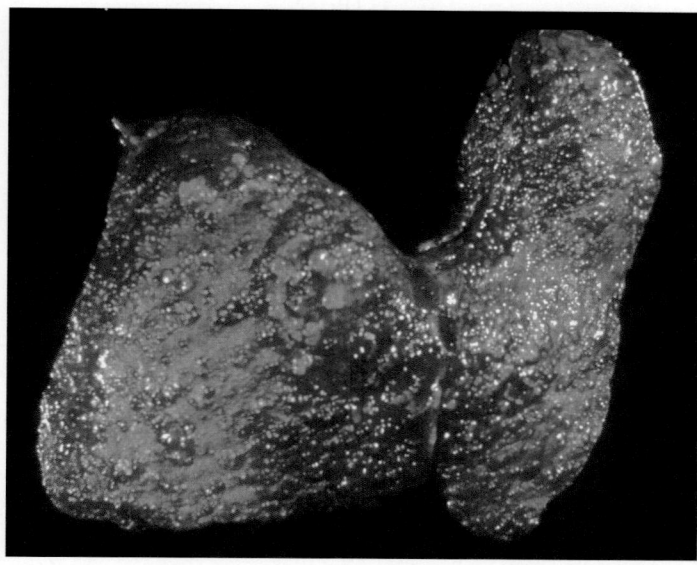

Figure 14-32 Alcoholic cirrhosis. The surface of the liver displays innumerable small, regular nodules.

distention, and jaundice. It is diagnosed by the history and physical examination, radiographic studies, blood studies demonstrating elevated liver enzymes and bilirubin, liver scan, and biopsy to determine extent of damage. Treatment includes prohibiting alcohol intake, nutrition therapy, and diuretics to reduce fluid. Liver transplant is the only cure.

hepatitis   Inflammation of the liver is termed **hepatitis**. Hepatitis is either viral or nonviral. Nonviral forms result from environmental toxins or drugs that adversely affect the liver, causing hepatitis. Viral forms have been categorized according to the six types that have been identified: A, B, C, D, E, and G. Each is abbreviated accordingly: hepatitis A virus (HAV), hepatitis B virus (HBV), hepatitis C virus (HCV), hepatitis D virus (HDV), hepatitis E virus (HEV), and hepatitis G virus (HGV). The three most common types are HAV, HBV, and HCV. Viral hepatitis now ranks as a major public health problem in industrialized nations.

- Hepatitis A, also known as infectious hepatitis, is transmitted through a fecal–oral route because it results from the ingestion of water or food contaminated with virus-infected feces.
- Hepatitis B is called serum hepatitis because the virus is transmitted through contact with infected blood, blood products, or body fluids.
- Hepatitis C, formerly referred to as non-A, non-B hepatitis, is transmitted through contaminated blood transfusion before 1990 (when testing began) or by sharing of contaminated needles among intravenous drug users. It can also be transmitted by needles used for body piercing or tattooing and from mother to fetus.
- Hepatitis D occurs in individuals already infected with hepatitis B, and its transmission is the same as hepatitis B.
- Hepatitis E is also transmitted via the fecal–oral route and occurs chiefly in the tropics.
- Hepatitis G is the most recently described hepatitis form. It occurs primarily in Asia, Africa, and South America.

Hepatitis is diagnosed through a hepatitis profile that identifies hepatitis antibodies. Hepatitis is treated symptomatically with plenty of bed rest. Immunoglobulin may be administered to lessen the severity of the disease. Vaccines are available against hepatitis A and hepatitis B.

KEY TERM	Definition
cirrhosis (si-ROH-sis)	chronic, progressive liver disease characterized by the replacement of hepatocytes with scar tissue
hepatitis (hep-uh-TYE-tis)	liver inflammation

KEY TERM PRACTICE: *Liver Disorders*

1. _____ is a chronic, progressive liver disease characterized by the replacement of hepatocytes with scar tissue.

2. The medical term for liver inflammation is _____ and is derived from the word part _____ for *liver* and the word part _____ for *inflammation*.

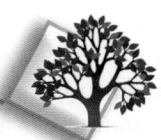

LIFE SPAN

The digestive system changes throughout life, beginning with its formation during embryonic development. By the eighth gestational week, a continuous tube runs from mouth to anus. Glandular organs develop as outpouchings of this tube.

Oral cavity changes are evident with age. During the first few years of life, primary teeth appear. They are later replaced by permanent teeth, starting around age 7 years. Dentition development is extremely variable. Some infants may be born with an erupted tooth, whereas some children may not develop their secondary teeth until they are in their teens. Childhood dentition is shown in **Figure 14-3A**.

Common age-associated changes include the wearing down of enamel and dentin, a decline in the number of taste buds, and decreased saliva production. Tooth loss and poor-fitting dentures are familiar complaints in the elderly and can lead to loss of appetite and subsequent malnutrition. Esophageal, gastric, and intestinal motility also lessen with age. Diminished intrinsic factor and HCl production are commonplace. Nutrient absorption is decreased because of impaired blood flow and motility. Although constipation is associated with old age, this is a myth. Age-related constipation is not caused by an aging GI tract but rather by lifestyle factors such as a low-fiber diet, decreased fluid intake, dehydration, and/or physical immobility.

Hepatocyte regeneration in the liver decreases, resulting in diminished liver size and weight. Liver function remains intact and underlying pathology generally causes alterations. Liver blood flow decreases with age, thereby affecting drug metabolism.

Other glandular organs may or may not demonstrate age-associated transformation. Anatomical pancreas changes consist of fatty acid deposits, fibrosis, and atrophy, but dysfunction is abnormal. No observable gallbladder changes accompany aging.

COMMON Abbreviations

Abbreviation	Term
Ach	acetylcholine
ADA	American Diabetes Association, American Dietetic Association
AN	anorexia nervosa
$BaSO_4$	barium sulfate
BE	barium enema
BM	bowel movement
BMI	body mass index
BMR	basal metabolic rate
BUN	blood, urea, nitrogen
C	carbon
cal	calorie
CBD	common bile duct
CCK	cholecystokinin
CDC	Centers for Disease Control and Prevention
CDR	Commission on Dietetic Registration
CF	cystic fibrosis
CHO	carbohydrate
$C_6H_{12}O_6$	glucose
CRF	chronic renal failure
CT	computerized tomography
ESRD	end-stage renal disease
ESWL	extracorporeal shock wave lithotripsy
GERD	gastroesophageal reflux disease
GI	gastrointestinal
HAV	hepatitis A virus
HBV	hepatitis B virus
HCl	hydrochloric acid
HCV	hepatitis C virus
HDV	hepatitis D virus
HEV	hepatitis E virus
HGV	hepatitis G virus
HSV-1	herpes simplex virus 1
IBD	inflammatory bowel disease
IBS	irritable bowel syndrome
kcal	kilocalorie
LD	licensed dietitian
LES	lower esophageal sphincter

continued

continued from page 735

Abbreviation	Term
MRI	magnetic resonance imaging
NHANES	National Health and Nutrition Examination Survey
NCHS	National Center for Health Statistics
NG	nasogastric
NSAID	nonsteroidal anti-inflammatory drug
PEM	protein-energy malnutrition
PKU	phenylketonuria
RD	registered dietitian
R/O	rule out
TMJ	temporomandibular joint
UGIS	upper gastrointestinal series

COMMON ABBREVIATIONS EXERCISES

1. CF is the abbreviation for _____.

2. PKU is the abbreviation for _____.

3. The abbreviation for temporomandibular joint is _____.

4. CCK is the abbreviation for _____.

5. The abbreviation for barium sulfate is _____.

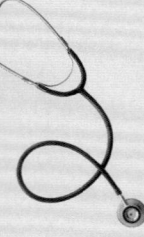

Case Study

Mr. Tom Lynn is a 67-year-old male with diabetes and end-stage renal disease (ESRD) who has just started hemodialysis. ESRD is characterized by scarred, atrophied kidneys with little to no function resulting from chronic renal failure (CRF). Unfortunately, it is a common manifestation of diabetes mellitus. Hemodialysis (hee-moh-dye-AL-i-sis) involves cleansing the blood through a semipermeable membrane. Dialysis refers to "the separation of substances in fluid." When the kidneys can no longer filter the blood, an artificial means in the form of hemodialysis is necessary to exchange the patient's "dirty" electrolyte-laden blood with clean, electrolyte-balanced blood.

continued

continued from page 736

As a newcomer to dialysis, Mr. Lynn must meet with Jane, the RD, to determine his nutrient needs while suffering from CRF. Actual nutrient amounts are highly individualized, and renal diets are challenging. The following table identifies the dietary nutrient parameters for a patient such as Mr. Lynn who is receiving hemodialysis.

Nutrient	Amount
energy (kcal/kg)	30–35
protein (g/kg)	1.2–1.4
fluid (mL)	500–750 plus daily urine output; 1,000 if anuric
sodium (g)	2–3
potassium (g/kg)	3–4
phosphorus (mg/g protein)	12–15
calcium (mg)	1,000–1,500

Mr. Lynn weighs 236 lb (107.04 kg). His medication list includes a specially formulated renal vitamin supplement and a phosphate binder to help maintain serum phosphorus between 4.5 and 6.0 mg/dL.

Case Study Questions

Select the best answer to each of the following questions.

1. **Hemodialysis refers to _____.**
   a. urine cleansing
   b. blood cleansing
   c. blood transfusion
   d. electrolyte equilibrium

2. **Sodium, potassium, phosphorus, and calcium are known collectively as _____.**
   a. organic compounds
   b. minerals
   c. electrolytes
   d. b and c

Calculate the answer for each of the following questions.

3. **To maintain a constant weight of 236 lb (107.04 kg), Mr. Lynn's energy requirements are determined by using the guidelines identified for a renal diet. If there are 2.2 kg per pound, what is his weight in kilograms? _____**

4. **What are Mr. Lynn's energy requirements in calories per kilogram?**
   _____

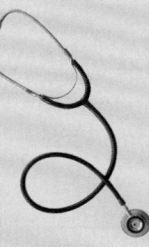

Real World Report

After Mr. Lynn had received dialysis for 5 months, Jane discussed the results of the latest report with him. The goals of nutrition therapy are to delay renal failure progression, prevent the toxic buildup of metabolic wastes, maintain the best possible nutrition status, and improve the patient's well-being.

MONTHLY HEMODIALYSIS—NUTRITIONAL STATUS LABORATORY REPORT

Patient Name:	Tom Lynn
Age:	67 years
Date:	August 30–September 30, 2011
Dry Weight:	95.70 kg
Dialysis Regimen:	M, W, F 12:30–17:30

Test (acceptable range)	Patient Results	Low	Normal	High
BUN (8–20 mg/dL)	10		X	
albumin (3.5–5.0 g/kg)	3.9		X	
potassium (3.5–6.0 g/kg)	6.6			X
phosphorus (4.5–6.0 mg/g protein)	7.4			X
calcium (9.5–11.5 mg)	9.5		X	
glucose (80–120 mg/dL)	102		X	
average fluid gain (2–4 lb [0.9–1.8 kg])	6.4		X	

Real World Report Questions

The following exercises review the medical terms used in the preceding medical report. Three terms may be unfamiliar: BUN (blood, urea, nitrogen) is a waste product of protein metabolism. Albumin is a blood protein used in clotting and warding off infection. Average fluid gain is the amount of fluid gained between dialysis treatments.

1. In which categories are Mr. Lynn's laboratory values abnormal? _____

2. On the day of the laboratory studies, what did Mr. Lynn weigh in kilograms? _____

3. According to the report, what was Mr. Lynn's average fluid gain between visits? _____

4. Potassium, phosphorus, and calcium are classified as _____.

5. Define glucose. _____

Review and Application

Multiple-Choice Questions

Select the best answer to each of the following questions.

1. The conversion of food into usable forms by the body is termed _____.
   a. digestion
   b. deglutition
   c. mastication
   d. defecation

2. The yellowish-green alkaline fluid that is secreted by the liver and stored in the gallbladder is called _____.
   a. chyme
   b. pulp
   c. bile
   d. dentin

3. The propelling movements by which food and digestive products move through the intestines is termed _____.
   a. mixing
   b. chyme
   c. propulsion
   d. peristalsis

4. _____ are the units of energy in food.
   a. Basal metabolic rates
   b. Calories
   c. Saccharides
   d. Catalysts

5. Organic compounds containing C, H, and O are called _____.
   a. vitamins
   b. minerals
   c. amino acids
   d. carbohydrates

6. Inorganic ions ingested for health and physiological functions are _____.
   a. fats
   b. fatty acids
   c. minerals
   d. vitamins

7. _____ is the storage form of glucose in muscle tissue.
   a. Sucrose
   b. Glycerol
   c. Glycogen
   d. Protein

8. A _____ is a ball of chewed food formed in the mouth.
   a. bolus
   b. pulp
   c. chyme
   d. dentin

9. Salivary glands located beneath the tongue are the _____.
   a. parotid glands
   b. submandibular glands
   c. sublingual glands
   d. masseter glands

10. The calcified substance covering a tooth crown is _____.
    a. cementum
    b. pulp
    c. dentin
    d. enamel

11. The three primary parts of a tooth are _____.
    a. crown, bone, and pulp
    b. root, neck, and crown
    c. root canal, periodontal ligament, and gingivae
    d. pulp cavity, cementum, and enamel

12. Excessive leanness due to muscle wasting is termed _____.
    a. emaciation
    b. bulimia
    c. anorexia
    d. marasmus

13. _____ is the medical term for inactive peristalsis that causes intestinal obstruction.
    a. Colitis
    b. Phenylketonuria
    c. Ileus
    d. Hernia

14. Folds in the stomach are termed _____.
    a. plicae
    b. rugae
    c. sphincters
    d. villi

15. The enzyme that breaks down fat is _____.
    a. lipase
    b. salivary amylase
    c. alcohol dehydrogenase
    d. nuclease

16. The _____ cells are pancreatic cells that secrete insulin.
    a. alpha   b. acinar   c. beta   d. delta

17. The duct formed by the union of the left hepatic duct and the right hepatic duct is the _____ duct.
    a. cystic   b. common hepatic   c. common bile   d. central

18. The _____ duct exits the gallbladder.
    a. common hepatic   b. common bile   c. cystic   d. pancreatic

19. _____ is the formation of glycogen from glucose, whereas _____ is the breaking down of glycogen back into glucose.
    a. Glycogenesis,   b. Glycogenolysis,   c. Glycogenesis,   d. Gluconeogenesis,
       glycogenolysis   glycogenesis   gluconeogenesis   glycogenesis

20. Inflammation of the gallbladder is known as _____.
    a. cholelithiasis   b. chylomicrons   c. cholecystokinin   d. cholecystitis

21. Microscopic, hair-like intestinal structures that increase the intestinal absorptive surface area are termed _____.
    a. lacteals   b. brush border   c. microvilli   d. micelles

22. _____ is the medical term for belching.
    a. Eructation   b. Bruxism   c. Flatus   d. Borborygmi

23. Small projections on the tongue are called _____.
    a. papillae   b. villi   c. microvilli   d. lobules

24. The section of the large intestine beginning at the cecum is the _____.
    a. anus   b. colon   c. rectum   d. anal canal

25. The hardened film of saliva, mucus, bacteria, and food on a tooth surface is called _____.
    a. gingiva   b. plaque   c. periodontal disease   d. oral leukoplakia

26. The _____ is the large intestine section between the sigmoid colon and the anal canal.
    a. rectum   b. anus   c. transverse colon   d. ascending colon

27. Identify the correct order of structures through which food travels in the GI tract. _____
    a. pharynx → esophagus → small intestine → stomach → large intestine
    b. esophagus → pharynx → small intestine → stomach → large intestine
    c. pharynx → esophagus → stomach → small intestine → large intestine
    d. esophagus → pharynx → stomach → small intestine → large intestine

28. This section of the small intestine is the location of most chemical digestion and nutrient absorption. _____
    a. duodenum   b. jejunum   c. ileum   d. ilium

29. The _____ is the largest visceral organ and functions in metabolism, digestion, and bile secretion.
    a. pancreas   b. small intestine   c. stomach   d. liver

30. A slow-healing sore on the surface of an organ or tissue resulting from a loss of tissue is called a(n) _____.
    a. hernia   b. abscess   c. ulcer   d. thrush

31. Gastric cells are found in the _____.
    a. stomach   b. colon   c. intestine   d. mouth

32. Hematochezia refers to _____.
    - a. mucus discharged from the rectum
    - b. passage of bloody stools
    - c. a bloody colon
    - d. hemorrhoids

33. Which term does not belong? _____
    - a. dyspepsia
    - b. colic
    - c. flatulence
    - d. truss

Word Parts Exercises

Using the following word parts, form a medical term for each definition. Each word part is used only once.

cec-	enter-	-itis
chol-	gastro-	-ology
-ectomy	gastro-	-pathy
-emia	hepat-	

34. stomach disease _____

35. inflammation of the cecum _____

36. surgical removal of the liver _____

37. presence of bile in the blood _____

38. study of the stomach and intestines _____

Matching Exercises

Match the disorder with its description.

_____ 39. anorexia nervosa

_____ 40. pancreatitis

_____ 41. phenylketonuria

_____ 42. primary malnutrition

_____ 43. marasmus

a. inflammation of the pancreas
b. lack of eating for fear of gaining weight
c. poor health resulting from an inadequate diet
d. severe malnutrition in infants and young children
e. hereditary metabolic disorder with phenylalanine hydroxylase deficiency

Match the disorder with its description.

_____ 44. strangulated hernia

_____ 45. diverticulitis

_____ 46. diverticulosis

_____ 47. celiac disease

_____ 48. irritable bowel syndrome

a. intestinal disease of gluten intolerance
b. presence of diverticula
c. inflammation of diverticula
d. alternating attacks of constipation and diarrhea
e. protrusion of intestine interfering with blood flow and fecal passage

Match the disorder with its description.

_____ 49. cirrhosis

_____ 50. dental caries

_____ 51. hiatal hernia

_____ 52. peptic ulcer

_____ 53. abscess

a. tooth decay or cavities
b. pus-filled cavity
c. chronic, scarred liver disease
d. protrusion of the stomach through the esophageal hiatus
e. sore on the upper GI tract membrane

Match the sign or symptom with its description

_____ 54. anorexia

_____ 55. halitosis

_____ 56. colic

_____ 57. melena

_____ 58. dysphagia

a. attack of abdominal pain caused by colonic spasms
b. loss of appetite
c. bad-smelling breath
d. difficulty swallowing
e. passage of dark, sticky feces

Match the sign or symptom with its description

_____ 59. gingivitis

_____ 60. peritonitis

_____ 61. steatorrhea

_____ 62. regurgitation

_____ 63. emaciation

a. excessive leanness caused by muscle wasting
b. greasy, fatty feces
c. inflammation of membrane lining the abdomen
d. inflammation of the gums
e. backflow of digestive juice into the esophagus

Match the clinical test or diagnostic procedure with its description.

_____ 64. barium enema

_____ 65. barium swallow

_____ 66. cholecystogram

_____ 67. cholangiogram

_____ 68. esophagoscopy

a. endoscopic examination of the esophagus
b. introduction of barium sulfate into the rectum and colon for diagnostic
   x-ray evaluation through the anus for diagnostic purposes
c. x-ray study of pharynx and esophagus after ingesting barium sulfate
d. x-ray of the gallbladder
e. radiograph of the bile ducts after dye introduction

Match the treatment with its description.

_____ 69. cholecystectomy

_____ 70. hemorrhoidectomy

_____ 71. truss

_____ 72. colostomy

_____ 73. herniorrhaphy

a. pressure-applying pad to support hernias
b. surgical repair of a hernia
c. artificial opening from the colon to the exterior
d. surgical removal of the gallbladder
e. surgical removal of hemorrhoids

Definitions

Define the following terms.

74. hepatomegaly _____

75. appendectomy _____

76. nutrients _____

77. root canal _____

78. gingivectomy _____

Provide a medical term for the following definitions.

79. swallowing _____

80. chewing _____

81. gums _____

82. belching, burping _____

Alternate Terms

Give an alternate term for each of the following terms.

83. fever blister _____

84. regional enteritis _____

85. canines _____

86. heartburn _____

87. premolars _____

88. canker sore _____

Spelling

Identify the correctly spelled term in each set.

89. _____
   a. kwashiorkor
   b. kwasiorkor
   c. kwashiorcor
   d. kwasshiorkor

90. _____
   a. esophagoscopy
   b. esofagoscopy
   c. esophigoscopy
   d. esophogoscopy

91. _____
   a. Vallsalva maneuver
   b. Valsalva maneuver
   c. Valselve maneuver
   d. Velsalva maneuver

92. _____
   a. accult
   b. ocult
   c. occalt
   d. occult

93. _____
   a. nasea
   b. nausa
   c. nauza
   d. nausea

94. _____
   a. flatulance
   b. flatalence
   c. flatulence
   d. flatullence

95. _____
   a. dafecation
   b. defecation
   c. defecetion
   d. deffecation

96. _____
   a. diarhea
   b. diarea
   c. diarrhea
   d. diarrhhea

Unscramble

Unscramble the letters to form a medical term.

97. robmigyrob _____

98. ntianicehrolgic _____

99. tagiilno _____

100. sitthepia _____

101. stiloic _____

102. aheinr _____

Abbreviations

Provide the term for the abbreviations and then define the terms.

103. CHO = _____

104. BMR = _____

105. IBS = _____

106. HAV = _____

107. IBD = _____

Analogies

Provide a medical term to complete a meaningful analogy.

108. Premolars are to bicuspids as canines are to _____.

109. Primary teeth are to _____ teeth as secondary teeth are to permanent teeth.

Short Answer

Answer the following questions.

110. A patient has been losing weight and experiencing bouts of vomiting. A barium swallow test showed the presence of the barium swallow still in the stomach 12 hours after ingestion. Provide an explanation for this occurrence.

_____

111. A patient has been diagnosed with lactose intolerance. Her physician explains that she may still enjoy milk products if she ingests commercially prepared lactase drops whenever she eats foods containing lactose. Why would lactase drops alleviate her symptoms?

_____

Labeling

Label the structures in the following diagram.

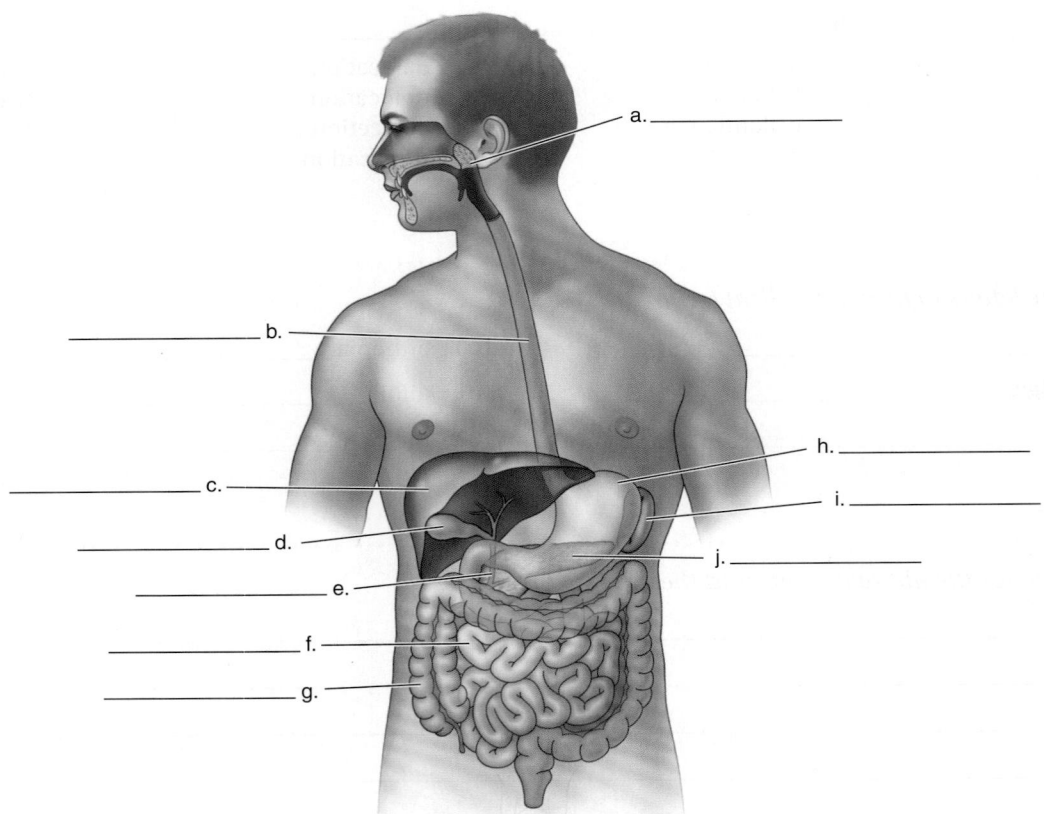

Word Search

Find the medical terms hidden in the puzzle.

R	N	H	H	P	N	W	P	E	S	I	C	B
I	E	Q	G	I	L	A	D	C	N	N	T	W
S	G	D	T	A	N	U	H	D	O	C	H	K
M	E	N	D	C	P	Y	P	S	I	I	R	K
A	E	L	R	A	M	P	U	D	S	S	U	A
D	F	E	U	E	L	G	E	P	E	O	S	I
M	A	V	L	B	A	B	F	N	H	R	H	D
S	W	E	V	H	O	X	L	N	D	S	N	R
G	R	P	P	J	Y	L	E	L	A	I	O	A
E	G	O	E	M	E	S	I	S	A	Z	X	C
Z	S	S	N	I	M	A	T	I	V	G	P	H
E	N	U	T	R	I	T	I	O	N	K	F	N
X	M	P	Z	S	E	C	E	F	A	A	W	T

adhesions
appendix
cardia
chyme
dentin
emesis
esophagus
feces
gallbladder
incisors
lobules
nutrition
pancreas
pulp
thrush
vitamins

Vocabulary Review

Review the key terms from this chapter, study the spelling and pronunciation of each term, and write its definition in the space provided. Listen to the audio available for most terms at http://thepoint.lww.com/nath2e and pronounce each term for yourself. Then check the box when you feel confident that you know the definition and can pronounce the term correctly.

Key Term	Pronunciation	Definition
❏ **abdominal hernia**	(ab-DOM-i-nul HUR-nee-uh)	
❏ **abscess**	(AB-ses)	
❏ **absorption**		
❏ **adhesions**	(ad-HEE-zhunz)	
❏ **alimentary canal**	(al-i-MEN-tuh-ree)	
❏ **amino acids**	(uh-MEE-noh)	
❏ **amylase**	(AM-il-ace)	
❏ **anal canal**		
❏ **anorexia**	(an-oh-RECK-see-uh)	
❏ **anorexia nervosa (AN)**	(an-oh-RECK-see-uh nur-VOH-suh)	
❏ **antacid**		
❏ **antibiotic**		
❏ **anticholinergics**	(an-tee-koh-lin-UR-jicks)	
❏ **anus**	(AY-nus)	

Key Term	Pronunciation	Definition
❏ aphtha	(AF-thuh)	
❏ appendicitis	(a-pen-di-SIGH-tis)	
❏ appendix		
❏ ascending colon	(KOH-lun)	
❏ barium enema (BE)	(BAIR-ee-um EN-e-muh)	
❏ barium swallow	(BAIR-ee-um)	
❏ basal metabolic rate (BMR)	(met-uh-BOL-ick)	
❏ bicuspids	(bye-KUS-pidz)	
❏ bile		
❏ body		
❏ bolus	(BOH-lus)	
❏ borborygmi	(bor-boh-RIG-migh)	
❏ bruxism	(BRUK-sizm)	
❏ bulimia	(bew-LIM-ee-uh)	
❏ calorie (cal)	(KAL-oh-ree)	
❏ carbohydrate		
❏ cardia	(KAHR-dee-uh)	
❏ catalysts	(KAT-uh-lists)	
❏ cecum	(SEE-kum)	
❏ celiac disease	(SEE-lee-ack)	
❏ cementum	(se-MEN-tum)	
❏ chemical digestion		
❏ cholangiogram	(kohl-AN-jee-oh-gram)	
❏ cholecystectomy	(koh-lee-sis-TECK-toh-mee)	
❏ cholecystitis	(koh-lee-sis-TIGH-tis)	
❏ cholecystogram	(kohl-ee-SIS-toh-gram)	
❏ cholelithiasis	(koh-lee-li-THIGH-uh-sis)	
❏ chyme	(KIME)	
❏ cirrhosis	(si-ROH-sis)	
❏ cold sores		
❏ colic	(KOL-ick)	
❏ colitis	(koh-LYE-tis)	
❏ colon	(KOH-lun)	
❏ colonoscopy	(KOH-lun-OS-kuh-pee)	
❏ colorectal cancer		
❏ colostomy	(koh-LOS-tuh-mee)	
❏ common bile duct (CBD)		
❏ common hepatic duct	(he-PAT-ick)	
❏ constipation		

Key Term	Pronunciation	Definition
❏ **Crohn disease**	(KROHN)	
❏ **crown**		
❏ **cryosurgery**	(krye-oh-SUR-juh-ree)	
❏ **cuspids**	(KUS-pidz)	
❏ **cystic duct**		
❏ **cystic fibrosis (CF)**	(SIS-tick figh-BROH-sis)	
❏ **deciduous teeth**	(de-SID-yoo-us)	
❏ **defecation**	(def-e-KAY-shun)	
❏ **deglutition**	(dee-gloo-TISH-un)	
❏ **dental caries**	(KAIR-eez)	
❏ **dentin**	(DEN-tin)	
❏ **descending colon**	(KOH-lun)	
❏ **diarrhea**	(dye-uh-REE-uh)	
❏ **digestion**		
❏ **diverticulitis**	(dye-vur-tick-yoo-LYE-tis)	
❏ **diverticulosis**	(dye-vur-tick-yoo-LOH-sis)	
❏ **diverticulum**	(dye-vur-TICK-yoo-lum)	
❏ **duodenal ulcer**	(dew-oh-DEE-nul UL-sur)	
❏ **duodenum**	(dew-oh-DEE-num)	
❏ **dyspepsia**	(dis-PEP-see-uh)	
❏ **dysphagia**	(dis-FAY-jee-uh)	
❏ **electrolytes**	(ee-LECK-troh-lites)	
❏ **emaciation**	(ee-may-see-AY-shun)	
❏ **emesis**	(EM-eh-sis)	
❏ **enamel**		
❏ **endoscope**	(EN-doh-skope)	
❏ **enzymes**		
❏ **eructation**	(ee-ruck-TAY-shun)	
❏ **esophageal hiatus**	(ee-sof-uh-JEE-ul high-AY-tus)	
❏ **esophageal varices**	(ee-sof-uh-JEE-ul VAIR-i-seez)	
❏ **esophagus**	(ee-SOF-uh-gus)	
❏ **extracorporeal shock wave lithotripsy (ESWL)**	(ecks-truh-kor-POH-ree-ul SHOCK WAVE lith-oh-TRIP-see)	
❏ **fecal incontinence**	(FEE-kul in-KON-ti-nence)	
❏ **fecal occult blood test**	(FEE-kul)	
❏ **feces**	(FEE-seez)	
❏ **flatulence**	(FLAT-yoo-lents)	
❏ **flexure**	(FLECK-shur)	
❏ **fundus**	(FUN-dus)	

Key Term	Pronunciation	Definition
❏ gallbladder		
❏ gallstones		
❏ gastric ulcer	(GAS-trick UL-sur)	
❏ gastroenteritis	(gas-troh-en-tur-EYE-tis)	
❏ gastroesophageal reflex disease (GERD)	(gas-troh-ee-sof-uh-JEE-ul)	
❏ gingiva	(JIN-ji-vuh)	
❏ gingivitis	(jin-ji-VYE-tis)	
❏ gluconeogenesis	(gloo-koh-nee-oh-JEN-e-sis)	
❏ glycogenesis	(glye-koh-JEN-e-sis)	
❏ glycogenolysis	(glye-koh-jen-OL-i-sis)	
❏ halitosis	(hal-i-TOH-sis)	
❏ heartburn		
❏ hematochezia	(hee-muh-toh-KEE-zee-uh)	
❏ hemorrhoidectomy	(hem-oh-roid-ECK-tuh-mee)	
❏ hemorrhoids	(HEM-uh-roidz)	
❏ hepatic portal vein	(he-PAT-ick)	
❏ hepatitis	(hep-uh-TYE-tis)	
❏ hepatocytes	(HEP-a-toh-sites)	
❏ hernia	(HUR-nee-uh)	
❏ herniorrhaphy	(hur-nee-OR-uh-fee)	
❏ hiatal hernia	(high-AY-tul HUR-nee-uh)	
❏ ileocecal valve	(il-ee-oh-SEE-kul)	
❏ ileum	(IL-ee-um)	
❏ ileus	(IL-ee-us)	
❏ immunosuppressant	(im-yoo-noh-suh-PRES-unt)	
❏ incisors	(in-SIGH-zurz)	
❏ inflammatory bowel disease (IBD)		
❏ ingestion	(in-JES-chun)	
❏ inguinal hernia	(ING-gwi-nul HUR-nee-uh)	
❏ intrinsic factor		
❏ irritable bowel syndrome (IBS)		
❏ jejunum	(je-JOO-num)	
❏ kwashiorkor	(kwah-shee-OR-kor)	
❏ laparoscope	(LAP-uh-roh-skope)	
❏ large intestine	(in-TES-tin)	
❏ ligation	(lye-GAY-shun)	
❏ lipase	(LIP-ace)	
❏ lipids	(LIP-ids)	

Key Term	Pronunciation	Definition
❏ liver		_____
❏ lobules	(LOB-yoolz)	_____
❏ lower esophageal sphincter	(ee-sof-uh-JEE-ul SFINK-tur)	_____
❏ malocclusion	(mal-oh-KLOO-zhun)	_____
❏ marasmus	(muh-RAZ-mus)	_____
❏ mastication	(mas-ti-KAY-shun)	_____
❏ McBurney point		_____
❏ mechanical digestion		_____
❏ melena	(me-LEE-nuh)	_____
❏ metabolism	(muh-TAB-oh-liz-um)	_____
❏ microvilli	(migh-kroh-VIL-eye)	_____
❏ minerals		_____
❏ molars	(MOH-lurz)	_____
❏ nasogastric (NG) tube	(nay-zoh-GAS-trick)	_____
❏ nausea	(NAW-zee-uh)	_____
❏ neck		_____
❏ necrotizing ulcerative gingivitis	(NECK-roh-tize-ing UL-sur-uh-tiv jin-ji-VYE-tis)	_____
❏ nutrients		_____
❏ nutrition		_____
❏ obesity		_____
❏ occult		_____
❏ oral leukoplakia	(lew-koh-PLAY-kee-uh)	_____
❏ orthodontics	(or-thoh-DON-ticks)	_____
❏ pancreas	(PAN-kree-us)	_____
❏ pancreatic duct	(pan-kree-AT-ick)	_____
❏ pancreatic juice	(pan-kree-AT-ick)	_____
❏ pancreatitis	(pan-kree-uh-TYE-tis)	_____
❏ papillae	(pa-PIL-ee)	_____
❏ parotid glands	(puh-ROT-id)	_____
❏ pepsin	(PEP-sin)	_____
❏ peptic ulcers	(PEP-tick UL-surs)	_____
❏ periodontal disease	(perr-ee-oh-DON-tul)	_____
❏ peristalsis	(perr-i-STAL-sis)	_____
❏ peritoneum	(perr-i-toh-NEE-um)	_____
❏ peritonitis	(perr-i-toh-NIGH-tis)	_____
❏ permanent teeth		_____
❏ phenylketonuria (PKU)	(fen-il-kee-toh-NEW-ree-uh)	_____
❏ plaque	(PLACK)	_____

Key Term	Pronunciation	Definition
❏ primary malnutrition		_____
❏ protein		_____
❏ pulp		_____
❏ pyloric sphincter	(pye-LOH-rick SFINK-tur)	_____
❏ pylorus	(pye-LOR-us)	_____
❏ pyrosis	(pye-ROH-sis)	_____
❏ rebound pain		_____
❏ rectum	(RECK-tum)	_____
❏ reducible hernia	(re-DEW-si-bul HUR-nee-uh)	_____
❏ regional enteritis	(en-tur-EYE-tis)	_____
❏ regurgitation	(ree-gur-ji-TAY-shun)	_____
❏ root canal		_____
❏ roots		_____
❏ rugae	(ROO-gee)	_____
❏ salivary glands	(SAL-i-verr-ee)	_____
❏ secondary malnutrition		_____
❏ serum gastrin test	(SEER-um GAS-trin)	_____
❏ sigmoid colon	(SIG-moid KOH-lun)	_____
❏ sigmoidoscopy	(sig-moy-DOS-koh-pee)	_____
❏ small intestine	(in-TES-tin)	_____
❏ spastic colon	(SPAS-tick KOH-lun)	_____
❏ steatorrhea	(stee-uh-toh-REE-uh)	_____
❏ stomach		_____
❏ strangulated hernia	(HUR-nee-uh)	_____
❏ sublingualglands	(sub-LING-gwul)	_____
❏ submandibular glands	(sub-man-DIB-yoo-lur)	_____
❏ temporomandibular joint (TMJ) syndrome	(tem-puh-roh-man-DIB-yoo-lur)	_____
❏ thrush		_____
❏ transverse colon	(KOH-lun)	_____
❏ truss		_____
❏ ulcer	(UL-sur)	_____
❏ ulcerative colitis	(UL-sur-uh-tiv koh-LYE-tis)	_____
❏ upper gastrointestinal series (UGIS)		_____
❏ uvula	(YOO-vew-luh)	_____
❏ Valsalva maneuver	(vahl-SAHL-vuh)	_____
❏ villi	(VIL-eye)	_____
❏ vitamins		_____

Answers

Word Grouping Exercises

Definition	Word Part	Definition	Word Part
appendix	appendico-	milk	galact-, galacto-
abdomen, belly	celio-, celo-	mouth	A. stom-, stomat-, stomato- B. oro-
anus, rectum	proct-, procto-	palate	palato-
bile	A. bili- B. chol-, chole-, cholo-	pancreas	pancreat-, pancreatico-, pancreato-, pancreo-
cecum	cec-, ceco-	peritoneum (abdominopelvic cavity lining)	peritoneo-
cheek	bucco-	pharynx	pharyng-, pharyngo-
chyle (milky fluid taken up by intestines)	chyl-, chylo-	pylorus, muscular opening	pylor-, pyloro-
colon	colo-	rectum	rect-, recto-
compound containing —NH₂	amino-	saliva, salivary glands	sial-, sialo-
duodenum	duoden-, duodeno-	salivary glands, saliva	ptyal-, ptyalo-
eating, devouring	-phagia	sigmoid, S-shaped	sigmoid-, sigmoido-
enzyme	-ase	starch	amyl-, amylo-
glucose, sugar	gluco-, glyco-	stomach	gastr-, gastro-
head	cephal-, cephalo-	stone, calculus	lith-, litho-
hernia	hernio-	sugar	sacchar-, sacchari-, saccharo-
ileum	ileo-	tongue	A. gloss-, glosso- B. linguo-
intestine	enter-, entero-	teeth, dental	dent-, denti-, dento-
jejunum	jejun-, jejuno-	uvula	uvul-, uvulo-
lipid, fat	lip-, lipo-	worm, worm-like	vermi-
liver	hepat-, hepato-		

Word Building Exercises

Word Part	Meaning	Common or Known Word	Example Medical Term
amino-	compound containing —NH₂	amino acid	amino acid
-ase	enzyme	lactase	maltase
bucco-	cheek	buccinator	buccal phase
cephal-, cephalo-	head	cephalic	cephalic phase
chol-, chole-, cholo-	bile	cholesterol	cholecystokinin
colo-	colon	colon	colon

Word Part	Meaning	Common or Known Word	Example Medical Term
dent-, denti-, dento-	teeth, dental	dentist	dentition
duoden-, duodeno-	duodenum	duodenum	duodenum
galact-, galacto-	milk	galactose	galactose
gastr-, gastro-	stomach	gastritis	gastric juice
gluco-, glyco-	glucose, sugar	glucose	gluconeogenesis
hepat-, hepato-	liver	hepatitis	hepatocytes
hernio-	hernia	herniated	herniorrhaphy
lip-, lipo-	lipid, fat	liposuction	lipase
pancreat-, pancreatico-, pancreato-, pancreo-	pancreas	pancreas	pancreatic
pharyng-, pharyngo-	pharynx	pharyngitis	pharyngeal phase
proct-, procto-	anus, rectum	proctologist	proctologist
sacchar-, sacchari-, saccharo-	sugar	saccharine	monosaccharide

Key Term Practice

Digestive System Preview

1. chemical digestion; mechanical digestion
2. alimentary canal
3. Digestion
4. peristalsis
5. Enzymes

Oral Cavity

1. papilla; papillae
2. uvula
3. below; tongue; sublingual
4. deglutition
5. bolus

Teeth

1. incisors, cuspids (canines), bicuspids (premolars), and molars
2. Cementum
3. gingiva
4. Enamel
5. crown

Esophagus

1. esophagus
2. esophageal hiatus
3. lower esophageal sphincter

Stomach

1. The four regions are the cardia, fundus, body, and pylorus.
2. Intrinsic factor
3. Rugae
4. Pepsin
5. eructation

Small Intestine

1. duodenum, jejunum, and ileum
2. microvillus, microvilli
3. villus, villi
4. small intestine

Pancreas

1. pancreas
2. pancreatic juice
3. pancreatic duct

Liver and Gallbladder

1. common bile duct (CBD)
2. glycogenolysis; *glyco-;-lysis*
3. Gluconeogenesis; *gluco-;neo-;-genesis*
4. hepatocytes; *hepato-;-cytes*
5. gallbladder

Large Intestine

1. ascending colon, transverse colon, descending colon, and sigmoid colon
2. defecation
3. feces
4. appendix
5. rectum

Nutrition

1. amino acids
2. carbohydrates, lipids, proteins, vitamins, minerals, water
3. Nutrition
4. basal metabolic rate (BMR)
5. calorie

Oral Cavity Disorders

1. thrush
2. oral leukoplakia; *oral*; *leuko-*
3. Aphtha
4. malocclusion
5. Halitosis

Ulcers

1. ulcer
2. gastric; *gastr-*
3. antacid
4. heartburn; pyrosis
5. Regurgitation

Appendicitis

1. diarrhea
2. Appendicitis
3. Rebound pain
4. nausea
5. McBurney point

Gallbladder Disorders

1. cholelithiasis
2. Cholangiogram
3. colic
4. cholecystitis; *chole-*;*-itis*
5. cholecystectomy; *chole-*;*-ectomy*

Pancreas Disorders

1. *pancreat-*; inflammation; pancreatitis
2. anorexia
3. cystic fibrosis (CF)
4. nasogastric (NG) tube

Eating, Nutritional, and Metabolic Disorders

1. Bulimia
2. primary malnutrition
3. secondary malnutrition
4. Emaciation
5. Anorexia nervosa (AN)

Gastroesophageal Disorders

1. gastroesophageal reflux disease
2. esophageal varices
3. upper gastrointestinal series (UGIS)
4. dysphagia
5. endoscope

Hernias

1. hiatal hernia
2. herniorrhaphy; hernia
3. truss
4. inguinal hernia
5. reducible hernia

Small Intestine Diseases

1. gastroenteritis; *gastro-*; *enter-*; *-itis*
2. steatorrhea
3. Celiac disease

Large Intestine Disorders

1. *peritoneo-*;*-itis*; peritonitis
2. cryosurgery
3. diverticulum, diverticula
4. Adhesions
5. hemorrhoidectomy

Colon Disorders

1. colitis; *colo-*;*-itis*
2. colonoscopy
3. dyspepsia
4. barium enema (BE)
5. Irritable bowel syndrome (IBS)

Liver Disorders

1. Cirrhosis
2. hepatitis; *hepat-*;*-itis*

Common Abbreviations Exercises

1. CF = cystic fibrosis
2. PKU = phenylketonuria
3. temporomandibular joint = TMJ
4. CCK = cholecystokinin
5. Barium sulfate = $BaSO_4$

Case Study

1. b is the correct answer.
   - a is incorrect because *hemo-* refers to "blood" and *dialysis* refers to the "separation of substances in a fluid."
   - c is incorrect because no blood is being transfused, which involves the administration of blood from one person into the bloodstream of another person; Mr. Lynn's own blood is being removed, cleansed, and returned to him.
   - d is incorrect because although electrolyte balance is achieved through hemodialysis, the equilibrium is short-lived; Mr. Lynn would have to be on continuous dialysis to maintain that balance.
2. d is the correct answer.
   - a is incorrect because organic compounds contain carbon; sodium, potassium, phosphorus, and calcium are inorganic elements.
3. Mr. Lynn weighs 107.27 kg, which is calculated by dividing 236 lb by 2.2 kg: 236/2.2 = 107.27.
4. Mr. Lynn's energy requirements are between 3,218.10 and 3,754.45 cal. The energy parameters for Mr. Lynn are 30 to 35 cal/kg, and his weight is 107.27 kg: $107.27 \times 30 = 3{,}218.10$ for the lower limit and $107.27 \times 35 = 3{,}754.45$ for the upper limit.

Real World Report

1. potassium, phosphorus, and average fluid gain—all are too high
2. 95.70 kg
3. 6.4 lb. (2.9 kg)
4. minerals or electrolytes
5. a simple carbohydrate with the chemical formula $C_6H_{12}O_6$; the body's primary fuel source

Review and Application

1. a	13. c	25. b	37. cholemia
2. c	14. b	26. a	38. gastroenterology
3. d	15. a	27. c	39. b
4. b	16. c	28. b	40. a
5. d	17. b	29. d	41. e
6. c	18. c	30. c	42. c
7. c	19. a	31. a	43. d
8. a	20. d	32. b	44. e
9. c	21. c	33. d	45. c
10. d	22. a	34. gastropathy	46. b
11. b	23. a	35. cecitis	47. a
12. a	24. b	36. hepatectomy	48. d

49. c
50. a
51. d
52. e
53. b
54. b
55. c
56. a
57. e
58. d
59. d
60. c
61. b
62. e
63. a
64. b
65. c
66. d
67. e
68. a
69. d
70. e
71. a
72. c
73. b
74. hepatomegaly = enlargement of liver
75. appendectomy = removal of appendix
76. nutrients = chemical substances in food that include carbohydrates, proteins, lipids, vitamins, minerals, and water
77. root canal = tooth cavity in the root containing pulp, nerves, and blood vessels
78. gingivectomy = excision of gum tissue
79. swallowing = deglutition
80. chewing = mastication
81. gums = gingivae
82. belching, burping = eructation
83. cold sores
84. Crohn disease
85. cuspids
86. pyrosis
87. bicuspids

88. aphtha
89. a
90. a
91. b
92. d
93. d
94. c
95. b
96. c
97. borborygmi
98. anticholinergic
99. ligation
100. hepatitis
101. colitis
102. hernia
103. CHO = carbohydrate; organic compound containing carbon, hydrogen, and oxygen and includes sugar, starch, and cellulose
104. BMR = basal metabolic rate; quantity of energy the body expends performing basic physiological tasks
105. IBS = irritable bowel syndrome; condition characterized by recurrent pain with constipation or diarrhea or alternating attacks of constipation and diarrhea
106. HAV = hepatitis A virus; causative agent for viral hepatitis A
107. IBD = inflammatory bowel disease; general term for bowel disorders that cause irritation, swelling, and tenderness
108. cuspids
109. deciduous
110. The barium sulfate is not able to exit the stomach because of an obstruction, most likely at the pyloric sphincter. So, the stomach contents remain in the stomach. This would explain the vomiting; and because no nutrients are absorbed across the gastric mucous membrane, this provides an explanation for the weight loss as well.
111. The lactase drops supply the missing enzyme, lactase, which is necessary for the digestion of milk sugar. Hence, the patient may still eat milk products as long as she takes the required enzyme.

Labeling

a. salivary gland   b. esophagus   c. liver

d. gallbladder   e. common bile duct   f. small intestine

g. large intestine   h. stomach   i. spleen

j. pancreas

Word Search

R	N	H	H	P	N	W	P	E	S	I	C	B
I	E	Q	G	I	L	A	D	C	N	N	T	W
S	G	D	T	A	N	U	H	D	O	C	H	K
M	E	N	D	C	P	Y	P	S	I	I	R	K
A	E	L	R	A	M	P	U	D	S	S	U	A
D	F	E	U	E	L	G	E	P	E	O	S	I
M	A	V	L	B	A	B	F	N	H	R	H	D
S	W	E	V	H	O	X	L	N	D	S	N	R
G	R	P	P	J	Y	L	E	L	A	I	O	A
E	G	O	E	M	E	S	I	S	A	Z	X	C
Z	S	S	N	I	M	A	T	I	V	G	P	H
E	N	U	T	R	I	T	I	O	N	K	F	N
X	M	P	Z	S	E	C	E	F	A	A	W	T

adhesions
appendix
cardia
chyme
dentin
emesis
esophagus
feces
gallbladder
incisors
lobules
nutrition
pancreas
pulp
thrush
vitamins

Vocabulary Review

Key Term	Definition	Key Term	Definition
abdominal hernia	abnormal protrusion of an organ through the abdominal wall	**antacid**	agent that neutralizes acid
abscess	pus-filled cavity created by bacterial infection and inflammation	**antibiotic**	medicine that inhibits bacterial growth or kills bacteria
absorption	passage of nutrients from the digestive tract into the blood or lymph for distribution to body	**anticholinergics**	drugs that block or neutralize the effects of the neurotransmitter acetylcholine (Ach)
adhesions	intestinal bands of scar tissue	**anus**	opening to the exterior through which feces exit the body
alimentary canal	digestive tube from the mouth to the anus	**aphtha**	white oral ulcer of unknown cause; also called a canker sore
amino acids	the building blocks of proteins	**appendicitis**	inflammation of the appendix with severe pain
amylase	starch-breaking enzyme	**appendix**	small worm-like lymphatic structure projecting from and opening into the cecum
anal canal	portion of the large intestine between the rectum and the anus	**ascending colon**	section of the large intestine from the cecum to the right colic (hepatic) flexure
anorexia	loss of appetite	**barium enema (BE)**	the infusion of barium sulfate into the rectum and colon for diagnostic x-ray evaluation of the lower intestinal tract
anorexia nervosa (AN)	psychological disorder characterized by not eating because of morbid fear of weight gain		

Key Term	Definition	Key Term	Definition
barium swallow	radiographic study of the pharynx and esophagus after swallowing barium sulfate	**cold sores**	small painful blisters in the mouth or on the surrounding lips caused by herpes simplex virus 1 (HSV-1); also called a fever blister
basal metabolic rate (BMR)	quantity of energy the body expends performing basic physiological tasks	**colic**	attack of abdominal pain caused by colonic spasms
bicuspids	teeth with two points; also called premolars	**colitis**	inflammation of the colon
bile	yellowish-green alkaline fluid secreted by the liver and passed into the duodenum	**colon**	main part of large intestine, beginning at the cecum and ending at the rectum
body	largest region of stomach between the fundus and the pylorus	**colonoscopy**	visual examination of the colon using a colonoscope
bolus	ball of chewed food	**colorectal cancer**	general term for various cancers within the colon and/or rectum
borborygmi	rumbling or gurgling noises produced by movement of gas and/or fluid in the GI tract	**colostomy**	surgical construction of an artificial opening between the colon and the exterior
bruxism	unconscious habit of clenching and grinding the teeth that occurs during sleep or in stressful situations and leads to excessive wear on the teeth	**common bile duct (CBD)**	duct formed by the union of the cystic duct and the hepatic duct
		common hepatic duct	duct formed by the union of the left hepatic duct and right hepatic duct
bulimia	psychological disorder characterized by binge eating and self-induced purging; also called bulimia nervosa	**constipation**	difficulty emptying the bowels or infrequent bowel movements
calorie (cal)	the energy value in food	**Crohn disease**	chronic inflammatory disorder of the intestines, usually affecting the terminal ileum, but possibly affecting other parts of the gastrointestinal tract; also called regional enteritis
carbohydrate	organic compound containing carbon, hydrogen, and oxygen and includes sugar, starch, and cellulose		
cardia	smallest stomach area adjacent to the esophagus	**crown**	exposed part of a tooth
catalysts	chemicals that speed up chemical reactions without being changed or used up in the process	**cryosurgery**	surgery in which extremely cold temperature is applied to destroy tissue or stop bleeding
cecum	pouch where the large intestine begins	**cuspids**	teeth with only one point; also called canines
celiac disease	malabsorption disorder caused by gluten sensitivity that hinders the digestive system's ability to metabolize fat; also called celiac sprue	**cystic duct**	duct of the gallbladder
		cystic fibrosis (CF)	hereditary disease associated with dysfunction of the exocrine glands and respiratory structures
cementum	thin layer of bony tissue covering the dentin of the roots and neck of a tooth	**deciduous teeth**	the 20 early teeth that are shed and replaced by permanent teeth; also called primary teeth
chemical digestion	the breaking down of food by enzymes		
		defecation	bowel movement
cholangiogram	x-ray of the bile ducts after introduction of a contrast dye	**deglutition**	swallowing
		dental caries	cavities or tooth decay
cholecystectomy	surgical removal of the gallbladder	**dentin**	calcified substance underneath the tooth enamel
cholecystitis	inflammation of the gallbladder		
cholecystogram	x-ray of the gallbladder	**descending colon**	section of the large intestine between the left colic (splenic) flexure and the sigmoid colon
cholelithiasis	presence of calculi in the gallbladder or bile ducts; also called gallstones		
		diarrhea	increased frequency of watery feces
chyme	semisolid paste formed in the stomach that is a mixture of gastric juice and food	**digestion**	the conversion of food into usable substances through the actions of enzymes and movements
cirrhosis	chronic, progressive liver disease characterized by the replacement of hepatocytes with scar tissue		
		diverticulitis	inflammation of the diverticula

Key Term	Definition
diverticulosis	presence of diverticula (abnormal pouches in the bowel)
diverticulum	abnormal pouch or sac opening from the intestine
duodenal ulcer	sore on the duodenum lining
duodenum	first section of small intestine beginning at the stomach
dyspepsia	indigestion
dysphagia	difficulty swallowing
electrolytes	minerals (ions) dissolved in solution and circulating in body fluids
emaciation	excessive leanness caused by muscle wasting
emesis	vomiting
enamel	calcified substance covering the tooth's crown
endoscope	fiberoptic scope used for viewing inside the body
enzymes	proteins that promote biochemical reactions
eructation	belching, burping
esophageal hiatus	opening in the diaphragm for the esophagus to pass through
esophageal varices	twisted, swollen veins in the esophagus
esophagus	muscular tube connecting the pharynx to the stomach
extracorporeal shock wave lithotripsy (ESWL)	fragmentation of stones using ultrasound shock waves so that the pulverized pieces can pass naturally
fecal incontinence	inability to control defecation
fecal occult blood test	analysis of feces to determine the abnormal presence of blood in the stool
feces	solid waste matter eliminated from the bowel during defecation
flatulence	excessive amount of gas in the GI tract
flexure	bend
fundus	dome-shaped stomach region
gallbladder	sac-like organ on the undersurface of the liver that stores bile
gallstones	presence of calculi in the gallbladder or bile ducts; also called cholelithiasis
gastric ulcer	sore on the stomach lining with inflammation
gastroenteritis	inflammation of the mucous membrane of both the stomach and intestine; also called traveler's diarrhea
gastroesophageal reflex disease (GERD)	regurgitation of acidic gastric juice into the esophagus
gingiva	mucous membrane surrounding the teeth; also called the gum

Key Term	Definition
gingivitis	inflammation of the gingivae (gums) around the roots of the teeth
gluconeogenesis	glucose formation from noncarbohydrates, such as proteins and fats
glycogenesis	glycogen formation from glucose
glycogenolysis	breaking down glycogen into glucose
halitosis	bad-smelling breath
heartburn	burning or warm sensation felt just below the sternum that results from regurgitation of gastric juice into the esophagus; another term for pyrosis
hematochezia	passage of bloody stools
hemorrhoidectomy	surgical removal of hemorrhoids
hemorrhoids	painful varicose veins in the lower rectum or anal wall
hepatic portal vein	vessel that delivers blood from the digestive system to the liver
hepatitis	liver inflammation
hepatocytes	liver cells
hernia	abnormal protrusion of an organ through the wall of its cavity
herniorrhaphy	surgical repair of a hernia
hiatal hernia	protrusion of the stomach through the esophageal hiatus (opening in diaphragm)
ileocecal valve	circular muscle (sphincter) between the ileum and the cecum
ileum	last section of small intestine, leading to the large intestine
ileus	obstruction of the intestines (or inactive peristalsis) causing failure to pass feces
immunosuppressant	drug that inhibits the immune response
incisors	front cutting teeth (four in upper jaw, four in lower jaw)
inflammatory bowel disease (IBD)	general term for bowel disorders that cause irritation, swelling, and tenderness
ingestion	taking food into the body; eating
inguinal hernia	abnormal protrusion of an organ through the inguinal canal in the groin region
intrinsic factor	substance secreted by stomach cells that promotes the absorption of vitamin B_{12} in the small intestine
irritable bowel syndrome (IBS)	condition characterized by recurrent pain with constipation or diarrhea or alternating attacks of constipation and diarrhea
jejunum	middle section of small intestine; location of most chemical digestion and nutrient absorption

Key Term	Definition
kwashiorkor	malnutrition in children characterized by ascites and caused by deficiency of calories in general and of protein in particular
laparoscope	instrument used to view the inside of the body through a small incision
large intestine	portion of the intestine between the small intestine and the anus that forms, stores, and expels waste matter
ligation	tying a bleeding vessel with a knotted surgical ligature
lipase	fat-breaking enzyme
lipids	organic nutrients consisting of fats and oils
liver	largest visceral organ that secretes bile and plays a role in many metabolic functions
lobules	functional units of liver that contain hepatocytes
lower esophageal sphincter	circular band of muscle between the stomach and the esophagus that prevents backflow of stomach contents into the esophagus
malocclusion	abnormal positioning of the upper and lower teeth when closing the jaw
marasmus	malnutrition in infants and young children characterized by loss of subcutaneous fat and wrinkled skin and caused by prolonged nutritional deficiency
mastication	chewing
McBurney point	site of extreme tenderness over the appendix, indicating appendicitis
mechanical digestion	the breaking down of food by forces of movement
melena	passage of dark, sticky feces containing partly digested blood
metabolism	all chemical and physical activity in the body, consisting of anabolism (building processes) and catabolism (breakdown processes)
microvilli	hair-like projections that increase the absorptive surface area of intestines
minerals	inorganic ions functioning as electrolytes
molars	teeth that grind and pulverize food
nasogastric (NG) tube	small tube inserted through the nose to the stomach for feeding purposes
nausea	unsettled feeling in the stomach with the urge to vomit
neck	area between the crown and the root of a tooth
necrotizing ulcerative gingivitis	painful ulcerative condition of the mouth caused by normal mouth microorganisms
nutrients	chemical substances in food that include carbohydrates, proteins, lipids, vitamins, minerals, and water
nutrition	branch of science that deals with nutrients in health and disease
obesity	body weight 20% or more in excess of ideal weight for a person's sex and height
occult	hidden and only detectable by chemical or microscopic evaluation
oral leukoplakia	abnormal thickening and whitening of mucous membranes in the mouth
orthodontics	dentistry concerned with the prevention and correction of teeth irregularities
pancreas	gland with endocrine and exocrine functions sandwiched between the stomach and the small intestine
pancreatic duct	pancreas excretory tube emptying into the duodenum
pancreatic juice	alkaline secretion from the pancreas that contains digestive enzymes
pancreatitis	pancreas inflammation
papillae	small projections on the tongue
parotid glands	salivary glands in front of and below the external ears
pepsin	a protein-digesting enzyme
peptic ulcers	sores in the digestive tract caused by excessive secretion of acid and the digestive action of pepsin
periodontal disease	pathology of the tissues that surround the neck and root of a tooth, including the underlying bone
peristalsis	progressive waves of involuntary muscle contractions in the digestive tract
peritoneum	membrane that lines the abdominopelvic cavity and covers the internal organs contained within the cavity
peritonitis	inflammation of the peritoneum
permanent teeth	the 32 adult teeth; also called the secondary teeth
phenylketonuria (PKU)	hereditary metabolic disorder characterized by a deficiency of phenylalanine hydroxylase
plaque	hardened film of saliva, mucus, bacteria, and food residue on the tooth surface
primary malnutrition	poor health resulting from an inadequate diet
protein	a dietary compound made of amino acids
pulp	soft interior of the tooth
pyloric sphincter	circular muscle enclosing pylorus between the stomach and the small intestine
pylorus	region of the stomach opening into the small intestine

Key Term	Definition
pyrosis	burning or warm sensation felt just below the sternum that results from regurgitation of gastric juice into the esophagus; another term for heartburn
rebound pain	soreness that is greater at a site after the pressure to that site has been removed
rectum	section of the large intestine between the sigmoid colon and the anal canal
reducible hernia	abnormal protrusion of an organ through the wall of its cavity that can be physically manipulated back into normal position
regional enteritis	chronic inflammatory disorder of the intestines, usually affecting the terminal ileum, but possibly affecting other parts of the gastrointestinal tract; also called Crohn disease
regurgitation	backflow of digestive juice into the esophagus
root canal	tooth cavity in the root containing pulp, nerves, and blood vessels
roots	parts of teeth embedded in tissue that anchor teeth to bone
rugae	stomach folds that allow the stomach to distend
salivary glands	exocrine structures that secrete saliva
secondary malnutrition	poor health resulting from a disease process that makes a normally healthy diet inadequate
serum gastrin test	test for levels of the gastric and intestinal hormone, gastrin, in blood serum
sigmoid colon	section of the large intestine between the descending colon and the rectum
sigmoidoscopy	visual examination of the sigmoid colon and rectum using a sigmoidoscope
small intestine	segment of gastrointestinal tract between stomach and large intestine involved with nutrient absorption
spastic colon	nonspecific term used to describe symptoms such as abdominal pain, flatulence, and alternating diarrhea with constipation thought to occur as a result of increased muscular function of the colon

Key Term	Definition
steatorrhea	greasy, fatty feces
stomach	organ in which food is stored after swallowing and that aids in mechanical and chemical digestion
strangulated hernia	interruption of blood flow in an abnormal protrusion of the intestine, possibly leading to fecal obstruction and gangrene
sublingual glands	salivary glands beneath the tongue
submandibular glands	salivary glands below the mandible (lower jaw)
temporo-mandibular joint (TMJ) syndrome	inflammation of the temporal bone and mandible articulation characterized by limited jaw movement and pain
thrush	*Candida albicans* fungal infection of the mouth characterized by white patches
transverse colon	section of the large intestine between the right colic (hepatic) flexure and the left colic (splenic) flexure
truss	pad attached to a belt that applies pressure to a reduced hernia to prevent recurrence or to prevent the increase in size of a hernia
ulcer	slow-healing sore on the surface of an organ or tissue resulting from loss of tissue
ulcerative colitis	chronic disease of unknown cause characterized by ulceration of the colon and rectum with rectal bleeding, inflammation, abdominal pain, and diarrhea
upper gastrointestinal series (UGIS)	x-rays of the esophagus, stomach, and duodenum after swallowing barium sulfate
uvula	fleshy appendage hanging from the soft palate at the entrance to the throat
Valsalva maneuver	action of exhaling when the mouth and nostrils are closed, increasing internal pressure and causing a hernia to become more pronounced
villi	finger-like projections from the interior intestinal wall
vitamins	essential organic nutrients necessary for normal metabolism

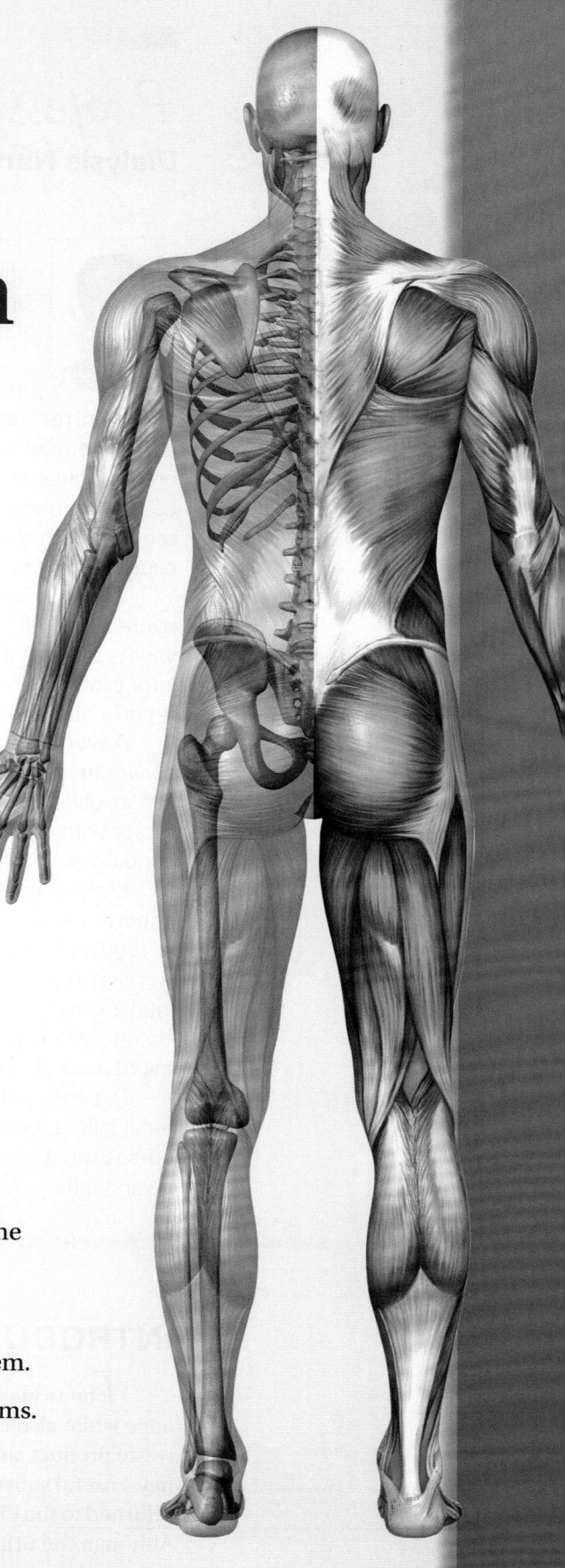

C H A P T E R 15

Urinary System

O B J E C T I V E S

After completing this chapter, you should be able to:

1. State the meanings of word parts related to the urinary system.

2. Identify the organs of the urinary system.

3. Cite the primary functions of each organ in the system.

4. Trace the pathway of urine through the urinary system.

5. Define common signs, symptoms, and treatments of various urinary system diseases.

6. Explain clinical tests and diagnostic procedures related to the urinary system.

7. Describe anatomical and physiological alterations throughout the life span.

8. Define common abbreviations related to the urinary system.

9. Define terms used in medical reports involving the urinary system.

10. Correctly define, spell, and pronounce the chapter's medical terms.

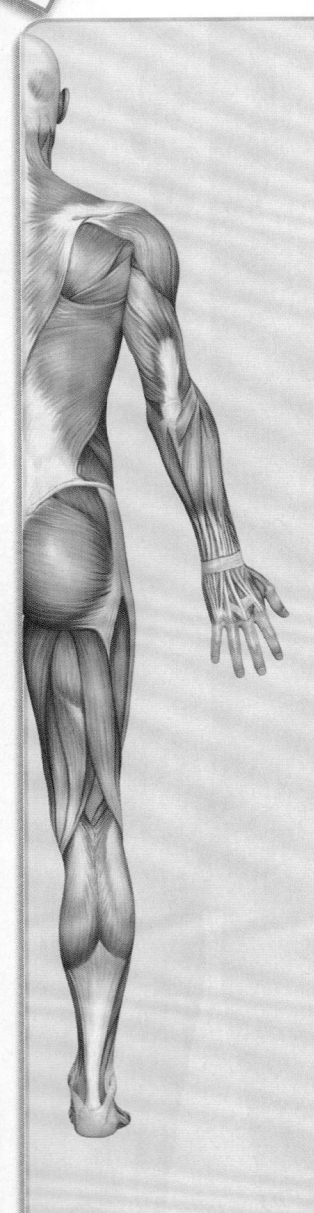

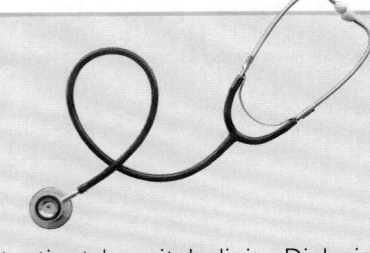

Professional Profile

Dialysis Nurse

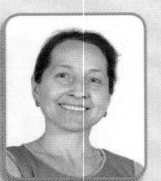

I'm Debbie, a dialysis nurse in an outpatient hospital clinic. Dialysis involves cleansing the blood when the kidneys are no longer functioning to capacity, and it is a necessary treatment for patients with kidney failure. A typical dialysis schedule for a patient is three times per week.

To be a dialysis nurse, I had to complete the requirements for the registered nurse (RN) degree, pass the required licensure examination, and then receive advanced training in urology, the study of the urogenital system. Dialysis nurses work closely with nephrologists, physicians specializing in kidney disorders. Patients receiving dialysis treatment are in various stages of renal distress, usually from the ravages of diseases like diabetes. As a dialysis nurse, I must carefully monitor both the dialysis equipment and the patient who is receiving treatment, because blood pressure and other vital signs fluctuate during the procedure.

I consult with the doctor to analyze the patient's kidney function and the effectiveness of the dialysis treatment. I must also gather the relevant information from a variety of tests. The patient's age, urinary output, weight, blood pressure, blood chemistry profiles, and urinalysis information are all important to the evaluation. Diagnostic reports often come from the radiologist's office.

A working knowledge of medical terminology that goes beyond the kidney is necessary in my job. For example, diabetes, which affects a majority of dialysis patients, can involve almost every body system. As a dialysis nurse, I must be able to communicate with other health care professionals in various medical specialties about patient conditions.

Dialysis nurses educate patients about kidney anatomy and physiology, citing the importance of blood pressure monitoring, because the kidneys play an important role in regulating blood pressure. The role of nutrition is also important, so those of us working in a dialysis clinic need to be able to explain the importance of limiting protein intake when kidney function is compromised. I also explain how kidney function can change with age and how it can be affected by various diseases and conditions that might arise as a person gets older.

Patients on dialysis are generally quite sick, and the death rate is high as a result of renal failure. Once the kidneys begin to fail, other body systems follow suit. So dialysis nurses must be prepared to work with patients who are subject to both a high morbidity and a high mortality rate.

INTRODUCTION

*T*he urinary system plays an important role in maintaining fluid and electrolyte balance while also ridding the body of physiological wastes, toxins, and drugs. Urine is a main waste product, and its formation begins with blood. As blood circulates through the two kidneys, useful substances are separated from useless ones. The substances the body can use are returned to the bloodstream and the remainder becomes urine for excretion outside the body. Although the urinary system has coordinated activities with other body systems, the kidneys begin the job of urine formation, and the ureters, bladder, and urethra complete the job of urine elimination.

The genital and urinary organs are collectively known as the genitourinary system. Abnormalities of this system are usually the result of primary kidney (renal) disorders or are secondary to a systemic disease, such as diabetes. Clinical and laboratory diagnostics are used to evaluate genitourinary pathology, which generally exhibits particular signs and symptoms. This chapter describes the basic anatomy and physiology of the urinary system and provides information relevant to disorders of this system.

MEDICAL TERM PARTS

Word Parts

Medical term prefixes, suffixes, and combining forms related to the urinary system are introduced in this section.

Word Part	Meaning
azo-	nitrogen
cyst-, cysti-, cysto-	bladder
glyco-	sugar
hem-, hema-	blood
hydr-, hydro-	water
juxta-	adjacent
keto-	containing a ketone group (chemical compound)
lith-, -lith, litho-	stone
meato-	passage
micturit-	urinated
nephr-, nephro-	kidney
noct-	night
olig-, oligo-	few, little
papillo-	small, rounded projection
prox-, proxi-, proximo-	nearest, next to
-ptosis	drooping, sinking down
pyel-, pyelo-	pelvis
pyo-	pus
reni-, reno-	kidney
scler-, sclero-	hard
ure-, uro-	urine
uretero-	related to ureter (urinary tube)
urethr-, urethro-	urethra
-uria	present in urine
urin-, urino-	urine
vas-, vaso-	blood vessel

Word Grouping Exercises

Using the *Medical Term Parts* table, identify the prefix, suffix, or combining form for each of the following definitions. The first one has been done as an example.

Definition	Word Part
drooping, sinking down	-ptosis
adjacent	
bladder	
blood	
blood vessel	
containing a ketone group (chemical compound)	
few, little	
hard	
kidney	A. B.
nearest, next to	
night	
nitrogen	
passage	
pelvis	
present in urine	
pus	
related to ureter (urinary tube)	
small, rounded projection	
stone	
sugar	
urethra	
urinated	
urine	A. B.
water	

Word Building Exercises

Word parts introduced in the *Medical Term Parts* section are listed in the following table. For this exercise, first supply the meaning of each word part, then use the word part to build a word you already know. The word you list under *Common or Known Word* does not have to be a medical term; a commonly used word is fine. Be sure, however, that the word correctly reflects the intended meaning. The first one has been done as an example. Check your answers in a dictionary.

Word Part	Meaning	Common or Known Word	Example Medical Term
prox-, proxi-, proximo-	*nearest, next to*	*proximity*	proximal convoluted tubule
cyst-, cysti-, cysto-			cystitis
glyco-			glycosuria
hem-, hema-			hematuria
hydr-, hydro-			hydronephritis
juxta-			juxtamedullary
lith-, -lith, litho-			lithotripsy
reni-, reno-			renin
scler-, sclero-			sclerosis
ure-, uro-			urine
uretero-			ureter
urethr-, urethro-			urethritis
urin-, urino-			urinary

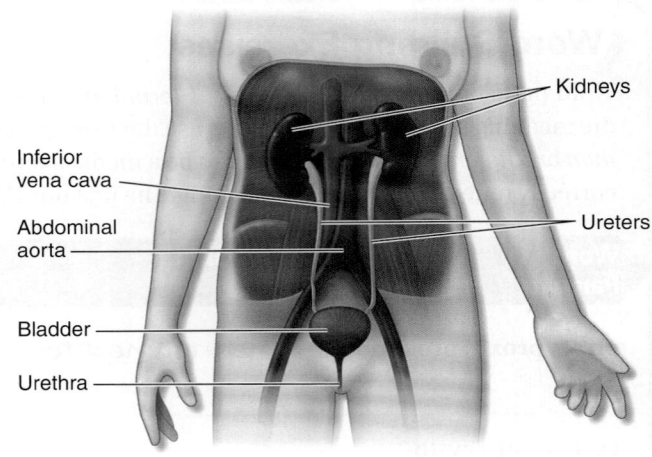

Figure 15-1 Anterior view of the urinary system organs after removal of the abdominal organs.

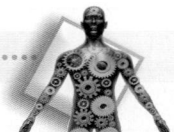

ANATOMY AND PHYSIOLOGY

Urinary System Preview

The urinary system is the body's blood filtering plant. It consists of two bean-shaped kidneys, a pair of tubular ureters, a sac-like bladder, and a urethra (**Figure 15-1**). The **kidneys** are paired organs whose main functions are to purify blood, control fluid and ion levels, and excrete wastes in urine. Every few minutes, the kidneys filter all the blood in the body, and your entire blood supply is filtered about 360 times per day. The kidneys also regulate blood pressure and play a role in red blood cell production.

Paired tubes called **ureters** transport urine from the kidneys to the bladder. Serving as a reservoir, the **urinary bladder** is an expandable sac that stores urine before **micturition** (urination). The canal leading from the bladder to the exterior is the **urethra** (*urethrae* = plural).

The system regulates body fluids and blood composition by four processes: filtration, reabsorption, secretion, and excretion. The kidneys are key organs. They allow the body to retain what it needs by filtering substances from the blood. In **filtration**, blood is filtered by the kidneys, resulting in a *filtrate*. During **reabsorption**, water and solutes, such as glucose, proteins, and sodium, are absorbed into the blood again from the filtrate. The kidneys are also involved with secretion. **Secretion** refers to the process of producing a substance in the kidneys and then discharging it.

Filtration, reabsorption, and secretion ensure that the blood returning to the body from the kidneys contains the essential components. The remaining fluid that the body cannot use becomes urine, which is excreted. **Excretion** is the process whereby wastes are eliminated from the body. Your kidneys excrete approximately 1 to 2 L (4.25 to 8.5 cups) of fluid per day.

KEY TERM	Definition
kidneys	paired organs whose main functions are to purify blood, control fluid and ion levels, and excrete wastes in urine
ureters (yoo-REE-turz)	paired tubes that transport urine from the kidneys to the bladder
urinary bladder	expandable sac that stores urine
micturition (mick-choo-RISH-un)	urination

continued

continued from page 766

KEY TERM	Definition
urethra (yoo-REE-thruh)	canal leading from the bladder to the exterior
filtration	process by which the kidneys filter blood
reabsorption	process by which water and solutes are removed from the filtrate in the kidneys and returned to the bloodstream
secretion	process of producing a substance in the kidneys and then discharging it
excretion	process by which wastes are eliminated from the body

KEY TERM PRACTICE: *Urinary System Preview*

1. Name the four processes by which body fluids and blood composition are regulated. _____

2. The _____ are paired organs whose main functions are to purify blood, control fluid and ion levels, and excrete wastes in urine.

3. The _____ are paired tubes that transport urine from the kidneys to the bladder.

4. The canal leading from the bladder to the exterior is called the _____.

5. The expandable sac that stores urine prior to micturition is known as the _____.

Kidneys

The kidneys are bean-shaped organs about 11 cm (4.3 in.) long, 5 cm (2 in.) wide, and 3 cm (1.2 in.) thick, posterior to the peritoneum, lying on either side of the vertebral column between T_{12} and L_3. The left kidney is slightly higher than the right kidney because of the placement of the liver within the cavity. Both fat and connective tissue hold the kidneys firmly in place against the muscles of the back.

Kidneys are rich in blood vessels, which are important for the kidneys' work of removing wastes and retaining substances that are needed. Blood flow into the kidneys begins with the **renal arteries** that branch off the abdominal aorta, and ends with the **renal veins**, vessels that carry blood out of the kidneys to the inferior vena cava. The **hilum**, marked by the renal artery, renal vein, and ureters, is the region where structures enter or exit the kidney.

Kidney anatomy is relatively complex. The primary structures are the renal cortex, renal medulla, renal pyramids, renal papillae, calyces, and renal pelvis. The **renal cortex** is the outer region of the kidney, and the **renal medulla** is the innermost region of the kidney. **Renal pyramids** are cone-shaped divisions in the renal medulla. The tips of the renal pyramids form the **renal papillae**, which empty urine into the **calyces** (*calyx* = singular), cup-shaped structures that drain into the renal pelvis. The **renal pelvis** is a funnel-shaped region that serves as a reservoir for urine before it flows into the ureter (**Figure 15-2**).

Nephrons are the functional units of the kidney. Each kidney contains approximately 1.25 million of these microscopic structures, and if the nephrons were lined up end to end, they would stretch 50 to 75 miles (80 to 121 kilometers). Each nephron consists of a renal corpuscle and a renal tubule. The **renal corpuscle** consists of the glomerulus and the glomerular capsule. The cluster of capillaries is called the **glomerulus**, and it is surrounded by the sac-like **glomerular** (Bowman) **capsule**. Blood enters the glomerulus at the afferent arteriole and exits

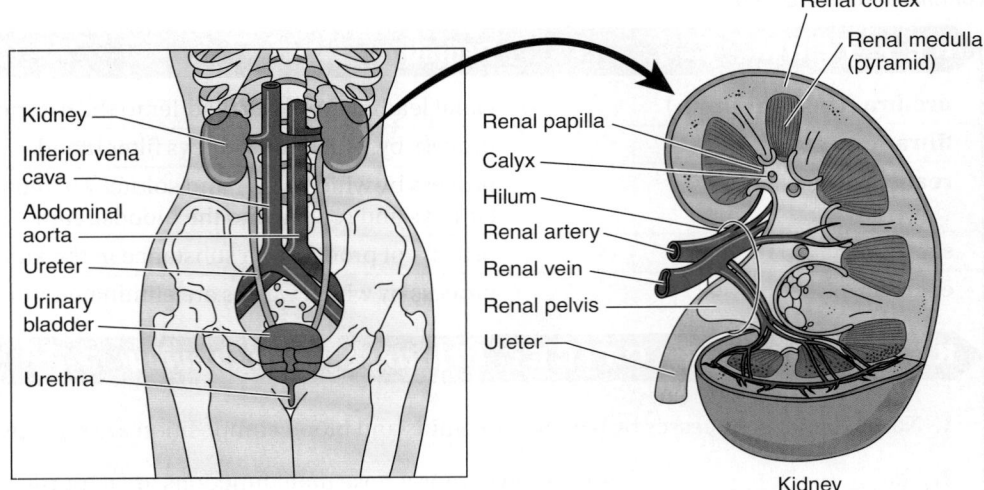

Figure 15-2 Cross-section of the left kidney.

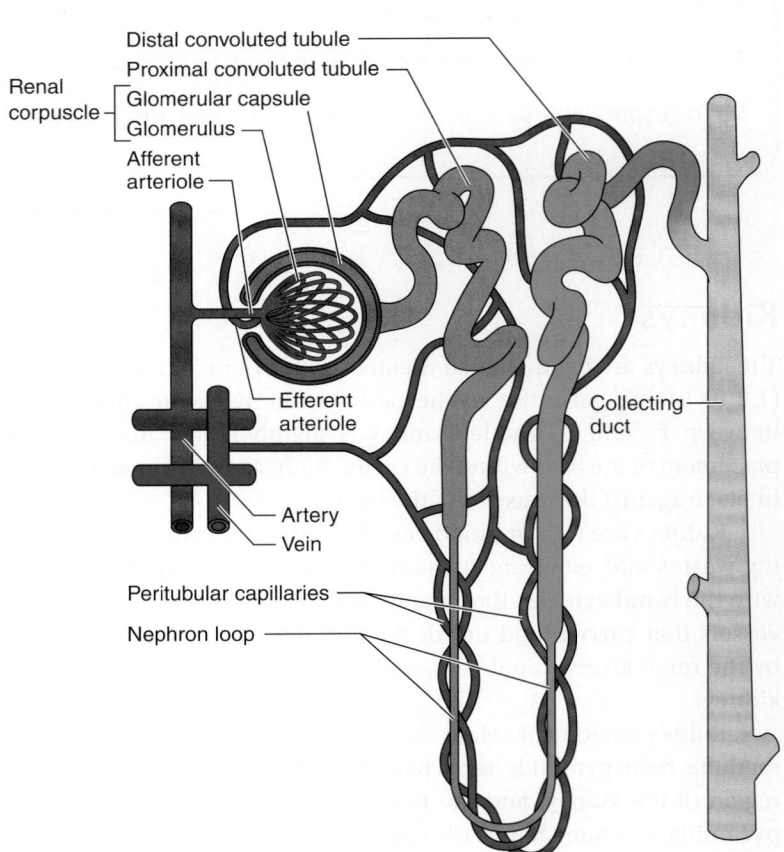

Figure 15-3 A representative nephron.

it at the efferent arteriole. The **renal tubule** is a coiled tube that leads away from the glomerular capsule and empties into the renal pelvis. It is involved in the formation of urine. The parts of the renal tubule are named as follows (in order from the glomerular capsule to the renal pelvis): proximal convoluted tubule, descending limb, nephron loop (loop of Henle), ascending limb, and the distal convoluted tubule. The formed urine then enters the collecting duct. Peritubular capillaries surround the renal tubule (**Figure 15-3**).

KEY TERM	Definition
renal (REE-nul) **arteries**	blood vessels that carry blood from the abdominal aorta into the kidneys
renal (REE-nul) **veins**	blood vessels that carry blood from the kidneys into the inferior vena cava
hilum (HIGH-lum)	area for the entrance and exit of structures
renal cortex (REE-nul KOR-tecks)	outer region of the kidney
renal medulla (REE-nul me-DUL-uh)	inner region of the kidney
renal (REE-nul) **pyramids**	cone-shaped divisions of the renal medulla
papillae (pap-PIL-ee)	tips of each renal pyramid
calyces (KAY-li-seez)	cup-like structures that drain into the renal pelvis
renal pelvis	funnel-shaped region that serves as a reservoir for urine before it flows into the ureter
nephrons (NEF-ronz)	functional units of the kidney consisting of the renal corpuscle and renal tubule
renal corpuscle (REE-nul KOR-pus-ul)	structure composed of the glomerulus and the surrounding glomerular capsule
glomerulus (gloh-MERR-yoo-lus)	capillary cluster in the renal corpuscle
glomerular (gloh-MERR-yoo-lur) **capsule**	sac surrounding the kidney glomerulus; also called Bowman capsule
renal tubule (REE-nul TEW-bewl)	coiled tube that leads away from the glomerular capsule and empties into the renal pelvis that is involved in urine formation

KEY TERM PRACTICE: *Kidneys*

1. The outer region of the kidney is termed the _____, and the innermost region is called the _____.

2. The functional units of the kidney are the _____.

3. _____ carry blood *into* the kidneys and _____ carry blood *out* of the kidneys.

4. _____ are the cone-shaped divisions of the renal medulla.

5. The funnel-shaped region that serves as a reservoir for urine before it flows into the ureter is known as the _____.

Ureters, Bladder, and Urethra

Ureters are tubular structures about 30 cm (12 in.) long that transport urine from each kidney to the bladder. They move urine by **peristalsis**, a progression of rhythmic, wave-like contractions.

The urinary bladder is a muscular organ that stores urine before micturition. It is located within the pelvic cavity, posterior to the pubic bone. In males, the bladder is located posteriorly against the rectum, and the prostate gland attaches to the urinary bladder. In females, the urinary bladder contacts the walls of the uterus and vagina. This explains why pregnant women feel the urge to urinate more frequently than usual.

The urinary bladder is composed of transitional epithelial tissue, which allows the organ to stretch, and the **detrusor muscle**, which contracts to empty the bladder during urination. Folds within the bladder, called rugae, disappear as the bladder fills. When the bladder volume reaches 200 to 300 mL (6.6 to 10 oz), stretch receptors initiate a nerve impulse, and you feel an urge to urinate. The bladder's two entrances from the ureters and one exit to the urethra form a triangular region referred to as the **trigone**. The neck is the region surrounding the urethral opening.

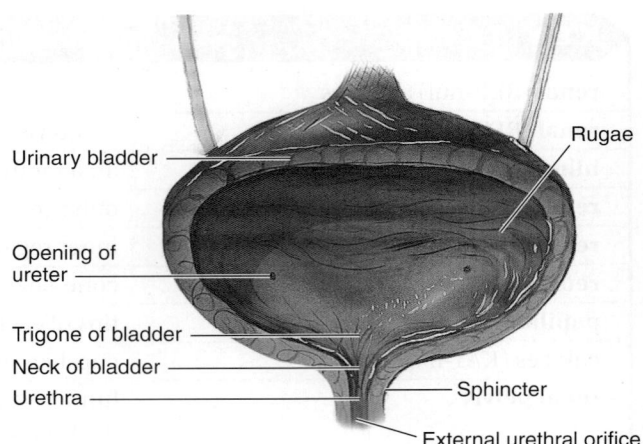

Figure 15-4 The urinary bladder.

The last structure in the urinary system is the urethra. It provides a passageway for urine to exit the body. The urethra in females is considerably shorter than that in males. Female urethrae are 2.5 to 5 cm (1 to 2 in.) long, whereas male urethrae are 17.5 to 20 cm (7 to 8 in.) long. In males, the urethra is also part of the reproductive system. During male ejaculation, a sphincter closes the opening to the bladder, enabling the urethra to transport and propel only semen.

Urethral structures include the external urethral sphincter, the internal urethral sphincter, and the external urethral orifice. A **sphincter** is a circular muscle surrounding an opening. The external sphincter can be consciously controlled. The **external urethral orifice** is the opening to the outside (**Figure 15-4**). In males, the orifice is located at the tip of the penis, and in females, it is found between the labia minora of the external genitals.

KEY TERM	Definition
peristalsis (perr-i-STAL-sis)	waves of smooth muscle contractions that propel substances through a structure, such as urine along the ureters
detrusor (dee-TROO-ser) **muscle**	muscle forming the urinary bladder
trigone (TRYE-gohn)	triangular region of the bladder marked by three openings: the two entrances of the ureters and the exit to the urethra
sphincter (SFINK-tur)	muscular ring that contracts to close off an opening in the body
external urethral orifice (ECKS-tur-nul yoo-REE-thrul OR-i-fis)	opening in urethra to outside

KEY TERM PRACTICE: *Ureters, Bladder, and Urethra*

1. The opening in the urethra to the outside is known as the _____.

2. The triangular area on the inner surface of the bladder marked by the openings to the ureters and urethra is termed the _____.

3. A _____ is a muscular ring that contracts to close off an opening in the body.

4. The _____ is the muscle forming the urinary bladder.

5. The term for waves of smooth muscle contractions that propel substances through a structure, such as urine along the ureters, is _____.

Kidney Physiology and Urine Formation

Hormones, chemical messengers secreted into the bloodstream, are critical to kidney physiology. Three important hormones associated with the kidney are erythropoietin (EPO), antidiuretic hormone (ADH), and aldosterone. The enzyme renin, secreted by juxtaglomerular cells in the renal corpuscle, is also an important substance released from the kidneys.

Erythropoietin (EPO) is a hormone released by the kidneys that stimulates red blood cell production in the red bone marrow. When tissue oxygen levels fall, EPO will be secreted to increase the rate of red blood cell production. Remember that red blood cells carry oxygen, so if more red blood cells are produced, more cells will be available to deliver critical oxygen to tissues.

Cells in the hypothalamus of the brain produce **antidiuretic hormone (ADH)**, which is stored and released by the posterior pituitary gland. This hormone promotes water reabsorption in the kidneys and thus causes water retention in the body. When blood or body fluid volume decreases or blood pressure drops, ADH is released. In so doing, fluid volume increases (remember that the fluid part of blood is plasma) and blood pressure is returned to normal.

Aldosterone is a physiologically important steroid hormone produced by the cortex of the adrenal glands. Aldosterone controls salt and water balance by stimulating sodium retention and water conservation in the kidney. When aldosterone levels increase, sodium is conserved. Wherever sodium goes, water follows, so urine output decreases. To help you remember the function of aldosterone, think about sodium as being a component of salt. The letters *s, a, l,* and *t* are found in *al*dosterone.

Renin is an enzyme released from certain kidney cells (juxtaglomerular cells) when there is a drop in renal blood flow. It regulates blood pressure through a complicated mechanism called the renin-angiotensin system that ultimately affects systemic blood pressure.

Each part of the renal tubules plays a critical role in maintaining fluid balance, primarily through reabsorption. Most nutrients are reabsorbed at the proximal convoluted tubule, that segment of the tube closest to the glomerulus. Depending on the body's need, the kidneys reabsorb water, and either reabsorb or secrete sodium, potassium, hydrogen, and bicarbonate ions. These ions are electrolytes, elements important for body functions. Fluid and electrolytes that are not retained become urine.

The kidneys form either concentrated or dilute urine. Urine contains about 95% water and 5% solids. Factors affecting urine volume include fluid intake, diet (particularly caffeine, which acts as a diuretic), environmental temperature, humidity, emotional state, respiratory rate, and body temperature. Metabolic wastes are the by-products of cellular activities and are removed from the blood and eliminated in the urine through excretion. The kidneys are also responsible for activating vitamin D, which is essential for the absorption of calcium.

KEY TERM	Definition
erythropoietin (e-rith-roh-POY-e-tin) **(EPO)**	renal hormone that stimulates red blood cell production in the red bone marrow
antidiuretic hormone (ADH) (an-tee-DYE-yoo-ret-ick HOR-mohn)	hormone made by the hypothalamus and secreted by the posterior pituitary gland to cause water retention, thereby elevating blood pressure
aldosterone (al-DOS-ter-ohn)	hormone that stimulates the kidneys to retain sodium and so regulates water and salt balance
renin (REE-nin)	enzyme released by certain kidney cells to regulate blood pressure when there is a drop in renal blood flow

continued

continued from page 771

KEY TERM PRACTICE: *Kidney Physiology and Urine Formation*

1. _____ is an enzyme released by certain kidney cells that is important for blood pressure regulation.

2. _____ is a hormone that stimulates the kidneys to retain sodium and so regulates water and salt balance.

3. _____ is a renal hormone that stimulates red blood cell production in the red bone marrow.

4. The hormone made by the hypothalamus and secreted by the posterior pituitary gland to cause water retention, thereby elevating blood pressure, is known as _____.

THE CLINICAL DIMENSION

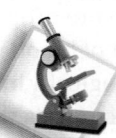

Alterations of renal and urinary tract function have profound systemic effects because the urinary system cleanses the body's blood and creates urine from those products not needed by the body. Disease recognition is often made possible by examining the urine. Several steps are involved in diagnosing disorders of the urinary system, but the first is usually a common urinalysis. Other disorders are accompanied by characteristic signs and symptoms such as back pain, difficulty urinating, discolored urine, and/or itching when urinating. Pathologies that can be determined by urinalysis include infection, kidney malfunction, diabetes, and liver disease. After initial examination of the urine, the clinician may then order more complex clinical tests and diagnostic procedures to identify the underlying disease or condition. Once the pathology has been determined, appropriate treatments can be used. This section describes various pathologies, along with their signs, symptoms, clinical tests, diagnostic procedures, and treatments, related to the urinary system.

Urinalysis

Urinalysis (UA) is the examination and analysis of urine. Physical, chemical, and microscopic characteristics of urine are determined by urinalysis. Physical characteristics include the following: pH, osmotic concentration (osmolarity), water content, color, odor, turbidity, and specific gravity. A urinalysis may also show urinary casts and crystals or the presence of bacteria. Additionally, urinalysis also identifies specific components within the following categories: nutrients and metabolites, nitrogenous wastes, ions, and blood cells. **Table 15-1** shows the general characteristics and typical values obtained from a standard urinalysis. Nutrients and metabolites (by-products of metabolism) in very low amounts are found in urine. Ions are common components of urine, but blood cells and bacteria are not normally found in urine. Normal urine should be clear and sterile with an average pH of 6.0. Filtration, reabsorption, and secretion determine the components found in urine, so the urinalysis is a good tool for assessing kidney function. Urine can be tested by dipstick method, and microscopic examination requires using the sediment of urine (**Figure 15-5**).

- *pH:* Acidity and alkalinity are determined on the pH scale, which measures the concentration of free hydrogen ions (H^+). The scale ranges from 0 to 14, where 0 indicates extremely acidic, 7 indicates neutral, and 14 indicates extremely alkaline (basic). The average pH value for urine is slightly acidic at 6.0; however, the normal range is 4.6 to 8.0. Values <4.5 may be caused by high-protein diets or uncontrolled diabetes mellitus. Individuals who have a diet rich in vegetables or who have severe anemia may have urine pH values >8.0.

TABLE 15-1

GENERAL URINALYSIS

	Normal Values	Comments
Characteristics		
pH	4.5–8.0	Alkaline = renal tubule disorder Acidic = respiratory or metabolic acidosis
Osmotic concentration (osmolarity)	855–1335 mOsm/L	Indicates dehydration or overhydration
Water content	93%–97%	Indicates dehydration or overhydration
Color	Pale yellow	Colorless = overhydration; red = hematuria; orange = bile present
Odor	Varies with composition	Changes with diet and medications
Turbidity	Clear	Cloudy = pus or bacteria present
Specific gravity	1.003–1.030	Elevated with dehydration, fever
Bacterial count	None (sterile)	Present during infection
Casts	Found in urine sediment	High number indicates renal disease
Crystals	Found in urine sediment	High number indicates kidney stones
Nutrients and Metabolites (mg/dL)		
Amino acids	0.188	Indicative of renal tubule function
Glucose	0.009	Present in diabetes mellitus
Ketones (mcg/dL)	17	Indicates starvation or abnormal carbohydrate metabolism; used to monitor patients with diabetes
Lipids	0.002	Increased with kidney disease
Proteins	0.000	Excess in glomerular disease
Nitrogenous Wastes (mg/dL)		
Ammonia	60	By-product of amino acid metabolism
Bilirubin	0	Abnormal finding; indicates liver disease or biliary obstruction
Creatinine	150	By-product of creatine phosphate breakdown in skeletal muscles
Urea	1,800	Most abundant organic waste; by-product of amino acid metabolism
Uric acid	40	Waste from RNA recycling
Ions (mEq/L)		
Bicarbonate (HCO_3^-)	1.9	Varies with diet, urine pH
Chloride (Cl^-)	110–250	Varies with diet
Potassium (K^+)	25–100	Varies with diet, urine pH, hormones
Sodium (Na^+)	40–220	Varies with diet, urine pH, hormones
Blood Cells		
Red blood cells (RBCs)	0.00	Indicates vascular damage; infection
White blood cells (WBCs)	0.00	Indicates renal infection or inflammation; pyuria

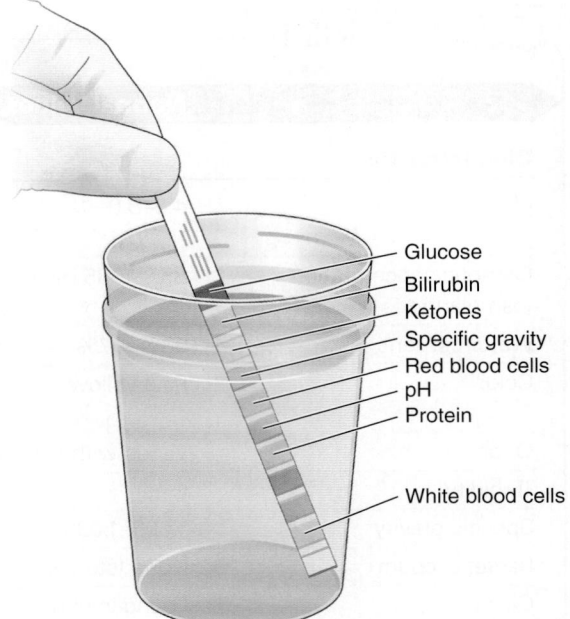

Glucose
Bilirubin
Ketones
Specific gravity
Red blood cells
pH
Protein

White blood cells

Figure 15-5 Fresh or refrigerated urine tested by dipstick method. Microscopic examination of urinary sediment is a separate task.

- *Osmotic concentration (osmolarity):* Osmotic concentration, also called **osmolarity**, refers to the total concentration of dissolved substances in a solution.
- *Water content:* Urine is normally 93% to 97% water. The concentration of urine changes throughout the day. That is, you can excrete a small volume of concentrated urine or a large volume of dilute urine, depending on diet, activity level, fluid intake, or other factors. For this reason, clinicians may analyze urine over a 24-hour period, instead of relying on one urine sample.
- *Color:* The normal color range for urine is pale yellow to amber; but color depends on diet, vitamin intake, and medications. The yellow urinary pigment, **urochrome**, affects the tint. Diet and medications can also significantly affect the color of urine.
- *Odor:* Urine has a slight odor, which depends on diet, nutritional status, diseases, and drug intake.
- *Turbidity:* **Turbidity** refers to the clarity of urine and is affected by suspended particles. Normal urine should not be cloudy.
- *Specific gravity:* **Specific gravity (sp. gr.)** is the density of urine compared to that of water, which has a specific gravity of 1.000. It is measured using a hydrometer. Values for urine specific gravity range from 1.010 to 1.035. The value varies according to fluid intake and disease. Low specific gravity may be the result of increased fluid intake or severe renal damage, whereas a high specific gravity could be caused by decreased fluid intake, loss of fluids, uncontrolled diabetes mellitus, or severe anemia.

Chemical characteristics of urine are measures of solutes, sediment, ketone bodies (by-products of fat metabolism), glucose and protein levels, salts, and ions.

A renal threshold for glucose exists, and glucose must reach a certain level in the blood before it is excreted. However, small amounts of glucose may be present in the urine after a big meal or when an individual is experiencing stress. Excreted glucose, termed **glycosuria** or **glucosuria**, is often an indication of disease, generally diabetes mellitus.

Large amounts of protein molecules are abnormal components of urine, yet a very small quantity may be present because diet and disease can affect urine protein levels. Patients with severe anemia usually excrete protein. Protein in the urine is known as **proteinuria**. When the primary protein is albumin, it is called **albuminuria**.

Microscopic tests are used to determine bacterial counts, the presence of casts (protein clumps), crystals (end products of food metabolism), and other substances that are not visible to the naked eye. Casts and crystals are precipitates found in urine sediment. Indications of a urinary tract infection (UTI) include bacteria or blood cells in the urine. **Bacteriuria** is the presence of bacteria in the urine. The common bacterium *Escherichia coli* is frequently the culprit. **Hematuria** (blood in the urine) is also a sign of a bacterial infection, injury, or disease of the urinary system. An elevated white blood cell count indicates **pyuria** (pus in the urine) and the presence of a urinary tract infection.

KEY TERM	Definition
urinalysis (yoor-i-NAL-i-sis) **(UA)**	examination and analysis of urine
osmolarity (oz-moh-LAIR-i-tee)	total concentration of dissolved substances in a solution; also called osmotic concentration
urochrome (YOOR-oh-krome)	yellow pigment in urine
turbidity (tur-BID-i-tee)	refers to the clarity of a liquid
specific gravity (sp. gr.)	measure of the density of the urine compared to that of water
glycosuria (glye-koh-SOO-ree-uh)	glucose in the urine; another term for glucosuria
glucosuria (gloo-koh-SOO-ree-uh)	glucose in the urine; another term for glycosuria
proteinuria (proh-tee-NEW-ree-uh)	protein in the urine
albuminuria (al-bew-mi-NEW-ree-uh)	protein, specifically albumin, in the urine
bacteriuria (back-teer-ee-YOO-ree-uh)	presence of bacteria in the urine
hematuria (hee-muh-TYOO-ree-uh)	presence of blood in the urine
pyuria (pigh-YOO-ree-uh)	presence of pus in the urine

KEY TERM PRACTICE: *Urinalysis*

1. Give the two terms meaning glucose in the urine. _____

2. What are the two terms that mean protein in the urine? _____

3. _____ is the medical term for bacteria in the urine.

4. _____ is the medical term for blood in the urine.

5. The examination of urine is known as _____ and is derived from the word part _____ for *urine*.

General Kidney Disorders

Inflammation of the kidney may involve the nephron or another specific region.

nephritis   **Nephritis** is a general term for inflammation of the kidneys caused by infection, degenerative disease, or disease of the blood vessels. Acute nephritis is frequently the result of drug-induced reactions, and chronic nephritis is caused by underlying kidney disease.

pyelitis   The term **pyelitis** describes generalized inflammation of the renal pelvis. It is sometimes caused by bacterial infection.

hydronephrosis   **Hydronephrosis** is a condition characterized by dilation of the pelvis and calyces of one or both kidneys (**Figure 15-6**). Its cause is generally an obstruction of the ureters, which creates an accumulation of urine in the renal collecting system and subsequent high pressure within the kidney. It may be a congenital disorder or may also result from neuromuscular problems, pregnancy, or some other unknown reason. Usually, the obstruction develops over weeks or months, although acute hydronephrosis also occurs. The obstruction can lead to infection or renal failure if not treated.

nephroptosis   **Nephroptosis** (floating kidney) is a condition in which the kidney drops out of its normal position due to loss of supporting adipose tissue. Wasting diseases, anorexia nervosa, and starvation, in which the fatty deposits surrounding the kidney are diminished, may cause it.

renal calculi   Kidney stones formed by the concentration of excessive calcium, mineral salts, cholesterol, or uric acid are called **renal calculi** (**Figure 15-7**). Their size and numbers vary. For example, a single stone may be the size of a grain of sand or large enough to fill the renal pelvis, called a staghorn calculus. The cause is unknown, but there appears to be a hereditary tendency toward their development.

Symptoms include flank (lumbar region) pain, **urgency** (strong desire to urinate), and hematuria. Hematuria is marked by a reddish color in urine. The diagnosis is made through kidney, ureter, bladder (KUB) radiographic studies; urinalysis; intravenous pyelogram (IVP); or intravenous urogram (IVU).

In a **KUB radiographic study,** the patient is injected with a contrast dye that is taken up within the vascular kidneys, ureters, and bladder, enabling kidney vessel functioning and obstructions to be visualized on a renogram. In addition to the KUB, the **intravenous pyelogram (IVP)**

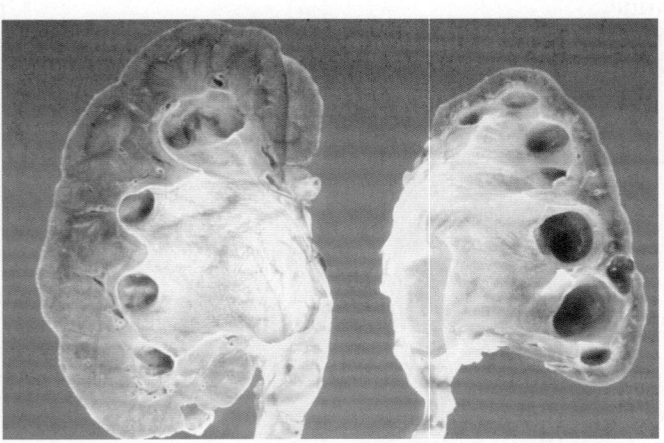

Figure 15-6 Hydronephrosis. Bilateral urinary tract obstruction has led to dilation of the ureters, pelves, and calyces. The kidney on the right shows severe atrophy.

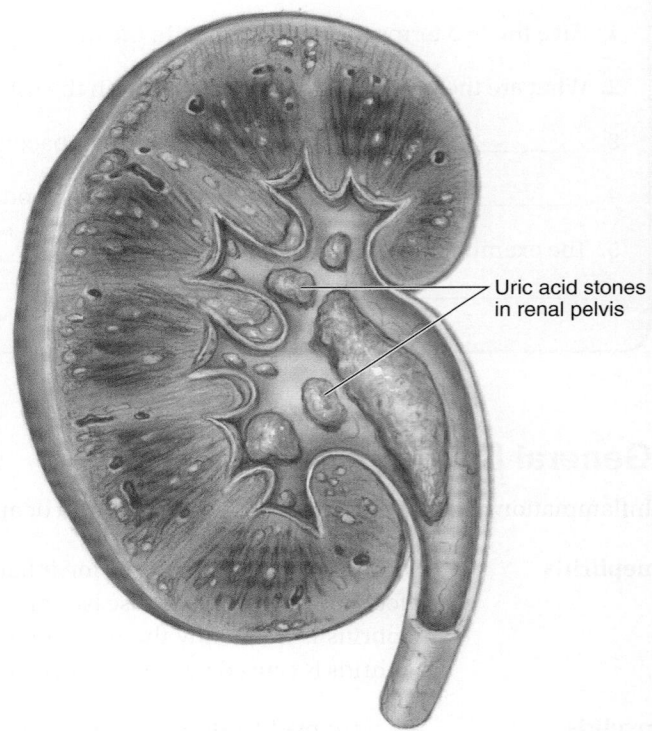

Uric acid stones in renal pelvis

Figure 15-7 Renal calculi.

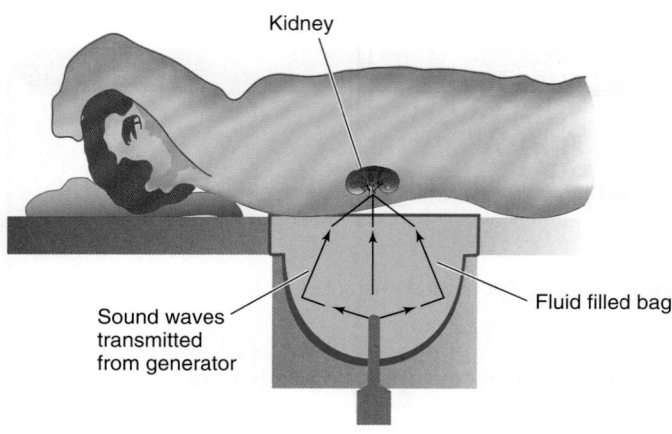

Kidney

Sound waves
transmitted
from generator

Fluid filled bag

Figure 15-8 Extracorporeal shock wave lithotripsy. (Note that the kidney is not drawn anatomically correct, but is for visualization purposes only.)

provides x-ray images of the kidney pelvis and ureter. This procedure involves the injection of a contrast dye into a vein. As the material travels through the bloodstream, it will eventually enter the highly vascular kidneys, where the contrast material can be seen on an x-ray. Similarly, the **intravenous urogram (IVU)** provides a radiograph of the entire urinary tract after infusion with a contrast dye.

Treatment of renal calculi may involve **extracorporeal shock wave lithotripsy (ESWL)**, whereby a patient is submerged in water or the patient lies on top of a cushion while sound waves are delivered to the kidney region in an effort to crush the stones to allow for natural passage (**Figure 15-8**). **Lithotripsy**, a procedure in which stones are crushed by mechanical force, laser, or focused sound energy, is another treatment option for kidney stones.

KEY TERM	Definition
nephritis (ne-FRYE-tis)	inflammation of the kidneys
pyelitis (pye-eh-LYE-tis)	inflammation of the kidney pelvis
hydronephrosis (high-droh-nuh-FROH-sis)	dilation of the renal pelvis and calyces of one or both kidneys
nephroptosis (NEF-rop-toh-sis)	condition in which the kidney drops out of its normal position due to loss of supporting adipose tissue; also called floating kidney
renal calculi (REE-nul KAL-kew-lye)	kidney stones
urgency	strong desire to urinate
KUB radiographic (RAY-dee-oh-graf-ick) **study**	procedure in which a contrast dye is injected into the blood and taken up by the urinary system (kidneys, ureters, and bladder) to be visualized through a renogram
intravenous pyelogram (IVP) (in-truh-VEE-nus PYE-e-loh-gram)	procedure in which a contrast dye is injected into a vein to be excreted by the kidneys to permit x-ray visualization of the renal pelvis and ureter
intravenous urogram (IVU) (in-truh-VEE-nus YOOR-oh-gram)	radiograph of the entire urinary tract after infusion with a contrast dye
extracorporeal (ecks-truh-kor-POH-ree-ul) **shock wave lithotripsy** (lith-oh-TRIP-see) **(ESWL)**	procedure in which sound waves are transmitted to the kidneys to break apart renal calculi
lithotripsy (lith-oh-TRIP-see)	procedure in which stones are crushed by mechanical force, laser, or focused sound energy

continued

continued from page 777

KEY TERM PRACTICE: *General Kidney Disorders*

1. The medical term for kidney stones is _____.

2. The word part *nephr-* means _____, and the word part *-itis* means _____; so _____ is the medical term for inflammation of the kidney.

3. The procedure in which stones are crushed by mechanical force, laser, or focused sound energy is termed _____, derived from the word part _____ for *stone*.

4. The condition in which the kidney drops out of its normal position due to loss of supporting adipose tissue is known as _____, and is derived from the word part _____ for *kidney* and the word part _____ for *drooping*.

5. _____ is the strong desire to urinate.

Glomerular Disorders

glomerulonephritis

Inflammation of the glomeruli, typically caused by an immune response, is termed **glomerulonephritis**.

Acute glomerulonephritis is characterized by hematuria and proteinuria. Some forms occur 1 to 2 weeks after a bacterial, viral, or other pathogenic infection. Although the microorganisms do not invade the kidney, the antigen–antibody complexes formed as part of the body's immune response become trapped in the glomerular capillaries, creating obstructions.

Diagnosis is usually made by patient history, physical examination, urinalysis, KUB, and possibly blood tests. Hematological findings indicate an elevated blood urea nitrogen level and hypoalbuminemia. **Blood urea nitrogen (BUN)** is a diagnostic test performed to determine the amount of urea present in the blood. An increase in urea blood levels (uremia) indicates malfunctioning kidneys. Uremia can lead to unconsciousness or death. **Hypoalbuminemia** is low blood albumin (protein) concentration due to albumin loss in the holes of damaged glomeruli.

Available treatment consists of antibiotic therapy if infection persists and the administration of diuretics to promote **diuresis** (excessive urine excretion). This reduces edema and hypertension (high blood pressure).

Chronic (developing and progressing slowly) glomerulonephritis begins asymptomatically and is not caused by an infection, although antigen–antibody immune complexes form. Disease progression leads to **oliguria** (scanty urine output), proteinuria, hematuria, and edema. Later stages are characterized by renal failure, hypertension, and azotemia. **Azotemia** (also called **uremia**) is an abnormal increase in the concentration of urea and other nitrogenous substances in the blood. Diagnosis protocols are the same as for acute glomerulonephritis. Treatment is aimed at controlling hypertension and elevated urea levels.

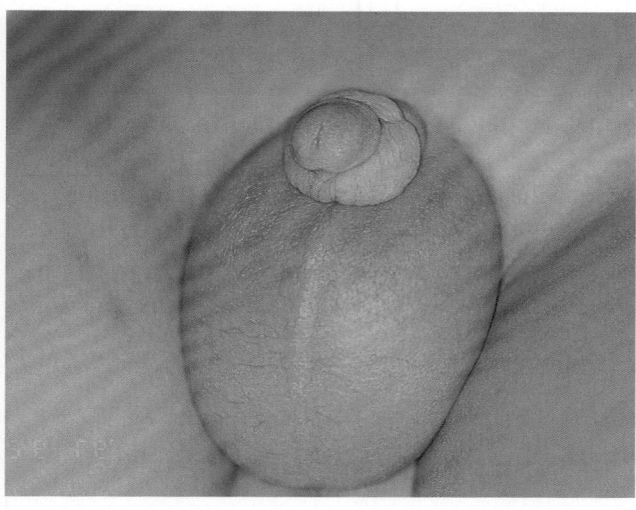

Figure 15-9 Scrotal swelling in a 7-year-old with nephrotic syndrome.

nephrotic syndrome   In **nephrotic syndrome**, the basement membrane of renal glomeruli is damaged. It occurs as a result of another existing disorder, such as glomerulonephritis, diabetes mellitus, systemic lupus erythematosus (an autoimmune disease), a renal vein blood clot, or exposure to toxins. Nephrotic syndrome is characterized by degenerative renal lesions, proteinuria, hypoproteinemia, generalized edema, and labial (in females) or scrotal (in males) swelling (**Figure 15-9**).

Tests of glomerular function evaluate the **glomerular filtration rate (GFR)**, the speed of filtrate formation (blood filtering) by the glomerulus. A clearance test can determine the GFR by monitoring plasma and renal concentrations of the protein creatinine. A **creatinine clearance test** is used to evaluate the glomerular filtration rate by measuring the clearance (removal from the blood) of creatinine. Creatinine, the end product of creatine metabolism, is excreted by the kidneys at a constant rate. This test can determine how well the glomeruli are functioning.

KEY TERM	Definition
glomerulonephritis (gloh-merr-yoo-loh-nef-RIGH-tis)	inflammation of the glomeruli
blood urea (YOO-ree-uh) **nitrogen (BUN)**	diagnostic test to determine the amount of urea present in the blood
hypoalbuminemia (high-poh-al-bew-min-EE-mee-uh)	low blood albumin (protein) concentration
diuresis (dye-yoo-REE-sis)	excessive urine excretion
oliguria (ol-i-GOO-ree-uh)	scanty urine production
azotemia (az-oh-TEE-mee-uh)	abnormal increase in the concentration of urea and other nitrogenous substances in the blood; also called uremia
uremia (yoo-REE-mee-uh)	abnormal increase in the concentration of urea and other nitrogenous substances in the blood; also called azotemia
nephrotic (ne-FROT-ick) **syndrome**	degenerative renal lesions resulting from damage to the basement membrane of the glomeruli

continued

continued from page 779

KEY TERM	Definition
glomerular (gloh-MERR-yoo-lur) **filtration rate (GFR)**	the rate at which blood is filtered by the glomerulus
creatinine clearance test	test used to determine the glomerular filtration rate by measuring the clearance of creatinine

KEY TERM PRACTICE: *Glomerular Disorders*

1. _____ is described as degenerative renal lesions resulting from damage to the basement membrane of the glomeruli.

2. The rate at which blood is filtered at the glomerulus is known as the _____.

3. Inflammation of the glomeruli is called _____.

4. This test is used to determine the amount of urea present in the blood. _____

5. An abnormal increase in the concentration of urea and other nitrogenous substances in the blood is termed _____ or _____, derived from the word part _____ for *nitrogen.*

Kidney Function Disorders

renal failure

Renal failure is a significant decline in kidney function resulting in uremia. Two types of renal failure exist: acute and chronic. Acute renal failure (ARF) is characterized by a rapid decrease in kidney functioning and is usually triggered by an acute disease process. Conversely, chronic renal failure (CRF) is characterized by diminished kidney function that declines over months to years. The three stages of CRF are early, second, and third stage. The early stage is marked by renal impairment. Renal insufficiency (kidney function at 25%) characterizes the second stage, and the third stage is characterized by end-stage renal disease.

end-stage renal disease (ESRD)

Renal failure may progress to **end-stage renal disease (ESRD)**. This is the final phase of kidney disease, occurring when less than 10% of normal renal function remains. **Anuria**, absence of urine formation, is common. It is characterized by the inability of the kidneys to filter the body's blood because of progressive nephron destruction, a drop in glomerular filtration rate, and a rise in BUN. These changes lead to uremia, represented by toxic waste retention, **hyperuricemia** (elevated blood levels of uric acid), anorexia, nausea, vomiting, and pruritus (itching). An obvious physical manifestation is **uremic frost**, in which the skin appears powdery from urea and uric acid salt deposits excreted in sweat. The condition is fatal if not treated and involves dialysis (an artificial means of filtering the blood, discussed in the next section) and dietary management. In some cases, treatment may include administration of erythropoietin to increase red blood cell production and alleviate anemia.

KEY TERM	Definition
renal (REE-nul) **failure**	significant decline in kidney function resulting in uremia
end-stage renal (REE-nul) **disease (ESRD)**	final phase of kidney disease marked by the inability of the kidneys to filter the body's blood and produce urine
anuria (an-YOO-ree-uh)	absence of urine formation
hyperuricemia (high-pur-yoo-ri-SEE-mee-uh)	elevated uric acid levels in the blood
uremic (yoo-REE-mick) **frost**	urea and uric acid salt deposits excreted in sweat as a result of uremia, giving the skin a powdery appearance

KEY TERM PRACTICE: *Kidney Function Disorders*

1. _____ is a significant decline in kidney function resulting in uremia.

2. Elevated uric acid levels in the blood is known as _____.

3. The term for urea and uric acid salt deposits excreted in sweat as a result of uremia, giving the skin a powdery appearance, is _____.

4. _____ is absence of urine formation.

5. _____ is the final phase of kidney disease marked by the inability of the kidneys to filter the body's blood and produce urine.

IN THE NEWS: Hemolytic Uremic Syndrome

Hemolytic uremic syndrome (HUS) is a disorder characterized by acute renal failure and is often caused by infection with *Escherichia coli*, an extremely pathogenic bacterium. The Centers for Disease Control and Prevention (CDC) report that 5% to 10% of children who become ill from the bacterium develop HUS. Moreover, 90% of HUS cases develop in children under age 3 years. This disease is characterized by sudden onset of gastrointestinal bleeding, hematuria, oliguria, and azotemia. Blood vessel walls become damaged by the bacterium's toxin, and the highly vascular kidneys begin to malfunction. Sadly, 1 in 20 children will die as a result of multiple organ failure. Of the individuals who survive, 1 in 3 will sustain permanent kidney damage, and 1 in 10 will develop complications such as hypertension or recurring seizures.

How do you contract *E. coli* infection? Eating food contaminated with *E. coli* is the primary way of contracting *E. coli*. In 2006, an epidemic of harmful *E. coli* emerged in the United States due to contaminated spinach. In June 2009, Nestle Toll House cookie dough was linked to an outbreak of *E. coli* O157:H7 in the United States, which sickened 70 people in 30 states. In May 2011, there was an *E. coli* O104:H4 outbreak in Europe. At least 18 people died, presumably from hemolytic uremic syndrome. Two decades ago the main culprit in *E. coli* outbreaks was *E. coli* O157:H7, but the number of outbreaks from this strain have greatly diminished since then only to be replaced by newer, more virulent strains, such as *E. coli* O104:H4.

The emergence of these new strains is a vivid reminder of just how adaptable nature is. When a pathogen attacks, scientists develop medicines and other countermeasures to fight the disease. Nature responds with its own modifications to overcome the human countermeasures and the battles go on.

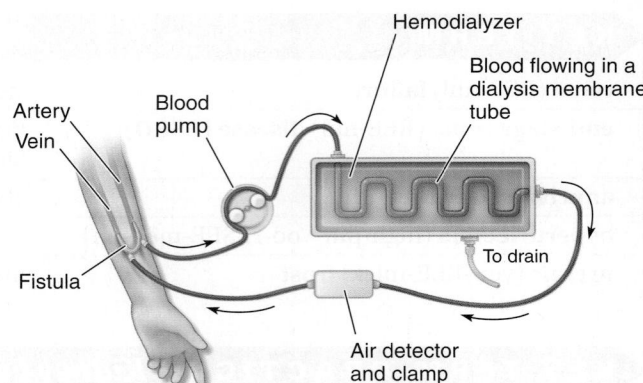

Figure 15-10 Dialysis cleans the blood for the kidneys.

Dialysis and Kidney Transplants

When the kidneys can no longer filter the blood and form urine, either a method of artificial kidney function (dialysis) is necessary or a kidney transplant is required. **Dialysis** (hemodialysis) is a procedure in which a machine called a **hemodialyzer** is used to filter the blood of unwanted substances that are normally removed by healthy kidneys. The hemodialyzer cleanses the blood by exposing the blood to dialyzing fluid (dialysate) across a semipermeable (dialysis) membrane. Before dialysis treatment, an internal **fistula** (passage connecting an artery and a vein) is surgically created (usually in the arm) for dialysis access. At the fistula site, blood passes from the body to a machine equipped with a semipermeable membrane for filtering. The cleansed blood is then returned to the body. This procedure is generally done at a hospital or clinic three times per week and usually takes 4 to 5 hours each session (**Figure 15-10**).

Peritoneal dialysis (PD) is another form of dialysis in which dialysate diffused across a peritoneal membrane filters toxins. The dialysate enters the peritoneal cavity through a permanent catheter. Wastes diffuse into the fluid, which is then drained and replaced with new dialysis fluid. There are three types of peritoneal dialyses: continuous ambulatory peritoneal dialysis (CAPD), continuous cycling peritoneal dialysis (CCPD), and intermittent peritoneal dialysis (IPD).

A **kidney transplant** involves surgically placing a kidney from a donor into a recipient. In a typical transplant case, the transplanted kidney is placed in the recipient's pelvic cavity, and the renal artery is sutured to the internal iliac artery. The renal artery and the renal vein of the donor kidney are connected to the recipient's renal artery and renal vein, and the lower end of the donor ureter is connected to the recipient's bladder. The recipient's diseased kidney may or may not be removed. The transplanted kidney in the recipient, as well as the remaining kidney in the donor, will hypertrophy and function fully.

KEY TERM	Definition
dialysis (dye-AL-i-sis)	procedure in which a machine (hemodialyzer) is used to replace normal kidney functions; also called hemodialysis
hemodialyzer (hee-moh-DYE-uh-lye-zur)	machine that acts as an artificial kidney during dialysis
fistula (fist-YOO-luh)	surgically created passage that connects an artery and a vein
peritoneal dialysis (PD) (perr-i-toh-NEE-ul dye-AL-i-sis)	filtration procedure using a dialysis solution in the peritoneal cavity to filter blood
kidney transplant	operation in which a donor kidney is placed into a recipient

continued

continued from page 782

KEY TERM PRACTICE: *Dialysis and Kidney Transplants*

1. A surgically created passage connecting an artery and a vein is termed a _____.

2. A _____ occurs when a donor kidney is placed into a recipient.

3. _____ is the procedure used to replace normal kidney functions.

4. The _____ is the machine that acts as an artificial kidney during dialysis.

5. A filtration procedure using a dialysis solution in the peritoneal cavity to filter blood is called _____.

Diabetes

Two types of diabetes exist: diabetes insipidus and diabetes mellitus.

diabetes insipidus	**Diabetes insipidus** is an endocrine disorder caused by inadequate secretion of antidiuretic hormone (ADH) from the posterior pituitary gland or by ADH insensitivity. With ADH insensitivity, the kidneys (primarily the collecting ducts) do not respond to the action of ADH. Its effects on the urinary system include chronic excretion of very large amounts of pale, dilute urine of low specific gravity. The nephrons are unable to absorb water back into the bloodstream, so the water increases urine volume. This excessive excretion of urine is termed **polyuria** and leads to dehydration and extreme thirst (**polydipsia**; *dipsa* = thirst). (**Figure 15-11**).
diabetes mellitus (DM)	**Diabetes mellitus (DM)** is a chronic disorder of carbohydrate metabolism caused by pancreatic dysfunction or insulin insensitivity. The associated **nephropathy** (kidney disease) is characterized by glycosuria, hyperglycemia (increased blood glucose concentrations), polyuria, and polydipsia. Complications include glomerulosclerosis, urinary retention, renal hypertension, proteinuria, and urinary tract infection. **Glomerulosclerosis** is described as hardening or scarring of the renal glomeruli. In **urinary retention**, the kidneys continue to make urine, but the urine remains in the bladder and is not excreted. Increased blood pressure as a result of kidney disease is termed **renal hypertension**.

KEY TERM	Definition
diabetes insipidus (dye-uh-BEE-teez in-SIP-i-dus)	disorder resulting from ADH deficiency or ADH insensitivity
polyuria (pol-ee-YOO-ree-uh)	excessive excretion of urine
polydipsia (pol-ee-DIP-see-uh)	extreme thirst
diabetes mellitus (DM) (dye-uh-BEE-teez mel-EYE-tus)	disorder of carbohydrate metabolism due to pancreatic dysfunction or insulin insensitivity
nephropathy (ne-FROP-uth-ee)	kidney disease

continued

continued from page 783

KEY TERM	Definition
glomerulosclerosis (gloh-merr-yoo-loh-skle-ROH-sis)	hardening or scarring of the renal glomeruli
urinary (YOOR-i-nerr-ee) **retention**	inability to urinate
renal hypertension (REE-nul high-pur-TEN-shun)	increased blood pressure due to kidney disease

KEY TERM PRACTICE: *Diabetes*

1. The term _____ refers to hardening of the renal glomeruli, and is derived from the word part _____ for *hard*.

2. The medical term used to describe the inability to discharge urine is _____.

3. The medical term for kidney disease is _____ and is derived from the word part _____ for *kidney* and the word part _____ for *disease*.

4. _____ is the medical term for extreme thirst.

5. _____ is the excessive excretion of urine.

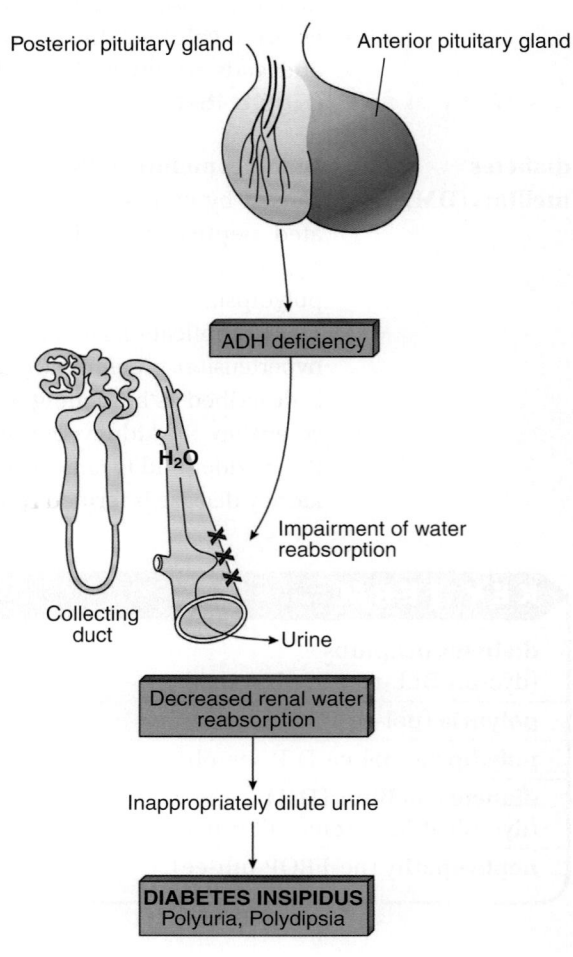

Figure 15-11 The mechanism of diabetes insipidus.

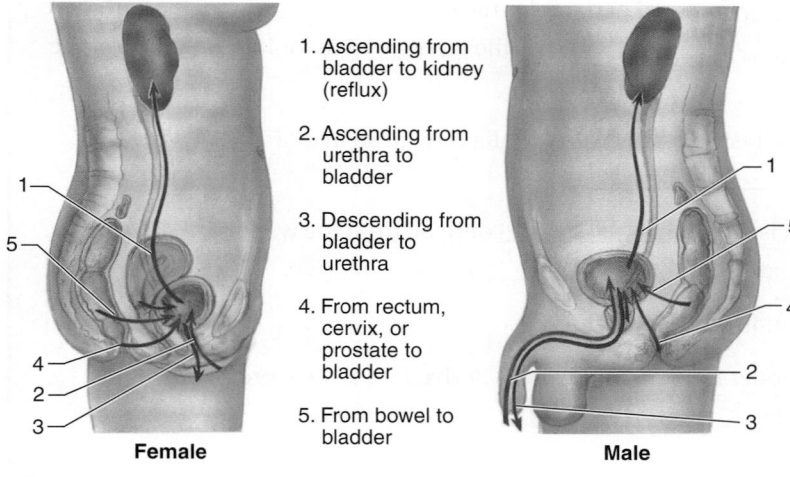

1. Ascending from bladder to kidney (reflux)

2. Ascending from urethra to bladder

3. Descending from bladder to urethra

4. From rectum, cervix, or prostate to bladder

5. From bowel to bladder

Female

Male

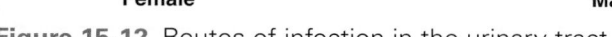

Figure 15-12 Routes of infection in the urinary tract.

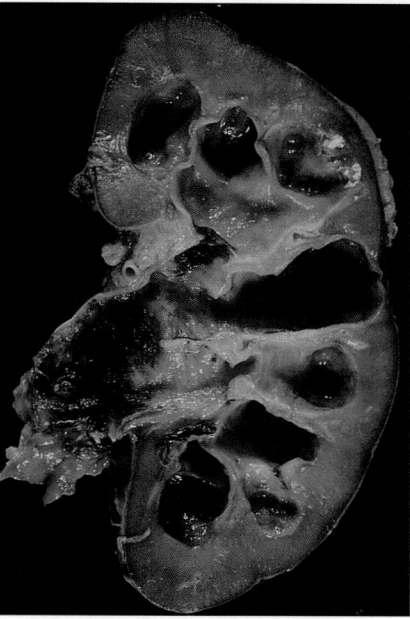

Figure 15-13 Chronic pyelonephritis. There is marked expansion of calyces caused by inflammatory destruction of papillae, with atrophy and scarring of the overlying cortex.

Urinary Tract Infections

urinary tract infection (UTI) A microbial infection, usually bacterial, of any part of the urinary system is termed a **urinary tract infection (UTI)**. Routes of infection in the urinary tract are shown in **Figure 15-12**. Signs and symptoms include flank pain, urgency, intense burning or pain while urinating (**dysuria**), hematuria, and pyuria. **Pyelonephritis**, an inflammation of the kidneys, renal pelvis, and associated connective tissue, is a urinary tract infection that has reached the renal pelvis (**Figure 15-13**). Diagnosis is made through patient history, physical examination, and urinalysis from a clean-catch urine specimen. To obtain a **clean-catch urine specimen**, the person urinates slightly to flush the external genitalia of resident bacteria, then places a specimen cup under the urine stream to collect a sample.

Three other common lower urinary tract disorders are generally caused by a microbial infection: **cystitis** (urinary bladder inflammation), **ureteritis** (ureter inflammation), and **urethritis** (inflammation of the urethra).

KEY TERM	Definition
urinary (YOOR-i-nerr-ee) **tract infection (UTI)**	infection of the kidneys, ureters, bladder, and/or urethra
dysuria (dis-YOO-ree-uh)	painful, burning sensation while urinating
pyelonephritis (pye-eh-loh-ne-FRYE-tis)	inflammation of the kidneys, renal pelvis, and associated connective tissue
clean-catch urine specimen	urine sample obtained after urinating slightly to flush the external genitalia

continued

continued from page 785

KEY TERM	Definition
cystitis (sis-TYE-tis)	inflammation of the bladder
ureteritis (yoo-ree-ter-EYE-tis)	inflammation of the ureter
urethritis (yoo-ree-THRYE-tis)	inflammation of the urethra

KEY TERM PRACTICE: *Urinary Tract Infections*

1. The word part *pyelo-* refers to _____, the word part *nephr-* means _____, and the word part *-itis* means _____; so _____ is the medical term for inflammation of the kidney.

2. A urine sample obtained after urinating slightly to flush the external genitalia is referred to as a _____.

3. The medical term for inflammation of the urethra is _____ derived from the word part _____ for *urethra* and the word part _____ for *inflammation*.

4. _____ is a painful, burning sensation while urinating.

5. _____ is the medical term for bladder inflammation and is derived from the word part _____ for *bladder* and the word part _____ for *inflammation*.

Inherited and Congenital Kidney Disorders

epispadias A congenital (existing at time of birth) malformation in which the urethra opens on the upper aspect (dorsum) of the penis instead of centrally with the glans penis is called **epispadias**. Epispadias rarely occurs in females and is marked by the urethral opening too far anteriorly at the clitoris.

hypospadias Another congenital defect is hypospadias. **Hypospadias** in males is characterized by the urethral orifice being at the ventral surface of the penis instead of the tip. In females, the urethral opening is located at the vagina.

phimosis Stenosis (narrowing) of the prepuce (foreskin) on the penis is referred to as **phimosis**. The foreskin cannot be drawn back to uncover the penis, so it may interfere with normal urination. It often leads to irritation and infection (**Figure 15-14**).

polycystic kidney disease **Polycystic kidney disease** is an inherited disease in which normal kidney tissue becomes replaced with multiple grape-like cysts that compress normal tissue, preventing normal functioning (**Figure 15-15**). The cysts progressively develop in both kidneys. Signs and symptoms include flank pain, hematuria, proteinuria, polyuria, nocturia (waking from sleep to urinate), urinary tract infection, hypertension, and calculi. These may not appear until adulthood. Definitive diagnosis is made through patient history, urinalysis, and intravenous pyelogram. There is no cure, and treatment options include dialysis and kidney transplant. This is an example of an end-stage renal disease.

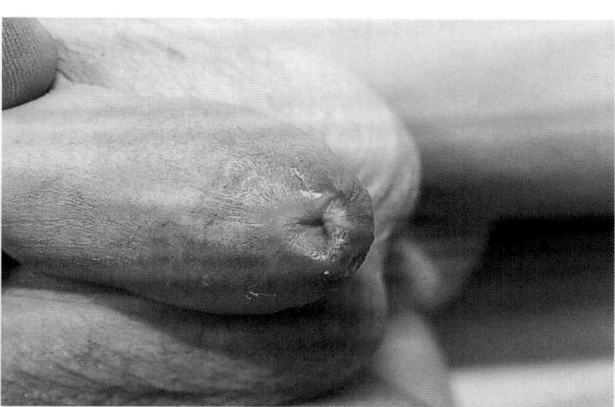

Figure 15-14 With phimosis the foreskin cannot be retracted over the tip.

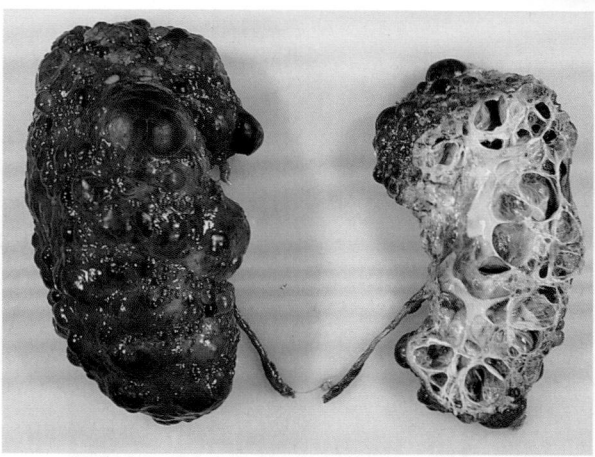

Figure 15-15 Polycystic disease. The kidney is enlarged, and the normal tissue is almost entirely replaced by cysts of varying size.

KEY TERM	Definition
epispadias (ep-i-SPAY-dee-us)	congenital defect in which the urethral opening is located on the penis upper aspect (dorsum) in males or clitoris in females
hypospadias (high-poh-SPAY-dee-us)	congenital defect in which the urethral opening is located on the penis ventral surface in males or vagina in females
phimosis (figh-MOH-sis)	narrowing of the penis foreskin preventing it from being drawn back to uncover the penis tip
polycystic (pol-ee-SIS-tick) **kidney disease**	inherited disorder in which normal kidney tissue is replaced with multiple cysts that compress normal tissue and prevent kidney functioning

KEY TERM PRACTICE: *Inherited and Congenital Kidney Disorders*

1. _____ is the medical term for the inherited kidney disorder in which normal kidney tissue is replaced with multiple cysts that compress normal tissue and prevent kidney functioning.

2. Identify two congenital defects of the urethral opening. _____

3. The term used to describe a narrowing of the penile foreskin is _____.

Cancer

renal adenocarcinoma   **Renal adenocarcinoma** (also called renal cell carcinoma) is cancer of the kidney. The cancer, which accounts for 2% of all cancers in adults, often metastasizes (spreads) to the bones and lungs. It affects males at twice the rate of females, typically appearing in middle age, and cigarette smoking may cause it. Classic signs and symptoms include hematuria, weight loss, and flank pain. Diagnosis is made through laboratory tests, radiographic studies, renal biopsy, KUB, magnetic resonance imaging (MRI), ultrasonography, or computed tomography (CT) scan. These diagnostic procedures enable the clinician to stage (identify disease progression of) the tumor.

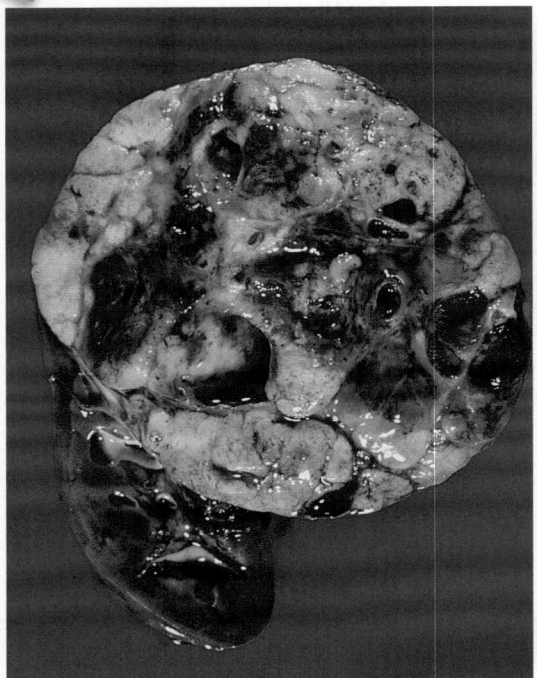

Figure 15-16 Wilms tumor. A cross-section of a pale tan neoplasm is attached to a residual portion of the kidney.

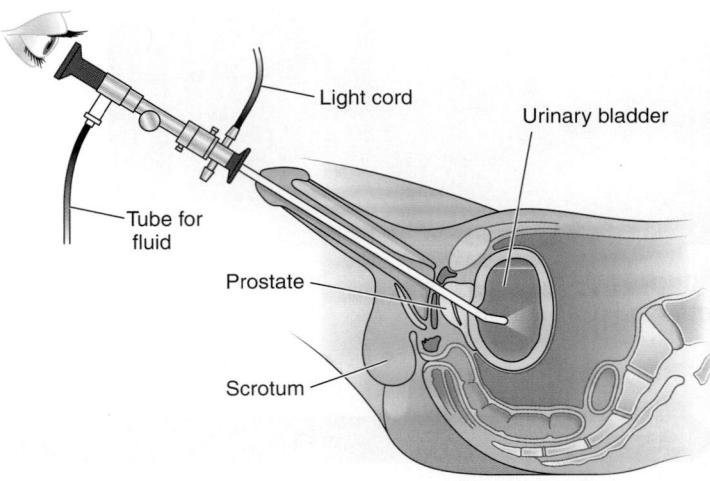

Figure 15-17 Cystoscopy. A lighted cystoscope is introduced into the bladder of a male subject. Sterile fluid is used to inflate the bladder.

Nephrectomy, surgical removal of the kidney, is the preferred treatment because this type of cancer responds poorly to radiation and chemotherapy. An individual can function nearly normally with only one kidney provided the remaining kidney is healthy.

Wilms tumor

Wilms tumor (nephroblastoma) is a cancer of the kidneys that typically affects young children (**Figure 15-16**). Wilms is an eponym referring to Dr. Max Wilms, the German physician who first described the disorder. It responds well to therapy and may be treated with surgery, radiation, or chemotherapy.

urinary bladder cancer

Urinary bladder cancer is malignant growth of cells in the urinary bladder. The first sign is usually hematuria. Initial diagnosis is made by the history and physical examination, urinalysis, and x-rays. It is confirmed by biopsy using a **cystoscope**, an instrument for viewing the bladder interior (**Figure 15-17**). Treatment depends on the growth, size, and location of the tumor.

KEY TERM	Definition
renal adenocarcinoma (REE-nul ad-eh-noh-kahr-si-NOH-muh)	kidney cancer; also called renal cell carcinoma
nephrectomy (ne-FRECK-toh-mee)	surgical removal of a kidney
Wilms (vilms) **tumor**	cancer of the kidneys that typically affects young children; also called nephroblastoma
urinary bladder cancer	malignant cell growth in the urinary bladder
cystoscope (SIS-toh-skope)	medical instrument used for viewing the urinary bladder interior

continued

continued from page 788

KEY TERM PRACTICE: *Cancer*

1. Renal cell carcinoma is one term for kidney cancer. What is another term? _____

2. _____ cancer of the kidneys typically affects young children.

3. A _____ is a medical instrument used for viewing the urinary bladder interior and is derived from the word part _____ for *bladder*.

4. The surgical removal of a kidney is termed _____ and comes from the word part _____ for *kidney* and the word part _____ for *removal of a structure*.

5. _____ is malignant cell growth in the urinary bladder.

Urinary Bladder Disorders

interstitial cystitis (IC)   **Interstitial cystitis (IC)** is a chronic bladder condition in which the bladder connective tissue is inflamed. Signs and symptoms include urgency, frequency, and incontinence. **Frequency** describes the act of urinating often, and **incontinence** is the inability to consciously control urination. **Kegel exercises**, the alternate contracting and re-laxing of pelvic floor muscles, are used to treat urinary incontinence. The goal of the exercises is to improve sphincter muscle tone by strengthening the pelvic floor muscles. Dr. Arnold Kegel, a California physician, began advocating such exercises during the late 1940s.

enuresis   A disorder that affects children is **enuresis**, involuntary nighttime bedwetting.

bladder neck obstruction (BNO)   Blockage of the bladder exit, termed **bladder neck obstruction (BNO)**, occurs as a result of disease or anatomical abnormality.

neurogenic bladder   **Neurogenic bladder** (neuropathic bladder) describes neurological deficits resulting in urinary bladder dysfunctions such as inconti-nence and retention. A common way for people with neurogenic bladders that do not empty normally to void (empty) their blad-ders is by **bladder catheterization**, a procedure in which a tube, attached to a collection bag, is placed through the urethra into the bladder to assist in bladder emptying. A Foley catheter is a urethral catheter with a retaining balloon (**Figure 15-18**).

bladder stones   **Bladder stones** (bladder calculi) are urinary tract calculi in the uri-nary bladder. Throughout human history, this was the primary form of urinary tract stone disease, and is even mentioned in the Hippo-cratic oath. Bladder stones are not as common as renal and ureteral stones and are now typically seen in patients with neurogenic blad-ders, urinary tract reconstruction, or obstruction. Bladder stones are treated with lithotripsy and lasers.

ruptured bladder   **Ruptured bladder** results from any disruption of the bladder wall. Traumatic injuries are a common cause, such as a car accident in which the seatbelt across the abdomen causes the rupture. Surgical treatment is necessary.

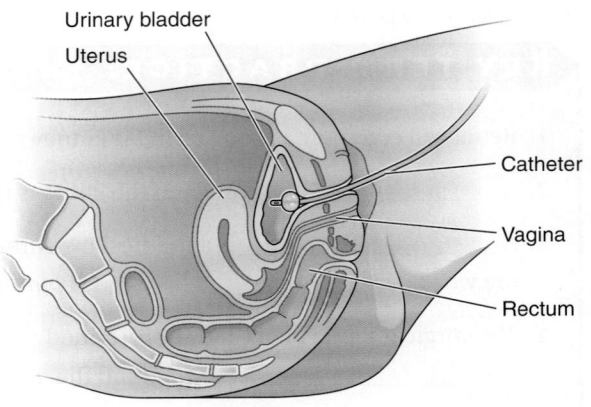

Figure 15-18 An indwelling (Foley) catheter in place in the female bladder.

KEY TERM	Definition
interstitial cystitis (IC) (in-tur-STISH-ul sis-TYE-tis)	chronic bladder condition in which the urinary bladder connective tissue is inflamed
frequency	urinating often
incontinence (in-KON-ti-nunce)	inability to control urination
Kegel exercises	alternate contraction and relaxation of pelvic floor muscles used to strengthen and tone these muscles for the treatment of incontinence
enuresis (en-yoo-REE-sis)	involuntary nighttime bedwetting, particularly in children
bladder neck obstruction (BNO)	blockage of the urinary bladder outlet
neurogenic (new-roh-JEN-ick) **bladder**	urinary bladder dysfunction resulting from impaired nervous system functioning
bladder catheterization	procedure in which a tube, attached to a collection bag, is placed through the urethra into the bladder to assist in bladder emptying
bladder stones	calculi in the urinary bladder
ruptured bladder	disruption of the bladder wall

KEY TERM PRACTICE: *Urinary Bladder Disorders*

1. Involuntary nighttime bedwetting is called _____.

2. The inability to control urination is termed _____.

3. Calculi in the urinary bladder are commonly called _____.

4. _____ is a chronic bladder condition in which the urinary bladder connective tissue is inflamed.

5. Urinary bladder dysfunction resulting from impaired nervous system functioning is termed _____.

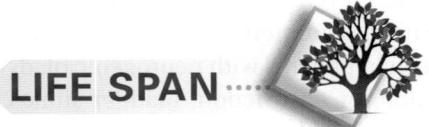

LIFE SPAN

Development of the urinary system begins during the third week of embryonic life. Excretory function of the system begins as early as the sixth week in utero, and urine formation, which occurs during the third month of fetal life, contributes to the surrounding amniotic fluid. Other portions of the system continue to develop throughout the remainder of the pregnancy.

The number of nephrons is fixed at birth. Recent research has correlated low nephron number to hypertension, thereby suggesting that this disease can be predicted at birth. Newborns typically will not urinate until 12 to 24 hours after birth. Infant urine is dilute with little urea because all the protein (from which urea is derived) is being used for growth processes. Immature kidneys are also less able to maintain fluid and electrolyte balance, and for this reason, infections, diarrhea, dehydration, or malnutrition can rapidly develop into a serious condition.

At birth, the infant's ureters are shorter than those found in an adult. The kidneys reach their full size during adolescence. Furthermore, between birth and adolescence, the kidneys increase in weight 10-fold.

Age affects the urinary system. Some changes go unnoticed, but others may impede normal physiological functioning. Beginning around age 20, the kidney cell numbers diminish so that by age 80, the kidney mass has declined by about one-third. Fortunately, there is considerable organ reserve to compensate for this loss. As a person ages, kidney function decreases due to the decline in functional nephrons. Aged kidneys appear grainy and scarred as a result of increasing fibrous connective tissue on the renal capsule. Furthermore, there is a reduction in the glomerular filtration rate that can be attributed to glomeruli atrophy, replacement of normal tissue with connective tissue, or unraveling of the coiled capillaries. Renal tubules may accumulate fat, affecting reabsorption and secretion. Medications also remain longer in the circulation as a result of diminished renal activity.

A reduced sensitivity to ADH, which leads to dehydration, also occurs as a person ages, and there may be difficulty with the micturition reflex (the automatic coordinated response controlling urination). Also, the ureters, bladder, and urethra lose elasticity with aging. Common disorders in the elderly include incontinence, urinary tract infections, renal calculi, and prostate disorders in males. Prostate disorders in men can lead to urinary retention.

COMMON *Abbreviations*

Abbreviation	Term
ADH	antidiuretic hormone
ARF	acute renal failure
BNO	bladder neck obstruction
BUN	blood urea nitrogen
CAPD	continuous ambulatory peritoneal dialysis
CCPD	continuous cycling peritoneal dialysis
CDC	Centers for Disease Control and Prevention
CRF	chronic renal failure
CT	computerized tomography
DM	diabetes mellitus
EPO	erythropoietin
ESRD	end-stage renal disease
ESRF	end-stage renal failure
ESWL	extracorporeal shock wave lithotripsy

continued

continued from page 791

Abbreviation	Term
GFR	glomerular filtration rate
H·	hydrogen ion
HUS	hemolytic uremic syndrome
IC	interstitial cystitis
IPD	intermittent peritoneal dialysis
IVP	intravenous pyelogram
IVU	intravenous urogram
KUB	kidneys, ureters, and bladder
MRI	magnetic resonance imaging
PD	peritoneal dialysis
RN	registered nurse
sp. gr.	specific gravity
UA	urinalysis
UTI	urinary tract infection
VCUG	voiding cystourethrogram

COMMON ABBREVIATIONS EXERCISES

1. ADH is the abbreviation for _____.

2. The abbreviation for urinary tract infection is _____.

3. ESRD is the abbreviation for _____.

4. The abbreviation for specific gravity is _____.

5. KUB stands for _____.

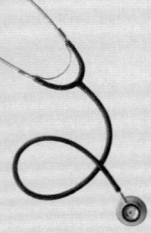

Case Study

Mr. Green's primary-care physician sent him to the nephrologist. Mr. Green, age 65 years, who has type 2 diabetes (insulin-dependent diabetes mellitus), lives alone. He has been retired for the past 15 years. The physician performed a cursory physical examination and took notes pertaining to Mr. Green's immediate history.

While taking the medical history, the doctor discovered several key factors critical to making a diagnosis. For the past 2 weeks, Mr. Green has been complaining of a backache in the right lower

continued

continued from page 792

flank. He stated that he had not been engaged in any physical activity and primarily sits and watches television all day. He had been taking aspirin to ease the pain, but it did not work. He was not sure how much aspirin he had taken, but he thought it was perhaps four pills a day, and he was uncertain of the dosage. Mr. Green stated that he has been urinating more frequently than usual. Furthermore, he is experiencing pain and a burning sensation while urinating. Physical examination revealed the following information:

- Height: 5 ft 10 in.
- Weight: 233 lb
- Blood pressure: 160/120 mm Hg
- Temperature: 99°F
- Respiration rate: 26/min
- Pulse: 80 bpm

The nephrologist ordered an IVP and KUB study, and a blood glucose stick and urinalysis were performed. The results from the blood and urine tests were obtained immediately. The blood glucose test indicated a glucose concentration of 200 mg/dL. The urinalysis indicated the following:

Test	Test Result
color	red
pH	3.0
specific gravity	1.050
glucose	positive
protein	negative

The nephrologist made a diagnosis of uncontrolled diabetes mellitus and UTI. Antibiotic therapy and nutrition education were prescribed. No further action would be taken until the results of the IVP and KUB were known.

Case Study Questions

Select the best answer to each of the following questions.

1. **Mr. Green stated he had pain in the right lower flank. In medical language, this region is called the right _____ region.**
   a. umbilical
   b. cervical
   c. sacral
   d. lumbar

2. **The source of Mr. Green's pain is likely his _____.**
   a. latissimus dorsi muscle
   b. abdominal aorta
   c. right kidney
   d. spleen

3. **Painful, burning urination is a classic sign of _____.**
   a. a urinary tract infection (UTI)
   b. renal calculi
   c. ureters calculi
   d. renal carcinoma

4. **The urinalysis revealed a red color. This may indicate _____.**
   a. blood in the urine
   b. eating beets
   c. a bacterial infection
   d. a and c

continued

continued from page 793

5. **Normal urine pH is 4.6 to 8.0, but Mr. Green's urine had a pH of 3.0. This may indicate _____.**
   a. a normal result
   b. uncontrolled diabetes mellitus
   c. hemoglobin in the urine
   d. anemia

6. **Mr. Green's urine had a specific gravity of 1.050. A specific gravity above 1.035 is considered high. Among the causes of a high specific gravity is/are _____.**
   a. loss of fluids
   b. uncontrolled diabetes mellitus
   c. increased fluid intake
   d. a and b

7. **Mr. Green tested positive for glucose in the urine. This condition is known as _____.**
   a. hematuria
   b. oliguria
   c. anuria
   d. glucosuria

8. **The IVP test was ordered because it could detect _____.**
   a. a renal calculus
   b. a pulled muscle
   c. hematuria
   d. gout

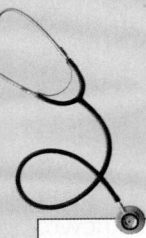

Real World Report

Debbie received a copy of Mr. Green's KUB and IVP reports. She and the nephrologist evaluated the results.

UROLOGY EXAMINATION

Patient name:	John Green
Age:	65 years
Date:	November 15, 2011

KUB

The bowel gas pattern appears unremarkable. Multiple bladder calculi are noted.

IVP WITH TOMOGRAMS (SECTIONAL RADIOGRAPHS)

After injection of contrast dye, there is prompt excretion of contrast dye by both kidneys. A large left renal cyst is noted. This was confirmed with ultrasound of the left kidney. Both ureters show evidence of obstructive uropathy. The bladder again shows multiple bladder calculi. Some of the calculi are probably in the bladder diverticula. A postvoid study shows a moderate amount of residual contrast dye in the bladder.

continued

continued from page 794

IMPRESSION

1. Multiple bladder calculi.

2. Large left renal cyst.

Dictated by: Sally Wright

This document has been reviewed and electronically approved

Real World Report Questions

The following exercises review the medical terms used in the preceding medical report.

1. What are bladder calculi? _____

2. The tests revealed hematuria.

   a. The word part *hemat-* means _____

   b. The word part *-uria* means _____

   c. The term *hematuria* means _____

3. What word in the report technically translates as "disorder of the urinary tract"?

_____

Review and Application

Multiple–Choice Questions

Select the best answer to each of the following questions.

1. The hollow chambers within the kidneys are called _____.
   a. vestibules   b. sinuses   c. hila   d. capsules

2. The word part *nephr-* means _____, and the word part *-osis* means _____.
   a. kidney; condition of   b. renin; pathology of   c. urine; inflammation of   d. nephron; condition of

3. Surgical removal of a kidney is termed _____.
   a. lithotomy   b. lithotripsy   c. nephrectomy   d. pyelotomy

4. The _____ delivers urine to the outside.
   a. urinary tubule   b. papillary duct   c. ureter   d. urethra

5. The structure connecting the kidney to the bladder is the _____.
   a. renal tubule   b. papillary duct   c. ureter   d. urethra

6. Hormones affecting the kidney include all of the following *except* _____.
   a. adrenocorticotropic hormone (ACTH)   b. antidiuretic hormone (ADH)   c. aldosterone   d. renin

7. The term used to describe rhythmic, wave-like contractions of smooth muscle is _____.
   a. wave summation   b. segmentation   c. filtration   d. peristalsis

8. The muscle forming the bladder is the _____.
   a. extensor   b. detrusor   c. trigone   d. sphincter

9. Sugar in the urine is aptly named _____.
   a. glycosuria   b. glucosuria   c. hypoglycemia   d. a and b

10. The triangular region of the urinary bladder that is formed from the openings of the urethra and ureters is the _____.
    a. trapezium   b. terminal   c. trigone   d. transitional epithelium

11. The final phase of kidney disease is termed _____.
    a. end-stage renal disease (ESRD)   b. end-stage kidney malfunctioning   c. acute glomerulonephritis   d. a and b

12. The urethral _____ is a circular muscle surrounding the external urethral orifice.
    a. circularis   b. sphincter   c. muscularis   d. serosa

13. A test of the physical, chemical, and microscopic composition of urine is termed _____.
    a. urinalysis   b. turbidity   c. urine probe   d. osmolarity

14. Kidneys and the urinary system perform the jobs of _____.
    a. filtration, dialysis, and reabsorption   b. filtration, reabsorption, and secretion   c. dialysis, reabsorption, and excretion   d. secretion, dialysis, and excretion

15. Within the kidneys, erythropoietin and renin are _____.
    a. secreted   b. excreted   c. filtered   d. removed

16. What is the correct order of structures within the nephron, beginning with the proximal convoluted tubule (PCT)? _____
    a. PCT → distal convoluted tubule → descending limb → loop of nephron → ascending limb
    b. PCT → loop of nephron → distal convoluted tubule → ascending limb → descending limb
    c. PCT → ascending limb → loop of nephron → descending limb → distal convoluted tubule
    d. PCT → descending limb → loop of nephron → ascending limb → distal convoluted tubule

17. Whenever an ion is reabsorbed in the convoluted tubule, this means that the particular ion will be _____.
    a. removed from the blood and excreted to the outside
    b. retained by the blood to be excreted to the outside
    c. retained in the blood to remain for use by the body
    d. removed from the blood to be excreted as urine

18. The secretion of antidiuretic hormone will _____ during times of dehydration, thereby _____ urine output to ensure water balance.
    a. increase; increasing   b. decrease; decreasing   c. decrease; increasing   d. increase; decreasing

19. ADH targets the distal convoluted tubule to promote water _____.
    a. reabsorption   b. secretion   c. excretion   d. filtration

20. Aldosterone, produced by the adrenal cortex, stimulates sodium _____.
    a. secretion   b. excretion   c. filtration   d. retention

21. If sodium is retained in the body, _____ automatically is too.
    a. water   b. hydrogen   c. calcium   d. vitamin D

22. Extracorporeal shock wave lithotripsy (ESWL) is used to destroy _____.
    a. renal calculi   b. renal ptosis   c. bacteriuria   d. nephrons

23. A pyelogram is used to assess the _____.
    a. renal artery   b. renal vein   c. glomerulus   d. renal pelvis and ureter

24. Bacteria in the urethra often cause _____.
    a. calculi   b. pyeloliths   c. urinary tract infections (UTIs)   d. bladder cancer

25. Females are more prone to urinary tract infections than males because _____.
    a. females usually sit to urinate, thus bacteria enter the urinary tract from an infected toilet seat
    b. males usually stand to urinate, thus there is relatively little risk of the penis being infected from a contaminated toilet seat
    c. after urinating, women must wipe, therefore contributing to infection
    d. the female urethra is shorter than the male urethra, thus enabling bacteria to enter the urinary tract more readily

26. The micturition reflex leads to the act of _____.
    a. urinating   b. filtering   c. childbirth   d. swallowing

27. Physical characteristics of urine include all of the following *except* _____.
    a. color   b. turbidity   c. osmolarity   d. pH

28. Increased levels of nitrogenous waste products, causing _____, result from kidney _____.
    a. hypoalbuminemia; disease   b. hypospadias; nephritis   c. uremia; failure   d. proteinemia; failure

29. As a person ages, kidney function declines as a result of _____.

    a. kidney ptosis   b. a decrease in the number   c. increased sensitivity   d. incontinence
                             of functional nephrons   to ADH

30. The term that best describes a scanty urine production is _____.

    a. oliguria   b. anuria   c. dysuria   d. polyuria

31. Inflammation of the kidney pelvis is termed _____.

    a. nephritis   b. pyelitis   c. polycystitis   d. pyelonephritis

32. After urinating, Ginger noticed that her urine appeared to have sand-like particles in it. The debris could possibly be _____.

    a. bacteria   b. viruses   c. sand   d. renal calculi deposits

33. Your neighbor tells you that her doctor diagnosed her as having hematuria and a UTI. You ask about her urine, and she tells you that it was _____.

    a. red and clear   b. yellow and clear   c. red and turbid   d. green and turbid

34. Gabbi has been dieting and states that she has never felt better. She has noticed that she urinates only about once per day, though. The dietitian tells her that she needs to drink more fluids. Gabbi needs to take in more liquids to _____.

    a. reduce her sodium   b. increase her   c. gain fluids that are   d. avoid the risk of
       sensitivity   sodium sensitivity   lost through urination   dehydration

Word Parts Exercises

Define the following word parts.

35. *olig-* _____

36. *azo-* _____

37. *-ptosis* _____

38. *-lith* _____

39. *-uria* _____

Matching Exercises

Match the following terms with the correct definition. Each term is used only once.

_____ 40. inflammation of the urethra

_____ 41. sugar in the urine

_____ 42. kidney cancer in children

_____ 43. inability to void urine because the kidneys fail to produce urine

_____ 44. blood in the urine

_____ 45. narrowing of penis foreskin

_____ 46. involuntary nighttime bedwetting, particularly in children

a. Wilms tumor
b. suppression
c. hematuria
d. phimosis
e. enuresis
f. glycosuria
g. urethritis

Match the disorder with its description.

_____ 47. glomerulonephritis

_____ 48. renal failure

_____ 49. polyuria

_____ 50. diabetes mellitus

_____ 51. pyuria

a. significant decline in kidney functioning
b. excessive excretion of urine
c. inflammation of the glomeruli
d. pus in the urine
e. disorder of carbohydrate metabolism

Match the sign or symptom with its description.

_____ 52. anuria

_____ 53. hematuria

_____ 54. oliguria

_____ 55. glucosuria

_____ 56. nocturia

a. scanty urine production
b. purposeful nighttime urination
c. glucose in the urine
d. blood in the urine
e. absence of urine formation

Match the clinical test or diagnostic procedure with its description.

_____ 57. nephrectomy

_____ 58. urinalysis

_____ 59. dialysis

_____ 60. lithotripsy

_____ 61. creatinine clearance test

a. focused sound energy, laser, or mechanical force to crush kidney stones
b. examination of urine
c. surgical removal of a kidney
d. used to assess GFR
e. blood cleansing by artificial means

Use the following terms to complete the statements. Each term is used only once.

a. glomerulus
d. kidneys
g. cortex
j. glomerular capsule

b. nephron
e. excretion
h. retroperitoneal
k. detrusor

c. urine
f. filtration
i. hilum
l. erythropoietin

62. The hormone _____ is necessary for the production of red blood cells.

63. The _____ is the sac surrounding the glomerulus.

64. The _____ is the muscle forming the urinary bladder.

65. _____ is the end product of kidney filtration.

66. The outer portion, or _____, forms the kidney shell.

67. The organs responsible for filtering the blood are the _____.

68. _____ is the process whereby metabolic wastes are removed from the blood.

69. The functional unit of the kidney is the _____.

70. Moving wastes outside the body is termed _____.

71. If an organ is located _____, it means it is attached to the posterior wall of the abdominal body cavity.

72. The region called the _____ describes the point where vessels enter an organ.

73. The _____ is a capillary cluster in the renal corpuscle.

Definitions

Define the following terms.

74. calyces _____

75. urochrome _____

76. secretion _____

77. filtration _____

78. excretion _____

Provide a medical term for the following definitions.

79. hormone made by the hypothalamus and secreted by the posterior pituitary gland to cause water retention, thereby elevating blood pressure _____

80. procedure in which a tube, attached to a collection bag, is placed through the urethra into the bladder to assist in bladder emptying _____

81. renal hormone that stimulates red blood cell production in the red bone marrow _____

82. opening in urethra to outside _____

83. cone-shaped divisions of the renal medulla _____

Alternate Terms

Give an alternate term for each of the following terms.

84. uremia _____

85. hemodialysis _____

86. glycosuria _____

87. floating kidney _____

88. renal cell carcinoma _____

89. nephroblastoma _____

Spelling

Identify the correctly spelled term in each set.

90. _____
   a. aldosterone
   b. eldosterone
   c. aldesteron
   d. alldosterone

91. _____
   a. hemachuria
   b. hematuria
   c. hemouria
   d. hematouria

92. _____
   a. incontinance
   b. incontinence
   c. incontinnence
   d. inkontinence

93. _____
   a. pappillae
   b. pappila
   c. papillae
   d. pupillae

94. _____
   a. reenul
   b. renul
   c. rennal
   d. renal

Unscramble

Unscramble the letters to form a medical term.

95. naler sivlep _____

96. tgnrioe _____

97. lraen snive _____

98. aiursyd _____

Abbreviations

Provide the term for the abbreviations and then define the terms.

99. KUB _____

100. ESRD _____

101. IVP _____

102. UA _____

103. BUN _____

Analogies

Provide a medical term to complete a meaningful analogy.

104. Bacteria are to bacteriuria as pus is to _____.

105. Excessive thirst is to polydipsia as excessive urination is to _____.

Short Answer

Answer the following questions.

106. Two college students, Kelsey and Marcy, are discussing a party they attended over the weekend. Kelsey said, "Whenever I drink a couple beers, I have to go to the bathroom at least five times that night. According to what I learned in my medical terminology class, I think I am secreting too much ADH." Marcy tells her she is wrong, because going to the bathroom so often after drinking a few beers is a clear indication that she is not secreting ADH. Who is correct and why? _____

107. Katie tells you that she has a pain in her right, lower back. She does not know why her back hurts because she has not done any strenuous activity. She slept comfortably but the pain began that morning while she was showering. What may be the source of this pain? _____

108. Sasha complains that she has had severe back pain for several days. She then states that the pain mysteriously disappeared after she urinated. Provide a plausible explanation for this phenomenon. _____

109. You are a safe driver, always wear your seat belt, but are in a hurry to make it home for Thanksgiving break. The Wednesday before the holiday, you realize that you have been riding in the automobile for several hours, have drunk three cups of coffee, and have not stopped to urinate. All of a sudden, the car crashes. You arrive at the emergency room with no injuries except a ruptured bladder. Provide a plausible explanation for the ruptured bladder. _____

110. Your doctor has asked for a routine urine sample. After her initial inspection, she notices an unusual color and odor. She asks if you have been megadosing on multivitamins and eating an overabundance of green, leafy vegetables. What may have prompted these questions? _____

Labeling

Label the structures in the following diagram.

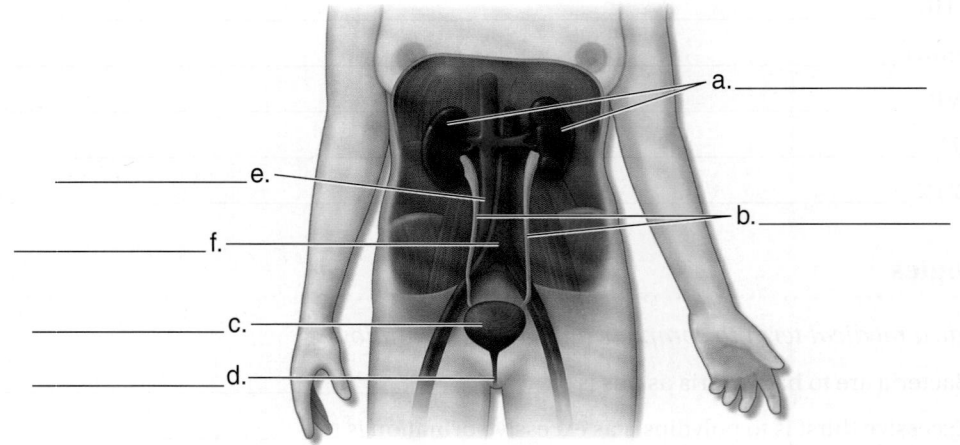

Word Search

Find the medical terms hidden in the puzzle.

A	P	I	X	X	C	K	K	P	R	K	H	P	Y
G	R	T	R	X	Q	H	N	K	E	N	T	L	L
Z	T	H	U	O	F	I	S	U	A	C	A	H	L
S	I	X	T	R	N	D	Q	Q	B	P	P	Z	V
C	I	W	Z	E	B	W	M	T	S	R	D	V	S
N	J	S	R	C	R	I	L	L	O	F	M	T	U
E	B	Y	L	S	L	U	D	K	R	T	U	W	L
P	K	R	X	A	A	N	K	I	P	W	L	V	U
H	C	N	O	I	T	I	R	U	T	C	I	M	R
R	B	D	Q	A	D	S	J	G	I	Y	H	Q	E
O	I	Y	J	N	X	Y	I	Y	O	A	J	O	M
N	S	R	E	T	E	R	U	R	N	M	L	W	O
S	T	Y	U	B	U	W	Y	F	E	P	T	M	L
O	S	M	O	L	A	R	I	T	Y	P	G	X	G

glomerulus
hilum
kidneys
micturition
nephrons
osmolarity
peristalsis
reabsorption
renin
turbidity
ureters
urethra

Vocabulary Review

Review the key terms from this chapter, study the spelling and pronunciation of each term, and write its definition in the space provided. Listen to the audio available for most terms at http://thepoint.lww.com/nath2e and pronounce each term for yourself. Then check the box when you feel confident that you know the definition and can pronounce the term correctly.

Key Term	Pronunciation	Definition
❏ **albuminuria**	(al-bew-mi-NEW-ree-uh)	_____
❏ **aldosterone**	(al-DOS-ter-ohn)	_____
❏ **antidiuretic hormone (ADH)**	(an-tee-DYE-yoo-ret-ick HOR-mohn)	_____
❏ **anuria**	(an-YOO-ree-uh)	_____
❏ **azotemia**	(az-oh-TEE-mee-uh)	_____
❏ **bacteriuria**	(back-teer-ee-YOO-ree-uh)	_____
❏ **bladder catheterization**		_____
❏ **bladder neck obstruction (BNO)**		_____
❏ **bladder stones**		_____
❏ **blood urea nitrogen (BUN)**	(YOO-ree-uh)	_____
❏ **calyces**	(KAY-li-seez)	_____
❏ **clean-catch urine specimen**		_____
❏ **creatinine clearance test**		_____
❏ **cystitis**	(sis-TYE-tis)	_____
❏ **cystoscope**	(SIS-toh-skope)	_____
❏ **detrusor muscle**	(dee-TROO-ser)	_____
❏ **diabetes insipidus**	(dye-uh-BEE-teez in-SIP-i-dus)	_____
❏ **diabetes mellitus (DM)**	(dye-uh-BEE-teez mel-EYE-tus)	_____
❏ **dialysis**	(dye-AL-i-sis)	_____
❏ **diuresis**	(dye-yoo-REE-sis)	_____
❏ **dysuria**	(dis-YOO-ree-uh)	_____
❏ **end-stage renal disease (ESRD)**	(REE-nul)	_____
❏ **enuresis**	(en-yoo-REE-sis)	_____
❏ **epispadias**	(ep-i-SPAY-dee-us)	_____
❏ **erythropoietin (EPO)**	(e-rith-roh-POY-e-tin)	_____
❏ **excretion**		_____
❏ **external urethral orifice**	(ECKS-tur-nul yoo-REE-thrul OR-i-fis)	_____
❏ **extracorporeal shock wave lithotripsy (ESWL)**	(ecks-truh-kor-POH-ree-ul) (lith-oh-TRIP-see)	_____

Key Term	Pronunciation	Definition
❑ **filtration**		_____
❑ **fistula**	(fist-YOO-luh)	_____
❑ **frequency**		_____
❑ **glomerular capsule**	(gloh-MERR-yoo-lur)	_____
❑ **glomerular filtration rate (GFR)**	(gloh-MERR-yoo-lur)	_____
❑ **glomerulonephritis**	(gloh-merr-yoo-loh-nef-RIGH-tis)	_____
❑ **glomerulosclerosis**	(gloh-merr-yoo-loh-skle-ROH-sis)	_____
❑ **glomerulus**	(gloh-MERR-yoo-lus)	_____
❑ **glucosuria**	(gloo-koh-SOO-ree-uh)	_____
❑ **glycosuria**	(glye-koh-SOO-ree-uh)	_____
❑ **hematuria**	(hee-muh-TYOO-ree-uh)	_____
❑ **hemodialyzer**	(hee-moh-DYE-uh-lye-zur)	_____
❑ **hilum**	(HIGH-lum)	_____
❑ **hydronephrosis**	(high-droh-nuh-FROH-sis)	_____
❑ **hyperuricemia**	(high-pur-yoo-ri-SEE-mee-uh)	_____
❑ **hypoalbuminemia**	(high-poh-al-bew-min-EE-mee-uh)	_____
❑ **hypospadias**	(high-poh-SPAY-dee-us)	_____
❑ **incontinence**	(in-KON-ti-nunce)	_____
❑ **interstitial cystitis (IC)**	(in-tur-STISH-ul sis-TYE-tis)	_____
❑ **intravenous pyelogram (IVP)**	(in-truh-VEE-nus PYE-e-loh-gram)	_____
❑ **intravenous urogram (IVU)**	(in-truh-VEE-nus YOOR-oh-gram)	_____
❑ **Kegel exercises**		_____
❑ **kidney transplant**		_____
❑ **kidneys**		_____
❑ **KUB radiographic study**	(RAY-dee-oh-graf-ick)	_____
❑ **lithotripsy**	(lith-oh-TRIP-see)	_____
❑ **micturition**	(mick-choo-RISH-un)	_____
❑ **nephrectomy**	(ne-FRECK-toh-mee)	_____
❑ **nephritis**	(ne-FRYE-tis)	_____
❑ **nephrons**	(NEF-ronz)	_____
❑ **nephropathy**	(ne-FROP-uth-ee)	_____
❑ **nephroptosis**	(NEF-rop-toh-sis)	_____
❑ **nephrotic syndrome**	(ne-FROT-ick)	_____
❑ **neurogenic bladder**	(new-roh-JEN-ick)	_____
❑ **oliguria**	(ol-i-GOO-ree-uh)	_____
❑ **osmolarity**	(oz-moh-LAIR-i-tee)	_____
❑ **papillae**	(pap-PIL-ee)	_____

Key Term	Pronunciation	Definition
❏ peristalsis	(perr-i-STAL-sis)	_____
❏ peritoneal dialysis (PD)	(perr-i-toh-NEE-ul dye-AL-i-sis)	_____
❏ phimosis	(figh-MOH-sis)	_____
❏ polycystic kidney disease	(pol-ee-SIS-tick)	_____
❏ polydipsia	(pol-ee-DIP-see-uh)	_____
❏ polyuria	(pol-ee-YOO-ree-uh)	_____
❏ proteinuria	(proh-tee-NEW-ree-uh)	_____
❏ pyelitis	(pye-eh-LYE-tis)	_____
❏ pyelonephritis	(pye-eh-loh-ne-FRYE-tis)	_____
❏ pyuria	(pigh-YOO-ree-uh)	_____
❏ reabsorption		_____
❏ renal adenocarcinoma	(REE-nul ad-eh-noh-kahr-si-NOH-muh)	_____
❏ renal arteries	(REE-nul)	_____
❏ renal calculi	(REE-nul KAL-kew-lye)	_____
❏ renal corpuscle	(REE-nul KOR-pus-ul)	_____
❏ renal cortex	(REE-nul KOR-tecks)	_____
❏ renal failure	(REE-nul)	_____
❏ renal hypertension	(REE-nul high-pur-TEN-shun)	_____
❏ renal medulla	(REE-nul me-DUL-uh)	_____
❏ renal pelvis		_____
❏ renal pyramids	(REE-nul)	_____
❏ renal tubule	(REE-nul TEW-bewl)	_____
❏ renal veins	(REE-nul)	_____
❏ renin	(REE-nin)	_____
❏ ruptured bladder		_____
❏ secretion		_____
❏ specific gravity (sp. gr.)		_____
❏ sphincter	(SFINK-tur)	_____
❏ trigone	(TRYE-gohn)	_____
❏ turbidity	(tur-BID-i-tee)	_____
❏ uremia	(yoo-REE-mee-uh)	_____
❏ uremic frost	(yoo-REE-mick)	_____
❏ ureteritis	(yoo-ree-ter-EYE-tis)	_____
❏ ureters	(yoo-REE-turz)	_____
❏ urethra	(yoo-REE-thruh)	_____
❏ urethritis	(yoo-ree-THRYE-tis)	_____
❏ urgency		_____

Key Term	Pronunciation	Definition
❏ urinalysis (UA)	(yoor-i-NAL-i-sis)	_____
❏ urinary bladder		_____
❏ urinary bladder cancer		_____
❏ urinary retention	(YOOR-i-nerr-ee)	_____
❏ urinary tract infection (UTI)	(YOOR-i-nerr-ee)	_____
❏ urochrome	(YOOR-oh-krome)	_____
❏ Wilms tumor	(vilms)	_____

Answers

Word Grouping Exercises

Definition	Word Part	Definition	Word Part
drooping, sinking down	-ptosis	pelvis	pyel-, pyelo-
adjacent	juxta-	present in urine	-uria
bladder	cyst-, cysti-, cysto-	pus	pyo-
blood	hem-, hema-	related to ureter (urinary tube)	uretero-
blood vessel	vas-, vaso-	small, rounded projection	papillo-
containing a ketone group (chemical compound)	keto-	stone	lith-, -lith, litho-
few, little	olig-, oligo-	sugar	glyco-
hard	scler-, sclero-	urethra	urethr-, urethro-
kidney	A. nephr-, nephro- B. reni-, reno-	urinated	micturit-
nearest, next to	prox-, proxi-, proximo-	urine	A. ure-, uro- B. urin-, urino-
night	noct-	water	hydr-, hydro-
nitrogen	azo-		
passage	meato-		

Word Building Exercises

Word Part	Meaning	Common or Known Word	Example Medical Term
prox-, proxi-, proximo-	nearest	proximity	proximal convoluted tubule
cyst-, cysti-, cysto-	bladder	cystic	cystitis
glyco-	sugar	glycogen	glycosuria
hem-, hema-	blood	hemoglobin	hematuria
hydr-, hydro-	water	hydrogen	hydronephritis
juxta-	adjacent	juxtaposition	juxtamedullary

Word Part	Meaning	Common or Known Word	Example Medical Term
lith-, -lith, litho-	stone	lithograph	lithotripsy
reni-, reno-	kidney	renal	renin
scler-, sclero-	hard	sclera	sclerosis
ure-, uro-	urine	urine	urine
uretero-	related to ureter (urinary tube)	ureter	ureter
urethr-, urethro-	urethra	urethra	urethritis
urin-, urino-	urine	urine	urinary

Key Term Practice

Urinary System Preview

1. The four processes are filtration, reabsorption, secretion, and excretion
2. ureters
3. urethra
4. urinary bladder

Kidneys

1. renal cortex; renal medulla
2. nephrons
3. Renal arteries; renal veins
4. Renal pyramids
5. renal pelvis

Ureters, Bladder, and Urethra

1. external urethral orifice
2. trigone
3. sphincter
4. detrusor muscle
5. peristalsis

Kidney Physiology and Urine Formation

1. Renin
2. Aldosterone
3. Erythropoietin (EPO)
4. antidiuretic hormone (ADH)

Urinalysis

1. glycosuria; glucosuria
2. proteinuria; albuminuria
3. Bacteriuria
4. Hematuria
5. urinalysis; *urin-*

General Kidney Disorders

1. renal calculi
2. kidney; inflammation; nephritis
3. lithotripsy; *litho-*
4. nephroptosis; *nephro-*; *-ptosis*
5. Urgency

Glomerular Disorders

1. Nephrotic syndrome
2. glomerular filtration rate (GFR)
3. glomerulonephritis
4. blood urea nitrogen (BUN)
5. uremia; azotemia; *azo-*

Kidney Function Disorders

1. Renal failure
2. hyperuricemia
3. uremic frost
4. Anuria
5. End-stage renal disease (ESRD)

Dialysis and Kidney Transplants

1. fistula
2. kidney transplant
3. Dialysis
4. hemodialyzer
5. peritoneal dialysis

Diabetes

1. glomerulosclerosis; *scler-*
2. urinary retention
3. nephropathy; *nephro-*; *-pathy*
4. Polydipsia
5. Polyuria

Urinary Tract Infections

1. pelvis; kidney; inflammation; pyelonephritis
2. clean-catch urine specimen
3. urethritis; *urethr-*; *-itis*
4. Dysuria
5. Cystitis; *cyst-*; *-itis*

Inherited and Congenital Kidney Disorders

1. Polycystic kidney disease
2. epispadias; hypospadias
3. phimosis

Cancer

1. renal adenocarcinoma
2. Wilms
3. cystoscope; *cysto-*
4. nephrectomy; *nephr-*; *-ectomy*
5. Urinary bladder cancer

Urinary Bladder Disorders

1. enuresis
2. incontinence
3. bladder stones
4. Interstitial cystitis (IC)
5. neurogenic bladder

Common Abbreviations Exercises

1. ADH = antidiuretic hormone
2. urinary tract infection = UTI
3. ESRD = end-stage renal disease
4. specific gravity = sp. gr.
5. KUB = kidneys, ureters, and bladder

Case Study

1. d is the correct answer.
   - a is incorrect because umbilical describes the anterior navel region.
   - b is incorrect because cervical describes the neck region.
   - c is incorrect because sacral describes the lower central backregion.
2. c is the correct answer.
   - a is incorrect because he had not been engaged in any sort of physical activity that may have pulled or stretched his muscle.
   - b is incorrect because the abdominal aorta runs centrally throughout the abdominal cavity.
   - d is incorrect because the spleen is located in the left hypochondriac region, just above the left kidney.
3. a is the correct answer.
   - b is incorrect because burning during urination is a classic sign of bacterial infection not renal calculi.
   - c is incorrect because burning during urination is a classic sign of bacterial infection not ureter calculi.
   - d is incorrect because burning during urination is a classic sign of bacterial infection not renal carcinoma.
4. d is the correct answer.
   - b is incorrect because beets will cause the urine to have a reddish brown color.
5. b is the correct answer.
   - a is incorrect because the normal urine pH range is 4.6 to 8.0.
   - c is incorrect because the urine would appear red. Furthermore, when a high volume of blood is lost, it may result in anemia, which would elevate the pH.
   - d is incorrect because in anemic states, the pH is elevated.

6. d is the correct answer.
   - c is incorrect because increased fluids leads to a low specific gravity.
7. d is the correct answer.
   - a is incorrect because hematuria is the term for blood in the urine.
   - b is incorrect because oliguria is the term for scanty urine output.
   - c is incorrect because anuria is the term for absence of urination.
8. a is the correct answer.
   - b is incorrect because an IVP does not detect a pulled muscle. Soft tissue injuries are more appropriately diagnosed by other measures.
   - c is incorrect because an IVP does not detect hematuria, which would be determined through microscopic examination of the urine.
   - d is incorrect because an IVP does not detect gout, which is characterized by severe joint pain and uric acid crystals in the blood.

Real World Report

1. bladder stones
2. a. blood; b. urine; c. blood in the urine
3. uropathy, a disorder involving the urinary tract

Review And Application

1. b	25. d	49. b
2. a	26. a	50. e
3. c	27. d	51. d
4. d	28. c	52. e
5. c	29. b	53. d
6. a	30. a	54. a
7. d	31. b	55. c
8. b	32. d	56. b
9. d	33. c	57. c
10. c	34. d	58. b
11. a	35. few, little	59. e
12. b	36. nitrogen	60. a
13. a	37. drooping, sinking down	61. d
14. b	38. stone	62. l
15. a	39. present in urine	63. j
16. d	40. g	64. k
17. c	41. f	65. c
18. d	42. a	66. g
19. a	43. b	67. d
20. d	44. c	68. f
21. a	45. d	69. b
22. a	46. e	70. e
23. d	47. c	71. h
24. c	48. a	72. i

73. a

74. calyces = cup-like structures that drain into the renal pelvis

75. urochrome = yellow pigment in urine

76. secretion = process of producing a substance in the kidneys and then discharging it

77. filtration = process by which the kidneys filter blood

78. excretion = process by which wastes are eliminated from the body

79. antidiuretic hormone (ADH)

80. bladder catheterization

81. erythropoietin (EPO)

82. external urethral orifice

83. renal pyramids

84. azotemia

85. dialysis

86. glucosuria

87. nephroptosis

88. renal adenocarcinoma

89. Wilms tumor

90. a

91. b

92. b

93. c

94. d

95. renal pelvis

96. trigone

97. renal veins

98. dysuria

99. KUB = kidneys, ureters, bladder; simple abbreviation for the kidneys, ureters, and bladder

100. ESRD = end-stage renal disease; final phase of kidney disease marked by the inability of the kidneys to filter the body's blood and produce urine

101. IVP = intravenous pyelogram; procedure in which a contrast dye is injected into a vein to be excreted by the kidneys to permit x-ray visualization of the renal pelvis and ureter

102. UA = urinalysis; examination of the urine

103. BUN = blood urea nitrogen; diagnostic test to determine the amount of urea present in the blood

104. pyuria

105. polyuria

106. ADH is secreted by the body to conserve water. Therefore, it is secreted during times of dehydration or when the body is lacking fluids. If Kelsey had been drinking a few beers, she obviously had plenty of fluid intake and would not be secreting ADH. Thus Marcy is correct: ADH secretion is suppressed when the body has plenty of circulating fluid.

107. Katie's pain is probably not muscle related if she has not been engaged in physical activity. Although she may have pulled a muscle by twisting or turning unnaturally, her pain may be the result of a kidney problem. Katie describes her pain at the location where the kidneys are found. Kidney pain frequently indicates an infection or kidney stones, called renal calculi.

108. Sasha may have been suffering from pain secondary to a kidney stone (renal calculus). She may have passed (excreted) the stone while urinating, thus the source of the pain was removed.

109. The accident occurred while the bladder was full. In a normal, seated position, the lap seat belt rests on the abdomen at the point of the urinary bladder. Because of the increased pressure on the full bladder, the lap belt was able to rupture the bladder. The lesson to be learned is to take frequent breaks while driving to empty the bladder and thus thwart the possibility of rupturing the bladder should you get in an accident.

110. Water-soluble vitamins are excreted in the urine. If you are megadosing on them, the body cannot make use of them all and will excrete the excesses. Vitamins in the urine have an unpleasant odor. Many plant pigments found in green, leafy vegetables are not broken down in the body and are frequently excreted in the urine, giving the urine a darker color. Although eating these vegetables is not detrimental to one's health, and in fact is beneficial, the urine will appear to have a deeper color instead of the characteristic pale yellow color.

Labeling

a. kidneys   **b.** ureters   **c.** bladder

d. urethra   **e.** inferior vena cava   **f.** abdominal aorta

Word Search

A	P	I	X	X	C	K	K	P	R	K	H	P	Y
G	R	T	R	X	Q	H	N	K	E	N	T	L	L
Z	T	H	U	O	F	I	S	U	A	C	A	H	L
S	I	X	T	R	N	D	Q	Q	B	P	P	Z	V
C	I	W	Z	E	B	W	M	T	S	R	D	V	S
N	J	S	R	C	R	I	L	L	O	F	M	T	U
E	B	Y	L	S	L	U	D	K	R	T	U	W	L
P	K	R	X	A	A	N	K	I	P	W	L	V	U
H	C	N	O	I	T	I	R	U	T	C	I	M	R
R	B	D	Q	A	D	S	J	G	I	Y	H	Q	E
O	I	Y	J	N	X	Y	I	Y	O	A	J	O	M
N	S	R	E	T	E	R	U	R	N	M	L	W	O
S	T	Y	U	B	U	W	Y	F	E	P	T	M	L
O	S	M	O	L	A	R	I	T	Y	P	G	X	G

glomerulus
hilum
kidneys
micturition
nephrons
osmolarity
peristalsis
reabsorption
renin
turbidity
ureters
urethra

Vocabulary Review

Key Term	Definition	Key Term	Definition
albuminuria	protein, specifically albumin, in the urine	bladder neck obstruction (BNO)	blockage of the urinary bladder outlet
aldosterone	hormone that stimulates the kidneys to retain sodium and so regulates water and salt balance	bladder stones	calculi in the urinary bladder
		blood urea nitrogen (BUN)	diagnostic test to determine the amount of urea present in the blood
antidiuretic hormone (ADH)	hormone made by the hypothalamus and secreted by the posterior pituitary gland to cause water retention, thereby elevating blood pressure	calyces	cup-like structures that drain into the renal pelvis
		clean-catch urine specimen	urine sample obtained after urinating slightly to flush the external genitalia
anuria	absence of urine formation	creatinine clearance test	test used to determine the glomerular filtration rate by measuring the clearance of creatinine
azotemia	abnormal increase in the concentration of urea and other nitrogenous substances in the blood; also called uremia		
		cystitis	inflammation of the bladder
bacteriuria	presence of bacteria in the urine	cystoscope	medical instrument used for viewing the urinary bladder interior
bladder catheterization	procedure in which a tube, attached to a collection bag, is placed through the urethra into the bladder to assist in bladder emptying	detrusor muscle	muscle forming the urinary bladder
		diabetes insipidus	disorder resulting from ADH deficiency or ADH insensitivity

Key Term	Definition	Key Term	Definition
diabetes mellitus (DM)	disorder of carbohydrate metabolism due to pancreatic dysfunction or insulin insensitivity	hydronephrosis	dilation of the renal pelvis and calyces of one or both kidneys
dialysis	procedure in which a machine (hemodialyzer) is used to replace normal kidney functions; also called hemodialysis	hyperuricemia	elevated uric acid levels in the blood
		hypoalbuminemia	low blood albumin (protein) concentration
diuresis	excessive urine excretion	hypospadias	congenital defect in which the urethral opening is located on the penis ventral surface in males or vagina in females
dysuria	painful, burning sensation while urinating		
end-stage renal disease (ESRD)	final phase of kidney disease marked by the inability of the kidneys to filter the body's blood and produce urine	incontinence	inability to control urination
		interstitial cystitis (IC)	chronic bladder condition in which the urinary bladder connective tissue is inflamed
enuresis	involuntary nighttime bedwetting, particularly in children	intravenous pyelogram (IVP)	procedure in which a contrast dye is injected into a vein to be excreted by the kidneys to permit x-ray visualization of the renal pelvis and ureter
epispadias	congenital defect in which the urethral opening is located on the penis upper aspect (dorsum) in males or clitoris in females		
		intravenous urogram (IVU)	radiograph of the entire urinary tract after infusion with a contrast dye
erythropoietin (EPO)	renal hormone that stimulates red blood cell production in the red bone marrow	Kegel exercises	alternate contraction and relaxation of pelvic floor muscles used to strengthen and tone these muscles for the treatment of incontinence
excretion	process by which wastes are eliminated from the body	kidney transplant	operation in which a donor kidney is placed into a recipient
external urethral orifice	opening in urethra to outside	kidneys	paired organs whose main functions are to purify blood, control fluid and ion levels, and excrete wastes in urine
extracorporeal shock wave lithotripsy (ESWL)	procedure in which sound waves are transmitted to the kidneys to break apart renal calculi		
		KUB radiographic study	procedure in which a contrast dye is injected into the blood and taken up by the urinary system (kidneys, ureters, and bladder) to be visualized through a renogram
filtration	process by which the kidneys filter blood		
fistula	surgically created passage that connects an artery and a vein		
frequency	urinating often	lithotripsy	procedure in which stones are crushed by mechanical force, laser, or focused sound energy
glomerular capsule	sac surrounding the kidney glomerulus; also called Bowman capsule		
glomerular filtration rate (GFR)	the rate at which blood is filtered by the glomerulus	micturition	urination
		nephrectomy	surgical removal of a kidney
glomerulonephritis	inflammation of the glomeruli	nephritis	inflammation of the kidneys
glomerulosclerosis	hardening or scarring of the renal glomeruli	nephrons	functional units of the kidney consisting of the renal corpuscle and renal tubule
glomerulus	capillary cluster in the renal corpuscle	nephropathy	kidney disease
		nephroptosis	condition in which the kidney drops out of its normal position due to loss of supporting adipose tissue; also called floating kidney
glucosuria	glucose in the urine; another term for glycosuria		
glycosuria	glucose in the urine; another term for glucosuria		
hematuria	presence of blood in the urine	nephrotic syndrome	degenerative renal lesions resulting from damage to the basement membrane of the glomeruli
hemodialyzer	machine that acts as an artificial kidney during dialysis		
hilum	area for the entrance and exit of structures	neurogenic bladder	urinary bladder dysfunction resulting from impaired nervous system functioning

Key Term	Definition	Key Term	Definition
oliguria	scanty urine production	renal tubule	coiled tube that leads away from the glomerular capsule and empties into the renal pelvis that is involved in urine formation
osmolarity	total concentration of dissolved substances in a solution; also called osmotic concentration		
papillae	tips of each renal pyramid	renal veins	blood vessels that carry blood from the kidneys into the inferior vena cava
peristalsis	waves of smooth muscle contractions that propel substances through a structure, such as urine along the ureters		
		renin	enzyme released by certain kidney cells to regulate blood pressure when there is a drop in renal blood flow
peritoneal dialysis (PD)	filtration procedure using a dialysis solution in the peritoneal cavity to filter blood		
		ruptured bladder	disruption of the bladder wall
phimosis	narrowing of the penis foreskin preventing it from being drawn back to uncover the penis tip	secretion	process of producing a substance in the kidneys and then discharging it
		specific gravity (sp. gr.)	measure of the density of the urine compared to that of water
polycystic kidney disease	inherited disorder in which normal kidney tissue is replaced with multiple cysts that compress normal tissue and prevent kidney functioning	sphincter	muscular ring that contracts to close off an opening in the body
		trigone	triangular region of the bladder marked by three openings: the two entrances of the ureters and the exit to the urethra
polydipsia	extreme thirst		
polyuria	excessive excretion of urine		
proteinuria	protein in the urine		
pyelitis	inflammation of the kidney pelvis	turbidity	refers to the clarity of a liquid
pyelonephritis	inflammation of the kidneys, renal pelvis, and associated connective tissue	uremia	abnormal increase in the concentration of urea and other nitrogenous substances in the blood; also called azotemia
pyuria	presence of pus in the urine		
reabsorption	process by which water and solutes are removed from the filtrate in the kidneys and returned to the bloodstream	uremic frost	urea and uric acid salt deposits excreted in sweat as a result of uremia, giving the skin a powdery appearance
renal adenocarcinoma	kidney cancer; also called renal cell carcinoma	ureteritis	inflammation of the ureter
		ureters	paired tubes that transport urine from the kidneys to the bladder
renal arteries	blood vessels that carry blood from the abdominal aorta into the kidneys	urethra	canal leading from the bladder to the exterior
renal calculi	kidney stones	urethritis	inflammation of the urethra
renal corpuscle	structure composed of the glomerulus and the surrounding glomerular capsule	urgency	strong desire to urinate
		urinalysis (UA)	examination and analysis of urine
renal cortex	outer region of the kidney	urinary bladder	expandable sac that stores urine
renal failure	significant decline in kidney function resulting in uremia	urinary bladder cancer	malignant cell growth in the urinary bladder
renal hypertension	increased blood pressure due to kidney disease	urinary retention	inability to urinate
renal medulla	inner region of the kidney	urinary tract infection (UTI)	infection of the kidneys, ureters, bladder, and/or urethra
renal pelvis	funnel-shaped region that serves as a reservoir for urine before it flows into the ureter	urochrome	yellow pigment in urine
		Wilms tumor	cancer of the kidneys that typically affects young children; also called nephroblastoma
renal pyramids	cone-shaped divisions of the renal medulla		

CHAPTER 16

Reproductive Systems

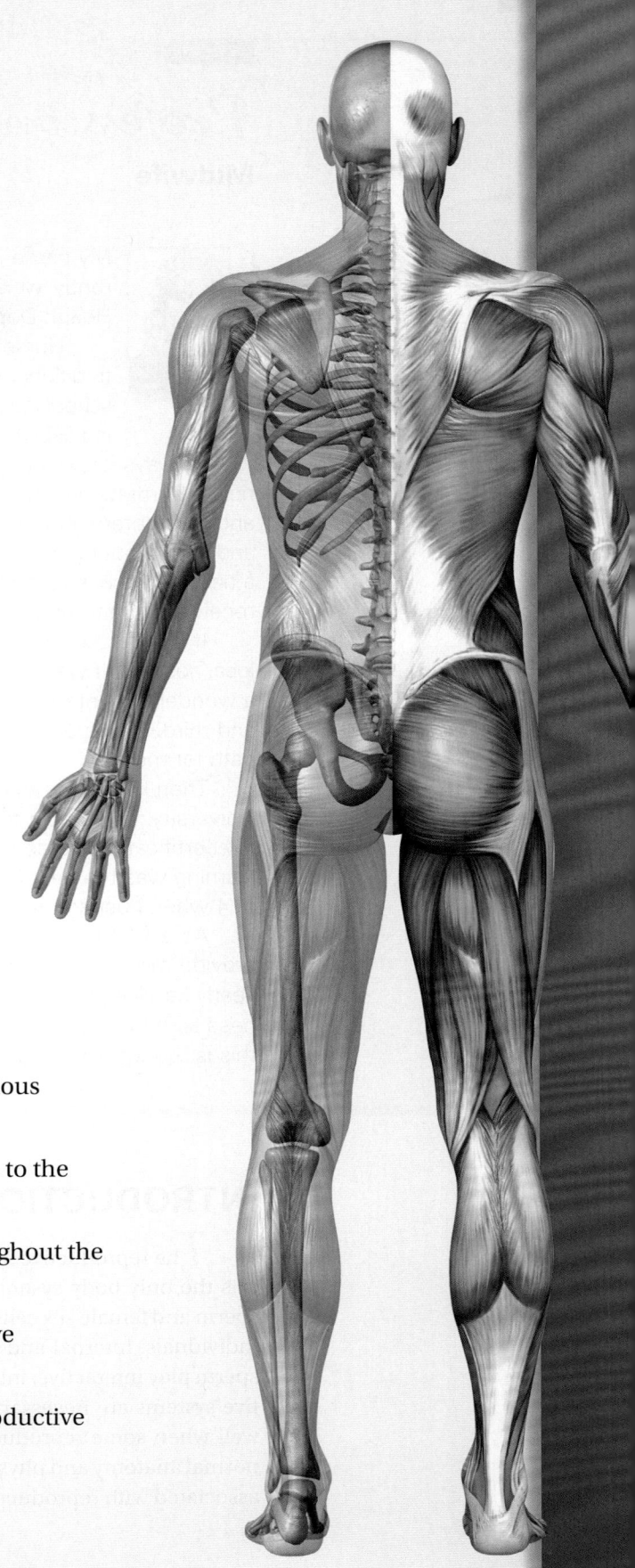

OBJECTIVES

After completing this chapter, you should be able to:

1. Define the meanings of word parts related to the reproductive systems.

2. Identify organs of the male and female reproductive systems.

3. Cite a function of each reproductive organ.

4. Describe available birth control methods and practices.

5. Define common signs, symptoms, and treatments of various reproductive system diseases.

6. Describe clinical tests and diagnostic procedures related to the reproductive systems.

7. Describe anatomical and physiological alterations throughout the life span.

8. Define common abbreviations related to the reproductive systems.

9. Define terms used in medical reports involving the reproductive systems.

10. Correctly define, spell, and pronounce the chapter's medical terms.

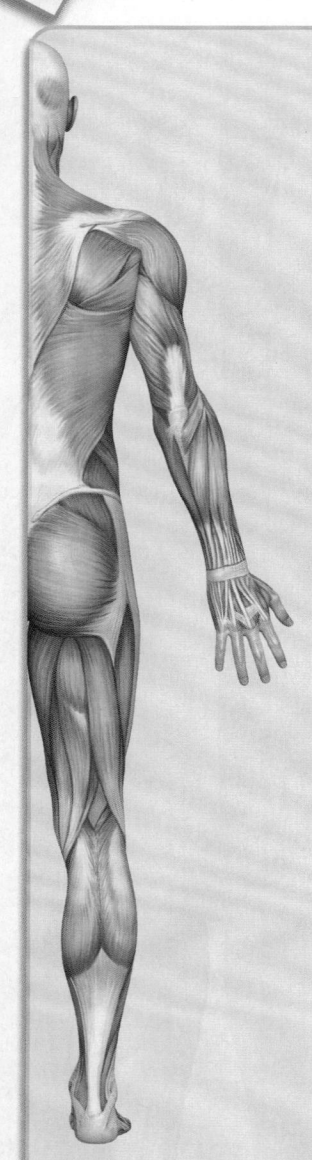

Professional Profile

Midwife

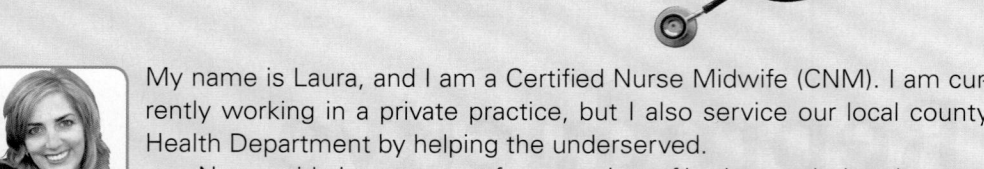

My name is Laura, and I am a Certified Nurse Midwife (CNM). I am currently working in a private practice, but I also service our local county Health Department by helping the underserved.

Nurse midwives can start from a variety of backgrounds, but the most traditional route is being a nurse first. As for myself, I went to nursing school right out of high school. I received my Bachelor of Science in Nursing (BSN) and registered nurse (RN) degrees at a small private college.

I always knew that I wanted to help people, but saw my calling during my obstetrics (OB) rotation in school clinicals. An amazing mom was giving birth to her first child and was determined to have natural childbirth. As a student, my role was to observe and assist, but not perform any nursing duties. It was very empowering to watch such a natural process take place, and to see this mom so empowered by the support she received from the nursing staff.

It didn't take too long for me to find a position in Labor and Delivery at a small local hospital. It was there that my husband and I had three all-natural childbirths. I had a wonderful obstetrician with my first baby, but a nurse midwife attended the second and third. It was at that point I knew for certain that nurse midwifery was the career path for me.

Then I attended the oldest nurse midwifery school in the nation, Frontier Nursing University. I was able to enroll and utilize their distance-learning program. I obtained my certificate in nurse midwifery and a Master of Science in Nursing (MSN). Distance learning was the best option for me, because I had three small children under the age of 4 when I began the program.

As a CNM, I touch so many lives in so many different aspects. Of course we provide evidence-based care throughout the childbearing years, but we also provide yearly services to all women regardless of age and birthing status. We are taught wellness care through our nursing backgrounds, not disease-based care. For many CNMs, this is more than just a career—it is something we were born to do.

INTRODUCTION

*T*he reproductive system is responsible for the continuation of the human species, and it is the only body system that differs significantly between the sexes. Male sex cells called sperm and female sex cells known as oocytes carry the genetic information that creates unique individuals. Internal and external structures, accessory glands and organs, and oocytes and sperm play interactive, interdependent roles in the process. Despite the fact that the reproductive systems are necessary for propagating human life, men and women can function quite well when some reproductive organs must be removed for medical reasons. In addition to normal anatomy and physiology, the signs, symptoms, diagnostic tests and clinical procedures associated with reproductive pathology are described in this chapter.

MEDICAL TERM PARTS

Word Parts

Medical term prefixes, suffixes, and combining forms related to the reproductive systems are introduced in this section.

Word Part	Meaning
acro-	tip, end
andro-	man, masculine
arch-, arche-, archi-	primitive, ancestral
balan-, balano-	glans penis
-cele	swelling, hernia
cervic-, cervico-	cervix, neck
colp-, colpo-	vagina
crypt-, crypto-	hidden, concealed
embry-, embryo-	embryo
-genesis	origin, beginning process
gyn-, gyne-, gyneco-, gyno-	female, woman
hyster-, hystero-	uterus
labio-	lips
leio-, lio-	smooth
mammil-, mammili-	nipple
mammo-	breast
mast-, masto-	breast
meato-	passage
meno-	menses, menstruation
metr-, metra-, metro-	uterus
olig-, oligo-	few, too few
oo-	egg, ovary
oophor-, oophoro-	ovary
orchi-, orchido-, orchio-	testes
ovari-, ovario-	ovary
ovi-, ovo-	egg
pelvi-, pelvio-, pelvo-	pelvis
perineo-	perineum
proct-, procto-	rectum or anus
prostat-, prostato-	prostate gland
salping-, salpingo-	uterine tube
sperma-, spermato-, spermo-	sperm, seed, semen, spermatozoa
-spermia	condition of spermatozoa or semen
uter-, utero-	uterus
vagin-, vagino-	vagina

Word Grouping Exercises

Using the *Medical Term Parts* table, identify the prefix, suffix, or combining form for each of the following definitions. The first one has been done as an example.

Definition	Word Part
man, masculine	*andro-*
breast	A. B.
cervix, neck	
condition of spermatozoa or semen	
egg	
egg, ovary	
female, woman	
few, too few	
glans penis	
hidden, concealed	
lips	
menses, menstruation	
nipple	
origin, beginning process	
ovary	A. B.
passage	
pelvis	
perineum	
primitive, ancestral	
prostate gland	
rectum or anus	
smooth	
sperm, seed, semen, spermatozoa	
swelling, hernia	
testes	
tip, end	
uterine tube	
uterus	A. B. C.
vagina	A. B.

Word Building Exercises

Word parts introduced in the *Medical Term Parts* section are listed in the following table. For this exercise, first supply the meaning of each word part, then use the word part to build a word you already know. The word you list under *Common or Known Word* does not have to be a medical term; a commonly used word is fine. Be sure, however, that the word correctly reflects the intended meaning. The first one has been done as an example. Check your answers in a dictionary.

Word Part	Meaning	Common or Known Word	Example Medical Term
arch-, arche-, archi-	*primitive, ancestral*	*archeology*	menarche
andro-			androgens
cervic-, cervico-			cervical cancer
crypt-, crypto-			cryptorchidism
embry-, embryo-			embryonic
-genesis			oogenesis
gyn-, gyne-, gyneco-, gyno-			gynecomastia
hyster-, hystero-			hysterectomy
mammil-, mammili-			mammilla
mammo-			mammary gland
meato-			urethral meatus
meno-			menopause
orchi-, orchido-, orchio-			orchiectomy
ovari-, ovario-			ovarian
ovi-, ovo-			oviduct
pelvi-, pelvio-, pelvo-			pelvic examination
proct-, procto-			proctocele
prostat-, prostato-			prostatitis
sperma-, spermato-, spermo-			spermiogenesis
uter-, utero-			uterus
vagin-, vagino-			vaginitis

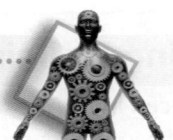

ANATOMY AND PHYSIOLOGY

Reproductive Systems Preview

Human **reproduction** (procreation) is the total process by which organisms produce offspring. During the process, genetic material is sexually passed from one generation to the next by forming a new person. An organ, such as the male testis (*testes* = plural) and female ovary (*ovaries* = plural), that produces sex cells is called a **gonad**. These sex cells, whether male sperm or female oocytes, are known as **gametes**. **Sperm**, also called *spermatozoa*, contain the genetic information to be transmitted by the male to the oocyte. Sperm is both the singular and the plural form of the term. *Spermatozoon* is the singular form of *spermatozoa*. An **oocyte** contains the female genetic information. In addition to gonads, basic structures of the reproductive system in both sexes include ducts, accessory glands, and external genitalia. The reproductive anatomy of each sex is described in this chapter.

KEY TERM	Definition
reproduction	total process by which organisms produce offspring; also known as procreation
gonad (GOH-nad)	organ such as the testis or ovary that produces sex cells
gametes (GAM-eets)	sex cells (sperm and oocytes)
sperm	sex cells that contain the male genetic information; also called spermatozoa
oocyte (OH-oh-site)	sex cell that contains the female genetic information

KEY TERM PRACTICE: *Reproductive Systems Preview*

1. _____ are sex cells, also called sperm and oocytes.

2. An organ, such as the testis or ovary, which produces sex cells, is termed a _____.

3. The total process by which organisms produce offspring is termed _____.

4. Female sex cells are referred to as _____, while male sex cells are termed _____.

Male Reproductive System Overview

Major structures of the male reproductive system are shown in **Figure 16-1**. Main organs include the testes (testicles), scrotum, penis, accessory glands and organs, and ducts. Accessory glands and organs secrete fluids. Ducts transport, receive, and store gametes. **Testes** also called **testicles**, are the paired male gonads located in the scrotum. **Seminiferous tubules** of the testes are the site of sperm formation (**spermatogenesis**). Cells between the seminiferous tubules, called **interstitial cells**, secrete the male hormone testosterone. The **scrotum** is a fleshy sac hanging from the pelvic region that encloses the testes. The visible exterior ridge joining the two halves of the scrotum is called the **raphe**, derived from the Greek word for *seam*. The **penis** is the external organ of sexual intercourse and urination.

A major gland is the **prostate**, a round, fluid-secreting organ surrounding the urethra, just inferior to the bladder. The prostate is the largest accessory gland of the male reproductive system. It secretes a milky fluid that is discharged by ducts into the urethra prior to ejaculation. Hormones from the hypothalamus, anterior pituitary gland, and testes control male reproductive functions.

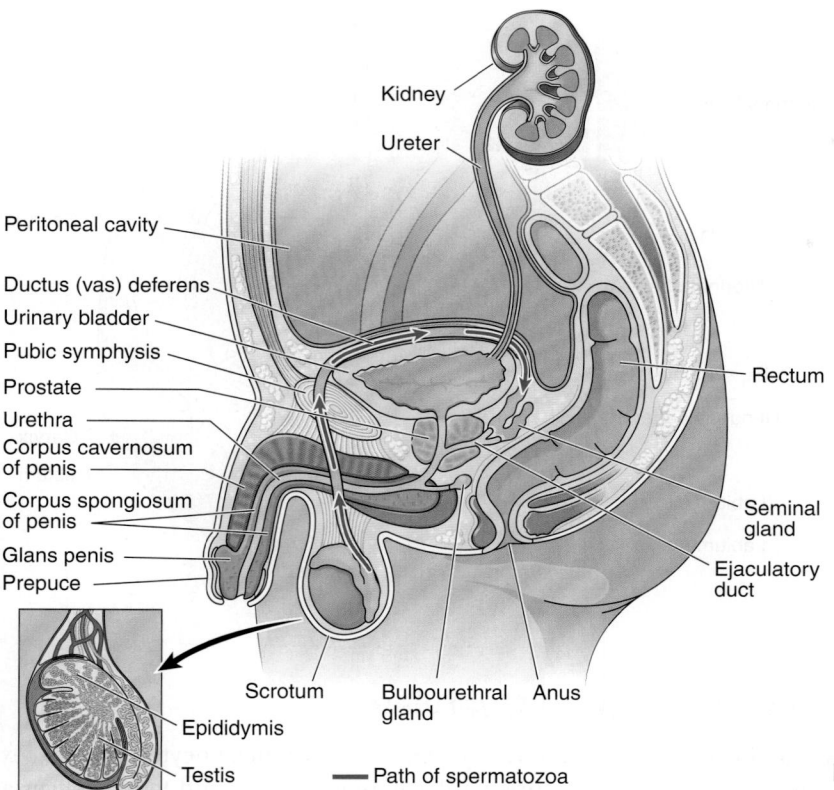

Kidney

Ureter

Peritoneal cavity

Ductus (vas) deferens
Urinary bladder
Pubic symphysis
Prostate
Urethra
Corpus cavernosum
of penis
Corpus spongiosum
of penis
Glans penis
Prepuce

Rectum

Seminal
gland

Ejaculatory
duct

Scrotum   Bulbourethral   Anus
gland

Epididymis

Testis   —— Path of spermatozoa

Figure 16-1 The male
reproductive system.

KEY TERM	Definition
testes (TES-teez)	paired male gonads located in the scrotum; also called testicles
testicles (TES-ti-kulz)	paired male gonads located in the scrotum; also called testes
seminiferous tubules (sem-ih-NIF-ur-us TOO-byulz)	site of sperm formation in the testes
spermatogenesis (sper-muh-toh-JEN-eh-sis)	process of sperm formation
interstitial cells (in-ter-STISH-ul CELLS)	cells between the seminiferous tubules that secrete testosterone
scrotum (SKROH-tum)	fleshy sac that encloses the testes
raphe (RAY-fee)	visible ridge joining the two halves of the scrotum
penis	male organ of sexual intercourse and urination
prostate (PROS-tate)	round, fluid-secreting organ surrounding the urethra that secretes a milky fluid

KEY TERM PRACTICE: *Male Reproductive System Overview*

1. The _____ is a fleshy sac that encloses the testes.

2. A round, fluid-secreting organ surrounding the urethra that secretes a milky fluid is the _____.

3. _____ is the process of sperm formation and is derived from the word part _____ for *semen, spermatozoa*, and the word part _____ for *beginning process*.

4. The _____ is the male organ of sexual intercourse and urination.

5. The paired male gonads located in the scrotum are known as the _____ or _____.

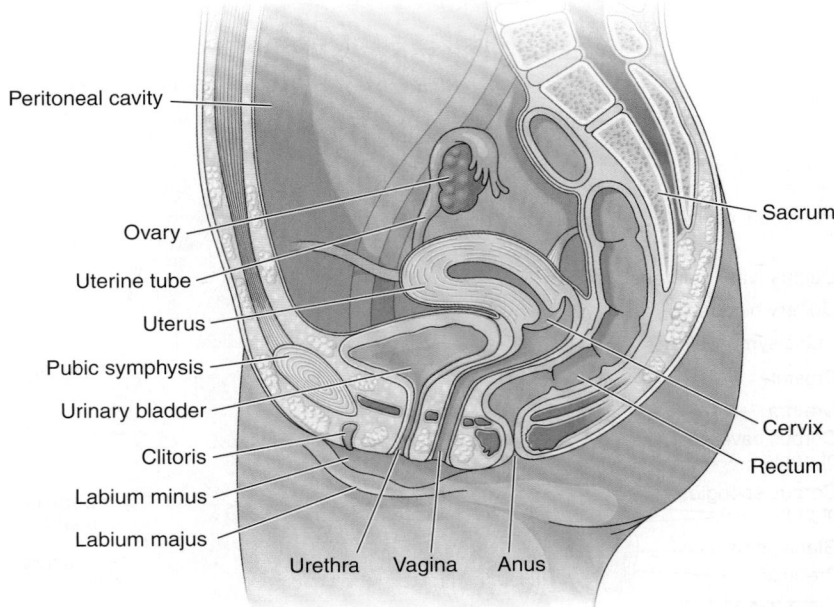

Figure 16-2 The female reproductive system.

Female Reproductive System Overview

The primary purposes of the female reproductive system are to produce oocytes, secrete sex hormones, receive sperm from the male, nourish a developing embryo and fetus, deliver a baby, and nurse an infant. These functions are accomplished through the actions of several organs, including paired mammary glands, ovaries, and uterine tubes; the single uterus and vagina; and the external genitalia (labium majus and labium minus) (**Figure 16-2**).

The **mammary glands** are milk-producing structures within the breasts composed of a network of ducts leading to the nipple. The **ovaries** are paired glands that produce oocytes and female sex hormones. Two narrow tubes that serve as a passageway from the ovaries to the uterus are termed **uterine tubes**. These tubes are also called the oviducts or fallopian tubes. The **uterus**, or womb, is the hollow muscular organ in the pelvic region in which a developing embryo or fetus is nourished before birth. An *embryo* is the early developmental stage that begins at conception and ends at the eighth week of gestation. From the eighth week until birth, the developing human is referred to as a *fetus*. In the absence of pregnancy, the uterine lining is shed monthly during menstruation. The **vagina** is a muscular tube connecting the uterus to the outside.

The **perineum** is the region surrounding the urogenital and anal openings. In females, it is found between the **vulva** (the external genitals) and the anus. *Vulva* is a Latin term for wrapper or covering. In males, the perineum is between the scrotum and the anus. Hormones from the hypothalamus, anterior pituitary gland, ovaries, and uterus control female reproductive functions.

KEY TERM	Definition
mammary (MAM-uh-ree) **glands**	milk-producing structures within the breasts composed of a network of ducts leading to the nipple
ovaries (OH-vur-eez)	paired glands that produce oocytes and female sex hormones
uterine (YOO-tur-in) **tubes**	narrow tubes that serve as a passageway from the ovaries to the uterus; also called oviducts or fallopian tubes

continued

continued from page 822

KEY TERM	Definition
uterus (YOO-tur-us)	the hollow muscular organ in the pelvic region in which a developing embryo or fetus is nourished before birth
vagina (vuh-JYE-nuh)	muscular tube connecting the uterus to the outside
perineum (perr-i-NEE-um)	region between the anus and the vulva in females and between the anus and the scrotum in males
vulva (VUL-vuh)	female external genitals

KEY TERM PRACTICE: *Female Reproductive System Overview*

1. The muscular tube connecting the uterus to the outside is the _____.

2. The term for female external genitals is _____.

3. Paired glands that produce oocytes and female sex hormones are _____.

4. _____ are milk-producing structures within the breasts composed of a network of ducts leading to the nipple.

5. The _____ is the region between the anus and the vulva in females; it is also the region between the anus and the scrotum in males.

The Testes and Male Accessory Glands

The testes are a pair of oval-shaped structures located within the scrotum. Before the testes can become fully functional, they must drop from the pelvic cavity. During development, a fibrous cord called the gubernaculum testis connects the fetal testis to the developing scrotum and guides the descent of each testicle to its permanent position.

Each testis is partitioned into lobules, which contain tubules. The seminiferous tubules are approximately 800 tightly coiled structures, in which spermatogenesis takes place. Connected to the posterior surface of each testis is an elongated structure consisting of coiled tubes called the **epididymis** (*epididymides* = plural). The epididymides can be felt through the skin of the scrotum. As the start of the reproductive tract, their functions include storing and maturing sperm, and transporting sperm between the testis and the ductus deferens.

Each **ductus deferens** (also called the **vas deferens**) begins at the tail of the epididymis and is a muscular tube connecting the epididymis with the ejaculatory duct. The **ejaculatory duct** is a short passageway that empties into the urethra. The **spermatic cord** encloses the ductus deferens, arteries, veins, lymphatics, and nerves in each testis and travels through the inguinal canal, connecting the testicles to the abdominal cavity (**Figure 16-3**).

Accessory glands include the seminal glands (seminal vesicles), prostate, and bulbourethral glands. The **seminal glands,** also called *seminal vesicles*, are paired glands that secrete seminal fluid into the ejaculatory duct. The prostate is about 4 cm (1.6 in.) in diameter and produces a slightly acidic fluid. Other fluid-secreting glands, located at the base of the penis just inferior to the prostate, are the paired **bulbourethral glands,** also called Cowper glands (see **Figure 16-1**). The name describes their location at the bulb of the urethra. The fluid they secrete lubricates the tip of the penis just before the ejaculation of semen. **Semen** is

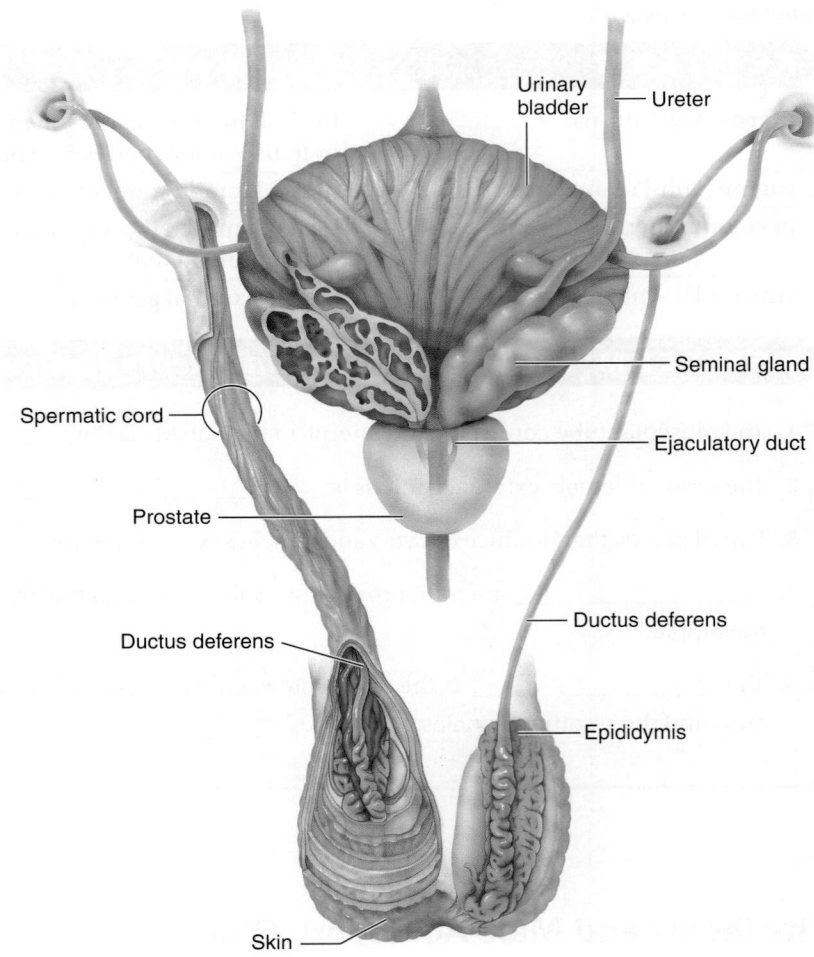

Urinary bladder

Ureter

Seminal gland

Spermatic cord

Ejaculatory duct

Prostate

Ductus deferens

Ductus deferens

Epididymis

Skin

Figure 16-3 The testes and their relationship to the urinary bladder, and prostate.

the thick, yellowish-white fluid containing sperm. Semen is also referred to as *ejaculate* or *seminal fluid*.

To summarize, the structures secreting substances that make up semen are the testes, epididymides, prostate, bulbourethral glands, and seminal glands. The duct pathway from the testes to the urethra is as follows:

seminiferous tubules → epididymides → ductus deferens → ejaculatory duct → urethra

Two muscles are associated with the scrotum: the dartos muscle and the cremaster muscle. Contraction of the dartos muscle elevates the testes and normal muscle tone causes wrinkling of the scrotal skin. Contraction of the cremaster muscle during sexual arousal or as a response to decreased temperature pulls the testes closer to the body. Regulating scrotal temperature is important, because the temperature required for normal sperm formation is approximately 2°F below normal body temperature. For this reason, sperm are produced in the testes, which are located outside the pelvic cavity where the temperature is cooler. Through the contraction or relaxation of the cremaster and dartos muscles, the temperature of the testicles can be regulated: When air or body temperature rises, the muscles relax and the testes move away from the body; when the temperature falls, the muscles contract and the testes move closer to the body. Males can be sterile, incapable of inducing pregnancy, if the temperature of the testes is too high to produce viable sperm.

KEY TERM	Definition
epididymis (ep-i-DID-i-mis)	elongated structure consisting of coiled tubes connected to the posterior surface of each testis that transports sperm between the testis and the ductus deferens
ductus deferens (DUCK-tus DEF-uh-renz)	tube connecting the epididymis and the ejaculatory duct; also called the vas deferens
vas deferens (VAS DEF-uh-renz)	tube connecting the epididymis and the ejaculatory duct; also called the ductus deferens
ejaculatory duct (eh-JACK-yoo-luh-tor-ee DUKT)	short passageway between the ductus deferens and the urethra
spermatic (spur-MAT-ick) **cord**	paired structure that encloses the ductus deferens, blood vessels, nerves, and lymphatic vessels in each testis
seminal (SEM-ih-nul) **glands**	paired glands that secrete semen into the ejaculatory duct; also called the seminal vesicles
bulbourethral (bul-boh-yoo-REE-thrul) **glands**	pair of glands located at the base of the penis just inferior to the prostate gland; also called Cowper glands
semen (SEE-mun)	fluid of the male reproductive organs that contains sperm; also called ejaculate or seminal fluid

KEY TERM PRACTICE: *The Testes and Male Accessory Glands*

1. The glands located at the base of the penis just inferior to the prostate gland are termed the _____ or Cowper glands.

2. The elongated structure consisting of coiled tubes connected to the posterior surface of each testis that transports sperm between the testis and ductus deferens is the _____.

3. _____ is the fluid of the male reproductive organs that contains sperm and is also known as ejaculate or seminal fluid.

4. Paired glands, also called seminal vesicles, that secrete semen into the ejaculatory duct are the _____.

5. The _____ is a short passageway between the ductus deferens and the urethra.

The Penis

The penis functions in both the urinary and the reproductive systems. In addition to urination, the penis is the external male organ of sexual intercourse (**coitus**). The urethra is the central tube within the penis and has two jobs: As part of the urinary system, it carries urine from the bladder out of the body; as part of the reproductive system, it transports semen during ejaculation. During ejaculation, a sphincter seals the urethral opening at the bladder so that only semen is ejaculated from an erect penis. The urethra is divided into three regions, named according to its location: prostatic, membranous, and spongy.

The three regions of the penis are the root, body (shaft), and glans. The *root* is the portion that attaches the penis to the body wall. The majority of the penis is called the *body* or *shaft* and is composed of three columns of erectile tissue that run the length of the penis. Erectile tissue is capable of filling with blood under pressure to swell and become stiff, resulting in **erection**. The three columns are the paired **corpora cavernosa** and a single **corpus spongiosum**. *Corpora*

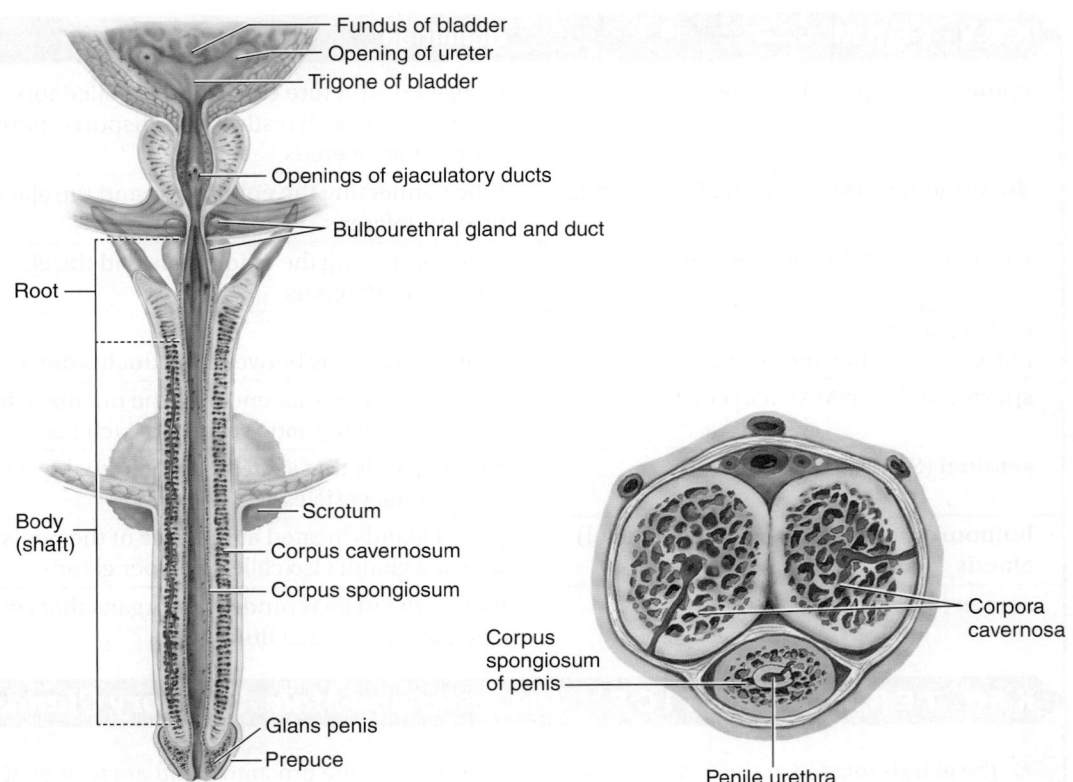

Figure 16-4 (A) A sagittal section of the penis. (B) The penis in cross-section.

is the plural form of the word *corpus,* and the corpora cavernosa are two columns of tissues. Associate the *s* in *single* with the *s* in corpu*s* *s*pongiosum to remember that it is a single column of erectile tissue. The **glans penis** surrounds the external urethral orifice (urethral opening) and forms the rounded tip of the penis.

The last penile structure is the **prepuce,** or foreskin, the loose fold of skin covering the penis tip in uncircumcised males (**Figure 16-4**). **Circumcision** is a surgery to remove the prepuce (foreskin). Circumcision is performed on many infants in the United States, but this practice is continually debated.

KEY TERM	Definition
coitus (KOH-i-tus)	sexual intercourse
erection	enlarged and stiffened state of the penis due to erectile tissue filling with blood
corpora cavernosa (KOR-poh-ruh kav-ur-NOH-suh)	two cylinders of erectile tissue in the penis
corpus spongiosum (KOR-pus spon-jee-OH-sum)	single cylinder of erectile tissue surrounding the urethra in the penis
glans (GLANZ) **penis**	region surrounding the external urethral orifice that forms the rounded tip of the penis
prepuce (PREE-poos)	fold of skin covering the glans penis in uncircumcised males; also called the foreskin
circumcision (sur-kum-SIZH-un)	surgery to remove the prepuce (foreskin) from the penis

continued

continued from page 826

KEY TERM PRACTICE: *The Penis*

1. Identify the three columns of erectile tissue making up the penis. _____

2. _____ is the medical term for sexual intercourse.

3. _____ is the surgery performed to remove the prepuce.

4. The medical term for the foreskin on the penis is _____.

5. The _____ is the region that surrounds the external urethral orifice and forms the rounded tip of the penis.

Male Reproductive Hormones

Several hormones are responsible for male reproductive functions and secondary sexual characteristics. **Secondary sexual characteristics** are features that develop at puberty but are not directly concerned with reproduction. For example, facial hair is a secondary sexual characteristic of males. Other secondary sexual characteristics in both sexes include voice changes, body hair distribution, and adipose tissue patterns.

Primary male hormones stimulate gamete development and sex hormone secretion. **Follicle-stimulating hormone (FSH)** is secreted by the anterior pituitary gland to stimulate spermatogenesis. **Luteinizing hormone (LH)**, from the anterior pituitary gland, acts with FSH to stimulate testosterone secretion by the interstitial cells in the testes. **Testosterone** is a male steroid hormone responsible for the development of secondary sexual characteristics and the maintenance of accessory glands of reproduction.

KEY TERM	Definition
secondary sexual characteristics	traits that develop at puberty but are not directly concerned with reproduction, such as voice changes, body hair distribution, and adipose tissue patterns
follicle (FOL-i-kul) **-stimulating hormone (FSH)**	anterior pituitary gland hormone stimulating spermatogenesis in testes
luteinizing (LOO-tee-in-eye-zing) **hormone (LH)**	anterior pituitary gland hormone that stimulates testosterone secretion
testosterone (tes-TOS-tur-ohn)	principal hormone secreted by cells in the testes

KEY TERM PRACTICE: *Male Reproductive Hormones*

1. _____ is the principal hormone secreted by cells in the testes.

2. Traits that develop at puberty but are not directly concerned with reproduction are termed _____.

3. _____ is the hormone secreted by the anterior pituitary gland that stimulates testosterone secretion.

4. The anterior pituitary gland hormone that stimulates spermatogenesis is known as _____.

Spermatozoa (Sperm)

Spermatogenesis is the formation and development of spermatozoa in the testes. Together, both testes produce approximately 300 million sperm daily. This process involves mitosis (somatic or nonsex cell division), meiosis I and II (gamete cell division), and **spermiogenesis** (physical maturation of sperm). Each spermatozoon begins as a diploid **spermatogonium** (sperm stem cell) with 46 individual chromosomes. Meiosis I is the next step in gamete cell division and results in two haploid secondary spermatocytes with 23 chromosomes each. In other words, the **diploid** (containing 46 chromosomes) sperm stem cell divides to become two **haploid** cells with 23 chromosomes. Diploid cells have two matched sets of chromosomes (23 pairs or 46 total) in the cell nucleus, one set from each parent. Haploid cells have a single set of unpaired chromosomes. During meiosis II, the secondary spermatocytes divide into four haploid spermatids. The last phase, spermiogenesis, results in four physically mature spermatozoa (sperm) (**Figure 16-5**). The stages are shown here:

spermatogonium → primary spermatocyte → 2 secondary spermatocytes →
4 spermatids → 4 spermatozoa

A physically mature spermatozoon has four different regions, aptly named the head, neck, middle piece, and tail. The head contains the nucleus and chromosomes. At the tip of the head is the **acrosome**, which contains enzymes necessary to penetrate and fertilize an oocyte. The neck attaches the middle piece to the head. The middle piece contains the mitochondria, which provide the spermatozoon's energy in the form of ATP. The tail is a **flagellum** that propels the spermatozoon (**Figure 16-6**). The spermatozoon is the only cell in the human body with a flagellum. The flagellum's whip-like motion moves the sperm about 4 mm (0.15 in.) per minute.

Male **fertility**, the ability to reproduce, is influenced by sperm factors. For example, sperm number, shape, and motility (movement) are important in the reproductive process. Not only must the sperm be perfectly shaped and quite motile, but there must also be many of them for fertilization. Too few sperm results in not enough being able to make the journey to the awaiting oocyte. Once in the vagina, spermatozoa undergo an activation process called **capacitation** in which physical changes on the sperm surface enable it to penetrate and fertilize an oocyte.

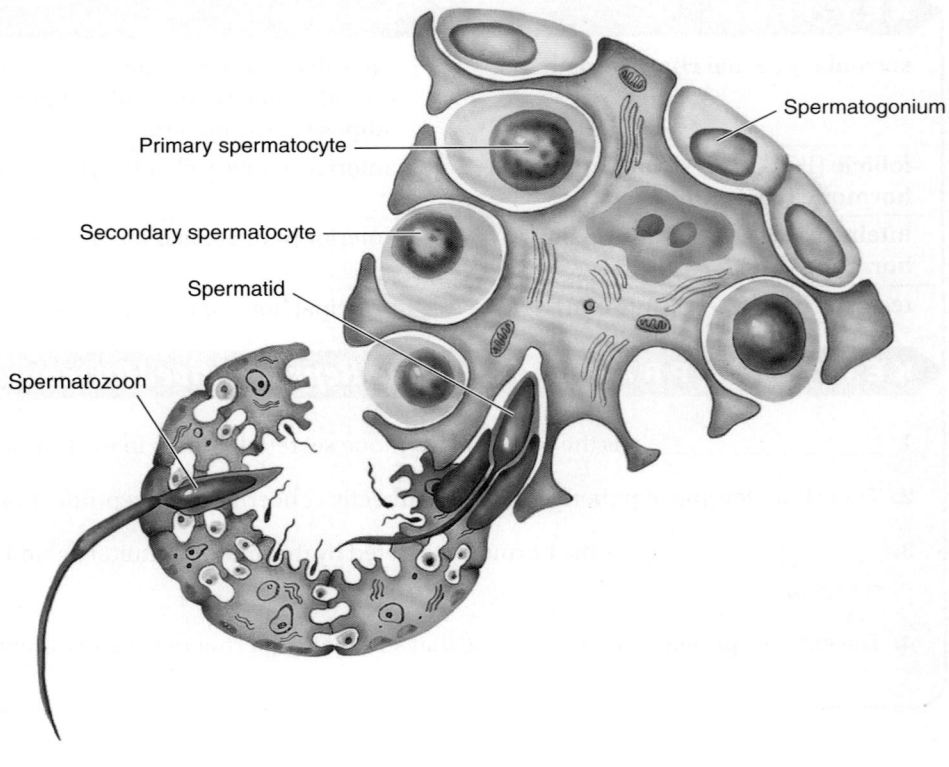

Spermatogonium

Primary spermatocyte

Secondary spermatocyte

Spermatid

Spermatozoon

Figure 16-5 The stages of spermatogenesis.

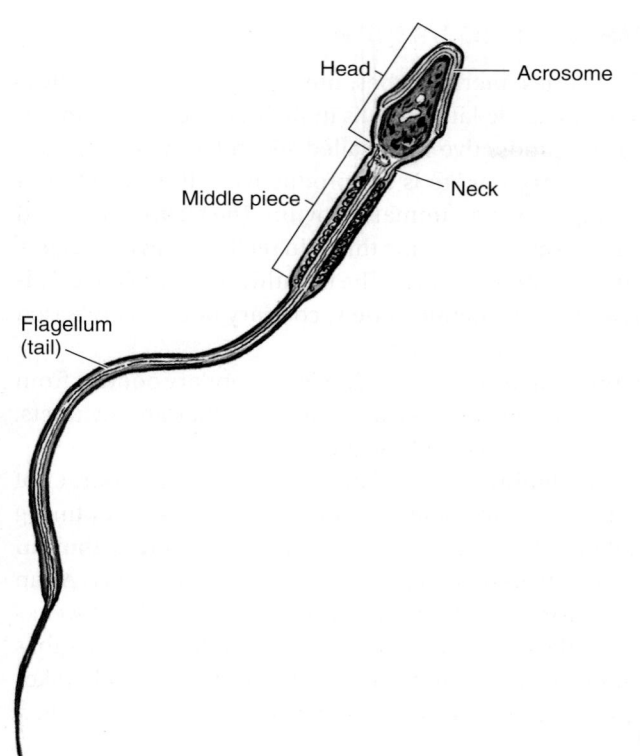

Head
Acrosome
Neck
Middle piece
Flagellum
(tail)

Figure 16-6 The regions
of a mature sperm.

KEY TERM	Definition
spermiogenesis (sper-mee-oh-JEN-eh-sis)	stage of spermatogenesis during which a sperm matures
spermatogonium (spur-muh-toh-GOH-nee-um)	sperm stem cell that gives rise to a mature sperm
diploid (DIP-loid)	containing 23 pairs or 46 chromosomes
haploid (HAP-loid)	containing 23 single, unpaired chromosomes
acrosome (ACK-roh-sohm)	structure at the end of a sperm that releases enzymes enabling the sperm to penetrate and fertilize an oocyte
flagellum (fla-JEL-um)	tail on spermatozoon
fertility	ability to reproduce by bringing about fertilization
capacitation (kuh-pas-ih-TAY-shun)	activation process that allows sperm to successfully fertilize an oocyte

KEY TERM PRACTICE: *Spermatozoa (Sperm)*

1. The tail on a spermatozoon is called a _____.

2. _____ is the activation process that allows sperm to successfully fertilize an oocyte.

3. The stage of spermatogenesis during which a sperm matures is known as _____ and is derived from the word part _____ for *origin*.

4. _____ means that a cell contains 23 single, unpaired chromosomes.

5. A _____ is a sperm stem cell that gives rise to a mature sperm and is derived from the word part _____ for *spermatozoa*.

Ovaries, Uterine Tubes, Uterus, and Vagina

Female reproductive organs include the ovaries, uterine tubes, uterus, and vagina. The ovaries are paired oval-shaped organs located near the lateral walls in the pelvic cavity. They secrete hormones and produce and release reproductive cells called secondary oocytes, from the word part *oo-* for *egg* or *ovary*. A **secondary oocyte** is a reproductive cell released from the ovary during ovulation and can be thought of as an immature ovum. The terms *oocyte* and *ovum* are oftentimes incorrectly exchanged to mean the same thing. In reality, an **ovum** (*ova* = plural) is produced after fertilization of the secondary oocyte. The monthly release of a secondary oocyte from the ovary is termed **ovulation**. Generally, one secondary oocyte is released from one ovary one month, and from the other ovary the next.

Uterine tubes are two narrow structures that provide a conduit for secondary oocytes from the ovaries to the uterus. Alternate names for uterine tubes are fallopian tubes and oviducts. Uterine tubes are about the diameter of a strand of cooked spaghetti.

Regions of the uterine tube include the fimbriae and infundibulum. A fringed border of finger-like projections called **fimbriae** at the opening of the uterine tubes assists in capturing a recently released secondary oocyte and bringing it into the uterine tubes. The **infundibulum** is the funnel-shaped opening of the uterine tubes encircling the top portion of the ovary. A gap exists between the uterine tubes and the ovaries, thus there is no physical connection. Sweeping ciliary action and peristalsis help secondary oocyte movement through the uterine tubes toward the uterus. Fertilization, the union of sperm and secondary oocyte, normally takes place in the uterine tubes by "upstream swimming" sperm. The normal time for the secondary oocyte to reach the uterus is 3 to 4 days.

The uterus is a hollow, muscular organ located between the urinary bladder and the rectum. Several ligaments hold the uterus in place. It serves as the site of implantation of a fertilized secondary oocyte, protects and sustains embryonic and fetal life, plays a role in childbirth, and serves as the source of menstrual flow in nonpregnant females.

The uterus has three layers. The outer perimetrium is an incomplete tissue layer that does not cover the **cervix**, the portion of the uterus that dips into the vagina. The middle muscular layer is called the myometrium (*myo* = muscle). The glandular membrane making up the inner layer of the uterine wall is termed the **endometrium**. The superficial part of the endometrium is shed during menstruation. The central, dome-shaped portion of the uterus opposite the cervix is the **fundus** (**Figure 16-7**).

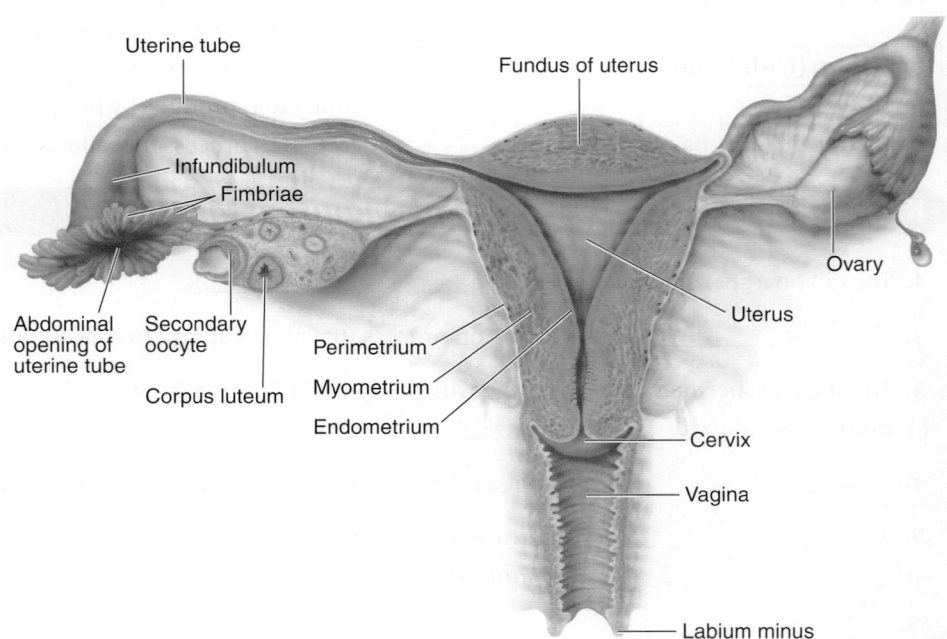

Figure 16-7 The ovaries, uterine tubes, uterus, and vagina.

The vagina is a muscular canal, 7.6 to 9 cm (3 to 3.5 in.) long, located posterior to the urethra. It connects the cervix to the outside. The **hymen** is a thin fold of mucous membrane covering the entrance to the vagina. It ruptures for a variety of reasons, such as sexual intercourse or tampon use, and it is often absent, even in virgins. Functions of the vagina include receiving the penis during coitus, serving as a passageway for menstrual fluids, and acting as the "birth canal" for a fetus during childbirth.

KEY TERM	Definition
secondary oocyte (OH-oh-site)	reproductive cell released from the ovary during ovulation
ovum (OH-vum)	functional secondary oocyte after fertilization
ovulation (ov-yoo-LAY-shun)	monthly release of a secondary oocyte from the ovary
fimbriae (FIM-bree-ee)	fringe-like processes on the outer extremity of the infundibulum of the uterine tube
infundibulum (in-fun-DIB-yoo-lum)	funnel-shaped opening of the uterine tube that encircles the ovary
cervix (SUR-vicks)	section of the uterus that dips into the vagina
endometrium (en-doh-MEE-tree-um)	glandular membrane lining the uterus
fundus (FUN-dus)	dome-shaped region of the uterus opposite the vaginal opening
hymen (HIGH-men)	thin fold of mucous membrane covering the entrance to the vagina

KEY TERM PRACTICE: *Ovaries, Uterine Tubes, Uterus, and Vagina*

1. The release of a secondary oocyte from the ovary is termed _____.

2. The _____ is a thin fold of mucous membrane that covers the entrance to the vagina.

3. The reproductive cell released from the ovary during ovulation is called a _____.

4. The glandular membrane lining the uterus is known as the _____, and is derived from the word part _____ for *inner* and the word part _____ for *uterus*.

5. An _____ is a fertilized secondary oocyte.

Vulva

Vulva, which literally means *wrapper*, is the collective term used to describe the female external genitals. These genitals are the mons pubis, two pairs of fleshy folds called the labia majora and labia minora, the clitoris, the vestibule, the vaginal and urethral orifices, and the greater and lesser vestibular glands. The **mons pubis** is the prominence caused by a pad of fat that overlies the pubic symphysis in females. At puberty, it becomes covered in pubic hair. The **labia majora** (*labium majus* = singular) are two thick outer folds of skin that form the lateral borders and surround the clitoris, the urethral opening, and the opening of the vagina. The **labia minora** (*labium minus* = singular) are two small folds of skin that lie immediately inside the labia majora and protect the vaginal and urethral openings. The **clitoris** is highly sensitive erectile tissue that responds to sexual stimulation. It is located at the front junction of the labia minora and is richly supplied with sensory nerve endings.

The central space between the labia minora is the **vestibule**. The vaginal and urethral orifices are the openings to the vagina and urethra, respectively (**Figure 16-8**). Lubricating glands associated with the vestibule are the mucus-secreting glands known as the **lesser vestibular glands** and **greater vestibular glands** (Bartholin glands). The greater vestibular glands have the same embryologic origin as the bulbourethral glands in the male.

Figure 16-8 Structures of the vulva.

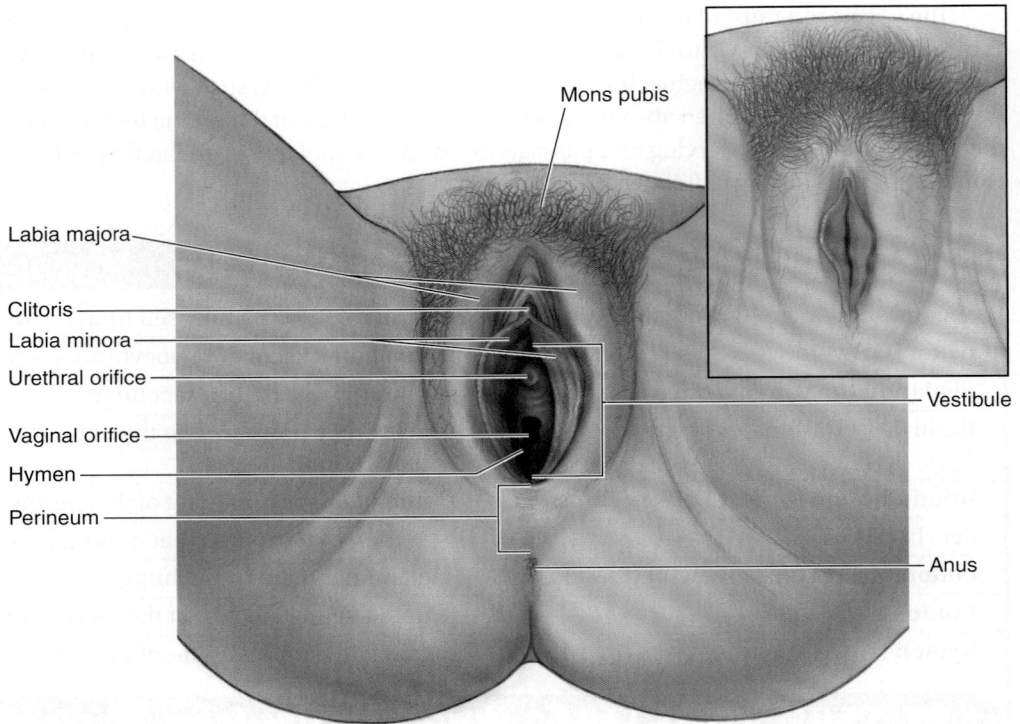

KEY TERM	Definition
mons pubis (PEW-bis)	prominence caused by a pad of fat that overlies the pubic symphasis in females
labia majora (LAY-bee-uh muh-JOR-uh)	two thick outer folds of skin that form the lateral borders and surround the clitoris, the urethral opening, and the opening of the vagina
labia minora (LAY-bee-uh muh-NOR-uh)	two small folds of skin that lie immediately inside the labia majora and protect the vaginal and urethral openings
clitoris (KLIT-oh-ris)	highly sensitive erectile tissue located at the junction of the labia minora
vestibule (VES-ti-bewl)	central space between the labia minora
lesser vestibular (ves-TIB-yoo-lur) **glands**	mucus-secreting glands between the openings of the vagina and urethra
greater vestibular (ves-TIB-yoo-lur) **glands**	mucus-secreting glands located on either side of the lower part of the vagina; also called Bartholin glands

KEY TERM PRACTICE: *Vulva*

1. The structure that is supplied with sensory nerve endings that respond to sexual stimulation and is located at the junction of the labia minora is termed the _____.

2. Mucus-secreting glands, also called Bartholin glands, that are located on either side of the lower part of the vagina are the _____.

3. The _____ is a prominence caused by a pad of fat that overlies the pubic symphasis in females.

4. The _____ are mucus-secreting glands between the openings of the vagina and urethra.

5. _____ are two small folds of skin that lie immediately inside the labia majora and protect the vaginal and urethral openings.

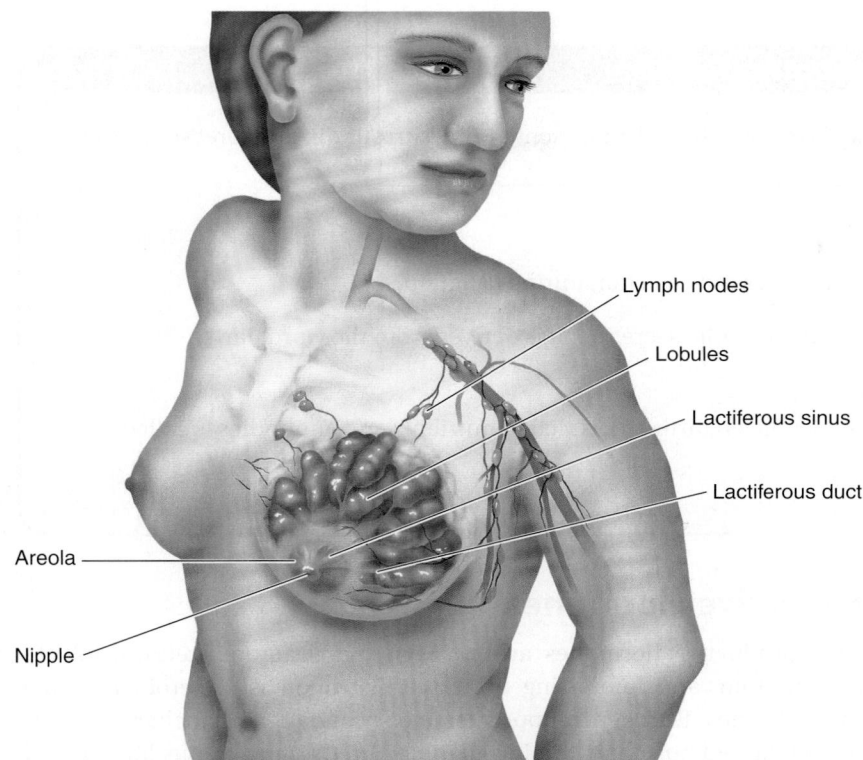

Lymph nodes

Lobules

Lactiferous sinus

Lactiferous duct

Areola

Nipple

Figure 16-9 Frontal view of the mammary glands.

Mammary Glands

Mammary glands are modified sweat glands within the breasts. Their function is **lactation**, the production of milk. External parts include the areola and nipple. The **areola** is the small, circular pigmented area around the nipple. The nipple marks the breast center and serves as the outlet for the lactiferous (milk-secreting) ducts when breast-feeding.

The glandular tissue is separated into lobes that contain secretory lobules. Lactiferous ducts exiting the secretory lobules form 15 to 20 expanded chambers called lactiferous sinuses that converge on the nipple surface (**Figure 16-9**). Hormones associated with lactation are prolactin and oxytocin. **Prolactin (PRL)** stimulates milk secretion, and **oxytocin (OXT)** stimulates milk ejection.

Breast-feeding involves nourishing an infant with milk from the mammary glands. **Colostrum**, or "first milk," is a thin, white fluid secreted after giving birth and before the production of true milk. This secretion is rich in protein, antibodies, fat-soluble vitamins, and minerals.

KEY TERM	Definition
lactation (lack-TAY-shun)	production of milk
areola (ah-REE-oh-luh)	pigmented ring surrounding the nipple
prolactin (proh-LACK-tin) **(PRL)**	hormone that stimulates milk secretion
oxytocin (ock-si-TOH-sin) **(OXT)**	hormone that stimulates milk ejection
colostrum (koh-LOS-trum)	first milk from a mother's breasts after she has given birth that is rich in nutrients and antibodies

continued

continued from page 833

KEY TERM PRACTICE: *Mammary Glands*

1. What are the singular and plural forms of the term describing the pigmented ring surrounding the breast nipple?

   _____

2. Milk production is termed _____.

3. _____ is the hormone that stimulates milk ejection during lactation.

4. _____ is the hormone that stimulates milk secretion; it is derived from the word part _____ for *milk*.

5. The first milk from a mother's breasts after she has given birth that is rich in nutrients and antibodies is called _____.

Female Reproductive Hormones

The primary female reproductive hormones are estrogen, progesterone, relaxin, follicle-stimulating hormone, inhibin, and luteinizing hormone. **Estrogen** is a steroid hormone produced mainly in the ovaries. Estrogen supports female secondary sexual characteristics. **Progesterone** is another steroid hormone, but it is manufactured by the corpus luteum (yellow mass of tissue that forms in the ovary after ovulation). Progesterone prepares the uterus for embryo implantation and the mammary glands for lactation.

   Relaxin is a hormone produced by the corpus luteum that relaxes the pelvic ligaments and pubic symphysis during pregnancy. Follicle-stimulating hormone (FSH) stimulates oocyte formation in females. The ovary secretes inhibin to halt the anterior pituitary gland's production of FSH. Luteinizing hormone (LH), secreted by the pituitary gland, targets the ovary, triggering ovulation.

KEY TERM	Definition
estrogen (ES-troh-jen)	female steroid hormone produced mainly in the ovaries that is responsible for the development of female secondary sexual characteristics
progesterone (proh-JES-tur-ohn)	steroid hormone manufactured by the corpus luteum that is essential for pregnancy and lactation
relaxin (ree-LACK-sin)	hormone that causes relaxation of the pelvic ligaments and pubic symphysis during pregnancy

KEY TERM PRACTICE: *Female Reproductive Hormones*

1. _____ is the female steroid hormone produced mainly in the ovaries that is responsible for the development of female secondary sexual characteristics.

2. _____ is a steroid hormone manufactured by the corpus luteum that is essential for pregnancy and lactation.

3. The hormone that causes relaxation of the pelvic ligaments and pubic symphysis during pregnancy is _____.

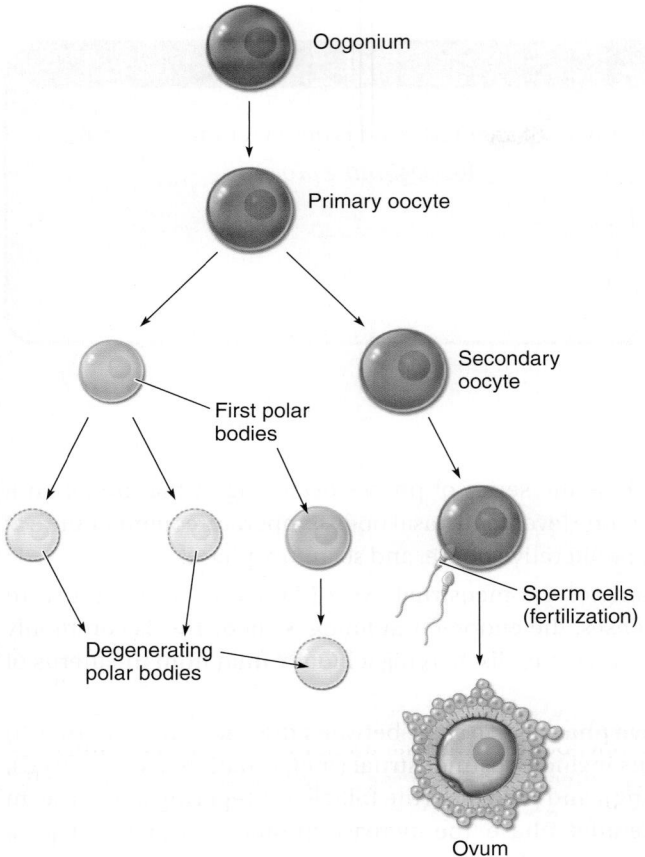

Figure 16-10 The stages of oogenesis.

Oogenesis

Oogenesis is the formation and development of the oocyte. Oogenesis begins with an **oogonium**, a stem cell in the ovaries that is formed before birth. A series of stages completes its transformation into a mature ovum. Many stages mirror those of spermatogenesis. The process involves mitosis (somatic or nonsex cell division) and meiosis (gamete cell division). The end result is a mature secondary oocyte capable of fertilization. If fertilization occurs, a mature ovum is formed (**Figure 16-10**). The stages can be summarized as follows:

oogonium → primary oocyte → first polar body and secondary oocyte → meiosis will be completed in the secondary oocyte if fertilization occurs, forming an ovum

A sac within the ovary called a **follicle** holds the immature egg cells. Every month, follicles enlarge until one fluid-filled follicle outpaces the others, ruptures, and releases a secondary oocyte from an ovary. This oocyte is about the size of a grain of sand and can be seen without a microscope. In the female, all mitotic divisions are complete before birth. For this reason, a female infant is born with the maximum number of potential ova she will ever have. At birth, the infant has approximately 2 million immature oocytes that remain in a state of suspended development, but by puberty that number drops to about 400,000 or less.

KEY TERM	Definition
oogenesis (oh-oh-JEN-e-sis)	the formation and development of the oocyte
oogonium (oh-oh-GOH-nee-um)	a stem cell that gives rise to an oocyte
follicle (FOL-i-kul)	sac within the ovary that holds immature egg cells

continued

continued from page 835

KEY TERM PRACTICE: *Oogenesis*

1. _____ is the term for the formation and development of an oocyte and is derived from the word part _____ for *egg* and the word part _____ for *beginning process*.

2. The sac within the ovary that holds immature egg cells is called the _____.

3. An _____ is a stem cell that gives rise to an oocyte.

The Menstrual Cycle

The **menstrual cycle** or **uterine cycle** is the series of phases occurring in the uterus on a 28-day rotation. During this time, hormone levels and basal body temperature (temperature at rest) change. The phases are menses, proliferative phase, and secretory phase.

1. *Menses* **Menses** marks the beginning of the menstrual cycle (days 1–7). The Latin word *mensis* means "month." During menses, the endometrial lining is shed. This is commonly called **menstruation**, the monthly process of discharging a bloody fluid from the uterus of a nonpregnant female.

2. *Proliferative phase* The **proliferative phase** is the stage between the end of menses (day 8) and ovulation (day 14). Other terms include postmenstrual (menstruation just occurred), estrogenic (estrogen levels are rising), and follicular (the follicle is preparing to release an oocyte) phases. During the proliferative phase, the increase in blood estrogen causes a growth of small, spiraling arteries on the endometrial wall and an increase in endometrial water content. In essence, the body is preparing the uterus for implantation and nurturing a developing embryo and fetus. Ovulation (day 14) marks the release of a secondary oocyte.

3. *Secretory phase* The **secretory phase** (days 15–28) occurs between ovulation and the onset of the next menses. It is also called the premenstrual (it is occurring just before the next menstrual cycle), postovulatory (ovulation has just occurred), or luteal (the corpus luteum secretes progesterone to sustain endometrial development) phase. During this phase, progesterone levels rise and would be sustained if a pregnancy occurred. Without pregnancy, progesterone levels fall, and the cycle begins again.

The cycle is illustrated in **Figure 16-11**.

Terms associated with the menstrual cycle include menarche, perimenopause, and menopause. **Menarche** is the first menstrual cycle of a young woman. It typically occurs during puberty, some time between the ages of 8 and 17 years. Vaginal secretions change from alkaline to acidic with menarche.

The transitional period leading to menopause is termed **perimenopause**. Perimenopause is the 3- to 5-year period prior to menopause during which estrogen levels begin to drop. **Menopause** is the permanent cessation of menstrual cycles. The average age of onset is between 45 and 50 years. The characteristic "hot flashes" result from a sharp increase in FSH and LH concentrations and a decrease in estrogen concentrations.

Hormone replacement therapy (HRT) is the administration of sex hormones to women after menopause. HRT is used to reduce signs and symptoms associated with menopause such as hot flashes, emotional fluctuations, and bone loss. The decision to treat with HRT is made after careful consideration and weighing the benefits versus the side effects. Note that there is considerable controversy surrounding the use of HRT, because some research

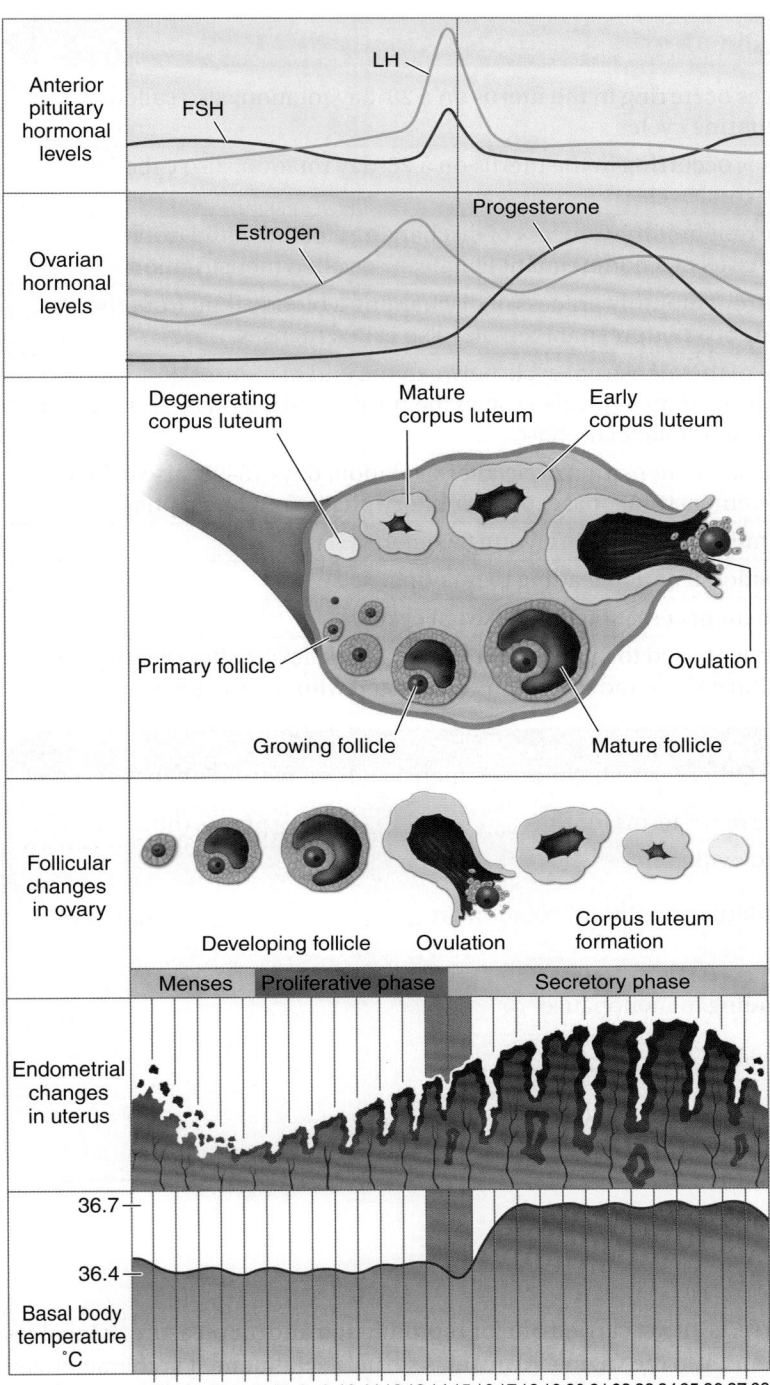

Anterior pituitary hormonal levels

LH

FSH

Ovarian hormonal levels

Estrogen

Progesterone

Degenerating corpus luteum

Mature corpus luteum

Early corpus luteum

Primary follicle

Ovulation

Growing follicle

Mature follicle

Follicular changes in ovary

Developing follicle

Ovulation

Corpus luteum formation

Menses | Proliferative phase | Secretory phase

Endometrial changes in uterus

36.7

36.4

Basal body temperature °C

Day   1 2 3 4 5 6 7 8 9 10 11 12 13 14 15 16 17 18 19 20 21 22 23 24 25 26 27 28

Figure 16-11 The menstrual cycle.

has shown that the adverse side effects are too great to warrant its use. Therapy is highly individualized and may require modification, but standard protocols suggest using estrogen-only pills in women without a uterus and a combination estrogen–progesterone pill for women with an intact uterus. Hormone replacement therapy is contraindicated in some females with estrogen-dependent tumors, history of blood clots, or certain other medical conditions.

KEY TERM	Definition
menstrual (MEN-stroo-ul) **cycle**	phases occurring in the uterus on a 28-day rotation; also called the uterine cycle
uterine (YOO-tur-in) **cycle**	phases occurring in the uterus on a 28-day rotation; also called the menstrual cycle
menses (MEN-seez)	recurrent monthly process of discharging a bloody fluid from the uterus of a nonpregnant female; also called menstruation
menstruation (men-stroo-AY-shun)	recurrent monthly process of discharging a bloody fluid from the uterus of a nonpregnant female; also called menses
proliferative (proh-LIF-ur-uh-tiv) **phase**	stage of the menstrual cycle between the end of menses and ovulation, days 8–14; also called the postmenstrual phase, estrogenic phase, and follicular phase
secretory (se-KREE-tuh-ree) **phase**	stage of the menstrual cycle after ovulation, days 15–28; also called the premenstrual phase, postovulatory phase, and luteal phase
menarche (me-NAHR-kee)	first menstrual cycle of a young woman
perimenopause (per-ih-men-OH-pawz)	transitional period leading to menopause
menopause (MEN-oh-pawz)	permanent cessation of menstrual cycles
hormone replacement therapy (HRT)	treatment used to maintain female hormone levels after menopause to reduce signs and symptoms associated with menopause

KEY TERM PRACTICE: *The Menstrual Cycle*

1. Postmenstrual, estrogenic, and follicular phases are other terms for the _____ phase, the stage of the menstrual cycle between the end of menses and ovulation.

2. Two terms describing the phases occurring in the uterus on a 28-day rotation are _____ and _____.

3. _____ is the transitional period leading to menopause.

4. The first menstrual cycle of a young woman is termed _____.

5. _____ is the permanent cessation of menstrual cycles.

Sexual Intercourse

Coitus, or sexual intercourse, is an act carried out for reproduction and/or pleasure. It involves the insertion of an erect penis into the vagina. **Arousal** is sexual excitement. It is characterized by stimulation from the parasympathetic (breed-and-feed) division of the nervous system, resulting in erection of the penis and clitoris and increased secretion from reproductive glands.

Intercourse occurs by the sexual response cycle: arousal, erection, lubrication, emission, ejaculation, orgasm, and detumescence. In males, erection is characterized by blood accumulating in the erectile tissues, causing the penis to swell and stiffen. In females, vaginal tissues become engorged with blood and swell. Male lubrication involves secretion from the bulbourethral glands. In females, the greater and lesser vestibular glands secrete mucus to reduce friction of moving parts during intercourse.

Emission and ejaculation occur only in males. **Emission** involves peristaltic contractions that push fluid and sperm into the urethra. **Ejaculation** is the ejection of semen from the penis during orgasm. During ejaculation, rhythmic contractions force semen to the outside.

Orgasm, or climax, is the peak of sexual excitement characterized by intense psychological and physiological responses in both the male and the female. There is intense muscle tightening around the genitalia accompanied by pleasurable waves of tingling sensations throughout the body. In the female, the uterus, uterine tubes, and vagina contract rhythmically.

Detumescence is the gradual reduction of swelling as the blood exits erectile tissues. Erection subsides in the male. In the female, blood leaves the vagina and clitoris and pleasant sensations diminish.

KEY TERM	Definition
arousal	sexual excitement
emission (ee-MISH-un)	discharge of semen into the male urethra
ejaculation (ee-jack-yoo-LAY-shun)	sudden ejection of semen from the penis during orgasm
orgasm (OR-gaz-um)	period of greatest sexual intensity; also called climax
detumescence (dee-tew-MES-unce)	diminished swelling in erectile organs after orgasm as the blood exits erectile tissues

KEY TERM PRACTICE: *Sexual Intercourse*

1. _____ involves the discharge of semen into the male urethra, and _____ is the expulsion of this semen from the penis.

2. _____ is characterized by diminished swelling in erectile organs after orgasm.

3. The period of greatest sexual intensity is termed _____.

4. The medical term for sexual excitement is _____.

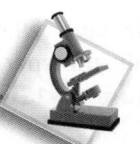

THE CLINICAL DIMENSION

The reproductive system undergoes considerable changes throughout life. Individuals are usually well aware of their reproductive system, but some serious pathologies can be hidden, displaying no signs or symptoms. Unlike other systems, males and females may have different pathological conditions because males and females have different reproductive organs. Some infectious diseases affect both males and females. This section considers pathologies, sexually transmitted disease, and birth control methods.

Penis and Testes Disorders

hypospadias   A congenital anomaly of the penis in which the urethra opens on the ventral surface is termed **hypospadias** (**Figure 16-12B**).

epispadias   In **epispadias**, another congenital condition, the urethral opening is located on the penis dorsal surface. Surgery is required to correct the abnormal locations (**Figure 16-12C**).

Figure 16-12 Normal and abnormal urethral openings: **(A)** normal urethral opening; **(B)** hypospadias; **(C)** epispadias.

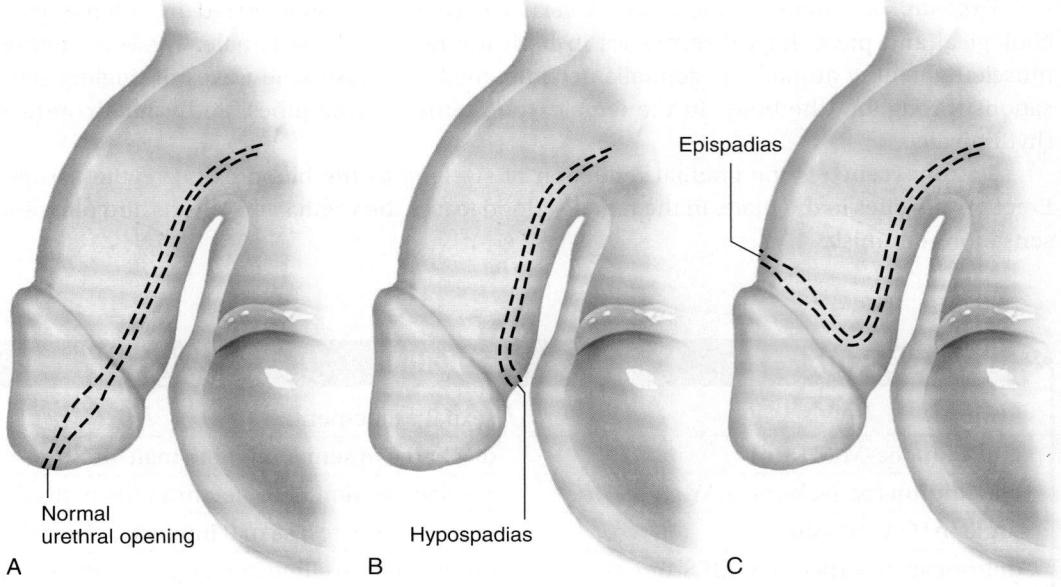

Epispadias

Normal urethral opening

A

Hypospadias

B

C

erectile dysfunction (ED) or impotence

Erectile dysfunction (ED) or **impotence** is the inability to achieve or maintain a penile erection long enough for intercourse. Its causes are complex and can involve, among other things, the brain, hormones, emotions, nerves, blood vessels, heart disease, obesity, diabetes, high blood pressure, stress, fatigue, trauma, and medications. It is diagnosed through a complete physical examination and history that includes investigation of medicinal side effects. The treatments depend on the underlying cause and are aimed at causing a sustainable erection. Options include medications that enhance the effects of nitric oxide, which relaxes muscles in the penis and increases blood flow, enabling an erection. Common medicines are sildenafil (Viagra), tadalafil (Cialis), or vardenafil (Levitra). If medications do not work, penis pumps, penile implants, and blood vessel surgery may be options.

hydrocele

Hydrocele refers to an accumulation of serous fluid in the testis or within the spermatic cord. It often causes swelling of the scrotum (**Figure 16-13**). Hydroceles that are present at birth generally resolve

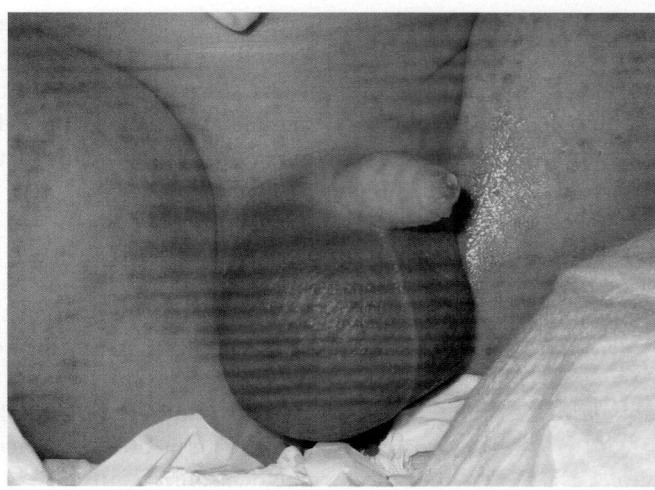

Figure 16-13 Infant with a hydrocele.

within 1 year. If the hydrocele persists after 1 year, surgical treatment is necessary. Hydroceles affecting adults result from the inability of the scrotal tissue to absorb fluid. They are caused by trauma, infection, or tumor, or they may be idiopathic (of unknown cause) in nature. The size of the enlargement ranges from slightly larger than the testis to the size of a grapefruit. Diagnosis is confirmed by ultrasonography. Treatment in the adult involves aspirating the fluid and injecting a sclerosing agent to prevent recurrence.

varicocele

A **varicocele** is swelling in one testicle or both caused by swelling of the veins in the spermatic cord, giving a "bag of worms" appearance (**Figure 16-14**). The distention of the testicular veins can lead to lowered sperm counts because the blood causes an increased temperature.

testicular torsion

Testicular torsion is a disorder in which the spermatic cord rotates, producing ischemia (inadequate blood supply) of the testis (**Figure 16-15**). Signs and symptoms include testicular pain and swelling. The condition can affect males at any point in life but is most common in newborns and adolescents. Onset is either spontaneous or may follow physical exertion or injury. An initial urinalysis is performed to rule out infection. The diagnosis is confirmed by ultrasonography. Immediate treatment by manual manipulation or surgical fixation is necessary to preserve testicular function.

orchitis

Orchitis is inflammation of one or both testes. Causes include trauma and bacterial or viral infection, especially with *Rubulavirus*, the pathogen of mumps. Severe cases result in atrophy of the affected testis. If both testes are affected, orchitis can lead to sterility. Signs and symptoms are swelling, tenderness, pain, and flu-like indicators. Diagnosis is made by the history and physical examination and a urinalysis that identifies the causative agent. Antibiotics are used to treat orchitis. A scrotal support may also be necessary to alleviate discomfort.

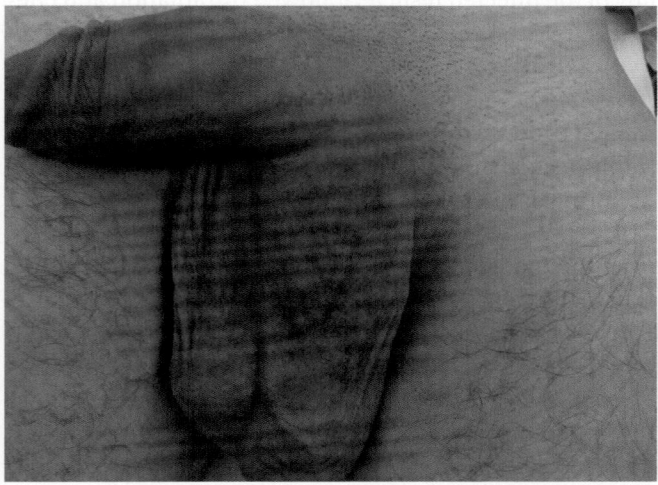

Figure 16-14 Varicocele with "bag of worms" appearance within the testicle.

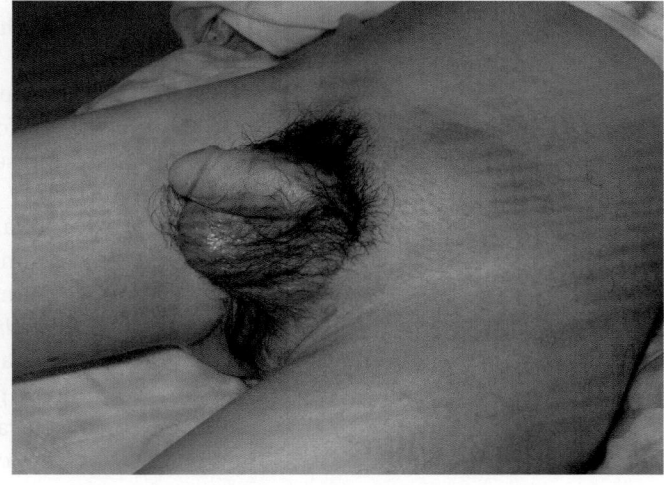

Figure 16-15 Adolescent with testicular torsion.

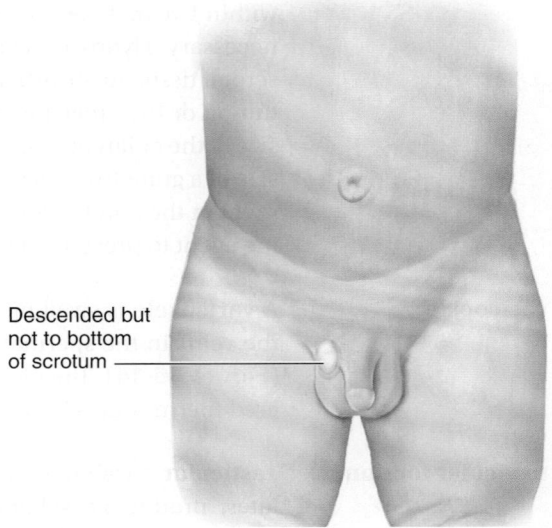

Descended but
not to bottom
of scrotum

Figure 16-16 Cryptorchidism.

cryptorchidism

Cryptorchidism is failure of one or both testes to descend into the scrotum (**Figure 16-16**). It is a common birth defect affecting the male genitalia. In most cases, the cryptorchid testis descends within the first year of life. An undescended testis requires an **orchiopexy**, surgical treatment to free and implant the testicle into the scrotum. Untreated, the male is more susceptible to testicular torsion, inguinal hernia, testicular cancer, and sterility.

testicular cancer

Testicular cancer is malignant growth in the testicles. It has an unknown cause but is associated with cryptorchidism, inguinal hernia during childhood, and having had mumps. Testicular cancer is rare, accounting for 1% of all cancers in men, but it is the most common type of cancer in men ages 20 to 35 years.

Its primary sign and symptom is a painless testicular lump. It is diagnosed by palpation and a biopsy confirming cancer. It is treated by orchiectomy of the infected testicle, followed by radiation and chemotherapy. The surgical removal of one or both testes is termed an **orchiectomy** or **castration**.

Prompt treatment is necessary to prevent spread to the lymphatic system. Prognosis is good if diagnosed and treated early. Men should perform monthly testicular self-examinations (TSEs) to detect the presence of abnormal growths.

epididymitis

Inflammation of the epididymis is known as **epididymitis**. It results from a urinary tract infection (UTI) or sexually transmitted disease. Common disease-causing agents are *Neisseria gonorrhoeae, Chlamydia trachomatis, Escherichia coli,* and members of the *Staphylococcus* and *Streptococcus* genera. Epididymitis is diagnosed by the history and physical examination, urinalysis indicating bacterial presence, and elevated white blood cell count. It is treated with antibiotics and analgesics. If left untreated, it can lead to sterility.

KEY TERM	Definition
hypospadias (high-poh-SPAY-dee-us)	congenital disorder characterized by the penile urethral opening being located on the ventral surface
epispadias (ep-ih-SPAY-dee-us)	congenital disorder characterized by the penile urethral opening being located on the dorsal surface
erectile (ee-RECK-tile) **dysfunction (ED)**	the inability to achieve or maintain a penile erection long enough for intercourse; also called impotence
impotence (IM-puh-tens)	the inability to achieve or maintain a penile erection long enough for intercourse; also called erectile dysfunction (ED)
hydrocele (HIGH-droh-seel)	accumulation of serous fluid in the testis or within the spermatic cord
varicocele (VAIR-ih-koh-seel)	swelling in one testicle or both caused by swelling of the veins in the spermatic cord
testicular (tes-TICK-yoo-lur) **torsion**	rotation of the spermatic cord that causes an interruption in the blood supply to the tissue
orchitis (or-KIGH-tis)	inflammation of one or both testes
cryptorchidism (kript-OR-kid-iz-um)	failure of one or both testes to descend into the scrotum
orchiopexy (or-kee-oh-PECK-see)	surgical treatment of an undescended testicle by freeing it and implanting it into the scrotum
testicular (tes-TICK-yoo-lur) **cancer**	malignant cell growth in the testis
orchiectomy (or-kee-ECK-tuh-mee)	surgical removal of one or both testes; also called castration
castration	surgical removal of one or both testes; also called orchiectomy
epididymitis (ep-i-did-i-MIGH-tis)	inflammation of the epididymis

KEY TERM PRACTICE: *Penis and Testes Disorders*

1. The word part _____ refers to *testes*, and the word part *-itis* means _____; so the medical term for inflammation of the testes is _____.

2. The surgical removal of one or both testes is termed _____ or _____.

3. _____ is the inability to achieve or maintain a penile erection long enough for intercourse; also called impotence.

4. Inflammation of the epididymis is termed _____.

5. Failure of one or both testes to descend into the scrotum is called _____ and is derived from the word part _____ for *hidden* and the word part _____ for *testes*.

Prostate Disorders

Pathology of the prostate ranges from inflammation and hyperplasia to cancer.

prostatitis   Inflammation of the prostate is termed **prostatitis**. Its cause may be bacterial, viral, or unknown. Men may be asymptomatic or experience pain and burning while urinating (dysuria). Prostatitis primarily affects men over age 50 years. It is diagnosed by urinalysis and digital rectal examination. A **digital rectal examination (DRE)** is an evaluative procedure involving direct palpation of the prostate with the fingers (digits) through the rectum to examine for swelling or growths (**Figure 16-17**). Treatment options

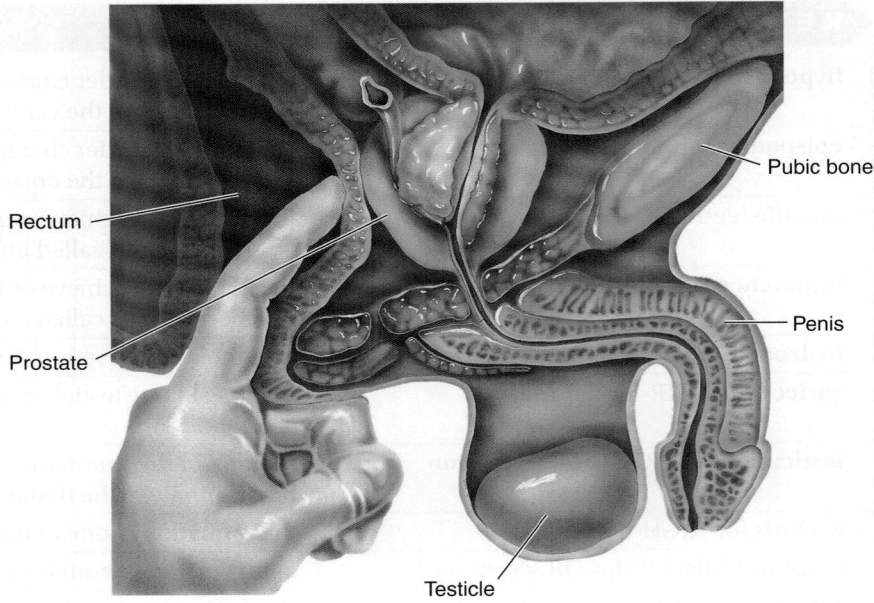

Rectum

Prostate

Pubic bone

Penis

Testicle

Figure 16-17 Digital rectal examination of the prostate. (Gloves are worn.)

include antimicrobics, analgesics, and increased fluid intake. Prognosis for the acute form is good. Chronic prostatitis leads to urinary tract infections, urethral obstruction, and urinary retention.

benign prostatic hyperplasia (BPH)

Benign prostatic hyperplasia (BPH) is a condition characterized by prostate enlargement and is common in men over age 50 years. The cause is not known, but it is associated with age-related metabolic and endocrine changes, and it does not evolve into cancer. Signs and symptoms include difficulty with starting urination, inability to maintain a steady urine stream, urinary retention, and frequent urination. The anatomical location of the prostate itself contributes to urinary system problems because the urethra runs through the gland's center.

BPH is diagnosed by the history and physical examination, DRE, intravenous pyelogram (IVP)—a kidney function test—and cystoscopy. Treatments include prostate gland massage, catheterization, drug therapy to relax the prostate muscles, surgery, and antibiotics to prevent the spread of infection. If the kidneys become involved, BPH can lead to pyelonephritis, hydronephrosis, and uremia.

prostate cancer

Prostate cancer, malignant neoplasia in the prostate gland, is the leading cause of cancer death among men. Seventy-three years is the average age of diagnosis. If affects less than 1% of the male population younger than age 50 years, 16% of men between the ages of 60 and 64 years, and 83% of men 65 years and older. Data from autopsies show that two-thirds of men over age 80 died *with* (not of) prostate cancer. Prostate cancer often metastasizes (spreads) to the bones before it is diagnosed.

The cause of prostate cancer is unknown, but dietary fat is associated with onset and may dictate its aggressiveness. The cancer may also be linked to a genetic predisposition. Signs and symptoms, if present, are interrupted urine flow, difficulty starting or stopping urine stream, urinary retention, pain or burning while urinating, and hematuria (blood in the

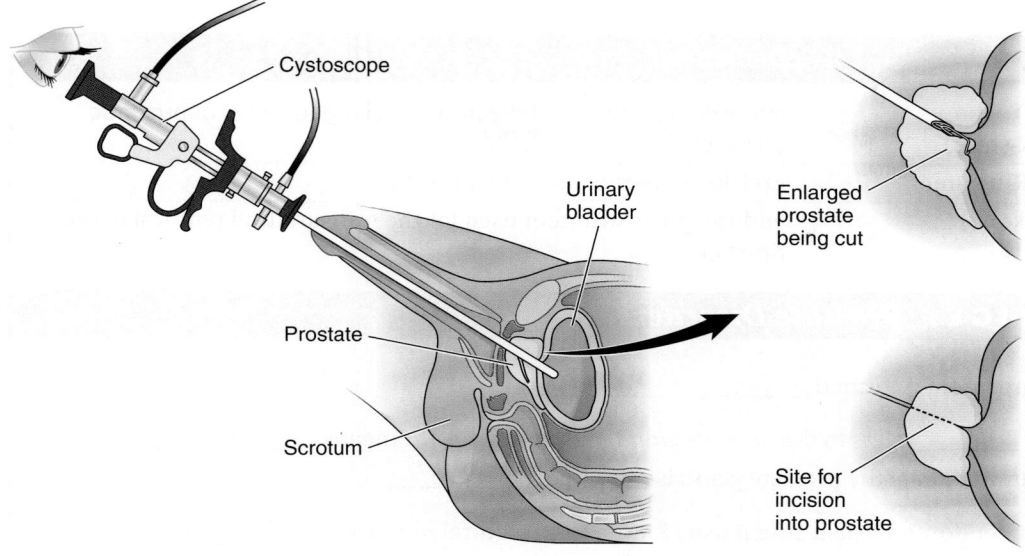

Cystoscope

Urinary
bladder

Prostate

Scrotum

Enlarged
prostate
being cut

Site for
incision
into prostate

Figure 16-18 Transure-thral resection of the prostate (TURP).

urine). The history and physical examination, DRE, ultrasound, and el-evated prostate-specific antigen levels in the blood diagnose the cancer. A biopsy is used for confirmation. The **prostate-specific antigen (PSA) test** measures the serum level of this normal protein (prostate-specific anti-gen) of the prostate. Increased levels occur with age, but greatly increased levels are associated with prostate cancer.

Treatment depends on the disease stage. If the man is over age 65 years when the cancer is discovered, often no treatment is administered because he will probably die of other causes before the disease progresses, so close monitoring or "watchful waiting" is used. Other options include hormonal therapy, orchiectomy to reduce hormone levels, transurethral resection of the prostate, prostatectomy, radiation, and chemotherapy. **Transurethral resection (TUR)** is the endoscopic removal of the prostate gland for re-lief of prostatic obstruction (**Figure 16-18**). It is also called a transure-thral resection of the prostate (TURP). The surgical removal of part or all of the prostate is called **prostatectomy**. It is performed through the ure-thral canal using a special endoscopic instrument called a cystoscope or **resectoscope**. The prognosis is poor if the disease has metastasized.

Prostate cancer screening is prudent. Men ages 40 years and over should have yearly DREs; and PSA levels should be checked annually in men 50 years and older. Screenings may be discontinued at age 70 years, because the disease is not as aggressive at this point.

KEY TERM	Definition
prostatitis (pros-tuh-TYE-tis)	prostate gland inflammation
digital rectal examination (DRE)	manual examination of the prostate through the rectum
benign prostatic hyperplasia (BPH) (pros-TAT-ick high-pur-PLAY-zhuh)	noncancerous prostate enlargement
prostate (PROS-tate) **cancer**	malignant cell growth of the prostate gland
prostate-specific antigen (PROS-tate-spuh-SIF-ick AN-ti-jen) **(PSA) test**	measures the circulating blood levels of prostate-specific antigen

continued

continued from page 845

KEY TERM	Definition
transurethral resection (TUR) (trans-yoo-REE-thrul ree-SECK-shun)	endoscopic removal of the prostate gland for relief of prostatic obstruction
prostatectomy (pros-tuh-TECK-tuh-mee)	excision of part or all of the prostate
resectoscope (ree-SECK-tuh-skope)	endoscopic instrument used for the transurethral removal of the prostate

KEY TERM PRACTICE: *Prostate Disorders*

1. Noncancerous prostate enlargement is termed _____.

2. The word part _____ refers to the *prostate gland*, the word part *-itis* means _____; so the medical term for inflammation of the prostate gland is _____.

3. A _____ is an endoscopic instrument used for the transurethral removal of the prostate.

4. Malignant cell growth of the prostate gland is called _____.

5. A _____ is the excision of part or all of the prostate and is derived from the word part _____ for *prostate gland* and the word part _____ for *surgical removal of a structure.*

Female Pelvic Disorders

endometriosis

A fairly common disorder of the female reproductive system is **endometriosis**, a condition characterized by the presence of endometrial tissue in abnormal locations such as the uterine wall, ovaries, or extragenital sites. The misplaced islands of endometrium imitate the menstrual cycle and cause pain at the locale. The underlying cause is not known. **Dysmenorrhea**, which involves abdominal pain, cramping, and difficult menstruation, is a hallmark of the condition. Heavy menses and pelvic pain during intercourse are also evident. The condition is diagnosed by pelvic examination and laparoscopy. **Laparoscopy** is the examination of the internal organs of the abdomen using a tube-shaped instrument called a laparoscope that is passed through the abdominal wall.

The **pelvic examination** is one method for assessing the internal pelvic organs and adnexa in both males and females. In general, **adnexa** are appendages attached to structures. In gynecology, adnexa refer to the appendages of the uterus, including the uterine tubes, ovaries, and ligaments, holding the uterus in place. Four types of pelvic examinations are vaginal examination, bimanual palpation of the uterus, rectovaginal examination in females, and bimanual palpation of the prostate and adnexa in males. The index and middle finger are inserted into the vagina in the vaginal examination. Bimanual palpation of the uterus combines the vaginal examination with manual palpation of the external pelvic region to feel the uterus and adnexa (**Figure 16-19**). The rectovaginal examination is accomplished by inserting the middle finger into the rectum and the index finger into the vagina and applying pressure to the pelvic region with the other hand. In men, bimanual palpation of the prostate and adnexa involves

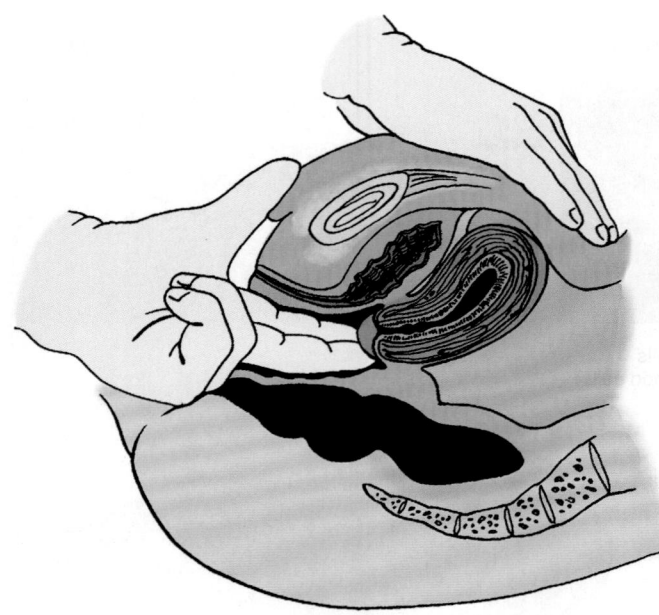

Figure 16-19 Bimanual examination of the uterus and adnexa.

inserting the index and middle fingers into the rectum while palpating the pelvic region with the other hand.

Treatment of endometriosis is necessary to prevent infertility, ectopic (outside uterus) pregnancy, and spontaneous abortion. Conservative measures involve hormone administration. Invasive action includes dilation and curettage, **hysterectomy** (surgical removal of the uterus), and bilateral salpingo-oophorectomy. The surgical treatment in which the cervix is expanded to allow access to the uterus with a curette to scrape away endometrial tissue is called a **dilation and curettage (D&C)**. The medical term describing the excision of the uterine tube and ovary is **salpingo-oophorectomy**. Excision of both uterine tubes and ovaries is termed bilateral salpingo-oophorectomy (BSO). Pregnancy, nursing, and menopause often cause symptom remission of endometriosis.

pelvic inflammatory disease (PID)

Pelvic inflammatory disease (PID) is inflammation of the female pelvic structures (endometrium, uterine tubes, and pelvic peritoneum) typified by abdominal pain, fever, and cervix tenderness. It is caused by infection from a variety of microbes, most notably *Neisseria gonorrhoeae,* the causative agent of gonorrhea. It is more common in **nulliparous** (never having borne a child) women. Intrauterine device use also increases the risk. Signs and symptoms are fever, chills, malaise, foul-smelling vaginal discharge, and abdominal pain.

This pathology is diagnosed by pain during vaginal examination, Gram stain to determine the causative agent, laparoscopy, and ultrasound to detect abnormalities. A **Gram stain** is a differential staining procedure that identifies bacteria as either gram-positive (G^+) or gram-negative (G^-) according to the dye absorbed by the bacterial cell wall. Gram-positive organisms retain the blue color of crystal violet; G^- microbes appear pink because they do not retain the crystal violet dye (**Figure 16-20**). It is important to know the Gram reaction so that appropriate antibiotics can be administered because some

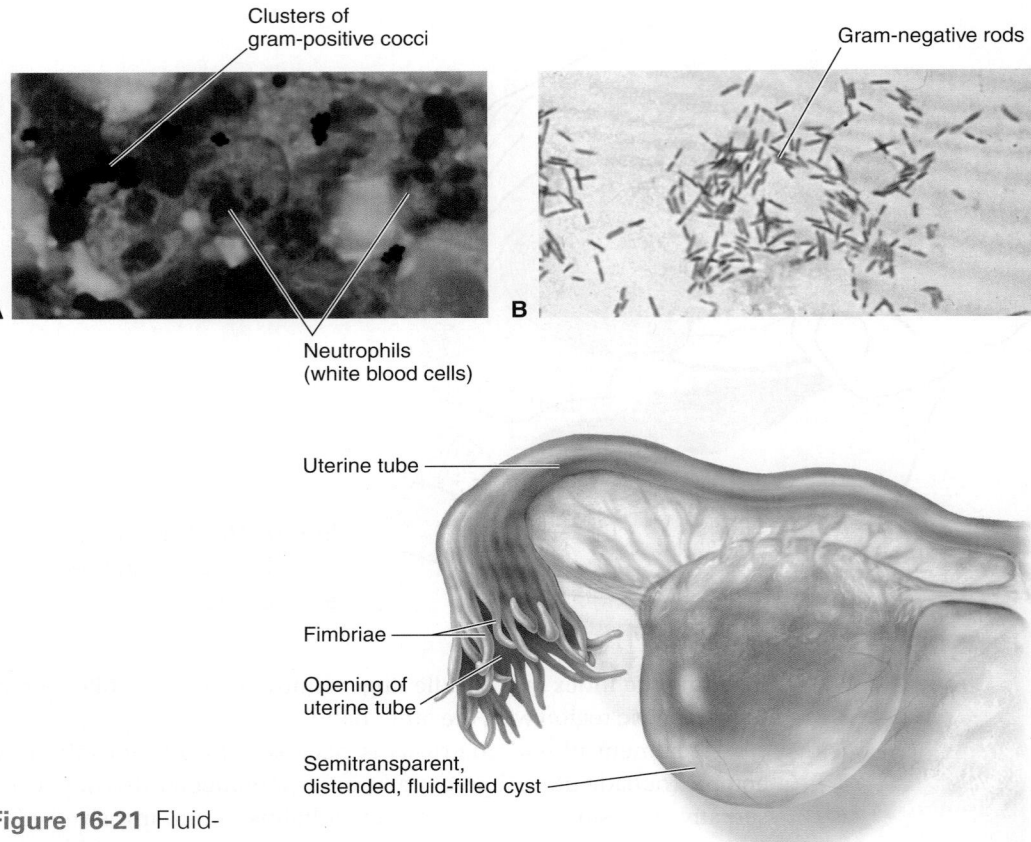

Clusters of
gram-positive cocci

Gram-negative rods

Figure 16-20 (A) Gram-positive cocci (*Staphylococcus aureus*) in pus (large, dark-red globules are white cell nuclei). **(B)** Gram-negative bacilli, or rods (*Escherichia coli*), from a culture plate.

A

B

Neutrophils
(white blood cells)

Uterine tube

Fimbriae

Opening of
uterine tube

Semitransparent,
distended, fluid-filled cyst

Figure 16-21 Fluid-filled ovarian cyst.

antibiotics target G⁺ organisms, others G⁻ organisms, and still others cover both types. Aggressive antibiotic therapy to combat the infection and analgesics for pain relief are used to treat PID. Early therapeutic intervention is necessary to prevent peritonitis or widespread infection, especially septicemia (systemic blood infection).

ovarian cysts

An ovarian condition that afflicts some women is **ovarian cysts**, which are fluid-filled sacs forming on or near the ovaries (**Figure 16-21**). Symptoms may not be present initially, but with time the increased cyst size may cause pain, swelling, and urinary retention if the bladder is affected. Two types exist: nonneoplastic (benign) and neoplastic (cancerous). Ovarian cysts are diagnosed by ultrasonography and laparoscopy. If necessary, benign cysts may be drained, but generally, no treatment is required. Neoplastic cysts are removed and appropriate follow-up treatment is given.

premenstrual syndrome (PMS) and premenstrual dysphoric disorder (PMDD)

Premenstrual syndrome (PMS) is a condition of unknown origin characterized by emotional and physical manifestations, including headache, fatigue, irritability, breast tenderness, and joint pain. It occurs only in ovulating women a few days before the onset of menstruation when estrogen levels peak, and it subsides when the menstrual period begins. It is diagnosed by physical examination and history that includes a record of symptoms matched to the menstrual cycle. Chronic depression must be ruled out. About 80% of menstruating women ages 25 to 40 experience symptoms of PMS. It is estimated that 5% to 10% have severe emotional symptoms with impaired domestic, occupational, and social functioning. When PMS is accompanied by these symptoms, which persist after the onset of menstruation, it is known as **premenstrual dysphoric disorder (PMDD)**. Therapy varies among individuals but is aimed at treating the signs and symptoms associated with bloating, anxiety, and depression that appear shortly before menstruation. Abnormal serotonin metabolism may trigger the mood and anxiety symptoms. Exercise, calcium supplements, reduced caffeine and sodium intake, analgesics, and diuretics may help minimize the physical signs and symptoms.

KEY TERM	Definition
endometriosis (en-doh-mee-tree-OH-sis)	presence of functional endometrial tissue outside the uterus
dysmenorrhea (dis-men-oh-REE-uh)	difficult and painful menstruation
laparoscopy (lap-uh-ROS-kuh-pee)	examination of the internal organs of the abdomen using a tube-shaped instrument called a laparoscope that is passed through the abdominal wall
pelvic (PEL-vick) **examination**	manually palpating and examining the vagina, uterus, rectum, and accessory organs and structures
adnexa (ad-NECK-suh)	appendages of the uterus, including the ovaries, uterine tubes, and uterine ligaments, that hold the uterus in place
hysterectomy (his-tur-ECK-tuh-mee)	surgical removal of the uterus
dilation and curettage (kewr-e-TAHZH) **(D&C)**	gynecological procedure in which the cervix is widened and the uterus is scraped
salpingo-oophorectomy (sal-pin-goh-oh-oh-foh-RECK-toh-mee)	removal of the uterine tube and ovary
pelvic (PEL-vick) **inflammatory disease (PID)**	inflammation of the reproductive organs that, if untreated, can cause infertility
nulliparous (nul-IP-uh-rus)	having never given birth to a child
Gram stain	differential stain used to identify microbes according to the dye retained within the bacterial cell wall
ovarian (oh-VAIR-ee-un) **cysts**	fluid-filled sacs on or near the ovaries
premenstrual (pree-MEN-stroo-ul) **syndrome (PMS)**	group of signs and symptoms experienced by some women in the days preceding menstruation
premenstrual dysphoric (pree-MEN-stroo-ul dis-FOR-ick) **disorder (PMDD)**	premenstrual syndrome accompanied by emotional symptoms with impaired functioning that persists after the onset of menstruation

KEY TERM PRACTICE: *Female Pelvic Disorders*

1. A gynecological procedure in which the cervix is widened and the uterus is scraped is called _____.

2. The condition in which endometrial tissue appears outside the uterus is termed _____.

3. PMS accompanied by emotional symptoms with impaired functioning that persists after the onset of menstruation is termed _____.

4. The surgical removal of the uterus is known as a _____ and is derived from the word part _____ for *uterus* and the word part _____ for *removal of*.

5. The _____ is a differential stain used to identify microbes according to the dye retained within the bacterial cell wall.

Female Cancers

Cancers affecting the female reproductive organs include breast, cervical, endometrial, labial or vulvar, ovarian, and vaginal. Although considered primarily a female cancer, breast cancer also affects men but to a much lesser extent.

breast cancer

Breast cancer, malignant tumors of mammary tissue, occurs primarily in females; however, 1,200 new cases are reported each year in American men. It involves a strong genetic predisposition. Other linked factors include exposure to high estrogen levels, having borne no children, and experiencing a late first pregnancy. Breast cancer usually develops as a single, small, hard, painless nodule. The advanced stage is marked by skin dimpling and nipple discharge. Measures to detect the cancer as quickly as possible are key. These include regular mammograms and monthly breast self-examinations (BSEs). **Mammography**, which is radiographic examination of breast tissue, is used for the initial diagnosis. It may be performed with contrast dye injected into mammary ducts. It is recommended that a baseline mammogram be taken between ages 35 and 39 years; thereafter, regular mammograms are suggested as part of routine health care. As of 2011, the American Cancer Society recommends yearly mammograms for women starting at age 40. The false-negative (the mammogram is interpreted as having no pathology when abnormality does exist) rate is approximately 10%. For this reason, management of a palpable nodule must be based on clinical grounds. Confirmation of disease is provided by biopsy. Treatment includes surgery (lumpectomy or mastectomy), radiation, and chemotherapy.

The surgical removal of a breast is termed **mastectomy**. Reconstructive surgery generally follows the procedure. One such restorative procedure is the **transverse rectus abdominis myocutaneous (TRAM) flap** in which an abdominal muscle (rectus abdominis) is threaded under the abdominal and thoracic cavities to the mastectomy site (**Figure 16-22**). Nipple reconstruction can also be completed after TRAM flap surgery. Systemic treatments include chemotherapy, hormone therapy, and biological therapy. Common drugs include Soltamox (tamoxifen) (used in premenopausal women) and Arimidex (anastrozole), Aromasin (exemestane), and Femara (letrozole) (used in postmenopausal women). Tamoxifen is used to block the growth of breast cancer by interfering with the effects of estrogen in breast tissue. Anastrozole, exemestane, and letrozole work by lowering estrogen levels to help shrink tumors and slow their growth. The 5-year survival rate is over 90% if caught early enough.

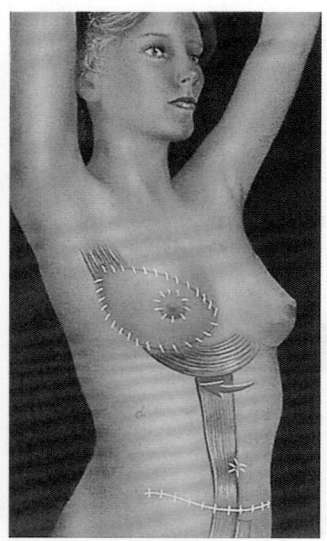

Figure 16-22 Breast reconstruction using the TRAM flap. The flap of the rectus abdominis muscle is tunneled through the abdomen to the breast area.

cervical cancer

Malignant neoplasms of the cervix are called **cervical cancer**. Cervical cancer is associated with human papillomavirus (HPV) infection. In addition, cigarette smoking has also been implicated as a causative factor. Watery, bloody, foul-smelling vaginal discharge and bleeding between periods or after intercourse are the main signs. It is easily diagnosed with a Pap smear or **Pap test**, a procedure in which cells are scraped from the cervix and viewed in stained smears. The cells are then determined to be in five classes based on their characteristics. When abnormal cells are found, excision of a cone-shaped section of cervical tissue, called a **conization**, is often performed (**Figure 16-23**). The cells can then be cultured or examined histologically.

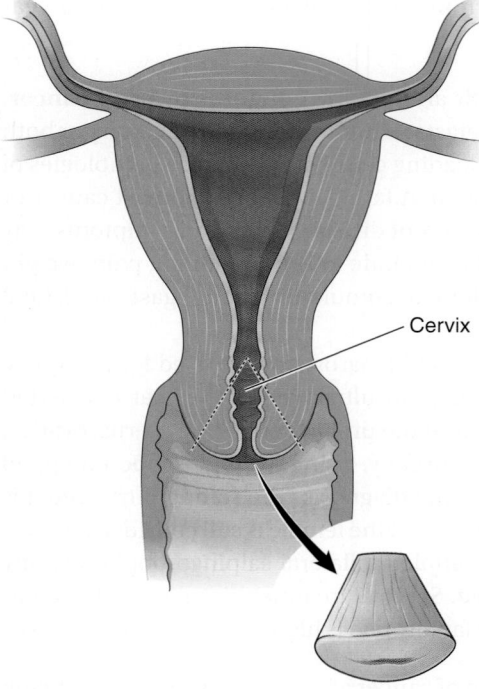

Cervix

Cone biopsy

Figure 16-23 Conization.

Surgery, radiation, cryosurgery, electrocoagulation, and laser ablation are common treatments. Immunization with Gardasil vaccine protects against four types of HPV. The vaccine is currently available for young men and women ages 9 to 26 years. **Cryosurgery** involves the localized freezing of diseased tissues without significant harm to adjacent structures. The use of an electrical device that destroys tissue is termed **electrocoagulation**. **Laser ablation** is the surgical removal of tissue via a laser instrument that uses radiation of optical frequencies. The prognosis is excellent if treated in the early stages.

endometrial cancer   Cancer of the endometrium (uterine lining), usually occurring after menopause, is termed **endometrial cancer**. This cancer is associated with estrogen replacement therapy (ERT), early menarche, late menopause, hypertension, diabetes mellitus, obesity, and use of tamoxifen (drug that inhibits the actions of estrogen). It occurs most often in women who have never been pregnant. Signs and symptoms are abnormal vaginal bleeding, pain in the pelvic area, and unexplained abnormal vaginal discharge. Diagnosis is made by the history and physical examination, pelvic examination, and biopsy. A total hysterectomy with radiation is the usual treatment for endometrial cancer. The prognosis is good if the cancer is detected in the early stages.

vulvar cancer
or labial cancer   **Vulvar cancer** or **labial cancer** is a disease in which cancer forms in tissues of the vulva (labia)—usually the outer labia majora. Human papillomavirus (HPV) infection and older age increase the risk. Signs and symptoms include bleeding or itching, a lump in the vulva, and tenderness in the surrounding area. Vulvar cancer is diagnosed by the history and physical examination, D&C, and biopsy for confirmation.

Treatments include vulvectomy and radiation therapy. The 5-year survival rate is 60%.

ovarian cancer

Another form of cancer with an unknown origin is **ovarian cancer**, which is characterized by metastatic tumors found in one ovary or both ovaries. Ovarian cancer is a leading cause of death from pathologies of the female reproductive system. A familial history of breast cancer or ovarian cancer increases the risk of disease. Signs and symptoms may be absent. When present, they include lower abdominal pain, weight loss, ascites (abdominal fluid accumulation), and gastrointestinal disturbances.

Transvaginal sonography and laparoscopy are used for diagnosis. **Transvaginal sonography** uses an ultrasonic probe that is inserted into the vagina. Echograms from the probe identify the uterus, ovaries, and ovarian structures. Laparoscopy, using an endoscope equipped with biopsy forceps, confirms the diagnosis. The standard treatment is removal of only the diseased ovary if the female is still considering bearing children. Otherwise, a complete bilateral salpingo-oophorectomy or hysterectomy is performed. Surgical treatment is followed by radiation and chemotherapy. The fatality rate is high if it is not detected early.

vaginal cancer

Vaginal cancer is a rare form of cancer affecting the vagina. Age (being age 60 years or older) and exposure to diethylstilbestrol (DES) before birth increase the risk of developing vaginal cancer. In the 1950s, DES was given to some women to prevent miscarriages. The main signs and symptoms are bleeding or discharge not related to menstruation, pain during sexual intercourse, pain in the pelvic area, and a lump in the vagina. It is treated by surgery, radiation therapy, and chemotherapy. Radiosensitizers (drugs that make cancer cells more sensitive to radiation therapy) are new types of treatment being tested in clinical trials.

KEY TERM	Definition
breast cancer	malignant tumors of mammary tissue
mammography (ma-MOG-ruh-fee)	x-ray examination of the breast
mastectomy (mas-TECK-tuh-mee)	surgical removal of a breast
transverse rectus abdominis myocutaneous (trans-VERS RECK-tus ab-DOM-in-us migh-oh-kew-TAY-nee-us) **(TRAM) flap**	surgical procedure to reconstruct the breast region after mastectomy using the rectus abdominis muscle, which is threaded under the abdominal and thoracic cavities to the mastectomy site
cervical (SUR-vi-kul) **cancer**	malignant neoplasms of the cervix
Pap test	test used to detect precancerous or cancerous cells of the cervix; also called a Pap smear
conization (kohn-ih-ZAY-shun)	removal of a cone-shaped section of tissue, most notably from the cervix
cryosurgery (krye-oh-SUR-juh-ree)	surgery in which low temperatures are applied to tissues to seal or remove them
electrocoagulation (ee-leck-troh-koh-ag-yoo-LAY-shun)	the use of an electrical device to destroy tissue
laser ablation (ab-LAY-shun)	removal of tissue with a laser

continued

continued from page 852

KEY TERM	Definition
endometrial (en-doh-MEE-tree-ul) **cancer**	malignant cells of the uterine endometrium
vulvar (VUL-vur) **cancer**	malignant cells of the folds surrounding the female genitalia; also called labial cancer
labial (LAY-bee-ul) **cancer**	malignant cells of the folds surrounding the female genitalia; also called vulvar cancer
ovarian (oh-VAIR-ee-un) **cancer**	malignant tumor of the ovary or ovaries
transvaginal sonography (trans-VAJ-i-nul suh-NOG-ruh-fee)	procedure for obtaining echograms of the uterus, ovaries, and ovarian structures
vaginal (VAJ-i-nul) **cancer**	malignant cells of the vagina

KEY TERM PRACTICE: *Female Cancers*

1. Give the two terms for malignant tumors in the folds surrounding the female genitalia. _____

2. The word part _____ means *breast*, and the word part *-ectomy* means _____; so the surgical removal of a breast is termed _____.

3. The surgical procedure to reconstruct the breast region after mastectomy using the rectus abdominis muscle, which is threaded under the abdominal and thoracic cavities to the mastectomy site, is known as a _____.

4. Removal of tissue with a laser is called _____.

5. _____ is an x-ray examination of the breast.

Female Benign Tumors

Leiomyomas and fibroids are the most common types of benign tumors of the female reproductive system.

leiomyoma

A **leiomyoma** is a benign neoplasm derived from smooth muscle, like that found in the myometrium of the uterus.

uterine fibroids

Uterine fibroids are benign tumors of the muscle and fibrous tissue of the uterus (**Figure 16-24**). Signs and symptoms include heavy menstrual periods, cramping, painful sex, abdominal distention, and an urge

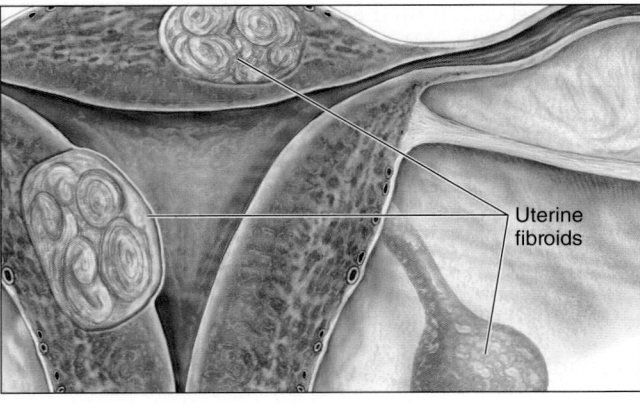

Figure 16-24 Uterine fibroids.

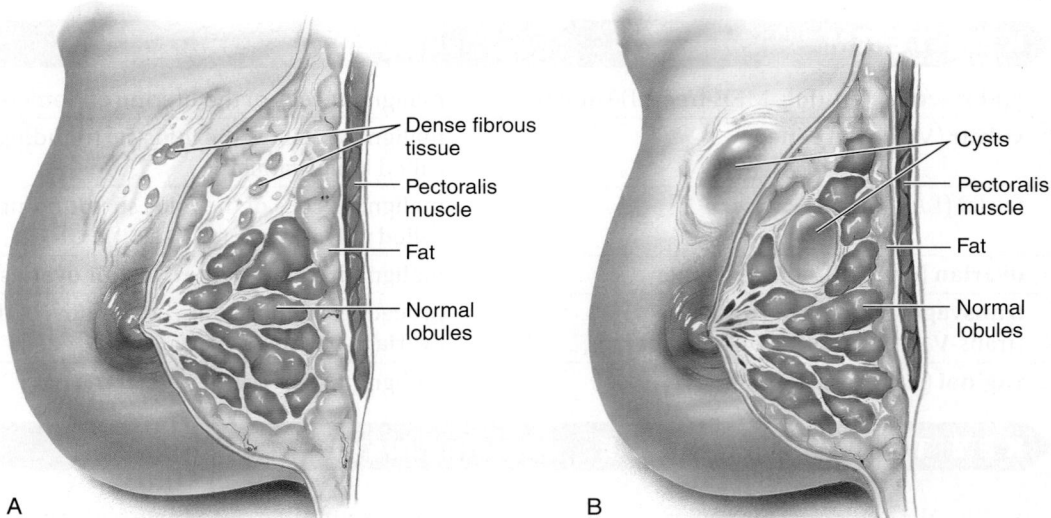

Figure 16-25 Fibrocystic breast changes:
(A) fibrosis; **(B)** cysts.

A

B

to urinate. Treatment depends on the severity and includes hormone therapy to shrink fibroid size or hysterectomy.

fibrocystic breast changes

The term **fibrocystic breast changes**, formerly called fibrocystic breast disease, refers to a common noncancerous breast condition that affects women between 30 and 40 years of age. There are two types of breast changes: fibrosis (lumps that are firm and hard) and cysts (fluid-filled sacs) (**Figure 16-25**). Common signs and symptoms are breast swelling or thickening, lumps within the breast, breast tenderness, and pain. The primary sign is a cyst that fluctuates in size throughout the menstrual cycle. A persistent lump is often the only sign. It is diagnosed by mammography and biopsy. Treatments include wearing a support bra to ease discomfort, taking over-the-counter pain relievers for pain, and restricting caffeine intake, because caffeine appears to influence the cyst development. Oral contraceptives are often prescribed for women with severe symptoms. Limiting salt intake was once suggested, but studies have not confirmed the benefit of sodium restriction with regard to fibrocystic breast changes.

KEY TERM	Definition
leiomyoma (lye-oh-migh-OH-muh)	benign neoplasm derived from uterine smooth muscle
uterine fibroids (FIGH-broidz)	benign tumors of the muscle and fibrous tissue of the uterus
fibrocystic (figh-broh-SIS-tick) **breast changes**	noncancerous breast condition that is characterized by fibrosis (lumps that are firm and hard) or cysts (fluid-filled sacs)

KEY TERM PRACTICE: *Female Benign Tumors*

1. A benign neoplasm derived from uterine smooth muscle is called a _____, a term made up of the word part _____ for *smooth*, the word part _____ for *muscle*, and the word part _____ for *tumor*.

2. Benign fibrous tumors of the muscle and fibrous tissue of the uterus are termed _____.

3. The term _____ refers to a noncancerous breast condition that is characterized by fibrosis or cysts.

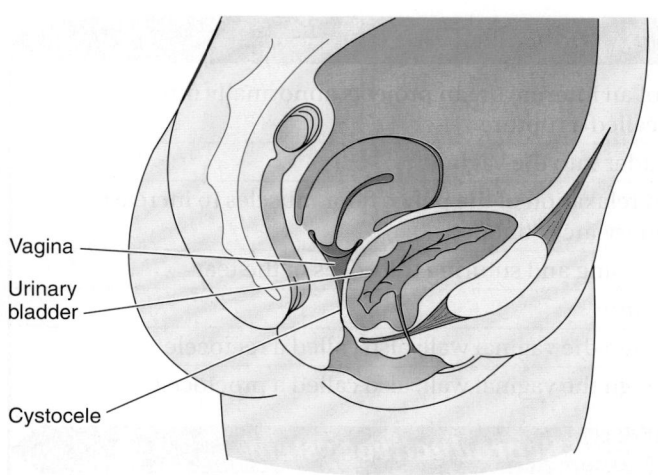

Figure 16-26 Cystocele. The bladder has herniated into the anterior wall of the vagina.

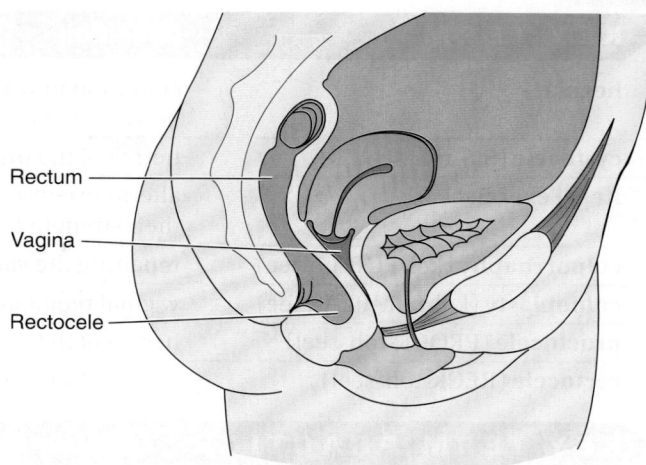

Figure 16-27 Rectocele. The posterior of the vagina is herniated.

Hernias of the Female Reproductive System

hernias
A **hernia** is a condition in which part of an internal organ projects abnormally through a body wall or cavity. Hernias are also called ruptures.

cystocele
A herniation of the urinary bladder into the vagina is termed a **cystocele** (**Figure 16-26**). It results from trauma or weakened pelvic muscles and ligaments. Pregnancy, labor, and aging are associated with cystocele development. Signs and symptoms include pelvic pressure, urinary frequency, urgency, and incontinence. It is diagnosed by the history and physical examination.

Treatment involves Kegel exercises, estrogen therapy to improve muscle tone, or colporrhaphy. With **Kegel exercises**, an individual voluntarily contracts and relaxes the pelvic floor muscles to strengthen muscle tissue and also voluntarily starts and stops urine flow several times during urination. Practicing Kegel exercises can alleviate urinary leakage that results from weakened pelvic floor muscles. Repairing the vagina by excising and suturing the edges of the tear is called **colporrhaphy**, and vaginal surgical repair that involves restructuring is known as **colpoplasty**.

proctocele or **rectocele**
A **proctocele** or **rectocele** is herniation of the rectum into the vagina (**Figure 16-27**). Proctoceles are caused by weakened vaginal walls resulting from trauma, pregnancy, or childbirth. Fecal incontinence, flatulence, and difficulty emptying the bowels are common signs. A complete history and physical examination are generally all that is necessary for the diagnosis. Treatment consists of a colpoplasty. When a simultaneous rectocele and cystocele operation is performed, it is referred to as an anterior and posterior (A&P) repair.

KEY TERM	Definition
hernia	condition in which part of an internal organ projects abnormally through a body wall or cavity; also called a rupture
cystocele (SIS-toh-seel)	hernia of the urinary bladder into the vagina
Kegel exercises	alternate contraction and relaxation of the pelvic floor muscles to increase their strength to treat urinary incontinence
colporrhaphy (kol-POR-uh-fee)	repairing the vagina by excising and suturing the edges of the tear
colpoplasty (kol-poh-PLAS-tee)	vaginal repair and restructure
proctocele (PROCK-toh-seel)	hernia of the rectum through the vaginal wall; also called a rectocele
rectocele (RECK-toh-seel)	hernia of the rectum through the vaginal wall; also called a proctocele

KEY TERM PRACTICE: *Hernias of the Female Reproductive System*

1. Vaginal repair and restructure is termed a _____ and is derived from the word part _____ for "vagina" and the word part _____ for "restructuring a body part."

2. Give two terms that mean a hernia of the rectum through the vaginal wall. _____

3. A _____ is a hernia of the urinary bladder into the vagina; it comes from the word part _____ for *bladder* and the word part _____ for *hernia*.

4. The term for alternate contraction and relaxation of the pelvic floor muscles to increase their strength to treat urinary incontinence is _____.

5. Repairing the vagina by excising and suturing the edges of the tear is termed a _____.

Infertility and Sterility

Nearly 90% of couples attempting pregnancy are able to do so within 1 year of having regular, unprotected sex. Two closely related terms with fine nuances of distinction are infertility and sterility, conditions affecting both males and females. The terms are frequently used interchangeably. Diagnosis is based on the history and physical examination. Treatment for both infertility and sterility, if available, depends on the underlying cause.

infertility **Infertility** is the diminished ability or inability to produce offspring in either the male or the female. Female infertility is characterized by the inability to conceive. A common cause is failure to ovulate due to low hormone output or from endometriosis. Male infertility is marked by the inability of sperm to fertilize an oocyte. Other causes are structural anomalies, such as scar tissue and varicocele (discussed below); sexually transmitted diseases; antisperm antibodies; and low sperm count (oligospermia).

Forms of infertility are diagnosed by the history and physical examination, semen analysis, hormone level evaluation, and laparoscopy to rule out uterine or uterine tube abnormalities. A **semen analysis** measures sperm count, motility, morphology (shape), and volume of semen produced. Decreased sperm numbers and semen volume, abnormal sperm shape, and impaired movement are associated with infertility.

sterility **Sterility** refers to the inability to conceive in the female or the inability to induce conception in the male. Female sterility is due to inadequacy in structure or function. A frequent cause of female sterility is blocked uterine tubes. Male sterility may be associated with impotence or **oligospermia** (low sperm count). Sterility can also be medically induced. For example, the removal of reproductive organs or the administration of drugs that prevent adequate hormone secretion (known as chemical sterility) renders a person sterile. Infertility is not as irreversible as sterility.

KEY TERM	Definition
infertility	diminished ability or inability to produce offspring in either the male or the female
semen (SEE-mun) **analysis**	test that measures the volume of semen and sperm number, morphology, and motility
sterility	inability to conceive in the female or the inability to induce conception in the male
oligospermia (ol-ih-goh-SPER-mee-uh)	low sperm count

KEY TERM PRACTICE: *Infertility and Sterility*

1. _____ is the diminished ability or inability to produce offspring in either the male or the female.

2. The medical term for a low sperm count is _____ and is derived from the word part _____ for *few, deficiency* and _____ for *condition of spermatozoa.*

3. A test that measures the volume of semen and sperm number, morphology, and motility is called a _____.

4. The inability to conceive in the female or the inability to induce conception in the male is termed _____.

Infections

Pathological states caused by microorganisms that can be acquired by means other than sexual intercourse are described in this section.

candidiasis   **Candidiasis** is a fungal disease caused by *Candida albicans* (**Figure 16-28**). This is the same yeast infection that causes **vaginitis** (vaginal inflammation). Itching, burning, and vaginal discharge are common signs and symptoms. Prolonged antibiotic use predisposes females to this infection, which is diagnosed

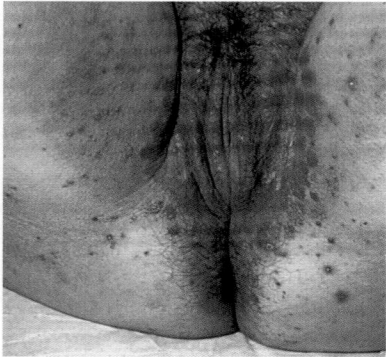

Figure 16-28 Cutaneous candidiasis.

by the clinical picture. Oral and cream antifungal medications are used to treat it. Individuals taking antibiotics are encouraged to eat yogurt daily to keep intestinal microorganisms in balance, thereby thwarting possible yeast infections.

toxic shock syndrome (TSS) — Toxic shock syndrome (TSS) is an acute, potentially fatal systemic disease caused by *Staphylococcus* infection. It occurs most often in menstruating women who use superabsorbent tampons. Superabsorbent tampons have been implicated because they create an environment conducive to bacterial growth and bacterial toxin release in the vagina. TSS involves circulatory failure and is characterized by widespread homeostatic imbalances as a reaction to the bacterial toxins. Common signs and symptoms are fever, rash, hypotension, gastrointestinal upset, and neuromuscular disturbances. It is diagnosed by physical examination, history of tampon use, and accompanying elevated liver enzymes. The condition is treated with antibiotics and fluids to increase blood pressure. It is recommended that tampons be changed every 4 to 6 hours to prevent TSS.

KEY TERM	Definition
candidiasis (kan-dih-DYE-uh-sis)	vaginal yeast infection caused by *Candida albicans* fungus
vaginitis (vaj-ih-NIGH-tis)	vaginal inflammation
toxic shock syndrome (TSS)	circulatory failure associated with tampon use and the growth of toxin-producing staphylococcal bacteria

KEY TERM PRACTICE: *Infections*

1. The disease associated with tampon use that has systemic effects is _____.

2. _____ is a vaginal yeast infection caused by a fungus.

3. Inflammation of the vagina is termed _____.

Sexually Transmitted Diseases (STDs)

Sexually transmitted diseases (STDs) or venereal diseases (VDs) — Sexually transmitted diseases (STDs), or venereal diseases (VDs), are contagious infections acquired during sexual contact. STDs are also called *sexually transmitted infections* (STIs). They are spread by contact with body fluids such as semen and vaginal secretions and by anal or oral sex. More than 50 STDs have been identified, and it is possible to have more than one simultaneously. Public health measures are aimed at education and prevention strategies. STDs are a major public health concern because 19 million new cases are reported annually in the United States. Moreover, approximately 25% of college students are infected with an STD, and the three most common STDs on college campuses are genital human papillomavirus (HPV) infection, chlamydia, and genital herpes. To prevent STDs, patients are advised to follow the ABCs for prevention: A is for abstinence, B is for be faithful, and C is for condom. Common STDs and the organisms that cause them are listed in **Table 16-1**.

TABLE 16-1

COMMON SEXUALLY TRANSMITTED DISEASES

Disease	Organism	Remarks
AIDS	HIV	First reported in the United States in 1981
Chancroid	*Haemophilus ducreyi*	Causes genital ulcers; found primarily in lesser-developed countries
Chlamydia	*Chlamydia trachomatis*	Most frequently reported STD in the United States
Genital herpes	Herpes simplex virus type 1 (HSV-1) Herpes simplex virus type 2 (HSV-2)	Both cause genital herpes; most cases caused by HSV-2
Genital human papillomavirus (HPV) infection	Human papillomavirus (HPV)	Most common STD in the United States more than 40 types
Gonorrhea	*Neisseria gonorrhoeae*	Multiplies easily in reproductive tract
Syphilis	*Treponema pallidum*	Untreated syphilis affects all body systems; full course can develop over years
Trichomoniasis	*Trichomonas vaginalis*	Most common curable STD in women
Viral hepatitis type B (HBV) Viral hepatitis type C (HCV)	*Hepadnaviridae* *Flaviviridae*	Seven different types of viral hepatitis; HBV and HCV are the two most common types

AIDS

AIDS is caused by infection with HIV, a retrovirus that causes immune system failure. Initially there are no symptoms, but flu-like symptoms occur approximately 6 weeks after an infection and mark early illness. The asymptomatic period may last up to 10 years because the virus remains latent. HIV infects certain cells (macrophages and lymphocytes) of the immune system, thereby hampering the body's protective response and allowing the development of other infections and cancer, notably Kaposi sarcoma.

AIDS is actually an advanced HIV infection, which is transmitted via contact with HIV in blood, semen, and vaginal secretions. Other major modes of transmission are by needle sharing among HIV-infected drug users and from mother to infant at childbirth. Preventive measures include abstinence from sexual intercourse, condom use, and refraining from needle sharing. There is no cure, but life can be prolonged through medications.

chancroid

An acute, localized venereal disease caused by *Haemophilus ducreyi* is termed **chancroid**. It is characterized by painful, ragged ulcers called

chancres, lymph node enlargement, and pus formation 7 to 10 days after sexual intercourse with an infected person (**Figure 16-29**). A Gram stain is done to confirm the causative organism. Treatment consists of antibiotics and sexual abstinence throughout the course of therapy.

chlamydia

Chlamydia is a bacterial infection caused by the bacterium *Chlamydia trachomatis*. In women, it is often a silent STD because females are frequently asymptomatic and may transmit the disease unknowingly. Symptoms appear in men within 1 to 3 weeks after exposure about 75% of the time. It is the leading cause of pelvic inflammatory disease (PID) in women.

Signs and symptoms of chlamydia when apparent in females are thick vaginal discharge, genital burning and itching, abdominal pain, and **dyspareunia** (painful sexual intercourse; *pareunos* = lying beside). Males experience penile discharge, genital burning and itching, urethritis, and scrotal swelling. Enlarged lymph nodes are noted in both sexes, as are possible lesions within the genitourinary tract. Newborns can contract chlamydia from infected mothers during birth. Antigen-specific serologic studies and the Giemsa stain (which identifies blood particles) are used for diagnosis. Initial treatment involves antibiotic injections for both partners and a course of oral antibiotics. Prompt treatment is necessary.

genital herpes

Vesicles on the genitals caused by the herpes simplex virus type 1 (HSV-1) or herpes simplex virus type 2 (HSV-2) are called **genital herpes** (**Figure 16-30**). Most cases are caused by HSV-2. The virus often remains in a latent state in the nervous system between flare-ups and has a tendency to recur at irregular intervals. The virus enters the body through interruptions in mucous membranes. Painful genital sores and blister-like lesions around and in genitals are common. The person may also experience flu-like symptoms. All infected people are contagious during outbreaks, and some individuals, called "shedders," are contagious even when no symptoms or outward signs are present. In the United States, one out of every five individuals ages

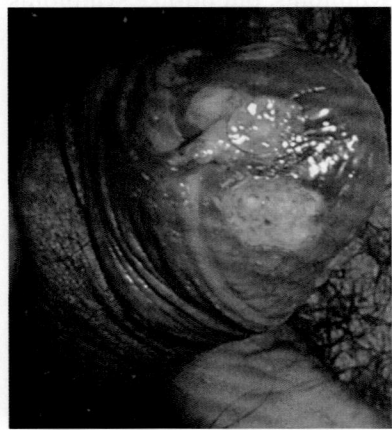

Figure 16-29 Chancroid. This patient has multiple painful ulcers on the glans penis.

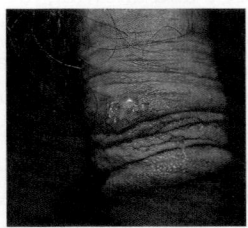

Figure 16-30 Vesicles of genital herpes (HSV-2) on the penis.

12 years and over is infected with the virus. Diagnosis is made by the presence of the characteristic lesions and a tissue culture identifying the virus. There is no cure, and the virus remains in certain nerve cells for life. Antiviral medications reduce the duration and frequency of outbreaks.

Genital herpes is associated with cervical cancer. Pregnant women can pass the virus to their unborn children, particularly if the woman's first episode occurs during pregnancy. If an outbreak that is not the first episode occurs during pregnancy, the risk of infection to the child during delivery is low. If an outbreak occurs during labor and delivery and the lesions are present in or near the birth canal, the infection can be passed to the newborn. For this reason, infected pregnant women are advised against vaginal births.

genital human papillomavirus (HPV) infection

Warts on the external genitalia, anus, vagina, and cervix characterize **genital human papillomavirus (HPV) infection** (**Figure 16-31**). However, most people with HPV do not develop signs, and in 90% of cases, the body's immune system clears the infection within 2 years. It is the most common STD in the United States and has been linked to the development of cervical cancer. Diagnosis is confirmed by the presence of warts and isolation of the virus. There is no cure, but a vaccine, Gardasil, is available to prevent the four most common types of HPV and must be given in three injections. Gardasil is given to males and females ages 9 to 26 years and is most effective when given before a person's first sexual experience.

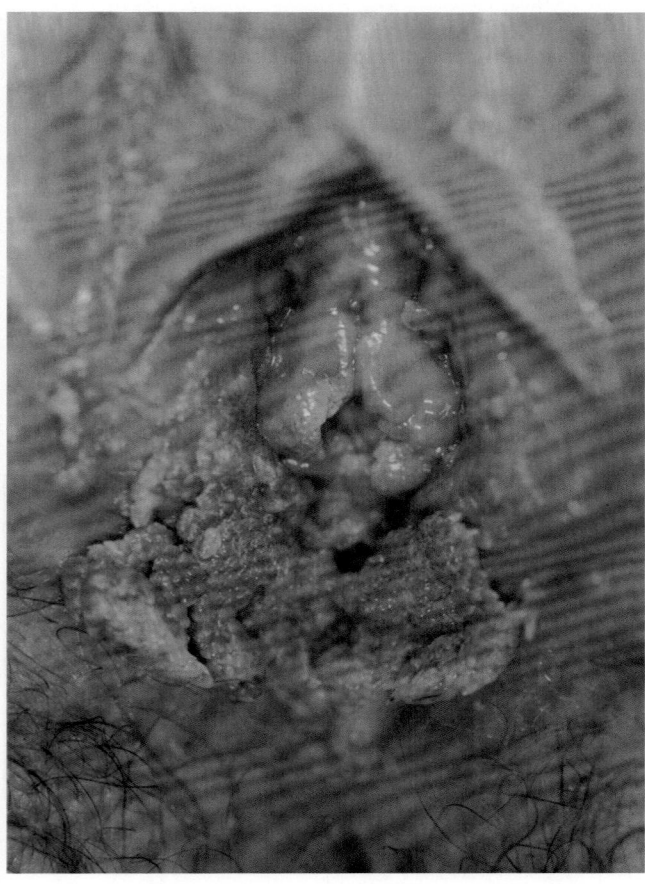

Figure 16-31 Vaginal and perineal genital warts of human papillomavirus (HPV).

gonorrhea

Gonorrhea is a venereal disease caused by the bacterium *Neisseria gonorrhoeae*. The most common signs and symptoms are a discharge from the vagina or penis and painful or difficult urination (**Figure 16-32**). Complications include PID, ectopic pregnancy, and infertility.

Gonorrhea can become a systemic infection. Eye infections can lead to blindness. Newborns can acquire this STD from infected mothers during a vaginal birth. For this reason, erythromycin antibiotic salve is routinely applied to the eyes of all infants at birth.

Gram stain is used to identify the causative agent. This disease is treated with antibiotics; however, antibiotic-resistant strains of gonorrhea are increasing. Untreated forms can also lead to blindness. The prognosis is good with treatment.

syphilis

Syphilis is a systemic infection caused by the *Treponema pallidum* spirochete. Lesions occur in any tissue or vascular body organ. It produces various clinical pictures and symptoms characteristic of other diseases. Painless, contagious local lesions called chancres appear on male and female genitalia (**Figure 16-33**).

Syphilis has primary, secondary, and tertiary stages. During the primary stage, the microbe multiplies and spreads to the lymph nodes and bloodstream. The chancre disappears within 4 to 6 weeks with or without treatment. Primary lesions heal and a latent (secondary) period lasting from 1 to 40 years follows with subclinical or asymptomatic manifestations. The tertiary stage is marked by gumma invasion of vascular organs and the central nervous system, which can lead to blood vessel damage, blindness, emotional instability, hallucinations, and insanity. A **gumma** is a mass of rubber-like necrotic (dead) tissue. Another word for gumma is **syphiloma**, and the terms are interchangeable. During the tertiary stage, the individual is no longer infectious. Diagnosis is made by the *T. pallidum* immobilization (TPI) test, which detects a particular antibody in a patient with syphilis, and/or other serum antibody tests. It is critical to treat syphilis with penicillin G or an alternative antibiotic in the early stages to prevent irreversible damage.

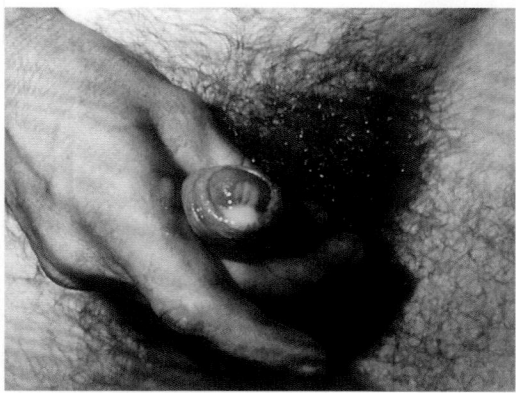

Figure 16-32 Urethral discharge associated with gonorrhea. This discharge may vary in color and amount and is accompanied by burning during urination.

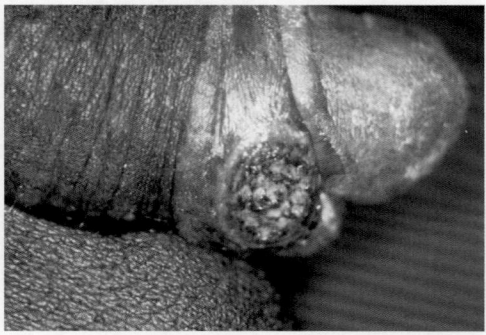

Figure 16-33 Chancre of primary syphilis.

trichomoniasis   An infection caused by the protozoan *Trichomonas vaginalis* is termed **trichomoniasis**. Most cases are asymptomatic, allowing the disease to spread unknowingly. Signs and symptoms, when present, include urethritis, dysuria, and vaginitis with green-yellow discharge. Diagnosis is made by isolating the causative agent in the urine or through microscopic examination of vaginal secretions. Antiprotozoal drugs are administered to both partners until the infection is completely eradicated. Failure to complete the treatment regimen leads to "Ping-Pong" vaginitis because the infection goes back and forth between one infected partner and the other.

viral hepatitis   **Viral hepatitis** in an inflammation of the liver caused by at least seven immunologically unrelated viruses: hepatitis A virus, hepatitis B virus, hepatitis C virus, hepatitis D virus, hepatitis E virus, and hepatitis G virus. Hepatitis B virus (HBV) and hepatitis C virus (HCV) are the two most common types and are spread by contact with the blood or body fluids of an infected person. Infection with HBV and HCV may lead to acute or chronic liver disease. In some cases, cirrhosis and cancer result. A vaccine is available for HBV, but not for HCV.

KEY TERM	Definition
sexually transmitted diseases (STDs)	contagious infections acquired during sexual contact; also called venereal diseases (VDs) or sexually transmitted infections (STIs)
venereal (ve-NEER-ee-ul) **diseases (VDs)**	contagious infections acquired during sexual contact; also called sexually transmitted diseases (STDs) or sexually transmitted infections (STIs)
acquired immunodeficiency (im-yoo-noh-dee-FISH-un-see) **syndrome (AIDS)**	caused by infection with or sexually transmitted infections HIV, a retrovirus that causes immune system failure
chancroid (SHANK-roid)	sexually transmitted disease characterized by painful, ragged ulcers at the infection site
chancres (SHANK-urz)	skin lesions or ulcers at the point where the pathogen enters the body
chlamydia (kla-MID-ee-uh)	sexually transmitted disease caused by the bacterium *Chlamydia trachomatis*
dyspareunia (dis-puh-ROOH-nee-uh)	painful sexual intercourse
genital herpes (HUR-peez)	sexually transmitted disease caused by the herpes simplex virus type 2 (HSV-2)
genital human papillomavirus (HPV) infection	warts on the genitalia or in the anus region caused by human papilloma virus (HPV)
gonorrhea (gon-uh-REE-uh)	sexually transmitted disease caused by *Neisseria gonorrhoeae*
syphilis (SIF-ih-lis)	sexually transmitted disease caused by *Treponema pallidum*
gumma (GUM-uh)	rubbery tumor that occurs in the tertiary stage of syphilis; also called a syphiloma
syphiloma (sif-ih-LOH-muh)	rubbery tumor that occurs in the tertiary stage of syphilis; also called a gumma
trichomoniasis (trick-oh-moh-NIGH-uh-sis)	sexually transmitted disease caused by the protozoan *Trichomonas vaginalis*
viral hepatitis (VIGH-rul hep-uh-TIGH-tis)	inflammation of the liver caused by at least seven immunologically unrelated viruses

continued

continued from page 863

KEY TERM PRACTICE: *Sexually Transmitted Diseases*

1. Name the advanced disease caused by infection with HIV. _____

2. Contagious infections acquired during sexual contact are termed _____ or _____.

3. The sexually transmitted disease caused by the protozoan *Trichomonas vaginalis* is _____.

4. A rubbery tumor that occurs in the tertiary stage of syphilis is known as a _____ or a _____.

5. _____ is painful sexual intercourse.

Birth Control Methods

The deliberate limiting of the number of children born by means of contraception is termed *birth control* (BC). **Contraception** is a way of avoiding pregnancy, using either artificial methods such as condoms and birth control pills, or natural methods, such as avoiding sex during the woman's fertile period (fertility awareness). Common birth control methods are described in this section, and **Table 16-2** compares the effectiveness of several birth control methods for females and males.

TABLE 16-2 — THE EFFECTIVENESS OF VARIOUS BIRTH CONTROL METHODS

Effectiveness as Measured by Number of Pregnancies per 100 Women	Females	Males
<1	• Birth control patch • Implant • Intrauterine device (IUD) • Sterilization (tubal ligation)	• Sterilization (vasectomy)
2–9	• Birth control pills (BCPs) • Injection • Vaginal ring	
15–24	• Cervical cap • Diaphragm • Female condom • Sponge • Condom	• Condom • Withdrawal (Pull-out method)
25	• Fertility awareness • Spermicide	
Percent Effective	**Emergency Contraception (Morning-After Pill)**	
89%	Taken within 72 hours of unprotected sex	
Less effective	Taken up to 120 hours after unprotected sex	

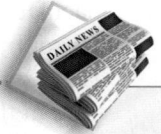

IN THE NEWS: Male Birth Control from an Indonesian Plant

To date there are only two male contraceptives: condoms and vasectomy. Both of these have problems because not all men like condoms and vasectomies are generally irreversible. Why isn't there a drug or hormonal method for men? The reason is that there are several problems to be overcome, such as the sheer number of sperm that have to be controlled, the stringent safety standards that have to be met, and finding a method that men will actually use.

Surprisingly, a plant in Indonesia may solve the issues. The plant, gandarusa, has been used for its medicinal qualities as a stress reducer or to "soothe the nerves." Over time an interesting side effect was found: reduced male fertility.

Since 1987, research on animals has found it safe to use, so human clinical trials have just recently begun. The active ingredient from the plant does not change male hormones; instead, it affects the chemistry of the enzyme on the tip of each spermatozoon so that no sperm can pierce the outer wall of the oocyte. Without the ability to penetrate an oocyte, fertilization cannot occur. Another important finding is that the effect of the drug wears off within 2 months after it is no longer taken, thus restoring fertility. If it reaches final FDA approval, the only hurdle remains with men. That is, will they actually use it?

abstinence	**Abstinence** is refraining from penile–vaginal intercourse.
birth control implant	A **birth control implant** is a matchstick-sized rod containing progesterone that suppresses ovulation. This birth control implant is inserted by a health care professional in the brachial region of the arm. It can be removed at any time and is effective for up to 3 years.
birth control injection	A **birth control injection** is an intramuscular hormone shot of Depo-Provera (medroxyprogesterone acetate) that is administered every 3 months to females. It works by suppressing ovulation.
birth control patch	The **birth control patch** is a thin, beige plastic patch that resembles a square bandage that sticks to the skin. The patch releases the same hormones (estrogen and progesterone) that are found in birth control pills and works by preventing ovulation. A new patch is placed on the skin once a week for three consecutive weeks, followed by a patch-free week.
birth control pills (BCPs) or oral contraceptives (OCTs)	**Birth control pills (BCPs)**, also called **oral contraceptives (OCTs)**, are tablets taken daily to manipulate the female hormone cycle so that ovulation does not occur. They usually contain a combination of estrogen and progesterone. Oral contraceptives are known to reduce the risk of ovarian cysts and cancer, endometrial cancer, and benign breast disease—an added benefit. In women taking birth control pills, there is less iron-deficiency anemia, rheumatoid arthritis, endometriosis, dysmenorrhea, and premenstrual syndrome symptoms.
condom	A **male condom** is a close-fitting sheath that covers the penis to prevent pregnancy or the spread of a sexually transmitted disease by capturing

ejaculated semen (**Figure 16-34**). They are commonly called rubbers or prophylactics. The **female condom** is a pouch with flexible rings on each end that is inserted into the vagina. The ring at the closed end stays in the vagina, and the open-ended ring remains just outside the vagina (or anus) during intercourse (**Figure 16-35**). As in the male condom, the female condom collects the ejaculate, preventing it from entering the female reproductive tract.

fertility awareness–based method (FAM)

The **fertility awareness–based method (FAM)** is a form of contraception in which sexual intercourse is avoided on days that ovulation may be occurring or when a woman is most likely to conceive (when the oocyte is still in the uterine tube). It is also called natural family planning.

intrauterine device (IUD)

An **intrauterine device (IUD)** is a small, T-shaped device that is inserted into the uterus (**Figure 16-36**). Its mechanism of action remains unclear, but its presence stimulates prostaglandin production that ultimately changes the chemical composition of uterine secretions and lowers the chances of fertilization and implantation. ParaGard and Mirena IUDs affect the way sperm move, and the progesterone in the Mirena IUD prevents ovulation.

sponge

The female **sponge** is a plastic foam sponge containing spermicide that is inserted into the vagina to prevent pregnancy. Because the sponge blocks the cervix, it prevents sperm from entering the uterus. It also contains **spermicide**, a substance that prevents pregnancy by destroying sperm. Spermicides can be use alone or in combination with other birth control methods and are available in creams, foams, gels, and suppositories.

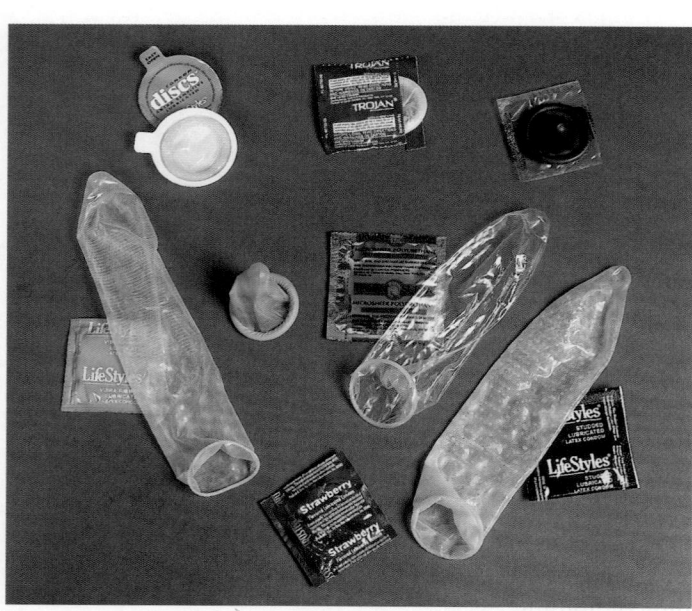

Figure 16-34 Male condoms are made of various materials (natural membrane, latex, polyurethane) and are sold in a wide variety of colors, shapes, and textures.

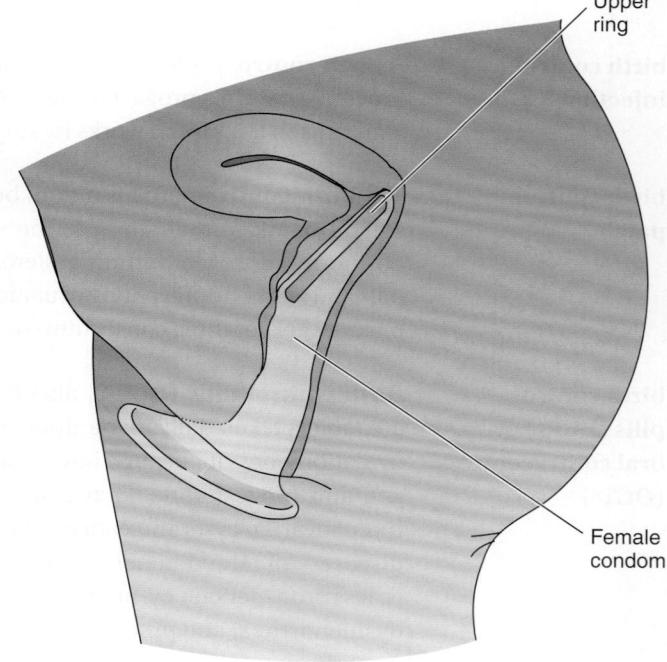

Upper ring

Female condom

Figure 16-35 Female condom. The upper ring keeps the condom in place.

sterilization   **Sterilization** is a surgical procedure that prevents a person from reproducing by removing all or part of the reproductive organs. Tubal ligation and vasectomy are two common surgical procedures that make the female (tubal ligation) or male (vasectomy) sterile.

tubal ligation   A sterilization technique in which a woman's uterine tubes are surgically blocked by cutting, cautery, or a plastic or metal device to prevent oocytes from entering the uterus is called a **tubal ligation** (**Figure 16-37**). The oocytes are released, but cannot reach the uterus or incoming sperm. Instead, they degenerate and are absorbed by the body.

vasectomy   A surgical operation that prevents sperm from being ejaculated is termed a **vasectomy** (**Figure 16-38**). A vasectomy involves cutting and removing a small segment (about 1 cm) of the vas (ductus) deferens from each testis. The ends are then tied and/or cauterized, making it impossible for sperm to travel from the epididymis to the distal portions of the reproductive tract. Sperm that are produced then degenerate in the epididymides.

vaginal barriers   **Vaginal barriers** are physical blockades that prevent sperm from entering the uterus. Examples include a **diaphragm**, a dome-shaped silicone cup placed inside the vagina at the entrance to the uterus and a

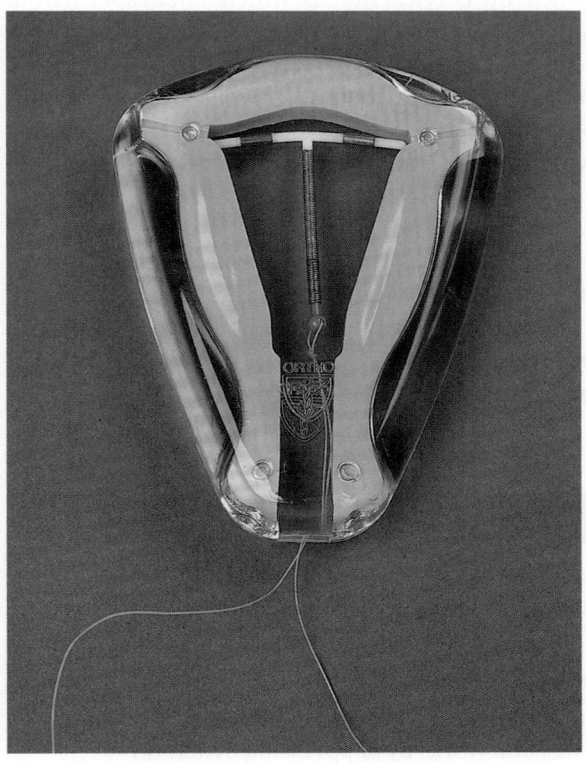

Figure 16-36 A plastic model of the uterus illustrating the location and orientation of the Copper T-380A IUD. Note the two string filaments protruding through the cervix of this model. These are trimmed after a doctor inserts the device.

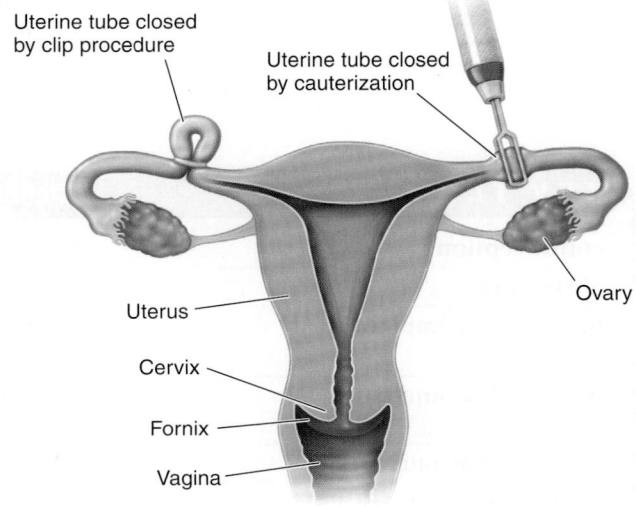

Uterine tube closed by clip procedure

Uterine tube closed by cauterization

Ovary

Uterus

Cervix

Fornix

Vagina

Figure 16-37 Two different procedures for tubal ligation.

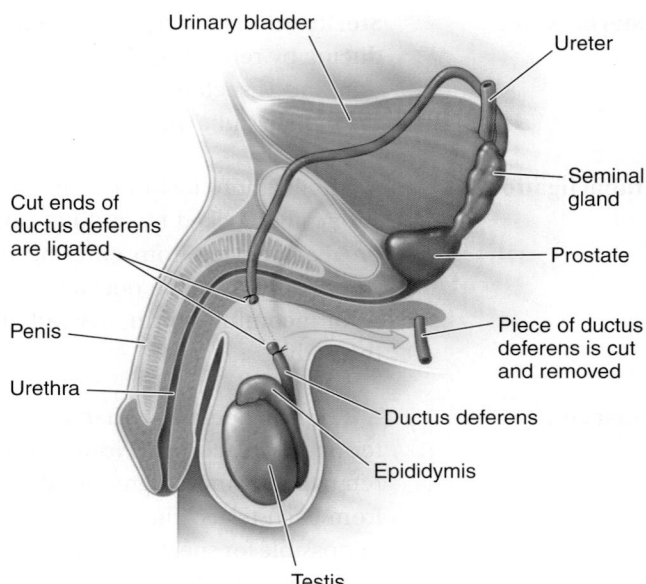

Figure 16-38 Vasectomy.

Labels in figure: Urinary bladder; Ureter; Seminal gland; Prostate; Cut ends of ductus deferens are ligated; Penis; Piece of ductus deferens is cut and removed; Urethra; Ductus deferens; Epididymis; Testis

similar device called the **cervical cap**. This tight-fitting device is placed inside the vagina and fitted tightly over the entrance to the cervix. A **vaginal ring** is a hormone-releasing barrier that is placed in the vagina once a month for 3 weeks to prevent ovulation. The NuvaRing also causes thickening of the cervical mucus, which blocks sperm from entering the uterus.

withdrawal method The **withdrawal method** (pull-out method) involves the man pulling the penis out of the vagina before ejaculating. It is estimated that 35 million couples worldwide use this method, which is the oldest form of birth control.

morning-after pill The **morning-after pill**, also called emergency contraception, is used to prevent pregnancy up to 5 days (120 hours) after unprotected sex. The morning-after pill contains hormones that (1) prevent ovulation, (2) thicken the cervical mucus to block sperm, and (3) thin the lining of the uterus to prevent implantation of the fertilized egg.

KEY TERM	Definition
contraception	way of avoiding pregnancy using either artificial or natural methods
abstinence	refraining from penile–vaginal intercourse
birth control implant	matchstick-sized rod containing progesterone inserted in the brachial region of the arm that suppresses ovulation
birth control injection	intramuscular hormone shot of Depo-Provera that is administered every 3 months to females that works by suppressing ovulation
birth control patch	thin patch worn on the skin that releases hormones to prevent ovulation
birth control pills (BCPs)	tablets taken daily to manipulate the female hormone cycle so that ovulation does not occur; also called oral contraceptives (OCTs)

continued

continued from page 8868

KEY TERM	Definition
oral contraceptives (OCTs) (OR-ul kon-truh-SEP-tivs)	tablets taken daily to manipulate the female hormone cycle so that ovulation does not occur; also called birth control pills (BCPs)
male condom	close-fitting sheath that covers the penis
female condom	pouch with flexible rings on each end that is inserted into the vagina
fertility awareness–based method (FAM)	form of contraception in which sexual intercourse is avoided on days that ovulation may be occurring or when a woman is most likely to conceive; also called natural family planning
intrauterine (in-truh-YOO-tur-in) **device (IUD)**	small, T-shaped device that is inserted into the uterus to prevent pregnancy
sponge	plastic foam sponge containing spermicide that is inserted into the vagina to prevent pregnancy
spermicide	substance that prevents pregnancy by destroying sperm
sterilization	surgical procedure that prevents a person from reproducing by removing all or part of the reproductive organs
tubal ligation (lye-GAY-shun)	sterilization technique in which a woman's uterine tubes are surgically blocked by cutting, cautery, or a plastic or metal device to prevent oocytes from entering the uterus
vasectomy (vas-ECK-tuh-mee)	excision of a small segment of the vas (ductus) deferens used to produce male sterility
vaginal (VAJ-i-nul) **barriers**	physical blockades that prevent sperm from entering the uterus
diaphragm (DYE-uh-fram)	dome-shaped device worn at the uterine entrance during intercourse to prevent conception
cervical (SUR-vi-kul) **cap**	tight-fitting device worn over the entrance to the cervix to prevent conception
vaginal ring	hormone-releasing barrier that is placed in the vagina once a month for 3 weeks to prevent ovulation
withdrawal method	birth control method that involves the man pulling the penis out of the vagina before ejaculating; also called the pull-out method
morning-after pill	tablet used to prevent pregnancy up to 5 days (120 hours) after unprotected sex; also called emergency contraception

KEY TERM PRACTICE: *Birth Control Methods*

1. Which form of birth control is used strictly by males? _____

2. Name three birth control measures that involve no pharmacological agents, devices, or surgery._____

3. Surgical blocking of the uterine tubes is termed _____.

4. A _____ is a substance that prevents pregnancy by destroying sperm and is derived from the word part _____ for *spermatozoa* and the word part _____, which means *agent that kills*.

5. Tablets taken daily to manipulate the female hormone cycle so that ovulation does not occur are known as _____ or _____.

LIFE SPAN

The reproductive system begins to form early in embryonic development. The gonads form from gonadal ridges in the mesoderm during the fifth week of gestation. Adjacent structures called mesonephric (Wolffian) ducts and paramesonephric (müllerian) ducts, respectively, form male and female reproductive structures.

In regard to gender determination, male embryonic sex cells contain a large X chromosome and a smaller Y chromosome. Females have two large X chromosomes. The sex-determining region of the Y chromosome (SRY) initiates the male pattern of development during the seventh embryonic week. Developing nurse cells, which support spermatogenesis, secrete a hormone, müllerian-inhibiting substance (MIS), that halts the development of female reproductive structures. By week 8, interstitial cells begin secreting testosterone and stimulating male reproductive structures.

The female uterus, uterine tubes, and vagina are formed from the paramesonephric ducts. The gonads develop into ovaries in the absence of SRY.

Sexual differentiation occurs around the eighth week when some male embryonic testosterone is converted to dihydrotestosterone (DHT). Dihydrotestosterone promotes urethral, prostate, scrotum, and penis development. Female embryos lack DHT, so the clitoris, labia minora, labia majora, and vestibule form.

Anatomical testicular and ovarian changes occur before birth. At 2 months before delivery, the testes of males descend toward the scrotum. In females, the ovaries move down into the pelvic cavity. The reproductive system remains in a latent state from birth until the onset of puberty. Puberty, which occurs some time between the ages of 10 and 15 years, is characterized by the development of secondary sexual characteristics in both sexes and the onset of menstruation in females. Hormones drive the psychological and physiological changes that occur.

Males and females differ significantly in terms of reproductive functional capacity. Women have a limited time of fertility between menarche and menopause. For 1 to 2 years after the onset of menses, ovulation occurs in only about 10% of the cycles. Thereafter, regular ovulatory cycles continue until menopause. It is currently thought that there is no male equivalent to menopause, but some research indicates men may actually experience something akin to menopause.

The aging female reproductive system experiences a great amount of change. Between ages 40 and 50 years, estrogen secretion decreases, leading to permanent cessation of menstrual periods. Reproductive organs also atrophy, but there is no correlation between loss of reproductive function and sexual desire because libido (sexual drive) is maintained throughout life.

The aging male reproductive system has less profound changes than the female. Testosterone production declines around age 55 years, but males retain the ability to produce sperm until age 80 or 90 years. Sperm production in the aging male does have some consequences. For example, it takes 20 to 25 minutes for the sperm of young men to travel up the uterine tubes, but it takes 2.5 days for the sperm of men in their 70s to make this same journey.

Enlargement of the prostate is a common age-related condition often causing polyuria, nocturia, and postvoiding dribbling. Research suggests that nearly all elderly men will experience some enlargement of the prostate gland.

COMMON Abbreviations

Abbreviation	Term
ACNM	American College of Nurse Midwives
AIDS	acquired immunodeficiency syndrome
A&P repair	anterior and posterior repair
BC	birth control
BCP	birth control pill
BPH	benign prostatic hyperplasia
BSE	breast self-examination
BSN	Bachelor of Science in nursing
BSO	bilateral salpingo-oophorectomy
CIS	carcinoma in situ
CNM	certified nurse midwife
D&C	dilation and curettage
DES	diethylstilbestrol
DHT	dihydrotestosterone
DRE	digital rectal examination
ED	erectile dysfunction
ERT	estrogen replacement therapy
FAM	fertility awareness–based method
FDA	Food and Drug Administration
FSH	follicle-stimulating hormone
G^-	gram-negative
G^+	gram-positive
HBV	hepatitis B virus
HIV	human immunodeficiency virus
HPV	human papillomavirus
HRT	hormone replacement therapy
HSV-2	herpes simplex virus type 2
IUD	intrauterine device
IVP	intravenous pyelogram
LH	luteinizing hormone
MEAC	Midwifery Education Accreditation Council
MIS	müllerian-inhibiting substance
OB	obstetrics
OCPs	oral contraceptive pills
OCT	oral contraceptive

continued

continued from page 871

Abbreviation	Term
OXT	oxytocin
PID	pelvic inflammatory disease
PMDD	premenstrual dysphoric disorder
PMS	premenstrual syndrome
PRL	prolactin
PSA	prostate-specific antigen
SRY	sex-determining region of the Y chromosome
STD	sexually transmitted disease
STI	sexually transmitted infection
TPI test	*Treponema pallidum* immobilization test
TRAM flap	transverse rectus abdominis myocutaneous flap
TSE	testicular self-examination
TSS	toxic shock syndrome
TUR	transurethral resection
TURP	transurethral resection of the prostate
UTI	urinary tract infection
VD	venereal disease

COMMON ABBREVIATIONS EXERCISES

1. VD is the abbreviation for _____.

2. The abbreviation for obstetrics is _____.

3. TSS is the abbreviation for _____.

4. The abbreviation for transverse rectus abdominis myocutaneous flap is _____.

5. IUD is the abbreviation for _____.

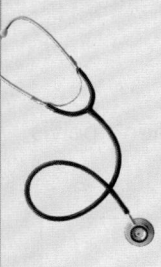

Case Study

Carla Saschen is a 39-year-old nulliparous woman who arrived at Laura's office for a routine physical examination, including a complete pelvic and breast examination. Clinical information revealed a complaint of nipple discharge and pelvic pain. A right breast mass was discovered during mammary palpation. Ms. Saschen uses an IUD. The pelvic examination was unremarkable. Mammograms and pelvis and transvaginal ultrasound studies were ordered.

The results of mammography studies indicated heterogeneously dense fibroglandular tissue dispersed to the superior lateral aspect of each breast. There was no definitive evidence of malignancy or microcalcification. Benign-appearing lymph nodes were also noted in the right axilla. The results of the ultrasound studies were not yet known.

Case Study Questions

Select the best answer to each of the following questions.

1. **Nipple discharge is _____.**
   a. normal
   b. abnormal in nulliparous women
   c. normal depending on day in menstrual cycle
   d. nothing to cause concern

2. **The word *nulliparous* refers to _____.**
   a. having borne no children
   b. having borne at least one child
   c. being premenopause
   d. having had a hysterectomy

3. **The phrase "benign appearing lymph nodes in the right axilla" refers to _____.**
   a. noncancerous nodes in adjacent lymphatic structures
   b. cancer of lymph nodes
   c. noncancerous nodes in the hip region
   d. an inconclusive mammography

4. **Why were pelvis and transvaginal ultrasound studies ordered?**
   _____
   a. The source of the pelvic pain required further study.
   b. Nipple discharge is associated with pelvic pain.
   c. Mammography revealed abnormal endometrium.
   d. All of the above are correct.

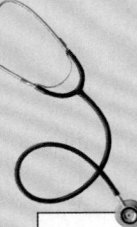

Real World Report

Laura's office received the medical report from the imaging department for Carla Saschen's pelvis and transvaginal ultrasound studies.

IMAGING DEPARTMENT

NAME:	Carla Saschen
AGE:	39 years
TEST:	Pelvis and transvaginal ultrasound
DATE ORDERED:	06/07/2010
ATTENDING:	J. R. Baum, MD
DOB:	05/22/1971
CLINICAL NOTES:	Pelvic pain; patient with IUD
EXAM DATE:	06/07/2010
REFERRING:	B. E. Rosen, DO

PELVIS AND TRANSVAGINAL ULTRASOUND

Real-time ultrasound evaluation of the pelvis was performed using both the transabdominal and the transvaginal approach. The patient's urinary bladder is not well distended, thus limiting transabdominal imaging.

Estimation of uterine size is approximately 9.5 × 4.5 × 6.8 cm. The intrauterine device is visualized within the endometrium. The endometrial lining measures 8–9 mm in thickness. There is no endometrial fluid. Incidental note is made of an 8-mm nabothian cyst.

Both ovaries were visualized, with the right measuring 3.6 × 2.7 × 2.4 cm and the left 2.3 × 2.6 × 1.9 cm. There are bilateral adnexal cysts. The larger on the right measured 2.6 cm. That on the left measured 1.8 cm. There was no free pelvic fluid.

IMPRESSION

Bilateral adnexal cysts, the larger being on the right. Appropriate positioning of the intrauterine device within the endometrial canal.

DICTATED BY: S. K. Lowell, MD

Real World Report Questions

The following exercises review the medical terms used in the preceding medical report. One term that may be new to you is nabothian cyst. A nabothian (na-BOH-thee-un) cyst develops when a mucous gland of the cervix is obstructed.

1. Endometrial lining refers to the _____.

a. outer layer of the uterus

b. inner layer of the vagina

c. middle layer of the vagina

d. inner layer of the uterus

2. IUD is the abbreviation for _____.

3. Identify the location of the 8-mm nabothian cyst.

_____

4. Explain what is meant by bilateral adnexal cysts.

_____

Review and Application

Multiple-Choice Questions

....

Select the best answer to each of the following questions.

1. The term that means "producing offspring" is _____.
   a. reproduction   b. gametogenesis   c. spermiogenesis   d. oogenesis

2. _____ is a general term used to describe an ovary or testis.
   a. Gonad   b. Gamete   c. Ovum   d. Reproduction

3. Identify the organ that is *not* part of the female reproductive system. _____
   a. uterine tube   b. ovary   c. prostate   d. vagina

4. Which of the following features is associated with the testes? _____
   a. fimbriae   b. median raphe   c. infundibulum   d. penis

5. The canal leading from the uterus to the exterior is the _____.
   a. urethra   b. uterine tube   c. rectum   d. vagina

6. Spermatozoa production is termed _____.
   a. fertility   b. spermatogenesis   c. spermatid   d. flagellum

7. Pairs of glands located at the base of the penis just inferior to the prostate gland are the _____.
   a. bulbourethral glands   b. corpora cavernosa   c. corpus spongiosum   d. paraurethral glands

8. The formation and development of the oocyte is termed _____.
   a. oogonium   b. ovulation   c. oogenesis   d. orchiopexy

9. This structure serves as an exit for both urine and semen. _____
   a. ejaculatory duct   b. prepuce   c. urethra   d. prostate gland

10. The paired glands that produce oocytes and female sex hormones are the _____.
    a. mammary glands   b. breasts   c. uterine tubes   d. ovaries

11. An alternate term for sexual intercourse is _____.
    a. erection   b. ejaculation   c. climax   d. coitus

12. The _____ is a functional secondary oocyte after fertilization.
    a. ovum   b. ovary   c. infundibulum   d. spermatocyte

13. The transitional period leading to female menopause is _____.
    a. menarche   b. menstruation   c. detumescence   d. perimenopause

14. Which of the following terms refers to an activation process that allows sperm to successfully fertilize an oocyte? _____
    a. capacitation   b. meiosis   c. fertilization   d. none of these

15. Surgical blocking of the uterine tubes is termed _____.
    a. vaginal barrier   b. intrauterine device   c. tubal ligation   d. vasectomy

16. _____ is a hormone that causes pelvic relaxation.
    a. Progesterone   b. Relaxin   c. Progesterone   d. Estrogen

17. Vaginal inflammation is termed _____ from the word part _____, which refers to the *vagina* and the suffix *-itis* meaning *inflammation*.
    a. oophoritis; *oo-* b. salpingitis; *salping-* c. vaginitis; *vagin-* d. orchitis; *orch-*

18. Orchitis is inflammation of the _____.
    a. ovary b. uterine tube c. prostate d. testis

19. Another term for a bag or sac is a/an _____.
    a. follicle b. secondary oocyte c. egg d. sperm

20. The fringe-like processes on the outer extremity of the uterine tube are called _____.
    a. fimbriae b. raphe c. scrotum d. infundibulum

21. The _____ is the term describing phases occurring in the uterus on a 28-day rotation.
    a. oogenesis b. uterine cycle c. spermatogenesis d. vas deferens

22. Circumcision is the procedure in which the _____ is removed from the _____.
    a. foreskin; prepuce b. prepuce; foreskin c. prepuce; glans penis d. glans penis; prepuce

23. _____ is the cessation of menstrual cycles.
    a. Menarche b. Menses c. Menstruation d. Menopause

24. _____ is the onset of menstruation and marks the very first menstrual cycle occurring during puberty.
    a. Menarche b. Oogenesis c. Menopause d. Ovulation

25. Sexual intercourse is also known as _____.
    a. orgasm and climax b. coitus and climax c. coitus d. climax and arousal

26. The culmination of sexual excitement is termed _____.
    a. orgasm b. arousal c. lubrication d. a and b

27. Male glands include _____.
    a. bulbourethral and ejaculatory b. bulbourethral and seminal vesicles c. Cowper and spermatic d. ejaculatory and urethra

28. Female glands include _____.
    a. lesser vestibular and greater vestibular b. mons pubis c. clitoris and Bartholin d. greater vestibular and clitoris

Word Parts Exercises

Using the following word parts, form a medical term for each definition. Each word part is used only once.

-cele	-celeo
-ectomy	-itis
leio-	-myoma
ophor-	recto-
varico-	vagin-

29. inflammation of the vagina _____

30. benign tumor of the uterine smooth muscle _____

31. swelling of the veins in the scrotal spermatic cord _____

32. hernia of the rectum through the vaginal wall _____

33. removal of an ovary _____

Matching

Match the disorder with its description.

_____ 34. uterine fibroids

_____ 35. vulvar cancer

_____ 36. leiomyomas

_____ 37. pelvic inflammatory disease

_____ 38. ovarian cysts

a. benign tumors composed of smooth muscle and fibrous tissue
b. benign neoplasm derived from uterine smooth muscle
c. inflammation of the female reproductive organs
d. fluid-filled sacs found on or near the ovaries
e. labial cancer

Match the disorder with its description.

_____ 39. infertility

_____ 40. impotence

_____ 41. prostate cancer

_____ 42. chancroid

_____ 43. syphilis

a. erectile dysfunction
b. malignant cell growth in the prostate gland
c. STD caused by *T. pallidum*
d. diminished ability to produce offspring
e. STD caused by *H. ducreyi*

Match the sign or symptom with its correct definition.

_____ 44. oligospermia

_____ 45. dyspareunia

_____ 46. chancre

_____ 47. syphiloma

_____ 48. orchitis

a. testes inflammation
b. rubbery tumor as a result of syphilis
c. painful sexual intercourse
d. low sperm count
e. ulcer associated with syphilis

Match the clinical test or diagnostic procedure with its correct definition.

_____ 49. digital rectal examination

_____ 50. Gram stain

_____ 51. transrectal ultrasonography

_____ 52. Pap test

_____ 53. mammography

a. clinical test in which cells scraped from the cervix are cultured
b. x-ray examination of the breast tissue
c. manual examination of the prostate through the rectum
d. differential staining technique used to identify bacteria
e. method of obtaining echograms through a probe inserted into the rectum

Match the treatment with its key description.

_____ 54. colporrhaphy

_____ 55. hysterectomy

_____ 56. birth control implant

_____ 57. orchiectomy

_____ 58. prostatectomy

a. matchstick-sized rod containing progesterone that is inserted in the brachial region of the arm to suppress ovulation
b. castration; surgical removal of the testicle(s)
c. surgical removal of the uterus
d. removal of the prostate gland
e. vaginal suture

Match the medical term with its correct definition.

_____ 59. epispadias

_____ 60. leukorrhea

_____ 61. mastectomy

_____ 62. epididymitis

_____ 63. hypospadias

a. inflammation of the epididymis
b. urethral opening being located on the penile dorsal surface
c. urethral opening being located on the penile ventral surface
d. surgical removal of a breast
e. thick, white vaginal discharge

Match the birth control method with its definition.

_____ 64. oral contraceptives

_____ 65. diaphragm

_____ 66. cervical cap

_____ 67. sterilization

_____ 68. intrauterine device

a. tight-fitting device worn at the cervical entrance
b. device worn by the female at the uterine opening during sexual intercourse
c. birth control pills
d. T-shaped device placed in the uterus
e. procedure that makes one unable reproduce

Definition

Define the following terms.

69. areola _____

70. cryptorchidism _____

71. cystocele _____

72. conization _____

73. electrocoagulation _____

Provide a medical term for the following definitions.

74. way of avoiding pregnancy using either artificial or natural methods _____

75. surgery in which low temperatures freeze tissue _____

76. STD caused by the herpes simplex virus _____

77. STD caused by *C. trachomatis* _____

78. cancer of unknown origin affecting the labia or vulva _____

Alternate Terms

Give an alternate term for each of the following terms.

79. birth control pills _____

80. orchiectomy _____

81. vas deferens _____

82. impotence _____

83. natural family planning _____

Spelling

Identify the correctly spelled term in each set.

84. _____

a. colostrum
b. colostrom
c. collostrum
d. collostrom

85. _____

a. chanchre
b. kanchre
c. chankre
d. chancre

86. _____

a. yoorethra
b. urithra
c. urethra
d. urrethra

87. _____

a. perrineum
b. perineum
c. perinium
d. perenium

88. _____

a. ogenesis
b. oogenesis
c. oogenisis
d. oogeneses

Unscramble

Unscramble the letters to form a medical term.

89. nipes _____

90. rutseu _____

91. creetino _____

92. tiiletyfr _____

93. sciitlro _____

Abbreviations

Provide the term for the abbreviations and then define the terms

94. BPH = _____

95. FAM = _____

96. ED = _____

97. PID = _____

98. D&C = _____

Analogies

Provide a medical term to complete a meaningful analogy.

99. Oviducts are to _____ as scrotal sac is to scrotum.

100. _____ glands are to breasts as _____ are to testes.

101. _____ is to menstrual cycle as prepuce is to foreskin.

102. _____ are to OCTs as rubbers are to condoms.

Short Answer

Answer the following question.

103. A couple is having difficulty conceiving a child. Semen analysis reveals oligospermia. The fertility specialist suggests that the man wear boxer shorts instead of tight-fitting briefs. Provide a plausible explanation for this recommendation.

_____

Labeling: Part 1

Label the structures in the following diagram.

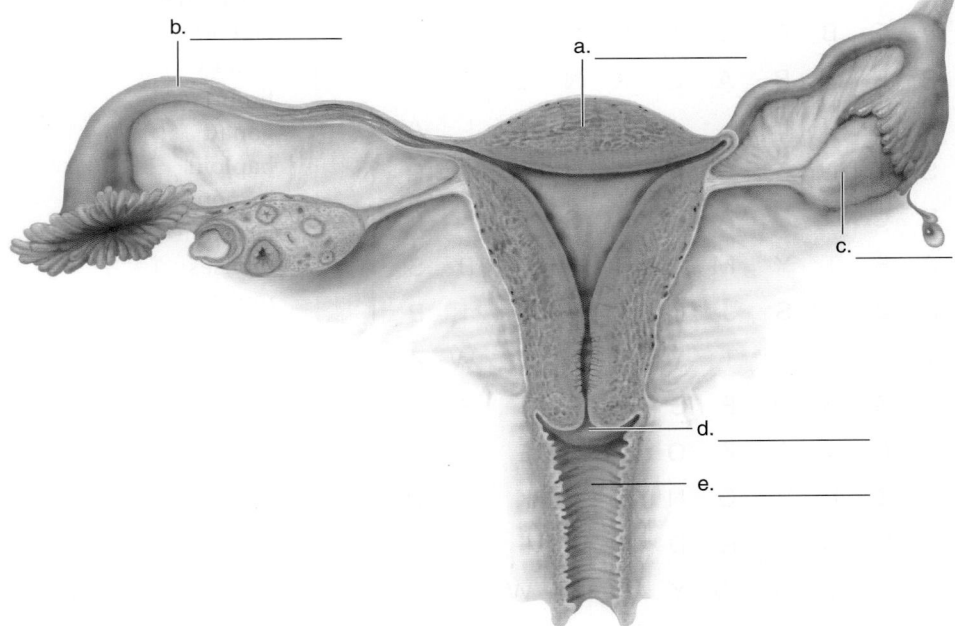

b. _____

a. _____

c. _____

d. _____

e. _____

Labeling: Part 2

Label the structures in the following diagram.

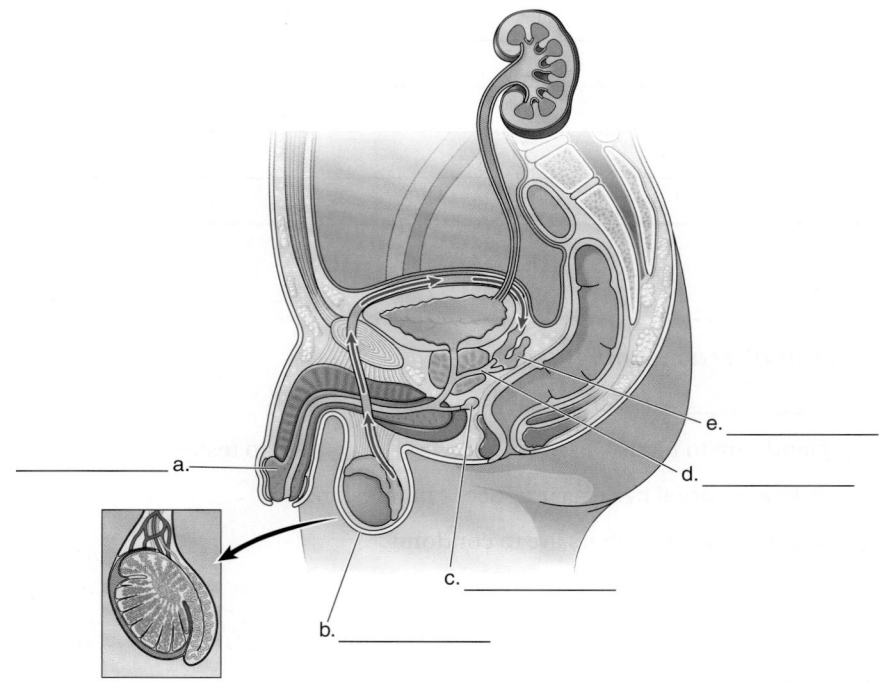

a. _____

b. _____

c. _____

d. _____

e. _____

Word Search

Find the medical terms hidden in the puzzle.

A	E	D	I	O	L	P	A	H	F	H	F	N	E	A	D
S	L	Q	W	K	S	O	P	I	Y	O	O	B	R	X	J
M	G	O	L	A	X	T	M	M	M	I	G	W	E	E	R
M	R	O	E	I	G	B	E	D	T	L	O	V	C	N	D
M	T	E	V	R	R	N	B	A	G	X	N	E	T	D	Y
H	D	R	P	I	A	V	L	I	J	E	A	X	I	A	Q
H	E	I	A	S	Y	U	L	E	R	G	D	G	O	H	N
C	N	E	L	E	C	Y	H	A	I	I	G	F	N	D	D
E	E	H	P	A	R	T	Y	M	C	R	H	P	B	S	A
E	H	E	J	J	Z	T	S	J	E	T	J	K	J	P	I
U	F	E	R	T	I	L	I	T	Y	N	A	V	W	Z	R
C	O	I	T	U	S	A	Q	F	S	K	S	T	X	H	F
F	Z	T	Y	W	Q	V	C	Z	O	K	W	E	I	A	Z
B	T	A	J	E	Z	L	V	Q	N	S	H	K	S	O	A
Y	U	M	E	Q	V	U	O	R	D	M	J	F	Z	M	N
X	M	X	C	E	G	V	U	W	Y	F	J	W	T	M	W

adnexa
areola
cervix
coitus
ejaculation
erection
fertility
fimbriae
gonad
haploid
hymen
lactation
menses
raphe
sperm
vulva

Vocabulary Review

Review the key terms from this chapter, study the spelling and pronunciation of each term, and write its definition in the space provided. Listen to the audio available for most terms at http://thepoint.lww.com/nath2e and pronounce each term for yourself. Then check the box when you feel confident that you know the definition and can pronounce the term correctly.

Key Term	Pronunciation	Definition
❑ abstinence		
❑ acquired immunodeficiency syndrome (AIDS)	(im-yoo-noh-dee-FISH-un-see)	
❑ acrosome	(ACK-roh-sohm)	
❑ adnexa	(ad-NECK-suh)	
❑ areola	(ah-REE-oh-luh)	
❑ arousal		
❑ benign prostatic hyperplasia (BPH)	(pros-TAT-ick high-pur-PLAY-zhuh)	
❑ birth control implant		
❑ birth control injection		
❑ birth control patch		
❑ birth control pills (BCPs)		
❑ bulbourethral glands	(bul-boh-yoo-REE-thrul)	
❑ breast cancer		
❑ candidiasis	(kan-dih-DYE-uh-sis)	
❑ capacitation	(kuh-pas-ih-TAY-shun)	
❑ castration		
❑ cervical cancer	(SUR-vi-kul)	
❑ cervical cap	(SUR-vi-kul)	
❑ cervix	(SUR-vicks)	
❑ chancres	(SHANK-urz)	
❑ chancroid	(SHANK-roid)	
❑ chlamydia	(kla-MID-ee-uh)	
❑ circumcision	(sur-kum-SIZH-un)	
❑ clitoris	(KLIT-oh-ris)	
❑ coitus	(KOH-i-tus)	
❑ colostrum	(koh-LOS-trum)	
❑ colpoplasty	(kol-poh-PLAS-tee)	
❑ colporrhaphy	(kol-POR-uh-fee)	
❑ conization	(kohn-ih-ZAY-shun)	
❑ contraception		

Key Term	Pronunciation	Definition
❏ corpora cavernosa	(KOR-poh-ruh kav-ur-NOH-suh)	_____
❏ corpus spongiosum	(KOR-pus spon-jee-OH-sum)	_____
❏ cryosurgery	(krye-oh-SUR-juh-ree)	_____
❏ cryptorchidism	(kript-OR-kid-iz-um)	_____
❏ cystocele	(SIS-toh-seel)	_____
❏ detumescence	(dee-tew-MES-unce)	_____
❏ diaphragm	(DYE-uh-fram)	_____
❏ digital rectal examination (DRE)		_____
❏ dilation and curettage (D&C)	(kewr-e-TAHZH)	_____
❏ diploid	(DIP-loid)	_____
❏ ductus deferens	(DUCK-tus DEF-uh-renz)	_____
❏ dysmenorrhea	(dis-men-oh-REE-uh)	_____
❏ dyspareunia	(dis-puh-ROOH-nee-uh)	_____
❏ ejaculation	(ee-jack-yoo-LAY-shun)	_____
❏ ejaculatory duct	(eh-JACK-yoo-luh-tor-ee DUKT)	_____
❏ electrocoagulation	(ee-leck-troh-koh-ag-yoo-LAY-shun)	_____
❏ emission	(ee-MISH-un)	_____
❏ endometrial cancer	(en-doh-MEE-tree-ul)	_____
❏ endometriosis	(en-doh-mee-tree-OH-sis)	_____
❏ endometrium	(en-doh-MEE-tree-um)	_____
❏ epididymis	(ep-i-DID-i-mis)	_____
❏ epididymitis	(ep-i-did-i-MIGH-tis)	_____
❏ epispadias	(ep-ih-SPAY-dee-us)	_____
❏ erectile dysfunction (ED)	(ee-RECK-tile)	_____
❏ erection		_____
❏ estrogen	(ES-troh-jen)	_____
❏ female condom		_____
❏ fertility		_____
❏ fertility awareness–based method (FAM)		_____
❏ fibrocystic breast changes	(figh-broh-SIS-tick)	_____
❏ fimbriae	(FIM-bree-ee)	_____
❏ flagellum	(fla-JEL-um)	_____
❏ follicle	(FOL-i-kul)	_____
❏ follicle-stimulating hormone (FSH)	(FOL-i-kul)	_____
❏ fundus	(FUN-dus)	_____

Key Term	Pronunciation	Definition
❏ gametes	(GAM-eets)	_____
❏ genital herpes	(HUR-peez)	_____
❏ genital human papillomavirus (HPV) infection		_____
❏ glans penis	(GLANZ)	_____
❏ gonad	(GOH-nad)	_____
❏ gonorrhea	(gon-uh-REE-uh)	_____
❏ Gram stain		_____
❏ greater vestibular glands	(ves-TIB-yoo-lur)	_____
❏ gumma	(GUM-uh)	_____
❏ haploid	(HAP-loid)	_____
❏ hernia		_____
❏ hormone replacement therapy (HRT)		_____
❏ hydrocele	(HIGH-droh-seel)	_____
❏ hymen	(HIGH-men)	_____
❏ hypospadias	(high-poh-SPAY-dee-us)	_____
❏ hysterectomy	(his-tur-ECK-tuh-mee)	_____
❏ impotence	(IM-puh-tens)	_____
❏ infertility		_____
❏ infundibulum	(in-fun-DIB-yoo-lum)	_____
❏ interstitial cells	(in-ter-STISH-ul CELLS)	_____
❏ intrauterine device (IUD)	(in-truh-YOO-tur-in)	_____
❏ Kegel exercises		_____
❏ labial cancer	(LAY-bee-ul)	_____
❏ labia majora	(LAY-bee-uh muh-JOR-uh)	_____
❏ labia minora	(LAY-bee-uh muh-NOR-uh)	_____
❏ lactation	(lack-TAY-shun)	_____
❏ laparoscopy	(lap-uh-ROS-kuh-pee)	_____
❏ laser ablation	(ab-LAY-shun)	_____
❏ leiomyoma	(lye-oh-migh-OH-muh)	_____
❏ lesser vestibular glands	(ves-TIB-yoo-lur)	_____
❏ luteinizing hormone (LH)	(LOO-tee-in-eye-zing)	_____
❏ male condom		_____
❏ mammary glands	(MAM-uh-ree)	_____
❏ mammography	(ma-MOG-ruh-fee)	_____
❏ mastectomy	(mas-TECK-tuh-mee)	_____
❏ menarche	(me-NAHR-kee)	_____

Key Term	Pronunciation	Definition
❏ menopause	(MEN-oh-pawz)	_____
❏ menses	(MEN-seez)	_____
❏ menstrual cycle	(MEN-stroo-ul)	_____
❏ menstruation	(men-stroo-AY-shun)	_____
❏ mons pubis	(PEW-bis)	_____
❏ morning-after pill		_____
❏ nulliparous	(nul-IP-uh-rus)	_____
❏ oligospermia	(ol-ih-goh-SPER-mee-uh)	_____
❏ oocyte	(OH-oh-site)	_____
❏ oogenesis	(oh-oh-JEN-e-sis)	_____
❏ oogonium	(oh-oh-GOH-nee-um)	_____
❏ oral contraceptives (OCTs)	(OR-ul kon-truh-SEP-tivs)	_____
❏ orchiectomy	(or-kee-ECK-tuh-mee)	_____
❏ orchiopexy	(or-kee-oh-PECK-see)	_____
❏ orchitis	(or-KIGH-tis)	_____
❏ orgasm	(OR-gaz-um)	_____
❏ ovarian cancer	(oh-VAIR-ee-un)	_____
❏ ovarian cysts	(oh-VAIR-ee-un)	_____
❏ ovaries	(OH-vur-eez)	_____
❏ ovulation	(ov-yoo-LAY-shun)	_____
❏ ovum	(OH-vum)	_____
❏ oxytocin (OXT)	(ock-si-TOH-sin)	_____
❏ Pap test		_____
❏ pelvic examination	(PEL-vick)	_____
❏ pelvic inflammatory disease (PID)	(PEL-vick)	_____
❏ penis		_____
❏ perimenopause	(per-ih-men-OH-pawz)	_____
❏ perineum	(perr-i-NEE-um)	_____
❏ premenstrual dysphoric disorder (PMDD)	(pree-MEN-stroo-ul dis-FOR-ick)	_____
❏ premenstrual syndrome (PMS)	(pree-MEN-stroo-ul)	_____
❏ prepuce	(PREE-poos)	_____
❏ proctocele	(PROCK-toh-seel)	_____
❏ progesterone	(proh-JES-tur-ohn)	_____
❏ prolactin (PRL)	(proh-LACK-tin)	_____
❏ proliferative phase	(proh-LIF-ur-uh-tiv)	_____

Key Term	Pronunciation	Definition
❏ prostate	(PROS-tate)	
❏ prostate cancer	(PROS-tate)	
❏ prostatectomy	(pros-tuh-TECK-tuh-mee)	
❏ prostate-specific antigen (PSA) test	(PROS-tate spuh-SIF-ick AN-ti-jen)	
❏ prostatitis	(pros-tuh-TYE-tis)	
❏ raphe	(RAY-fee)	
❏ rectocele	(RECK-toh-seel)	
❏ relaxin	(ree-LACK-sin)	
❏ reproduction		
❏ resectoscope	(ree-SECK-tuh-skope)	
❏ salpingo-oophorectomy	(sal-pin-goh-oh-oh-foh-RECK-toh-mee)	
❏ scrotum	(SKROH-tum)	
❏ secondary oocyte	(OH-oh-site)	
❏ secondary sexual characteristics		
❏ secretory phase	(se-KREE-tuh-ree)	
❏ semen	(SEE-mun)	
❏ semen analysis	(SEE-mun)	
❏ seminal glands	(SEM-ih-nul)	
❏ seminiferous tubules	(sem-ih-NIF-ur-us TOO-byulz)	
❏ sexually transmitted diseases (STDs)		
❏ sperm		
❏ spermatic cord	(spur-MAT-ick)	
❏ spermatogenesis	(sper-muh-toh-JEN-eh-sis)	
❏ spermatogonium	(spur-muh-toh-GOH-nee-um)	
❏ spermicide		
❏ spermiogenesis	(sper-mee-oh-JEN-eh-sis)	
❏ sponge		
❏ sterility		
❏ sterilization		
❏ syphilis	(SIF-ih-lis)	
❏ syphiloma	(sif-ih-LOH-muh)	
❏ testes	(TES-teez)	
❏ testicles	(TES-ti-kulz)	
❏ testicular cancer	(tes-TICK-yoo-lur)	
❏ testicular torsion	(tes-TICK-yoo-lur)	

Key Term	Pronunciation	Definition
❏ testosterone	(tes-TOS-tur-ohn)	_____
❏ toxic shock syndrome (TSS)		_____
❏ transverse rectus abdominis myocutaneous (TRAM) flap	(trans-VERS RECK-tus ab-DOM-in-us migh-oh-kew-TAY-nee-us)	_____
❏ transurethral resection (TUR)	(trans-yoo-REE-thrul ree-SECK-shun)	_____
❏ transvaginal sonography	(trans-VAJ-i-nul suh-NOG-ruh-fee)	_____
❏ trichomoniasis	(trick-oh-moh-NIGH-uh-sis)	_____
❏ tubal ligation	(lye-GAY-shun)	_____
❏ uterine cycle	(YOO-tur-in)	_____
❏ uterine fibroids	(FIGH-broidz)	_____
❏ uterine tubes	(YOO-tur-in)	_____
❏ uterus	(YOO-tur-us)	_____
❏ vagina	(vuh-JYE-nuh)	_____
❏ vaginal barriers	(VAJ-i-nul)	_____
❏ vaginal cancer	(VAJ-i-nul)	_____
❏ vaginal ring		_____
❏ vaginitis	(vaj-ih-NIGH-tis)	_____
❏ varicocele	(VAIR-ih-koh-seel)	_____
❏ vas deferens	(VAS-DEF-uh-renz)	_____
❏ vasectomy	(vas-ECK-tuh-mee)	_____
❏ venereal diseases (VDs)	(ve-NEER-ee-ul)	_____
❏ vestibule	(VES-ti-bewl)	_____
❏ viral hepatitis	(VIGH-rul hep-uh-TIGH-tis)	_____
❏ vulva	(VUL-vuh)	_____
❏ vulvar cancer	(VUL-vur)	_____
❏ withdrawal method		_____

Answers

Word Grouping Exercises

Definition	Word Part	Definition	Word Part
man, masculine	andro-	condition of spermatozoa or semen	-spermia
breast	A. mammo- B. mast-, masto-	egg	ovi-, ovo-
cervix, neck	cervic-, cervico-	egg, ovary	oo-

Definition	Word Part	Definition	Word Part
embryo	embry-, embryo-	primitive, ancestral	arch-, arche-, archi-
female, woman	gyn-, gyne-, gyneco-, gyno-	prostate gland	prostat-, prostato-
few, too few	olig-, oligo-	rectum or anus	proct-, procto-
glans penis	balan-, balano-	smooth	leio-, lio-
hidden, concealed	crypt-, crypto-	sperm, seed, semen, spermatozoa	sperma-, spermato-, spermo-
lips	labio-	swelling, hernia	-cele
menses, menstruation	meno-	testes	orchi-, orchido-, orchio-
nipple	mammil-, mammili-	tip, end	acro-
origin, beginning process	-genesis	uterine tube	salping-, salpingo-
ovary	A. oophor-, oophoro- B. ovari-, ovario-	uterus	A. hyster-, hystero- B. metr-, metra-, metro- C. uter-, utero-
passage	meato-	vagina	A. colp-, colpo- B. vagin-, vagino-
pelvis	pelvi-, pelvio-, pelvo-		
perineum	perineo-		

Word Building Exercises

Word Part	Meaning	Common or Known Word	Example Medical Term
arch-, arche-, archi-	primitive, ancestral	archeology	menarche
andro-	man, masculine	androgynous	androgens
cervic-, cervico-	cervix, neck	cervical region	cervical cancer
crypt-, crypto-	hidden, concealed	cryptic	cryptorchidism
embry-, embryo-	embryo	embryo	embryonic
-genesis	origin, beginning process	histogenesis	oogenesis
gyn-, gyne-, gyneco-, gyno-	female, woman	gynecologist	gynecomastia
hyster-, hystero-	uterus	hysterectomy	hysterectomy
mammil-, mammili-	nipple	mammilla	mammilla
mammo-	breast	mammogram	mammary gland
meato-	passage	auditory meatus	urethral meatus
meno-	menses, menstruation	menstruation	menopause
orchi-, orchido-, orchio-	testes	orchitis	orchiectomy
ovari-, ovario-	ovary	ovarian cancer	ovarian
ovi-, ovo-	egg	oviparous	oviduct
pelvi-, pelvio-, pelvo-	pelvis	pelvis	pelvic examination
proct-, procto-	rectum or anus	proctologist	proctocele
prostat-, prostato-	prostate gland	prostate	prostatitis
sperma-, spermato-, spermo-	sperm, seed, semen, spermatozoa	sperm	spermiogenesis
uter-, utero-	uterus	uterus	uterus
vagin-, vagino-	vagina	vagina	vaginitis

Key Term Practice

Reproductive Systems Preview

1. Gametes
2. gonad
3. reproduction
4. oocytes; sperm

Male Reproductive System Overview

1. scrotum
2. prostate
3. Spermatogenesis; *spermato-*; *-genesis*
4. penis
5. testes; testicles

Female Reproductive System Overview

1. vagina
2. vulva
3. ovaries
4. Mammary glands
5. perineum

The Testes and Male Accessory Glands

1. bulbourethral glands
2. epididymis
3. Semen
4. seminal glands
5. ejaculatory duct

The Penis

1. corpora cavernosum and corpus spongiosum
2. Coitus
3. Circumcision
4. prepuce
5. glans penis

Male Reproductive Hormones

1. Testosterone
2. secondary sexual characteristics
3. Luteinizing hormone (LH)
4. follicle-stimulating hormone (FSH)

Spermatozoa (Sperm)

1. flagellum
2. Capacitation
3. spermiogenesis; *-genesis*
4. Haploid
5. spermatogonium; *spermato-*

Ovaries, Uterine Tubes, Uterus, and Vagina

1. ovulation
2. hymen
3. secondary oocyte
4. endometrium; *endo-*; *metr-*
5. ovum

Vulva

1. clitoris
2. greater vestibular glands
3. mons pubis
4. lesser vestibular glands
5. Labia minora

Mammary Glands

1. singular = areola; plural = areolae
2. lactation
3. Oxytocin (OXT)
4. Prolactin (PRL); *lact-*
5. colostrum

Female Reproductive Hormones

1. Estrogen
2. Progesterone
3. relaxin

Oogenesis

1. Oogenesis; *oo-*; *-genesis*
2. follicle
3. oogonium

The Menstrual Cycle

1. proliferative
2. menstrual cycle; uterine cycle
3. Perimenopause
4. menarche
5. Menopause

Sexual Intercourse

1. Emission; ejaculation
2. Detumescence
3. orgasm
4. arousal

Penis and Testes Disorders

1. *orchi-*; inflammation; orchitis
2. orchiectomy; castration
3. Erectile dysfunction (ED)
4. epididymitis
5. cryptorchidism; *crypt-*; *orchi-*

Prostate Disorders

1. benign prostatic hyperplasia (BPH)
2. *prostat-*; inflammation; prostatitis
3. resectoscope
4. prostate cancer
5. prostatectomy; *prostat-*; *-ectomy*

Female Pelvic Disorders

1. dilation and curettage (D&C)
2. endometriosis
3. premenstrual dysphoric disorder (PMDD)
4. hysterectomy; *hyster-*; *-ectomy*
5. Gram stain

Female Cancers

1. vulvar cancer and labial cancer
2. *mast-*; removal of; mastectomy
3. transverse rectus abdominis myocutaneous (TRAM) flap
4. laser ablation
5. Mammography

Female Benign Tumors

1. leiomyoma; *leio-*; *myo-*; *-oma*
2. uterine fibroids
3. fibrocystic breast changes

Hernias of the Female Reproductive System

1. colpoplasty; *colpo-*; *-plasty*
2. proctocele and rectocele
3. cystocele; *cysto-*; *-cele*
4. Kegel exercises
5. colporrhaphy

Infertility and Sterility

1. Infertility
2. oligospermia; *oligo-*; *-spermia*
3. semen analysis
4. sterility

Infections

1. toxic shock syndrome (TSS)
2. Candidiasis
3. vaginitis

Sexually Transmitted Diseases

1. AIDS
2. sexually transmitted diseases (STDs); venereal diseases (VDs)
3. trichomoniasis
4. gumma; syphiloma
5. Dyspareunia

Birth Control Methods

1. vasectomy
2. abstinence, fertility awareness–based method (FAM), and withdrawal method
3. tubal ligation
4. spermicide; *sperma-*; *-cide*
5. birth control pills (BCPs); oral contraceptives (OCTs)

Common Abbreviations Exercises

1. VD = venereal disease
2. obstetrics = OB
3. TSS = toxic shock syndrome
4. transverse rectus abdominis myocutaneous flap = TRAM flap
5. IUD = intrauterine device

Case Study

1. b is the correct answer.
   - a and c are incorrect because nipple discharge is not normal in women who are not breast-feeding.
   - d is incorrect because nipple discharge is an abnormal condition in nonlactating women. Thus, further investigation is warranted.
2. a is the correct answer.
   - b, c, and d are incorrect because these phrases do not define nulliparous.
3. a is the correct answer.
   - b is incorrect because the lymph nodes appeared benign, or not a threat to life or long-term health.
   - c is incorrect because the axilla refers to the armpit, not the hip region.
   - d is incorrect because the mammogram provides a good subsequent reading, although the 10% false-negative rate for mammography must be considered.
4. a is the correct answer.
   - b is incorrect because there is no known association with nipple discharge and pelvic pain. Furthermore, the purpose of these tests is to view pelvic and vaginal structures.
   - c is incorrect because mammography is used to study breast tissue, not endometrial (uterine) tissue.
   - d is incorrect because only a is correct.

Real World Report

1. d
2. intrauterine device
3. The cysts are found in the cervix because they are distentions of the mucous (nabothian) glands of the uterine cervix.
4. Bilateral adnexal cysts are closed, abnormal sacs attached to both the right and the left ovaries. *Adnexal* means that they are adjoined to anatomical parts.

Review and Application

1. a	18. d	35. e	52. a
2. a	19. a	36. b	53. b
3. c	20. a	37. c	54. e
4. b	21. b	38. d	55. c
5. d	22. c	39. d	56. a
6. b	23. d	40. a	57. b
7. a	24. a	41. b	58. d
8. c	25. c	42. e	59. b
9. c	26. a	43. c	60. e
10. d	27. b	44. d	61. d
11. d	28. a	45. c	62. a
12. a	29. vaginitis	46. e	63. c
13. d	30. leiomyoma	47. b	64. c
14. a	31. varicocele	48. a	65. b
15. c	32. rectocele	49. c	66. a
16. b	33. oophorectomy	50. d	67. e
17. c	34. a	51. e	68. d

69. areola = pigmented ring surrounding the nipple
70. cryptorchidism = failure of one or both testes to descend into the scrotum
71. cystocele = hernia of the urinary bladder into the vagina
72. conization = removal of a cone-shaped section of tissue, most notably from the cervix
73. electrocoagulation = cauterizing tissue to stop bleeding
74. contraception
75. cryosurgery
76. genital herpes
77. chlamydia
78. vulvar cancer
79. oral contraceptives (OCTs)
80. castration
81. ductus deferens
82. erectile dysfunction (ED)
83. fertility awareness–based method (FAM)
84. a
85. d
86. c
87. b
88. b
89. penis
90. uterus
91. erection
92. fertility
93. clitoris
94. BPH = benign prostatic hyperplasia; noncancerous prostate enlargement
95. FAM = fertility awareness–based method; form of contraception in which sexual intercourse is avoided on days that ovulation may be occurring or when a woman is most likely to conceive; also called natural family planning
96. ED = erectile dysfunction; the inability to achieve or maintain a penile erection long enough for intercourse; also called impotence
97. PID = pelvic inflammatory disease; inflammation of the reproductive organs that, if untreated, can cause infertility
98. D&C = dilation and curettage; gynecological procedure in which the cervix is widened and the uterus is scraped
99. uterine tubes
100. mammary; testicles
101. uterine cycle
102. BCPs
103. Normal sperm development requires that the temperature be approximately 2°F cooler than body temperature. Thus, boxer shorts will allow the testicles to drop down farther from the pelvic region and allow the sperm to develop in a slightly cooler environment, away from the groin area.

Labeling: Part 1

a. fundus of uterus
b. uterine tube
c. ovary
d. cervix
e. vagina

Labeling: Part 2

a. glans penis
b. scrotum
c. bulbourethral gland
d. ejaculatory duct
e. seminal gland

Word Search

A	E	D	I	O	L	P	A	H	F	H	F	N	E	A	D
S	L	Q	W	K	S	O	P	I	Y	O	O	B	R	X	J
M	G	O	L	A	X	T	M	M	I	G	W	E	E	R
M	R	O	E	I	G	B	E	D	T	L	O	V	C	N	D
M	T	E	V	R	R	N	B	A	G	X	N	E	T	D	Y
H	D	R	P	I	A	V	L	I	J	E	A	X	I	A	Q
H	E	I	A	S	Y	U	L	E	R	G	D	G	O	H	N
C	N	E	L	E	C	Y	H	A	I	I	G	F	N	D	D
E	E	H	P	A	R	T	Y	M	C	R	H	P	B	S	A
E	H	E	J	J	Z	T	S	J	E	T	J	K	J	P	I
U	F	E	R	T	I	L	I	T	Y	N	A	V	W	Z	R
C	O	I	T	U	S	A	Q	F	S	K	S	T	X	H	F
F	Z	T	Y	W	Q	V	C	Z	O	K	W	E	I	A	Z
B	T	A	J	E	Z	L	V	Q	N	S	H	K	S	O	A
Y	U	M	E	Q	V	U	O	R	D	M	J	F	Z	M	N
X	M	X	C	E	G	V	U	W	Y	F	J	W	T	M	W

adnexa
areola
cervix
coitus
ejaculation
erection
fertility
fimbriae
gonad
haploid
hymen
lactation
menses
raphe
sperm
vulva

Vocabulary Review

Key Term	Definition	Key Term	Definition
abstinence	refraining from penile–vaginal intercourse	**birth control injection**	intramuscular hormone shot of Depo-Provera that is administered every 3 months to females that works by suppressing ovulation
AIDS	caused by infection with HIV, a retrovirus that causes immune system failure	**birth control patch**	thin patch worn on the skin that releases hormones to prevent ovulation
acrosome	structure at the end of a sperm that releases enzymes enabling the sperm to penetrate and fertilize an oocyte	**birth control pills (BCPs)**	tablets taken daily to manipulate the female hormone cycle so that ovulation does not occur; also called oral contraceptives (OCTs)
adnexa	appendages of the uterus, including the ovaries, uterine tubes, and uterine ligaments, that hold the uterus in place	**bulbourethral glands**	pair of glands located at the base of the penis just inferior to the prostate gland; also called Cowper glands
areola	pigmented ring surrounding the nipple	**breast cancer**	malignant tumors of mammary tissue
arousal	sexual excitement	**candidiasis**	vaginal yeast infection caused by *Candida albicans* fungus
benign prostatic hyperplasia (BPH)	noncancerous prostate enlargement	**capacitation**	activation process that allows sperm to successfully fertilize an oocyte
birth control implant	matchstick-sized rod containing progesterone inserted in the brachial region of the arm that suppresses ovulation	**castration**	surgical removal of one or both testes; also called orchiectomy

Key Term	Definition	Key Term	Definition
cervical cancer	malignant neoplasms of the cervix	**dyspareunia**	painful sexual intercourse
cervical cap	tight-fitting device worn over the entrance to cervix to prevent pregnancy	**ejaculation**	sudden ejection of semen from the penis during orgasm
cervix	section of the uterus that dips into the vagina	**ejaculatory duct**	short passageway between the ductus deferens and the urethra
chancres	skin lesions or ulcers at the point where the pathogen enters the body	**electrocoagulation**	the use of an electrical device to destroy tissue
chancroid	sexually transmitted disease characterized by painful, ragged ulcers at the infection site	**emission**	discharge of semen into the male urethra
chlamydia	sexually transmitted disease caused by the bacterium *Chlamydia trachomatis*	**endometrial cancer**	malignant cells of the uterine endometrium
circumcision	surgery to remove the prepuce (foreskin) from the penis	**endometriosis**	presence of functional endometrial tissue outside the uterus
clitoris	highly sensitive erectile tissue located at the junction of the labia minora	**endometrium**	glandular membrane lining the uterus
coitus	sexual intercourse	**epididymis**	elongated structure consisting of coiled tubes connected to the posterior surface of each testis that transports sperm between the testis and the ductus deferens
colostrum	first milk from a mother's breasts after she has given birth that is rich in nutrients and antibodies		
colpoplasty	vaginal repair and restructure	**epididymitis**	inflammation of the epididymis
colporrhaphy	repairing the vagina by excising and suturing the edges of the tear	**epispadias**	congenital disorder characterized by the penile urethral opening being located on the dorsal surface
conization	removal of a cone-shaped section of tissue, most notably from the cervix	**erectile dysfunction (ED)**	the inability to achieve or maintain a penile erection long enough for intercourse; also called impotence
contraception	way of avoiding pregnancy using either artificial or natural methods	**erection**	enlarged and stiffened state of the penis due to erectile tissue filling with blood
corpora cavernosa	two cylinders of erectile tissue in the penis	**estrogen**	female steroid hormone produced mainly in the ovaries that is responsible for the development of female secondary sexual characteristics
corpus spongiosum	single cylinder of erectile tissue surrounding the urethra in the penis		
cryosurgery	surgery in which low temperatures are applied to tissues to seal or remove them	**female condom**	pouch with flexible rings on each end that is inserted into the vagina
cryptorchidism	failure of one or both testes to descend into the scrotum	**fertility**	ability to reproduce by bringing about fertilization
cystocele	hernia of the urinary bladder into the vagina	**fertility awareness–based method (FAM)**	form of contraception in which sexual intercourse is avoided on days that ovulation may be occurring or when a woman is most likely to conceive; also called natural family planning
detumescence	diminished swelling in erectile organs after orgasm as the blood exits erectile tissues		
diaphragm	dome-shaped device worn at the uterine entrance during intercourse to prevent conception	**fibrocystic breast changes**	noncancerous breast condition that is characterized by fibrosis (lumps that are firm and hard) or cysts (fluid-filled sacs)
digital rectal examination (DRE)	manual examination of the prostate through the rectum	**fimbriae**	fringe-like processes on the outer extremity of the infundibulum of the uterine tube
dilation and curettage (D&C)	gynecological procedure in which the cervix is widened and the uterus is scraped		
		flagellum	tail on spermatozoon
diploid	containing 23 pairs or 46 chromosomes	**follicle**	sac within the ovary that holds immature egg cells
ductus deferens	tube connecting the epididymis and the ejaculatory duct; also called the vas deferens	**follicle-stimulating hormone (FSH)**	anterior pituitary gland hormone stimulating spermatogenesis in testes
dysmenorrhea	difficult and painful menstruation	**fundus**	dome-shaped region of the uterus opposite the vaginal opening

Key Term	Definition	Key Term	Definition
gametes	sex cells (sperm and oocytes)	Kegel exercises	alternate contraction and relaxation of the pelvic floor muscles to increase their strength to treat urinary incontinence
genital herpes	sexually transmitted disease caused by the herpes simplex virus type 2 (HSV-2)	labial cancer	malignant cells of the folds surrounding the female genitalia; also called vulvar cancer
genital human papillomavirus (HPV) infection	warts on the genitalia or in the anus region caused by human papilloma virus (HPV)	labia majora	two thick outer folds of skin that form the lateral borders and surround the clitoris, the urethral opening, and the opening of the vagina
glans penis	region surrounding the external urethral orifice that forms the rounded tip of the penis	labia minora	two small folds of skin that lie immediately inside the labia majora and protect the vaginal and urethral openings
gonad	organ such as the testis or ovary that produces sex cells	lactation	production of milk
gonorrhea	sexually transmitted disease caused by *Neisseria gonorrhoeae*	laparoscopy	examination of the internal organs of the abdomen using a tube-shaped instrument called a laparoscope that is passed through the abdominal wall
Gram stain	differential stain used to identify microbes according to the dye retained within the bacterial cell wall	laser ablation	removal of tissue with a laser
greater vestibular glands	mucus-secreting glands located on either side of the lower part of the vagina; also called Bartholin glands	leiomyoma	benign neoplasm derived from uterine smooth muscle
gumma	rubbery tumor that occurs in the tertiary stage of syphilis; also called a syphiloma	lesser vestibular glands	mucus-secreting glands between the openings of the vagina and urethra
haploid	containing 23 single, unpaired chromosomes	luteinizing hormone (LH)	anterior pituitary gland hormone that stimulates testosterone secretion
hernia	condition in which part of an internal organ projects abnormally through a body wall or cavity; also called a rupture	male condom	close-fitting sheath that covers the penis
hormone replacement therapy (HRT)	treatment used to maintain female hormone levels after menopause to reduce signs and symptoms associated with menopause	mammary glands	milk-producing structures within the breasts composed of a network of ducts leading to the nipple
hydrocele	accumulation of serous fluid in the testis or within the spermatic cord	mammography	x-ray examination of the breast
hymen	thin fold of mucous membrane covering the entrance to the vagina	mastectomy	surgical removal of a breast
		menarche	first menstrual cycle of a young woman
hypospadias	congenital disorder characterized by the penile urethral opening being located on the ventral surface	menopause	permanent cessation of menstrual cycles
hysterectomy	surgical removal of the uterus	menses	recurrent monthly process of discharging a bloody fluid from the uterus of a nonpregnant female; also called menstruation
impotence	the inability to achieve or maintain a penile erection long enough for intercourse; also called erectile dysfunction (ED)	menstrual cycle	phases occurring in the uterus on a 28-day rotation; also called the uterine cycle
infertility	diminished ability or inability to produce offspring in either the male or the female	menstruation	recurrent monthly process of discharging a bloody fluid from the uterus of a nonpregnant female; also called menses
infundibulum	funnel-shaped opening of the uterine tube that encircles the ovary	mons pubis	prominence caused by a pad of fat that overlies the pubic symphysis in females
interstitial cells	cells between the seminiferous tubules that secrete testosterone	morning-after pill	tablet used to prevent pregnancy up to 5 days (120 hours) after unprotected sex; also called emergency contraception
intrauterine device (IUD)	small T-shaped device that is inserted into the uterus to prevent pregnancy	nulliparous	having never given birth to a child

Key Term	Definition	Key Term	Definition
oligospermia	low sperm count	progesterone	steroid hormone manufactured by the corpus luteum that is essential for pregnancy and lactation
oocyte	sex cell that contains the female genetic information	prolactin (PRL)	hormone that stimulates milk secretion
oogenesis	the formation and development of the oocyte	proliferative phase	stage of the menstrual cycle between the end of menses and ovulation, days 8–14; also called the postmenstrual phase, estrogenic phase, and follicular phase
oogonium	a stem cell that gives rise to an oocyte		
oral contraceptives (OCTs)	tablets taken daily to manipulate the female hormone cycle so that ovulation does not occur; also called birth control pills (BCPs)	prostate	round, fluid-secreting organ surrounding the urethra that secretes a milky fluid
orchiectomy	surgical removal of one or both testes; also called castration	prostate cancer	malignant cell growth of the prostate gland
orchiopexy	surgical treatment of an undescended testicle by freeing it and implanting it into the scrotum	prostatectomy	excision of part or all of the prostate
		prostate-specific antigen (PSA) test	measures the circulating blood levels of prostate-specific antigen
orchitis	inflammation of one or both testes	prostatitis	prostate gland inflammation
orgasm	period of greatest sexual intensity; also called climax	raphe	visible ridge joining the two halves of the scrotum
ovarian cancer	malignant tumor of the ovary or ovaries	rectocele	hernia of the rectum through the vaginal wall; also called a proctocele
ovarian cysts	fluid-filled sacs on or near the ovaries		
ovaries	paired glands that produce oocytes and female sex hormones	relaxin	hormone that causes relaxation of the pelvic ligaments and pubic symphysis during pregnancy
ovulation	monthly release of a secondary oocyte from the ovary		
ovum	functional secondary oocyte after fertilization	reproduction	total process by which organisms produce offspring; also known as procreation
oxytocin (OXT)	hormone that stimulates milk ejection		
Pap test	test used to detect precancerous or cancerous cells of the cervix; also called a Pap smear	resectoscope	endoscopic instrument used for the transurethral removal of the prostate
		salpingo-oophorectomy	removal of the uterine tube and ovary
pelvic examination	manually palpating and examining the vagina, uterus, rectum, and accessory organs and structures	scrotum	fleshy sac that encloses the testes
		secondary oocyte	reproductive cell released from the ovary during ovulation
pelvic inflammatory disease (PID)	inflammation of the reproductive organs that, if untreated, can cause infertility	secondary sexual characteristics	traits that develop at puberty but are not directly concerned with reproduction, such as voice changes, body hair distribution, and adipose tissue patterns
penis	male organ of sexual intercourse and urination		
perimenopause	transitional period leading to menopause	secretory phase	stage of the menstrual cycle after ovulation, days 15–28; also called the premenstrual phase, postovulatory phase, and luteal phase
perineum	region between the anus and the vulva in females and between the anus and the scrotum in males		
premenstrual dysphoric disorder (PMDD)	premenstrual syndrome accompanied by emotional symptoms with impaired functioning that persists after the onset of menstruation	semen	fluid of the male reproductive organs that contains sperm; also called ejaculate or seminal fluid
		semen analysis	test that measures the volume of semen and sperm number, morphology, and motility
premenstrual syndrome (PMS)	group of signs and symptoms experienced by some women in the days preceding menstruation	seminal glands	paired glands that secrete semen into the ejaculatory duct; also called the seminal vesicles
prepuce	fold of skin covering the glans penis in uncircumcised males; also called the foreskin		
proctocele	hernia of the rectum through the vaginal wall; also called a rectocele	seminiferous tubules	site of sperm formation in the testes

Key Term	Definition	Key Term	Definition
sexually transmitted diseases (STDs)	contagious infections acquired during sexual contact; also called venereal diseases (VDs) or sexually transmitted infections (STIs)	trichomoniasis	sexually transmitted disease caused by the protozoan *Trichomonas vaginalis*
sperm	sex cells that contain the male genetic information; also called spermatozoa	tubal ligation	sterilization technique in which a woman's uterine tubes are surgically blocked by cutting, cautery, or a plastic or metal device to prevent oocytes from entering the uterus
spermatic cord	paired structure that encloses the ductus deferens, blood vessels, nerves, and lymphatic vessels in each testis	uterine cycle	phases occurring in the uterus on a 28-day rotation; also called the menstrual cycle
spermatogenesis	process of sperm formation	uterine fibroids	benign tumors of the muscle and fibrous tissue of the uterus
spermatogonium	sperm stem cell that gives rise to a mature sperm	uterine tubes	narrow tubes that serve as a passageway from the ovaries to the uterus; also called oviducts or fallopian tubes
spermicide	substance that prevents pregnancy by destroying sperm	uterus	the hollow muscular organ in the pelvic region in which a developing embryo or fetus is nourished before birth
spermiogenesis	stage of spermatogenesis during which a sperm matures	vagina	muscular tube connecting the uterus to the outside
sponge	plastic foam sponge containing spermicide that is inserted into the vagina to prevent pregnancy	vaginal barriers	physical blockades that prevent sperm from entering the uterus
sterility	inability to conceive in the female or the inability to induce conception in the male	vaginal cancer	malignant cells of the vagina
sterilization	surgical procedure that prevents a person from reproducing by removing all or part of the reproductive organs	vaginal ring	hormone-releasing barrier that is placed in the vagina once a month for 3 weeks to prevent ovulation
syphilis	sexually transmitted disease caused by *Treponema pallidum*	vaginitis	vaginal inflammation
syphiloma	rubbery tumor that occurs in the tertiary stage of syphilis; also called a gumma	varicocele	swelling in one testicle or both caused by swelling of the veins in the spermatic cord
testes	paired male gonads located in the scrotum; also called testicles	vas deferens	tube connecting the epididymis and the ejaculatory duct; also called the ductus deferens
testicles	paired male gonads located in the scrotum; also called testes	vasectomy	excision of a small segment of the vas (ductus) deferens used to produce male sterility
testicular cancer	malignant cell growth in the testis	venereal diseases (VDs)	contagious infections acquired during sexual contact; also called sexually transmitted diseases (STDs) or sexually transmitted infections (STIs)
testicular torsion	rotation of the spermatic cord that causes an interruption in the blood supply to the tissue		
testosterone	principal hormone secreted by cells in the testes	vestibule	central space between the labia minora
toxic shock syndrome (TSS)	circulatory failure associated with tampon use and the growth of toxin-producing staphylococcal bacteria	viral hepatitis	inflammation of the liver caused by at least seven immunologically unrelated viruses
transverse rectus abdominis myocutaneous (TRAM) flap	surgical procedure to reconstruct the breast region after mastectomy using the rectus abdominis muscle, which is threaded under the abdominal and thoracic cavities to the mastectomy site	vulva	female external genitals
		vulvar cancer	malignant cells of the folds surrounding the female genitalia; also called labial cancer
transurethral resection (TUR)	endoscopic removal of the prostate gland for relief of prostatic obstruction	withdrawal method	birth control method that involves the man pulling the penis out of the vagina before ejaculating; also called the pull-out method
transvaginal sonography	procedure for obtaining echograms of the uterus, ovaries, and ovarian structures		

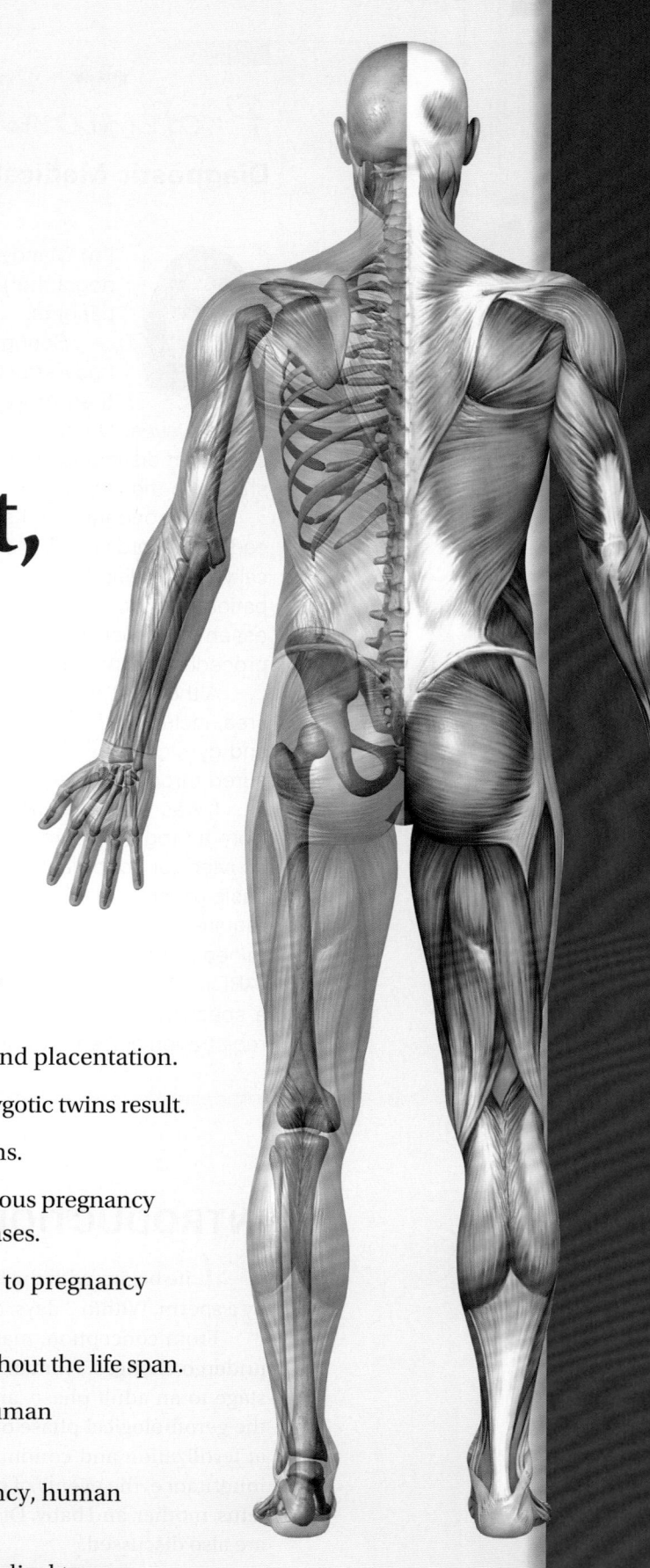

CHAPTER

17

Pregnancy, Human Development, and Child Health

OBJECTIVES

After completing this chapter, you should be able to:

1. Define the meaning of word parts related to pregnancy, human development, and child health.

2. Define key terms significant to fertilization, gestation, and placentation.

3. Explain how multiple births, monozygotic twins, and dizygotic twins result.

4. Define genes, chromosomes, inheritance, and mutations.

5. Define common signs, symptoms, and treatments of various pregnancy and human development disorders, and childhood diseases.

6. Explain clinical tests and diagnostic procedures related to pregnancy and childhood disorders.

7. Describe anatomical and physiological alterations throughout the life span.

8. Define common abbreviations related to pregnancy, human development, and child health.

9. Define terms used in medical reports involving pregnancy, human development, and child health.

10. Correctly define, spell, and pronounce the chapter's medical terms.

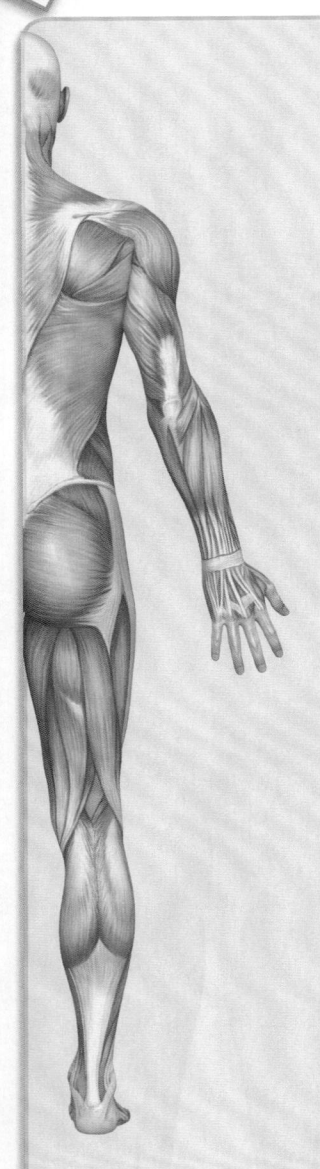

Professional Profile

Diagnostic Medical Sonographer

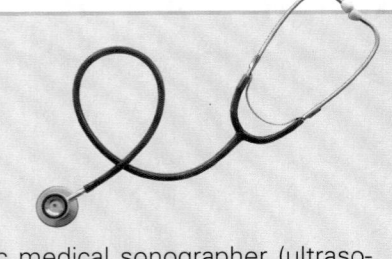

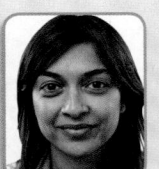

I'm Mandy, and I work as a diagnostic medical sonographer (ultrasonographer). A hospital employs me to perform diagnostic testing on patients.

Sonography uses sound waves to generate images of internal body structures. To do this, I spread a gel across the skin surface and then move a transducer across the area. The gel aids in transmitting sound waves. During the scanning procedure, I view the screen and look for subtle clues that distinguish unhealthy tissue from normal tissue. I then select images to be shown to the physician.

As a sonographer, I spend a great deal of time with patients—explaining the procedure, recording the medical history, and setting up the equipment. My job is physically demanding because I must stand all day while assisting with lifting and moving patients to the desired positions for the best pictures. Good communication skills are essential, especially because patients are usually apprehensive about the diagnostic procedure or the results that may be revealed.

Although I have been cross-trained to perform ultrasound on nearly every body area, including the abdomen, brain, and cardiovascular system, I most enjoy obstetric and gynecological sonography. Fetal health, growth, and status can be directly measured through ultrasonography.

I was educated at a vocational school, where I earned an associate's degree from a program accredited by the Joint Review Committee on Education in Diagnostic Medical Sonography. My coursework included classes in anatomy and physiology, basic physics, medical ethics, medical terminology, and patient care. Licensure is not required, but the hospital that employs me requires certification. To that end, I obtained registration through the American Registry of Diagnostic Medical Sonographers (ARDMS) by passing a general physics and instrumentation examination, along with a specialty examination in obstetrics/gynecology and abdominal viewing. I keep my registration current by completing 30 hours of continuing education every 3 years.

INTRODUCTION

Life begins with the fertilization of a secondary oocyte, recently released from the ovary, by a sperm. Within 3 days, the fertilized egg, called a zygote, implants itself on the uterine wall.

From conception, marked by the beginning of pregnancy, to death, humans constantly undergo changes. Human development is the progression in maturation from an embryonic stage to an adult phase, and lifespan development encompasses the prenatal stage through the gerontological phase of life. This chapter focuses primarily on the stages of life beginning at fertilization and continuing to childhood. Along with a summary of human genetics and inheritance, the events of pregnancy are described, including the transformations of embryo, fetus, mother, and baby. Disorders of pregnancy, labor, delivery, newborn infants, and children are also discussed.

MEDICAL TERM PARTS

Word Parts

Medical term prefixes, suffixes, and combining forms related to pregnancy, human development, and child health are introduced in this section.

Word Part	Meaning
allant-, allanto-	allantois (a fetal membrane), allantoid, sausage-shaped
amnio-	amnion (innermost embryonic membrane)
-blast	immature precursor cell
blasto-	process of budding
chorio-	membrane, fetal membrane, chorion (outermost embryonic membrane)
embry-, embryo-	embryo
encephal-, encephalo-	brain
episio-	vulva
heter-, hetero-	other, different
homo-	same, alike
karyo-	nucleus
lact-, lacti-, lacto-	milk
mening-, meningo-	meninges
mes-, meso-	middle
ped-, pedi-, pedo-	child
phen-, pheno-	appearance
talo-	talus, ankle
terato-	malformed
troph-, tropho-	food, nutrition
zyg-, zygo-	joining

Word Grouping Exercises

Using the *Medical Term Parts* table, identify the prefix, suffix, or combining form for each of the following definitions. The first one has been done as an example.

Definition	Word Part
food, nutrition	*troph-, tropho*
allantois (a fetal membrane), allantoid, sausage-shaped	
amnion (innermost embryonic membrane)	
appearance	

continued

continued from page 899

Definition	Word Part
brain	
child	
embryo	
immature precursor cell	
joining	
malformed	
membrane, fetal membrane, chorion (outermost embryonic membrane)	
meninges	
middle	
milk	
nucleus	
other, different	
process of budding	
same, alike	
talus, ankle	
vulva	

 ## Word Building Exercises

Word parts introduced in the *Medical Term Parts* section are listed in the following table. For this exercise, first supply the meaning of each word part, then use the word part to build a word you already know. The word you list under *Common or Known Word* does not have to be a medical term; a commonly used word is fine. Be sure, however, that the word correctly reflects the intended meaning. The first one has been done as an example. Check your answers in a dictionary.

Word Part	Meaning	Common or Known Word	Example Medical Term
amnio-	*amnion (innermost embryonic membrane)*	*amniotic fluid*	amniocentesis
-blast			trophoblast
embry-, embryo-			embryology
episio-			episiotomy
heter-, hetero-			heterozygous
homo-			homozygous

continued

continued from page 900

Word Part	Meaning	Common or Known Word	Example Medical Term
mening-, meningo-			meningocele
mes-, meso-			mesoderm
ped-, pedi-, pedo-			pediatrics
phen-, pheno-			phenotype
talo-			talipes equinovarus
zyg-, zygo-			zygote

ANATOMY AND PHYSIOLOGY

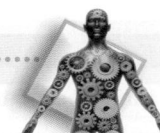

Pregnancy, Human Development, and Child Health Preview

Comprehension of human development requires a basic understanding of general terms such as fertilization, zygote, placenta, embryo, fetus, and gestation. **Fertilization** is the process that begins with penetration of the secondary oocyte by the sperm, forming an ovum (**Figure 17-1**). Once fertilized, the cell is referred to as a **zygote**. Ovaries are the sites of secondary oocyte release, and fertilization usually takes place within the uterine tubes. The zygote makes its way to the uterus, where implantation occurs and the placenta is formed to become the home of embryonic and future fetal growth and development. The **placenta** is a vascular organ that

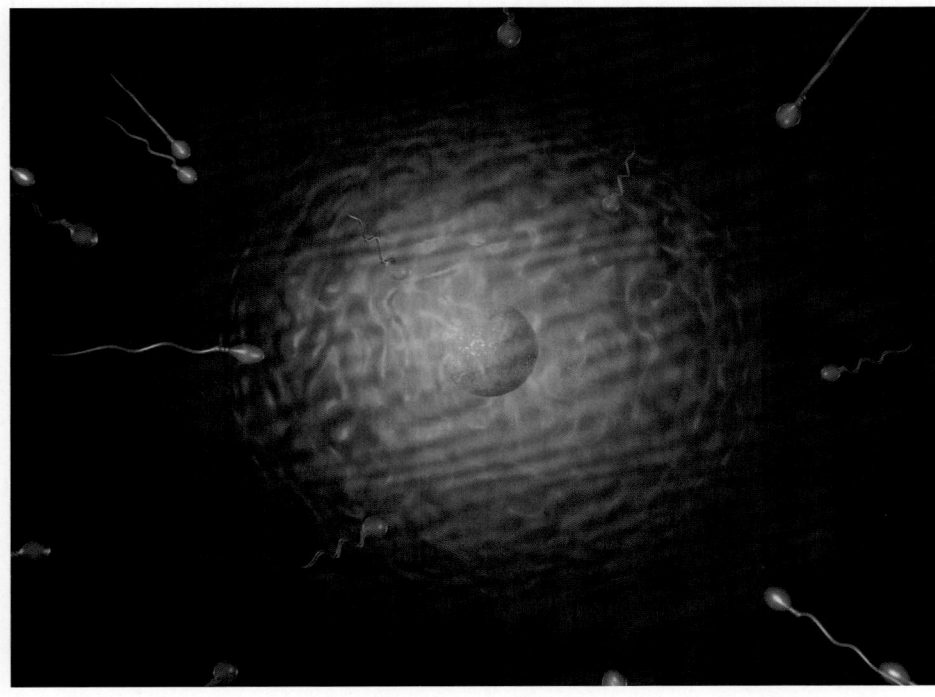

Figure 17-1 Secondary oocyte with approaching sperm.

develops inside the uterus to supply food and oxygen to the developing human through the **umbilical cord**, a structure containing two arteries and one vein that connects the embryo or fetus with the placenta

The term **embryo** describes a developing human in the early stages from fertilization to the end of the eighth week. Thereafter, it is called a **fetus**. **Gestation** (pregnancy) is the time spent in the womb, or in medical terms, *in utero*. When gestation is complete, the fetus is normally delivered by way of the vagina. After delivery, the baby is called a *neonate*, until the end of the first month.

Life expectancy is the average number of years a person born today can expect to live under current conditions. In the United States, the life expectancy at birth for the total population is 77.5 years. (These data are from 2003, the most recent available.) Life expectancy varies worldwide and by ethnicity, gender, and socioeconomic status.

Life span is the length of time that a member of a particular species can remain alive and is the extreme limit of our longevity. The human lifespan appears to be fixed at approximately 100 years, but some individuals have lived to be 120, and Jeanne Calment of France died in 1997 at the age of 122. She is still the longest-lived person.

KEY TERM	Definition
fertilization	union of the male sperm and the female secondary oocyte
zygote (ZYE-gote)	fertilized ovum; cell formed from the union of a sperm and secondary oocyte
placenta (pluh-SEN-tuh)	a vascular organ of pregnancy that develops on the wall of the uterus to supply food and oxygen to the embryo/fetus through the umbilical cord
umbilical (um-BIL-i-kul) cord	connecting stalk between the embryo or fetus and the placenta that contains two arteries and one vein
embryo (EM-bree-oh)	product of conception from the moment of fertilization to the end of the eighth gestational week
fetus (FEE-tus)	developing human from week 9 of gestation until birth
gestation (jes-TAY-shun)	period of development from fertilization until birth; also called pregnancy
life expectancy	the average number of years a person born today can expect to live
life span	length of time that a member of a particular species can remain alive and is the extreme limit of our longevity

KEY TERM PRACTICE: *Pregnancy, Human Development, and Child Health Preview*

1. A fertilized ovum is known as a _____.

2. After fertilization, the developing human is called an _____ until the ninth week of gestation.

3. _____ is the length of time that a member of a particular species can remain alive and is the extreme limit of our longevity.

4. _____ is the medical term describing the union of the male sperm and the female secondary oocyte.

5. The _____ is a vascular organ of pregnancy that develops on the wall of the uterus to supply food and oxygen to the embryo/fetus through the umbilical cord.

Fertilization and Implantation

A male or female reproductive cell—sperm or oocyte—is known as a **gamete**. Their union during fertilization forms a zygote. Fertilization usually takes place in the uterine tube, where sperm penetration of the oocyte is facilitated by an enzyme released from the sperm head (acrosome). An outer layer surrounding the oocyte contains a sperm receptor site that allows only one sperm to fertilize it.

The resulting zygote, now called an ovum, contains 23 pairs of chromosomes—one set from each gamete—and is genetically unique. Inheritance is discussed later in the chapter.

The zygote is genetically complete. It then becomes a pre-embryo and undergoes cell division as it travels through the uterine tube toward the uterus. By the time the pre-embryo arrives in the uterus, about 5 or 6 days later, it is a mass of cells called a **blastocyst** (**Figure 17-2**).

The stage at which the blastocyst becomes attached to the endometrium of the uterus is termed **implantation**. It usually implants on the upper posterior uterine wall between days 7 and 10 after fertilization. Enzymes digest a hole in the endometrium for attachment. Germ layers—endoderm, ectoderm, and mesoderm—form and eventually give rise to all other body tissues and organs.

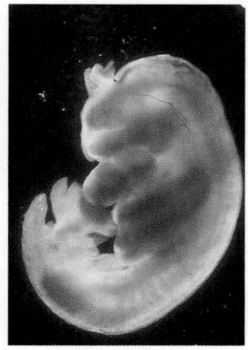

Figure 17-2
Blastocyst at 7 to 8 days after fertilization.

KEY TERM	Definition
gamete (GAM-eet)	male or female reproductive cell (sperm or oocyte)
blastocyst (BLAS-toh-sist)	mass of cells that implants on the endometrium after fertilization
implantation	attachment of the blastocyst to the endometrium

KEY TERM PRACTICE: *Fertilization and Implantation*

1. The term for a male or female reproductive cell is _____.

2. _____ is attachment of the blastocyst to the endometrium.

3. A mass of cells that implants on the endometrium after fertilization is called a _____.

Placenta Formation and Gestation

The germ layers form four nourishing and protecting membranes outside the embryo, known as extraembryonic membranes. These include the yolk sac (endoderm and mesoderm), the amnion (ectoderm and mesoderm), the allantois (endoderm and mesoderm), and the chorion (mesoderm). As the layers continue to grow, blood vessels appear in the chorion and begin forming the placenta. The placenta serves as the organ of metabolic exchange between the mother and the embryo/fetus. It is a structure about 16 cm (6 in.) in diameter and nearly 2 cm (1 in.) thick. At birth it weighs about 1.3 lb (600 g). It is formed partly by maternal tissue and partially by embryonic tissue. Although blood does not flow between these layers, other substances are able to diffuse across the membrane. There is no mixing of maternal and fetal blood.

Extraembryonic membranes play a role in placenta formation and the nurturing of the developing human. The yolk sac is a thin membrane that surrounds the embryo, forming blood cells and giving rise to sex cells. The **amnion** is the innermost fetal membrane, forming a fluid-filled sac that encircles the developing embryo/fetus and contains amnionic fluid. The word *amnionic* means "related to the amnion," but its synonym is amnio*t*ic, spelled with a *t* instead of an *n*. Both spellings are correct.

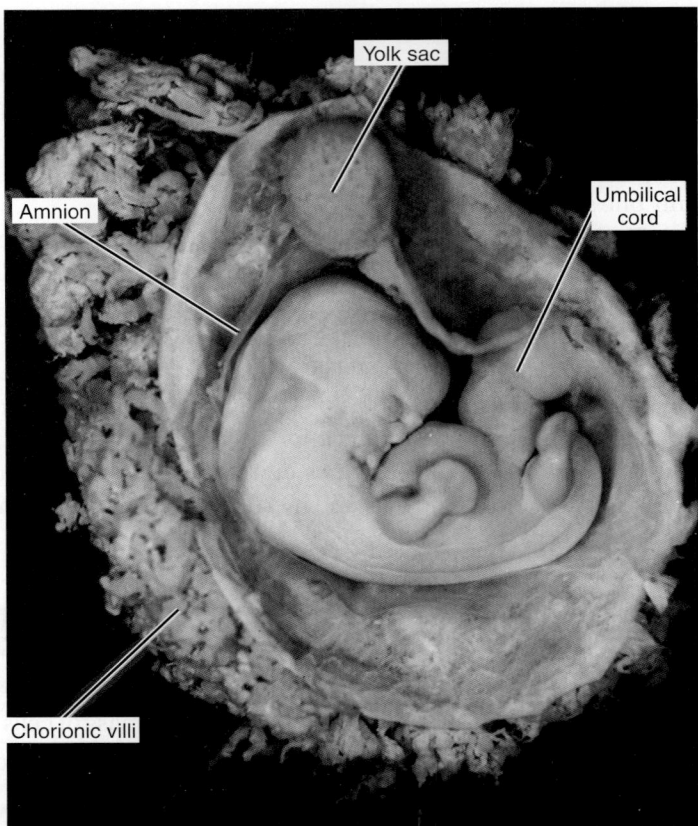

Figure 17-3 Human embryo (13 mm, sixth week) showing the yolk sac in the chorionic cavity.

The **allantois** is a membranous sac that forms the umbilical blood vessels. The **chorion** is the outermost membrane, containing a dense concentration of blood vessels. It contacts the uterine wall and becomes part of the placenta. Vascular projections from its outer surface, called **chorionic villi**, move into the wall to form the placenta. The umbilical cord is a structure connecting the embryo/fetus to the placenta. It consists of two umbilical arteries and one vein. It serves as the passageway for materials between the mother and the embryo/fetus (**Figure 17-3**).

During placenta formation and gestation, the developing embryo/fetus is most susceptible to injury from alcohol, cigarette smoking, drugs, ionizing radiation, lead, medications, mercury, and viruses. Substances such as these that cause **congenital** (present at birth) abnormalities are termed **teratogens**. **Teratology** is the scientific study of congenital malformations.

A group of blood tests designed to identify teratogenic diseases in pregnant women and neonates is known as the **TORCH series**. TORCH is an acronym for *t*oxoplasmosis, *o*ther infections, *r*ubella, *c*ytomegalovirus (CMV), and *h*erpes simplex virus (HSV). All of these diseases can cross the placenta and infect the fetus.

Once formed, the placenta has endocrine functions and secretes hormones. Placental hormones include human chorionic gonadotropin, human placental lactogen, estrogen, progesterone, and relaxin. **Human chorionic gonadotropin (hCG)** maintains high estrogen and progesterone levels, which are necessary to maintain the developing embryo during the early weeks of pregnancy. The common tool used to confirm pregnancy is a test for hCG in maternal blood or urine. This hormone appears in the maternal bloodstream and urine soon after zygote implantation. In-home pregnancy kits test for the presence of hCG in the urine. Maternal urine levels rise to around 500,000 international units within 24 hours of pregnancy. In-home urine tests are quite accurate but not as reliable as blood tests for detecting pregnancy. The

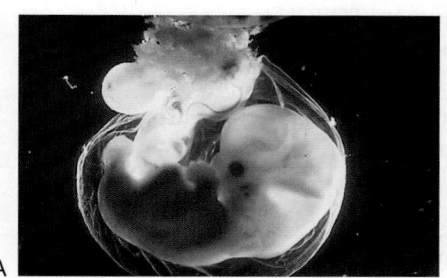

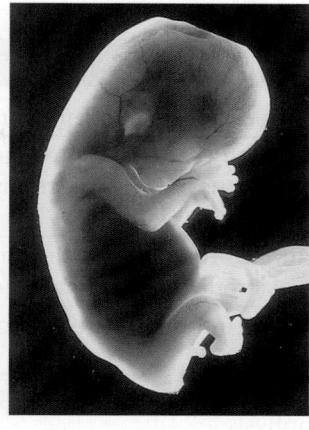

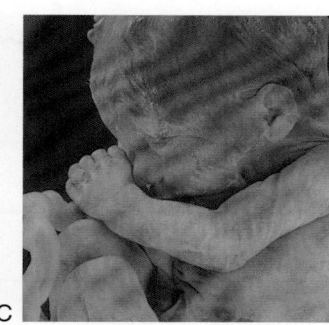

Figure 17-4 (A) Human embryo at 37 days.

(B) Human embryo at 41 days.

(C) Fetus between 12 and 15 weeks.

hormone is important during the first trimester to stimulate estrogen and progesterone; thereafter, the placenta secretes the necessary hormones to sustain pregnancy.

Human placental lactogen (hPL) is important to embryo/fetal growth during pregnancy. A deficiency of hPL during pregnancy leads to abnormal intrauterine and postnatal growth. The hPL test is a maternal blood test useful for evaluating placental function. Low values indicate fetal distress or possible miscarriage. Estrogen, progesterone, and placental lactogen maintain pregnancy by acting on uterine tissue. **Relaxin** relaxes the pubic symphysis and assists in dilation of the cervix near the end of pregnancy.

Growth of the embryo/fetus depends on a nutritive environment during pregnancy. Pregnancy is typically classified into trimesters, each 3 months in duration. Forty weeks serves as the gestational age of a full-term infant.

The first trimester is a period of embryological and early fetal development. At 4 weeks, the embryo is about the size of a pea. Organ formation begins by week 8, and the fetus develops recognizable arms and legs (**Figures 17-4 A** and **B**).

During the second trimester, organs and systems develop. By week 9, the fetus is the size of a strawberry. In this stage, the fetus begins to look distinctly human (**Figure 17-4C**). Hair, eyebrows, and eyelashes develop, and lanugo (fine, fetal hair) covers the skin. The mother can feel fetal movements, and the heartbeat can be auscultated (heard through a stethoscope).

The third trimester is a phase of rapid fetal growth. The fetus sleeps, wakes, sucks its thumb, and is easily startled during the period before birth.

KEY TERM	Definition
amnion (AM-nee-on)	innermost fetal membrane forming a fluid-filled protective sac
allantois (uh-lan-TOH-is)	membranous sac that forms the umbilical blood vessels
chorion (KOH-ree-on)	outermost fetal membrane that forms part of the placenta
chorionic villi (KOH-ree-on-ick VIL-eye)	vascular projections from the chorion's outer surface that move into the wall to form the placenta
congenital (kun-JEN-i-tul)	existing before or at birth, though not necessarily detected then
teratogens (TERR-uh-toh-jenz)	substances that alter the normal development of a fetus causing congenital abnormalities

continued

continued from page 905

KEY TERM	Definition
teratology (terr-uh-TOL-uh-jee)	scientific study of congenital malformations blood tests used to identify
TORCH series	teratogenic diseases in pregnant women; TORCH is an acronym for *t*oxoplasmosis, *o*ther infections, *r*ubella, *c*ytomegalovirus (CMV), and *h*erpes simplex virus (HSV).
human chorionic gonadotropin (hCG) (KOH-ree-on-ick goh-nad-oh-TROH-pin)	hormone originating in chorionic tissue that maintains estrogen and progesterone levels; its presence indicates pregnancy
human placental lactogen (hPL) (pluh-SEN-tul LACK-toh-jen)	hormone important to embryo/fetal growth
relaxin (ree-LACK-sin)	hormone secreted during pregnancy that causes relaxation of the pubic symphysis

KEY TERM PRACTICE: *Placenta Formation and Gestation*

1. Vascular projections from the outer surface of the chorion that form the placenta are termed

   _____.

2. The word part _____ means *malformed*, and the word part _____ means *the study of*; therefore, the study of substances that cause congenital malformations is known as _____.

3. _____ is a hormone secreted during pregnancy that causes relaxation of the pubic symphysis.

4. The outermost fetal membrane that forms part of the placenta is the _____.

5. The innermost fetal membrane forming a fluid-filled protective sac is known as the _____.

Pregnancy

During pregnancy, the maternal systems undergo significant changes. For example, maternal respiratory rate and blood volume increase, and nutritional requirements increase by 10% to 30%. The mammary glands and the uterus enlarge. In addition, the maternal filtration rate of the kidneys increases approximately 50%.

Gynecology (GYN) is the medical specialty concerned with female reproductive health. Many gynecologists also practice **obstetrics (OB)**, the branch of medicine concerned with the care of women during pregnancy, childbirth, and for some 6 weeks following delivery. An **obstetrician (OB)** is a physician specializing in pregnancy, delivering babies, and the care of women after childbirth. The act of giving birth is termed **parturition** (or childbirth), and the time from when contractions start to the baby's delivery is called **labor**. Both **postpartum** and **post partum** mean "after childbirth." Written as one word, *postpartum* is used as an adjective, as in *postpartum hemorrhage*. Written as two words, *post partum* is used as an adverb, as in *hemorrhage occurring post partum*.

Remarkable skin changes occur throughout pregnancy. These include chloasma, linea nigra, and striae gravidarum. Some are caused by hormonal changes induced by pregnancy. Dark coloration on the skin of the face caused by hormonal changes related to pregnancy is termed **chloasma**. It is commonly referred to as the "mask of pregnancy," and it is made worse by sunlight. The linea alba is a fibrous band running vertically along the entire length of the midline of the anterior abdomen. During pregnancy, this band becomes pigmented and appears as a black line called the **linea nigra**. **Striae gravidarum** is the medical term for stretch marks that occur during pregnancy on the abdomen, thighs, and breasts (**Figure 17-5**).

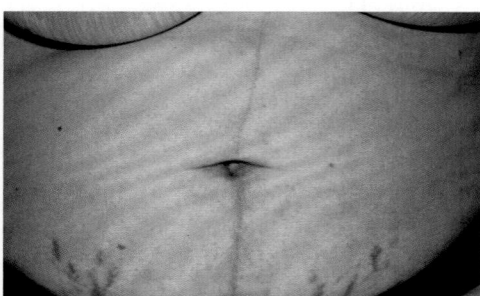

Figure 17-5 Linea nigra and striae gravidarum. The linea alba darkens during pregnancy, but the normal color usually returns after delivery. In contrast, although the purplish color of striae gravidarum will fade over time, the striae themselves are permanent.

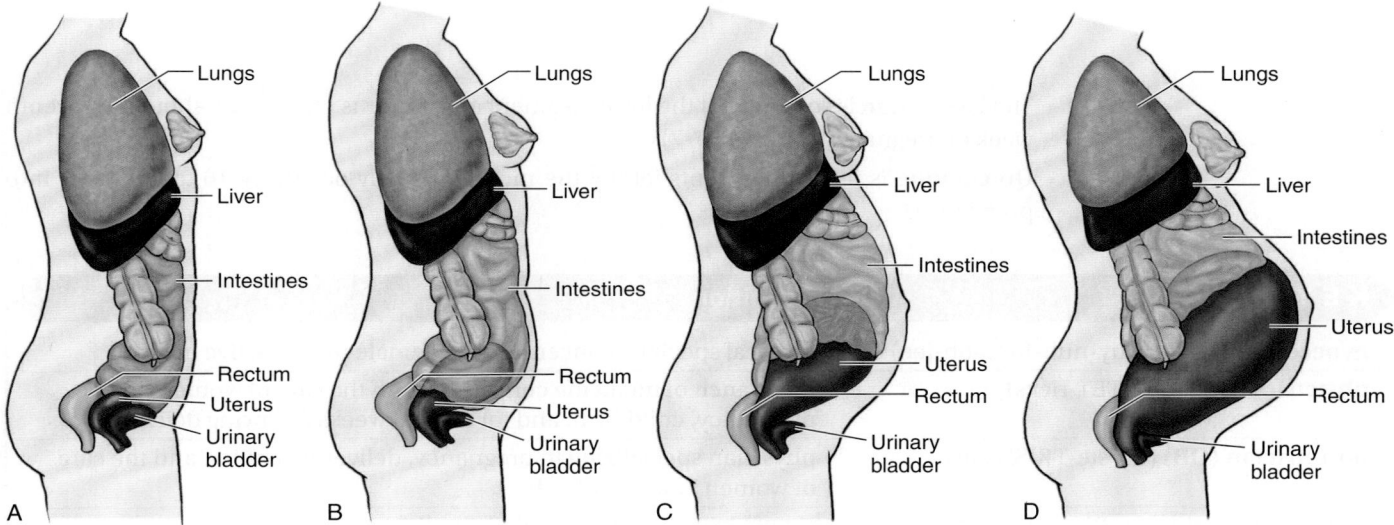

Figure 17-6 Uterine growth at **(A)** conception, **(B)** first trimester, **(C)** second trimester, and **(D)** third trimester.

(*Striae* refers to "line," and *gravid* means "pregnant.") Changes in the size of the uterus and the displacement of maternal organs are shown in **Figure 17-6**.

The formula used to calculate an infant's date of birth is known as **Nägele's rule**. The calculation involves subtracting 3 months from the beginning of the last normal menstrual period and then adding 7 days to that date. For example, if the last menstrual period began on December 20, count back 3 months to September 20. Then add 7 days to determine September 27 as the expected delivery date.

Pregnancy (gestation) is the period of development of the offspring. The average length of human gestation is 10 lunar months, 280 days, or 40 weeks. (A lunar month is 28 days.) This period is calculated from the onset of the last menstrual period and varies between 250 and 310 days. The **gestational age** is the age of the developing embryo/fetus computed from the first day of the last menstrual period to any point in time thereafter until birth.

Various signs indicate pregnancy:

- **Braxton Hicks contractions** are irregular and painless uterine contractions that occur with increasing frequency throughout pregnancy.

- The **Chadwick sign** is a bluish discoloration of the cervix and vagina around the sixth week of pregnancy. This sign results from increased blood flow to the pregnant uterus.

- The **Goodell sign** is a softening of the cervix, considered to be evidence of pregnancy. The cervix continues to soften or "ripen" as pregnancy progresses, appearing "mushy" just before birth.

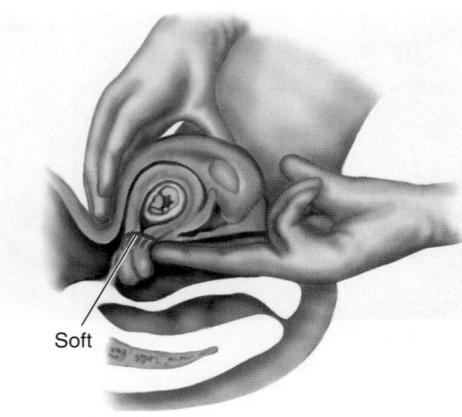

Figure 17-7 Hegar sign.

- The **Hegar sign** is softening of the lower segment of the uterus that occurs about the seventh week of pregnancy (**Figure 17-7**).
- **Quickening** is fetal movements felt by the mother, usually occurring 16 to 20 weeks into pregnancy.

KEY TERM	Definition
gynecology (GYN) (guy-nuh-KOL-oh-jee)	medical specialty concerned with female reproductive health
obstetrics (OB) (ob-STET-ricks)	the branch of medicine concerned with the care of women during pregnancy, childbirth, and for some 6 weeks following delivery
obstetrician (OB) (ob-ste-TRISH-un)	physician specializing in pregnancy, delivering babies, and the care of women after childbirth
parturition (pahr-tew-RISH-un)	act of giving birth; also called childbirth
labor	time from when contractions start to the baby's delivery
postpartum (pohst-PAR-tum)	adjective form that refers to the period immediately after childbirth
post partum (pohst PAR-tum)	adverb form that refers to the period immediately after childbirth
chloasma (kloh-AZ-muh)	dark coloration on the facial skin caused by pregnancy-induced hormonal changes
linea nigra (LIN-ee-uh NIGH-gruh)	dark line extending up the center of the abdomen of a pregnant woman
striae gravidarum (STRYE-ee grav-i-DAHR-um)	stretch marks seen in pregnancy
Nägele's (NAY-guh-leez) **rule**	formula used to calculate an infant's delivery date
pregnancy	period of development of the offspring; also called gestation
gestational (jes-TAY-shun-ul) **age**	age of the developing embryo/fetus computed from the first day of the last menstrual cycle to any point in time until birth
Braxton Hicks (BRACKS-tun HICKS) **contractions**	irregular and painless uterine contractions that occur with increasing frequency throughout pregnancy
Chadwick sign	bluish discoloration of the cervix and vagina around the sixth week of pregnancy
Goodell sign	softening of the cervix, indicative of pregnancy
Hegar (HAY-gar) **sign**	softening of the lower portion of the uterus occurring at about week 7 of pregnancy
quickening	fetal movements felt by the mother

continued

continued from page 908

KEY TERM PRACTICE: *Pregnancy*

1. The medical term for childbirth is _____.

2. An _____ is a physician who specializes in pregnancy, delivering babies, and the care of women after childbirth.

3. Fetal movements felt by the mother are known as _____.

4. _____ is a bluish discoloration of the cervix and vagina around the sixth week of pregnancy.

5. The formula used to calculate an infant's delivery date is termed _____.

Labor and Delivery

Medical terms associated with labor and delivery are numerous. Those describing the cervix or uterus include effacement, incompetent cervix, and lightening. **Effacement** describes the thinning out of the cervix just before or during labor. An **incompetent cervix** is a condition in which the cervix dilates prematurely before the fetus reaches full term. If not sutured until full-term pregnancy is achieved, incompetent cervix results in the premature expulsion of an embryo or fetus before it is viable. **Lightening** refers to the sinking or dropping of the fetus into the pelvic inlet. Lightening takes place during late pregnancy when the fetal head begins to descend into the mother's pelvis, reducing pressure on the mother's diaphragm during the last weeks before delivery.

An **abortion** is the expulsion of an embryo or fetus from the uterus before it can survive outside the womb. A distinction made between abortion and premature birth is that premature infants are those born after the stage of viability but before 37 weeks' gestation. Abortion may be either spontaneous (occurring from natural causes) or induced (medically caused). The lay term for abortion is miscarriage; however, this term is no longer accepted in clinical usage.

The exact mechanism that triggers the events of labor is not known, but there is a surge of oxytocin (OXT) that stimulates the contractions before, during, and after birth (for delivery of the placenta). The drug called Pitocin is artificial oxytocin and is often given to induce labor. In the medical vernacular it may be referred to as "vitamin P."

There are three stages of labor: dilation, expulsion, and placenta delivery (**Figure 17-8**). The first stage begins with contractions and cervical dilation. **Contractions** are tightenings of uterine muscles that occur at increasingly frequent intervals immediately before childbirth. Dilation of the cervix to about 10 cm (4 in.) occurs in the first stage of labor and is characterized by rupture of the amniochorionic membrane. This event is commonly known as having the pregnant woman's "water break." The average duration of the first stage is 8 hours.

During the second stage, or expulsion, contractions reach their maximum intensity and eventually push the baby out of the womb. Within 1 hour after delivery, placenta delivery (stage 3) occurs when the organ separates from the uterine wall and is ejected through the vagina. It is often referred to as "afterbirth." Approximately 1 to 2 hours after delivery, uterine tone returns.

The normal birth position, in which the baby's head enters the cervix and birth canal first is termed **vertex**. If the fetus does not rotate as normally occurs and presents feet or buttocks first, it is a **breech** birth (**Figure 17-9**). An **episiotomy**, a surgical incision made at the opening of the vagina to prevent undue laceration at delivery time, may be performed before a vaginal birth. The incision enlarges the vaginal opening to prevent tearing (**Figure 17-10**). Another term for episiotomy is *vaginoperineotomy*, a descriptive term denoting an incision in the vaginal and perineal regions.

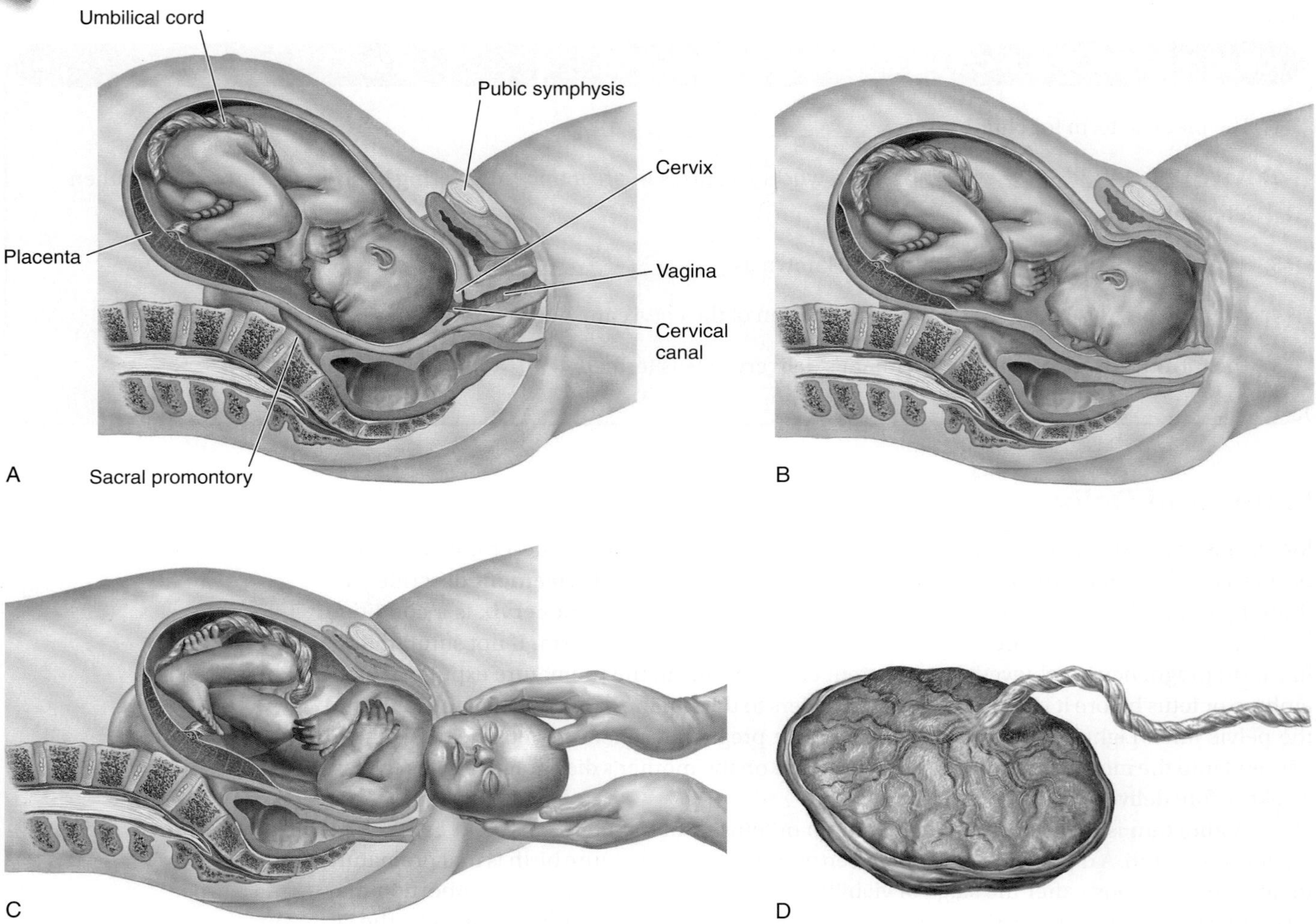

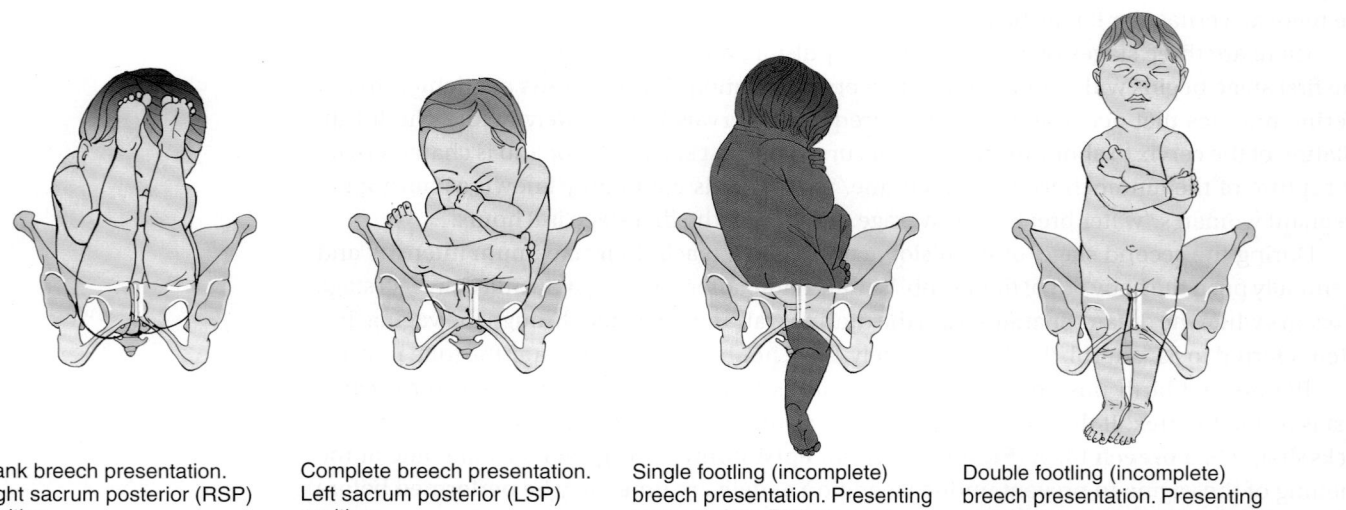

Figure 17-8 (A) Full term before labor. **(B)** Dilation stage. **(C)** Expulsion stage. **(D)** Placenta delivery.

Frank breech presentation. Right sacrum posterior (RSP) position.

Complete breech presentation. Left sacrum posterior (LSP) position.

Single footling (incomplete) breech presentation. Presenting part: one foot. Right sacrum anterior (RSA) position.

Double footling (incomplete) breech presentation. Presenting part: both feet. Sacrum posterior (SP) position.

Figure 17-9 Types of breech presentations.

Infants may be delivered by the natural route of the vagina or by a surgical procedure termed a cesarean section. Measurement of the inlet and outlet diameters of the pelvis, called **pelvimetry**, determines the feasibility of a vaginal childbirth. Sometimes during a vaginal birth, it may be necessary to use **obstetric forceps**, a large, double-bladed instrument resembling tongs that interlocks around the fetal head to facilitate delivery during a difficult labor (**Figure 17-11**).

A **cesarean section (C-section)** is delivery of a fetus through an abdominal and uterine incision. It is performed when the fetus's head is too large to fit through the pelvic girdle, when there is hemorrhage due to abruptio placentae or placenta previa (discussed later), with a breech or shoulder presentation, or when there is fetal and/or maternal distress (**Figure 17-12**). The history

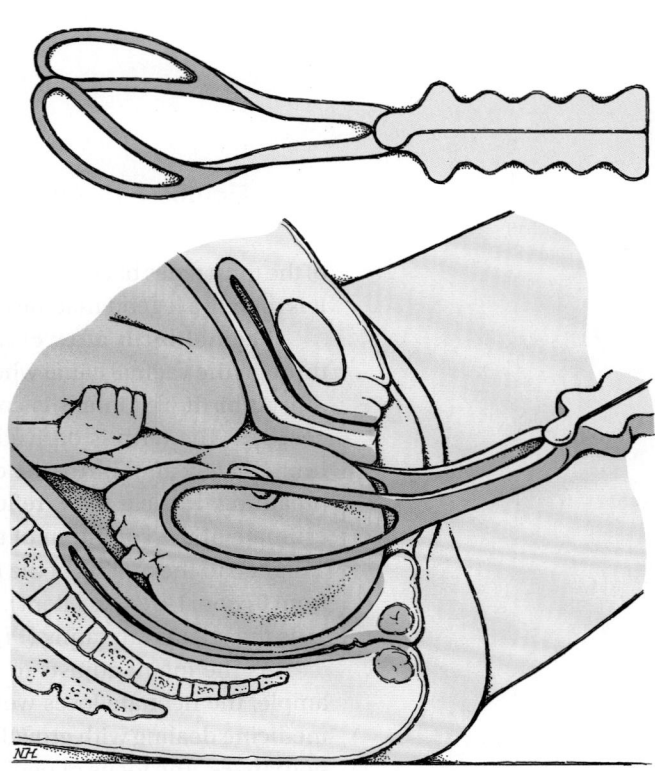

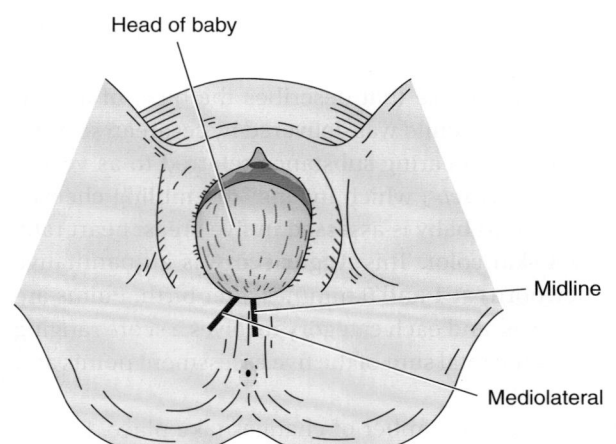

Figure 17-10 Position of episiotomy incision in a woman during second stage of labor. Baby's head is presenting in vaginal outlet (crowning).

Figure 17-11 Obstetrical forceps.

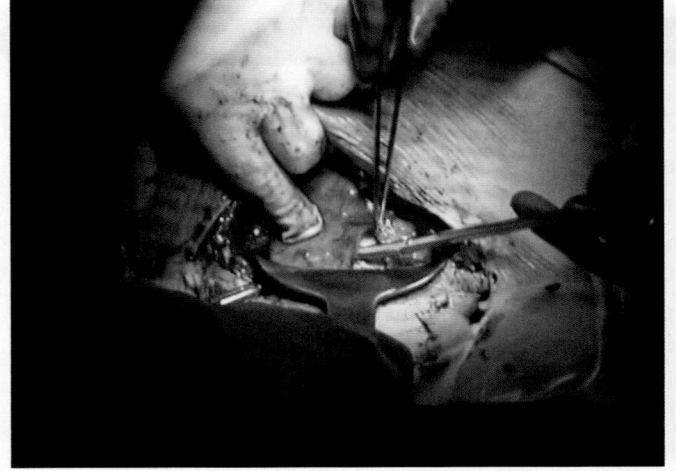

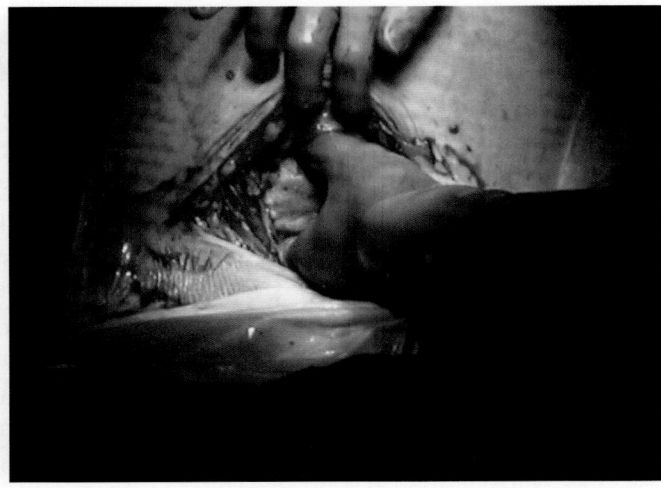

Figure 17-12 Cesarean section: **(A)** incision through the abdominal wall and uterus; **(B)** removal of the fetus from the uterus.

Apgar Scoring Chart			
	Score		
Sign	0	1	2
Heart rate	Absent	Slow (<100)	>100
Breathing	Absent	Slow, irregular; weak cry	Good; strong cry
Muscle tone	Flaccid	Some flexion of extremities	Well flexed
Reflex response			
Response to catheter in nostril	No response	Grimace	Cough or sneeze
or			
Slap of sole of foot	No response	Grimace	Cry and withdrawal of foot
Color	Blue, pale	Body pink, extremities blue	Completely pink

Figure 17-13 Apgar score.

of the term dates back to 715 BCE, when the practice was included under *lex cesarea*, Roman law. It is merely a legend that the procedure was performed at the birth of Julius Caesar in 100 BCE.

Vaginal birth after cesarean (VBAC) is the phrase that describes the birth of a child through the vaginal canal when the mother's previous child was delivered by cesarean section.

At birth, the infant is covered with a cheesy-appearing substance referred to as **vernix caseosa**. The term is derived from the word part *caseo-*, which means "resembling cheese." Immediately after birth, the condition of a newborn baby is assessed in five areas: heart rate, breathing, muscle tone, reflex response, and skin color. This **Apgar score** is a quantitative estimate of the condition of the neonate (newborn) at 1 and 5 minutes after birth. Points are assigned to the quality of the five assessment areas, and each category receives a score ranging from 0 (poor) to 2 (excellent). The Apgar score is the total sum of the five assessment points and 10 is the maximum rating (**Figure 17-13**).

As the infant adjusts to life outside the womb, a number of changes take place. For example, the neonate loses weight within the first 48 hours as fluid shifts occur. The branch of medicine dealing with growth and development of children from birth through adolescence is **pediatrics**. The focus of pediatrics is on care, prevention, and treatment of diseases. The word part *ped-* means "child," so a physician who specializes in pediatrics is a **pediatrician**.

KEY TERM	Definition
effacement (e-FACE-munt)	the thinning out of the cervix just before or during labor
incompetent cervix (in-KOM-puh-tunt SUR-vicks)	condition in which the cervix dilates prematurely before the fetus reaches full term
lightening	sinking or dropping of the fetus into the pelvic inlet
abortion	expulsion of an embryo or fetus from the uterus before it can survive outside the womb
contractions	tightenings of uterine muscles that occur at increasingly frequent intervals immediately before childbirth
vertex (VUR-tecks)	normal birth position of the fetus so that the crown of the head presents first in the cervix and the vaginal canal
breech	fetus positioned so the buttocks and/or feet present first in the cervix and vaginal canal

continued

continued from page 912

KEY TERM	Definition
episiotomy (eh-piz-ee-OT-oh-mee)	surgical incision made in the vagina to enlarge the opening and facilitate childbirth; also called a vaginoperineotomy
pelvimetry (pel-VIM-i-tree)	measurement of the inlet and outlet diameters of the pelvis to determine the feasibility of a vaginal childbirth
obstetric forceps (ob-STET-rick FOR-seps)	instrument resembling tongs used for grasping the fetus's head during delivery
cesarean (se-ZAIR-ee-un) **section (C-section)**	operation to deliver a baby by cutting through the mother's abdomen and uterus
vaginal (VAJ-i-nul) **birth after cesarean** (se-ZAIR-ee-un) **(VBAC)**	vaginal delivery of a baby when the previous birth was by cesarean section
vernix caseosa (VUR-nicks kay-see-OH-suh)	cheesy-appearing deposit on the surface of the fetus
Apgar score	score assessing the condition of a newborn baby in five key areas (heart rate, breathing, muscle tone, reflex response, and skin color)
pediatrics (pee-dee-AT-ricks)	branch of medicine dealing with the care and development of children and with the prevention and treatment of children's diseases
pediatrician (pee-dee-uh-TRISH-un)	physician specializing in the care and development of children and in the prevention and treatment of children's diseases

KEY TERM PRACTICE: *Labor and Delivery*

1. The word part _____ means *vulva* and the word part _____ refers to *incision*, so the surgical incision in the vulva to enlarge the opening and facilitate childbirth is termed _____.

2. A normal birth presentation is termed _____, and a birth in which any part except the head presents first in the cervix is called _____.

3. The score assessing the condition of a newborn baby in five key areas is known as an _____.

4. _____ is the measurement of the inlet and outlet diameters of the pelvis to determine the feasibility of a vaginal childbirth.

5. The expulsion of an embryo or fetus from the uterus before it can survive outside the womb is termed an _____.

Lactation

After delivery, nourishment is delivered to a breastfed newborn by lactation. **Lactation** is the production of milk in the breasts. Hormones influence this process, which is controlled by a positive feedback loop. As the infant suckles at the breast, this action causes secretion known as milk "let down," which in turn causes more infant suckling. Hormones manage this positive feedback loop. Prolactin (PRL), estrogen, and progesterone control milk secretion, and oxytocin causes milk ejection.

The yellowish fluid rich in antibodies and minerals secreted by a mother's breasts after giving birth and before the production of true milk is known as **colostrum**. This "first milk" is produced during the first 2 to 3 days after delivery; thereafter, breast milk is produced. Colostrum contains less fat than breast milk, is richer in protein, and it contains more antibodies, which confer immunity to the newborn. Colostrum also acts as a laxative, assisting in meconium expulsion. **Meconium** is the dark, greenish colored fecal material that collects in the intestines of an unborn baby. This first fecal discharge is composed of epithelial cells, mucus, and bile. The pasty material is expelled 3 to 4 days after birth. If any meconium is detected in the amniotic fluid, it is an indication of fetal distress.

A colostrum-like milk secretion sometimes occurs in the mammary glands of newborn infants of either sex 3 to 4 days after birth, and lasts 1 to 2 weeks. It is sometimes referred to as "witch's milk" and is the result of endocrine stimulation from the mother before birth.

KEY TERM	Definition
lactation (lack-TAY-shun)	production and secretion of breast milk
colostrum (koh-LOS-trum)	first milk produced by the mother's breasts after childbirth
meconium (mee-KOH-nee-um)	dark greenish fecal material that collects in the intestines of a newborn and is released shortly after birth

KEY TERM PRACTICE: *Lactation*

1. _____ is the production and secretion of breast milk; the term is derived from the word part _____, which means *milk*.

2. The first milk produced by lactating breasts is termed _____.

3. _____ is the dark greenish fecal material that collects in the intestines of a newborn and is released shortly after birth.

Artificial Fertilization and Multiple Births

Couples who have been unsuccessful in conceiving a child may choose in vitro fertilization. **In vitro fertilization (IVF)** is the process by which egg cells are fertilized by sperm outside the body. *In vitro* in Latin means literally "in glass," referring in this case to laboratory tools. A female's egg cells are retrieved from the uterine tube and placed in a small circular dish (Petri dish) with male sperm obtained from ejaculate. The cells are cultured and the subsequent zygote is then returned to the uterus for implantation. This artificial culturing medium mimics the natural process, but the zygote must be implanted into a human uterus to nurture a developing embryo and sustain life. Fertilization takes place in an artificial environment, thus popularizing the phrase "test tube baby"; however, this is inaccurate because the process actually occurs in a Petri dish. The first successful test tube baby, Louise Brown, was born in 1978. Physiologist Robert G. Edwards, who developed IVP, won the Nobel Prize in Medicine in 2010 for his achievement. Conversely, fertilization that occurs within the body is termed **in vivo fertilization**, from the Latin phrase that means "in a living being."

Women opting for in vitro fertilization are injected with pregnancy hormones before the zygote is introduced so that the uterus is prepared to nurture a developing embryo. Once implanted, the body recognizes the pregnancy and naturally produces the necessary hormones.

The terms twins, triplets, quadruplets, and quintuplets describe the birth of more than one child in a single pregnancy. Multiple births result when there is more than one fertilized ovum, a separation of zygotes in an early stage, or a division of a zygote at a very early stage. Identical (maternal) twins are **monozygotic twins**, a term used to describe two individuals derived from a single (*mono*) fertilized egg (*zygote*). Monozygotic twins are two individuals of the same sex and identical genetic makeup (**Figure 17-14A**). Twins derived from two zygotes

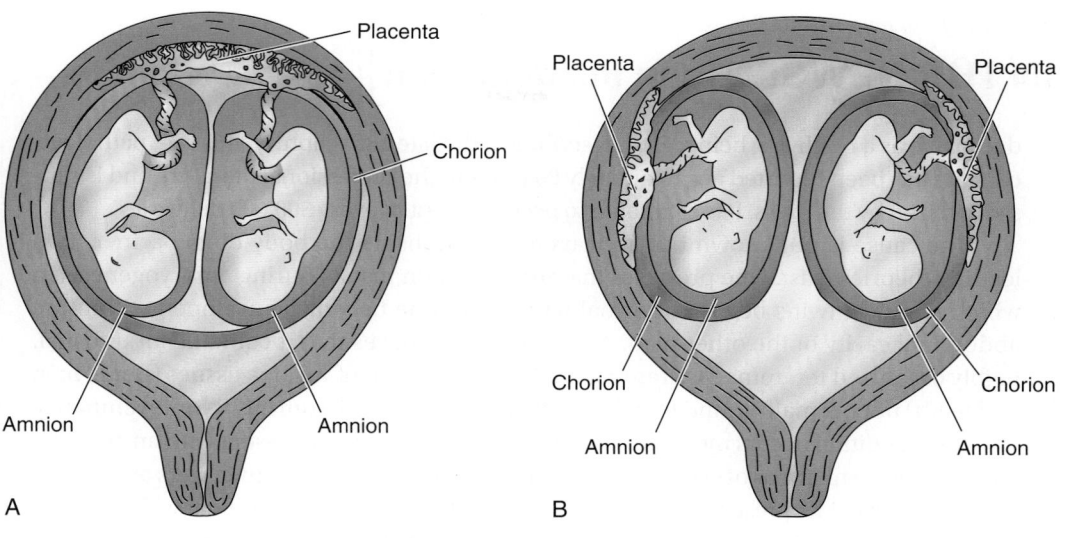

A

B

Figure 17-14 Multiple births: **(A)** monozygotic twins with one placenta, one chorion, and two amnia; **(B)** dizygotic twins with two placentas, two chorions, and two amnia.

are called **dizygotic twins** (fraternal twins). Two placentas are present with dizygotic twins, and the twins look no more alike than any other two siblings born at different times. For this reason, they can be the same or opposite sex (**Figure 17-14B**). Although the reason is not known, naturally occurring multiple births happen at a fairly predictable exponential rate. For example, twins are born at a rate of 1 per 89 births, triplets occur in 1 per 89^2 (or 7,921) births, quadruplets at 1 per 89^3 (or 704,969) births, and quintuplets at a rate of 1 per 89^4 births (or 62,742,241). Fertility medications enhance reproductive function by stimulating follicle development, so the incidence of multiple births increases in women who take fertility drugs.

KEY TERM	Definition
in vitro (VEE-troh) **fertilization (IVF)**	the process by which egg cells are fertilized by sperm outside the body
in vivo (VEE-voh) **fertilization**	fertilization occurring inside the body
monozygotic (mon-oh-zye-GOT-ick) **twins**	two individuals derived from a single fertilized egg; also called identical twins or maternal twins
dizygotic (dye-zye-GOT-ick) **twins**	two individuals derived from two zygotes; also called fraternal twins

KEY TERM PRACTICE: *Artificial Fertilization and Multiple Births*

1. Fraternal twins are also called _____ twins.

2. Two genetically identical individuals are termed _____.

3. _____ is fertilization occurring *inside* the body, while _____ is fertilization *outside* the body.

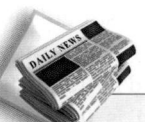

IN THE NEWS: A Twin Inside a Twin

It is a curiosity: A small, imperfectly formed fetus is contained within another fetus. Such cases generally capture the attention of the international news media because of the condition's bizarre nature. In this unusual condition, known as *fetus in fetu*, an abnormally formed fetal mass is contained within the abdomen of a normally developed fetus, and remains

continued

continued from page 915

IN THE NEWS: A Twin Inside a Twin

during life as a nonliving being. First described in the late 18th century, this rare pathological state has been reported approximately 80 times in the professional literature and is sensationalized by the press. It is estimated to occur in 1 out of every 500,000 deliveries.

The cause is not known but appears as a twin inside the body of its partner. Two leading theories exist. One proposes that the condition results during embryogenesis in which identical twins begin as normal fetuses but one becomes enveloped within the abdominal cavity of the other twin. The other theory poses that it could be an unusual, highly organized teratoma. A teratoma is a tumor made up of various tissues (bone, hair, and teeth) not normally found together and probably derived from embryonic remnants.

The condition occurs more commonly in males, who usually present with an abdominal mass by the first year of age, although cases have been reported in teenagers and adults. CT studies reveal its presence, typically located on the posterior abdominal wall. In some cases, the discovered mass has weighed as much as 4.4 lb (2 kg), and one was 30 cm (11.8 in.) in length! Descriptions are varied, ranging from well-developed extremities with hair covering the entire body to bone, cartilage, teeth, fat, and muscles found in masses of tissue.

Patients present with localized pain. Signs and symptoms include abdominal distention, vomiting, feeding difficulty, and dyspnea related to mass size. The fetus in fetu mass size can increase, causing hemorrhage. Intra-abdominal fetus in fetu is self-contained in a sac with no major vascular connections to the host. In cases in which the host is unaware of the mass, the fetus in fetu is attached to significant vessels and appears to grow with the host. CT scans confirm the presence of a vertebral column in the internal mass, a distinguishing feature of the condition. Chromosomal analyses are normal and identical to the host. Surgical excision of the mass is recommended because of the potential for impaired renal function and malignancy.

Developmental Stages

Life after birth proceeds through various phases. A newborn infant is termed a **neonate** during the first month of life. During this time, metabolism and oxygen consumption increase.

At birth, the first breath must be quite forceful because the infant's lungs are fluid-filled and collapsed. A recently discovered master gene may actually initiate the first breath, which should come within 30 seconds to 1 minute after delivery. Stored fat is the newborn's primary energy source for the first few days after birth. Wastes are also eliminated. During this time, the kidneys excrete relatively dilute urine. Furthermore, the neonate has a limited ability to regulate body temperature, so body temperature typically fluctuates.

The first year of life is called **infancy** or babyhood. Muscle coordination develops, and the head is still disproportionately large—approximately one-fourth the total body height. The infant birth weight doubles during the first 4 months, and it triples by 1 year.

Infancy is distinguished by several benchmarks. By the end of the second month, the infant is able to follow a moving object with his or her eyes. At 6 months, deciduous (first) teeth may appear, and by 12 to 18 months, the spinal lumbar curvature appears.

Childhood is the time between infancy and puberty. Although many changes occur during this period, two of the most profound are the establishment of bladder control and the development of the nervous system. **Puberty** is a sequence of events by which a child becomes a young adult. The onset of puberty is marked by increased production of gonadotropin-releasing hormone (GnRH), increased circulating levels of follicle-stimulating hormone (FSH) and luteinizing hormone (LH), and increased sensitivity of ovarian and testicular cells to FSH and LH. At puberty, the reproductive organs are functional. In girls, the first signs of puberty occur after age 8 with the process largely completed by age 16. Females generally begin menstruation by age 12. In boys, normal puberty begins at age 9 and is largely completed by age 18.

The period from puberty to adulthood is **adolescence**. **Adulthood** is the period of life after adolescence. The process of aging, termed **senescence**, describes all the changes that an individual undergoes after maturity. Senescence ends with death.

KEY TERM	Definition
neonate (NEE-oh-nate)	an infant age 1 month or younger; also called a newborn
infancy	the first year of life; also called babyhood
childhood	period of life between infancy and puberty
puberty	sequence of events by which a child becomes a young adult
adolescence	period of life from puberty to maturity
adulthood	period of life after adolescence
senescence (se-NES-ence)	process of aging

KEY TERM PRACTICE: *Developmental Stages*

1. _____ is the term for a newborn, derived from the word part _____ meaning *new*.

2. _____ describes the aging process.

3. The period of life between infancy and puberty is termed _____.

4. _____, also called babyhood, is the first year of life.

5. The sequence of events by which a child becomes a young adult is called _____.

Inheritance

An elementary understanding of gene and chromosome interaction is fundamental to understanding inheritance and genetic disorders. So, let's briefly turn our attention to genes, genotypes, phenotypes, chromosomes, and sex chromosomes. We are who we are because of the passage of genetic material in the form of DNA from one generation to the next. **Genes** are made up of DNA strands, and the genetic makeup of a person is the *genotype*. The genotype determines the *phenotype*, which are observable characteristics such as brown hair and green eyes. A **chromosome** is a rod-shaped structure located in a cell's nucleus that carries the genes. The transmission of genetically controlled characteristics and qualities from parent to offspring is called **inheritance**. Chromosomes carry the genes that determine not only sex (gender) but all the characteristics an individual inherits from his or her parents. A photomicrograph in which a cell's chromosomes are arranged according to size and classification is called a *karyotype* (**Figure 17-15**).

Human cells each contain 46 chromosomes, or 23 pairs of chromosomes. The chromosomes of the 23rd pair are called **sex chromosomes**, and these sex chromosomes (designated X and Y) are the pair that determines an individual's gender. Males are designated XY because their pair of sex chromosomes consist of one X chromosome and one Y chromosome; females are XX because they have two X chromosomes. The Y chromosome of the male sperm determines the sex of an offspring, and this chromosome is slightly smaller than the X chromosome. With respect to mature sperm cells, 50% possess an X chromosome and 50% a Y chromosome (**Figure 17-16**). It is interesting that sperm containing a Y chromosome swim faster than sperm with an X chromosome, perhaps because the Y chromosome is lighter.

Other terms related to genetics are dominant and recessive. *Dominant genes* control a particular trait, and their effects appear in the offspring's phenotype. Dominant genes inhibit

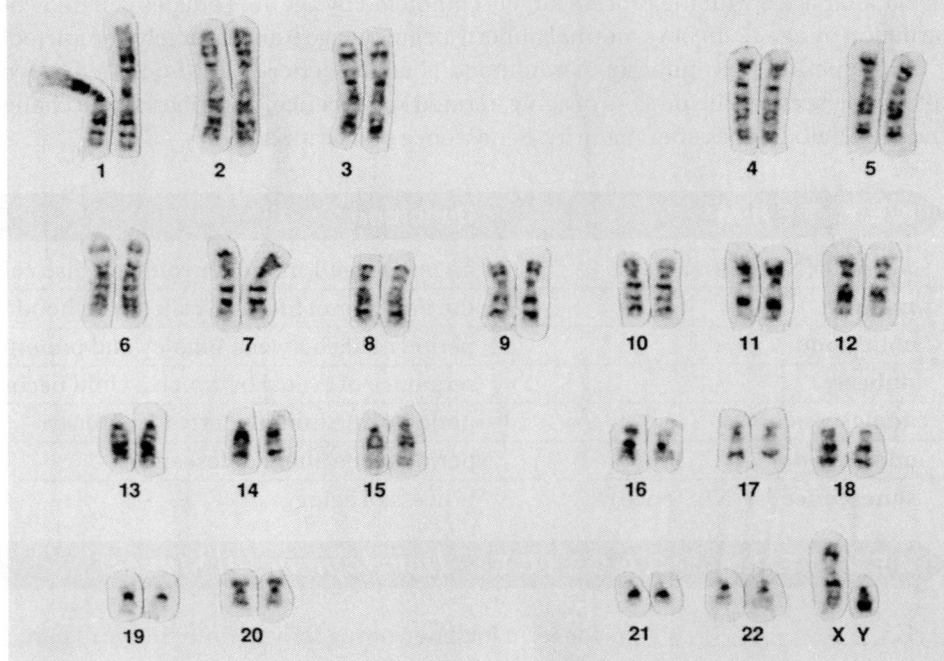

Figure 17-15 A karyotype of human chromosomes.

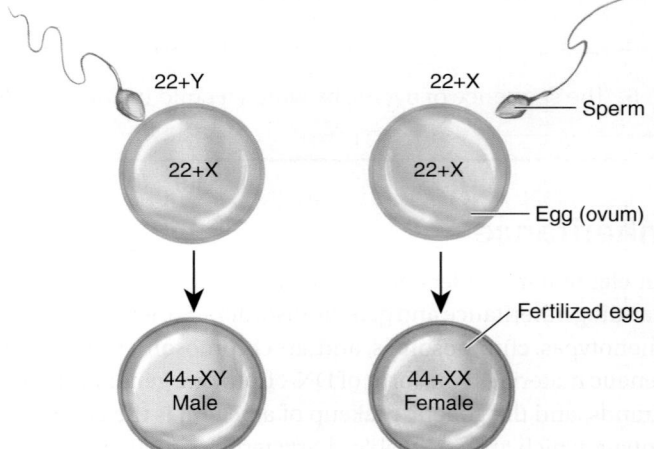

Figure 17-16 Inheritance of gender. Each ovum contains 22 autosomes (chromosomes that do not determine sex) and an X chromosome. Each spermatozoon (sperm) contains 22 autosomes and either an X chromosome or a Y chromosome. The gender of the zygote is determined at the time of fertilization by the combination of the sex chromosomes of the sperm (either X or Y) and the ovum (X).

the expression of recessive genes. A gene that is not expressed is termed a *recessive gene*. The effects of recessive genes do not appear in the offspring because the dominant gene masks them. As the name implies, **sex-linked inheritance** is a term for the traits that result from a gene located on either the X or Y chromosome. Males express more recessive sex-linked traits than females because they have only one X chromosome, and the Y chromosome contains fewer genes than the X chromosome. Red-green color blindness is an example of a sex-linked trait.

Another type of inheritance that pertains to the sex cells is holandric inheritance. The transmission of genes located on a segment of the Y chromosome for which there is no matching region on the X chromosome is known as **holandric inheritance** (also called Y-linked inheritance). These genetic traits are carried on the Y chromosome and therefore can be inherited only by males.

Mutations occurring at the genetic level often result in genetic disease. **Mutations** are random changes in genes caused by changes in the DNA. A mutation can be beneficial, harmful, or it can have neutral effects.

Genetic diseases are categorized into three main groups on the basis of the timing of the gene's expression. The first classification includes disorders with effects that occur during embryonic or fetal development. The newborn exhibits characteristics of the disease. Conditions that affect metabolic processes and that are expressed post partum make up the second group. An example of a postpartum effect is seen in phenylketonuria (PKU), a condition in which the body lacks the enzyme to metabolize phenylalanine. It is detected at birth. If left untreated, PKU results in developmental deficiencies, seizures, and tumors. Group three is reserved for conditions that have effects that appear during adolescence or adulthood. Examples include hypercholesterolemia and diabetes mellitus.

KEY TERM	Definition
genes	strands of DNA that function as hereditary units
chromosome	rod-shaped structure in the cell nucleus that carries the genes
inheritance	characteristics and qualities transmitted from parent to offspring through genes
sex chromosomes	23rd pair of chromosomes, designated X and Y, that determines gender
sex-linked inheritance	genetic traits that result from a gene located on either the X or Y chromosome
holandric (hol-AN-drick) **inheritance**	genetic traits carried on the Y chromosome inherited only by males; also called Y-linked inheritance
mutations	random changes in genes caused by changes in the DNA

KEY TERM PRACTICE: *Inheritance*

1. Traits that result from a gene located on either the X or Y chromosome are termed _____.

2. _____ are random changes in genes caused by changes in the DNA.

3. The term for characteristics and qualities transmitted from parent to offspring through genes is _____.

4. Also called Y-linked inheritance, the genetic traits carried on the Y chromosome and only inherited by males are known as _____.

5. A _____ is a rod-shaped structure in the cell nucleus that carries the genes.

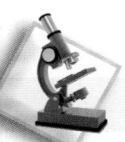

THE CLINICAL DIMENSION

Pathology associated with pregnancy, human development, and childhood results from various factors. Some of these factors are not known or fully understood. Abnormal conditions include disorders of pregnancy, congenital disorders, prematurity and related consequences, syndromes, and infectious childhood diseases.

Conditions of Pregnancy

gestational diabetes mellitus (GDM)   **Gestational diabetes mellitus (GDM)** is a condition in which pregnant women develop the inability to appropriately metabolize carbohydrates, resulting in hyperglycemia, commonly called high blood sugar. Polyuria (excessive urination), polydipsia (excessive thirst), and polyphagia (frequent eating), the classic signs of diabetes mellitus, are frequently absent with GDM, and women are often asymptomatic. For this reason pregnant women are routinely screened.

A common test evaluating circulating blood glucose levels is the **2-hour postprandial glucose test**. (The term *postprandial* means "occurring after a meal.") About 2 hours after ingesting a concentrated glucose solution, the glucose level of maternal blood is tested. Normal values are between 70 and 140 mg/dL. Elevated levels indicate possible diabetes mellitus.

Risk factors for GDM include a history of birthing babies over 10 pounds, obesity, maternal age over 30 years, family history of diabetes mellitus, and previous stillbirths. Although the condition resolves after delivery, women with GDM are at increased risk of developing type 2 diabetes later in life.

hydatidiform mole

A **hydatidiform mole** is a rare mass with swollen chorionic villi that forms inside the uterus at the beginning of a pregnancy (**Figure 17-17**). It is also known as molar pregnancy, derived from the word *molar* meaning "mass." Signs and symptoms include nausea, vomiting, vaginal bleeding, anemia, unusually large uterus for gestational period, absence of fetal heart sounds, edema, and hypertension. Elevated hCG levels and an ultrasound showing no fetal skeleton are used for diagnosis. Uterine suction and dilation and curettage are treatments. **Dilation and curettage (D&C)** is a surgical procedure in which the cervix is dilated and the uterine wall is scraped to remove extra tissue. The extracted tissue is examined for malignant cells. The woman is closely monitored for 1 year and advised against pregnancy during this time. When hCG levels and uterine tissue returns to normal, pregnancy may be attempted. In some cases, hysterectomy is necessary.

choriocarcinoma

A malignant, aggressive cancer of the uterus is **choriocarcinoma** (**Figure 17-18**). It originates in the cells of the chorion and may follow any type of pregnancy especially a hydatidiform mole. It requires surgical excision and chemotherapy.

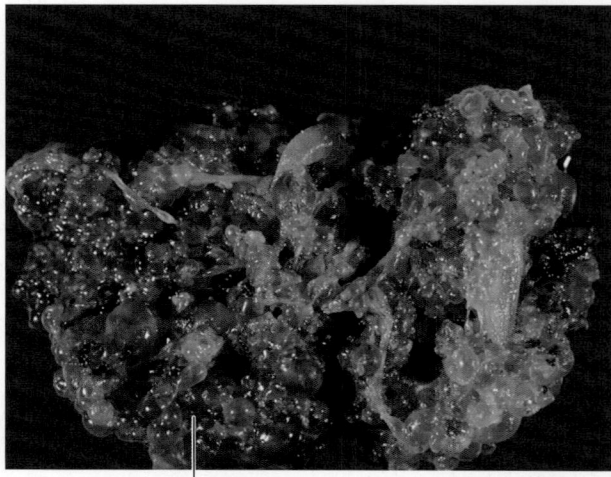

Figure 17-17 Hydatidiform mole. Note the grape-like swollen chorionic villi.

Grape-like edematous chorionic villi

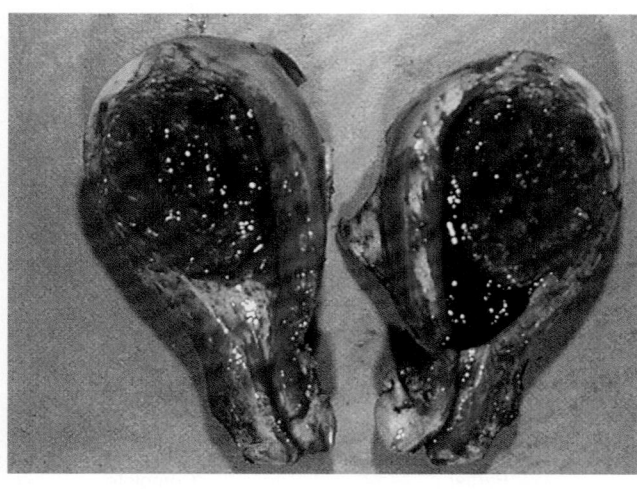

Figure 17-18 Choriocarcinoma. The endometrial cavity is filled with a soft, markedly hemorrhagic tumor.

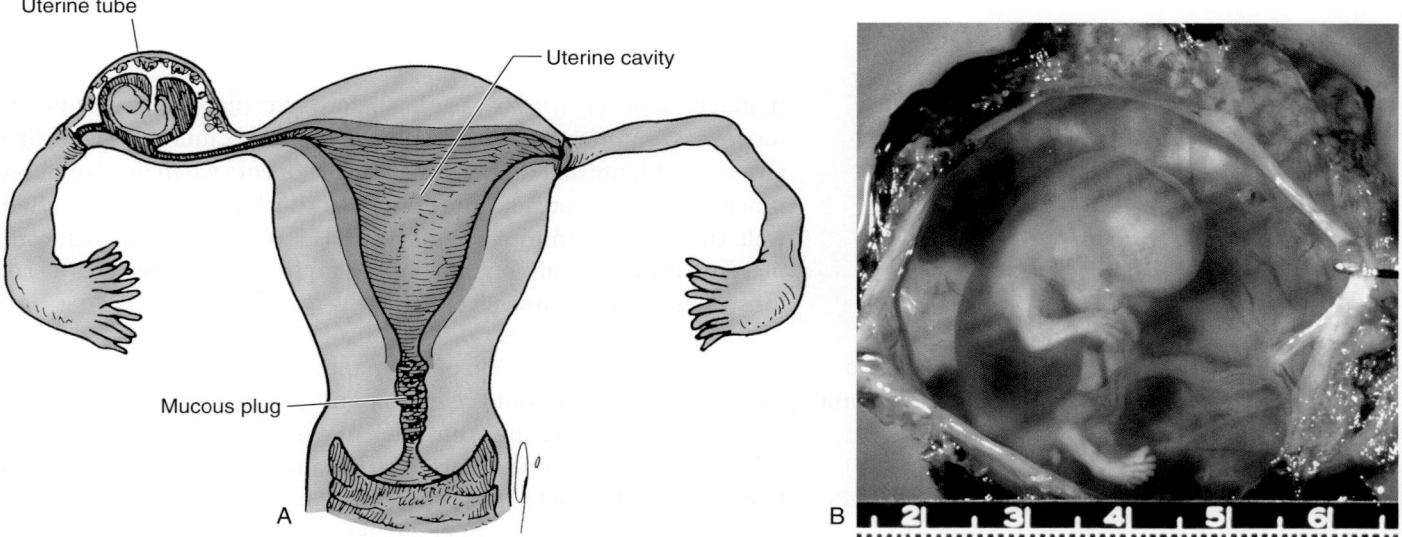

Uterine tube

Uterine cavity

Mucous plug

A

B

Figure 17-19 **(A)** An ectopic pregnancy located where the ampulla of the uterine tube narrows to join the isthmus. **(B)** An enlarged uterine tube has been opened to disclose a minute fetus.

chorioangioma	A benign tumor of the placental blood vessels is termed **chorioangioma**. It is usually of no clinical significance and expels with the placenta after childbirth.
ectopic pregnancy	In an extrauterine pregnancy, called an **ectopic pregnancy**, a fertilized ovum develops at an abnormal location outside the uterine cavity, often in the uterine tube (**Figures 17-19A and B**). Ectopic pregnancies are never viable and must be surgically removed. The risk increases in women who douche regularly and in those with pelvic inflammatory disease (PID). Nearly 95% of ectopic pregnancies occur in the uterine tube.
abruptio placentae	**Abruptio placentae** is the premature detachment of the placenta from the uterine wall. It usually occurs around month 5. Bleeding can lead to anemia, shock, or kidney failure. Fetal mortality rate is high.

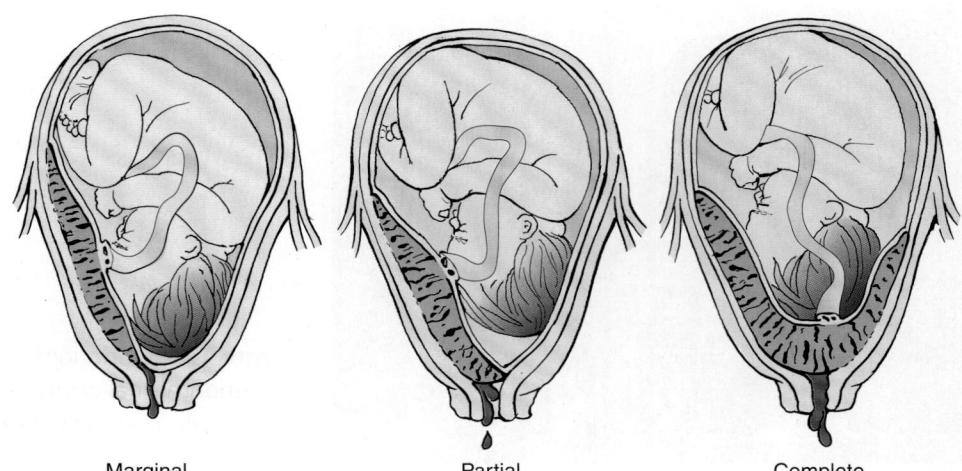

Figure 17-20 Three classifications of placenta previa.

Marginal   Partial   Complete

placenta previa	In **placenta previa** (*previa* = going before), the placenta is positioned too low, oftentimes over the opening of the cervix into the vagina, interfering with normal delivery of a baby. It occurs when implantation is near the cervix instead of the upper two-thirds portion of the uterine wall. Ultrasound confirms the diagnosis (**Figure 17-20**). Women with placenta previa remain on total bed rest until the fetus reaches a size for successful cesarean delivery.
preeclampsia and **eclampsia (toxemia of pregnancy)**	**Preeclampsia** is a condition of pregnancy characterized by hypertension, oftentimes with fluid retention and proteinuria (protein in the urine). It occurs after the 20th week of gestation. It may result from substances secreted by the placenta that cause dysfunction of the inner lining of blood vessels. It is a dangerous complication of pregnancy and may affect both the mother and fetus. **Eclampsia**, also called **toxemia of pregnancy**, is an acute, life-threatening complication of pregnancy. It is characterized by hypertension, proteinuria, edema, sodium retention, convulsions, and sometimes coma. It occurs in women who have developed preeclampsia disease occurring in the latter half of pregnancy. An emergency C-section may be ordered to save the life of the mother and/or fetus.
premature birth	A **premature birth** occurs when the infant is born after the stage of viability, but before 37 weeks' gestation. The infant also has a birth weight of at least 500 g (1.1 lb.). There is a difference between premature birth and abortion. Abortion occurs when an embryo or fetus is removed from the womb before its independent survival (viability) is possible.
stillbirth	A **stillbirth** occurs when a woman gives birth to an infant who has died before delivery.

KEY TERM	Definition
gestational diabetes mellitus (GDM) (jes-TAY-shun-ul dye-uh-BEE-teez muh-LYE-tus)	inability to metabolize carbohydrates, resulting in hyperglycemia, that occurs only during pregnancy
2-hour postprandial (pohst-PRAN-dee-ul) **glucose test**	test that determines blood glucose levels 2 hours after drinking a sugar solution
hydatidiform (high-duh-TID-ih-form) **mole**	rare mass that forms inside the uterus at the beginning of a pregnancy
dilation and curettage (kewr-e-TAHZH) **(D&C)**	surgical procedure involving expansion of the cervix and scraping of the uterus to remove extra tissue
choriocarcinoma (koh-ree-oh-kahr-si-NOH-muh)	malignant, aggressive cancer of the uterus originating from cells of the chorion
chorioangioma (koh-ree-oh-an-jee-OH-muh)	benign tumor of the placental blood vessels
ectopic (eck-TOP-ick) **pregnancy**	development of the fertilized egg outside the uterus
abruptio placentae (ab-RUP-tee-oh pluh-SEN-tee)	condition in which the placenta prematurely separates from the uterine wall
placenta previa (pluh-SEN-tuh PREE-vee-uh)	condition in which the placenta is positioned at the opening of the uterine cervix in the vagina, interfering with normal delivery
preeclampsia (pree-ih-KLAMP-see-uh)	condition of pregnancy characterized by hypertension, oftentimes with fluid retention and proteinuria
eclampsia (ih-KLAMP-see-uh)	acute, life-threatening complication of pregnancy characterized by hypertension, proteinuria, convulsions, and sometimes coma that occurs in women who have developed preeclampsia; also called toxemia of pregnancy
toxemia (tock-SEE-mee-uh) **of pregnancy**	acute, life-threatening complication of pregnancy characterized by hypertension, proteinuria, convulsions, and sometimes coma that occurs in women who have developed preeclampsia; also called eclampsia
premature birth	birth that occurs when the infant is born after the stage of viability, but before 37 weeks' gestation
stillbirth	birth of an infant who has died before delivery

KEY TERM PRACTICE: *Conditions of Pregnancy*

1. An acute, life-threatening complication of pregnancy characterized by hypertension, proteinuria, convulsions, and sometimes coma that occurs in women who have developed preeclampsia is known as _____ or _____.

2. A condition of pregnancy characterized by hypertension, oftentimes with fluid retention and proteinuria, is termed _____.

3. A _____ is the birth of an infant who has died before delivery.

4. The development of the fertilized egg outside the uterus is called an _____.

5. _____ is a condition in which the placenta is positioned at the opening of the uterine cervix in the vagina, interfering with normal delivery.

Genetic Disorders

albinism

Albinism is an inherited disorder characterized by the absence of melanin (dark pigment) in the hair, skin, and eyes (see **Figure 4-4**). It results from defective metabolism of tyrosine, the precursor molecule to melanin. It is associated with several ocular abnormalities and visual defects.

cystic fibrosis (CF)

A genetic disease, characterized by dysfunction of exocrine glands, is **cystic fibrosis (CF)**. Cystic fibrosis presents as a disease primarily of the digestive and respiratory systems as thick mucus clogs pancreatic ducts, intestines, and bronchi, often resulting in respiratory infections. The mucus is abnormally thick because of impaired chloride ion transport.

The gene for CF is found on chromosome 7. Research suggests that carriers (individuals with the gene for the trait but who are not affected by the disorder) are protected against cholera. Genetic counseling is indicated for couples who are carriers or who have a family history of CF.

severe combined immunodeficiency (SCID)

Severe combined immunodeficiency (SCID) is a disorder characterized by an absence of immunity. This leads to increased infections because of the poor immune response.

This disorder is treated with bone marrow stem cell transplants from a matched donor. If detected early enough, SCID may be curable. Unfortunately, because screening for SCID is not routine, the disease is frequently well advanced by the time it is diagnosed. In progressive cases, the child must live life in a sterile environment (plastic bubble) and typically dies young.

phenylketonuria (PKU)

Phenylketonuria (PKU) is a metabolic disorder in which there is a deficiency of an enzyme necessary for the metabolism of the amino acid, phenylalanine, to another important amino acid, tyrosine. This deficiency results in an accumulation of phenylalanine in the blood, tissues, and urine, impairing early neuronal development. Untreated forms lead to mental retardation, eczema (skin inflammation with itching), fair hair, and seizures.

Newborns are automatically screened by the **Guthrie test**, which detects the presence of phenylalanine in the blood. Treatment includes dietary monitoring of phenylalanine. Protein intake is restricted because this amino acid is a natural part of many proteins. Because diet sodas often contain phenylalanine, a warning for individuals with PKU appears on the label (see **Figure 14-22**).

Tay–Sachs disease

A genetic disease characterized by an abnormal lipid accumulation in the brain and nerves that leads to tissue damage is **Tay–Sachs disease**. It principally affects individuals of eastern European Jewish heritage. Tay–Sachs disease is caused by a deficiency of, or defect in, a particular enzyme. It results in loss of sight and other brain functions. Signs and symptoms appear within the first 3 to 6 months of age and include abnormal startle reaction, decreased axial muscle tone, and blindness. There is no cure. Death occurs at 3 to 5 years of age.

KEY TERM	Definition
albinism (AL-bi-niz-um)	hereditary absence of melanin in the hair, skin, and eyes
cystic fibrosis (CF) (SIS-tick-figh-BROH-sis)	hereditary disease of infancy affecting various exocrine glands and characterized by thick mucus that clogs ducts and airways
severe combined immunodeficiency (SCID)	congenital disorder characterized by an absence of immunity
phenylketonuria (PKU) (fen-il-kee-toh-NEW-ree-uh)	genetic disease in which the body lacks the enzyme to metabolize phenylalanine
Guthrie test	test that determines the level of phenylalanine in the serum of a neonate to detect PKU
Tay–Sachs (SACKS) **disease**	genetic disease marked by accumulation of lipids in nervous tissue affecting people of eastern European Jewish ancestry

KEY TERM PRACTICE: *Genetic Disorders*

1. Identify the genetic disease that results from the absence of the enzyme that metabolizes phenylalanine.
   _____

2. Name the genetic disease that is characterized by an accumulation of lipids in the nervous system and affects individuals of eastern European Jewish descent. _____

3. The _____ is a test that determines the level of phenylalanine in the serum of a neonate to detect PKU.

4. _____ is a hereditary absence of melanin in the hair, skin, and eyes.

5. A hereditary disease of infancy affecting various exocrine glands and characterized by thick mucus that clogs ducts and airways is termed _____.

Congenital Syndromes

A syndrome is a group of signs and symptoms that when considered together are characteristic of or indicate a specific disease or other disorder. Many syndromes are endocrine diseases but are described here because they are genetic disorders that are present at birth.

Several tests exist to detect congenital disease, including the α-fetoprotein serum test, amniocentesis, and chorionic villus sampling. Alpha (α)-fetoprotein (AFP) is a protein produced by a fetus that is present in the amniotic fluid and bloodstream of the mother. The **α-fetoprotein serum test** is used to identify possible congenital defects. Normal adult levels are below 40 ng/mL. α-fetoprotein peaks between the 16th and 18th gestational weeks. Elevated levels occur in women carrying fetuses with Down syndrome, anencephaly, and spina bifida.

An **amniocentesis** is a transabdominal procedure in which fluid is extracted from the amniotic sac. The test is done between the 15th and 18th gestational weeks to determine chromosomal abnormalities and the health, sex, and genetic constitution of a fetus by withdrawing fetal cells in the amniotic fluid through a needle inserted into the womb of the mother (**Figure 17-21**). Analysis of amniotic fluid is often used to look for Tay–Sachs disease, hemophilia, sickle cell anemia, and Down syndrome.

Another invasive procedure is **chorionic villus sampling (CVS)** or **chorionic villus biopsy (CVB)**, a prenatal test for genetic analysis that is carried out by examining cells from the villi of the chorion, which has the same DNA as the fetus (**Figure 17-22**). The tiny outgrowths (villi) are withdrawn through a needle inserted into the vagina under guided ultrasound. This test

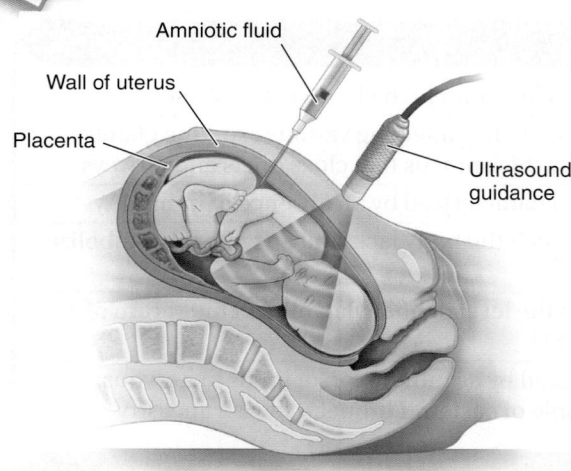

Figure 17-21 Amniocentesis is a test performed by withdrawing fetal cells from the amniotic fluid through a needle inserted into the womb of the mother.

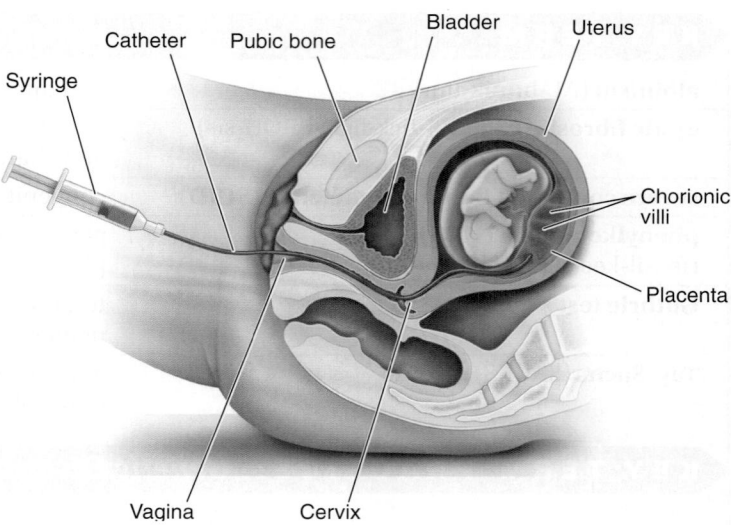

Figure 17-22 Chorionic villus sampling is a test performed by withdrawing cells from the villi of the chorion through a needle inserted into the vagina.

can be performed sooner than an amniocentesis (as soon as the second month of pregnancy), and the results are obtained faster than amniocentesis results. With CVS, there is danger that the amniotic sac will not seal and fluid leakage will occur, resulting in loss of pregnancy. The CVS test is also linked to limb abnormalities in the newborn.

Cri-du-chat syndrome

Cri-du-chat syndrome is a disorder characterized by problems of the larynx and nervous system. It is also called *cat's cry syndrome* because the cry of affected infants sounds like a meowing cat. Other signs and symptoms include difficulty swallowing and sucking; low birth weight; cognitive, speech, and motor delays; and unusual facial features. It is caused by deletion of the short arm of one of the number 5 chromosomes. The clinical picture, the presence of the characteristic cat-like cry, and a karyotype study demonstrating chromosomal abnormality lead to the diagnosis. The only treatment is supportive.

Down syndrome

Down syndrome, or trisomy 21, results from a chromosomal disorder. The syndrome is caused by trisomy of chromosome 21. Trisomy refers to the fact there is a triplet instead of a pair of chromosomes. Signs and symptoms include mild to severe mental retardation, multiple structure defects, and characteristic facial features such as small head with flat skull back, eye slant, low-set ears, simian line (horizontal crease) across the palm, and short stubby fingers (**Figures 17-23 A and B**). It is also associated with heart defects. It occurs more often in babies borne to women over age 35, and a mother's chance of producing a trisomic child increases dramatically just before menopause. Severe forms are diagnosed at birth, while milder forms are evident later. It can also be detected in utero using CVS or amniocentesis. The presence of white dots on the iris and a karyotype confirm the diagnosis. There is no cure. A multifaceted approach is used to enhance the quality of life and maximize motor skills and mental development. The life expectancy has improved because of surgical interventions for heart defects.

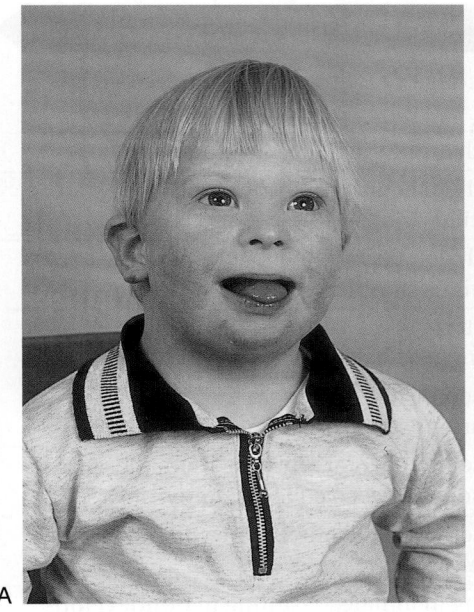
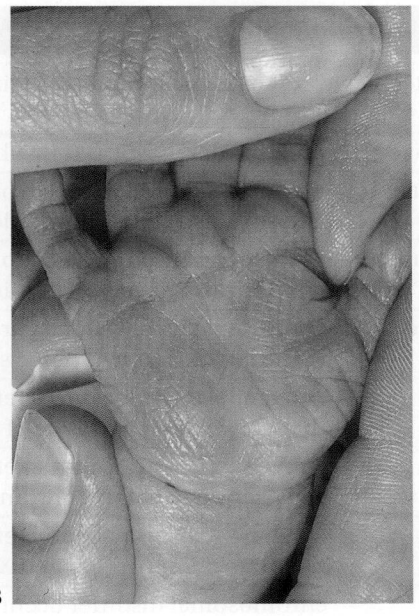

Figure 17-23 Typical features of a child with Down syndrome: **(A)** facial features; **(B)** horizontal palm crease (simian line).

Edwards syndrome

A syndrome caused by a triplet of chromosome 18 is **Edwards syndrome**, or trisomy 18. It results from a mistake in meiosis called nondisjunction (failure of paired chromosomes to separate during cell division). The incidence of Edwards syndrome increases as the mother's age of conception increases. Heart defects, kidney malformations, and other internal organ abnormalities are common, leading to a low survival rate. There is no cure and death usually occurs within 2 to 3 years.

Klinefelter syndrome

Klinefelter syndrome is a chromosomal disorder in which the individual has a chromosome count of 47 caused by an extra X chromosome (XXY sex chromosomes). The person is considered to be male, but the extra X chromosome leads to decreased testosterone production. The syndrome is characterized by a constellation of abnormal conditions, including hypogonadism (small testes) and gynecomastia (breast presence in males). Individuals with the syndrome are generally tall and thin and are sterile. The disease results from nondisjunction. History and physical examination provide the initial diagnosis. Semen analysis indicating lack of sperm production and a karyotype confirming the presence of an extra X chromosome provide conclusive evidence for the disorder. Treatment includes long-term hormone therapy starting at puberty and continued throughout life to maintain other normal physiological development and sexual function. Currently, no treatment exists to restore sperm production.

Turner syndrome

Turner syndrome is an inherited chromosomal disorder with a chromosome count of 45. The individual has a single female sex chromosome, referred to as monosomy, designated XO. The ovaries are not functional. The cause is nondisjunction of the X chromosome. The absence of one of the two X chromosomes results in an underdeveloped uterus, vagina, and breasts and causes infertility. The condition may not be recognized at birth. It is diagnosed by a karyotype demonstrating only one X chromosome instead of two. There is no treatment to restore fertility, but hormone therapy is prescribed to reduce other physiological signs and symptoms.

KEY TERM	Definition
α-fetoprotein (AL-fuh-fee-toh-PROH-teen) **serum test**	protein marker test for certain congenital defects
amniocentesis (am-nee-oh-sen-TEE-sis)	prenatal diagnostic test in which amniotic fluid is evaluated
chorionic villus (koh-ree-ON-ick VIL-us) **sampling (CVS)**	prenatal test used to detect birth defects by analyzing cells of the chorion; also called chorionic villus biopsy
chorionic villus (koh-ree-ON-ick VIL-us) **biopsy (CVB)**	prenatal test used to detect birth defects by analyzing cells of the chorion; also called chorionic villus sampling
cri-du-chat (kree–due–shah) **syndrome**	congenital defect with a characteristic cat-like cry caused by problems of the larynx and nervous system; also called cat's cry syndrome
Down syndrome	congenital disorder characterized by mild to severe mental retardation that occurs from a tripling of chromosome 21; also called trisomy 21
Edwards syndrome	congenital disorder characterized by several physical anomalies caused by a tripling of chromosome 18; also called trisomy 18
Klinefelter syndrome	congenital disorder characterized by male phenotype with an extra X chromosome, designated XXY
Turner syndrome	chromosomal disorder occurring in females resulting in nondevelopment of reproductive organs, designated XO

KEY TERM PRACTICE: *Congenital Syndromes*

1. What syndrome is characterized by each of the following genotypes?

   a. XXY _____

   b. XO _____

2. Provide an alternate medical term for each of the following syndromes.

   a. trisomy 18 _____

   b. trisomy 21 _____

3. The prenatal test used to detect birth defects by analyzing cells of the chorion is called _____ or _____.

4. _____ is a prenatal diagnostic test in which amniotic fluid is evaluated.

5. A congenital defect with a characteristic cat-like cry caused by problems of the larynx and nervous system is known as _____.

Nongenetic Syndromes

Two nongenetic syndromes are fetal alcohol syndrome and Reye syndrome. Both are caused by environmental factors.

fetal alcohol syndrome (FAS)   **Fetal alcohol syndrome (FAS)** is a condition involving a pattern of malformation that affects infants born to women who drank excessive amounts of alcohol during pregnancy. Various birth defects include facial abnormalities, strabismus (crossed eyes), and learning difficulties. Other common signs are small size for gestational age (SGA), microcephaly (small head), and mental retardation (**Figure 17-24**). The physical examination

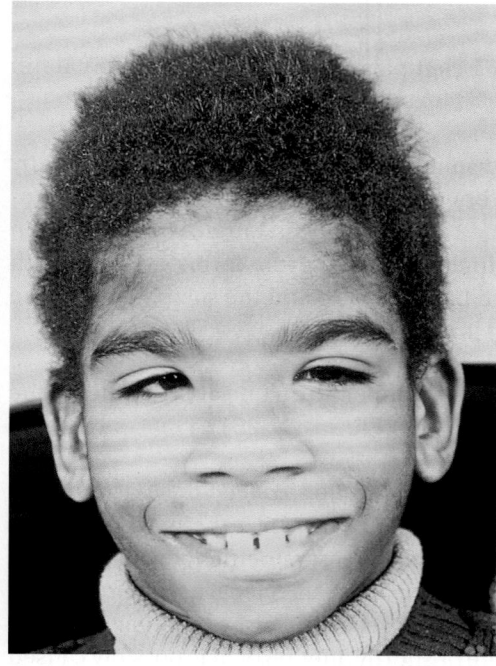

Figure 17-24 Fetal alcohol syndrome. Note the facial abnormalities and strabismus.

and a history of maternal alcohol abuse confirm the diagnosis. Damage to the brain is permanent, so treatment for children with FAS is supportive. Because no safe levels of alcohol intake in pregnant women have been established, pregnant females are advised to consume no alcohol.

Reye syndrome

Reye syndrome is an acute illness of childhood with unknown cause, which usually follows a respiratory, gastrointestinal, or varicella (chickenpox) infection. Signs include fever, encephalitis (brain swelling), and liver failure. It has been associated with aspirin use, but it also occurs when aspirin was not used. Early diagnosis is critical. History, physical examination, and elevated serum ammonia levels are used to diagnose it. Treatment includes hospitalization for medical management, surveillance, and rapid intervention. Because aspirin has been implicated with the onset of Reye syndrome, it is recommended that children not be given aspirin.

KEY TERM	Definition
fetal alcohol syndrome (FAS)	pattern of malformation found among children of mothers who abused alcohol while pregnant
Reye syndrome	acute childhood illness of unknown cause that follows a respiratory or varicella infection and results in encephalitis and liver failure

KEY TERM PRACTICE: *Nongenetic Syndromes*

1. The syndrome that affects children of mothers who consumed large quantities of alcohol while pregnant is

_____.

2. _____ is an acute illness of unknown cause that affects children after a bout of chickenpox or respiratory infection and results in encephalitis and liver failure.

Congenital Bone Disorders

Several congenital disorders affect bones, including cleft palate, cleft lip, developmental hip dysplasia, and talipes equinovarus.

cleft palate	**Cleft palate** is a congenital split in the roof of the mouth, caused by failure of embryonic facial bones to fuse. Cleft palate is a multifactorial genetic disorder affecting 1 in 10,000 births. Surgical repair as soon as possible is the best treatment. Mild to severe forms exist in which the division extends through both the hard and the soft palate into the nose, often resulting in cleft lip.
cleft lip	**Cleft lip** is a congenital split in the upper lip on one or both sides of the center associated with a cleft palate (**Figure 17-25**).
developmental hip dysplasia	**Developmental hip dysplasia** (also called *congenital hip dysplasia* [CHD]) is a birth defect of the hip joint in which the newborn's hips easily become dislocated. Signs include asymmetric folds in the thigh of a newborn with limited abduction of the affected leg. A shortened femur is evident when the knees are flexed. The cause is unknown, but the abnormality is obvious before or shortly after birth. It is possibly caused by ligament shortening that occurs from the maternal secretion of relaxin. Developmental hip dysplasia is more common in females and babies born breech. It is diagnosed by a positive Ortolani test, a physical assessment maneuver that detects hip dysplasia (**Figure 17-26**). Physical examination and x-rays confirm the diagnosis. It is treated by manipulation of the femoral head into the acetabulum. The joint may require splinting, casting, or surgery.

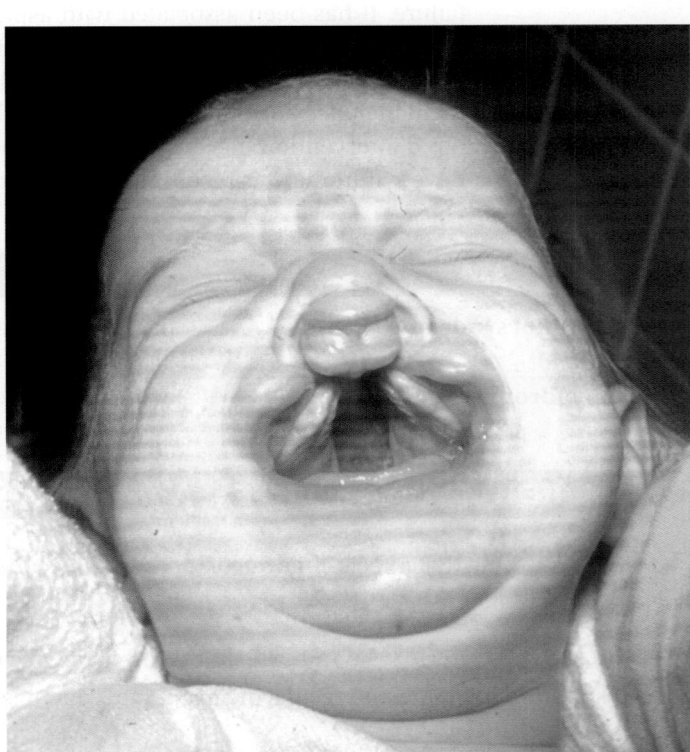

Figure 17-25 Cleft lip and cleft palate in an infant.

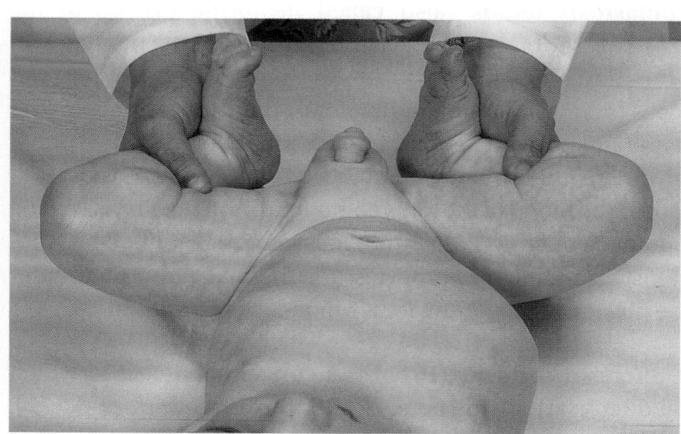

Figure 17-26 Examining the hips of a newborn using the Ortolani test.

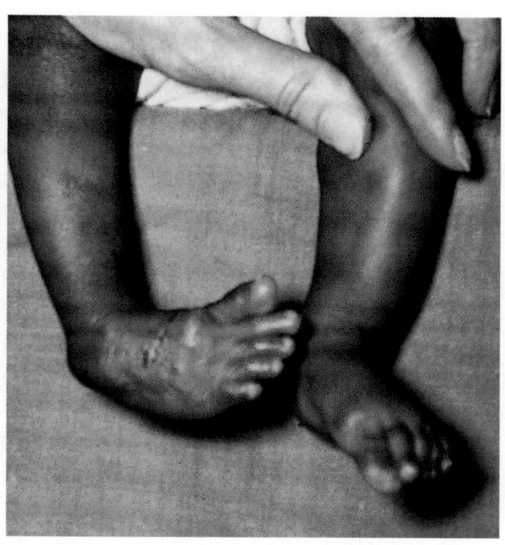

Figure 17-27 Talipes equinovarus.

talipes equinovarus or clubfoot

Talipes is the medical term for any deformity of the foot involving the talus bone. One form of talipes is **talipes equinovarus**, commonly called *clubfoot*. It is characterized by a foot that is rotated internally at the ankle (**Figure 17-27**). It affects 1 in every 1,000 births, and its cause is thought to be fetal position while in utero, but genetic factors have been implicated. It occurs in more males than females and, without treatment, the person must walk on the sides of their feet. Treatment options include casting, splinting, and orthopedic surgery if necessary.

KEY TERM	Definition
cleft palate	congenital split in the roof of the mouth, caused by failure of embryonic facial bones to fuse
cleft lip	congenital split in the upper lip on one or both sides of the center associated with a cleft palate
developmental hip dysplasia (dis-PLAY-zhuh)	birth defect of the hip joint in which the newborn's hips easily become dislocated; also called congenital hip dysplasia (CHD)
talipes (TAL-i-peez)	any deformity of the foot involving the talus bone
talipes equinovarus (TAL-i-peez ee-kwye-noh-VAY-rus)	congenital foot deformity in which the foot is rotated internally at the ankle; also called clubfoot

KEY TERM PRACTICE: *Congenital Bone Disorders*

1. A congenital split in the roof of the mouth, caused by failure of embryonic facial bones to fuse, is known as a

   _____.

2. Any deformity of the foot involving the talus bone is termed _____.

3. _____ is a congenital foot deformity in which the foot is rotated internally at the ankle.

4. A birth defect of the hip joint in which the newborn's hips easily become dislocated is called _____.

5. A congenital split in the upper lip on one or both sides of the center associated with a cleft palate is termed

   _____.

Congenital Blood and Cardiac Disorders

erythroblastosis fetalis or hemolytic disease of the newborn

Erythroblastosis fetalis (also called *hemolytic disease of the newborn*) is a serious blood disease of fetuses and neonates in which the antibodies produced by Rh⁻ mothers destroy the red blood cells (erythrocytes) of an Rh⁺ fetus. It can occur only in Rh⁺ fetuses and infants who are borne to Rh⁻ mothers who have previously given birth to an Rh⁺ child (or who have been sensitized to Rh⁺ blood). The blood of the fetus contains an antigen that is lacking in the mother's blood, so this stimulates maternal antibody formation against the infant's erythrocytes, and these maternal antibodies cross the placenta to enter the fetus's blood (see **Figure 10-18**).

patent ductus arteriosus (PDA)

Patent ductus arteriosus (PDA) is a congenital defect in which the fetal ductus arteriosus persists after birth (see **Figure 11-16**). (*Patent* means open.) The ductus arteriosus is a fetal structure that directs blood from the left pulmonary artery to the descending aorta. Its failure to close permits oxygenated blood to recirculate to the lungs instead of going to the rest of the body. A murmur with thrills (vibrations) when palpated confirms the diagnosis. Treatment consists of antiprostaglandin drugs to close the opening or surgery to correct the condition. It is common in premature infants.

atrial septal defect (ASD)

Atrial septal defect (ASD) is an abnormal opening between the left atrium and the right atrium that causes oxygenated arterial blood to be mixed with unoxygenated venous blood (see **Figure 11-15**). If the hole is small, the signs and symptoms are fatigue, dyspnea, and infections. A large hole is marked by cyanosis (blue coloration due to lack of oxygen), dyspnea (shortness of breath), and syncope (fainting). A murmur (blowing or roaring sound) can be heard with the stethoscope. Atrial septal defect is associated with premature birth and patent ductus arteriosus (failure of the fetal shunt connecting the pulmonary artery to the aorta arch to close). Surgery is needed to correct the condition.

coarctation of aorta

Narrowing of the aorta that causes partial blood flow obstruction is termed **coarctation of aorta** (see **Figure 11-14**). The condition results in increased left ventricular pressure and decreased blood pressure distal to the constriction. Signs and symptoms may not be evident until adolescence. When present, they include left ventricular failure, pulmonary edema, cyanosis, dyspnea, and tachycardia (increased heart rate). Surgical treatment is aimed at creating a clear passage within the aorta.

tetralogy of Fallot

The term *tetralogy* refers to "four related items." **Tetralogy of Fallot** is a congenital heart defect with a combination of four abnormalities (see **Figure 11-18**). The first is pulmonary stenosis, or tightening of the pulmonary valve. Right ventricular hypertrophy, which is caused by increased pressure in the right ventricle, is the second. Ventricular septal defect, an abnormal opening between the ventricles, is the third aberration; and an overriding aorta is the fourth. The overriding aorta is a displacement of the aorta so that it crosses (overrides) the ventricular septum and receives both venous and arterial blood. Infants born with the condition exhibit cyanosis because the atrial blood is not fully oxygenated; thus they appear blue. Hypoxia (low oxygen levels), tachycardia, tachypnea, and dyspnea are also present. It is diagnosed by the history and physical examination demonstrating finger and toe clubbing, delayed growth, and other signs common to the separate conditions. Surgical treatment is necessary.

transposition of great arteries

The reversal of the aorta and pulmonary artery that results in two closed-loop systems in the newborn is termed **transposition of great arteries**. In this condition, the aorta originates from the right (instead of the left) ventricle and the pulmonary artery originates from the left (instead of the right) ventricle. Neonates are cyanotic and have tachypnea. Heart failure ensues unless surgical measures are immediately initiated to correct the anomalies.

ventricular septal defect

Ventricular septal defect is a congenital defect of the heart septum between the left and right ventricles, characterized by an abnormal opening that allows blood to shunt from the higher pressure left ventricle to the lower pressure right ventricle (see **Figure 11-19**). It is heard as a murmur with a stethoscope. Signs include increased heart and respiratory rates and failure to gain weight. Surgery is necessary to correct the defect.

KEY TERM	Definition
erythroblastosis fetalis (e-rith-roh-blas-TOH-sis fee-TAY-lis)	blood disease in which maternal antibodies attack the developing red blood cells of the fetus; also called hemolytic disease of the newborn
patent ductus arteriosus (PDA) (DUCK-tus ahr-teer-ee-OH-sus)	presence of ductus arteriosus after birth that causes oxygenated blood to recirculate to the lungs instead of the rest of the body
atrial septal defect (ASD)	abnormal opening between the left atrium and right atrium
coarctation (koh-ark-TAY-shun) **of aorta** (ay-OR-tuh)	narrowing of the aorta causing blood flow obstruction
tetralogy (te-TRAL-uh-jee) **of Fallot** (fah-LOH)	congenital heart defect with four abnormalities
transposition of great arteries	rotation of the aorta and the pulmonary artery resulting in two closed-loop systems
ventricular (ven-TRICK-yoo-lur) **septal defect**	abnormal opening between the left ventricle and the right ventricle

KEY TERM PRACTICE: *Congenital Blood and Cardiac Disorders*

1. _____ is the congenital heart defect characterized by four cardiac anomalies, and is derived from the word part _____ meaning *four*.

2. An abnormal opening between the left atrium and the right atrium is termed _____.

3. The rotation of the aorta and the pulmonary artery resulting in two closed-loop systems is known as _____.

4. An abnormal opening between the left ventricle and the right ventricle is called _____.

5. The presence of ductus arteriosus after birth that causes oxygenated blood to recirculate to the lungs instead of the rest of the body is known as _____.

Congenital Neuromuscular System Disorders

Pathology of the nervous system tends to be serious. Several congenital nervous system disorders are described here.

anencephaly

A tragic condition in which a fetus or infant lacks the cerebrum, cerebellum, and flat bones of the skull is called **anencephaly** (**Figure 17-28**). Because these critical structures are absent, the fetus usually dies before birth, during the birth process, or shortly afterward. It results from a failure of the cephalic neural tube to close during the second or third week of prenatal development. There is a familial occurrence pattern, and the condition is more common in females. Ultrasound and increased α-fetoprotein (AFP) levels diagnose anencephaly before birth. There is no treatment.

cerebral palsy (CP)

Another congenital nervous system disorder is cerebral palsy. **Cerebral palsy (CP)** is a generic term for various types of non-progressive motor conditions causing physical disability that are present at birth or beginning in early childhood. Causes are both hereditary and acquired and involve damage to the motor control area of the brain. The classes depend on the cause and are grouped as intrauterine, natal, and early postnatal. Signs include paralysis (two, three, or four limbs), muscular weakness, abnormal body movements, and uncoordinated muscle movement (**Figure 17-29**). It is diagnosed by the clinical picture and accompanying neurological examination. There is no cure, so treatment is aimed at achieving maximum function. Palliative measures, muscle relaxants, and anticonvulsive drugs may be warranted.

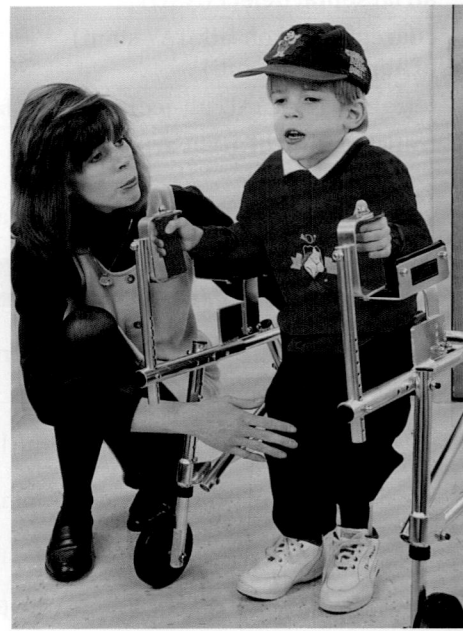

Figure 17-29 Neuromuscular weakness is a hallmark of cerebral palsy.

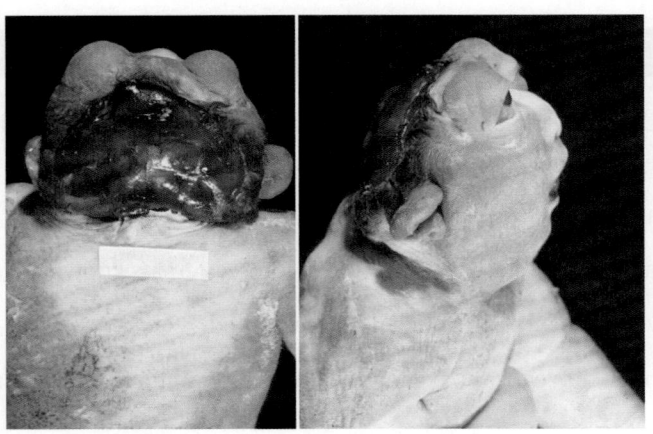

Figure 17-28 An infant with anencephaly.

hydrocephalus

Hydrocephalus is a condition marked by excessive cerebrospinal fluid (CSF) accumulation in the brain ventricles, enlarging the head and sometimes causing brain damage (see **Figure 7-17**). (The term *hydrocephalus* literally means "water on the brain.") It results from an obstruction in the subarachnoid space that prevents CSF from circulating or being properly absorbed. The abnormal increase in CSF around the brain results in infant head enlargement because the bones of the skull are still not fused. In addition to head enlargement, other signs and symptoms are bulging fontanelles (soft spots between infant skull bones), high-pitched crying, and abnormal leg muscle tone. Hydrocephalus is caused by fetal head trauma, blood clot, premature birth, and infection. The outward appearance and clinical picture lead to the initial diagnosis, which is confirmed by CT or MRI scans. Treatment involves the placement of shunts to drain the excess fluid. Shunt catheters are positioned to empty either into the peritoneal cavity (ventriculoperitoneal shunt) or the right atrium (ventriculoatrial shunt) (**Figures 17-30 A** and **B**).

spina bifida

Spina bifida occurs when one or more of the vertebral arches fails to close and a part of the spinal cord and its meninges protrudes through the opening. It results from incomplete closure of the neural tube. Partial or total paralysis of the lower body is common. The herniated (protruding) portion contains cerebrospinal fluid and sometimes nervous tissue. It occurs primarily in the lumbosacral region.

Spina bifida is associated with maternal exposure to ionizing radiation during embryonic and fetal life. It is diagnosed by amniocentesis revealing an elevated α-fetoprotein level. Prenatal ultrasonography is also useful for diagnosing purposes. Visual

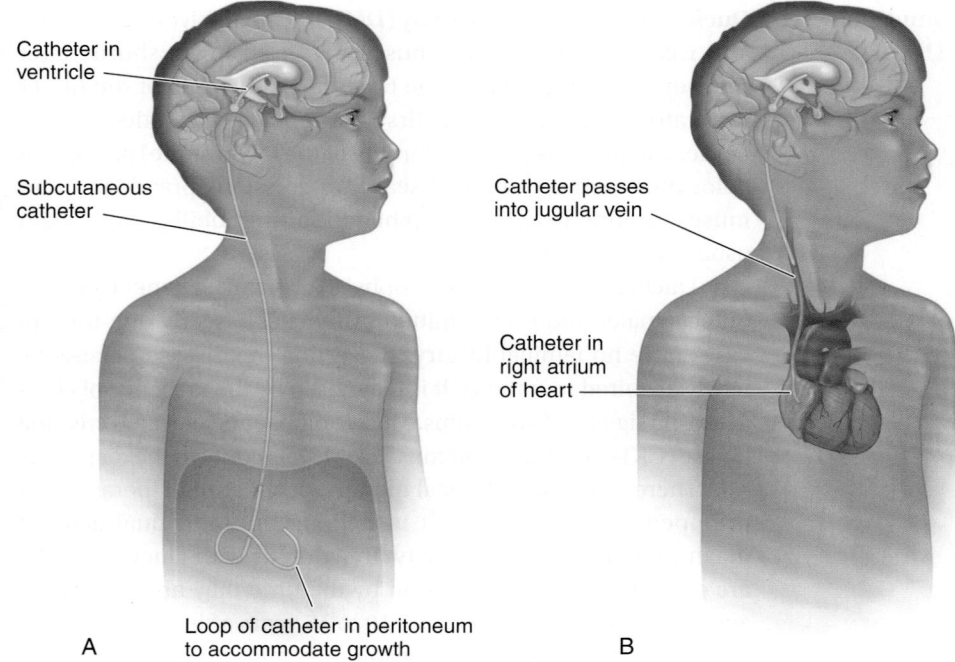

Catheter in ventricle

Subcutaneous catheter

Loop of catheter in peritoneum to accommodate growth

A

Catheter passes into jugular vein

Catheter in right atrium of heart

B

Figure 17-30 Shunt placements for the correction of hydrocephalus. **(A)** A ventriculoperitoneal shunt drains excess fluid from the lateral ventricle into the peritoneal cavity. **(B)** A ventriculoatrial shunt drains into the right atrium of the heart, where the excess fluid is pumped into the bloodstream.

inspection and x-ray examination after birth may reveal the disease. If the individual is asymptomatic, it may never be discovered.

The asymptomatic form is termed *spina bifida occulta* (hidden), and the only obvious sign may be a tuft of hair located on the skin overlying the defect. Some forms are treated by surgery.

meningocele

The protrusion of the meninges through an opening in the skull or vertebra to form a CSF-filled cyst is termed a **meningocele**. Skin overlying the region of defect may be tender (see **Figure 7-16**). The cause is unknown but may be influenced by genetic and environmental factors. It is diagnosed by physical examination and confirmed by radiographic studies. Surgery within 48 hours of birth is recommended to treat the deformity.

congenital megacolon or Hirschsprung disease

Congenital megacolon (also called *Hirschsprung disease*) is a disorder in which ganglionic cells of the enteric nervous system are missing from the colon, resulting in colon enlargement. The enteric nervous system is made up of ganglionic cells scattered throughout the intestines that control functions such as peristalsis and defecation. The disorder is characterized by the inability to defecate as a result of ganglion cell absence. The accumulation of feces causes colon enlargement, signified by the term *megacolon*. The first sign is the failure of meconium to be expelled. Other indications are a distended abdomen, failure to thrive, constipation, and vomiting. Congenital megacolon affects more males than females, and the risk increases with Down syndrome. It is diagnosed by history and physical examination and an x-ray of the bowel. Tissue biopsy confirms the absence of ganglionic cells. Treatment is surgical removal of the affected bowel portion and then reuniting the segments of functional bowel. A colostomy (temporary opening made in the abdomen to function as an anus) is necessary while the resectioned bowel heals. Untreated forms lead to impaired growth.

Duchenne muscular dystrophy (DMD)

Duchenne muscular dystrophy (DMD) is progressive degeneration and weakening of skeletal muscles with an onset shortly after birth or some time before age 6. It affects muscles of the upper respiratory and pelvic areas first. Fat replaces atrophied muscle tissue, and lordosis (inward curving of the lower spine) and spinal deformities are common. Disease progression spreads to other muscle groups resulting in debilitation, immobility, and death usually in adolescence.

Duchenne muscular dystrophy is an X-linked genetic disease (affects males and is transmitted by females). Nearly one-third of cases have no familial history, suggesting the disease persists by newly acquired mutations. It is diagnosed by the presence of characteristic signs and symptoms. Muscle biopsy and elevated creatine kinase (CK)—an enzyme in muscles—levels confirm the diagnosis.

There is no cure. Physical therapy, occupational therapy, and orthopedic appliances assist in helping the individual achieve maximum functioning capacity. Individuals with Duchenne MD are generally wheelchair bound by the time they are 12 years of age. The average survival rate is 10 to 15 years after disease onset. Death results from cardiac or respiratory failure.

KEY TERM	Definition
anencephaly (an-en-SEF-uh-lee)	condition in which a fetus or infant lacks the cerebrum, cerebellum, and flat bones of the skull
cerebral palsy (CP) (se-REE-brul PAWL-zee)	generic term for various types of nonprogressive motor conditions causing physical disability that are present at birth or beginning in early childhood
hydrocephalus (high-droh-SEF-uh-lus)	condition marked by excessive cerebrospinal fluid accumulation in the brain ventricles, enlarging the head and sometimes causing brain damage
spina bifida (SPYE-nuh BIH-fih-duh)	condition in which one or more of the vertebral arches fails to close and a part of the spinal cord and its meninges protrudes through the opening
meningocele (meh-NING-goh-seel)	cerebrospinal fluid–filled cyst formed from the protrusion of the meninges through an opening in the skull or vertebra
congenital megacolon	disorder in which ganglionic cells of the enteric nervous system are missing from the colon, resulting in colon enlargement; also called Hirschsprung disease
Duchenne (doo-SHAYN) **muscular dystrophy** (DIS-truh-fee) **(DMD)**	X-linked degenerative disease marked by skeletal muscle weakening with an onset shortly after birth or some time before age 6

KEY TERM PRACTICE: *Congenital Neuromuscular System Disorders*

1. The word part *an-* means _____ and the word part _____ refers to *the brain*, so _____ is absence of the brain.

2. The word part _____ means *water* and the word part *cephal-* means _____, so _____ is fluid accumulation on the brain causing the head to bulge.

3. A _____ is a CSF-filled cyst formed from the protrusion of the meninges through an opening in the skull or vertebra; it is derived from the word part _____ meaning *meninges*.

4. _____ is a generic term for various types of nonprogressive motor conditions causing physical disability that are present at birth or beginning in early childhood.

5. A condition in which one or more of the vertebral arches fails to close and a part of the spinal cord and its meninges protrudes through the opening is termed _____.

Premature Infant

premature infant   An infant born before the 37th gestational week is termed a **premature infant** (**Figure 17-31**). Within a health care setting, these infants are often referred to as *preemies*. There is a medical difference between babies born small and premature infants. **Small for gestational age (SGA)** infants are not premature, but rather designated as low-birth-weight infants. Oftentimes the cause of premature birth is unknown, and multiple fetuses account for 15% of all preterm births. Other conditions leading to preterm births include diabetes, heart disease, poor nutrition, uterine defects, and preeclampsia.

Because a premature infant's organs are not fully developed, they require special neonatal care. Premature infants often have several

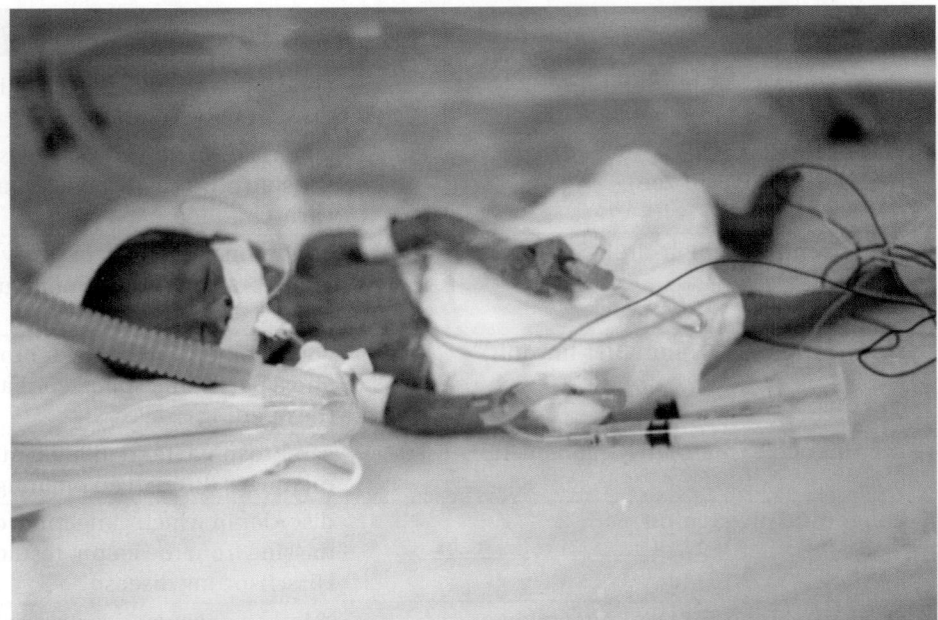

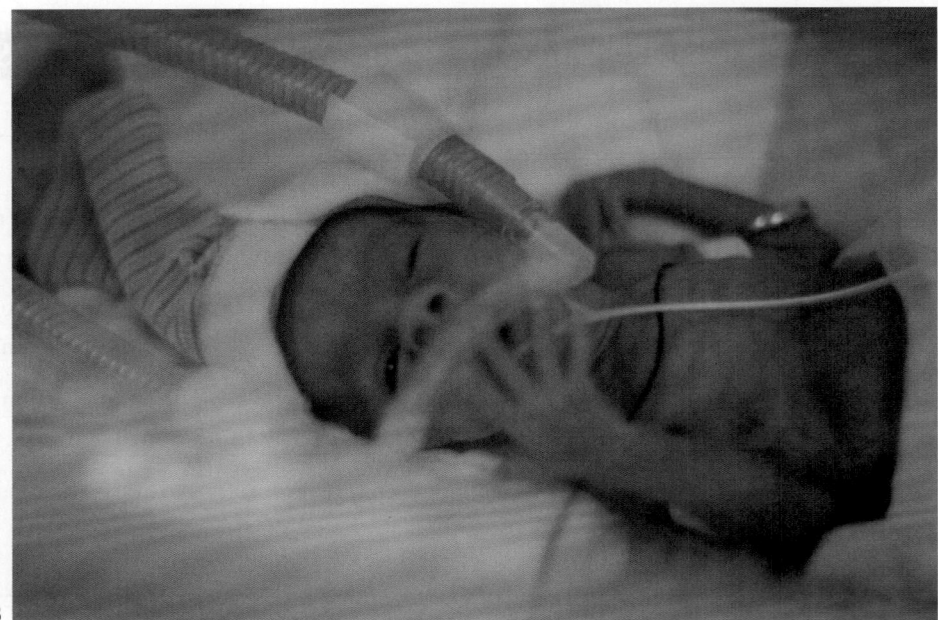

Figure 17-31 An infant born 15 weeks premature, at 25 weeks of gestation. **(A)** The infant at 2 weeks, weighing 1 lb (0.45 kg), 5.5 oz (162.7 mL). **(B)** The infant at 5 weeks, weighing 1 lb (0.45 kg) 11.5 oz (340.1 mL). Note the wedding ring encircling the infant's left arm.

coexisting conditions, and the treatment of each depends on the underlying cause. Airway management and pulmonary function need to be established. Supplemental oxygen flow that is required to sustain life often causes retinopathy of prematurity (ROP), a condition that can lead to blindness. Known measures to prevent premature births include adequate nutrition intake, appropriate prenatal care, no smoking or alcohol use, and addressing other known risk factors.

infant respiratory distress syndrome (IRDS)

Infant respiratory distress syndrome (IRDS) is a disease seen in premature neonates that is associated with reduced amounts of lung surfactant. It is characterized by respiratory distress, cyanosis, collapse of alveoli (tiny air sacs in the lungs), and loss of pulmonary surfactant (a natural substance that prevents alveoli from sticking together). Abnormal hyaline membrane (thin, clear membrane) lines alveoli and alveolar ducts when the disease persists longer than a few hours. For this reason it is also known as *hyaline membrane disease of the newborn.*

Signs and symptoms include nasal flaring, grunting respirations, and ineffective gas exchange. It is diagnosed by the heightened respiratory rate, which is a compensatory mechanism to increase gas exchange, and blood gas studies indicating the potential for poor tissue oxygenation. Chest x-rays demonstrate the presence of hyaline membranes.

Treatment involves restoring respiratory function as soon as possible, aerosol infusion of surfactant (lipoprotein that decreases surface tension to prevent alveoli from sticking together), or delivery of surfactant through an endotracheal tube to the pulmonary structures. Infants treated for IRDS are predisposed to developing bronchopulmonary dysplasia (discussed below).

Prevention is the best measure. When a premature birth is imminent, the mother may be injected with a corticosteroid to stimulate the fetus's surfactant-synthesizing system.

bronchopulmonary dysplasia (BPD)

A chronic pulmonary insufficiency affecting premature infants who required oxygen therapy is **bronchopulmonary dysplasia (BPD)**. It is typically seen in infants who required positive pressure ventilation (a form of mechanical ventilation) Signs are overinflated lungs and lobular emphysema that are revealed on chest x-rays. Other signs and symptoms include dyspnea, tachypnea (rapid breathing rate), wheezing, cyanosis, sternal retractions (sucking in of the skin around the ribs and top of the sternum), and cracking sounds heard through auscultation. The oxygen pressure delivered to the young lungs to sustain life irreversibly damages the bronchial tree. Abnormal arterial blood gases (ABGs), lung scarring, and decreased lung oxygen levels with increased lung carbon dioxide levels confirm the diagnosis.

Supportive treatment is given as new alveoli continue to develop until about age 8 years. Bronchodilators, nutrition, anti-inflammatory drugs, theophylline (vasodilator and smooth muscle relaxant that opens bronchial airways), anticholinergic drugs, and diuretics are given. Diuretics decrease fluid accumulation, thereby lessening the incidence of pulmonary hypertension (increased blood pressure in the pulmonary circuit). Nutritional demands increase because the infant expends a great deal of energy in the process of breathing. There are no preventive measures, but the infant should be weaned as early as possible from mechanical ventilation.

retinopathy of prematurity (ROP)

Premature infants placed in a high-oxygen environment are at risk of developing an oxygen-induced disease of the eye termed **retinopathy of prematurity (ROP)**. It is marked by abnormal replacement of the sensory retina with fibrous tissue and blood vessels. There are no obvious signs or symptoms, but retina-screening studies should be initiated in these infants beginning at 4 to 6 weeks. Because retina vessels develop around the 28th gestational week, premature infants born before this critical time are at the highest risk of developing ROP. The lower the birth weight and the more premature the infant is, the greater the possibility.

Careful monitoring of oxygen delivery is essential. Oxygen-saturation levels and titration concentrations should be adjusted to achieve the best possible outcome. Artificial lighting also increases the risk in premature infants. Ophthalmoscopic evaluation or scleral depression (procedure in which an instrument is slid behind the eyeball to view the retina) is used for diagnosis. Mild forms are self-limiting and the condition resolves with no further treatment. In other situations, laser therapy may be used to cauterize abnormal vasculature. Severe cases result in blindness.

necrotizing enterocolitis (NEC)

Necrotizing enterocolitis (NEC) is extensive ulceration (open sores) and necrosis (tissue death) of the ileum and colon in premature infants during the neonatal period. It is possibly due to intestinal ischemia and bacterial invasion. Signs and symptoms include feeding intolerance, distended abdomen, diarrhea, bloody stool, bile-colored vomit, and decreased or absent bowel sounds. Although the cause is unknown, it is thought to result from an abnormal defense response that allows normal bacteria to invade the intestinal mucosa. Blood shunts away from the intestines causing ischemia. Normal mucus production also diminishes, exposing the intestinal lumen.

Treatment is immediate and aggressive. The infant receives nothing by mouth (abbreviated NPO for *non per os*), gastric contents are emptied via nasogastric (NG) tube, and intravenous (IV) fluids with antibiotics are administered. Drinking breast milk confers some immunity. Close monitoring is essential because many infants die from NEC.

KEY TERM	Definition
premature infant	infant born before the 37th gestational week
small for gestational age (SGA)	refers to a low-birth weight infant who is not premature
infant respiratory (RES-pi-ruh-tohr-ee) **distress syndrome (IRDS)**	disease seen in premature neonates associated with reduced amounts of lung surfactant; also called hyaline membrane disease of the newborn
bronchopulmonary dysplasia (BPD) (brong-koh-PUL-moh-nair-ee dis-PLAY-zhuh)	a chronic pulmonary insufficiency affecting premature infants who required oxygen therapy
retinopathy (ret-i-NOP-uh-thee) **of prematurity (ROP)**	oxygen-induced disease of the eye marked by abnormal replacement of the sensory retina with fibrous tissue and blood vessels
necrotizing enterocolitis (NEC) (NECK-roh-tize-ing en-tur-oh-koh-LYE-tis)	extensive ulceration (open sores) and necrosis (tissue death) of the ileum and colon in premature infants during the neonatal period

KEY TERM PRACTICE: *Premature Infant*

1. An oxygen-induced disease of the eye blood vessels marked by abnormal replacement of the sensory retina with fibrous tissue and blood vessels is termed _____.

2. An infant born before the 37th gestational week is termed a _____ infant.

3. _____ is extensive ulceration (open sores) and necrosis (tissue death) of the ileum and colon in premature infants that occurs during the neonatal period.

4. _____ refers to a low-birth weight infant who is not premature.

5. _____ is a chronic pulmonary insufficiency affecting premature infants who required oxygen therapy.

Infectious Diseases of Childhood

Infectious diseases are caused by a microbial agent, such as a bacterium or virus, and can be passed from one person to another. Fortunately, **vaccines**, which are biological preparations that produce immunity, exist for many diseases that otherwise would cause illness. Through a rigorous immunization program that begins in infancy, people have become resistant to particular diseases. **Immunizations** and **vaccinations** are synonymous terms describing vaccines given to protect against certain diseases by stimulating an immune response through the activation of antibodies. The antibodies formed in response to the stimulation confer immunity against particular infectious agents.

Table 17-1 gives the recommended immunization schedule for persons ages 0 through 6 years. Diseases of children ages 0 through 6 years that are prevented through immunizations include:

- Hepatitis B
- Rotavirus
- Diphtheria, tetanus, pertussis
- *Haemophilus influenzae* type b
- Pneumonia
- Polio
- Influenza
- Measles, mumps, rubella
- Varicella
- Hepatitis A
- Meningitis

Table 17-2 gives the recommended immunization schedule for persons ages 7 through 18 years. Immunizations for this population include:

- Tetanus, diphtheria, pertussis
- Human papillomavirus (HPV)

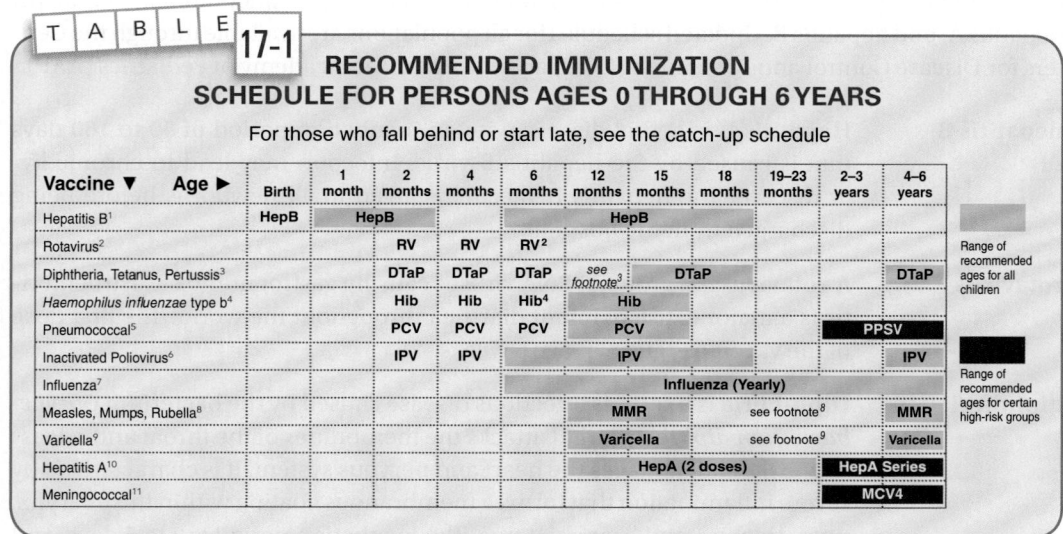

TABLE 17-1 RECOMMENDED IMMUNIZATION SCHEDULE FOR PERSONS AGES 0 THROUGH 6 YEARS

For those who fall behind or start late, see the catch-up schedule

Vaccine ▼ Age ▶	Birth	1 month	2 months	4 months	6 months	12 months	15 months	18 months	19–23 months	2–3 years	4–6 years	
Hepatitis B[1]	HepB	HepB				HepB						
Rotavirus[2]			RV	RV	RV[2]							Range of recommended ages for all children
Diphtheria, Tetanus, Pertussis[3]			DTaP	DTaP	DTaP	*see footnote*[3]	DTaP				DTaP	
Haemophilus influenzae type b[4]			Hib	Hib	Hib[4]	Hib						
Pneumococcal[5]			PCV	PCV	PCV	PCV				PPSV		
Inactivated Poliovirus[6]			IPV	IPV		IPV					IPV	Range of recommended ages for certain high-risk groups
Influenza[7]						Influenza (Yearly)						
Measles, Mumps, Rubella[8]						MMR		see footnote[8]			MMR	
Varicella[9]						Varicella		see footnote[9]			Varicella	
Hepatitis A[10]						HepA (2 doses)				HepA Series		
Meningococcal[11]										MCV4		

The Recommended Immunization Schedules for Persons Aged 0 Through 18 Years are approved by the Advisory Committee on Immunization Practices (**http://www.cdc.gov/vaccines/recs/acip**), the American Academy of Pediatrics (**http://www.aap.org**), and the American Academy of Family Physicians (**http://www.aafp.org**).

TABLE 17-2

RECOMMENDED IMMUNIZATION SCHEDULE FOR PERSONS AGES 17 THROUGH 18 YEARS

For those who fall behind or start late, see the schedule below and the catch-up schedule

Vaccine ▼ Age ▶	7–10 years	11–12 years	13–18 years	
Tetanus, Diphtheria, Pertussis[1]		Tdap	Tdap	Range of recommended ages for all children
Human Papillomavirus[2]	see footnote[2]	HPV (3 doses)(females)	HPV Series	
Meningococcal[3]	MCV4	MCV4	MCV4	
Influenza[4]	Influenza (Yearly)			Range of recommended ages for catch-up immunization
Pneumococcal[5]	Pneumococcal			
Hepatitis A[6]	HepA Series			
Hepatitis B[7]	Hep B Series			
Inactivated Poliovirus[8]	IPV Series			Range of recommended ages for certain high-risk groups
Measles, Mumps, Rubella[9]	MMR Series			
Varicella[10]	Varicella Series			

The Recommended Immunization Schedules for Persons Aged 0 Through 18 Years are approved by the Advisory Committee on Immunization Practices (**http://www.cdc.gov/vaccines/recs/acip**), the American Academy of Pediatrics (**http://www.aap.org**), and the American Academy of Family Physicians (**http://www.aafp.org**).

- Meningitis
- Influenza
- Pneumonia
- Hepatitis A
- Hepatitis B
- Polio
- Measles, mumps, rubella
- Varicella

Recommended vaccines for adults include influenza, tetanus, diphtheria, pertussis, varicella, human papillomavirus, herpes zoster, measles, mumps, rubella, pneumonia, meningitis, hepatitis A, and hepatitis B. Updated schedules for all populations are available through the Centers for Disease Control and Prevention (CDC) and the American Academy of Pediatrics (AAP).

hepatitis B	**Hepatitis B** is a viral disease with an incubation period of 50 to 160 days that is caused by the hepatitis B virus. Infection may lead to chronic liver disease. The hepatitis B vaccine is given to all newborns before being discharged from the hospital.
rotavirus	A **rotavirus** is a group of RNA viruses causing gastroenteritis. Gastroenteritis is a major cause of infant diarrhea throughout the world. The first dose of the vaccine is given at age 6 weeks.
diphtheria	**Diphtheria** is a serious infectious disease caused by the bacterium *Corynebacterium diphtheriae* that attacks the membranes of the throat and releases a toxin that damages the heart and nervous system. It is characterized by severe inflammation that forms a membranous coating within the pharynx, nose, trachea, and bronchial tree. The incubation period is 2 to 5 days, and the patient is contagious for 2 to 4 weeks. It is treated with antibiotics and has a high fatality rate, especially in unvaccinated children. The first dose of the vaccine is usually given at age 2 months.

tetanus	**Tetanus** is a disease marked by painful muscular contractions caused by a neurotoxin of *Clostridium tetani* acting on the central nervous system. Tetanus is characterized by extreme body stiffness and painful muscular spasms and contractions, especially around the neck and jaw, providing the foundation for the common term for the illness, *lockjaw*. Puncture wounds are the most common source because they are void of bacterial-killing oxygen. The incubation period is 3 to 21 days, but the onset of disease is usually within 8 days after infection. The history, physical examination, and clinical picture are enough to provide a diagnosis. Treatments include supportive care, muscle relaxants, and prompt wound cleaning with hydrogen peroxide. Vaccines containing tetanus antitoxin are available and boosters are administered every 10 years. A non-immunized person can be given tetanus immunoglobulin (TIG) within 72 hours of injury. The mortality rate is about 35%, thus immunization is important. The first dose of the vaccine is given at 2 months old.
pertussis	**Pertussis** (*tussis* = cough) is an acute inflammation of the larynx, trachea, and bronchi, caused by the bacterium *Bordetella pertussis*. It is characterized by recurrent bouts of violent coughing that continue until the breath is exhausted. The explosive sudden coughing attacks are followed by a sharp, shrill inhalation. The ending inhalation makes a "whooping" sound, so it is commonly referred to as *whooping cough*. It is spread by direct or indirect contact with nasopharyngeal secretions of an infected person. Diagnosis is based on the characteristic cough and the presence of *B. pertussis* in bacterial studies. Pertussis is treated with erythromycin antibiotic and palliative care (care that alleviates pain and symptoms without eliminating the cause). The first dose of pertussis vaccine is given at 2 months old.
Haemophilus influenzae **type b**	*Haemophilus influenzae* **type b** is a bacterial species that causes meningitis, pneumonia, and epiglottitis. The first dose of the vaccine is given to infants starting at 2 months old.
pneumonia	**Pneumonia** is an infection of the lungs that can cause mild to severe illness. It is characterized by cough, fever, fatigue, nausea, vomiting, shortness of breath, chills, and chest pain. It can be caused by bacteria, viruses, or fungi. The pneumococcal vaccine is given to infants starting at 2 months old.
polio	**Polio** (poliomyelitis) is an infectious viral disease that affects the nervous system, leading to muscle wasting (**Figure 17-32**). Between 1940 and 1950, 35,000 people per year contracted polio. As a result of diligent vaccination, polio has been eliminated in the United States. It still occurs in other parts of the world. Inactivated poliovirus vaccine is first given at 2 months of age.
influenza	**Influenza** is an acute respiratory infection caused by inhaling the influenza virus. It is characterized by sudden onset, chills, fever of short duration (3 to 4 days), headache, muscle aches, and a dry cough. It may be followed by a secondary bacterial infection that can last 10 days. Between 5% and 20% of the population gets the flu each year in the United States. The seasonal influenza vaccine is given at 6 months of age.
measles	**Measles** (rubeola) is a very contagious, acute viral disease characterized by inflammation of the respiratory membranes and red maculopapular

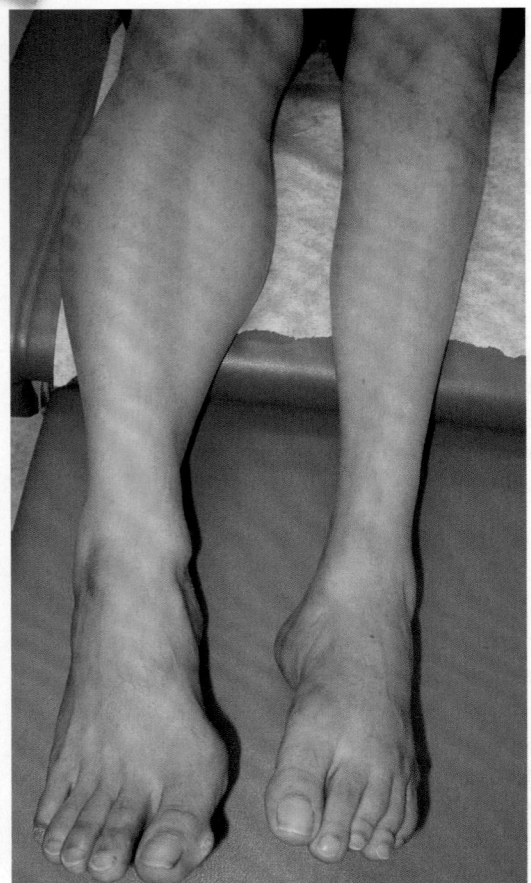

Figure 17-32 Polio leg wasting.

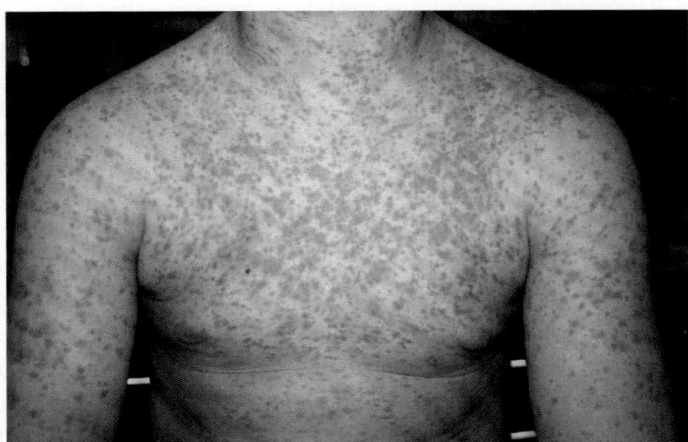

Figure 17-33 Measles.

skin eruptions. Signs and symptoms include a high temperature, sore throat, and bright red rash of small spots that spread, covering the entire body (**Figure 17-33**). The incubation period is 2 weeks. Then coryza (severe nasal congestion), cough, conjunctivitis, and Koplik spots appear. **Koplik spots** are tiny, gray-white areas on a bright red base occurring on the parotid salivary gland. Fever, chills, and the emergence of tiny rose-red eruptions mark days 3 and 4 of the infection. The rash gradually fades within 3 to 4 days, conferring lifetime immunity. As a direct result of vaccination, very few children in the United States get measles; however, worldwide, measles is still a significant cause of vaccine-preventable deaths in children. Vaccines for measles are given beginning at age 1.

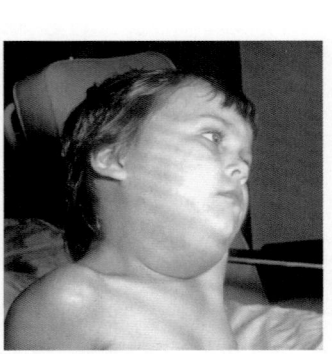

mumps

Figure 17-34 Young boy with mumps.

rubella

Mumps, also called *epidemic parotitis,* is an acute, communicable (contagious) viral disease characterized by fever and inflamed parotid salivary glands (**Figure 17-34**). Other organ tissues, notably the testes, pancreas, ovaries, and meninges, are often involved. Males have testicular tenderness. The virus is contracted by small drops of liquid in the air. It has an incubation period of 14 to 21 days; the patient is contagious for 1 to 7 days before swelling and up to 9 days past the characteristic signs. It is diagnosed by history and physical examination. Treatment is supportive. Lifelong immunity is conferred through active infection or vaccination. The mumps vaccine is given beginning at age 1.

An acute, viral, contagious disease characterized by fever, pale pink rash, and inflammation of cervical lymph nodes is termed **rubella** (**Figure 17-35**).

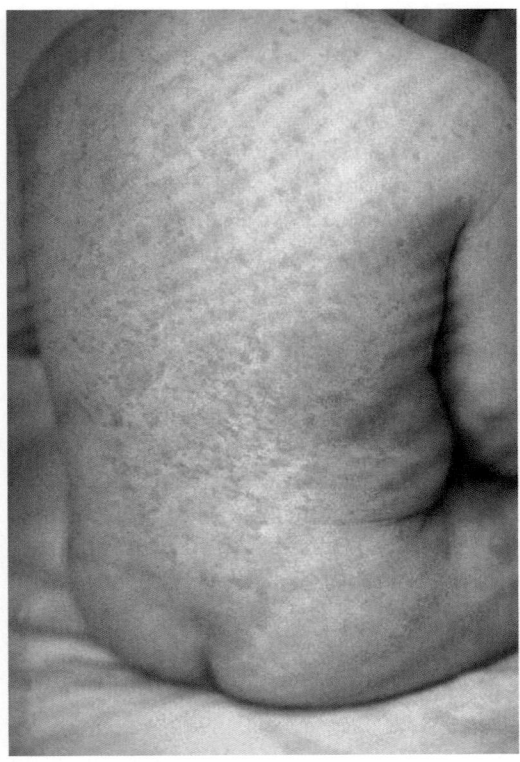

Figure 17-35 Rash of rubella on skin of a child's back.

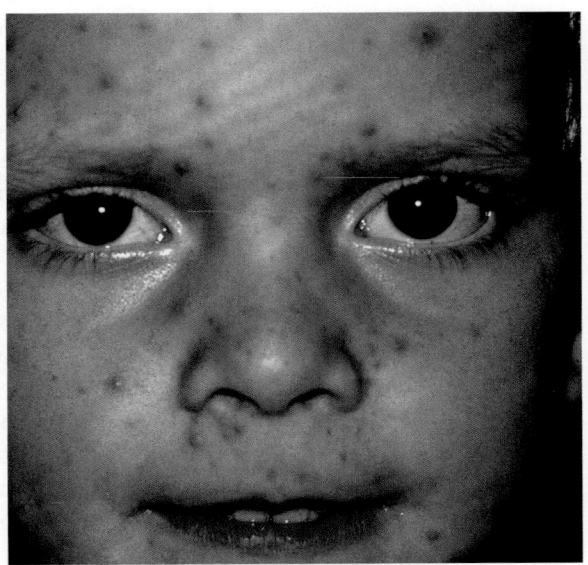

Figure 17-36 Chickenpox. Facial macules and papules in 5-year-old boy.

Other terms for this condition are epidemic roseola, German measles, and 3-day measles. It is associated with fetal abnormalities when a woman is infected during pregnancy. The reddish pink rash appears first on the face, and the person is contagious 1 week before eruption until 1 week after the rash appearance. The incubation period after exposure is 14 to 21 days. Active infection confers lifetime immunity. The clinical picture, history, and physical examination make the initial diagnosis. Diagnosis is confirmed by virology studies indicating rubella virus presence. Rubella is treated symptomatically. Vaccines are also available to prevent primary infection and the first dose is given at 1 year of age. Measles, mumps, and rubella vaccines are given in an MMR combination vaccination

chickenpox or varicella

The varicella-zoster virus (VZV) is a herpes virus that causes **chickenpox**, which is also known as **varicella**. Varicella is a highly contagious viral disease that causes an acute infection in unvaccinated children and young adults.

The contagion is spread by respiratory droplets or by contact with fluid from skin lesions. The virus has an incubation period of 14 to 17 days. **Incubation** refers to the development of an infection inside the body to the point at which the first signs of disease become apparent. A person is contagious 1 to 2 days before the appearance of the characteristic lesions to approximately 6 days after final eruptions. Signs are skin lesions that begin as red macules (small, pigmented spot), transform to papules (small, hard, round bumps), and eventually become fluid-filled vesicles (sacs) (**Figure 17-36**). The vesicles eventually crust and heal with no or slight scarring. Intense pruritus (itching) is a common symptom. The disease resolves in about 2 weeks, and the person then has lifetime immunity against chickenpox. It is diagnosed by the presence of macules and a history of virus exposure.

Treatment is supportive. Antiviral medications can lessen the severity of symptoms if the disease is discovered in the very early stages. A varicella vaccine is available and given to children beginning at age 1. Adolescents and adults receive the injection and a follow-up booster 4 to 8 weeks later. Shingles is caused by reactivation of the chickenpox virus, and is characterized by an eruption of groups of vesicles on one side of the body following the course of a nerve (see **Figure 4-31**). In many cases, the varicella-zoster virus has remained latent for years, following a primary chickenpox infection.

hepatitis A

Hepatitis A is a viral disease caused by hepatitis A virus characterized by fever, damage to the liver, and jaundice. It is transmitted by the fecal–oral route and is commonly seen in school-age children and young adults. Hepatitis A vaccine is given in two doses at least 6 months apart, beginning at age 1.

meningococcal meningitis

Meningococcal meningitis is an acute infectious disease of children and young adults caused by *Neisseria meningitidis* that infects the cerebrospinal fluid bathing the brain and spinal cord. It is characterized by fever, headache, photophobia (light sensitivity), vomiting, stiff neck, seizures, and coma. There are approximately 1,000 cases each year in the United States. About 15% of survivors will have long-term disabilities including deafness and brain damage. It is spread by person-to-person contact. The meningococcal vaccine can be given as early as age 2.

human papillomavirus (HPV)

Human papillomavirus (HPV) infection is the most common viral, sexually transmitted disease. A single unprotected contact with an infected person carries a 60% risk of infection. Certain strains cause genital warts and other strains are associated with cervical cancer. The HPV vaccine is recommended for the prevention of genital warts, cervical precancers, and cancers in females, and the first dose can be administered at age 11.

KEY TERM	Definition
vaccines (VACK-seenz)	biological preparations that are administered to stimulate the immune system to produce antibodies against a specific disease
immunizations	vaccines that provide immunity; also called vaccinations
vaccinations	vaccines that provide immunity; also called immunizations
hepatitis (hep-uh-TIGH-tus) **B**	viral disease caused by hepatitis B virus that may lead to chronic liver disease
rotavirus (roh-tuh-VYE-rus)	group of RNA viruses that cause gastroenteritis
diphtheria (dif-THEER-ee-uh)	serious infectious disease caused by *Corynebacterium diphtheriae* that attacks throat membranes and releases a toxin that damages the heart and nervous system
tetanus (TET-uh-nus)	disease marked by painful muscular contractions caused by a neurotoxin of *Clostridium tetani* acting on the central nervous system; also called lockjaw
pertussis (pur-TUS-is)	infectious respiratory bacterial disease that causes violent coughing spasms, caused by *Bordetella pertussis*; also called whooping cough
Haemophilus influenzae (hee-moh-FIH-lus in-flew-EN-zee) **type b**	bacterial species that causes meningitis, pneumonia, and epiglottitis
pneumonia (new-MOH-nee-uh)	infection of the lungs that can cause mild to severe illness

continued

continued from page 946

KEY TERM	Definition
polio (POH-lee-oh)	an infectious viral disease that affects the nervous system, leading to muscle wasting; abbreviated term for poliomyelitis
influenza (in-flew-EN-zuh)	acute respiratory infection caused by inhaling the influenza virus
measles	very contagious, acute viral disease characterized by fever and a red rash of small spots; also called rubeola
Koplik spots	small gray-white areas on a red background occurring on the parotid salivary gland that are characteristic of measles
mumps	acute, contagious disease that causes fever and swelling of the parotid salivary glands; also called epidemic parotitis
rubella (roo-BEL-uh)	highly contagious viral disease that causes swelling of the cervical lymph nodes and a skin rash; also called epidemic roseola, German measles, and 3-day measles
chickenpox	infectious disease caused by the varicella-zoster virus (VZV) characterized by small itching blisters; also called varicella
varicella (vair-i-SEL-uh)	infectious disease caused by the varicella-zoster virus (VZV) characterized by small itching blisters; also called chickenpox
incubation	phase of development of an infectious disease from the time of infection to the appearance of symptoms
hepatitis (hep-uh-TIGH-tus) **A**	viral disease caused by hepatitis A virus characterized by fever, damage to the liver, and jaundice
meningococcal meningitis (muh-ning-goh-COCK-ul men-in-JYE-tis)	acute infectious disease caused by *Neisseria meningitidis* that infects the cerebrospinal fluid bathing the brain and spinal cord
human papillomavirus (HPV) (pap-ih-LOH-muh-VYE-rus)	sexually transmitted viral disease that causes genital warts and is associated with cervical cancer

KEY TERM PRACTICE: *Infectious Diseases of Childhood*

1. Give the medical term for the childhood disease caused by *Bordetella pertussis.* _____

2. Give the medical term for chickenpox. _____

3. _____ are biological preparations that are administered to stimulate the immune system to produce antibodies against a specific disease.

4. An acute infectious disease by *Neisseria meningitidis* that infects the cerebrospinal fluid bathing the brain and spinal cord is termed _____.

5. _____ are small gray-white areas on a red background occurring on the parotid salivary gland that are characteristic of measles.

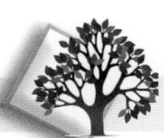

LIFE SPAN

This chapter focuses on the stages of life from a single cell to a fully functioning human. Numerous tests have been developed to chart developmental progress after birth. One such assessment is the Denver Developmental Screening Test (DDST), a standardized screening tool that assesses the developmental progress of children from birth through adolescence.

Psychologists and pediatricians use the test to evaluate gross motor skills, language proficiency, fine motor coordination, and social interactions. Statistical analyses are applied to identify patterns of developmental deficits.

Development phases are marked by periods of anatomical growth. During embryonic growth, the germ layers grow, and during the fetal stage, organs are established, but immature.

Prenatal development includes the formation of all body systems. The integumentary system is complete by the seventh gestational month. Epiphyseal cartilages, which are the growing regions of long bones, are formed by month 8. Muscle formation is nearly complete by month 6, although both muscle mass and muscle control increase throughout postnatal development. The nervous system is complete by month 6, but the sense organs are not completed until nearly the ninth gestation month. Brain development continues through adolescence. The endocrine and digestive systems are in place by the seventh gestational month, and entire respiratory system structures are not completed until nearly the ninth gestational month. Nephron formation in the urinary system and testicle descent in the male reproductive system are completed toward the end of the eighth month of gestation. The reproductive system may not be fully functional until puberty. At delivery, the head is disproportionately large and remains so for quite some time after birth.

General effects of aging are numerous and involve every body system. For example, nervous system changes include glaucoma and cataracts. Musculoskeletal effects are evidenced by a loss of skeletal muscle strength and shaggy-appearing bone margins, called lipping. The circulatory system loses efficiency, atherosclerosis becomes more apparent, skin is less elastic, and nephron numbers decline nearly 50% between the ages of 30 and 75 years. Although nothing can be done about getting old, healthy lifestyles can influence age-related disorders. We consider aging in the last chapter on gerontology.

COMMON Abbreviations

Abbreviation	Term
AAP	American Academy of Pediatrics
AFP	α-fetoprotein (alpha fetoprotein)
ARDMS	American Registry of Diagnostic Medical Sonographers
ASD	atrial septal defect
BPD	bronchopulmonary dysplasia
CDC	Centers for Disease Control and Prevention
CF	cystic fibrosis
CHD	congenital hip dysplasia
CK	creatine kinase
CMV	Cytomegalovirus
CNS	central nervous system
CP	cerebral palsy
C-section	cesarean section
CSF	cerebrospinal fluid
CT	computed tomography
CVB	chorionic villus biopsy

continued

continued from page 948

Abbreviation	Term
CVS	chorionic villus sampling
D&C	dilation and curettage
DDST	Denver Developmental Screening Test
DNA	deoxyribonucleic acid
DTP	diphtheria–tetanus–pertussis
EDC	estimated date of confinement
EFM	external fetal monitoring
FAS	fetal alcohol syndrome
FHR	fetal heart rate
FSH	follicle-stimulating hormone
GDM	gestational diabetes mellitus
GnRH	gonadotropin-releasing hormone
GYN	gynecology
hCG	human chorionic gonadotropin
hPL	human placental lactogen
HSV	herpes simplex virus
IRDS	infant respiratory distress syndrome
IV	intravenous
LH	luteinizing hormone
LMP	last menstrual period
MD	muscular dystrophy
MMR	measles, mumps, rubella
MRI	magnetic resonance imaging
NEC	necrotizing enterocolitis
NG	nasogastric
NPO	*non per os*; nothing by mouth
OB	obstetrician; obstetrics
OXT	oxytocin
PDA	patent ductus arteriosus
PG US	pregnancy ultrasound
PID	pelvic inflammatory disease
PKU	phenylketonuria
PRL	prolactin
ROP	retinopathy of prematurity
SCID	severe combined immunodeficiency
SGA	small for gestational age
TIG	tetanus immunoglobulin
TORCH series	*t*oxoplasmosis, *o*ther infections, *r*ubella, *c*ytomegalovirus (CMV), and *h*erpes simplex virus (HSV)
VBAC	vaginal birth after cesarean section
VZV	varicella-zoster virus

continued

continued from page 949

COMMON ABBREVIATIONS EXERCISES

1. The abbreviation for tetanus immunoglobulin is _____.

2. OB is the abbreviation for _____.

3. Identify the terms for the acronym TORCH. _____

4. ROP is the abbreviation for _____.

5. PKU is the abbreviation for _____.

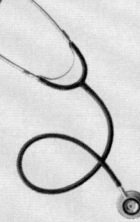

Case Study

Sabine Bauer is a 22-year-old female who presented in the OB/GYN office for prenatal care. Her last menstrual period (LMP) was February 14, 2011. Her appointment date was July 2, 2011. Pregnancy ultrasound revealed a single fetus in the vertex position. The fetal heart rate (FHR) was 147 beats per minute. The anteriorly located placenta was low lying, suggesting a probable placenta previa. Diagnostic ultrasound demonstrated a fetal spine, four-chamber heart, cord insertion, stomach, three-vessel cord, kidneys, and bladder. All were unremarkable. Estimated menstrual age was 20 weeks and 5 days. Estimated date of confinement (EDC), or the delivery date for a pregnant woman, was November 21, 2011. A small choroid plexus cyst measuring 6 by 4 mm was noted. The obstetrician recommended follow-up ultrasound for the low-lying placenta and choroid plexus cyst.

Case Study Questions

Select the best answer to each of the following questions.

1. **Mrs. Bauer's LMP was February 14, 2011. This means that _____.**
   a. she had been bleeding for about 5 months
   b. February 14, 2011 was the first day of her menstrual cycle
   c. February 14, 2011 was the last day of her menstrual cycle
   d. the baby was due on February 14, 2011

2. **The vertex position _____.**
   a. is a normal finding
   b. is an abnormal finding
   c. indicates a breech birth
   d. indicates that the baby will be born feet first

3. **Placenta previa is best described as a condition in which the _____.**
   a. placenta is implanted in the lower portion of the uterus, extending toward the cervix
   b. placenta is implanted in the upper portion of the uterus, extending toward the cervix.
   c. uterus is bicornuate.
   d. placenta contains more than one fetus.

4. **The ultrasound test confirmed the presence of a three-vessel cord. This refers to _____.**
   a. the spinal cord that contains nerves, arteries, and veins
   b. an umbilical cord with two arteries and one vein
   c. an umbilical cord with one artery and two veins
   d. a spermatic cord that contains ductus deferens, blood vessels, and lymphatic vessels

5. **How did the obstetrician arrive at November 21st as the EDC? _____**
   a. The Braxton Hicks formula was used.
   b. The Goodell sign was applied.
   c. The Chadwick sign was applied.
   d. Nägele's rule was used.

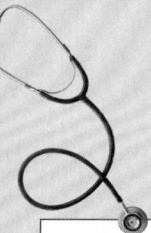

Real World Report

Mandy performed the follow-up pregnancy ultrasound (PG US) on Sabine Bauer. The ultrasound report follows.

IMAGING DEPARTMENT

NAME:	Sabine Bauer	DOB:	02/02/1989
AGE:	22 years		
DATEORD:	08/27/2011	EXAM DATE:	08/27/2011
TEST:	PG US	ORDPHYS:	K.K.Miner, MD

CLINICAL INFORMATION:

Follow-up for possible placenta previa and possible choroid plexus cyst.

PREGNANCY ULTRASOUND

Multiple ultrasonographic scans of the lower abdomen and pelvis were obtained and compared with previous examination of July 2, 2011. There is a single intrauterine pregnancy in cephalic presentation. The placenta lies anteriorly in unremarkable position. The previously described low-lying position of the placenta is no longer present on this examination.

Fetal cardiac and somatic motion were visible during the examination. An adequate amount of amniotic fluid is demonstrated.

There is a moderate dilation of the lateral ventricles, which was not observed on the previous examination. The previously described choroid plexus cyst cannot be positively identifiable on this examination.

The fetal measurement is consistent with a 28-week 4-day menstrual age.

IMPRESSION

1. A single intrauterine pregnancy in cephalic presentation. Anterior placenta is noted; the placental position is unremarkable on this examination.
2. There is mild to moderate dilation of the lateral ventricles, which was not observed on the previous study.
3. Sonogram reveals ultrasonographic menstrual age of 28 weeks, 4 days.
4. A repeat ultrasonographic examination in several weeks for reevaluation of the intracranial structures is recommended.

Real World Report Questions

The following exercises review the medical terms used in the preceding medical report.

1. Define single intrauterine pregnancy.

_____

2. Amniotic fluid refers to fluid _____.

  a. contained in the amniotic sac surrounding the fetus

  b. contained in the uterus that surrounds the fetus

  c. produced by the choroid plexus

  d. secreted by the mammary glands

3. Define cephalic presentation.

_____

4. The medical report used the terms *intrauterine* and *intracranial*. Define the following word parts.

  a. *intra-* _____

  b. *uter-* _____

  c. *crani-* _____

Review and Application

Multiple-Choice Questions

Select the best response to each of the following questions.

1. The organ in which a fetus develops is a/an _____.
   a. embryo   b. placenta   c. zygote   d. chorion

2. _____ is the number of years a particular individual can live.
   a. Lifespan   b. Life expectancy   c. Senescence   d. Life inheritance

3. An unborn offspring at gestational week 9 is termed a/an _____.
   a. zygote   b. embryo   c. fetus   d. ovum

4. The period of development from fertilization until birth is called _____.
   a. fertilization   b. development   c. growing   d. gestation

5. Male and female reproductive cells are _____.
   a. gametes   b. genes   c. chromosomes   d. embryos

6. The endoderm, ectoderm, and mesoderm make up _____.
   a. the uterine wall b. the germ layers   c. layers of the amnion   d. the allantois

7. The medical specialty concerned with female reproductive health is termed _____.
   a. gynecology   b. oogenesis   c. spermatogenesis   d. adolescence

8. A generic term for various types of nonprogressive motor conditions causing physical disability that are present at birth or beginning in early childhood is known as _____.
   a. Down syndrome   b. cerebral palsy (CP) c. hydrocephalus   d. varicella

9. _____ is a congenital split in the roof of the mouth.
   a. Cleft palate   b. Patent ductus arteriosus   c. Cleft lip   d. Coarctation of aorta

10. Agents that cause birth defects are termed _____.
    a. congenital producers   b. congenital enhancers   c. teratogens   d. mutations

11. Which term means "existing before or at birth?" _____
    a. teratogen   b. congenital   c. placental   d. gestation

12. The _____ is the outermost fetal membrane that forms part of the placenta.
    a. chorion   b. yolk sac   c. amnion   d. allantois

13. The _____ is the innermost fetal membrane.
    a. chorion   b. yolk sac   c. amnion   d. allantois

14. A physician specializing in the care and development of children is a/an _____.
    a. podiatrist   b. obstetrician   c. pediatrician   d. b and c

15. The period of life between puberty and maturity is _____.
    a. senescence   b. infancy   c. childhood   d. adolescence

16. Genetic traits carried on the Y chromosome inherited only by males is termed _____.

    a. holandric inheritance   b. genes   c. gametes   d. recessive

17. The period of life between infancy and puberty is called _____.

    a. adolescence   b. senescence   c. childhood   d. postpartum

18. The 23rd pair of chromosomes, designated X and Y, is called the _____.

    a. incomplete dominance pair   b. pair of sex chromosomes   c. pair of homozygous chromosomes   d. somatic cell pair

19. A genetic trait that results from a gene located on either the X or Y chromosome is termed _____.

    a. sex-linked inheritance   b. sex chromosomes   c. holandric inheritance   d. teratology

20. The cheesy-appearing deposit on the surface of the fetus is called _____.

    a. vernix   b. a zygote   c. vernix caseosa   d. parturition

21. The _____ is a mass of cells that implants on the endometrium after fertilization.

    a. blastocyst   b. chromosome   c. zygote   d. mutation

22. The connecting stalk between the embryo or fetus and the placenta that contains two arteries and one vein is the _____.

    a. placenta   b. chorion   c. umbilical cord   d. allantois

23. Which lists the developmental stages in order of youngest to oldest? _____

    a. infancy → neonate → adolescence → adulthood   b. neonate → infancy → childhood → adulthood   c. infancy → adolescence → childhood → adulthood   d. childhood → infancy → adolescence → neonate

Word Parts Exercises

Using the following word parts, form a medical term for each definition. Each word part is used only once.

amnio-   -cele   centesis   embryo-
embryo-   -logy   meningo-   -pathy

24. embryonic or congenital defect resulting in faulty development _____

25. study of the embryo and its development _____

26. procedure for withdrawing amniotic fluid for analysis _____

27. protrusion of the meninges through the skull or vertebra that forms a CSF-filled cyst _____

Matching Exercises

Match the disorder with its description.

_____ 28. severe combined immunodeficiency disease (SCID)

_____ 29. cystic fibrosis (CF)

_____ 30. patent ductus arteriosus (PDA)

_____ 31. spina bifida

_____ 32. tetanus

a. hereditary disease affecting various exocrine glands
b. presence of ductus arteriosus after birth
c. congenital disorder marked by a deficient immune system
d. painful muscle contractions caused by a neurotoxin
e. congenital disorder in which the spinal cord protrudes through an opening in the spinal column

Match the sign with its description.

_____ 33. lightening

_____ 34. linea nigra

_____ 35. chloasma

_____ 36. striae gravidarum

_____ 37. Braxton Hicks contractions

a. dark line extending up the abdomen of a pregnant woman
b. pregnancy stretch marks
c. dark coloration of facial skin caused by hormones of pregnancy
d. irregular and painless uterine contractions
e. dropping of the fetus into the pelvis

Match the clinical test or diagnostic procedure with its description.

_____ 38. hCG test

_____ 39. amniocentesis

_____ 40. 2-hour postprandial glucose test

_____ 41. TORCH series

_____ 42. chorionic villus sampling

a. blood test to identify teratogenic diseases in pregnant women
b. laboratory test to determine blood sugar levels
c. prenatal test evaluating extensions of the chorion
d. prenatal test evaluating fluid in the placenta
e. measures level of human chorionic gonadotropin in the blood or urine to detect pregnancy

Match the clinical test or diagnostic procedure with its description.

_____ 43. chorionic villus biopsy

_____ 44. Guthrie test

_____ 45. hPL test

_____ 46. α-fetoprotein

_____ 47. pelvimetry

a. blood test performed on the mother to evaluate placental function
b. prenatal test to detect defects by analyzing cells of the chorion
c. blood test used to detect phenylalanine
d. x-ray study to determine feasibility of a vaginal delivery
e. fetal protein test to detect fetal disorders

Match the term with its definition.

_____ 48. quickening

_____ 49. Chadwick sign

_____ 50. Hegar sign

_____ 51. Goodell sign

_____ 52. stillbirth

a. blue-violet color of the cervix and vagina during pregnancy
b. birth of a dead infant
c. softening of the cervix, which indicates pregnancy
d. softening of the lower uterus at week 7 of pregnancy
e. fetal movements felt by the mother

Match the pregnancy condition with its definition.

_____ 53. abruptio placentae

_____ 54. abortion

_____ 55. chorioangioma

_____ 56. eclampsia

_____ 57. choriocarcinoma

a. malignant tumor of the uterus
b. benign tumor of placental blood vessels
c. premature separation of the placenta from the uterus
d. illness of late pregnancy characterized by hypertension and convulsions
e. physiological expulsion of the fetus

Match the disease with its description.

_____ 58. mumps

_____ 59. rubella

_____ 60. diphtheria

_____ 61. measles

_____ 62. varicella

a. chickenpox; caused by VZV
b. disease caused by *C. diphtheriae*
c. viral disease characterized by a red rash of small spots
d. disease affecting the salivary glands
e. viral disease of the lymph nodes

Definitions

Define the following terms.

63. vertex _____

64. vernix caseosa _____

65. incompetent cervix _____

66. abortion _____

67. implantation _____

68. meningocele _____

Provide a medical term for the following definitions.

69. measurement of the inlet and outlet diameters of the pelvis to determine the feasibility of a vaginal childbirth

   _____

70. study of malformations caused by agents that bring about birth defects _____

71. hormone that causes relaxation of the pelvis _____

72. score assessing the condition of the neonate _____

73. branch of medicine dealing with the care of children _____

74. product of conception from the moment of fertilization to the end of the eighth gestational week _____

Alternate Terms

Give an alternate term for each of the following terms.

75. chickenpox _____

76. trisomy 21 _____

77. trisomy 18 _____

Spelling

Identify the correctly spelled term in each set.

78. _____
   a. allele
   b. allelle
   c. alelle
   d. aleal

79. _____
   a. genotype
   b. genotipe
   c. jenotype
   d. genetype

80. _____
   a. jestation
   b. gestetion
   c. gestasion
   d. gestation

81. _____
   a. line nigrea
   b. linea nigra
   c. linea nigera
   d. linee niger

Unscramble

Unscramble the letters to form a medical term.

82. pietocc _____

83. robtaoin _____

84. sinbimal _____

85. file yexcnactep _____

86. blora _____

Abbreviations

Provide the term for the abbreviations and then define the terms.

87. DTP = _____

88. BPD = _____

89. hCG = _____

90. EDC = _____

91. SGA = _____

92. PKU = _____

Analogies
··

Provide a medical term to complete a meaningful analogy.

93. Chorionic villus biopsy is to _____ as poliomyelitis is to _____.

94. Chickenpox is to _____ as measles is to _____.

Short Answer
··

Answer the following questions

95. Give the genotype of a male child. _____

96. Give the genotype of a female child. _____

97. Name the two structures that enable blood to avoid the nonfunctioning fetal lungs while the fetus is in the womb.

    _____

98. Is it possible for dizygotic twins to have two different biological fathers? Explain your answer. _____

99. Identify one similarity between an organism floating in outer space and an organism floating in utero. _____

100. Calculate the birth date of an infant whose mother's last menstrual period (LMP) was March 17. _____

Word Search
··

Find the medical terms hidden in the puzzle.

N	C	V	W	J	R	I	R	F	N	Q	C	Y	E	P
E	O	N	T	A	N	L	Z	O	O	O	O	C	P	D
M	O	I	O	D	G	D	I	A	Y	J	L	N	B	P
O	D	L	T	O	A	N	G	G	F	P	O	A	M	Z
S	M	B	S	A	M	D	O	F	R	E	S	F	Z	C
O	Z	M	T	A	Z	L	U	E	A	Q	T	N	M	B
M	I	E	O	S	O	I	G	L	Z	Q	R	I	L	O
O	V	T	M	C	P	N	L	R	T	G	U	N	H	C
R	O	V	E	U	A	E	G	I	K	H	M	I	W	C
H	S	N	D	N	O	U	C	E	T	L	O	T	N	U
C	Y	F	C	K	V	E	Z	R	N	R	I	O	O	P
G	Z	Y	G	O	T	E	J	T	O	E	E	B	D	K
P	O	S	T	P	A	R	T	U	M	F	S	F	I	R
M	U	I	N	O	C	E	M	U	R	D	O	M	Z	K
P	F	Q	M	S	Y	C	D	R	L	V	N	F	D	B

adulthood
amnion
chromosome
colostrum
fertilization
forceps
genes
gynecology
infancy
meconium
postpartum
pregnancy
zygote

Vocabulary Review

Review the key terms from this chapter, study the spelling and pronunciation of each term, and write its definition in the space provided. Listen to the audio available for most terms at http://thepoint.lww.com/nath2e and pronounce each term for yourself. Then check the box when you feel confident that you know the definition and can pronounce the term correctly.

Key Term	Pronunciation	Definition
❑ **2-hour postprandial glucose test**	(pohst-PRAN-dee-ul)	_____
❑ **abortion**		_____
❑ **abruptio placentae**	(ab-RUP-tee-oh pluh-SEN-tee)	_____
❑ **adolescence**		_____
❑ **adulthood**		_____
❑ **albinism**	(AL-bi-niz-um)	_____
❑ **allantois**	(uh-lan-TOH-is)	_____
❑ **α-fetoprotein serum test**	(AL-fuh-fee-toh-PROH-teen)	_____
❑ **amniocentesis**	(am-nee-oh-sen-TEE-sis)	_____
❑ **amnion**	(AM-nee-on)	_____
❑ **anencephaly**	(an-en-SEF-uh-lee)	_____
❑ **Apgar score**		_____
❑ **atrial septal defect (ASD)**		_____
❑ **blastocyst**	(BLAS-toh-sist)	_____
❑ **Braxton Hicks contractions**	(BRACKS-tun HICKS)	_____
❑ **breech**		_____
❑ **bronchopulmonary dysplasia (BPD)**	(brong-koh-PUL-moh-nair-ee dis-PLAY-zhuh)	_____
❑ **cerebral palsy (CP)**	(se-REE-brul PAWL-zee)	_____
❑ **cesarean section (C-section)**	(se-ZAIR-ee-un)	_____
❑ **Chadwick sign**		_____
❑ **chickenpox**		_____
❑ **childhood**		_____
❑ **chloasma**	(kloh-AZ-muh)	_____
❑ **chorioangioma**	(koh-ree-oh-an-jee-OH-muh)	_____
❑ **choriocarcinoma**	(koh-ree-oh-kahr-si-NOH-muh)	_____
❑ **chorion**	(KOH-ree-on)	_____
❑ **chorionic villi**	(KOH-ree-on-ick VIL-eye)	_____
❑ **chorionic villus biopsy (CVB)**	(koh-ree-ON-ick VIL-us)	_____

Key Term	Pronunciation	Definition
❏ chorionic villus sampling (CVS)	(koh-ree-ON-ick VIL-us)	_____
❏ chromosome		_____
❏ cleft lip		_____
❏ cleft palate		_____
❏ coarctation of aorta	(koh-ark-TAY-shun) (ay-OR-tuh)	_____
❏ colostrum	(koh-LOS-trum)	_____
❏ congenital	(kun-JEN-i-tul)	_____
❏ congenital megacolon		_____
❏ contractions		_____
❏ cri-du-chat syndrome	(kree-due-shah)	_____
❏ cystic fibrosis (CF)	(SIS-tick figh-BROH-sis)	_____
❏ developmental hip dysplasia	(dis-PLAY-zhuh)	_____
❏ dilation and curettage (D&C)	(kewr-e-TAHZH)	_____
❏ diphtheria	(dif-THEER-ee-uh)	_____
❏ dizygotic twins	(dye-zye-GOT-ick)	_____
❏ Down syndrome		_____
❏ Duchenne muscular dystrophy (DMD)	(doo-SHAYN) (DIS-truh-fee)	_____
❏ eclampsia	(ih-KLAMP-see-uh)	_____
❏ ectopic pregnancy	(eck-TOP-ick)	_____
❏ Edwards syndrome		_____
❏ effacement	(e-FACE-munt)	_____
❏ embryo	(EM-bree-oh)	_____
❏ episiotomy	(eh-piz-ee-OT-oh-mee)	_____
❏ erythroblastosis fetalis	(e-rith-roh-blas-TOH-sis fee-TAY-lis)	_____
❏ fertilization		_____
❏ fetal alcohol syndrome (FAS)		_____
❏ fetus	(FEE-tus)	_____
❏ gamete	(GAM-eet)	_____
❏ genes		_____
❏ gestation	(jes-TAY-shun)	_____
❏ gestational age	(jes-TAY-shun-ul)	_____
❏ gestational diabetes mellitus (GDM)	(jes-TAY-shun-ul dye-uh-BEE-teez muh-LYE-tus)	_____
❏ Goodell sign		_____
❏ Guthrie test		_____

Key Term	Pronunciation	Definition
❏ gynecology (GYN)	(guy-nuh-KOL-oh-jee)	_____
❏ Haemophilus influenzae type b	(hee-moh-FIH-lus in-flew-EN-zee)	_____
❏ Hegar sign	(HAY-gar)	_____
❏ hepatitis A	(hep-uh-TIGH-tus)	_____
❏ hepatitis B	(hep-uh-TIGH-tus)	_____
❏ holandric inheritance	(hol-AN-drick)	_____
❏ human chorionic gonadotropin (hCG)	(KOH-ree-on-ick goh-nad-oh-TROH-pin)	_____
❏ human papillomavirus (HPV)	(pap-ih-LOH-muh-VYE-rus)	_____
❏ human placental lactogen (hPL)	(pluh-SEN-tul LACK-toh-jen)	_____
❏ hydatidiform mole	(high-duh-TID-ih-form)	_____
❏ hydrocephalus	(high-droh-SEF-uh-lus)	_____
❏ immunizations		_____
❏ implantation		_____
❏ in vitro fertilization (IVF)	(VEE-troh)	_____
❏ in vivo fertilization	(VEE-voh)	_____
❏ incompetent cervix	(in-KOM-puh-tunt SUR-vicks)	_____
❏ incubation		_____
❏ infancy		_____
❏ infant respiratory distress syndrome (IRDS)	(RES-pi-ruh-tohr-ee)	_____
❏ influenza	(in-flew-EN-zuh)	_____
❏ inheritance		_____
❏ Klinefelter syndrome		_____
❏ Koplik spots		_____
❏ labor		_____
❏ lactation	(lack-TAY-shun)	_____
❏ life expectancy		_____
❏ lifespan		_____
❏ lightening		_____
❏ linea nigra	(LIN-ee-uh NIGH-gruh)	_____
❏ measles		_____
❏ meconium	(mee-KOH-nee-um)	_____
❏ meningocele	(meh-NING-goh-seel)	_____
❏ meningococcal meningitis	(muh-ning-goh-COCK-ul men-in-JYE-tis)	_____
❏ monozygotic twins	(mon-oh-zye-GOT-ick)	_____

Key Term	Pronunciation	Definition
❑ mumps		_____
❑ mutations		_____
❑ Nägele's rule	(NAY-guh-leez)	_____
❑ necrotizing enterocolitis (NEC)	(NECK-roh-tize-ing en-tur-oh-koh-LYE-tis)	_____
❑ neonate	(NEE-oh-nate)	_____
❑ obstetric forceps	(ob-STET-rick FOR-seps)	_____
❑ obstetrician (OB)	(ob-ste-TRISH-un)	_____
❑ obstetrics (OB)	(ob-STET-ricks)	_____
❑ parturition	(pahr-tew-RISH-un)	_____
❑ patent ductus arteriosus (PDA)	(DUCK-tus ahr-teer-ee-OH-sus)	_____
❑ pediatrician	(pee-dee-uh-TRISH-un)	_____
❑ pediatrics	(pee-dee-AT-ricks)	_____
❑ pelvimetry	(pel-VIM-i-tree)	_____
❑ pertussis	(pur-TUS-is)	_____
❑ phenylketonuria (PKU)	(fen-il-kee-toh-NEW-ree-uh)	_____
❑ placenta	(pluh-SEN-tuh)	_____
❑ placenta previa	(pluh-SEN-tuh PREE-vee-uh)	_____
❑ pneumonia	(new-MOH-nee-uh)	_____
❑ polio	(POH-lee-oh)	_____
❑ post partum	(pohst PAR-tum)	_____
❑ postpartum	(pohst-PAR-tum)	_____
❑ preeclampsia	(pree-ih-KLAMP-see-uh)	_____
❑ pregnancy		_____
❑ premature birth		_____
❑ premature infant		_____
❑ puberty		_____
❑ quickening		_____
❑ relaxin	(ree-LACK-sin)	_____
❑ retinopathy of prematurity (ROP)	(ret-i-NOP-uh-thee)	_____
❑ Reye syndrome		_____
❑ rotavirus	(roh-tuh-VYE-rus)	_____
❑ rubella	(roo-BEL-uh)	_____
❑ senescence	(se-NES-ence)	_____
❑ severe combined immunodeficiency (SCID)		_____
❑ sex chromosomes		_____

Key Term	Pronunciation	Definition
❑ sex-linked inheritance		
❑ small for gestational age (SGA)		
❑ spina bifida	(SPYE-nuh BIH-fih-duh)	
❑ stillbirth		
❑ striae gravidarum	(STRYE-ee grav-i-DAHR-um)	
❑ talipes	(TAL-i-peez)	
❑ talipes equinovarus	(TAL-i-peez ee-kwye-noh-VAY-rus)	
❑ Tay–Sachs disease	(SACKS)	
❑ teratogens	(TERR-uh-toh-jenz)	
❑ teratology	(terr-uh-TOL-uh-jee)	
❑ tetanus	(TET-uh-nus)	
❑ tetralogy of Fallot	(te-TRAL-uh-jee) (fah-LOH)	
❑ TORCH series		
❑ toxemia of pregnancy	(tock-SEE-mee-uh)	
❑ transposition of great arteries		
❑ Turner syndrome		
❑ umbilical cord	(um-BIL-i-kul)	
❑ vaccinations		
❑ vaccines	(VACK-seenz)	
❑ vaginal birth after cesarean (VBAC)	(VAJ-i-nul) (se-ZAIR-ee-un)	
❑ varicella	(vair-i-SEL-uh)	
❑ ventricular septal defect	(ven-TRICK-yoo-lur)	
❑ vernix caseosa	(VUR-nicks kay-see-OH-suh)	
❑ vertex	(VUR-tecks)	
❑ zygote	(ZYE-gote)	

Answers

Word Grouping Exercises

Definition	Word Part	Definition	Word Part
food, nutrition	troph-, tropho-	appearance	phen-, pheno-
allantois (a fetal membrane), allantoid, sausage-shaped	allant-, allanto-	brain	encephal-, encephalo-
amnion (innermost embryonic membrane)	amnio-	child	ped-, pedi-, pedo-

Definition	Word Part	Definition	Word Part
embryo	embry-, embryo-	milk	lact-, lacti-, lacto-
immature precursor cell	-blast	nucleus	karyo-
joining	zyg-, zygo-	other, different	heter-, hetero-
malformed	terato-	process of budding	blasto-
membrane, fetal membrane, chorion (outermost embryonic membrane)	chorio-	same, alike	homo-
meninges	mening-, meningo-	talus, ankle	talo-
middle	mes-, meso-	vulva	episio-

Word Building Exercises

Word Part	Meaning	Common or Known Word	Example Medical Term
amnio-	amnion (innermost embryonic membrane)	amniotic fluid	amniocentesis
-blast	immature precursor cell	osteoblast	trophoblast
embry-, embryo-	embryo	embryo	embryology
episio-	vulva	episiotomy	episiotomy
heter-, hetero-	other, different	heterosexual	heterozygous
homo-	same, alike	homosexual	homozygous
mening-, meningo-	meninges	meninges	meningocele
mes-, meso-	middle	mesosphere	mesoderm
ped-, pedi-, pedo-	child	pedophile	pediatrics
phen-, pheno-	appearance	phenomena	phenotype
talo-	talus, ankle	talon	talipes equinovarus
zyg-, zygo-	joining	zygomatic arch	zygote

Key Term Practice

Pregnancy, Human Development, and Child Health Preview

1. zygote
2. embryo
3. Lifespan
4. Fertilization
5. placenta

Fertilization and Implantation

1. gamete
2. Implantation
3. blastocyst

Placenta Formation and Gestation

1. chorionic villi
2. *terato-*, *-ology*; teratology
3. Relaxin
4. chorion
5. amnion

Pregnancy

1. parturition
2. obstetrician
3. quickening
4. Chadwick sign
5. Nägele's rule

Labor and Delivery

1. *episio-, -otomy*; episiotomy
2. vertex; breech
3. Apgar score
4. Pelvimetry
5. abortion

Lactation

1. Lactation; *lact-*
2. colostrum
3. Meconium

Artificial Fertilization and Multiple Births

1. dizygotic twins
2. monozygotic twins
3. In vivo fertilization; in vitro fertilization (IVF)

Developmental Stages

1. Neonate; *neo-*
2. Senescence
3. childhood
4. Infancy
5. puberty

Inheritance

1. sex-linked inheritance
2. Mutations
3. inheritance
4. holandric inheritance
5. chromosome

Conditions of Pregnancy

1. eclampsia; toxemia of pregnancy
2. preeclampsia
3. stillbirth
4. ectopic pregnancy
5. Placenta previa

Genetic Disorders

1. phenylketonuria (PKU)
2. Tay–Sachs disease
3. Guthrie test
4. Albinism
5. cystic fibrosis (CF)

Congenital Syndromes

1. a. Klinefelter syndrome; b. Turner syndrome
2. a. Edwards syndrome; b. Down syndrome
3. chorionic villus sampling (CVS); chorionic villus biopsy (CVB)
4. Amniocentesis
5. cri-du-chat syndrome

Nongenetic Syndromes

1. fetal alcohol syndrome (FAS)
2. Reye syndrome

Congenital Bone Disorders

1. cleft palate
2. talipes
3. Talipes equinovarus
4. developmental hip dysplasia
5. cleft lip

Congenital Blood and Cardiac Disorders

1. Tetralogy of Fallot; *tetra-*
2. atrial septal defect
3. transposition of great arteries
4. ventricular septal defect
5. patent ductus arteriosus

Congenital Neuromuscular System Disorders

1. without; *encephal-*; anencephaly
2. *hydro-*; head; hydrocephalus
3. meningocele; *meningo-*
4. Cerebral palsy (CP)
5. spina bifida

Premature Infant

1. retinopathy of prematurity (ROP)
2. premature
3. Necrotizing enterocolitis (NEC)
4. Small for gestational age (SGA)
5. Bronchopulmonary dysplasia (BPD)

Infectious Diseases of Childhood

1. pertussis
2. varicella
3. Vaccines
4. meningococcal meningitis
5. Koplik spots

Common Abbreviations Exercises

1. tetanus immunoglobulin = TIG
2. OB = obstetrician; obstetrics
3. TORCH = *t*oxoplasmosis, *o*ther infections, *r*ubella, *c*ytomegalovirus (CMV), and *h*erpes simplex virus (HSV)
4. ROP = retinopathy of prematurity
5. PKU = phenylketonuria

Case Study

1. b is the correct answer.
   - a is incorrect because the ultrasound indicated a fairly normal pregnancy; there was no indication of spotting or bleeding, and LMP refers to the first day of the last menstrual period.
   - c is incorrect because LMP refers to the first day of the last menstrual period, not the last day.
   - d is incorrect because the baby's due date was November 21, 2011, as indicated in the report.
2. a is the correct answer.
   - b is incorrect because the vertex (head-first) position is a normal finding.
   - c is incorrect because the vertex position is normal; breech birth means the fetus is positioned with feet or buttocks first, which is abnormal.
   - d is incorrect because feet first indicates a breech birth, the reverse of the normal vertex position.
3. a is the correct answer.
   - b is incorrect because placenta previa is a condition in which implantation occurs in the lower, not the upper, portion of the uterus.
   - c is incorrect because a bicornuate uterus refers to a uterus with two horns, something not indicated in the report and not the definition of placenta previa.
   - d is incorrect because the report revealed a single fetus, and placenta previa relates to abnormal implantation in the uterus.
4. b is the correct answer.
   - a is incorrect because spinal cord structures are not described as a three-vessel cord. Moreover, there are more than three nerves, arteries, and veins contained within the spinal cord.
   - c is incorrect because the fetal umbilical cord contains two arteries and one vein, not one artery and two veins; anything else is an abnormal finding.
   - d is incorrect because the report relates to the umbilical cord; the spermatic cord contains spermatic vessels, nerves, lymphatic vessels, and the ductus deferens.
5. d is the correct answer.
   - a is incorrect because Braxton Hicks refers to contractions not a formula.
   - b is incorrect because the Goodell sign is a softening of the cervix, which indicates pregnancy; it is not a formula used to determine expected delivery date.
   - c is incorrect because the Chadwick sign is the characteristic blue-violet color of the cervix and vagina around the sixth week of pregnancy; it is not a formula used to determine infant arrival date.

Real World Report

1. There is one fetus contained within the uterus/womb.
2. a
3. The fetus is in the vertex position with the head pointing downward toward the cervix.
4. a. within, inside; b. uterus, uterine; c. cranium, head

Review and Application

1. b
2. a
3. c
4. d
5. a
6. b
7. a
8. b
9. d
10. c
11. b
12. a
13. c
14. c
15. d

16. a
17. c
18. b
19. a
20. c
21. a
22. c
23. b
24. embryopathy
25. embryology
26. amniocentesis
27. meningocele
28. c
29. a
30. b

31. e
32. d
33. e
34. a
35. c
36. b
37. d
38. e
39. d
40. b
41. a
42. c
43. b
44. c
45. a

46. e
47. d
48. e
49. a
50. d
51. d
52. b
53. c
54. e
55. b
56. d
57. a
58. d
59. e
60. b

61. c
62. a
63. vertex = normal birth position of the fetus so that the crown of the head presents first in the cervix and the vaginal canal
64. vernix caseosa = cheesy appearing deposit on the surface of the fetus
65. incompetent cervix = condition in which the cervix dilates prematurely before the fetus reaches full term
66. abortion = expulsion of an embryo or fetus from the uterus before it can survive outside the womb
67. implantation = attachment of the blastocyst to the endometrium
68. meningocele = cerebrospinal fluid–filled cyst formed from the protrusion of the meninges through an opening in the skull or vertebra
69. pelvimetry
70. teratology
71. relaxin
72. Apgar score
73. pediatrics
74. embryo
75. varicella
76. Down syndrome
77. Edwards syndrome
78. a
79. a

80. d
81. b
82. ectopic
83. abortion
84. albinism
85. life expectancy
86. labor
87. DTP = diphtheria–tetanus–pertussis; diphtheria toxoid, tetanus toxoid, pertussis vaccine
88. BPD = bronchopulmonary dysplasia; a chronic pulmonary insufficiency affecting premature infants who required oxygen therapy
89. hCG = human chorionic gonadotropin; hormone originating in chorionic tissue that maintains estrogen and progesterone levels; its presence indicates pregnancy
90. EDC = estimated date of confinement; the delivery date for a pregnant woman
91. SGA = small for gestational age; refers to a low-birth-weight infant who is not premature
92. PKU = phenylketonuria; genetic disease in which the body lacks the enzyme to metabolize phenylalanine
93. chorionic villus sampling; polio
94. varicella; rubeola
95. XY
96. XX
97. foramen ovale; ductus arteriosus

98. Yes, dizygotic twins could have different biological fathers. Dizygotic twins result from the fertilization of two separate female eggs. If two oocytes were released and fertilized by sperm from two separate men, dizygotic twins with different biological fathers could result.

99. Life in utero and life in space are both characterized by a sense of weightlessness, and both are marked by a connection: The baby has an umbilical cord connecting it to the uterus, and an astronaut has a tether connecting him or her to the spacecraft.

100. December 24

Word Search

```
N  C  V  W  J  R  I  R  F  N  Q  C  Y  E  P
E  O  N  T  A  N  L  Z  O  O  O  O  C  P  D
M  O  I  O  D  G  D  I  A  Y  J  L  N  B  P
O  D  L  T  O  A  N  G  G  F  P  O  A  M  Z
S  M  B  S  A  M  D  O  F  R  E  S  F  Z  C
O  Z  M  T  A  Z  L  U  E  A  Q  T  N  M  B
M  I  E  O  S  O  I  G  L  Z  Q  R  I  L  O
O  V  T  M  C  P  N  L  R  T  G  U  N  H  C
R  O  V  E  U  A  E  G  I  K  H  M  I  W  C
H  S  N  D  N  O  U  C  E  T  L  O  T  N  U
C  Y  F  C  K  V  E  Z  R  N  R  I  O  O  P
G  Z  Y  G  O  T  E  J  T  O  E  E  B  D  K
P  O  S  T  P  A  R  T  U  M  F  S  F  I  R
M  U  I  N  O  C  E  M  U  R  D  O  M  Z  K
P  F  Q  M  S  Y  C  D  R  L  V  N  F  D  B
```

adulthood
amnion
chromosome
colostrum
fertilization
forceps
genes
gynecology
infancy
meconium
postpartum
pregnancy
zygote

Vocabulary Review

Key Term	Definition
2-hour postprandial glucose test	test that determines blood glucose levels 2 hours after drinking a sugar solution
abortion	expulsion of an embryo or fetus from the uterus before it can survive outside the womb
abruptio placentae	condition in which the placenta prematurely separates from the uterine wall
adolescence	period of life from puberty to maturity
adulthood	period of life after adolescence
albinism	hereditary absence of melanin in the hair, skin, and eyes
allantois	membranous sac that forms the umbilical blood vessels

Key Term	Definition
α-fetoprotein serum test	protein marker test for certain congenital defects
amniocentesis	prenatal diagnostic test in which amniotic fluid is evaluated
amnion	innermost fetal membrane forming a fluid-filled protective sac
anencephaly	condition in which a fetus or infant lacks the cerebrum, cerebellum, and flat bones of the skull
Apgar score	score assessing the condition of a newborn baby in five key areas (heart rate, breathing, muscle tone, reflex response, and skin color)

Key Term	Definition	Key Term	Definition
atrial septal defect (ASD)	abnormal opening between the left atrium and right atrium	**congenital**	existing before or at birth, though not necessarily detected then
blastocyst	mass of cells that implants on the endometrium after fertilization	**congenital megacolon**	disorder in which ganglionic cells of the enteric nervous system are missing from the colon, resulting in colon enlargement; also called Hirschsprung disease
Braxton Hicks contractions	irregular and painless uterine contractions that occur with increasing frequency throughout pregnancy	**contractions**	tightenings of uterine muscles that occur at increasingly frequent intervals immediately before childbirth
breech	fetus positioned so the buttocks and/or feet present first in the cervix and vaginal canal	**cri-du-chat syndrome**	congenital defect with a characteristic cat-like cry caused by problems of the larynx and nervous system; also called cat's cry syndrome
bronchopulmonary dysplasia (BPD)	a chronic pulmonary insufficiency affecting premature infants who required oxygen therapy	**cystic fibrosis (CF)**	hereditary disease of infancy affecting various exocrine glands and characterized by thick mucus that clogs ducts and airways
cerebral palsy (CP)	generic term for various types of nonprogressive motor conditions causing physical disability that are present at birth or beginning in early childhood	**developmental hip dysplasia**	birth defect of the hip joint in which the newborn's hips easily become dislocated; also called congenital hip dysplasia (CHD)
cesarean section (C-section)	operation to deliver a baby by cutting through the mother's abdomen and uterus	**dilation and curettage (D&C)**	surgical procedure involving expansion of the cervix and scraping of the uterus to remove extra tissue
Chadwick sign	bluish discoloration of the cervix and vagina around the sixth week of pregnancy	**diphtheria**	serious infectious disease caused by *Corynebacterium diphtheriae* that attacks throat membranes and releases a toxin that damages the heart and nervous system
chickenpox	infectious disease caused by the varicella-zoster virus (VZV) characterized by small itching blisters; also called varicella	**dizygotic twins**	two individuals derived from two zygotes; also called fraternal twins
childhood	period of life between infancy and puberty	**Down syndrome**	congenital disorder characterized by mild to severe mental retardation that occurs from a tripling of chromosome 21; also called trisomy 21
chloasma	dark coloration on the facial skin caused by pregnancy-induced hormonal changes		
chorioangioma	benign tumor of the placental blood vessels	**Duchenne muscular dystrophy (DMD)**	X-linked degenerative disease marked by skeletal muscle weakening with an onset shortly after birth or some time before age 6
choriocarcinoma	malignant, aggressive cancer of the uterus originating from cells of the chorion	**eclampsia**	acute, life-threatening complication of pregnancy characterized by hypertension, proteinuria, convulsions, and sometimes coma that occurs in women who have developed preeclampsia; also called toxemia of pregnancy
chorion	outermost fetal membrane that forms part of the placenta		
chorionic villi	vascular projections from the chorion's outer surface that move into the wall to form the placenta		
chorionic villus biopsy (CVB)	prenatal test used to detect birth defects by analyzing cells of the chorion; also called chorionic villus sampling	**ectopic pregnancy**	development of the fertilized egg outside the uterus
chorionic villus sampling (CVS)	prenatal test used to detect birth defects by analyzing cells of the chorion; also called chorionic villus biopsy	**Edwards syndrome**	congenital disorder characterized by several physical anomalies caused by a tripling of chromosome 18; also called trisomy 18
chromosome	rod-shaped structure in the cell nucleus that carries the genes	**effacement**	the thinning out of the cervix just before or during labor
cleft lip	congenital split in the upper lip on one or both sides of the center associated with a cleft palate		
cleft palate	congenital split in the roof of the mouth, caused by failure of embryonic facial bones to fuse	**embryo**	product of conception from the moment of fertilization to the end of the eighth gestational week
coarctation of aorta	narrowing of the aorta causing blood flow obstruction		
colostrum	first milk produced by the mother's breasts after childbirth		

Key Term	Definition
episiotomy	surgical incision made in the vagina to enlarge the opening and facilitate childbirth; also called a vaginoperineotomy
erythroblastosis fetalis	blood disease in which maternal antibodies attack the developing red blood cells of the fetus; also called hemolytic disease of the newborn
fertilization	union of the male sperm and the female secondary oocyte
fetal alcohol syndrome (FAS)	pattern of malformation found among children of mothers who abused alcohol while pregnant
fetus	developing human from week 9 of gestation until birth
gamete	male or female reproductive cell (sperm or oocyte)
genes	strands of DNA that function as hereditary units
gestation	period of development from fertilization until birth; also called pregnancy
gestational age	age of the developing embryo/fetus computed from the first day of the last menstrual cycle to any point in time until birth
gestational diabetes mellitus (GDM)	inability to metabolize carbohydrates, resulting in hyperglycemia, that occurs only during pregnancy
Goodell sign	softening of the cervix, indicative of pregnancy
Guthrie test	test that determines the level of phenylalanine in the serum of a neonate to detect PKU
gynecology (GYN)	medical specialty concerned with female reproductive health
Haemophilus influenzae **type b**	bacterial species that causes meningitis, pneumonia, and epiglottitis
Hegar sign	softening of the lower portion of the uterus occurring at about week 7 of pregnancy
hepatitis A	viral disease caused by hepatitis A virus characterized by fever, damage to the liver, and jaundice
hepatitis B	viral disease caused by hepatitis B virus that may lead to chronic liver disease
holandric inheritance	genetic traits carried on the Y chromosome inherited only by males; also called Y-linked inheritance
human chorionic gonadotropin (hCG)	hormone originating in chorionic tissue that maintains estrogen and progesterone levels; its presence indicates pregnancy
human papillomavirus (HPV)	sexually transmitted viral disease that causes genital warts and is associated with cervical cancer
human placental lactogen (hPL)	hormone important to embryo/fetal growth

Key Term	Definition
hydatidiform mole	rare mass that forms inside the uterus at the beginning of a pregnancy
hydrocephalus	condition marked by excessive cerebrospinal fluid accumulation in the brain ventricles, enlarging the head and sometimes causing brain damage
immunizations	vaccines that provide immunity; also called vaccinations
implantation	attachment of the blastocyst to the endometrium
in vitro fertilization (IVF)	the process by which egg cells are fertilized by sperm outside the body
in vivo fertilization	fertilization occurring inside the body
incompetent cervix	condition in which the cervix dilates prematurely before the fetus reaches full term
incubation	phase of development of an infectious disease from the time of infection to the appearance of symptoms
infancy	the first year of life; also called babyhood
infant respiratory distress syndrome (IRDS)	disease seen in premature neonates associated with reduced amounts of lung surfactant; also called hyaline membrane disease of the newborn
influenza	acute respiratory infection caused by inhaling the influenza virus
inheritance	characteristics and qualities transmitted from parent to offspring through genes
Klinefelter syndrome	congenital disorder characterized by male phenotype with an extra X chromosome, designated XXY
Koplik spots	small gray-white areas on a red background occurring on the parotid salivary gland that are characteristic of measles
labor	time from when contractions start to the baby's delivery
lactation	production and secretion of breast milk
life expectancy	the average number of years a person born today can expect to live
lifespan	length of time that a member of a particular species can remain alive and is the extreme limit of our longevity
lightening	sinking or dropping of the fetus into the pelvic inlet
linea nigra	dark line extending up the center of the abdomen of a pregnant woman
measles	very contagious, acute viral disease characterized by fever and a red rash of small spots; also called rubeola
meconium	dark greenish fecal material that collects in the intestines of a newborn and is released shortly after birth
meningocele	cerebrospinal fluid–filled cyst formed from the protrusion of the meninges through an opening in the skull or vertebra

Key Term	Definition	Key Term	Definition
meningococcal meningitis	acute infectious disease caused by *Neisseria meningitidis* that infects the cerebrospinal fluid bathing the brain and spinal cord	**placenta previa**	condition in which the placenta is positioned at the opening of the uterine cervix in the vagina, interfering with normal delivery
monozygotic twins	two individuals derived from a single fertilized egg; also called identical twins or maternal twins	**pneumonia**	infection of the lungs that can cause mild to severe illness
mumps	acute, contagious disease that causes fever and swelling of the parotid salivary glands; also called epidemic parotitis	**polio**	an infectious viral disease that affects the nervous system, leading to muscle wasting; abbreviated term for poliomyelitis
mutations	random changes in genes caused by changes in the DNA	**post partum**	adverb form that refers to the period immediately after childbirth
Nägele's rule	formula used to calculate an infant's delivery date	**postpartum**	adjective form that refers to the period immediately after childbirth
necrotizing enterocolitis (NEC)	extensive ulceration (open sores) and necrosis (tissue death) of the ileum and colon in premature infants during the neonatal period	**preeclampsia**	condition of pregnancy characterized by hypertension, oftentimes with fluid retention and proteinuria
neonate	an infant age 1 month or younger; also called a newborn	**pregnancy**	period of development of the offspring; also called gestation
obstetric forceps	instrument resembling tongs used for grasping the fetus's head during delivery	**premature birth**	birth that occurs when the infant is born after the stage of viability, but before 37 weeks' gestation
obstetrician (OB)	physician specializing in pregnancy, delivering babies, and the care of women after childbirth	**premature infant**	infant born before the 37th gestational week
obstetrics (OB)	the branch of medicine concerned with the care of women during pregnancy, childbirth, and for some 6 weeks following delivery	**puberty**	sequence of events by which a child becomes a young adult
parturition	act of giving birth; also called childbirth	**quickening**	fetal movements felt by the mother
		relaxin	hormone secreted during pregnancy that causes relaxation of the pubic symphysis
patent ductus arteriosus (PDA)	presence of ductus arteriosus after birth that causes oxygenated blood to recirculate to the lungs instead of the rest of the body	**retinopathy of prematurity (ROP)**	oxygen-induced disease of the eye marked by abnormal replacement of the sensory retina with fibrous tissue and blood vessels
pediatrician	physician specializing in the care and development of children and in the prevention and treatment of children's diseases	**Reye syndrome**	acute childhood illness of unknown cause that follows a respiratory or varicella infection and results in encephalitis and liver failure
pediatrics	branch of medicine dealing with the care and development of children and with the prevention and treatment of children's diseases	**rotavirus**	group of RNA viruses that cause gastroenteritis
pelvimetry	measurement of the inlet and outlet diameters of the pelvis to determine the feasibility of a vaginal childbirth	**rubella**	highly contagious viral disease that causes swelling of the cervical lymph nodes and a skin rash; also called epidemic roseola, German measles, and 3-day measles
pertussis	infectious respiratory bacterial disease that causes violent coughing spasms, caused by *Bordetella pertussis*; also called whooping cough	**senescence**	process of aging
		severe combined immunodeficiency (SCID)	congenital disorder characterized by an absence of immunity
phenylketonuria (PKU)	genetic disease in which the body lacks the enzyme to metabolize phenylalanine	**sex chromosomes**	23rd pair of chromosomes, designated X and Y, that determines gender
placenta	a vascular organ of pregnancy that develops on the wall of the uterus to supply food and oxygen to the embryo/fetus through the umbilical cord	**sex-linked inheritance**	genetic traits that result from a gene located on either the X or Y chromosome
		small for gestational age (SGA)	refers to a low-birth weight infant who is not premature

Key Term	Definition	Key Term	Definition
spina bifida	condition in which one or more of the vertebral arches fails to close and a part of the spinal cord and its meninges protrudes through the opening	**transposition of great arteries**	rotation of the aorta and the pulmonary artery resulting in two closed-loop systems
stillbirth	birth of an infant who has died before delivery	**Turner syndrome**	chromosomal disorder occurring in females resulting in nondevelopment of reproductive organs, designated XO
striae gravidarum	stretch marks seen in pregnancy	**umbilical cord**	connecting stalk between the embryo or fetus and the placenta that contains two arteries and one vein
talipes	any deformity of the foot involving the talus bone	**vaccinations**	vaccines that provide immunity; also called immunizations
talipes equinovarus	congenital foot deformity in which the foot is rotated internally at the ankle; also called clubfoot	**vaccines**	biological preparations that are administered to stimulate the immune system to produce antibodies against a specific disease
Tay–Sachs disease	genetic disease marked by accumulation of lipids in nervous tissue affecting people of eastern European Jewish ancestry	**vaginal birth after cesarean (VBAC)**	vaginal delivery of a baby when the previous birth was by cesarean section
teratogens	substances that alter the normal development of a fetus causing congenital abnormalities	**varicella**	infectious disease caused by the varicella-zoster virus (VZV) characterized by small itching blisters; also called chickenpox
teratology	scientific study of congenital malformations	**ventricular septal defect**	abnormal opening between the left ventricle and the right ventricle
tetanus	disease marked by painful muscular contractions caused by a neurotoxin of *Clostridium tetani* acting on the central nervous system; also called lockjaw	**vernix caseosa**	cheesy-appearing deposit on the surface of the fetus
tetralogy of Fallot	congenital heart defect with four abnormalities	**vertex**	normal birth position of the fetus so that the crown of the head presents first in the cervix and the vaginal canal
TORCH series	blood tests used to identify teratogenic diseases in pregnant women; TORCH is an acronym for *t*oxoplasmosis, *o*ther infections, *r*ubella, *c*ytomegalovirus (CMV), and *h*erpes simplex virus (HSV)	**zygote**	fertilized ovum; cell formed from the union of a sperm and secondary oocyte
toxemia of pregnancy	acute, life-threatening complication of pregnancy characterized by hypertension, proteinuria, convulsions, and sometimes coma that occurs in women who have developed preeclampsia; also called eclampsia		

CHAPTER
18

Mental Health

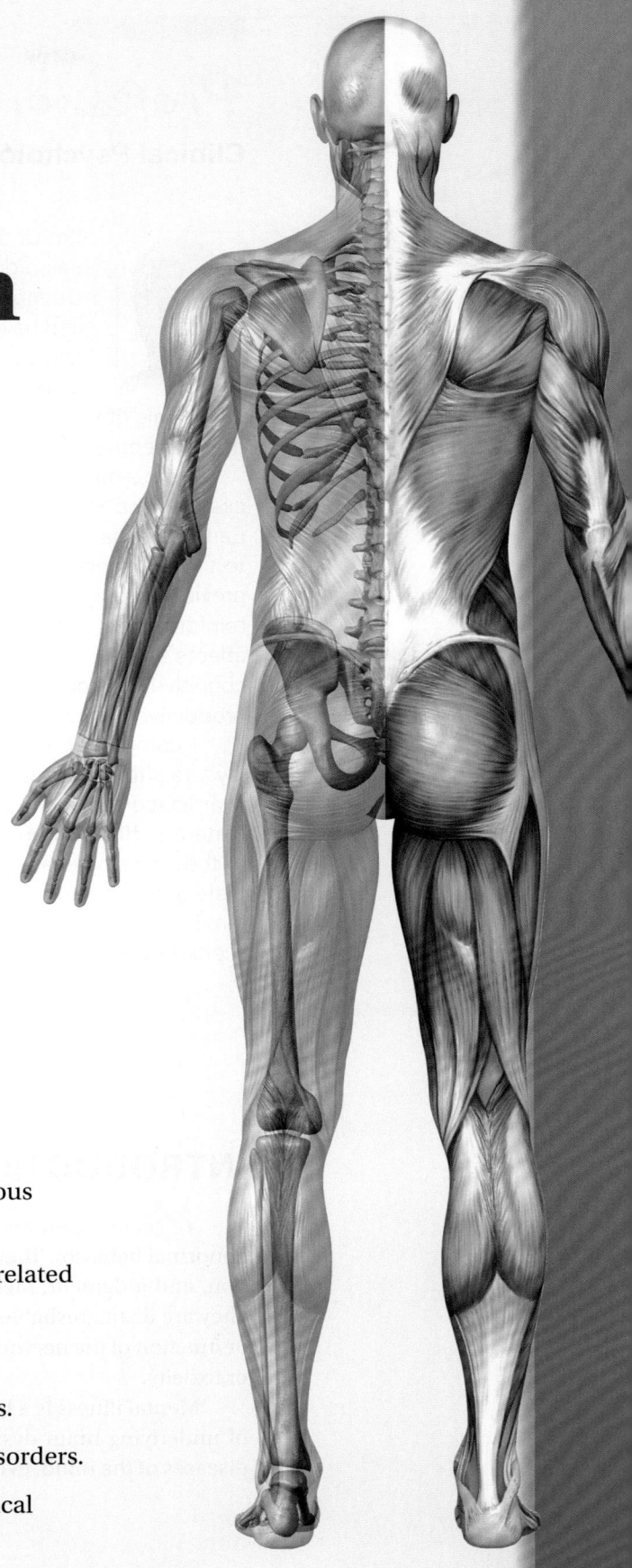

OBJECTIVES

After completing this chapter, you should be able to:

1. Define the meanings of word parts related to mental health.

2. Explain the function of neurotransmitters in normal and abnormal brain physiology.

3. Describe the role of each type of mental health professional.

4. Identify the significance of the *ICD-9-CM* and *DSM-IV-TR* publications in regard to mental disorders.

5. Characterize various mental disorders.

6. Explain different signs, symptoms, and treatments of various mental disorders.

7. Describe clinical tests, scales, and diagnostic procedures related to mental disorders.

8. Summarize mental disorders throughout the lifespan.

9. Define common abbreviations related to mental disorders.

10. Define terms used in medical reports involving mental disorders.

11. Correctly define, spell, and pronounce the chapter's medical terms.

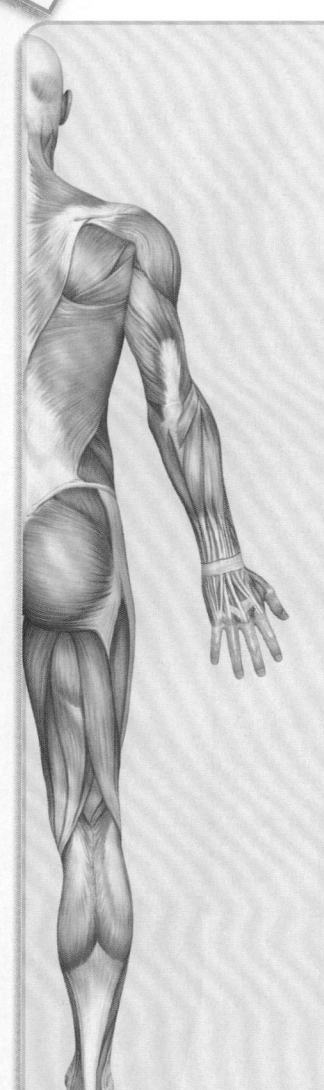

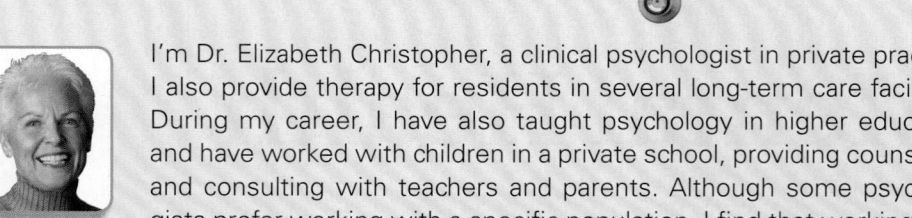

Professional Profile

Clinical Psychologist

I'm Dr. Elizabeth Christopher, a clinical psychologist in private practice. I also provide therapy for residents in several long-term care facilities. During my career, I have also taught psychology in higher education and have worked with children in a private school, providing counseling and consulting with teachers and parents. Although some psychologists prefer working with a specific population, I find that working with individuals of various ages is most rewarding and interesting. I practice from an eclectic perspective, using a variety of interventions based on the client's diagnosis.

From a historical perspective, psychologists have been providing psychotherapy to clients since Sigmund Freud, who was the first person to engage in the "talking cure." Early American psychologists focused on individual differences in people and adapting to the environment in which a person lives. The behavioral movement in psychology provided therapists with a structured plan to help people change their behavior, using reinforcement and punishment. Cognitive therapists focus on how a person's thinking affects their behavior. For example, many depressed people think their life is terrible. A cognitive therapist helps a person examine his or her life more logically, explore more productive behaviors, and eventually feel less depressed.

I completed a doctoral degree (Ph.D.) in clinical psychology, which took about 4 years after undergraduate schooling. This process included coursework, taking major examinations, writing a dissertation, and completing an internship. I needed to complete a sufficient number of internship hours before I could take the written portion of the licensing examination. After passing the written portion, I was required to complete another examination administered orally by the state. My specialty areas include family and individual therapy, geriatrics, and substance abuse. Before I can renew my license every 2 years, I must complete 24 hours of continuing education.

INTRODUCTION

Mental disorders are psychiatric conditions that affect brain function and often lead to abnormal behavior. There may be impaired intellectual function, including memory, orientation, and judgment. Mental disorders are associated with impairment in social functioning. They are distinguishable from neurological disorders, which are disturbances in the structure or function of the nervous system and result from developmental abnormality, disease, injury, or toxicity.

Mental illness is a broad term used to describe pathology of the mind with the inference of underlying brain dysfunction. It includes brain disease, with behavioral symptoms, and diseases of the mind, evidenced by abnormal behavior.

Detailed descriptions and definitions that could be used accurately to diagnose disorders are essential. An official nomenclature (system of names assigned to terms in the mental health field) that is applicable to a variety of clinical, educational, research, or statistical settings requiring uniform medical terminology has been established. The sources used are the *Diagnostic and Statistical Manual of Mental Disorders, Fourth Edition, Text Revision* (*DSM-IV-TR*) and *International Statistical Classification of Diseases and Related Health Problems, Ninth Edition, Clinical Modification* (*ICD-9-CM*). The *ICD-9-CM* provides standardized diagnostic codes for mental disorders, and the *DSM-IV-TR* gives descriptions and terms, and serves as the standard for clinicians by offering guidelines for various mental disorders. *DSM-IV-TR* revisions were facilitated by the growing body of research and the necessity for consistent nomenclature that could be used by clinicians and researchers alike. These books will be referred to as the *DSM* and the *ICD* throughout this chapter.

Authors of both volumes worked closely together to develop mutually beneficial texts. Codes and terms in both are compatible; thus, congruency exists between the manuals. The official coding systems of mental disorders in the *DSM* and the *ICD* are identical. This has aided considerably in studying, diagnosing, treating, and communicating about mental disorders. Mental conditions and related medical terms from these two sources are highlighted in this chapter.

MEDICAL TERM PARTS

Word Parts

Medical term prefixes, suffixes, and combining forms related to mental health are introduced in this section.

Word Part	Meaning
ap-, apo-	separated from, derived from
cata-	down, opposite
hypn-, hypno-	sleep, hypnosis
hyster-, hystero-	hysteria
log-, logo-	speech, words
-mania	obsession, compulsion
morph-, morpho-	form, shape
narco-	stupor, narcosis
neur-, neuri-, neuro-	nerve, nerve tissue
-phil, -phile, -philia, -philic	affinity for, craving for
-phobia	extreme or irrational fear
-phrenia	the mind
psych-, psyche-, psycho-	mind, mental, psychological
schiz-, schizo-	split, cleft
somat-, somato-	the body, bodily
thym-, thymi-, -thymia, thymo-	mind, soul, emotions

Word Grouping Exercises

Using the *Medical Term Parts* table, identify the prefix, suffix, or combining form for each of the following definitions. The first one has been done as an example.

Definition	Word Part
down, opposite	*cata-*
affinity for, craving for	
the body, bodily	
extreme or irrational fear	
form, shape	
hysteria	
the mind	
mind, mental, psychological	
mind, soul, emotions	
nerve, nerve tissue	
obsession, compulsion	
separated from, derived from	
sleep, hypnosis	
speech, words	
split, cleft	
stupor, narcosis	

Word Building Exercises

Word parts introduced in the *Medical Term Parts* section are listed in the following table. For this exercise, first supply the meaning of each word part, then use the word part to build a word you already know. The word you list under *Common or Known Word* does not have to be a medical term; a commonly used word is fine. Be sure, however, that the word correctly reflects the intended meaning. The first one has been done as an example. Check your answers in a dictionary.

Word Part	Meaning	Common or Known Word	Example Medical Term
cata-	*down, opposite*	*catabolic*	catatonic
hypn-, hypno-			hypnosis
hyster-, hystero-			hysteria
log-, logo-			logospasms
-mania			hypermania
morph-, morpho-			dysmorphophobia
narco-			narcolepsy

continued

continued from page 974

Word Part	Meaning	Common or Known Word	Example Medical Term
neur-, neuri-, neuro-			neurosis
-phil, -phile, -philia, -philic			pedophile
-phobia			agoraphobia
-phrenia			schizophrenia
psych-, psyche-, psycho-			psychology
schiz-, schizo-			schizophrenia
somat-, somato-			somatoform
thym-, thymi-, -thymia, thymo-			dysthymia

ANATOMY AND PHYSIOLOGY

The brain is the controlling center of the central nervous system (CNS). It is the foundation for personality, intellect, thinking, and behavior. At the same time, it maintains vital life systems and normal body functions.

Relative to mental functions, the **psyche** refers to the subjective aspects of the mind and self. The word part *psyche-* means "mind, mental, or psychological." Psyche is often used interchangeably with **mind**, which refers to the seat of consciousness and higher functions of the human brain. These higher functions include cognition, reasoning, and emotion. The mind generates thoughts, feelings, and ideas, and stores knowledge and memories.

Cognition is a generic term for the mental activities associated with thinking, learning, and memory. The **consciousness** is the state of being aware and responsive to the environment. An emotion, feeling, or mood associated with a thought is termed **affect**.

Brain physiology involves the role of neurotransmitters. **Neurotransmitters** are chemicals stored in synaptic vesicles that transfer "information" between different neurons. **Neurons** (nerve cells) are the basic functional units of the nervous system that transmit impulses. Neurotransmitters are produced by neuron endings and react with receptors on neighboring cells to produce a response. The neurotransmitter is released by one cell, called the presynaptic cell, crosses the synapse (gap), and stimulates or inhibits another cell, called the postsynaptic cell (**Figure 18-1**). One or several neurotransmitters may be released at any given time. These neurotransmitters are important in causing disorders resulting from neurobiological mechanisms. In fact, problems with neurotransmitters may contribute to mental disorders. Clinically important neurotransmitters are dopamine, epinephrine, γ-aminobutyric acid (GABA), norepinephrine, and serotonin.

Neuroimaging techniques can provide pictures of brain regions involved with certain pathologies. **Organic brain disease** is impaired functioning associated with recognizable,

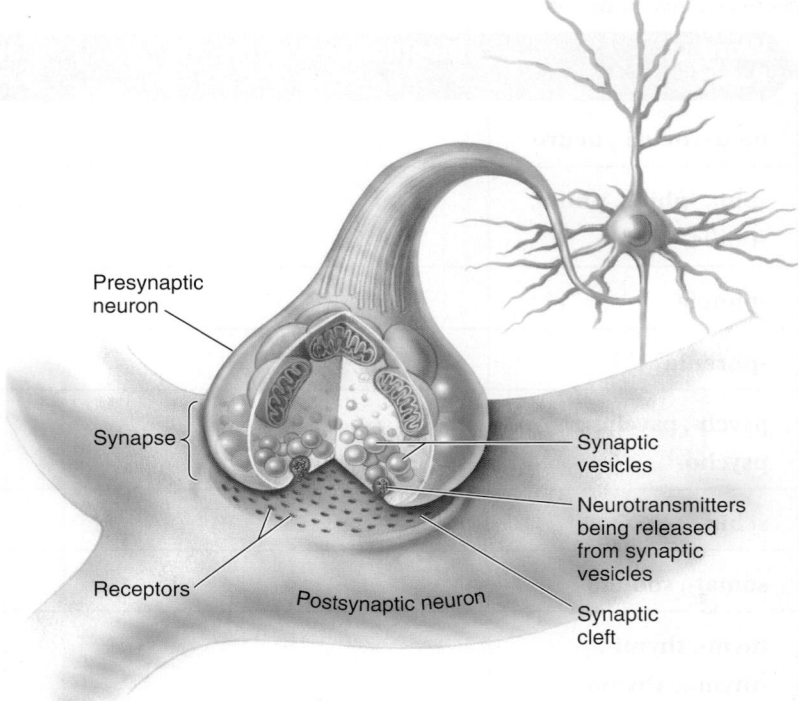

Presynaptic neuron

Synapse

Receptors

Postsynaptic neuron

Synaptic vesicles

Neurotransmitters being released from synaptic vesicles

Synaptic cleft

Figure 18-1 When a nerve impulse arrives in the presynaptic neuron, neurotransmitters are released in the synaptic cleft. The neurotransmitters then bind to specific receptors on the postsynaptic neuron.

structural changes in the brain. Organic brain diseases have a known or presumed physiological cause. Other brain dysfunction cannot be determined by viewing its anatomy.

In the study of mental disorders, a **neurosis** is a psychological or behavioral disorder with anxiety as the primary characteristic, whereas a **psychosis** (also called a *psychotic disorder*) is both a mental and a behavioral disorder causing gross distortion of reality, disorganized affective (emotional) response, and the inability to cope with ordinary demands of everyday life. Both neurotic and psychotic disorders can produce profound impairment in social functioning, and a person with a neurosis may be unable to perform daily activities.

The key and critical difference between a neurosis and a psychosis relates to something known as *reality testing*. Reality testing is the objective evaluation of an emotion or thought against real life. People with neurotic disorders can judge what is real and what is not. They may be completely disabled by the neurotic disorder, but their ability to evaluate reality is intact. In contrast, psychotic disorders always involve significant impairment in reality testing whereby the individual cannot trust his or her ability to provide accurate information regarding the world. A person with a psychotic disorder experiences hallucinations (perceptions of nonexisting stimuli) and/or delusions (false beliefs). Most affective disorders do not fall into the psychotic category. For example, most people with depression or mania are not psychotic (although they may be).

KEY TERM	Definition
psyche (SIGH-kee)	subjective aspects of the mind and self
mind	seat of consciousness and higher functions (cognition, reasoning, and emotion) of the human brain
cognition (kog-NISH-un)	generic term for the mental activities associated with thinking, learning, and memory

continued

continued from page 976

KEY TERM	Definition
consciousness	state of being aware and responsive to the environment
affect	an emotion, feeling, or mood associated with a thought
neurotransmitters (new-roh-trans-MIT-urz)	chemicals that transfer "information" between different neurons
neurons (NEW-ronz)	basic functional units of the nervous system that transmit impulses; also called nerve cells
organic brain disease	disease or impaired functioning with a definite structural alteration in the brain
neurosis (new-ROH-sis)	psychological or behavioral disorder with anxiety as the primary characteristic
psychosis (sigh-KOH-sis)	both a mental and a behavioral disorder causing gross distortion of reality, disorganized affective (emotional) response, and the inability to cope with ordinary demands of everyday life; also called psychotic disorder

KEY TERM PRACTICE: *Anatomy and Physiology*

1. _____ are chemicals that transfer "information" between different neurons.

2. A _____ is a psychological or behavioral disorder with anxiety as the primary characteristic.

3. The state of being aware and responsive to the environment is termed _____.

4. The _____ refers to the subjective aspects of the mind and self.

5. An emotion, feeling, or mood associated with a thought is known as _____.

Mental Health Professionals

More than 54 million Americans have a mental disorder, but fewer than 8 million seek treatment. Moreover, one in five children has a diagnosable mental, emotional, or behavioral disorder; however, 70% do not receive treatments. Another significant finding is that every year about half of primary care physician visits are the result of conditions caused or exacerbated by mental or emotional problems. Clearly, mental health issues are significant.

Psychotherapy is treatment of emotional, behavioral, personality, and psychiatric disorders by psychological means such as verbal or nonverbal communication with patients. It involves the use of interpersonal exchange between a therapist and a client with the goal of ultimately producing cognitive, affective, and behavioral change. No chemical or physical measures are used. **Counseling** is a therapeutic relationship in which a trained professional assists a person in solving and adjusting to problems and situations through dialogue and activities. Advice, opinion, and instruction are given to aid in the transition. **Counselors** are professionals who give advice on personal, social, health, or psychological problems. Psychologists, psychiatrists, and social workers who are licensed in the field often do counseling.

There are several educational paths for achieving a license to practice mental health therapy, and professionals often enter the field of mental health from a variety of educational backgrounds. Psychologists must usually complete a doctoral degree before they can take the licensing examination in their state to practice psychotherapy. Counselors and social workers need to complete only a master's degree to become licensed. Depending on the level of their license, some counselors and social workers may be limited in the types of disorders that they can treat and diagnoses they can make. For example, in Ohio, license levels include professional counselor (PC), professional clinical counselor (PCC), licensed social worker (LSW), licensed independent social worker (LISW), and psychologist. Other states may use similar or different titles.

School counselors and school psychologists are also licensed professionals in most states. They must complete a master's degree and take a licensing examination. School counselors work directly with children, individually or in groups. School psychologists provide assessment services and consult with parents and teachers to develop plans to help children succeed academically and socially.

Psychoanalysts are professionals who practice a method developed by Sigmund Freud for the exploration and synthesis of patterns in emotional thinking and for the treatment of a wide variety of disorders. Freudian psychoanalysis is rarely practiced in the United States today and has been replaced with more effective and fast-acting forms of psychotherapy.

The medical specialty that deals with the origins, diagnosis, prevention, and treatment of mental and behavioral disorders is termed **psychiatry**. Physicians (who hold an M.D. or D.O. degree) with postgraduate training in psychiatry are called **psychiatrists**.

Psychology is the science that studies the functions of the mind, including sensation, perception, memory, thought, learning, and behavior. The discipline is divided into professional practice (clinical psychology), scholarly discipline (academic psychology), and science (research psychology). Professionals with a state-issued license in psychology are termed **psychologists**. Psychologists generally hold doctorate degrees, such as a Ph.D., and are usually licensed to provide therapeutic services and/or work in academic settings. Unlike psychiatrists, most psychologists are not licensed to prescribe medications. However, a few states allow psychologists who pass a pharmacology examination to write prescriptions for medications. Quite often, psychologists and psychiatrists work together to treat mental illness. For example, a depressed client might see a psychiatrist who prescribes an antidepressant and follows up with periodic medication checks while at the same times the client may see a psychologist once a week for therapy and counseling. **Social workers** are professionals who provide help to people in need of social services, such as medical assistance or public assistance. Social workers try to improve their clients' quality of life. As a discipline, social work focuses on research, policy, and community development to advance the well-being of all individuals.

KEY TERM	Definition
psychotherapy (sigh-koh-THERR-uh-pee)	treatment of emotional, behavioral, personality, and psychiatric disorders by psychological means such as verbal or nonverbal communication with patients
counseling	therapeutic relationship in which a trained professional assists a person in solving and adjusting to problems and situations through dialogue and activities
counselors	professionals who give advice on personal, social, health, or psychological problems
psychoanalysts (sigh-koh-AN-uh-lists)	professionals who practice a method developed by Sigmund Freud for the exploration and synthesis of patterns in emotional thinking and for the treatment of a wide variety of disorders
psychiatry (sigh-KIGH-uh-tree)	medical specialty that deals with the origins, diagnosis, prevention, and treatment of mental and behavioral disorders
psychiatrists (sigh-KIGH-uh-trists)	physicians (who hold an M.D. or D.O. degree) trained in the diagnosis, treatment, and prevention of psychiatric disorders
psychology (sigh-KOL-uh-jee)	science that studies the functions of the mind, including sensation, perception, memory, thought, learning, and behavior

continued

continued from page 978

KEY TERM	Definition
psychologists (sigh-KOL-uh-jists)	professionals with a state-issued license in psychology who study and treat mental disorders
social workers	professionals who provide help to people in need of social services, such as medical assistance or public assistance

KEY TERM PRACTICE: *Mental Health Professionals*

1. A _____ practices psychiatry; a psychologist practices _____.

2. The word part *psycho-* refers to _____, and the treatment of mental disease by psychological methods is termed _____.

3. _____ are professionals who give advice on personal, social, health, or psychological problems.

4. _____ are professionals who provide help to people in need of social services, such as medical assistance or public assistance.

5. Professionals who practice a method developed by Sigmund Freud for the exploration and synthesis of patterns in emotional thinking and for the treatment of a wide variety of disorders are called _____.

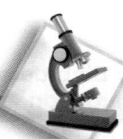

THE CLINICAL DIMENSION

This section provides a description of signs and symptoms of various disorders, tests and scales, diagnostic procedures, and treatments pertaining to mental disease. An overview of general pathology presents a sense of the magnitude of mind conditions while demonstrating that they are not trivial considerations. Pathological conditions are presented according to *DSM* headings and standard nomenclature.

Using the *Diagnostic and Statistical Manual of Mental Disorders* (*DSM*)

The handbook used by mental health professionals is published by the American Psychiatric Association and is called *Diagnostic and Statistical Manual of Mental Disorders (DSM)*. Currently in its fourth edition (*DSM-IV*), the next edition is scheduled to be released in 2013. Disorders in the *DSM* are categorized as mild, moderate, severe, in partial remission, in full remission, and prior history. These categorizations are called **severity and course specifiers**.

- *Mild* refers to few or no symptoms with minor impairment.
- *Moderate* means that there are symptoms and functional impairment.
- *Severe* describes symptoms with marked impairment in social or occupational functioning.
- *Partial remission* describes the situation in which some signs and symptoms remain in an individual for a condition that had previously met the criteria for a condition.
- *Full remission* means that there are no longer any signs or symptoms, but it is still clinically relevant to document the disorder.
- *Prior history* indicates that an individual was previously diagnosed with a disorder, but is now recovered.

The **multiaxial classification** is a procedure described in the *DSM* for the diagnosis of patients on five axes:

I. Psychiatric syndrome present

II. Patient's history of personality and developmental disorders

III. Possible nonmental medical disorder

IV. Severity of psychosocial stressors

V. Highest level of adaptive functioning in the past year.

This tool assists the clinician in developing a treatment plan and predicting an outcome. It also allows clinicians to note primary and secondary diagnoses and report them in clinical notes. The diagnostic codes are obtained from the *DSM* and the *International Classification of Diseases (ICD)*. (The *ICD* was discussed in Chapter 1.) An example multiaxial evaluation report form is shown in **Figure 18-2**. The vast majority of insurance companies require the information from these axes before approving treatments for the insured.

Multiaxial Evaluation Report Form

AXIS I: **Clinical Disorders**
Other Conditions That May Be a Focus of Clinical Attention

Diagnostic code   *DSM-IV* name

— — —.— —   _____
— — —.— —   _____
— — —.— —   _____

AXIS II: **Personality Disorders**
Mental Retardation

Diagnostic code   *DSM-IV* name

— — —.— —   _____
— — —.— —   _____

AXIS III: **General Medical Conditions**

ICD-9-CM code   *ICD-9-CM* name

— — —.— —   _____
— — —.— —   _____

AXIS IV: **Psychosocial and Environmental Problems**

Check:
___ Problems with primary support group   Specify: _____
___ Problems related to the social environment   Specify: _____
___ Educational problems   Specify: _____
___ Occupational problems   Specify: _____
___ Housing problems   Specify: _____
___ Economic problems   Specify: _____
___ Problems with access to health care services   Specify: _____
___ Problems related to interaction with the
       legal system/crime   Specify: _____
___ Other psychosocial and environmental problems   Specify: _____

AXIS V: **Global Assessment of Functioning Scale**

Score: ____ ____ ____
Time frame: _____

Figure 18-2 The multiaxial evaluation report form.

KEY TERM	Definition
severity and course specifiers	qualifiers (mild, moderate, severe, in partial remission, in full remission, and prior history) regarding specific mental health conditions
multiaxial classification	procedure described in the *DSM* for the diagnosis of patients on five axes

KEY TERM PRACTICE: *Using the Diagnostic and Statistical Manual of Mental Disorders (DSM)*

1. The procedure described in the *DSM* for the diagnosis of patients on five axes is termed _____.

2. Qualifiers—such as mild, moderate, severe, in partial remission, in full remission, and prior history—regarding specific mental health conditions in the *DSM* are known as _____.

Tests and Scales

Tests are a method of examination used to determine the presence or degree of a psychological or behavioral trait. **Scales** are standardized tests that measure psychological, personality, or behavioral characteristics. These evaluation tools are administered by professionals in the mental health field to assess individuals and develop treatment plans. This section focuses on commonly used tests and scales.

intelligence quotient (IQ)

An **intelligence quotient (IQ)** is a number representing a person's reasoning ability as compared to the statistical norm or average for his or her age. It is based on performance on a standardized problem-solving test. **Table 18-1** lists IQ scores with their representative descriptions.

Stanford-Binet intelligence scale

The **Stanford-Binet intelligence scale** (Stanford-Binet test) is a standardized test used to measure intelligence. This scale consists of a series of questions designed to assess cognitive abilities in children and adults. The test is administered by a clinically trained examiner and interpreted by a trained professional, usually a psychologist. The raw scores are based on the number of items

TABLE 18-1

IQ SCORES AND DESCRIPTIONS

Score	Description
>20	profound retardation
20–35	severe retardation
35–50	moderate retardation
50–70	mild retardation
70–90	dull normal
90–110	normal
110–125	superior
125–140	very superior
≥140	genius

answered by the test taker and are then converted into a standard age score. This score, which corresponds to a particular age group, is similar to the numerical rating used in the intelligence quotient. Thus the answers provided indicate the mental age of the test taker. An adult version, normalized against adult age levels, also exists.

Wechsler intelligence scales

The **Wechsler intelligence scales** are standardized tests for measuring general intelligence. Originally developed by psychologist David Wechsler in 1949, the scales are continually revised and updated. They are used to measure general intelligence in preschool children (Wechsler Preschool and Primary Scale of Intelligence), children (Wechsler Intelligence Scale for Children), and adults (Wechsler Adult Intelligence Scale).

Rorschach test

The **Rorschach test,** also called the inkblot test, is a psychological test of personality or mental state in which a person describes what he or she sees on a series of 10 standardized inkblots of various designs and colors, like the one in **Figure 18-3.** The responses indicate personality patterns, special interests, originality of thought, deviations of affect, and neurotic and psychotic tendencies. A trained professional scoring the test can also determine attitudes, emotions, and personality.

thematic apperception test (TAT)

The **thematic apperception test (TAT)** is a psychological test for exploring aspects of the personality using a set of pictures that suggest life situations from which the person constructs a story. *Apperception* means the "comprehension or assimilation of something in terms of previous experiences." The tool is designed to recall attitudes, feelings, and conflicts of personality that are then interpreted by a psychologist.

Minnesota Multiphasic Personality Inventory (MMPI)

The **Minnesota Multiphasic Personality Inventory (MMPI)** is a test of an individual's personality based primarily on responses to a questionnaire. The 550 true–false statements are coded on four validity scales (an index used to measure how well the test measures what it purports to measure) and 10 personality scales. The questionnaire is administered either individually or in a group setting. The MMPI is used widely for mental health screening.

Goodenough-Harris drawing test

The **Goodenough-Harris drawing test** is a brief test for assessing a person's level of intelligence based on how accurately drawn and how many elements are included when a child or adult is given a pencil and sheet of white paper and asked to draw a person (**Figure 18-4**). In 1926, it was originally called the Goodenough Draw-A-Man test by its developer, Florence Goodenough. The test was later revised by Dr. Dale Harris, and is currently known as the Goodenough-Harris drawing test.

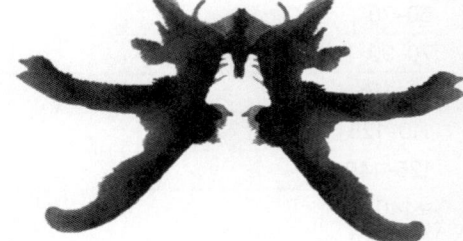

Figure 18-3 Rorschach test: an example of a picture used in testing.

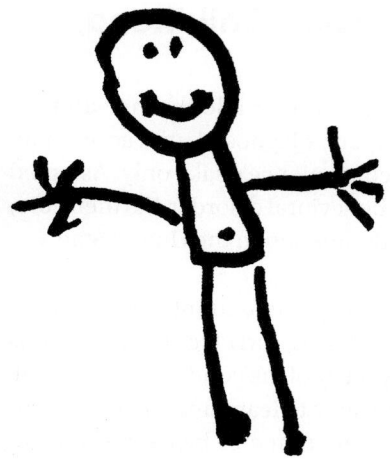

Figure 18-4 Goodenough-Harris drawing test: an 8-point drawing.

KEY TERM	Definition
scales	standardized tests that measure psychological, personality, or behavioral characteristics
intelligence quotient (IQ)	number representing a person's reasoning ability as compared to the statistical norm or average for his or her age
Stanford-Binet intelligence scale	standardized test used to measure intelligence; also called Stanford-Binet test
Wechsler intelligence scales	standardized tests for measuring general intelligence in preschoolers, children, and adults
Rorschach (ROR-shahk) **test**	test of personality or mental state based on a person's interpretation of standardized inkblots of various designs and colors; also called inkblot test
thematic apperception test (TAT)	test for exploring aspects of the personality in which the person is shown pictures of people in various situations and asked to describe what is happening
Minnesota Multiphasic Personality Inventory (MMPI)	standardized test that uses true–false questions to assess a person's personality
Goodenough-Harris drawing test	brief test for assessing a person's level of intelligence based on how accurately drawn and how many elements are included when a child or adult is given a pencil and sheet of white paper and asked to draw a person

KEY TERM PRACTICE: *Tests and Scales*

1. List two scales commonly used to assess intelligence. _____

2. The _____ is a test of personality or mental state based on a person's interpretation of standardized inkblots.

3. A test for exploring aspects of the personality in which a person is shown pictures of people in various situations and asked to describe what is happening is known as the _____.

4. The _____ is best described as a brief test for assessing a person's level of intelligence based on how accurately drawn and how many elements are included when a child or adult is given a pencil and sheet of white paper and asked to draw a person.

5. The _____ is a standardized test that uses true–false questions to assess a person's personality.

Disorders Usually First Diagnosed in Infancy, Childhood, or Adolescence

The disorders in this section first appear during infancy, childhood, or adolescence and are usually diagnosed during this period, but they may not be properly diagnosed until adulthood. For this reason, categorizing a mental disorder by age is for convenience's sake only. As noted previously, 20% of children may have a mental, emotional, or behavioral disorder. Furthermore, as many as 1 in 33 children and 1 in 8 adolescents may have depression in the United States.

mental retardation	**Mental retardation** is below average general intellectual functioning that is present at birth or during early life. The limitations of the disorder depend on the severity of the condition. In general, mental retardation limits the capacity to learn and to function independently. Primary mental retardation may be the result of familial or hereditary factors with no known brain **lesion** (structural change) or prenatal cause. Secondary mental retardation results from brain tissue damage or a chromosomal disorder; prenatal, maternal, or postnatally acquired infections; intoxication, trauma, or prematurity; disorders of growth, nutrition, or metabolism; and degenerative diseases, tumor, or major psychiatric disorders. These causes can also be associated with psychosocial/environmental deprivation. Any condition that interrupts or compromises blood, oxygen, or nutrient supply to the brain can result in neurological damage and subsequent mental retardation.

Mental retardation is classified as mild, moderate, severe, or profound. With the exception of Down syndrome, there may be no outward physical manifestations. Impaired intellectual and social growth is often the first indication. Delayed motor and communication skills lead to further evaluation. Observation of behaviors and confirmation of intelligence using standardized tests provide the initial diagnosis. Limitations in two of the following areas are necessary for diagnostic purposes: communication, home living, self-care, social and interpersonal skills, self-direction, and health and safety. Usually more than one test is used to confirm the diagnosis.

Underlying causes that respond to therapy are treated. Other treatment measures include providing occupational therapy (OT), physical therapy (PT), and psychotherapy to ensure the highest quality of life and to establish as much cognitive function as possible.

learning disorder (LD)	Formerly known as academic skills disorders, a **learning disorder (LD)** is any defect or disturbance in a child's ability to acquire skills in reading, writing, or arithmetic. Learning disorders are often complicated by behavioral disturbances resulting from feelings of inadequacy. The child may have normal to above normal intelligence and adequate educational opportunities, yet is hindered from learning basic skills or information at the same rate as most people of the same age.

Learning disorders have an unknown cause, but cognitive processing abnormalities have been implicated. Language barriers, lack of opportunity, poor teaching, inadequate schooling, and environmental and nutritional factors must be ruled out in the preliminary diagnosis. If the problem still persists, a learning disorder is assumed to be present. Treatment involves designing individual educational plans (IEPs) complete with specially formulated teaching techniques. Currently, one-on-one instruction appears to be the best method. Educational psychology has advanced research in this area.

stuttering

Communication disorders are characterized by the ineffective use of words to convey ideas or information. **Stuttering** is a kind of communication disorder demonstrated by the inability to say something with two or more syllables without repeating one syllable, straining unnaturally, or both. It is characterized by frequent repetitions or prolongations of sounds or syllables, impeding the speech pattern. The typical age of onset is between 2 and 7 years. Its cause is unknown, but it may have a genetic component because there appears to be a familial trend. Stuttering occurs more frequently in males. **Anxiety** (overwhelming sense of apprehension) and nervousness seem to be major factors in the persistence of stuttering.

After hearing difficulties have been ruled out, the diagnosis of stuttering is based on observed patterns of speech cadence disturbance. Speech therapy and not drawing attention to the speaker's disorder while talking are treatments.

pervasive developmental disorders

Pervasive developmental disorders are characterized by severe, persistent, and all-encompassing impairment in several areas of development, including social, communication, and behavior.

autism

Autism is an example of a pervasive developmental disorder. **Autism** is a form of behavior and thinking observed in young children in which the child seems to concentrate on herself or himself without regard to other environmental influences. Manifestations are obvious within the first 3 years of life. Language usage, reaction to stimuli, interpretation of the world, and formation of relationships are not fully established and follow unusual patterns.

Signs and symptoms include excessive shyness, aloofness, withdrawal, introspection, and possible seizures. Proper communication and age-appropriate activities are not displayed. Children with autism often engage in obsessive behaviors including a preoccupation with objects and memorizing lists or facts. Children with autism perform nonfunctional rituals and are easily upset by trivial environmental changes.

Four primary symptoms are key characteristics of the disorder: language deficits, cognitive impairment, repetitive movements and body rocking, and social isolation. The cause is unknown, but an organically-based CNS dysfunction has been implicated. It occurs more commonly in males. Behavior observation—notably the four primary characteristics—leads to the diagnosis.

Cognitive-behavioral therapy that includes the child and family is prescribed to promote adaptive responses and skills to encourage self-sufficiency in the individual. **Cognitive-behavioral therapy (CBT)** is a form of treatment that combines traditional cognitive therapy techniques with methods taken from behavior therapy. The result is an intervention that seeks to change cognitions, or the way a person thinks, with the goal of behavioral change. **Behavior therapy** uses behavior-modification techniques in which a person's desirable responses are positively reinforced while undesirable behaviors are negatively rewarded.

Asperger disorder

Asperger disorder is another pervasive developmental disorder and is characterized by severe and enduring impairment in social skills and interests and by repetitive behaviors leading to impaired social and occupational functioning. There is no delay in language development. The impaired social and communication functions are not as severe as in autism. It was first diagnosed in 1944 by Austrian pediatrician Hans Asperger, who described children in his practice who lacked nonverbal communication skills.

attention deficit disorder (ADD)

Attention deficit disorder (ADD) is a disorder of attention, organization, and impulse control appearing in childhood and often persisting to adulthood. Hyperactivity may be a feature, but is not necessary for the diagnosis. This disorder is not identified in the *DSM*; however, it does have an *ICD* code.

attention deficit hyperactivity disorder (ADHD)

Attention deficit hyperactivity disorder (ADHD) is a type of attention deficit and disruptive behavior disorder characterized by a persistent pattern of inattention and/or increased activity and impulsivity. It is manifested at home, school, and in social situations with an onset before age 7. Children are often impatient, unable to do seat work in the classroom, and they avoid situations requiring attentive behavior. The cause is unknown, but a familial pattern exists. It is diagnosed by behavior observation and impaired function that directly results from the behavior. Behavior therapy that rewards appropriate behavior and discourages undesirable or inappropriate behavior is beneficial. Amphetamine drugs such as methylphenidate (Ritalin), dextroamphetamine (Dexedrine), and amphetamine-dextroamphetamine (Adderall) may be prescribed.

pica

A feeding and eating disorder of infancy or early childhood is **pica**, a desire for strange food or other substances of no nutritional value. (It may also occur in women during pregnancy as a result of emotional distress or malnutrition.) Examples of nonnutritive substances include clay, dirt, sand, and hair, but the ingested material typically varies with age. Eating material of no nutritious worth on a persistent basis for at least 1 month fulfills the criterion for pica diagnosis. The disorder seems to last for several months and then remits with no treatment.

tic disorders

Tic disorders are habitual, irresistible, repetitive movements that a person feels compelled to do. A **tic** is a sudden, rapid, recurrent, nonrhythmic, involuntary motor movement or vocalization. These motions can be voluntarily suppressed for only brief moments. Examples include throat clearing, excessive eye blinking, sniffing, or lip pursing. The movements are more pronounced when the person is under stress. There is no known cause.

Tourette disorder

Tourette disorder is a type of tic disorder characterized by multiple motor tics and one or more vocal tics. It is also known as *Gilles de la Tourette disease*. The disorder generally begins in late childhood and adolescence, but may start as early as 2 years old. Additional features include **echolalia** (involuntary parrot-like repetition of a word just spoken by another person), obscene utterances, and other compulsive acts that are present for more than 1 year. Vocal tics may include clicks, grunts, or snorts. Obsessive–compulsive behavior and attention deficit disorder may accompany this lifelong condition. The cause is unknown and the disorder affects more males than females. Observation confirms the diagnosis. Patients administered haloperidol (Haldol) have shown some improvement.

KEY TERM	Definition
mental retardation	below average general intellectual functioning that is present at birth or during early life
lesion (LEE-zhun)	structural change
learning disorder (LD)	any defect or disturbance in a child's ability to acquire skills in reading, writing, or arithmetic
stuttering	saying something haltingly and repeating sounds when attempting to pronounce words
anxiety (ang-ZYE-ih-tee)	overwhelming sense of apprehension
pervasive developmental disorders	disorders characterized by severe, persistent, and all-encompassing impairment in several areas of development, including social, communication, and behavior
autism (aw-TIZ-um)	disturbance in psychological development that is marked by mental introversion and concentration on self or one object
cognitive-behavioral therapy (CBT)	treatment whose goal is to change problem actions, manners, and cognition through conditioning, learning, and cognitive restructuring
behavior therapy	treatment that uses behavior-modification techniques in which a person's desirable responses are positively reinforced while undesirable behaviors are negatively rewarded
Asperger (AHS-pur-gur) **disorder**	disorder characterized by severe and enduring impairment in social skills and interests and by repetitive behaviors, leading to impaired social and occupational functioning
attention deficit disorder (ADD)	disorder of attention, organization, and impulse control appearing in childhood and often persisting to adulthood
attention deficit hyperactivity disorder (ADHD)	condition characterized by hyperactivity, inability to concentrate, and impulsive or inappropriate behavior
pica (PYE-kuh)	craving to eat substances that provide no nutritional value
tic disorders	habitual, irresistible, repetitive movements that a person feels compelled to do
tic	sudden, rapid, recurrent, nonrhythmic, involuntary motor movement or vocalization
Tourette disorder	tic disorder characterized by some combination of multiple twitches, involuntary vocal grunts, and obscene speech
echolalia (eck-oh-LAY-lee-uh)	involuntary parrot-like repetition of a word just spoken by another person

continued

continued from page 987

KEY TERM PRACTICE: *Disorders Usually First Diagnosed in Infancy, Childhood, or Adolescence*

1. An abnormal craving to eat substances containing no health benefit is termed _____

2. _____ disorder is characterized by some combination of multiple twitches, involuntary grunts, and obscene language.

3. A structural change in the brain that may cause a disorder is termed a _____.

4. _____ is the involuntary parrot-like repetition of a word just spoken by another person.

5. _____ is a disorder characterized by severe and enduring impairment in social skills and interests and by repetitive behaviors, leading to impaired social and occupational functioning.

Delirium, Dementia, and Amnestic and Other Cognitive Disorders

Delirium, dementia, and amnestic and other cognitive disorders are marked by a pronounced deficit in cognition caused by organic disease, medical conditions, chemical substances, or a combination of these. Amnestic disorders are characterized by disturbances in memory.

delirium
Delirium is an altered state of consciousness. It is characterized by confusion, disorientation, illusions, and hallucinations. It is caused by illness, medication, and toxic, structural, and metabolic disorders.

delusion
A **delusion** is a false belief maintained in the face of strong contradictory evidence. Fever, poisoning, metabolic disorders, or brain injury can cause it. Treatment involves addressing the underlying pathology along with pharmacological or behavioral therapy as appropriate.

dementia
Dementia is the progressive loss of cognitive and intellectual functions. Although these functions wane, other brain functions are often retained. The result of organic brain disease, it is characterized by confusion, disorientation, **apathy** (total lack of feeling or emotion), and stupor. Depending on the cause, the onset may be gradual or sudden.

amnesia
Amnesia is a loss of memory as a result of shock, injury, psychological disturbance, or medical disorder. The loss of memory could last minutes to months.

Alzheimer disease (AD)
Alzheimer disease (AD) is a progressive dementia with diffuse cerebral cortical atrophy, slender gyri, sulci and ventricle enlargement (see **Figure 7-13**), and microscopic snarls of protein called neurofibrillary tangles (**Figure 18-5**). It results in memory impairment and dementia manifested as confusion, visual–spatial disorientation, hampered judgment, delusions, and possible hallucinations. **Hallucinations** are sensory experiences of something not actually existing in the external world. These alterations in perception could be auditory (hearing nonexisting voices) or visual (seeing objects that are not there).

Alzheimer disease makes up 70% of all dementia cases. The onset is usually during late middle life, and death generally ensues within 5 to 10 years. It currently ranks as the fourth leading cause of death in the United States. Nearly all persons with Down syndrome who live past age 40 develop AD. Risk factors include advancing age, history of head injury, and not maintaining

Neurofibrillary
tangles

Normal neurons

Figure 18-5 Neurofibrillary tangles characteristic of Alzheimer disease are visible in this microscopic study.

mental stimulation throughout life. A familial history is noted in 10% of all cases and is linked to gene mutations.

Alzheimer disease is one of the most overdiagnosed and misdiagnosed disorders because of overlapping signs and symptoms and its similarity to other dementias. Diagnosis involves ruling out all other organic brain disorders. Magnetic resonance imaging (MRI) and computed tomography (CT) scans reveal brain changes, but the diagnosis can be confirmed only at autopsy by pathological studies that show neurofibrillary tangles and clumps of protein called amyloid deposits that cause senile plaques.

IN THE NEWS: Alzheimer Disease Present Physically but Not Psychologically

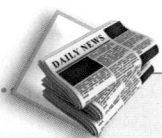

In Alzheimer disease, degenerated brain cells and β-amyloid (abnormal protein) create the core of senile plaques and neurofibrillary tangles. In fact, these are the hallmarks of diagnosing the disease postmortem. An interesting finding was made recently about these plaques and tangles in the brains of 19 nuns who demonstrated no outward manifestation of the disease.

The Nun Study is a longitudinal study conducted by David Snowdon at the University of Kentucky. More than 600 members of the School Sisters of Notre Dame religious congregation have donated their bodies to science. Annually, these sisters undergo cognitive and physical examinations and blood work, and all convent and medical records are examined. This group has become the largest brain donor group in the world so that Alzheimer disease could be studied.

At the autopsy of Sister Mary, age 101 years, the researchers uncovered plaques and tangles that would be expected in someone who in life showed signs of advanced Alzheimer disease. Sister Mary, however, was mentally and spiritually active, kept up with current affairs, and exhibited clear reasoning and thinking. Researchers noted 18 other nuns with similar medical profiles also exhibited brain pathology indicative of Alzheimer disease.

Dr. Snowden found that the nuns who showed Alzheimer signs only in their brains also had minimal stroke evidence. Nuns whose brains demonstrated both strokes and the changes of Alzheimer disease showed symptoms of dementia in 93% of cases. Although the reason is not clear, it is surmised that good nutrition, exercise, aspirin intake, and ongoing mental activity may help in preventing stroke, thereby staving off this form of dementia.

vascular dementia   **Vascular dementia**, also called multi-infarct dementia, is a step-like decline in intellectual function that results from an inadequate blood supply to the brain because of blocked blood vessels. In addition to cognitive deficits, there is evidence of cerebrovascular disease. The onset is usually gradual and symptoms progress as the disease advances. Signs and symptoms include apathy, disregard for personal hygiene, disorientation, depression, anxiety, restlessness, and sleeplessness. **Depression** is persistent extreme sadness, melancholy, or dejection that is unrealistic and out of proportion to the cause. The history and physical examination, along with arteriograms and vascular studies confirming occlusion, provide the diagnosis. The goal of pharmacological treatment is to increase blood flow to the brain. Endarterectomy, excision of deposits in the arteries, restores blood flow.

KEY TERM	Definition
delirium (de-LIRR-ee-um)	altered state of consciousness characterized by confusion, disorientation, illusions, and hallucinations
delusion (de-LEW-zhun)	false belief maintained in the face of strong contradictory evidence
dementia (de-MEN-shuh)	progressive loss of cognitive and intellectual functions
apathy (AP-uh-thee)	total lack of feeling or emotion
amnesia (am-NEE-zhuh)	loss of memory as a result of shock, injury, psychological disturbance, or medical disorder
Alzheimer disease	degenerative brain disorder that causes dementia, especially late in life
hallucinations (huh-lew-si-NAY-shuns)	sensory experiences of something not actually existing in the external world
vascular dementia (VAS-kew-lur de-MEN-shuh)	cognitive impairment caused by inadequate blood supply to the brain because of blocked blood vessels; also called multi-infarct dementia
depression	state of profound sadness that is unrealistic and out of proportion to the cause

KEY TERM PRACTICE: *Delirium, Dementia, and Amnestic and Other Cognitive Disorders*

1. Cognitive impairment that results from inadequate blood supply to the brain is known as _____.

2. Characteristics of _____ include neurofibrillary tangles, senile plaques, and dementia.

3. _____ are sensory experiences or perceptions of things with no basis in reality.

4. A _____ is a false belief maintained in the face of strong contradictory evidence.

5. Total lack of feeling or emotion is termed _____.

Substance Abuse

Substance-related disorders are associated with drug abuse, medication side effects, and toxin exposure. Nearly 15% of adults with a mental illness also have a co-occurring substance abuse disorder. Alcohol and prescription medications, such as benzodiazepines and various painkillers, are popular choices for drug abuse. In recent years, oxycodone (OxyContin), a CNS depressant that relieves pain, has become so popular among abusers that many pharmacies no longer keep it on site. Opiates, drugs that cause a feeling of euphoria, are also commonly abused. Furthermore, there is an ongoing debate about the addictive properties of caffeine and the likelihood of caffeine addiction. An **addiction** is a habitual psychological or physiological dependence on a substance.

alcoholism   **Alcoholism** is an addiction to alcohol (**Figure 18-6**). The excessive use interferes with health, interpersonal relations, or occupation. It is characterized by an increasing adaptation to the effects of alcohol such that increased amounts are required to achieve the same results. The abuse can lead to medical diseases such as cirrhosis, gastrointestinal cancers, pancreatitis, and peripheral neuropathy, as well as psychiatric disorders. About 30% of U.S. adults drink to excess at least occasionally, and 3% to 5% of women and 10% of men have chronic problems of excessive drinking. In 40% of alcoholics, the pattern of excessive drinking was evident before age 20. It appears as though personal history and environmental factors are at least as important as a genetic predisposition to developing alcoholism. Alcoholism decreases life expectancy by 15 years and costs the U.S. approximately $200 billion yearly.

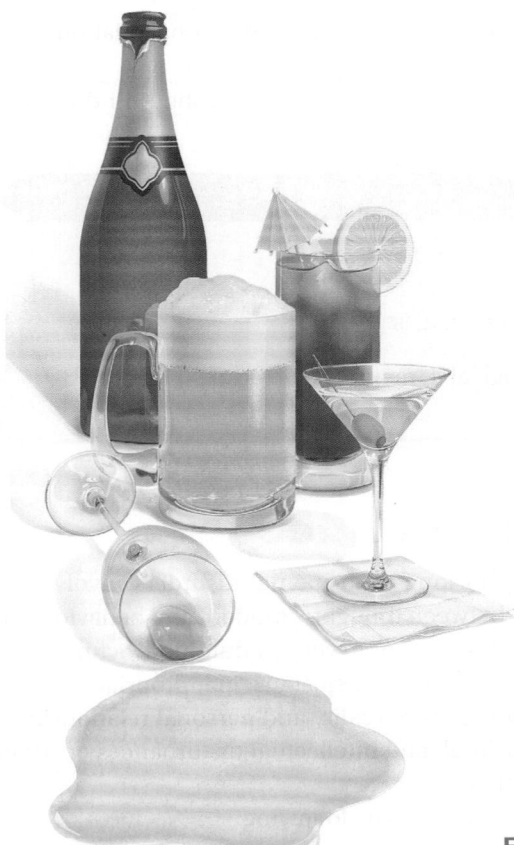

Figure 18-6 Common alcoholic beverages.

Alcohol withdrawal is often accompanied by **delirium tremens (DT)**, a form of delirium induced by the removal of alcohol after a prolonged period of intoxication. Agitation, tremors, hallucinations, delusions, fever, dilated pupils, sweating, and tachycardia characterize it. These also occur with barbiturate removal.

Alcohol is absorbed by the gastrointestinal tract, and the amount absorbed in the central nervous system is directly proportional to the blood alcohol concentration. Because women secrete less of the enzyme that metabolizes alcohol than men, women achieve higher blood levels of alcohol than men after drinking equivalent amounts of alcohol. Furthermore, the alcohol metabolism rate in the liver is constant. Thus, the liver metabolizes 10 to 15 mL of alcohol every hour. That is the equivalent of one 12-oz. beer, one 6-oz. glass of wine, or 1 oz. of 86-proof liquor per hour.

Alcoholism is diagnosed by the history and physical examination, which includes a questionnaire regarding frequency of alcohol use. Laboratory findings are also indicators. The γ-glutamyltransferase (GGT) blood analysis is a sensitive test that detects blood alcohol levels.

Treatment involves counseling, rehabilitation programs, and abstinence. Membership in Alcoholics Anonymous (AA) offers a treatment option that is often successful. AA is a fellowship of people addicted to alcohol who support one another to overcome their addiction.

KEY TERM	Definition
addiction (uh-DIK-shun)	habitual psychological or physiological dependence on a substance
alcoholism (AL-kuh-hol-iz-um)	an addiction to alcohol that interferes with health, interpersonal relations, or occupation
delirium tremens (DT) (de-LIRR-ee-um TREE-munz)	agitation, tremors, and hallucinations that are caused by alcohol withdrawal

KEY TERM PRACTICE: *Substance Abuse*

1. An addiction to alcohol is termed _____.

2. The term for agitation, tremors, and hallucinations caused by alcohol withdrawal is _____.

3. An _____ is a habitual psychological or physiological dependence on a substance.

Schizophrenia and Tardive Dyskinesia

schizophrenia

Schizophrenia is a group of long-term mental disorders involving a breakdown in the relation between thought, emotion, and behavior that typically begins during adolescence or in young adulthood. Schizophrenia is characterized by hallucinations, delusions, inappropriate actions and feelings, and a withdrawal from reality and personal relationships. Associated affective, behavioral, and intellectual disturbances occur in various degrees and combinations.

Types of schizophrenia include the following:

- **Catatonic-type schizophrenia** is characterized by frenzied motor activity, stupor, rigidity, and excitement.

- **Disorganized-type schizophrenia** is marked by incoherent, scattered delusions, dull feelings, social impairment, poor functioning and adaptation, and disorganized mannerisms.
- **Paranoid-type schizophrenia** is characterized by delusions of persecution and/or grandeur, hallucinations, and hostility.
- **Residual-type schizophrenia** is described as having at least one schizophrenic episode but currently without symptoms. Illogical thinking and odd behavior are still present.
- **Undifferentiated-type schizophrenia** is typified by disorganized behavior, incoherence, delusions, and hallucinations.

The cause of schizophrenia is thought to be malfunctioning of neuronal systems that use dopamine, serotonin, glutamate, and GABA as neurotransmitters. There may be an underlying genetic component in which a brain lesion is present in early life but does not manifest until adolescence or adulthood. Current theories focus on a genetic predisposition along with a possible prenatal viral infection (**Figure 18-7**).

People with schizophrenia display abnormal perceptions and content of thought. Schizophrenia is not "split personality," as popularly thought; that pathology is known as dissociative identity disorder. Schizophrenia is the most prevalent psychosis in America, affecting 2 million people (1% of the population). Approximately 25% of individuals with schizophrenia require custodial or institutional care, and 10% commit suicide. Signs and symptoms include confusion, odd behavior, disinterest in school or work, shortened attention span, memory deficits, diminished decision-making ability, **alogia** (inability to speak), **anhedonia** (chronic absence of pleasure in acts that were once normally pleasurable), **abulia** (inability to make a decision), delusions, auditory hallucinations, social withdrawal, and disorganized thinking.

Neurophysiological studies indicating generalized limbic lobe and prefrontal cortex abnormalities and a small thalamus indicate

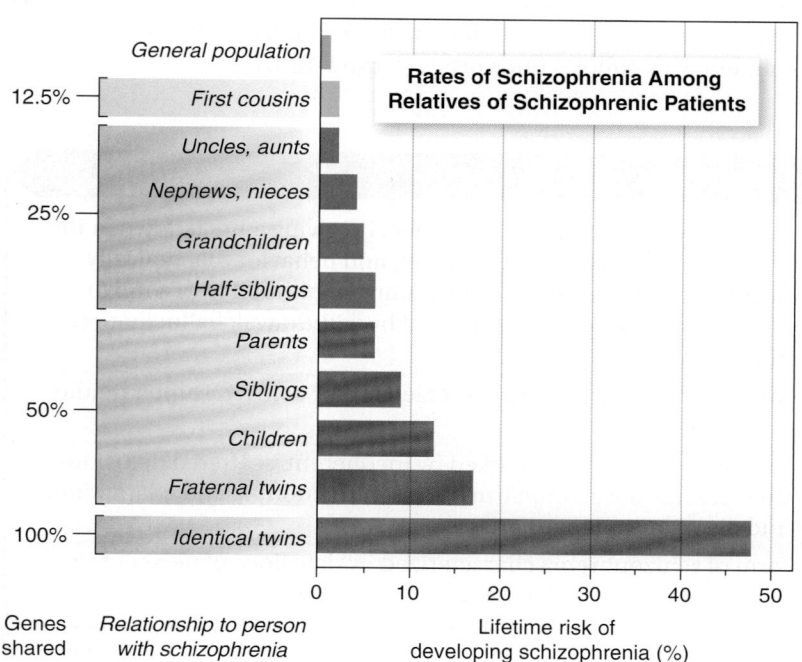

Figure 18-7 The familial nature of schizophrenia. The risk of schizophrenia increases with the number of shared genes, suggesting a genetic basis for the disease.

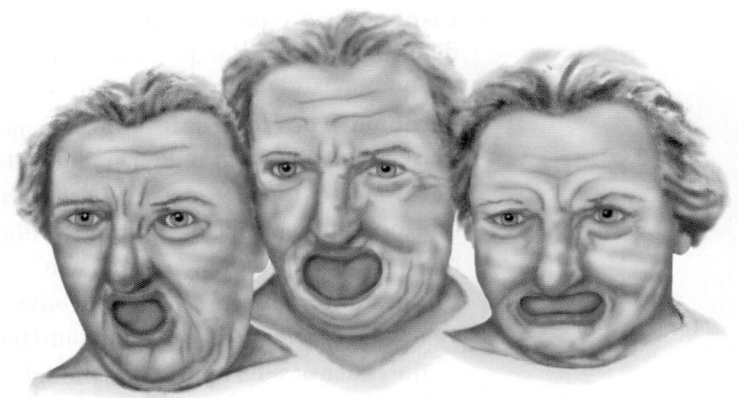

Figure 18-8 Tardive dyskinesia showing the bizarre movements that chiefly involve the face, mouth, jaw, and tongue.

schizophrenia. Brain imaging studies are inconsistent. Other tests that may assist in the diagnosis include the Rorschach test, TAT, and the MMPI. Schizophrenia is treated with intense psychotherapy, cognitive-behavioral therapy, and antipsychotic drugs. Inconsistent results have been achieved with cognitive-behavioral therapy. **Antipsychotic drugs** (antipsychotics) are a functional category of chemical agents helpful in the treatment of psychoses and thought disorders. Atypical antipsychotics are a newer class of drugs that exert their action by serotonergic blockade (stopping the actions of serotonin). Antipsychotics also counteract or alleviate the symptoms of some neuroses. These drugs include clozapine, olanzapine, quetiapine, and risperidone. Drugs shorten the episodes of acute psychosis, limit the need for institutional care, and reduce the risk of relapse. Unfortunately, patients frequently stop taking their medications, and it is estimated that only half of people with schizophrenia are receiving medical treatment or supervision at any given time.

tardive dyskinesia (TD) **Tardive dyskinesia (TD)** is a condition characterized by involuntary movements of the facial muscles and tongue that results from long-term treatment with antipsychotic drugs (**Figure 18-8**).

KEY TERM	Definition
schizophrenia (skit-soh-FREE-nee-uh)	group of long-term mental disorders involving a breakdown in the relation between thought, emotion, and behavior that typically begins during adolescence or in young adulthood with a mixture of signs and symptoms characterized by withdrawal, hallucinations, and delusions
catatonic-type schizophrenia (kat-uh-TON-ick-TIPE skit-soh-FREE-nee-uh)	form of schizophrenia with frenzied motor activity, stupor, rigidity, and excitement
disorganized-type schizophrenia (skit-soh-FREE-nee-uh)	form of schizophrenia marked by incoherent, scattered delusions, dull feelings, social impairment, poor functioning and adaptation, and disorganized mannerisms
paranoid-type schizophrenia (skit-soh-FREE-nee-uh)	form of schizophrenia characterized by delusions of persecution and/or grandeur, hallucinations, and hostility

continued

continued from page 994

KEY TERM	Definition
residual-type schizophrenia (skit-soh-FREE-nee-uh)	form of schizophrenia in which the individual has had at least one schizophrenic episode, but is currently without symptoms other than illogical thinking and odd behavior
undifferentiated-type schizophrenia (skit-soh-FREE-nee-uh)	form of schizophrenia typified by disorganized behavior, incoherence, delusions, and hallucinations
alogia (uh-LOH-jee-uh)	inability to speak
anhedonia (an-hee-DOH-nee-uh)	overall chronic absence of enjoyment in acts that used to be enjoyable
abulia (uh-BOO-lee-uh)	inability to make a decision
antipsychotic (an-tee-sigh-KOT-ick) drugs	chemical agents used to treat psychoses and thought disorders; also called antipsychotics
tardive dyskinesia (TD) (TAHR-div dis-ki-NEE-zhuh)	condition characterized by involuntary movements of the facial muscles and tongue that results from long-term treatment with antipsychotic drugs

KEY TERM PRACTICE: *Schizophrenia and Tardive Dyskinesia*

1. The condition characterized by involuntary movements of the facial muscles and tongue that results from long-term treatment with antipsychotic drugs is termed _____.

2. Catatonic, disorganized, paranoid, residual, and undifferentiated are various types of a condition called _____.

3. _____ is a group of long-term mental disorders involving a breakdown in the relation between thought, emotion, and behavior that typically begins during adolescence or in young adulthood with a mixture of signs and symptoms characterized by withdrawal, hallucinations, and delusions.

4. Chemical agents—also called antipsychotics—that are used to treat psychoses and thought disorders are known as _____.

5. The inability to make a decision is termed _____.

Mood Disorders

Mood is the pervasive feeling, tone, and internal emotional state of a person. Virtually every aspect of a person's behavior or his or her perception of events is influenced by mood.

mood disorders   **Mood disorders** are a group of mental ailments characterized by emotional disturbances that disrupt all other aspects of life. Mood disorders color the whole psychic life. Examples include major depression and bipolar disorder.

major depression   **Major depression** (major depressive disorder) is a psychological illness marked by sustained unhappiness and hopelessness, often with suicidal tendencies; anhedonia; sleep and appetite disturbances; and feelings of worthlessness and guilt. The individual often experiences a deep, persistent sadness. Major depression is the most common psychiatric disorder and is the leading cause of disability worldwide among people ages 5 years and older. Approximately 20 million Americans are affected yearly. About 10% of men and 25% of women will experience it at some point in their lives; and 15% to 30% of those afflicted commit suicide.

Risk factors for major depression include alcohol abuse, chronic physical illness, stress, social isolation, history of physical or sexual abuse, and family history of depression. The cause is an electrochemical malfunction of the limbic system resulting in metabolic disturbances of dopamine and serotonin. The limbic system is an area of the brain involved with motivation and mood. In addition, glial cell (supportive neuron) numbers are diminished in individuals with a familial history of depression. The diagnosis is based on a depressed mood and marked reduction or interest in pleasurable activities lasting at least 2 weeks. Furthermore, three or more of the following must also be present: weight loss or gain, increased or decreased sleep, increased or decreased level of psychomotor activity, fatigue, feelings of guilt or worthlessness, diminished ability to concentrate, and recurring thoughts of suicide or death. The Major Depression Inventory can also be used as a screening tool to detect major depressive disorder. This test is a self-report mood questionnaire developed by the World Health Organization and is beneficial because it can generate an *ICD* or *DSM* diagnosis of depression.

Antidepressants, drugs used to prevent or reduce depression, are used to treat it. These drugs include tricyclic antidepressants, selective serotonin reuptake inhibitors (SSRIs), monamine oxidase (MAO) inhibitors, and protriptyline. Cognitive-behavioral therapy is another form of treatment.

Electroconvulsive shock therapy and transcranial magnetic stimulation have demonstrated value in cases that do not respond to the other therapy options. Passing an electric current through the brain to produce convulsions and seizures is known as **electroconvulsive therapy (ECT)**. It is particularly useful in the treatment of depressive and severe psychiatric disorders. It is also known as electroshock therapy. The positive response rate for ECT is about 80%.

In **transcranial magnetic stimulation (TMS)**, a magnetic current is passed through the brain to stimulate nerve cells. Because TMS is a relatively new treatment for depression, further studies are needed to determine its full effectiveness.

dysthymic disorder

Another mood disorder, **dysthymic disorder**, is a chronically depressed mood that occurs for most of the day, more days than not, for at least 2 years. During the depressed state, at least two of the following symptoms must be present for diagnosis: poor appetite or overeating, insomnia or hypersomnia, low energy or fatigue, low self-esteem, poor concentration or difficulty making decisions, and feelings of hopelessness. Psychotherapy and antidepressants are courses of treatment.

bipolar disorder

Bipolar disorder is an affective disorder characterized by alternating periods of euphoria (mania) and depression. **Euphoria** is an exaggerated sense of physical and emotional well-being (happiness) that is usually not appropriate to the situation. Rapid speaking, fleeting ideas, insomnia, excessive energy, impaired judgment, delusions, and even hallucinations may mark the manic episodes. Indifference (flat affect), sadness, withdrawal, loss of appetite, and sleep disturbances characterize the depressive aspect. The cause is unknown, but thought to be the result of neurotransmitter alterations. The risk is greater if family members have the disorder. The history, physical examination, and psychological evaluation provide the diagnosis. The drug **lithium carbonate** is given for the manic phase, and antidepressants are administered for the depressive phase. Psychotherapy also provides benefit.

cyclothymic disorder   **Cyclothymic disorder** is a mental disorder characterized by noticeable, clinically significant mood swings that are unrelated to life events. The fluctuating mood disturbances involve many episodes of hypomania (a mild degree of mania) and depression, but to a lesser degree than in bipolar disorder. There is a 15% to 50% risk that the person will ultimately develop bipolar disorder.

seasonal affective disorder (SAD)   The main symptom of a seasonal pattern disorder is the onset and remission of major depressive episodes at characteristic times of the year. Most begin in fall or winter and remit in the spring. **Seasonal affective disorder (SAD)** is a seasonal pattern mood disorder occurring and resolving at the same time over a period of years. It frequently occurs in the winter and is characterized by morning hypersomnia, decreased energy, increased appetite, weight gain, and carbohydrate craving. These signs and symptoms fade or disappear in the spring. The incidence is greater in women than in men. Its cause is suggested to be increased melatonin secretion by the pineal gland because the disorder is more prevalent at higher latitudes and in areas of shortened sunlight hours. The hormone melatonin is released in response to darkness and suppressed by light. Exposure to artificial sunlight has shown some therapeutic merit.

KEY TERM	Definition
mood disorders	group of mental ailments characterized by emotional disturbances that disrupt all other aspects of life
major depression	psychological illness marked by sustained unhappiness and hopelessness, often with suicidal tendencies; also called major depressive disorder
antidepressants (an-tee-dee-PRES-unts)	drugs used in the treatment, alleviation, or prevention of depression
electroconvulsive therapy (ECT)	passage of a small electric current through the brain to treat mental disorders; also called electroshock therapy
transcranial magnetic stimulation (TMS)	passage of a magnetic current through the brain to treat mental disorders
dysthymic (dis-THIGH-mick) **disorder**	depressed mood for most of the day, for more days than not, for at least 2 years
bipolar (bye-POH-lur) **disorder**	disorder characterized by alternating periods of euphoria and severe depression

continued

continued from page 997

KEY TERM	Definition
euphoria (yoo-FOH-ree-uh)	exaggerated feeling of happiness
lithium carbonate (LITH-ee-um KAHR-buh-nate)	drug used to treat bipolar disorder
cyclothymic (sigh-kloh-THIGH-mick) **disorder**	mental disorder characterized by noticeable, clinically significant mood swings (hypomania and depression) that are unrelated to life events but to a lesser degree than bipolar disorder
seasonal affective disorder (SAD)	depression associated with the onset of winter and thought to be caused by decreasing amounts of daylight

KEY TERM PRACTICE: *Mood Disorders*

1. The disorder characterized by alternating periods of euphoria and severe depression is known as

   _____.

2. _____ is characterized by feelings of unhappiness in the winter that resolve in the spring.

3. _____ is a mental disorder characterized by noticeable, clinically significant mood swings (hypomania and depression) that are unrelated to life events but to a lesser degree than bipolar disorder.

4. An exaggerated feeling of happiness is termed _____.

5. Drugs used in the treatment, alleviation, or prevention of depression are known as _____.

Anxiety Disorders

anxiety disorders

Anxiety disorders are a group of interrelated mental illnesses involving anxious and apprehensive reactions to stress or in anticipation of a future event. Panic disorder, phobias, obsessive–compulsive disorder, post-traumatic stress disorder, and generalized anxiety disorder are common types.

panic disorder

Panic disorder is a condition in which the person suffers repeated panic attacks that come on suddenly and are overwhelming and uncontrollable, leading to total inaction or unreasonable acts. A panic attack is a sudden, overpowering feeling of fear or anxiety that prevents functioning. An attack is often triggered by a past or present source of anxiety. The extreme anxiety attack leads to total inaction or unreasonable acts. These recurrent attacks occur unpredictably. Signs include dyspnea (shortness of breath), dizziness, tingling, and anxiousness. The cause of panic disorders is not understood. Recent data have suggested that genetics appears to be a factor in many cases. This disorder affects 2% to 5% of the American population and is twice as common among women as men.

Treatments are psychotherapy, cognitive-behavioral therapy, hypnosis, and medication. **Hypnosis** is an artificially induced trancelike state of enhanced relaxation. While in this state, the person is highly susceptible to suggestions, is oblivious to all else, and responds readily to commands and questions from the hypnotist.

The scientific validity of hypnosis has been debated for two centuries and appears to run a cycle of acceptance and rejection.

phobias

Phobias are disproportionate, obsessive, persistent, and unrealistic fears of situations or objects. Specific types are named using a combining form expressing the object that inspires the fear. For example, the word part *aqua-* refers to "water," *-phobia* means "fear of," so the word *aquaphobia* is "fear of water." Many people who have a phobia realize the irrationality of their fear, but are powerless to prevent it.

Phobias are produced by the interaction of two factors: genetic predisposition and classical conditioning. Classical conditioning is a form of learning that occurs when two stimuli are repeatedly paired. In classical conditioning, a previously neutral stimulus becomes a conditioned stimulus when presented together with an unconditioned stimulus. There is clear evidence that phobias may be the result of inherited temperament traits or some other factor that is yet unknown. It is also now accepted that phobias are conditioned early in life, either vicariously or through direct experience. The feared object or situation is a conditioned stimulus that elicits CNS arousal and subsequent avoidance behavior. Treatments are highly individualized and may include psychotherapy, cognitive-behavioral therapy, hypnosis, and pharmaceutics. **Table 18-2** lists selected phobias and their descriptions.

obsessive–compulsive disorder (OCD)

Obsessive–compulsive disorder (OCD) is an anxiety disorder characterized by intrusive, unwanted thoughts that produce a rapid increase in anxiety. The anxiety leads the person to perform ritualistic behaviors (compulsions) in an attempt to reduce the anxiety. In OCD, the person cannot control his or her anxiety and is dominated by the repetitive impulses. The acts then become organized rituals such as hand washing and excessive neatness. This condition

TABLE 18-2

PHOBIAS

Term	Description
acrophobia	fear of heights
agoraphobia	fear of crowded or public places
arachnophobia	fear of spiders
claustrophobia	fear of confined space
gephyrophobia	fear of crossing a bridge
hemophobia	fear of blood
pathophobia	fear of disease
phobophobia	fear of developing a phobia
xenophobia	fear of strangers
zoophobia	fear of animals

affects 2% to 3% of Americans. Some theorize it is a response to severe stress, but others suggest genetic factors, frontal lobe abnormality, or neurotransmitter dysfunction. There is strong evidence that the prefrontal cortex of the brain is involved in OCD. A similar disorder, obsessive–compulsive personality disorder (OCPD), is characterized by perfectionism and rigidity.

Psychotherapy, hypnosis, stress reduction, relaxation techniques, biofeedback, exercise, and anxiolytics are treatments that may help. **Biofeedback** is a training technique that enables an individual to gain some voluntary control over autonomic body functions. Individuals using biofeedback techniques can learn to influence desired physiological responses such as lowering blood pressure, alleviating headaches, or achieving conscious management over normally involuntary body physiology. **Anxiolytic** drugs, which affect the neurotransmitter GABA and generally do not cause excessive sedation, are sometimes prescribed. Common drugs of this type are benzodiazepines and diazepam. However, the gold standard of treatment for OCD is called exposure and response prevention. **Exposure and response prevention (ERP)** is a form of cognitive therapy that involves exposing a person with OCD to the very thing that produces anxiety (such as germs or body fluids) and *not* allowing him or her to reduce the ensuing anxiety with any form of compulsive behavior. Research has found that with repeated exposures, obsessive thoughts decline.

post-traumatic stress disorder (PTSD)

Post-traumatic stress disorder (PTSD) is characterized by a group of symptoms that are displayed after a psychologically traumatic event. Signs and symptoms include numbed responsiveness to stimuli, cognitive dysfunction, and dysphoria that either appear within a short time of the event or have a delayed onset. The condition of feeling acutely hopeless, uncomfortable, and unhappy is termed **dysphoria**. The disorder may spontaneously resolve within 6 months.

Post-traumatic stress disorder is common among combat veterans and survivors of major physical trauma. Intrusive, recurring flashbacks to the event give evidence for diagnosis. Counseling, behavior therapy, and drugs for anxiety and depression are therapeutic measures.

generalized anxiety disorder (GAD)

Another type of anxiety disorder is **generalized anxiety disorder (GAD)**, characterized by chronic, repeated episodes of nervousness, agitation, and feelings that something negative is going to happen. The fear and dread are accompanied by autonomic changes such as diarrhea, hypertension (high blood pressure), and muscle tension. The most prevalent type of anxiety disorder, it affects more females than males, and occurs primarily in individuals ages 20 to 25 years. Treatment options consist of psychotherapy, hypnosis, relaxation techniques, biofeedback, physical exercise, and administration of anxiolytic drugs. Physical manifestations are treated symptomatically.

KEY TERM	Definition
anxiety (ang-ZYE-ih-tee) **disorders**	group of interrelated mental illnesses involving anxious and apprehensive reactions to stress or in anticipation of a future event
panic disorder	condition in which a person suffers repeated panic attacks that come on suddenly and are overwhelming and uncontrollable, leading to total inaction or unreasonable acts
hypnosis (hip-NOH-sis)	trancelike state of enhanced relaxation that is artificially induced
phobias (FOH-bee-uhz)	disproportionate, obsessive, persistent, and unrealistic fears of situations or objects
obsessive–compulsive disorder (OCD)	psychiatric disorder characterized by intrusive, unwanted thoughts and irresistible repetitive behaviors
biofeedback	a training technique that enables an individual to gain some voluntary control over autonomic body functions
anxiolytic (ANG-zee-oh-lit-ick)	drug that relieves anxiety
exposure and response prevention (ERP)	a form of cognitive therapy that involves exposing a person with OCD to the thing that produces anxiety and *not* allowing him or her to reduce the anxiety with any form of compulsive behavior
post-traumatic stress disorder (PTSD)	group of symptoms, such as sleep disturbances, flashbacks, and depression, that are displayed after a psychologically traumatic event
dysphoria (dis-FOH-ree-uh)	condition of feeling acutely hopeless, uncomfortable, and unhappy
generalized anxiety (ang-ZYE-ih-tee) **disorder (GAD)**	chronic, repeated episodes of nervousness, agitation, and feelings that something negative is going to happen

KEY TERM PRACTICE: *Anxiety Disorders*

1. Disproportionate, obsessive, persistent, and unrealistic fears of situations or objects are called

   _____.

2. _____ is a psychological condition affecting people who have witnessed or suffered a psychologically traumatic event.

3. _____ is a condition of feeling acutely hopeless, uncomfortable, and unhappy.

4. _____ is a form of cognitive therapy that involves exposing a person with OCD to the thing that produces anxiety and *not* allowing him or her to reduce the anxiety with any form of compulsive behavior.

5. A training technique that enables an individual to gain some voluntary control over autonomic body functions is termed _____.

Somatoform Disorders

somatoform disorder
A **somatoform disorder** is a group of mental disorders in which physical symptoms suggest a disorder, but there is no underlying physiological dysfunction or disease. *Soma* refers to "body"; therefore, these disorders with physiological signs and symptoms are the effect of the mind on the body. An alternate term is **psychosomatic disorder**. There is strong evidence linking psychological factors to the physiological mechanisms. Psychotherapy and medications to manage pain may offer benefit for somatoform disorders if no underlying pathology is discovered.

somatization disorder	**Somatization disorder** is characterized by the displacement of emotional conflicts onto the body. This results in various physical symptoms. Patients present with a complicated medical history and physical symptoms related to various organ systems. No organic foundation can be discovered. The onset is typically before age 30 years. The individual never experiences a symptom-free period lasting longer than 1 year and typically visits many physicians in pursuit of effective treatment. Treatment involves ruling out any underlying pathology and then treating the remaining symptoms appropriately.
conversion disorder	**Conversion disorder** is a psychological defense mechanism in which an unconscious emotional conflict is transformed into a physical disability. The affected body part may have symbolic meaning pertinent to the nature of the conflict. Physical signs and symptoms occur instead of anxiety. Symptoms may include blindness, deafness, paralysis, blurred vision, or numbness. Because no pathology can be determined, the disorder is treated symptomatically. (The *DSM* classifies conversion disorder as a somatoform disorder, whereas the *ICD* classifies it as a dissociative disorder. Dissociative disorders are discussed later in this chapter.)
pain disorder	**Pain disorder** is severe and long-lasting pain thought to be caused by psychological factors. The pain is so severe that it interferes with life activities, social functioning, and work. It often leads to depression. The disorder often occurs after an injury that caused the original pain. After treating the underlying cause, pain medications and therapy may be beneficial.
hypochondriasis	**Hypochondriasis** is a chronic condition characterized by a morbid concern for a person's own physical or mental health. The person believes he or she is suffering from some grave, bodily disease even though there are no pathological findings. The delusion is that one is suffering from a disease that does not exist. The person frequently searches the body for signs of pathology. For example, normal bumps and moles are immediately assumed to be symptomatic of cancer. It is also known as **hypochondria**. Many researchers now believe that hypochondriasis may be a form of OCD, and it responds well to ERP therapy.
body dysmorphic disorder	**Body dysmorphic disorder** is characterized by preoccupation with an imagined defect in appearance. It is also known as **dysmorphophobia**, which describes the condition as a morbid fear of being deformed.
hysteria	**Hysteria** is a malady with physical symptoms that seem better explained by psychological factors rather than underlying pathology. It is generally cured by psychotherapy alone.

KEY TERM	Definition
somatoform (soh-muh-TOH-form) **disorder**	group of mental disorders in which physical symptoms suggest a disorder, but there is no underlying physiological dysfunction or disease; also called psychosomatic disorder
psychosomatic (sigh-koh-soh-MAT-ick) **disorder**	group of mental disorders in which physical symptoms suggest a disorder, but there is no underlying physiological dysfunction or disease; also called somatoform disorder
somatization (soh-muh-ti-ZAY-shun) **disorder**	disorder in which emotional conflicts are projected onto the body and revealed as pathological states
conversion disorder	psychological defense mechanism in which an unconscious emotional conflict is transformed into a physical disability
pain disorder	severe and long-lasting pain thought to be caused by psychological factors
hypochondriasis (high-poh-kon-DRY-uh-sis)	chronic condition characterized by a morbid concern for a person's own physical or mental health accompanied by the conviction of having a serious disease without supportive evidence; also called hypochondria
hypochondria (high-poh-KON-dree-uh)	chronic condition characterized by a morbid concern for a person's own physical or mental health accompanied by the conviction of having a serious disease without supportive evidence; also called hypochondriasis
body dysmorphic (dis-MOR-fick) **disorder**	disorder in a normal-appearing person characterized by an abnormal fear of being deformed; also called dysmorphophobia
dysmorphophobia (dis-mor-foh-FOH-bee-uh)	disorder in a normal-appearing person characterized by an abnormal fear of being deformed; also called body dysmorphic disorder
hysteria	malady with physical symptoms that seem better explained by psychological factors rather than underlying pathology

KEY TERM PRACTICE: *Somatoform Disorders*

1. List two terms that mean a chronic condition characterized by a morbid concern for a person's own physical or mental health accompanied by the conviction of having a serious disease without supportive evidence.

   _____

2. The word part *hyster-* refers to _____; and the word _____ describes a malady with physical symptoms that seem better explained by psychological factors.

3. A psychological defense mechanism in which an unconscious emotional conflict is transformed into a physical disability is termed _____.

4. Severe and long-lasting pain thought to be caused by psychological factors is known as

   _____.

5. A group of mental disorders in which physical symptoms suggest a disorder, but there is no underlying physiological dysfunction or disease, is termed _____ or _____.

Factitious Disorders

factitious disorders	Physical and psychological signs and symptoms that are intentionally produced or feigned to gain attention and play the sick role are called **factitious disorders**. Two examples are Munchausen syndrome and Munchausen syndrome by proxy. The syndrome is named after Baron Karl F. H. von Munchausen, a German soldier and proverbial teller of exaggerated tales.
Munchausen syndrome	**Munchausen syndrome** is a personality disorder in which a patient presents with false symptoms or simulates acute illness to gain medical attention. The extent of the fabrication depends on the person's medical knowledge. Individuals are eager to undergo examinations, hospitalizations, diagnostic procedures, and therapeutic manipulations. When no underlying cause can be revealed, they often leave a health care facility without notice and seek attention at another institution.
Munchausen syndrome by proxy	**Munchausen syndrome by proxy** is a form of Munchausen syndrome in which symptoms are projected onto a child by a caregiver, usually the mother. The term *proxy* means "a person is acting as a substitute for somebody else." In this case, because of the child's supposed illness, the mother or caregiver gains the sympathy. It is considered a form of child maltreatment or abuse because the clinical signs are often induced by the caregiver. For example, emetic agents may be given to the child to induce unnecessary vomiting. The person may tamper with the child's medical specimens to create a need for further medical care. This leads to medical interventions and investigations. Occasionally, children are placed in danger as a result. Serious health consequences and death have been reported. The disorder is also known as **factitious illness by proxy**. The cause of both factitious disorders is not known. It is thought to be a form of attention-seeking behavior. A history of repeated hospitalizations, no underlying pathology, symptoms that do not match laboratory findings, and recurrent fabricated stories provide the diagnosis. The treatment is psychotherapy.

KEY TERM	Definition
factitious (fack-TISH-us) **disorder**	physical and psychological signs and symptoms that are intentionally produced or feigned to gain attention and play the sick role
Munchausen (MUN-chow-zun) **syndrome**	disorder in which a person pretends to have an illness to undergo testing or treatment or be admitted to a hospital
Munchausen (MUN-chow-zun) **syndrome by proxy**	disorder in which a caregiver harms a child, falsifies medical records, and/or tampers with laboratory specimens to create a situation requiring medical attention; also called factitious illness by proxy
factitious (fack-TISH-us) **illness by proxy**	disorder in which a caregiver harms a child, falsifies medical records, and/or tampers with laboratory specimens to create a situation requiring medical attention; also called Munchausen syndrome by proxy

continued

continued from page 1004

KEY TERM PRACTICE: *Factitious Disorders*

1. A _____ is characterized by physical and psychological signs and symptoms that are intentionally produced or feigned to gain attention and play the sick role.

2. The factitious disorder that is characterized by a person pretending to be sick to gain attention and hospital admission is termed _____.

3. A disorder in which a caregiver harms a child, falsifies medical records, and/or tampers with laboratory specimens to create a situation requiring medical attention is known as _____ or _____.

Dissociative Disorders

dissociative disorders   **Dissociative disorders** are a group of mental disorders characterized by disturbances in memory, identity, consciousness, or perception. Forms include dissociative amnesia, dissociative fugue, and dissociative identity disorder. Intense psychotherapy is the treatment for all forms.

dissociative amnesia   **Dissociative amnesia** is the inability to recall important personal information that goes beyond normal forgetfulness. The memory impairment is usually reversible. It can appear in any age group. The main symptom is a retrospective memory gap. Acute forms occur in response to natural disaster or severe trauma.

dissociative fugue   **Dissociative fugue** is the unexpected travel away from home or a person's usual place of daily activities, accompanied by the inability to recall some or all of the person's past. **Fugue** is a condition in which a person suddenly abandons a present activity or lifestyle and begins a new or different one for a period of time, often in a different city. Amnesia during the fugue period is reported, although earlier events are remembered and habits and skills are unaffected.

dissociative identity disorder   **Dissociative identity disorder** (formerly called multiple personality disorder) is the presence of two or more distinct personalities in the same person, sometimes without any one personality being aware of the other. The individual is unable to recall important personal information and memory gaps are common. Severe physical and sexual abuse during childhood have been linked to the disorder.

KEY TERM	Definition
dissociative disorders	group of mental disorders characterized by disturbances in memory, identity, consciousness, or perception
dissociative amnesia (am-NEE-zhuh)	inability to recall important personal information that goes beyond normal forgetfulness
dissociative fugue (fyoog)	unexpected travel away from home or a person's usual place of daily activities, accompanied by the inability to recall some or all of the person's past
fugue (fyoog)	condition in which a person suddenly abandons a present activity or lifestyle and begins a new or different one for a period of time, often in a different city
dissociative identity disorder	presence of two or more distinct personalities in the same person, sometimes without any one personality being aware of the other

KEY TERM PRACTICE: *Dissociative Disorders*

1. _____ refers to a condition in which a person suddenly abandons a present activity or lifestyle and begins a new or different one for a period of time, often in a different city.

2. _____ are a group of mental disorders characterized by disturbances in memory, identity, consciousness, or perception.

3. The inability to recall important personal information that goes beyond normal forgetfulness is termed _____.

4. Unexpected travel away from home or a person's usual place of daily activities, accompanied by the inability to recall some or all of the person's past, is called _____.

5. The presence of two or more distinct personalities in the same person, sometimes without any one personality being aware of the other is known as _____.

Sexual and Gender Identity Disorders

sexual dysfunction

Sexual dysfunction is a disturbance of sexual functioning with a psychological rather than a physical cause. Examples include impotence (inability to achieve penis erection), and premature ejaculation. Sexual activity, desire, arousal, and orgasm can be affected and are often a source of great distress and interpersonal difficulty. Psychotherapy and counseling are common forms of treatment.

paraphilias

Paraphilias are abnormal sexual desires involving nonhuman objects, the suffering or humiliation of oneself oneself, one's partner, children, or other nonconsenting persons. Examples of paraphilias include exhibitionism, fetishism, frotteurism, pedophilia, sexual masochism, sexual sadism, transvetic fetishism, and voyeurism. Treatment for paraphilias requires various forms of intense therapy.

exhibitionism

A compulsion to expose the genitals in public with the intent of provoking sexual interest in the viewer is termed **exhibitionism**.

fetishism

Fetishism is characterized by using a nonliving object (fetish) to produce sexual arousal. For example, the person may **masturbate**

(self-stimulate the genitals to produce orgasm) while smelling or fondling an item. It is diagnosed as a disorder if the behavior recurs over 6 months and impairs social and occupational functioning.

frotteurism

Frotteurism is the production of sexual excitement by rubbing against a nonconsenting person. The behavior occurs in crowded places where the frotteur can easily escape.

pedophilia

Pedophilia is abnormal sexual attraction to children by adults. The disorder usually begins in adolescence. Clinically, the sexual activity must be with a prepubescent child (age 13 years or younger). Furthermore, the pedophile must be at least 16 years of age and at least 5 years older than the child. Sexual desire fluctuates with the pedophile's stress level. Twice as many males as females are afflicted. If the behavior recurs over a period of at least 6 months, it is diagnosed as pedophilia.

sexual masochism

Sexual masochism is a sexual disorder in which a person experiences sexual pleasure by being abused, humiliated, or maltreated. The name is derived from two authors, Marquis de Sade and Leopold von Sacher-Masoch, who wrote on the subject.

sexual sadism

Sexual sadism is a sexual disorder in which a person derives sexual pleasure by inflicting abuse and maltreatment on the victim. It is named after Marquis de Sade, who confessed to being addicted to the practice.

transvetic fetishism

Transvetic fetishism is a paraphilia that involves cross-dressing by a male in women's clothes. Sexual arousal occurs when the male thinks of himself as a female while wearing the clothes. The disorder has only been described in heterosexual males.

voyeurism

Voyeurism is the practice of deriving sexual pleasure by looking ("peeping") at the naked body or genitals of unsuspecting individuals, usually strangers. Orgasm usually occurs by masturbation during the voyeuristic act or by recalling the memory of viewing the naked person.

gender identity disorder

A **gender identity disorder** is a conflict between a person's actual physical gender and the gender that the person identifies himself or herself to be. Throughout life, the individual identifies with and desires to be the other sex. Clinically significant impairment in functioning in the genetically assigned sex is apparent. Individuals often play the role of the other sex. It is also known as **transsexualism**. A transsexual is a person whose chromosomes, gonads, and other body markings are of one sex, but the individual identifies psychosocially with the other. Persons may routinely live and dress as a member of the opposite sex. The cause is unknown. It is diagnosed on the basis of two criteria that must both be present: There must be strong and persistent evidence of cross-gender identification, and there must be constant discomfort about one's assigned sex. A history of transsexual behaviors, along with a stated desire to live as the opposite sex, often leads to hormonal therapy and gender reassignment operations (**Figure 18-9**). *It should be noted that the proposed changes for the DSM-V, to be published in May 2013, will likely remove this entry as a diagnostic category.*

Figure 18-9 Surgical procedure and outcome of female-to-male gender reassignment surgery.

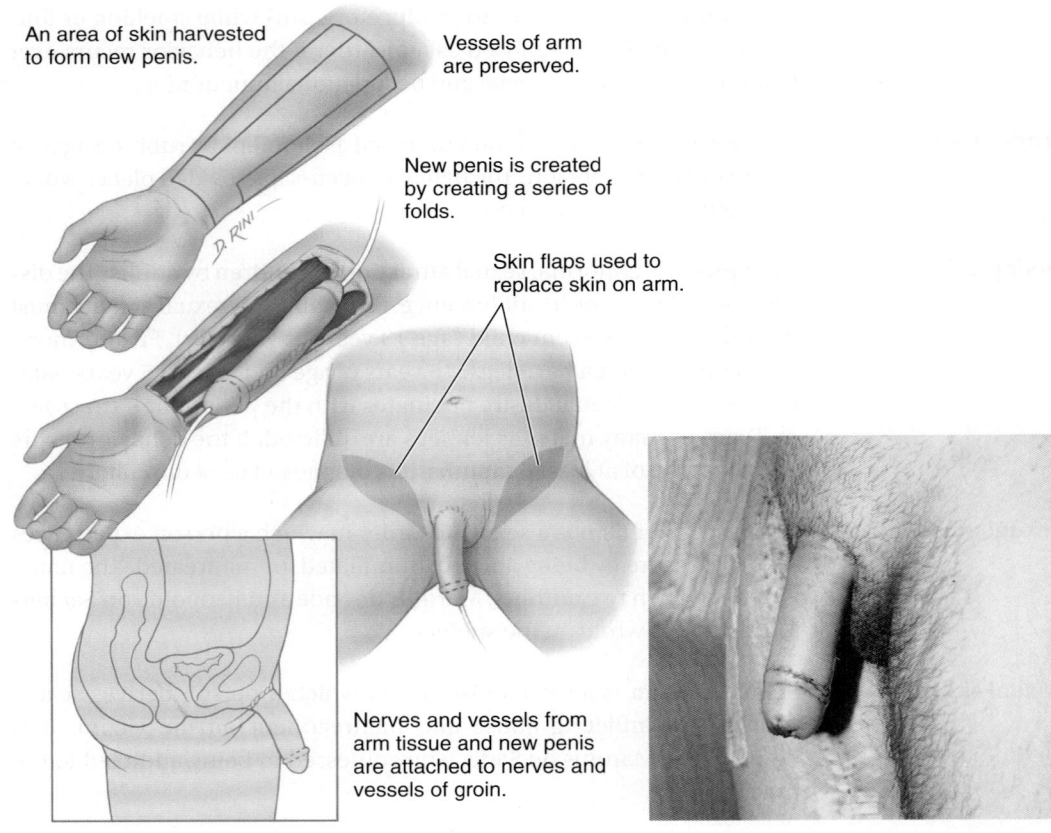

An area of skin harvested to form new penis.

Vessels of arm are preserved.

New penis is created by creating a series of folds.

Skin flaps used to replace skin on arm.

Nerves and vessels from arm tissue and new penis are attached to nerves and vessels of groin.

KEY TERM	Definition
sexual dysfunction	disturbance of sexual functioning with a psychological rather than a physical cause
paraphilias (pair-uh-FIL-ee-uhz)	abnormal sexual desires involving nonhuman objects, the suffering or humiliation of oneself, one's partner, children, or other nonconsenting persons
exhibitionism (eck-si-BISH-un-iz-um)	compulsion to expose the genitals in public with the intent of provoking sexual interest in the viewer
fetishism (FET-ish-iz-um)	the use of a nonliving object (fetish) to produce sexual arousal
masturbate (MAS-tur-bate)	to self-stimulate the genitals to produce orgasm
frotteurism (FROT-tur-iz-um)	production of sexual excitement by rubbing against a nonconsenting person
pedophilia (pee-doh-FIL-ee-uh)	abnormal sexual attraction to children by adults
sexual masochism (MAS-oh-kiz-um)	sexual disorder in which a person experiences sexual pleasure by being abused, humiliated, or maltreated
sexual sadism (SAD-iz-um)	sexual disorder in which a person derives sexual pleasure by inflicting abuse and maltreatment on the victim
transvetic fetishism (trans-VET-ick FET-ish-iz-um)	paraphilia that involves cross-dressing by a male in women's clothes
voyeurism (VOY-yur-izm)	practice of deriving sexual pleasure by looking ("peeping") at the naked body or genitals of unsuspecting individuals, usually strangers
gender identity disorder	conflict between a person's actual physical gender and the gender that the person identifies himself or herself to be; also called transsexualism
transsexualism (trans-SECK-shoo-ul-iz-um)	conflict between a person's actual physical gender and the gender that the person identifies himself or herself to be; also called gender identity disorder

continued

continued from page 1008

KEY TERM PRACTICE: *Sexual and Gender Identity Disorders*

1. The use of a nonliving object to produce sexual arousal is called _____.

2. The general term _____ describes abnormal sexual desires involving nonhuman objects, the suffering or humiliation of oneself, one's partner, children, or other nonconsenting persons.

3. To _____ is to self-stimulate the genitals to produce orgasm.

4. _____ describes the compulsion to expose the genitals in public with the intent of provoking sexual interest in the viewer.

5. The production of sexual excitement by rubbing against a nonconsenting person is termed _____.

Eating Disorders

Eating disorders are characterized by disturbances in eating behavior. Examples include anorexia nervosa and bulimia nervosa, which affect millions of Americans yearly, 85% to 90% of whom are teens and young adult women. Although obesity is a health condition of clinical significance, it is not associated with a psychological or behavioral syndrome, so it does not appear in *DSM*; however, it is included in the *ICD*.

anorexia nervosa (AN)   **Anorexia nervosa (AN)** is a disorder of unknown cause characterized by a profound aversion to food for fear of gaining weight and by an abnormal perception of body size and shape. The condition leads to emaciation, nutritional deficiencies, and even death. It is more common in women than in men. It has been defined as a compulsive pursuit of thinness at the expense of health. It is characterized by weight loss and body weight that is below 85% of normal weight for height. The distorted body image is accompanied by hyperactivity and, in women, by amenorrhea (absence of menstrual periods) as a result of low fat reserves. At least 50% of patients have persistent psychiatric problems—particularly with eating and sexuality—throughout life. The mortality rate is about 5%.

bulimia nervosa   Binge eating (uncontrolled rapid ingestion over short periods) and inappropriate compensatory measures to prevent weight gain characterize **bulimia nervosa**. The insatiable appetite and excessive food intake are followed by self-induced vomiting, diuretic or laxative use, fasting, and vigorous exercise to avoid gaining additional pounds. The self-induced vomiting causes tooth erosion from the acidity of the vomitus (**Figure 18-10**). Feelings of guilt, depression, and self-disgust are typical.

    Anorexia nervosa and bulimia nervosa are diagnosed by the complete history of the behavior and physical examination. Psychotherapy or counseling is the primary treatment method.

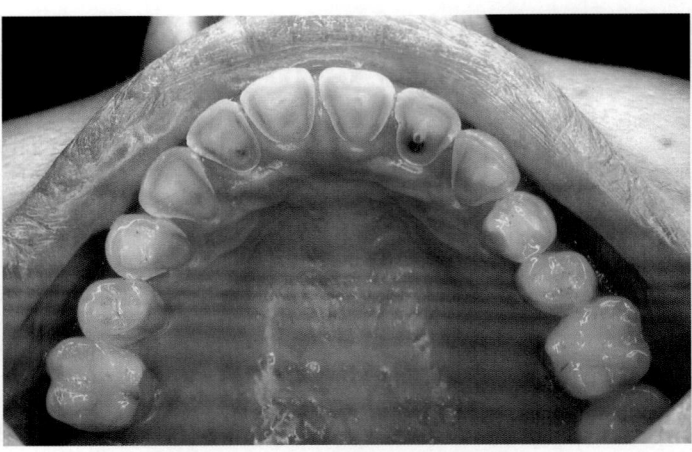

Figure 18-10 Severe erosion is evident on the lingual surfaces of maxillary teeth, especially the anterior teeth of this person with bulimia nervosa.

KEY TERM	Definition
anorexia nervosa (AN) (an-oh-RECK-see-uh nur-VOH-suh)	eating disorder characterized by extreme fear of becoming overweight that leads to dieting to the point of illness and sometimes death
bulimia nervosa (bew-LIM-ee-uh nur-VOH-suh)	eating disorder characterized by bouts of overeating that are followed by undereating, laxative use, or vomiting

KEY TERM PRACTICE: *Eating Disorders*

1. An eating disorder characterized by extreme fear of becoming overweight that leads to dieting to the point of illness and sometimes death is termed _____.

2. _____ is an eating disorder characterized by bouts of overeating that are followed by undereating, laxative use, or vomiting.

Sleep Disorders

Sleep disorders are listed in the *DSM* because they can produce significant impairment in cognitive, affective, and behavioral states, and thus negatively affect social functioning. Many cause profound alterations in daily physical and psychological functioning.

The average length of daily sleep for adults is 6 to 8 hours; children and adolescents require more. Sleep disorders are evaluated and assessed by **polysomnography**, the simultaneous and continuous monitoring of relevant normal and abnormal physiological activity during sleep. The instrument measures rapid eye movements (REMs)—the symmetrical, quick scanning movements of the eyes—which occur frequently during sleep in clusters for 5 to 60 minutes and are associated with dreaming.

The rest of the sleep time, the non-REM sleep cycle, is divided into four stages. Stage 1 is transitional and accounts for 5% of sleep. Stage 2 is deeper and occupies about 50% of sleep. Stages 3 and 4 are characterized as slow-wave deep sleep that makes up 10% to 20% of sleep.

dyssomnias and **parasomnias**

Sleep disorders are grouped by **dyssomnias**, abnormalities in the amount, quality, or timing of sleep, and **parasomnias**, abnormal behavioral or physiological events associated with sleep, sleep stages, or sleep–wake transitions. Examples of parasomnias are sleepwalking with no recollection of the event, seizures that cause a person to awaken, and nightmares with vivid recall. Parasomnias are organically, psychologically, or drug induced. Treatment is aimed at removing hindrances for sleepwalkers to prevent injury. Drugs such as diazepam (Valium) may be prescribed.

primary insomnia

Primary insomnia is characterized by the inability to sleep in the absence of external stimuli, such as noise or bright light. The cause may be pain, thyroid disorder, alcohol and caffeine ingestion, amphetamine use, anxiety, fear, or stress. Diagnosis is confirmed if the condition has continued for more than 1 month and interferes with normal functioning. Treatment consists of ruling out any possible underlying pathology, creating a favorable sleep environment, removing stimuli, instituting a regular bedtime, engaging in stress-relief activities, and exercising.

narcolepsy

Narcolepsy, also known as *paroxysmal sleep,* is a sleep disorder that usually appears in young adulthood. It is characterized by frequent brief bouts of deep sleep during the day and often disrupted sleep at night. It is sometimes accompanied by hallucinations and sleep paralysis. For no apparent reason, the person is plunged into REM sleep from a waking state. Narcolepsy occurs from a few seconds to 30 minutes. The onset is usually before age 25. Data suggest a strong genetic role in its cause. It is diagnosed by a history of repeated episodes. Treatment includes napping, establishing a routine bedtime, and administering low doses of amphetamines.

sleep apnea

Breathing-related sleep disorders are characterized by sleep disruption that leads to excessive sleepiness and interferes with activities of daily living. **Sleep apnea**, intermittent breathing cessation of short duration during sleep, is an example of a breathing-related sleep disorder. Snorting and gasping are common after periods of breathlessness. The frequent awakening results in daytime tiredness. The condition occurs more commonly in men than in women. Causes include obesity, hypertension, airway obstruction, and alcohol ingestion. Sleep history, daytime sleepiness, sleep laboratory studies, and accounts of others witnessing the event provide a diagnosis. Any underlying pathology should be treated.

If the condition persists, weight loss, continuous positive airway pressure therapy, uvulopalatopharyngoplasty, and drugs such as protriptyline (an antidepressant) and modafinil (a psychostimulant) are treatment options. **Continuous positive airway pressure (CPAP)** is a type of respiratory therapy in which airway pressure is maintained above atmospheric pressure throughout the respiratory cycle by means of a mechanical device. This form of treatment forces the airways to remain open (see **Figure 12-27**). **Uvulopalatopharyngoplasty (UPPP)** is a surgical procedure to remove portions of the uvula (V-shaped fleshy extension hanging above the tongue at the throat entrance), soft palate (back portion of the roof of the mouth), and the lining of the back of the throat to open the airway and create an obstructive-free passage. It is also known as *palatopharyngoplasty.* This procedure removes unnecessary tissue and improves signs and symptoms of snoring from all causes.

KEY TERM	Definition
polysomnography (pol-ee-som-NOG-ruh-fee)	monitoring of the physiological activities that occur during sleep
dyssomnias (dis-SOM-nee-uz)	abnormalities in the amount, quality, or timing of sleep
parasomnias (pair-uh-SOM-nee-uz)	abnormal behavioral or physiological events associated with sleep, sleep stages, or sleep–wake transitions
primary insomnia (in-SOM-nee-uh)	inability to sleep in the absence of external stimuli, such as noise or bright light, lasting longer than 1 month
narcolepsy (NAHR-koh-lep-see)	condition characterized by frequent, brief, uncontrollable bouts of deep sleep; also called paroxysmal sleep
sleep apnea (AP-nee-uh)	temporary cessation of breathing that occurs while a person sleeps
continuous positive airway pressure (CPAP)	respiratory therapy that maintains the air passages at a greater pressure than atmospheric pressure by means of a mechanical device to assist with the breathing cycle
uvulopalatopharyngoplasty (UPPP) (yoo-vyoo-loh-pal-uh-toh-fuh-RIN-goh-plas-tee)	surgical resection of unnecessary tissues of the soft palate and oropharyngeal region; also called palatopharyngoplasty

KEY TERM PRACTICE: *Sleep Disorders*

1. The medical term for abnormalities in the amount, quality, or timing of sleep is _____.

2. _____ is characterized by a temporary cessation of breathing during sleep.

3. _____ is the surgical resection of unnecessary tissues of the soft palate and oropharyngeal region.

4. The monitoring of the physiological activities that occur during sleep is termed _____.

5. Abnormal behavioral or physiological events associated with sleep, sleep stages, or sleep–wake transitions are known as _____.

Personality Disorders

personality disorders

Personality disorders are disorders characterized by attitudes or behaviors that cause difficulty in getting along with others or succeeding in the workplace or social situations. They are manifested by lifelong patterns of abnormal behavior or actions, rather than psychotic or neurotic disturbances. Impaired judgment, impulse control, and interpersonal functioning typify personality disorders.

The cause of personality disorders is unknown, although biological, social, and environmental factors have been implicated. Treatment is psychotherapy and family education to promote the best environment to achieve desired outcomes.

paranoid personality disorder

Paranoid personality disorder is characterized by the tendency to be hypersensitive and misinterpret the actions of others as deliberately harmful, demeaning, or threatening. This often interferes with the ability to maintain healthy interpersonal relationships because the actions of others are misunderstood as unreasonably suspicious.

schizoid personality disorder	The **schizoid personality disorder** is characterized by detachment and unresponsiveness. Traits include social withdrawal, emotional coldness or aloofness, and indifference to others. People with this type of personality disorder have difficulty expressing anger.
antisocial personality disorder	A refusal to accept the obligations and restraints imposed by society is characteristic of **antisocial personality disorder**. There is an enduring pattern of behavior with disregard for and violation of the rights and safety of others. The onset is before age 15. Early childhood signs include chronic lying, stealing, fighting, and truancy. Adolescent signs are unusually early or aggressive sexual behavior, excessive drinking, and illicit drug use. Excessive alcohol consumption and illicit drug use may persist into adulthood. Guilt is not expressed, and these individuals frequently do not learn from their mistakes. This diagnosis is commonly applied to serial killers.
borderline personality disorder	**Borderline personality disorder** is an enduring pattern that begins in early adulthood and is characterized by unstable interpersonal relationships, inappropriate anger, and impulsivity (acting on sudden urges). Individuals with the disorder express chronic feelings of emptiness or boredom and intolerance of being alone.
histrionic personality disorder	**Histrionic personality disorder** is characterized by excessive, dramatic, and shallow emotions; attention-seeking behavior; and demands for approval and reassurance. The pattern begins in childhood and endures into adulthood. People with this disorder need to be the center of attention.
narcissistic personality disorder	A pervasive pattern in adulthood of self-centeredness, self-importance, lack of empathy for others, sense of entitlement, and viewing others as objects to meet one's need characterize **narcissistic personality disorder**. The disorder is named for Narcissus, a beautiful youth in Greek mythology who falls in love with his own reflection in a pool.

KEY TERM	Definition
personality disorders	psychiatric disorders in attitude or behavior that cause difficulty in getting along with others or succeeding in the workplace or social situations
paranoid personality disorder	disorder marked by being unreasonably suspicious of other people and their thoughts and/or motives
schizoid (SKIZ-oid) **personality disorder**	disorder marked by detachment and unresponsiveness
antisocial personality disorder	disorder marked by the refusal to accept the obligations and restraints imposed by society
borderline personality disorder	enduring pattern that begins in early adulthood and is characterized by unstable interpersonal relationships, inappropriate anger, and impulsivity
histrionic (his-tree-ON-ick) **personality disorder**	disorder marked by excessive, dramatic, and shallow emotions, attention-seeking behavior, and demands for approval and reassurance
narcissistic (nahr-sih-SIS-tick) **personality disorder**	disorder marked by excessive self-admiration and self-centeredness

continued

continued from page 1013

KEY TERM PRACTICE: *Personality Disorders*

1. Psychiatric disorders in attitude or behavior that cause difficulty in getting along with others or succeeding in the workplace or social situations are termed _____.

2. Name the personality disorder characterized by excessive self-centered behavior. _____

3. _____ is an enduring pattern that begins in early adulthood and is characterized by unstable interpersonal relationships, inappropriate anger, and impulsivity.

4. _____ is a disorder marked by the refusal to accept the obligations and restraints imposed by society.

5. The disorder marked by being unreasonably suspicious of other people and their thoughts and/or motives is called _____.

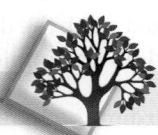

LIFE SPAN

Mental disorders can strike at any point in life. Those evident at birth are often readily identified. Others may be present at birth, but may not manifest until early childhood, adolescence, or adulthood. Research suggests that exposure to stress during puberty may cause physical changes that alter behavior and brain chemistry.

According to research in the United States, late-life depression affects approximately 6 million adults, but only 10% will receive treatment. At least 10% to 20% of widows or widowers develop clinically significant depression within 1 year of the death of a spouse. Older Americans are more likely to commit suicide than any other age group, albeit they constitute only 13% of the U.S. population. During 2002–2006 (the latest dates for which statistics were available from the Centers for Disease control and Prevention), the highest suicide rates for males ages 65 and older were among non-Hispanic whites, with 33.16 suicides per 100,000.

Several factors contribute to the development of mental disorders. There may be a genetic predisposition for mental illness, or prenatal and perinatal (from the 22nd week of gestation through the first 28 days after delivery) factors may also contribute, either solely or in conjunction with other issues. Viral infections and nutritional deficiencies occurring at a specific stage of development and growth may influence mental disorder development. Neuroanatomical alterations, neurotransmitter abnormalities, and neurochemical dysregulation at a later phase of life may cause mental illness. For example, dementias primarily affect the population over age 50, unless there is an underlying pathological condition that precipitates an earlier onset. Great variability exists among the various disorders. Much is still to be learned in this medical field, especially in terms of understanding the causes and in preventing and treating mental diseases.

COMMON Abbreviations

Abbreviation	Term
AA	Alcoholics Anonymous
AD	Alzheimer disease
ADD	attention deficit disorder
ADHD	attention deficit hyperactivity disorder
AN	anorexia nervosa
CBT	cognitive-behavioral therapy
CPAP	continuous positive airway pressure
CT	computed tomography
DSM-IV	*Diagnostic and Statistical Manual of Mental Disorders, Fourth Edition*
DT	delirium tremens
ECT	electroconvulsive therapy
EEG	electroencephalogram
ERP	exposure and response prevention
GABA	γ-aminobutyric acid
GAD	generalized anxiety disorder
GAF	global assessment of functioning
GGT	γ-glutamyltransferase
ICD-9	*International Statistical Classification of Diseases and Related Health Problems, Ninth Edition*
IEP	individual educational plan
IQ	intelligence quotient
LD	learning disorder
LISW	licensed independent social worker
LSW	licensed social worker
MAO	monamine oxidase
MDI	major depression inventory
MMPI	Minnesota Multiphasic Personality Inventory
MRI	magnetic resonance imaging
OCD	obsessive–compulsive disorder
OCPD	obsessive–compulsive personality disorder
OT	occupational therapy
PC	professional counselor
PCC	professional clinical counselor
PT	physical therapy
PTSD	post-traumatic stress disorder
REM	rapid eye movement
SAD	seasonal affective disorder

continued

continued from page 1015

Abbreviation	Term
SSRI	selective serotonin reuptake inhibitor
TAT	thematic apperception test
TD	tardive dyskinesia
TMS	transcranial magnetic stimulation
UPPP	uvulopalatopharyngoplasty

COMMON ABBREVIATIONS EXERCISES

1. TAT is the abbreviation for _____.

2. The abbreviation for obsessive–compulsive disorder is _____.

3. ADD is the abbreviation for _____.

4. The abbreviation for electroencephalogram is _____.

5. Tardive dyskinesia is abbreviated _____.

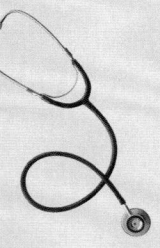

Case Study

Dr. Christopher began treating John Johnson, age 54. During the initial therapy session, John noted that he was recently divorced, but had been separated from his wife for 18 months. He had been living in a small apartment and seeing his children on weekends. Since the court date to finalize the divorce 1 month earlier, he reported not sleeping well or eating much, and described himself as feeling depressed most of the day every day. He was not eating because he felt nauseous and reported frequent upset stomach. He said he had lost about 10 lb (4.5 kg).

At work, his fellow computer programmers expressed concern because they noticed him staring at his computer monitor for long periods of time. He described himself as being unable to concentrate at work for the past couple weeks. He was surprised that he felt that way and is not certain if it is related to his divorce—because he had been separated from his wife for so long—or to a recent fight he had with his 16-year-old son, who no longer wants to visit him on weekends. John also mentioned that he did not feel like golfing with his friends and that he tended to spend a lot of time alone. He had never felt this way before in his life and decided he might need some help.

When Dr. Christopher asked him, John admitted that he had thought about suicide but had not thought about how or when he might kill himself.

continued

continued from page 1016

Case Study Questions

Select the best answer to each of the following questions.

1. **John was probably suffering from**
   _____.
   a. attention deficit hyperactivity disorder (ADHD)
   b. dysthymic disorder
   c. major depression
   d. anorexia nervosa

2. **John's recurrent thoughts of suicide are**
   _____.
   a. typical with major depression
   b. highly abnormal
   c. not worth paying attention to
   d. signs that he is ready to die

3. **The psychosocial stressors that may have contributed to John's depression include**
   _____.
   a. gastroenteritis
   b. the size of his apartment
   c. the fight he had with his son
   d. no exercise

4. **Part of a treatment plan for John might be**
   _____.
   a. a referral to a psychiatrist
   b. a referral to a family physician
   c. joint therapy with his son
   d. any of the above

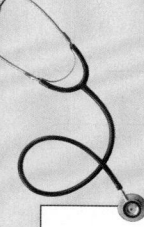

Real World Report

Dr. Christopher conducted a multiaxial evaluation to assess John's overall condition in five areas. This allowed her to create and develop a treatment plan.

MULTIAXIAL EVALUATION REPORT FORM

AXIS I: CLINICAL DISORDERS—OTHER CONDITIONS THAT MAY BE A FOCUS OF CLINICAL ATTENTION

Diagnostic Code	*DSM-IV* Name
296-22	major depressive disorder, single episode, moderate

AXIS II: PERSONALITY DISORDERS—MENTAL RETARDATION

Diagnostic Code	*DSM-IV* Name
none	

AXIS III: GENERAL MEDICAL CONDITIONS

ICD-9-CM Code	*ICD-9-CM* Name
558-9	gastroenteritis, acute

continued

continued from page 1017

AXIS IV: PSYCHOSOCIAL AND ENVIRONMENTAL PROBLEMS

X Problems with primary support group   Specify: divorce; conflict with child

X Occupational problems   Specify: difficulty concentrating & completing projects

AXIS V: GLOBAL ASSESSMENT OF FUNCTIONING SCALE

Score: 55

Time frame: past 2 weeks

Real World Report Questions

The following exercises review the medical terms used in the preceding medical report.

1. What is the *DSM* diagnostic code?

_____

2. What is the DSM axis I diagnostic name for John's mental disorder?

_____

_____

3. The report includes John's general medical condition.

a. The *ICD-9-CM* code is _____.

b. The *ICD-9-CM* name is _____.

4. List John's specific psychosocial and environmental problems.

_____

_____

Review and Application

Multiple-Choice Questions

Select the best answer to each of the following questions.

1. Psychological or behavioral disorders with anxiety as the primary characteristic are termed _____.
    a. neuroses   b. psychoses   c. panic disorders   d. cognition psychoses

2. Chemical messengers called _____ transmit impulses.
    a. drugs   b. enzymes   c. neurotransmitters   d. blood

3. A disease with a definite structural change in the brain tissue is known as _____.
    a. cognitive decline   b. organic brain disease c. neuropathy   d. mental disorder

4. Individuals with doctorate degrees, such as Ph.D.s, licensed to practice psychology are _____.
    a. psychiatrists   b. social workers   c. hypnotists   d. psychologists

5. One's _____ involves emotions, feelings, or mood.
    a. affect   b. neurons   c. psychiatry   d. consciousness

6. General wakefulness and responsiveness to the environment is termed _____.
    a. mind   b. affect   c. consciousness   d. psyche

7. Five coordinates used to assess mental disorders are part of the _____.
    a. intelligence quotient b. multiaxial classification   c. severity and course   d. signs and symptoms
                                                                specifiers

8. _____ are qualifiers regarding specific mental health conditions.
    a. Biofeedback techniques   b. Dementia   c. Stanford-Binet tests   d. Severity and course
                                                                                       specifiers

9. Trained professionals working with economically, physically, mentally, or socially disadvantaged people are called _____.
    a. alcoholics   b. bulimics   c. social workers   d. schizophrenics

10. _____ are professionals who give advice on personal, social, health, or psychological problems.
    a. Psychics   b. Counselors   c. Somnographers   d. Narcoleptics

11. A client wishes to receive therapy from an individual trained in Freudian psychology. A _____ is the professional most likely to be skilled in this area.
    a. psychoanalyst   b. counselor   c. social worker   d. neurosurgeon

12. An overwhelming sense of apprehension is termed _____.
    a. depression   b. grief   c. anxiety   d. denial

13. Brian engages in behaviors that are self-serving, and he has total disregard for any other person. This is an example of _____.
    a. obsessive–compulsive   b. panic disorder   c. narcissistic personality   d. panic disorder
       disorder (OCD)   disorder

14. Ryan has tried nearly every form of therapy to treat his major depression. As a last resort, his psychiatrist recommended _____, treatment that uses electricity to induce convulsions.
    a. biofeedback   b. electroshock   c. psychotherapy   d. hypnosis

Word Parts Exercises

Using the following word parts, form a medical term for each definition. Each word part is used only once.

gyne-   -phobia
patho-   -phobia
phobo-   -phobia
pyro-   -phobia
zoo-   -phobia

15. fear of developing a phobia _____

16. fear of fire _____

17. fear of animals _____

18. fear of women _____

19. fear of disease _____

Matching Exercises

Match the disorder with its description.

_____ 20. autism

_____ 21. mental retardation

_____ 22. vascular dementia

_____ 23. schizophrenia

_____ 24. obsessive–compulsive disorder (OCD)

a. disorder characterized by inescapable thoughts and excessive ritualistic behaviors
b. disorder characterized by mental introversion and concentration on oneself
c. below average intellectual function
d. psychological disturbance characterized by withdrawal, hallucinations, and delusions
e. cognitive impairment resulting from ischemia

Match the disorder with its description.

_____ 25. somatoform disorder

_____ 26. conversion disorder

_____ 27. cyclothymic disorder

_____ 28. sexual masochism

_____ 29. narcolepsy

a. significant mood swings that are unrelated to life events
b. symptoms without any underlying pathology
c. condition in which the person has uncontrollable bouts of sleep
d. person experiences sexual pleasure by being abused, humiliated, or maltreated
e. psychological defense mechanism in which an emotional conflict is transformed into a physical disability

Match the disorder with its description.

_____ 30. antisocial personality disorder

_____ 31. exhibitionism

_____ 32. histrionic personality disorder

_____ 33. paranoid-type personality disorder

_____ 34. schizoid personality disorder

a. disorder causing a compulsion to display one's genitals in public
b. disorder marked by being unreasonably suspicious of others and their motives
c. disorder marked by detachment and unresponsiveness
d. disorder marked by overdramatic reactions or behaviors
e. disorder marked by the refusal to accept the obligations and restraints imposed by society

Match the sign or symptom with its definition.

_____ 35. amnesia

_____ 36. dysphoria

_____ 37. euphoria

_____ 38. delusion

_____ 39. abulia

a. state of unhappiness
b. feeling of elation
c. inability to make a decision
d. memory loss
e. exhibiting false beliefs

Match the clinical test or diagnostic procedure with its description.

_____ 40. Goodenough-Harris drawing test

_____ 41. Minnesota Multiphasic
Personality Inventory (MMPI)

_____ 42. polysomnography

_____ 43. Rorschach test

_____ 44. Stanford-Binet intelligence scale

a. monitoring physiological activities that occur during sleep
b. assessing intelligence based on illustrating accuracy
c. test of mental state based on person's interpretation of standardized inkblots
d. test that uses true-false questions to assess personality
e. standardized test used to measure intelligence

Match the treatment with its description.

_____ 45. biofeedback

_____ 46. behavior therapy

_____ 47. hypnosis

_____ 48. antipsychotic drugs

_____ 49. psychotherapy

a. treatment goal is to change problem actions
b. technique for controlling automatic body functions
c. treatment of mental disorders by psychological methods
d. chemical agents used to treat psychoses
e. artificially induced sleep-like state used to invoke behavioral change

Match the term with its definition.

_____ 50. anhedonia

_____ 51. echolalia

_____ 52. euphoria

_____ 53. alogia

_____ 54. anxiety

a. overall chronic absence of joy
b. overwhelming sense of apprehension
c. inability to speak
d. echoing the words of others
e. abnormal happiness

Definitions

Define the following terms.

55. counseling _____

56. apathy _____

57. tic _____

58. mood disorders _____

59. masturbate _____

Provide a medical term for the following definitions.

60. disorder brought about by contrived or unnatural means _____

61. to pretend incapacitation or illness _____

62. state marked by extreme restlessness, confusion, and hallucinations _____

63. spasms of the tongue and facial muscles after withdrawal from antipsychotic drugs _____

64. group of disorders characterized by nervousness in response to an anticipated future event _____

Alternate Terms

Give an alternate term for each of the following terms.

65. multi-infarct dementia _____

66. palatopharyngoplasty _____

67. Stanford-Binet test _____

68. inkblot test _____

Spelling

Identify the correctly spelled term in each set.

69. _____
a. sychosomatic
b. psychosommatic
c. psykosomatic
d. psychosomatic

70. _____
a. hypochondria
b. hypokondria
c. hyphchondrea
d. hypechondria

71 _____
a. pysychiatry
b. psychiatry
c. psychoiatry
d. physchiatry

72. _____
a. hallucination
b. hallucinnation
c. hallusination
d. hallusincation

73. _____
a. abullia
b. ebullia
c. abulia
d. abbulia

Unscramble

Unscramble the letters to form a medical term.

74. timsaatziona _____

75. caip _____

76. atceff _____

77. gotonniic _____

78. echyps _____

Abbreviations

Provide the term for the abbreviations and then define the terms.

79. CPAP = _____

80. ADHD = _____

81. IQ = _____

82. TAT = _____

Analogies

Provide a medical term to complete a meaningful analogy.

83. Paroxysmal sleep is to _____ as _____ is to dysmorphophobia.

84. _____ is to factitious illness by proxy as _____ is to antipsychotics.

Short Answer

Answer the following questions.

85. A patient has arm paralysis for which no known physiological disturbance can be found. This is an example of _____.

86. A parent brings her child to the emergency room after purposely giving the child unnecessary medicine to make her vomit. The parent is happy that her child is ill and enjoys the attention. This is an example of _____.

Word Search

Find the medical terms hidden in the puzzle.

```
P  P  C  S  S  Q  W  D  Y  I  K  X  C  W  P
S  V  L  S  G  P  N  N  E  Q  B  O  Q  S  R
Y  H  D  E  X  I  I  T  S  L  G  H  Q  Y  T
C  J  T  N  M  R  P  J  I  N  L  B  X  S  F
H  Q  J  S  S  P  R  R  I  F  R  U  I  S  E
O  R  I  U  T  L  S  T  Z  A  X  G  P  V  Y
L  G  Q  O  Y  G  I  Y  M  I  O  T  G  H  V
O  R  J  I  O  O  M  N  C  L  T  D  X  F  Z
G  E  P  C  N  H  B  Z  O  H  N  Z  R  F  V
Y  H  J  S  U  D  N  H  J  Y  I  W  Z  X  M
D  C  P  N  C  X  C  O  W  R  E  A  W  W  I
G  Y  V  O  K  Y  O  M  I  R  W  M  T  Y  X
L  S  H  C  S  C  O  U  N  S  E  L  O  R  S
I  P  S  P  I  V  I  A  Q  I  E  R  T  L  Y
G  E  S  N  O  R  U  E  N  L  X  L  Q  G  C
```

cognition
consciousness
counselors
lesion
mind
neurons
psyche
psychiatry
psychologist
psychology

Vocabulary Review

Review the key terms from this chapter, study the spelling and pronunciation of each term, and write its definition in the space provided. Listen to the audio available for most terms at http://thepoint.lww.com/nath2e and pronounce each term for yourself. Then check the box when you feel confident that you know the definition and can pronounce the term correctly.

Key Term	Pronunciation	Definition
☐ **abulia**	(uh-BOO-lee-uh)	_____
☐ **addiction**	(uh-DIK-shun)	_____
☐ **affect**		_____
☐ **alcoholism**	(AL-kuh-hol-iz-um)	_____
☐ **alogia**	(uh-LOH-jee-uh)	_____
☐ **Alzheimer disease**		_____
☐ **amnesia**	(am-NEE-zhuh)	_____
☐ **anhedonia**	(an-hee-DOH-nee-uh)	_____
☐ **anorexia nervosa (AN)**	(an-oh-RECK-see-uh nur-VOH-suh)	_____
☐ **antidepressants**	(an-tee-dee-PRES-unts)	_____

Key Term	Pronunciation	Definition
❑ antipsychotic drugs	(an-tee-sigh-KOT-ick)	_____
❑ antisocial personality disorder		_____
❑ anxiety	(ang-ZYE-ih-tee)	_____
❑ anxiety disorders	(ang-ZYE-ih-tee)	_____
❑ anxiolytic	(ANG-zee-oh-lit-ick)	_____
❑ apathy	(AP-uh-thee)	_____
❑ Asperger disorder	(AHS-pur-gur)	_____
❑ attention deficit disorder (ADD)		_____
❑ attention deficit hyperactivity disorder (ADHD)		_____
❑ autism	(aw-TIZ-um)	_____
❑ behavior therapy		_____
❑ biofeedback		_____
❑ bipolar disorder	(bye-POH-lur)	_____
❑ body dysmorphic disorder	(dis-MOR-fick)	_____
❑ borderline personality disorder		_____
❑ bulimia nervosa	(bew-LIM-ee-uh nur-VOH-suh)	_____
❑ catatonic-type schizophrenia	(kat-uh-TON-ick-TIPE skit-soh-FREE-nee-uh)	_____
❑ cognition	(kog-NISH-un)	_____
❑ cognitive-behavioral therapy (CBT)		_____
❑ consciousness		_____
❑ continuous positive airway pressure (CPAP)		_____
❑ conversion disorder		_____
❑ counseling		_____
❑ counselors		_____
❑ cyclothymic disorder	(sigh-kloh-THIGH-mick)	_____
❑ delirium	(de-LIRR-ee-um)	_____
❑ delirium tremens (DT)	(de-LIRR-ee-um TREE-munz)	_____
❑ delusion	(de-LEW-zhun)	_____
❑ dementia	(de-MEN-shuh)	_____
❑ depression		_____
❑ disorganized-type schizophrenia	(skit-soh-FREE-nee-uh)	_____
❑ dissociative amnesia	(am-NEE-zhuh)	_____
❑ dissociative disorders		_____

Key Term	Pronunciation	Definition
❏ **dissociative fugue**	(fyoog)	_____
❏ **dissociative identity disorder**		_____
❏ **dysmorphophobia**	(dis-mor-foh-FOH-bee-uh)	_____
❏ **dysphoria**	(dis-FOH-ree-uh)	_____
❏ **dyssomnias**	(dis-SOM-nee-uz)	_____
❏ **dysthymic disorder**	(dis-THIGH-mick)	_____
❏ **echolalia**	(eck-oh-LAY-lee-uh)	_____
❏ **electroconvulsive therapy (ECT)**		_____
❏ **euphoria**	(yoo-FOH-ree-uh)	_____
❏ **exhibitionism**	(eck-si-BISH-un-iz-um)	_____
❏ **exposure and response prevention (ERP)**		_____
❏ **factitious disorder**	(fack-TISH-us)	_____
❏ **factitious illness by proxy**	(fack-TISH-us)	_____
❏ **fetishism**	(FET-ish-iz-um)	_____
❏ **frotteurism**	(FROT-tur-iz-um)	_____
❏ **fugue**	(fyoog)	_____
❏ **gender identity disorder**		_____
❏ **generalized anxiety disorder (GAD)**	(ang-ZYE-ih-tee)	_____
❏ **Goodenough-Harris drawing test**		_____
❏ **hallucinations**	(huh-lew-si-NAY-shuns)	_____
❏ **histrionic personality disorder**	(his-tree-ON-ick)	_____
❏ **hypnosis**	(hip-NOH-sis)	_____
❏ **hypochondria**	(high-poh-KON-dree-uh)	_____
❏ **hypochondriasis**	(high-poh-kon-DRY-uh-sis)	_____
❏ **hysteria**		_____
❏ **intelligence quotient (IQ)**		_____
❏ **learning disorder (LD)**		_____
❏ **lesion**	(LEE-zhun)	_____
❏ **lithium carbonate**	(LITH-ee-um KAHR-buh-nate)	_____
❏ **major depression**		_____
❏ **masturbate**	(MAS-tur-bate)	_____
❏ **mental retardation**		_____
❏ **mind**		_____

Key Term	Pronunciation	Definition
Minnesota Multiphasic Personality Inventory (MMPI)		
mood disorders		
multiaxial classification		
Munchausen syndrome	(MUN-chow-zun)	
Munchausen syndrome by proxy	(MUN-chow-zun)	
narcissistic personality disorder	(nahr-sih-SIS-tick)	
narcolepsy	(NAHR-koh-lep-see)	
neurons	(NEW-ronz)	
neurosis	(new-ROH-sis)	
neurotransmitters	(new-roh-trans-MIT-urz)	
obsessive–compulsive disorder (OCD)		
organic brain disease		
pain disorder		
panic disorder		
paranoid personality disorder		
paranoid-type schizophrenia	(skit-soh-FREE-nee-uh)	
paraphilias	(pair-uh-FIL-ee-uhz)	
parasomnias	(pair-uh-SOM-nee-uz)	
pedophilia	(pee-doh-FIL-ee-uh)	
personality disorders		
pervasive developmental disorders		
phobias	(FOH-bee-uhz)	
pica	(PYE-kuh)	
polysomnography	(pol-ee-som-NOG-ruh-fee)	
post-traumatic stress disorder (PTSD)		
primary insomnia	(in-SOM-nee-uh)	
psyche	(SIGH-kee)	
psychiatrists	(sigh-KIGH-uh-trists)	
psychiatry	(sigh-KIGH-uh-tree)	
psychoanalysts	(sigh-koh-AN-uh-lists)	
psychologists	(sigh-KOL-uh-jists)	
psychology	(sigh-KOL-uh-jee)	

Key Term	Pronunciation	Definition
❏ psychosis	(sigh-KOH-sis)	
❏ psychosomatic disorder	(sigh-koh-soh-MAT-ick)	
❏ psychotherapy	(sigh-koh-THERR-uh-pee)	
❏ residual-type schizophrenia	(skit-soh-FREE-nee-uh)	
❏ Rorschach test	(ROR-shahk)	
❏ scales		
❏ schizoid personality disorder	(SKIZ-oid)	
❏ schizophrenia	(skit-soh-FREE-nee-uh)	
❏ seasonal affective disorder (SAD)		
❏ severity and course specifiers		
❏ sexual dysfunction		
❏ sexual masochism	(MAS-oh-kiz-um)	
❏ sexual sadism	(SAD-iz-um)	
❏ sleep apnea	(AP-nee-uh)	
❏ social workers		
❏ somatization disorder	(soh-muh-ti-ZAY-shun)	
❏ somatoform disorder	(soh-muh-TOH-form)	
❏ Stanford-Binet intelligence scale		
❏ stuttering		
❏ tardive dyskinesia (TD)	(TAHR-div dis-ki-NEE-zhuh)	
❏ thematic apperception test (TAT)		
❏ tic		
❏ tic disorders		
❏ Tourette disorder		
❏ transcranial magnetic stimulation (TMS)		
❏ transsexualism	(trans-SECK-shoo-ul-iz-um)	
❏ transvetic fetishism	(trans-VET-ick FET-ish-iz-um)	
❏ undifferentiated-type schizophrenia	(skit-soh-FREE-nee-uh)	
❏ uvulopalatopharyngoplasty (UPPP)	(yoo-vyoo-loh-pal-uh-toh-fuh-RIN-goh-plas-tee)	
❏ vascular dementia	(VAS-kew-lur de-MEN-shuh)	
❏ voyeurism	(VOY-yur-izm)	
❏ Wechsler intelligence scales		

Answers

Word Grouping Exercises

Definition	Word Part	Definition	Word Part
down, opposite	cata-	mind, soul, emotions	thym-, thymi-, -thymia, thymo-
affinity for, craving for	-phil, -phile, -philia, -philic	nerve, nerve tissue	neur-, neuri-, neuro-
the body, bodily	somat-, somato-	obsession, compulsion	-mania
extreme or irrational fear	-phobia	separated from, derived from	ap-, apo-
form, shape	morph-, morpho-	sleep, hypnosis	hypn-, hypno-
hysteria	hyster-, hystero-	speech, words	log-, logo-
the mind	-phrenia	split, cleft	schiz-, schizo-
mind, mental, psychological	psych-, psyche-, psycho-	stupor, narcosis	narco-

Word Building Exercises

Word Part	Meaning	Common or Known Word	Example Medical Term
cata-	down, opposite	catabolic	catatonic
hypn-, hypno-	sleep, hypnosis	hypnotic	hypnosis
hyster-, hystero-	hysteria	hysteric	hysteria
log-, logo-	speech, words	logogram	logospasms
-mania	obsession, compulsion	mania	hypermania
morph-, morpho-	form, shape	morphology	dysmorphophobia
narco-	stupor, narcosis	narcotic	narcolepsy
neur-, neuri-, neuro-	nerve, nerve tissue	neuron	neurosis
-phil, -phile, -philia, -philic	affinity for, craving for	bibliophile	pedophile
-phobia	extreme or irrational fear	claustrophobia	agoraphobia
-phrenia	the mind	schizophrenia	schizophrenia
psych-, psyche-, psycho-	mind, mental, psychological	psychiatrist	psychology
schiz-, schizo-	split, cleft	schizophrenia	schizophrenia
somat-, somato-	the body, bodily	somatotype	somatoform
thym-, thymi-, -thymia, thymo-	mind, soul, emotions	thymic	dysthymia

Key Term Practice

Anatomy and Physiology

1. Neurotransmitters
2. neurosis
3. consciousness
4. psyche
5. affect

Mental Health Professionals

1. psychiatrist; psychology
2. mind, mental, psychological; psychotherapy
3. Counselors
4. Social workers
5. psychoanalysts

Using the *Diagnostic and Statistical Manual of Mental Disorders (DSM)*

1. multiaxial classification
2. severity and course specifiers

Tests and Scales

1. Stanford-Binet intelligence scale; Wechsler intelligence scales
2. Rorschach test
3. thematic apperception test (TAT)
4. Goodenough-Harris drawing test
5. Minnesota Multiphasic Personality Inventory (MMPI)

Disorders Usually First Diagnosed in Infancy, Childhood, or Adolescence

1. pica
2. Tourette
3. lesion
4. Echolalia
5. Asperger disorder

Delirium, Dementia, and Amnestic and Other Cognitive Disorders

1. vascular dementia
2. Alzheimer disease (AD)
3. Hallucinations
4. delusion
5. apathy

Substance Abuse

1. alcoholism
2. delirium tremens (DT)
3. addiction

Schizophrenia and Tardive Dyskinesia

1. tardive dyskinesia (TD)
2. schizophrenia
3. Schizophrenia
4. antipsychotic drugs
5. abulia

Mood Disorders

1. bipolar disorder
2. Seasonal affective disorder (SAD)
3. Cyclothymic disorder
4. euphoria
5. antidepressants

Anxiety Disorders

1. phobias
2. Post-traumatic stress disorder (PTSD)
3. Dysphoria
4. Exposure and response prevention (ERP)
5. biofeedback

Somatoform Disorders

1. hypochondriasis and hypochondria
2. hysteria; hysteria
3. conversion disorder
4. pain disorder
5. somatoform disorder; psychosomatic disorder

Factitious Disorders

1. factitious disorders
2. Munchausen syndrome
3. Munchausen syndrome by proxy; factitious illness by proxy

Dissociative Disorders

1. Fugue
2. Dissociative disorders
3. dissociative amnesia
4. dissociative fugue
5. dissociative identity disorder

Sexual and Gender Identity Disorders

1. fetishism
2. paraphilias
3. masturbate
4. Exhibitionism
5. frotteurism

Eating Disorders

1. anorexia nervosa (AN)
2. Bulimia nervosa

Sleep Disorders

1. dyssomnias
2. Sleep apnea
3. Uvulopalatopharyngoplasty
4. polysomnography
5. parasomnias

Personality Disorders

1. personality disorders
2. narcissistic personality disorder
3. Borderline personality disorder
4. Antisocial personality disorder
5. paranoid personality disorder

Common Abbreviations Exercises

1. TAT = thematic apperception test
2. obsessive-compulsive disorder = OCD
3. ADD = attention deficit disorder
4. electroencephalogram = EEG
5. tardive dyskinesia = TD

Case Study

1. c is the correct answer.
   - a is incorrect because his lack of attention at work is a new behavior, and if he had ADHD, he would have had attention problems his whole life.
   - b is incorrect because dysthymic disorder occurs for a period of at least 2 years.
   - d is incorrect because John's weight loss is probably the result of his stomach problems and his depression.
2. a is the correct answer.
   - b is incorrect because most people with depression have at least considered suicide as an option.
   - c is incorrect because any thoughts of suicide should be addressed.
   - d is incorrect because someone who is serious about suicide has a method and a plan to carry it out.
3. c is the correct answer.
   - a is incorrect because gastroenteritis is a physical issue.
   - b is incorrect because John did not mention that he felt uncomfortable in his apartment.
   - d is incorrect because lack of exercise is a physical issue.
4. d is the correct answer. Any of the options listed could be part of a treatment plan.

Real World Report

1. 296.22
2. major depression disorder, single episode, moderate
3. a. 558-9; b. gastroenteritis acute
4. divorce, conflict with child, difficulty concentrating and completing projects

Review and Application

1. a	14. b	27. a	40. b
2. c	15. phobophobia	28. d	41. d
3. b	16. pyrophobia	29. c	42. a
4. d	17. zoophobia	30. d	43. c
5. a	18. gynephobia	31. a	44. e
6. c	19. pathophobia	32. d	45. b
7. b	20. b	33. b	46. a
8. d	21. c	34. c	47. e
9. c	22. e	35. d	48. d
10. b	23. d	36. a	49. c
11. a	24. a	37. b	50. a
12. c	25. b	38. e	51. d
13. c	26. e	39. c	52. e

53. c
54. b
55. counseling = therapeutic relationship in which a trained professional assists a person in solving and adjusting to problems and situations through dialogue and activities
56. apathy = total lack of feeling or emotion
57. tic = sudden, rapid, recurrent, nonrhythmic, involuntary motor movement or vocalization
58. mood disorders = group of mental ailments characterized by emotional disturbances that disrupt all other aspects of life
59. masturbate = to self-stimulate the genitals to produce orgasm
60. factitious disorder
61. Munchausen syndrome
62. delirium
63. tardive dyskinesia
64. anxiety disorders
65. vascular dementia
66. uvulopalatopharyngoplasty
67. Stanford-Binet intelligence scale
68. Rorschach test
69. d
70. a
71. b
72. a
73. c
74. somatization
75. pica
76. affect
77. cognition
78. psyche
79. CPAP = continuous positive airway pressure; respiratory therapy that maintains the air passages at a greater pressure than atmospheric pressure by means of a mechanical device to assist with the breathing cycle
80. ADHD = attention deficit hyperactivity disorder; condition characterized by hyperactivity, inability to concentrate, and impulsive or inappropriate behavior
81. IQ = intelligence quotient; number representing a person's reasoning ability as compared to the statistical norm or average for his or her age
82. TAT = thematic apperception test; test for exploring aspects of the personality in which the person is shown pictures of people in various situations and asked to describe what is happening
83. narcolepsy; body dysmorphic disorder
84. Munchausen syndrome by proxy; antipsychotic drugs
85. hysteria
86. Munchausen syndrome by proxy

Word Search

P	P	C	S	S	Q	W	D	Y	I	K	X	C	W	P
S	V	L	S	G	P	N	N	E	Q	B	O	Q	S	R
Y	H	D	E	X	I	I	T	S	L	G	H	Q	Y	T
C	J	T	N	M	R	P	J	I	N	L	B	X	S	F
H	Q	J	S	S	P	R	R	I	F	R	U	I	S	E
O	R	I	U	T	L	S	T	Z	A	X	G	P	V	Y
L	G	Q	O	Y	G	I	Y	M	I	O	T	G	H	V
O	R	J	I	O	O	M	N	C	L	T	D	X	F	Z
G	E	P	C	N	H	B	Z	O	H	N	Z	R	F	V
Y	H	J	S	U	D	N	H	J	Y	I	W	Z	X	M
D	C	P	N	C	X	C	O	W	R	E	A	W	W	I
G	Y	V	O	K	Y	O	M	I	R	W	M	T	Y	X
L	S	H	C	S	C	O	U	N	S	E	L	O	R	S
I	P	S	P	I	V	I	A	Q	I	E	R	T	L	Y
G	E	S	N	O	R	U	E	N	L	X	L	Q	G	C

cognition
consciousness
counselors
lesion
mind
neurons
psyche
psychiatry
psychologist
psychology

Vocabulary Review

Key Term	Definition
abulia	inability to make a decision
addiction	habitual psychological or physiological dependence on a substance
affect	an emotion, feeling, or mood associated with a thought
alcoholism	an addiction to alcohol that interferes with health, interpersonal relations, or occupation
alogia	inability to speak
Alzheimer disease	degenerative brain disorder that causes dementia, especially late in life
amnesia	loss of memory as a result of shock, injury, psychological disturbance, or medical disorder
anhedonia	overall chronic absence of enjoyment in acts that used to be enjoyable
anorexia nervosa (AN)	eating disorder characterized by extreme fear of becoming overweight that leads to dieting to the point of illness and sometimes death
antidepressants	drugs used in the treatment, alleviation, or prevention of depression
antipsychotic drugs	chemical agents used to treat psychoses and thought disorders; also called antipsychotics
antisocial personality disorder	disorder marked by the refusal to accept the obligations and restraints imposed by society
anxiety	overwhelming sense of apprehension
anxiety disorders	group of interrelated mental illnesses involving anxious and apprehensive reactions to stress or in anticipation of a future event
anxiolytic	drug that relieves anxiety
apathy	total lack of feeling or emotion
Asperger disorder	disorder characterized by severe and enduring impairment in social skills and interests, and by repetitive behaviors, leading to impaired social and occupational functioning
attention deficit disorder (ADD)	disorder of attention, organization, and impulse control appearing in childhood and often persisting to adulthood
attention deficit hyperactivity disorder (ADHD)	condition characterized by hyperactivity, inability to concentrate, and impulsive or inappropriate behavior
autism	disturbance in psychological development that is marked by mental introversion and concentration on self or one object

Key Term	Definition
behavior therapy	treatment that uses behavior-modification techniques in which a person's desirable responses are positively reinforced while undesirable behaviors are negatively rewarded
biofeedback	a training technique that enables an individual to gain some voluntary control over autonomic body functions
bipolar disorder	disorder characterized by alternating periods of euphoria and severe depression
body dysmorphic disorder	disorder in a normal-appearing person characterized by an abnormal fear of being deformed; also called dysmorphophobia
borderline personality disorder	enduring pattern that begins in early adulthood and is characterized by unstable interpersonal relationships, inappropriate anger, and impulsivity
bulimia nervosa	eating disorder characterized by bouts of overeating that are followed by undereating, laxative use, or vomiting
catatonic-type schizophrenia	form of schizophrenia with frenzied motor activity, stupor, rigidity, and excitement
cognition	generic term for the mental activities associated with thinking, learning, and memory
cognitive-behavioral therapy (CBT)	treatment whose goal is to change problem actions, manners, and cognition through conditioning, learning, and cognitive restructuring
consciousness	state of being aware and responsive to the environment
continuous positive airway pressure (CPAP)	respiratory therapy that maintains the air passages at a greater pressure than atmospheric pressure by means of a mechanical device to assist with the breathing cycle
conversion disorder	psychological defense mechanism in which an unconscious emotional conflict is transformed into a physical disability
counseling	therapeutic relationship in which a trained professional assists a person in solving and adjusting to problems and situations through dialogue and activities
counselors	professionals who give advice on personal, social, health, or psychological problems
cyclothymic disorder	mental disorder characterized by noticeable, clinically significant mood swings (hypomania and depression) that are unrelated to life events but to a lesser degree than bipolar disorder

Key Term	Definition	Key Term	Definition
delirium	altered state of consciousness characterized by confusion, disorientation, illusions, and hallucinations	factitious disorder	disorder brought about by contrived and unnatural means
delirium tremens (DT)	agitation, tremors, and hallucinations that are caused by alcohol withdrawal	factitious illness by proxy	disorder in which a caregiver harms a child, falsifies medical records, and/or tampers with laboratory specimens to create a situation requiring medical attention; also called Munchausen syndrome by proxy
delusion	false belief maintained in the face of strong contradictory evidence		
dementia	progressive loss of cognitive and intellectual functions	fetishism	the use of a nonliving object (fetish) to produce sexual arousal
depression	state of profound sadness that is unrealistic and out of proportion to the cause	frotteurism	production of sexual excitement by rubbing against a nonconsenting person
disorganized-type schizophrenia	form of schizophrenia marked by incoherent, scattered delusions, dull feelings, social impairment, poor functioning and adaptation, and disorganized mannerisms	fugue	condition in which a person suddenly abandons a present activity or lifestyle and begins a new or different one for a period of time, often in a different city
dissociative amnesia	inability to recall important personal information that goes beyond normal forgetfulness	gender identity disorder	conflict between a person's actual physical gender and the gender that the person identifies himself or herself to be; also called transsexualism
dissociative disorders	group of mental disorders characterized by disturbances in memory, identity, consciousness, or perception	generalized anxiety disorder (GAD)	chronic, repeated episodes of nervousness, agitation, and feelings that something negative is going to happen
dissociative fugue	unexpected travel away from home or a person's usual place of daily activities, accompanied by the inability to recall some or all of the person's past	Goodenough-Harris drawing test	brief test for assessing a person's level of intelligence based on how accurately drawn and how many elements are included when a child or adult is given a pencil and sheet of white paper and asked to draw a person
dissociative identity disorder	presence of two or more distinct personalities in the same person, sometimes without any one personality being aware of the other		
		hallucinations	sensory experiences of something not actually existing in the external world
dysmorpho-phobia	disorder in a normal-appearing person characterized by an abnormal fear of being deformed; also called body dysmorphic disorder	histrionic personality disorder	disorder marked by excessive, dramatic, and shallow emotions, attention-seeking behavior, and demands for approval and reassurance
dysphoria	condition of feeling acutely hopeless, uncomfortable, and unhappy	hypnosis	trancelike state of enhanced relaxation that is artificially induced
dyssomnias	abnormalities in the amount, quality, or timing of sleep	hypochondria	chronic condition characterized by a morbid concern for a person's own physical or mental health accompanied by the conviction of having a serious disease without supportive evidence; also called hypochondriasis
dysthymic disorder	depressed mood for most of the day, for more days than not, for at least 2 years		
echolalia	involuntary parrot-like repetition of a word just spoken by another person		
electroconvulsive therapy (ECT)	passage of a small electric current through the brain to treat mental disorders; also called electroshock therapy	hypochondriasis	chronic condition characterized by a morbid concern for a person's own physical or mental health accompanied by the conviction of having a serious disease without supportive evidence; also called hypochondria
euphoria	exaggerated feeling of happiness		
exhibitionism	compulsion to expose the genitals in public with the intent of provoking sexual interest in the viewer	hysteria	malady with physical symptoms that seem better explained by psychological factors rather than underlying pathology
exposure and response prevention (ERP)	a form of cognitive therapy that involves exposing a person with OCD to the thing that produces anxiety and *not* allowing him or her to reduce the anxiety with any form of compulsive behavior	intelligence quotient (IQ)	number representing a person's reasoning ability as compared to the statistical norm or average for his or her age

Key Term	Definition	Key Term	Definition
learning disorder (LD)	any defect or disturbance in a child's ability to acquire skills in reading, writing, or arithmetic	**organic brain disease**	disease or impaired functioning with a definite structural alteration in the brain
lesion	structural change	**pain disorder**	severe and long-lasting pain thought to be caused by psychological factors
lithium carbonate	drug used to treat bipolar disorder	**panic disorder**	condition in which a person suffers repeated panic attacks that come on suddenly and are overwhelming and uncontrollable, leading to total inaction or unreasonable acts
major depression	psychological illness marked by sustained unhappiness and hopelessness, often with suicidal tendencies; also called major depressive disorder	**paranoid personality disorder**	disorder marked by being unreasonably suspicious of other people and their thoughts and/or motives
masturbate	to self-stimulate the genitals to produce orgasm	**paranoid-type schizophrenia**	form of schizophrenia characterized by delusions of persecution and/or grandeur, hallucinations, and hostility
mental retardation	below average general intellectual functioning that is present at birth or during early life	**paraphilias**	abnormal sexual desires involving non-human objects, the suffering or humiliation of oneself, one's partner, children, or other nonconsenting persons
mind	seat of consciousness and higher functions (cognition, reasoning, and emotion) of the human brain	**parasomnias**	abnormal behavioral or physiological events associated with sleep, sleep stages, or sleep–wake transitions
Minnesota Multiphasic Personality Inventory (MMPI)	standardized test that uses true–false questions to assess a person's personality	**pedophilia**	abnormal sexual attraction to children by adults
mood disorders	group of mental ailments characterized by emotional disturbances that disrupt all other aspects of life	**personality disorders**	psychiatric disorders in attitude or behavior that cause difficulty in getting along with others or succeeding in the workplace or social situations
multiaxial classification	procedure described in the *DSM* for the diagnosis of patients on five axes	**pervasive developmental disorders**	disorders characterized by severe, persistent, and all-encompassing impairment in several areas of development, including social, communication, and behavior
Munchausen syndrome	disorder in which a person pretends to have an illness to undergo testing or treatment or be admitted to a hospital	**phobias**	disproportionate, obsessive, persistent, and unrealistic fears of situations or objects
Munchausen syndrome by proxy	disorder in which a caregiver harms a child, falsifies medical records, and/or tampers with laboratory specimens to create a situation requiring medical attention; also called factitious illness by proxy	**pica**	craving to eat substances that provide no nutritional value
narcissistic personality disorder	disorder marked by excessive self-admiration and self-centeredness	**polysomnography**	monitoring of the physiological activities that occur during sleep
narcolepsy	condition characterized by frequent, brief, uncontrollable bouts of deep sleep; also called paroxysmal sleep	**post-traumatic stress disorder (PTSD)**	group of symptoms, such as sleep disturbances, flashbacks, and depression, that are displayed after a psychologically traumatic event
neurons	basic functional units of the nervous system that transmit impulses; also called nerve cells	**primary insomnia**	inability to sleep in the absence of external stimuli, such as noise or bright light, lasting longer than 1 month
neurosis	psychological or behavioral disorder with anxiety as the primary characteristic	**psyche**	subjective aspects of the mind and self
neurotransmitters	chemicals that transfer "information" between different neurons	**psychiatrists**	physicians (who hold an M.D. or D.O. degree) trained in the diagnosis, treatment, and prevention of psychiatric disorders
obsessive–compulsive disorder (OCD)	psychiatric disorder characterized by intrusive, unwanted thoughts and irresistible repetitive behaviors	**psychiatry**	medical specialty that deals with the origins, diagnosis, prevention, and treatment of mental and behavioral disorders

Key Term	Definition	Key Term	Definition
psychoanalysts	professionals who practice a method developed by Sigmund Freud for the exploration and synthesis of patterns in emotional thinking and for the treatment of a wide variety of disorders	severity and course specifiers	qualifiers (mild, moderate, severe, in partial remission, in full remission, and prior history) regarding specific mental health conditions
psychologists	professionals with a state-issued license in psychology who study and treat mental disorders	sexual dysfunction	disturbance of sexual functioning with a psychological rather than a physical cause
psychology	science that studies the functions of the mind, including sensation, perception, memory, thought, learning, and behavior	sexual masochism	sexual disorder in which a person experiences sexual pleasure by being abused, humiliated, or maltreated
psychosis	both a mental and a behavioral disorder causing gross distortion of reality, disorganized affective response, and the inability to cope with ordinary demands of everyday life; also called psychotic disorder	sexual sadism	sexual disorder in which a person derives sexual pleasure by inflicting abuse and maltreatment on the victim
psychosomatic disorder	group of mental disorders in which physical symptoms suggest a disorder, but there is no underlying physiological dysfunction or disease; also called somatoform disorder	sleep apnea	temporary cessation of breathing that occurs while a person sleeps
		social workers	professionals who provide help to people in need of social services, such as medical assistance or public assistance
psychotherapy	treatment of emotional, behavioral, personality, and psychiatric disorders by psychological means such as verbal or nonverbal communication with patients	somatization disorder	disorder in which emotional conflicts are projected onto the body and revealed as pathological states
residual-type schizophrenia	form of schizophrenia in which the individual has had at least one schizophrenic episode but is currently without symptoms other than illogical thinking and odd behavior	somatoform disorder	group of mental disorders in which physical symptoms suggest a disorder, but there is no underlying physiological dysfunction or disease; also called psychosomatic disorder
Rorschach test	test of personality or mental state based on a person's interpretation of standardized inkblots of various designs and colors; also called inkblot test	Stanford-Binet intelligence scale	standardized test used to measure intelligence; also called Stanford-Binet test
scales	standardized tests that measure psychological, personality, or behavioral characteristics	stuttering	saying something haltingly and repeating sounds when attempting to pronounce words
schizoid personality disorder	disorder marked by detachment and unresponsiveness	tardive dyskinesia (TD)	condition characterized by involuntary movements of the facial muscles and tongue that results from long-term treatment with antipsychotic drugs
schizophrenia	group of long-term mental disorders involving a breakdown in the relation between thought, emotion, and behavior that typically begins during adolescence or in young adulthood with a mixture of signs and symptoms characterized by withdrawal, hallucinations, and delusions	thematic apperception test (TAT)	test for exploring aspects of the personality in which the person is shown pictures of people in various situations and asked to describe what is happening
		tic	sudden, rapid, recurrent, nonrhythmic, involuntary motor movement or vocalization
		tic disorders	habitual, irresistible, repetitive movements that a person feels compelled to do
		Tourette disorder	tic disorder characterized by some combination of multiple twitches, involuntary vocal grunts, and obscene speech
seasonal affective disorder (SAD)	depression associated with the onset of winter and thought to be caused by decreasing amounts of daylight	transcranial magnetic stimulation (TMS)	passage of a magnetic current through the brain to treat mental disorders

Key Term	Definition	Key Term	Definition
transsexualism	conflict between a person's actual physical gender and the gender that the person identifies himself or herself to be; also called gender identity disorder	**vascular dementia**	cognitive impairment caused by inadequate blood supply to the brain because of blocked blood vessels; also called multi-infarct dementia
transvetic fetishism	paraphilia that involves cross-dressing by a male in women's clothes	**voyeurism**	practice of deriving sexual pleasure by looking ("peeping") at the naked body or genitals of unsuspecting individuals, usually strangers
undifferentiated-type schizophrenia	form of schizophrenia typified by disorganized behavior, incoherence, delusions, and hallucinations	**Wechsler intelligence scales**	standardized tests for measuring general intelligence in preschoolers, children, and adults
uvulopalato-pharyngoplasty (UPPP)	surgical resection of unnecessary tissues of the soft palate and oropharyngeal region; also called palatopharyngoplasty		

Pharmacology

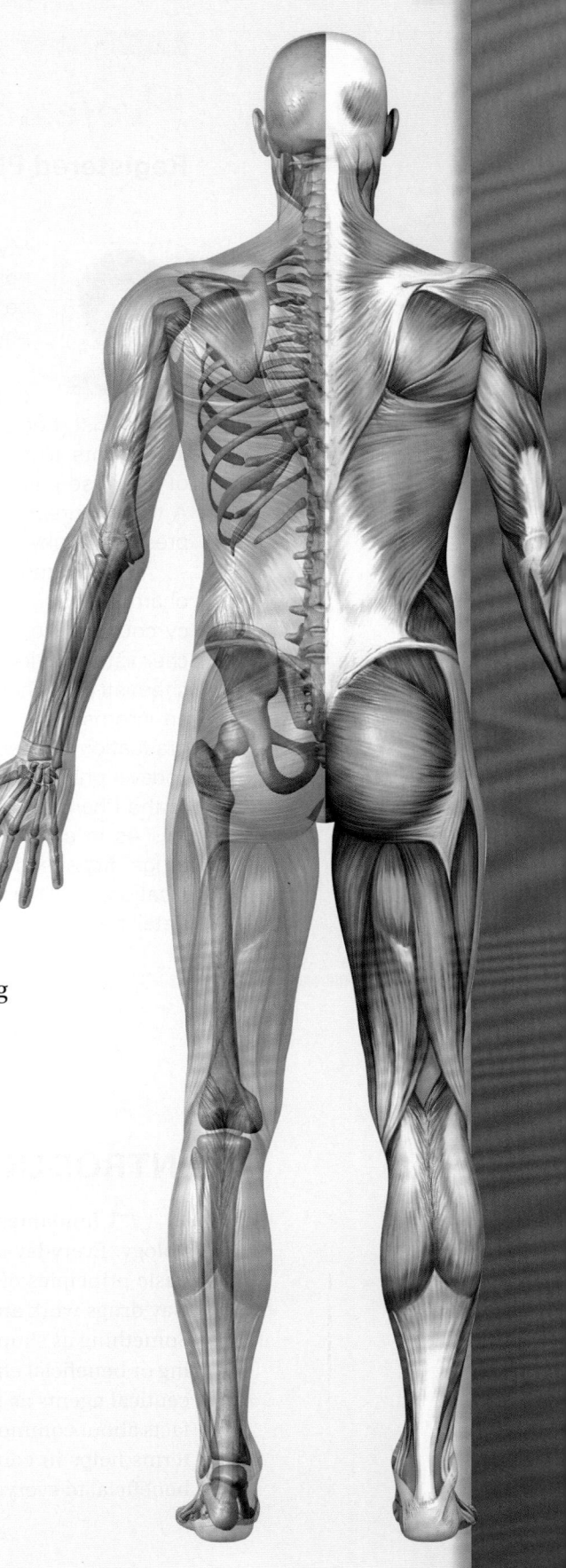

O B J E C T I V E S

After completing this chapter, you should be able to:

1. Define the meanings of word parts related to pharmacology.

2. Explain general principles of pharmacology.

3. Define basic pharmacological terms.

4. Describe the relationship between normal physiology and drug metabolism.

5. Identify drug treatments according to their classification.

6. Explain the necessity of altering dosage levels throughout the life span.

7. Define common abbreviations related to pharmacology.

8. Define terms used in medical reports involving pharmacology.

9. Correctly define, spell, and pronounce the chapter's medical terms.

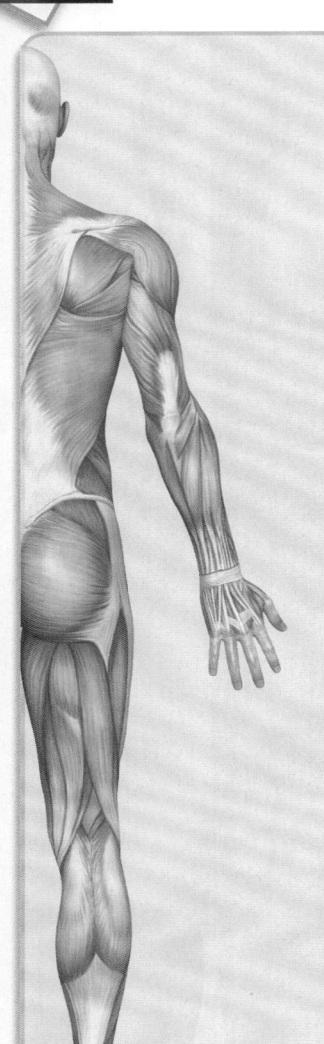

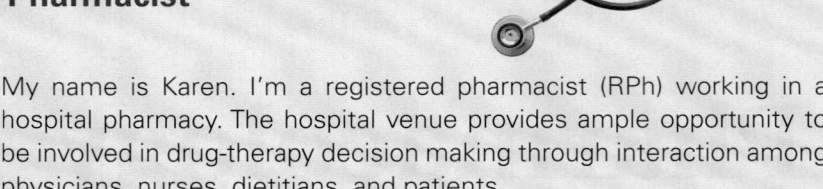

Professional Profile:
Registered Pharmacist

My name is Karen. I'm a registered pharmacist (RPh) working in a hospital pharmacy. The hospital venue provides ample opportunity to be involved in drug-therapy decision making through interaction among physicians, nurses, dietitians, and patients.

Understanding drug classes is critical for knowing clinical effects, drug compositions, and physical and chemical properties. As a hospital pharmacist, I do a considerable amount of drug compounding, which involves mixing ingredients to form tablets, capsules, ointments, and solutions. Regular evaluation of drug use patterns and outcomes for hospital patients is another aspect of the job. A monthly report summarizes the general use of each drug and the names of the prescribing physicians.

I graduated with a bachelor of science degree in pharmacy 15 years ago. The pharmacy program was 5 years of study. I spent the first 2 years taking prepharmacy courses like general biology and chemistry, anatomy and physiology, and organic chemistry. During the third and fourth years, I studied pharmaceutics, pharmaceutical chemistry, biochemical pharmacology, and pharmacy administration. The fifth year was an internship in which I worked under the direction of a licensed pharmacist. After graduation, I passed the state licensing examination and began work immediately. Today's pharmacy programs are different; most are 6-year doctoral programs, leading to the Pharm.D, or Doctor of Pharmacy.

As in all medical professions, I need to keep accurate, confidential records of drugs dispensed. This is a rewarding field requiring scientific aptitude, good communications skills, and a desire to help others. Pharmacy also requires close attention to detail because filling prescriptions directly affects the lives of others.

INTRODUCTION

A fundamental understanding of pharmacology begins with learning medical terminology. Everyday life is full of medicinal items, supplements, and terms. Knowledge of the basic principles of *pharmacology*, the science and study of drugs, and an awareness of the way drugs work are important for anyone, whether you work in the health care field or not. Something as simple as swallowing an aspirin from the medicine cabinet can have devastating or beneficial effects, depending on the individual. Previous chapters mentioned pharmaceutical agents as treatments for pathological conditions. This chapter focuses on a few key facts about common pharmaceutics and their classification. A working knowledge of medical terms helps in comprehending drug names that are new to you, and this understanding is beneficial to everyone.

MEDICAL TERM PARTS

Word Parts

Medical term prefixes, suffixes, and combining forms related to pharmacology are introduced in this section.

Word Part	Meaning
alge-, algesi-	pain
bacteri-, bacterio-	bacteria
chrys-, chryso-	gold
-cide	substance that kills
esthesio-	sensation, perception
iatro-	physicians, medicine, treatment
ino-	muscle fiber
pharmaco-	drugs
rect-, recto-	rectum
-stat	substance that keeps something from changing, flowing, or moving
top-, topo-	place, topical, local
tox-, toxi-, toxico-, toxo-	poison, toxin

Word Grouping Exercises

Using the *Medical Term Parts* table, identify the prefix, suffix, or combining form for each of the following definitions. The first one has been done as an example.

Definition	Word Part
bacteria	*bacteri-, bacterio-*
drugs	
gold	
muscle fiber	
pain	
physicians, medicine, treatment	
place, topical, local	
poison, toxin	
rectum	
sensation, perception	
substance that keeps something from changing, flowing, or moving	
substance that kills	

Word Building Exercises

Word parts introduced in the *Medical Term Parts* section are listed in the following table. For this exercise, first supply the meaning of each word part, then use the word part to build a word you already know. The word you list under *Common or Known Word* does not have to be a medical term; a commonly used word is fine. Be sure, however, that the word correctly reflects the intended meaning. The first one has been done as an example. Check your answers in a dictionary.

Word Part	Meaning	Common or Known Word	Example Medical Term
chrys-, chryso-	*gold*	*chrysanthemum*	chrysotherapy
alge-, algesi-			analgesia
bacteri-, bacterio-			bactericide
-cide			fungicide
esthesio-			anesthesia
pharmaco-			pharmacology
rect-, recto-			rectal
-stat			bacteriostatic
top-, topo-			topical
tox-, toxi-, toxico-, toxo-			toxicology

FUNDAMENTALS

Pharmacology Preview

The scope of health care is expanding, particularly with all the medicines currently available, so it is important to distinguish among the various terms related to this area of medicine. As the science and study of drugs, **pharmacology** includes the sources, chemistry, properties, nature, and actions of those drugs. Sources of drugs include plants, minerals, animals, bacteria, and laboratories for synthetically produced agents. A **pharmacologist** is a person who studies pharmacology.

Pharmacotherapy, or *chemotherapy*, is the use of drugs to treat disease. The branch of pharmacology dealing with active substances found in plants is called *pharmacognosy*. The growth of pharmacognosy is flourishing, as new plants and their medicinal merits are discovered. Furthermore, the nature of the human condition drives drug development so that disease can be prevented, treated, or eradicated. **Toxicology** is the study of poisons, including their source, chemical composition, action on the body, and antidotes.

Comparable to pharmacology, **pharmacy** is the practice of preparing and dispensing drugs. It is also another term for a drugstore. A **prescription (Rx)** is a written order by a medical practitioner that authorizes a patient to be provided medicine, treatment, or a medical

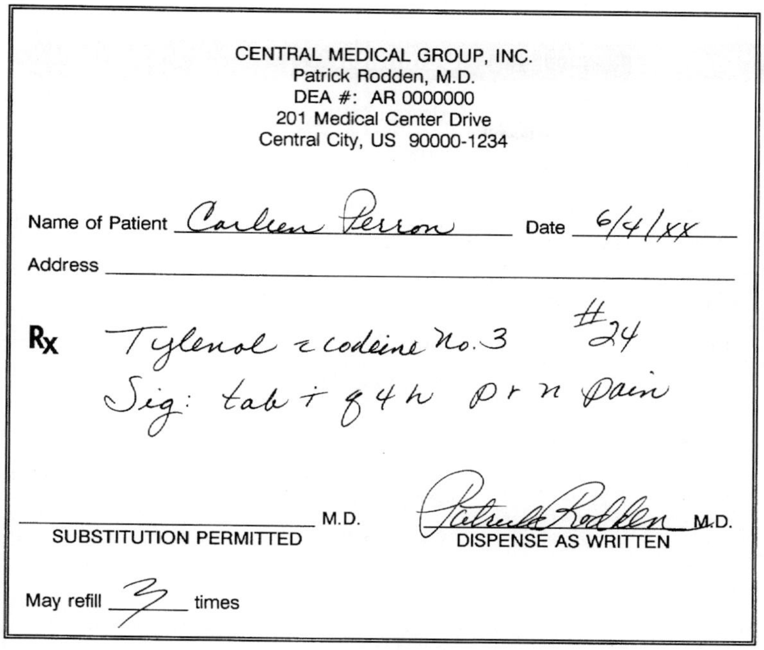

CENTRAL MEDICAL GROUP, INC.
Patrick Rodden, M.D.
DEA #: AR 0000000
201 Medical Center Drive
Central City, US 90000-1234

Name of Patient _Carleen Perron_   Date _6/4/xx_

Address _____

Rx   _Tylenol c̄ codeine No. 3_   _#24_
       Sig: tab ī q 4 h p̄ r n pain

_____ M.D.   _Patrick Rodden_ M.D.
SUBSTITUTION PERMITTED   DISPENSE AS WRITTEN

May refill __3__ times

Figure 19-1 A sample prescription.

device (**Figure 19-1**). The abbreviation _Rx_ is derived from the Latin for _recipe_ and literally means "take recipe." Prescription drugs can be dispensed only with an order from a licensed professional, such as a physician, and in some states nurse practitioners, psychologists, and optometrists. _Over-the-counter (OTC) drugs_ require no prescription.

The person trained and licensed to dispense medicinal drugs and advise on their use is a **pharmacist**. Medicinal drugs are known by two similar-sounding terms: **pharmaceuticals** and **pharmaceutics**.

Most instructional abbreviations commonly encountered on prescriptions and drug notes are derived from Latin terms. **Table 19-1** explains each abbreviation.

TABLE **19-1**

PRESCRIPTION ORDER ABBREVIATIONS

Abbreviation	Term	Definition
aa	_ana_	of each
a.c.	_ante cibos_	before meals
ad lib	_ad libitum_	as desired
a.m., AM	_ante meridiem_	before noon; morning
amt		amount
aq	_aqua_	water
bid	_bis in die_	twice a day
c̄	_cum_	with
cap, caps	capsula	capsule, capsules

continued

continued from page 1041

Abbreviation	Term	Definition
comp		compound
dil	*dilutus*	dilute
DAW		dispense as written
elix.		elixir
g		gram
gtt	*gutta*	drop
h, hr	*hora*	hour
IM		intramuscular
IV		intravenous
IVPB		intravenous piggyback
kg		kilogram (1 kg = 2.2 lb)
mcg		microgram
mEq		milliequivalent
mg		milligram
mL		milliliter
noct.	*nocte*	at night
non rep.	*non repetatur*	do not repeat; no refills
NPO	*non per os*	nothing by mouth
p.c.	*post cibum*	after meals
p.m., PM	*post meridiem*	afternoon
p.o., PO	*per os*	by mouth
PR	*per rectum*	by rectum
prn, PRN	*pro re nata*	as needed
pulv.	*pulvis*	powder
q	*quodque*	every
q.h.	*quaque hora*	every hour
q.i.d.	*quater in die*	four times a day
q.s.	*quantum satis*	sufficient quantity
s̄	*sine*	without
sig	*signa*	write on label
s.o.s.	*si opus sit*	if needed
stat	*statim*	immediately
supp	*suppositorium*	suppository
syr	*syrupus*	syrup
tab	*tabella*	tablet
tbsp		tablespoon (15 mL)
t.i.d.	*ter in die*	three times a day
tinct	*tinctura*	tincture
top.		topical
tsp		teaspoon (5 mL)
vo		verbal order

Many drugs have three different names: the generic name, the trade (brand) name, and the chemical name. A *generic name* is the scientific name or official name for a drug. A *trade name* or *brand name* is usually the trademark of a manufacturer for a particular product. As a proper noun, trade names (brand names) usually begin with capital letters. The *chemical name* indicates the chemical makeup of the drug or the drug's classification. For example, the three names used for a common drug used to treat peptic ulcers are cimetidine (generic name), Tagamet (trade name), and histamine (H_2) blocker (chemical name).

This chapter focuses on the various classifications of drugs, the way they work or their primary mechanism of action or function, and examples of commonly prescribed drugs. The fundamental principles of pharmacology are explained to teach medical terms associated with drugs and prescription orders.

KEY TERM	Definition
pharmacology (far-muh-KOL-uh-jee)	the science and study of drugs
pharmacologist (far-muh-KOL-uh-jist)	person who studies pharmacology
pharmacotherapy (far-muh-koh-THERR-uh-pee)	use of drugs to treat disease; also called chemotherapy
toxicology (tock-si-KOL-uh-jee)	study of poisons, including their source, chemical composition, action on the body, and antidotes
pharmacy (FAR-muh-see)	practice of preparing and dispensing drugs; it is also a drugstore
prescription (Rx)	written order by a medical practitioner that authorizes a patient to be provided medicine, treatment, or a medical device
pharmacist (FAR-muh-sist)	person trained and licensed to dispense medicinal drugs and advise on their use
pharmaceuticals (far-muh-SUE-ti-kulz)	medicinal drugs; also called pharmaceutics
pharmaceutics (far-muh-SUE-ticks)	medicinal drugs; also called pharmaceuticals

KEY TERM PRACTICE: *Pharmacology Preview*

1. An order of written instructions for supplying a medicine is called a _____.

2. The word part _____ means *drugs*, and the word part *-ology* means _____; so _____ means the study of drugs.

3. Medicinal drugs are known as _____ or _____.

4. The practice of preparing and dispensing drugs, or the place where drugs are purchased, is termed _____.

5. _____ is the study of poisons, including their source, chemical composition, action on the body, and antidotes; it is derived from the word part _____, which means *poison*.

Basic Pharmacology Terms

The actions of drugs on the body and the body's reaction to drugs are the center of pharmacology. **Drugs** are any substances other than food or water that are taken for medicinal purposes. **Pharmacodynamics** is the study of a drug's mechanism of action. The way that individuals react to drugs is highly variable. **Pharmacokinetics** (*kinesis* = movement) pertains to the drug's absorption, distribution, metabolism, and elimination.

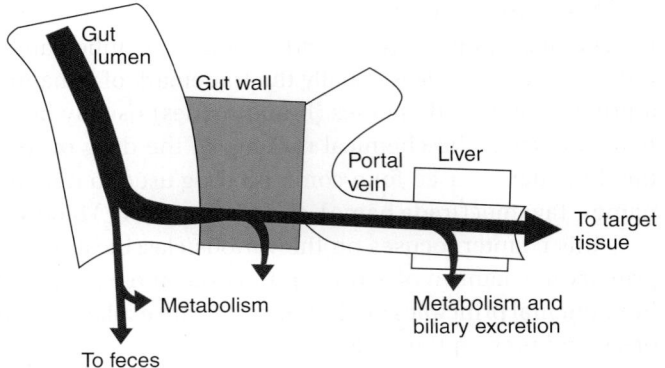

Figure 19-2 A drug encounters several barriers and sites of loss in its sequential movement from the gastrointestinal tract to the systemic circulation. The removal of a drug as it first passes through the gut wall and the liver further reduces the systemic bioavailability.

Pharmacodynamics and pharmacokinetics are critical to bringing about the drug's efficacy and potency. **Efficacy** is the ability of a drug to produce a desired result, and **potency** is the pharmacological strength of that drug measured by the amount needed to produce a certain effect. The **lethal dose (LD)** is the amount likely to cause death, and the **effective dose (ED)** is the dose required to produce desired effects.

Dosage levels can be described in terms of their effectiveness. For example, the **curative dose (CD)** is the amount of medication needed to cure disease or correct deficiency, whereas the **loading dose** is a single, large dose of a drug initially given to achieve the desired therapeutic level quicker than repeated small doses would. The **maintenance dose** (maintenance drug therapy) refers to the systemic dosage of medication required to maintain protection against exacerbation (increase in disease severity or symptoms).

For drugs to be effective, they must be readily accessible to the target tissue. **Bioavailability** is the degree to which a drug becomes available to target tissues after administration. A primary factor to consider in bioavailability is first-pass metabolism or first-pass effect. **First-pass metabolism** is the breakdown of the drug before it reaches the general circulation. The liver metabolizes drugs on their way from the gastrointestinal (GI) tract to the body's systemic circulation (**Figure 19-2**). After passing through the liver, the drug must still contain enough compound to be effective once it reaches its target tissue.

KEY TERM	Definition
drugs	substances other than food or water that are taken for medicinal purposes
pharmacodynamics (far-muh-koh-dye-NAM-icks)	the study of a drug's mechanism of action in the body
pharmacokinetics (far-muh-koh-ki-NET-icks)	pertains to the drug's absorption, distribution, metabolism, and elimination by the body
efficacy (EF-ih-kuh-see)	ability of a drug to produce a desired result
potency (POH-tun-see)	pharmacological strength of a drug measured by the amount needed to produce a certain effect
lethal dose (LD)	amount of drug that will likely cause death
effective dose (ED)	dose required to produce desired effects
curative (KYUR-uh-tiv) **dose (CD)**	amount of drug required to cure disease or correct a deficiency
loading dose	single, large dose of a drug initially given to achieve the desired therapeutic level quicker than repeated small doses would

continued

continued from page 1044

KEY TERM	Definition
maintenance dose	the systemic dosage of medication required to maintain protection against exacerbation; also called maintenance drug therapy
bioavailability (bye-oh-uh-vale-uh-BIL-ih-tee)	degree to which a drug becomes available to target tissues after administration
first-pass metabolism	breakdown of a drug in the liver before reaching the general circulation; also called the first-pass effect

KEY TERM PRACTICE: *Basic Pharmacology Terms*

1. The _____ is the amount of drug that will likely cause death.

2. _____ refers to the drug's absorption, distribution, metabolism, and elimination by the body.

3. _____ is the branch of pharmacology that deals with the drug's mechanism of action in the body.

4. The ability of a drug to produce a desired result is termed its _____.

5. The breakdown of a drug in the liver before reaching the general circulation is known as _____.

Drug Reactions, Regulations, and References

Before a drug can be marketed, it undergoes rigorous research and testing. During drug testing, the agent is compared with an inert substance known as a **placebo**, which contains no active ingredients. Placebos are given to patients participating in clinical trials to assess the performance of the actual new drug. The placebo effect is a sense of benefit felt by a patient that arises solely from the knowledge that treatment has been given. Despite scrupulous testing, a drug could still unfavorably affect a person. An **adverse drug reaction (ADR)** is any response to a drug that causes harm when the drug is given at its normal dosage and usage. An **iatrogenic** result is an inadvertent, adverse response brought on unintentionally by the drug, treatment, or health care provider. Sometimes these results occur because of medical mistakes or because the person has a particular, unknown sensitivity to a drug.

A **side effect** is a secondary, typically undesirable effect of a drug. It is technically an expanded application of the drug's normal actions. For instance, excessive bleeding that occurs after administration of an anticoagulant demonstrates a side effect that is an extension of the desired treatment, although it is not desired. In other cases, a side effect could be an unrelated, undesirable result due to drug administration. The development of Cushing disease after treatment with steroids is an example of a negative side effect.

A drug **contraindication** is any special symptom or circumstance that makes a particular treatment inadvisable. Contraindications are often seen when drugs interact. The effect of one drug may be modified (usually negatively) by another drug given simultaneously. Contraindications are also seen when a condition, such as pregnancy, renders a particular treatment imprudent. **Potentiation** means that the interaction between two or more drugs given together is greater than the sum of each acting separately. For example, alcohol potentiates the sedating effect of tranquilizers (medications that reduce anxiety) when the two are consumed together.

Terms directly related to the patient are addiction, compliance, regimen, palliative, and prophylactic. **Addiction** is a state of physiological or psychological dependence on a drug.

Compliance refers to the patient's willingness to conform to treatment and/or a prescribed regimen. A **regimen** is a prescribed recommended program of medication, diet, exercise, or other measures intended to improve health or stabilize a medical condition. A **palliative** is a medicine that treats symptoms only. The goal of palliative care is to relieve mental and physical pain when no cure is available. Last, a **prophylactic** is a drug that prevents the development of a disease. Taking antimalarial pills to prevent the development of malaria is an example of a prophylactic treatment.

In the United States, the government regulates the manufacture, distribution, and use of medications. This regulation guarantees that all drugs with the same name are of equal safety, strength, quality, and purity. The Food and Drug Administration (FDA), a part of the U.S. Department of Health and Human Services, ensures the safety of food and drugs in the United States. This agency enforces the Food, Drug, and Cosmetic Act (FDCA), which regulates the quality, purity, potency, effectiveness, safety, labeling, and packaging of foods, drugs, and cosmetics.

Another act, the Controlled Substances Act, regulates the prescribing, manufacturing, and dispensing of controlled substances. A **controlled substance** is a prescription medication or illegal drug. Controlled substances are assigned to one of five schedules, according to their:

- potential for or evidence of abuse,
- potential for physiological dependence,
- contribution to a public health risk,
- harmful pharmacological effect, or
- role as a precursor of other controlled substances.

Table 19-2 lists the drug schedules with examples.

TABLE 19-2 — DRUG SCHEDULES

Schedule	Potential for Abuse	Description	Example
I	High	• No current accepted medical use	Heroin, LSD, various amphetamines
II	High	• Current accepted medical use • Abuse leads to psychological or physical dependence • No telephone orders • Cannot be refilled	Cocaine, codeine, Demerol, Dilaudid, morphine; certain *Cannabis*, amphetamines, barbiturates
III	Medium—less than I or II	• Current accepted medical use • Moderate to low potential for physical dependence • Can be refilled • Five refills maximum • No prescription filled after 6 months of original prescription date	Opium, Vicodin, Tylenol with codeine; other narcotics, amphetamines, barbiturates
IV	Low—less than III	• Current accepted medical use • Limited potential for dependence • Can be refilled • Five refills maximum • No prescription filled after 6 months of original prescription date	Darvocet, Equanil, Librium, Valium, other barbiturates
V	Less than IV	• Current accepted medical use • Limited dependence possible • Can be refilled as authorized on the prescription by the prescribing practitioner • Some may not require a prescription	Donnagel-PG, Lomotil, Robitussin A-C

The Controlled Substances Act requires prescribers and dispensers to register with the Drug Enforcement Agency (DEA), pay a fee, receive a personal registration number (DEA number) that accompanies all prescriptions, and keep a record of all controlled drugs prescribed and dispensed. The DEA enforces the Controlled Substances Act.

Uniform drug formulations, or standards, have been established for the manufacture of like drugs from various pharmaceutical companies. Therefore, in the United States, a drug will have the same strength, quality, and purity regardless of place or manufacturer. The standard for preparing and dispensing drugs is outlined in the *United States Pharmacopeia (USP)*, an authorized publication that serves as the national **formulary**, a detailed collection of formulas for medicines. A *pharmacopeia* is a book or database that lists drugs used in medical practice and describes their composition, preparation, use, dosages, effects, and side effects. The federal government recognizes the *USP* as the official standard for all drugs dispensed in the United States. Over-the-counter medicines, such as vitamins and minerals, that conform to these standards are stamped *USP* on the label; however, many OTC products do not carry this stamp and may or may not meet these standards.

Drug references are available in many forms. The *Physicians' Desk Reference (PDR)* is published yearly and lists patient information approved by the FDA. This large book describes the efficacy, adverse effects, pharmacology, and proper use of drugs. The vast majority of the information is the same as that found in pharmaceutical inserts or circulars contained in drug packaging. Manufacturers pay to be listed in this text, which is divided into six sections.

KEY TERM	Definition
placebo (pluh-SEE-boh)	substance with no medicinal ingredients, yet the person may derive therapeutic effects
adverse drug reaction (ADR)	any response to a drug that causes harm when the drug is given at its normal dosage and usage
iatrogenic (eye-at-roh-JEN-ick)	inadvertent, adverse response brought on unintentionally by the drug, treatment, or health care provider
side effect	secondary, typically undesirable effect of a drug that is an expanded application of the drug's normal actions
contraindication (kon-truh-in-dih-KAY-shun)	any special symptom or circumstance that makes a particular treatment inadvisable
potentiation (poh-ten-shee-AY-shun)	interaction between two or more drugs given together is greater than the sum of each acting separately
addiction	state of physiological or psychological dependence on a drug
compliance	willingness to conform to treatment and/or a prescribed regimen
regimen (REJ-i-mun)	treatment plan directed at improving health
palliative (PAL-ee-uh-tiv)	drug that relieves or soothes symptoms but does not cure a disorder
prophylactic (proh-fih-LACK-tick)	drug that prevents the development of a disease
controlled substance	prescription medication or illegal drug
formulary (FOR-mew-lerr-ee)	detailed collection of formulas for medicines

continued

continued from page 1047

KEY TERM PRACTICE: *Drug Reactions, Regulations, and References*

1. _____ occurs when the interaction between two or more drugs given together is greater than the sum of each acting separately.

2. A drug that relieves or soothes symptoms but does not cure the disorder is called a _____.

3. An _____ effect occurs when the treatment itself causes patient harm; the term is derived from the word part _____, meaning "physicians, medicine, or treatment."

4. An _____ is a state of physiological or psychological dependence on a drug.

5. A detailed collection of formulas for medicines is termed a _____.

IN THE NEWS: Color Does Matter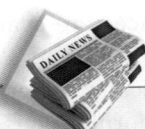

Does the color of medicinal pills matter? Surprisingly, the answer is a resounding "Yes!" The *BMJ* (*British Medical Journal*) reported that brightly colored stimulants achieve a higher response than duller colored pills of the exact same chemical composition. Further, they found that blue- and green-colored tranquilizing pills were more effective than brightly colored ones. One study actually found that patients given blue sleeping pills fell asleep faster and slept longer than patients given other pills. The reason for this is the placebo effect. Patients have their own expectations about medicines; when pills meet their expectations, the medication is more effective for them.

Furthermore, pills that taste "like medicine" are more effective even if the taste has nothing to do with the active ingredient. "We are beginning to understand how words and rituals change brain chemistry and circuitry," says Fabrizio Benedetti, a neuroscientist at the University of Turin, who has been in the forefront of placebo research during the past decade. The placebo effect is truly amazing.

THE CLINICAL DIMENSION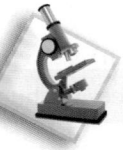

Routes of Administration

Physically introducing something into the body is termed *administration*. Several routes for administering drugs exist, and each differs in terms of bioavailability, the amount of unchanged drug reaching systemic circulation. There are advantages and disadvantages to each approach. Drugs are administered enterally (absorbed through the gastrointestinal tract), parenterally (given by injection), or percutaneously (absorbed through the skin or mucous membranes).

enteral administration	**Enteral administration** is a drug route by way of the gastrointestinal tract. Enteral routes include oral, nasogastric, sublingual, and buccal.
oral route	The most common, yet complicated, route is the oral route. The **oral route** is a convenient way to give a drug by mouth, but the amount of drug reaching the bloodstream is altered by

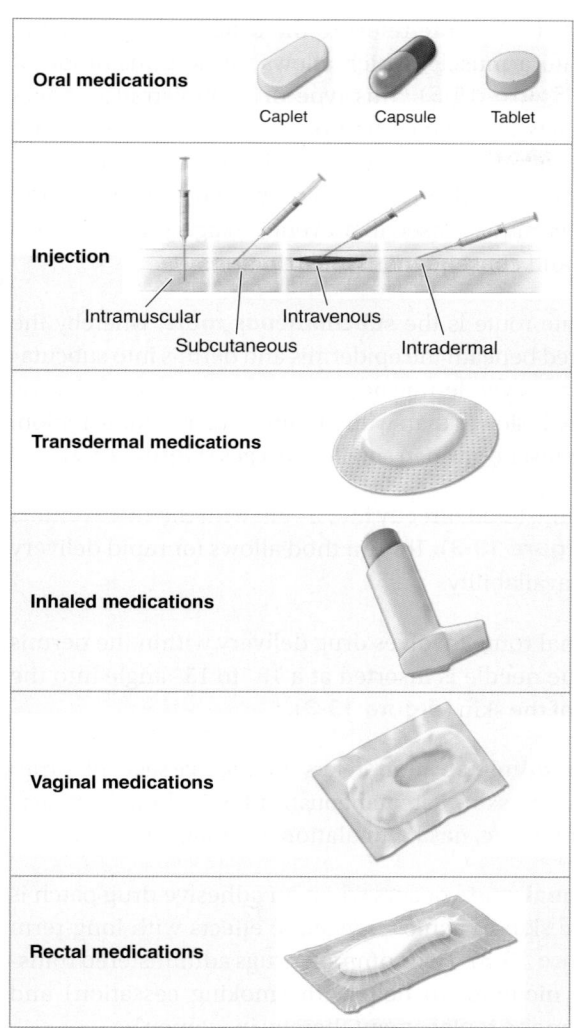

Oral medications	Caplet Capsule Tablet
Injection	Intramuscular Intravenous Subcutaneous Intradermal
Transdermal medications	
Inhaled medications	
Vaginal medications	
Rectal medications	

Figure 19-3 Several routes for administering drugs exist, and each differs in terms of the amount of drug reaching its target tissue.

first-pass metabolism (**Figure 19-3**). *Per os* means *by mouth*, and it is often charted as PO. Note that in charting, *non per os* (NPO) means "nothing by mouth."

nasogastric route   The **nasogastric route** involves drug delivery through the nasal passages and into the stomach. A flexible nasogastric tube is passed through the nose and into the stomach. It is used to feed a patient or remove gastric secretions.

sublingual route   With the **sublingual route**, delivery is beneath the tongue. There is immediate absorption, gastric enzymes do not destroy the drug, and there is no first-pass metabolism. Some medicines delivered by the sublingual route include nitroglycerin for chest pain (angina pectoris) and ergotamine tartrate for migraines.

buccal route   The **buccal route** refers to administration between the cheeks and gum. The drug is absorbed directly into the bloodstream, and first-pass metabolism is avoided.

parenteral administration   **Parenteral administration** refers to the introduction of a drug outside the intestines, by intramuscular, subcutaneous, intravenous, or intradermal injection.

intramuscular (IM) route

Intramuscular (IM) route refers to the drug being injected at a 90° angle into a muscle, which allows for administration of large doses (**Figure 19-3**). This type of administration offers long-term effects and avoids first-pass metabolism. A **Z-tract injection** is another IM technique in which the skin and subcutaneous tissue are displaced laterally before inserting the needle. The technique is used to prevent leakage along the track of the needle and consequent tissue irritation.

subcutaneous route

An intermediate route is the **subcutaneous route**, whereby the drug is delivered beneath the epidermis and dermis into subcutaneous tissue by a hypodermic needle inserted at a 45° angle. The absorption rate is slower than with intramuscular administration, and the drug must be given in smaller dosages (**Figure 19-3**).

intravenous (IV) route

A drug is administered directly into a vein with the **intravenous (IV) route** (**Figure 19-3**). This method allows for rapid delivery and 100% bioavailability.

intradermal route

The intradermal route involves drug delivery within the dermis of the skin. The needle is inserted at a 10° to 15° angle into the dermal layer of the skin (**Figure 19-3**).

percutaneous administration

Percutaneous administration refers to the passage of drugs through unbroken skin. Percutaneous routes include transdermal, ophthalmic, otic, nasal, inhalation, vaginal, and rectal.

transdermal route

The **transdermal route** occurs when an adhesive drug patch is applied to the skin to achieve systemic effects with long-term delivery (**Figure 19-3**). Two common drugs administered transdermally are nicotine (to help with smoking cessation) and estrogen (hormone replacement therapy in women).

ophthalmic route

The **ophthalmic route** is used when drops and ointments are administered directly into the eye.

otic route

The **otic route** is used to place drops directly into the ear canal. The patient normally lies on his/her side while administering ear drops.

nasal route

With the **nasal route**, medications are dropped or sprayed into the nose. Most nasal medications are over-the-counter preparations that shrink swollen, irritated nasal mucous membranes.

inhalation

With the **inhalation route**, the drug is inhaled and delivered directly to respiratory tissues (**Figure 19-3**). The bioavailability ranges from 5% to 100%. The drug must be in an aerosol or gas phase, and it is rapidly absorbed through the large surface area of the alveoli (air sacs) in the lungs.

vaginal route

The **vaginal route** is another method for drug delivery by a medicated suppository called a *pessary* (**Figure 19-3**). A suppository is a medicated preparation in the form of a cylinder that is inserted into the vagina, rectum, or urethra. As the suppository melts at body temperature, it is absorbed through the membranes.

rectal route

With the **rectal route**, the drug is delivered by suppository with 30% to near 100% bioavailability, and there is less first-pass metabolism (**Figure 19-3**).

KEY TERM	Definition
enteral (EN-tur-ul)	drug route by way of the gastrointestinal tract
oral route	administering a drug by mouth
nasogastric route	drug delivery through the nasal passages and into the stomach
sublingual (sub-LING-gwul) **route**	administering a drug beneath the tongue
buccal (BUCK-ul) **route**	administering a drug between the gum and cheek
parenteral (puh-REN-tur-ul) **administration**	introduction of a drug outside the intestines, by intramuscular, subcutaneous, intravenous, or intradermal injection
intramuscular (in-truh-MUS-kew-lur) **route**	administering a drug within a muscle
Z-tract injection	intramuscular technique in which the skin and subcutaneous tissue are displaced laterally before inserting the needle
subcutaneous (sub-kew-TAY-nee-us) **route**	administering a drug beneath the epidermis and dermis into subcutaneous tissue using a hypodermic needle
intravenous (IV) route	administering a drug directly into a vein
intradermal (in-truh-DUR-mul) **route**	administering a drug within the dermis
percutaneous (pur-kew-TAY-nee-us) **administration**	passage of drugs through unbroken skin
transdermal (trans-DUR-mul) **route**	administering a drug through unbroken skin by an adhesive patch
ophthalmic (off-THAL-mick) **route**	administering drops or ointments directly into the eye
otic (OH-tick) **route**	administering drops directly into the ear canal
nasal route	dropping or spraying medications into the nose
inhalation route	drug is inhaled and delivered directly to respiratory tissues
vaginal (VAJ-i-nul) **route**	administering a drug into the vagina using a medicated suppository
rectal (RECK-tul) **route**	administering a drug through the rectum

KEY TERM PRACTICE: *Routes of Administration*

1. This route is best described by administering drops directly into the ear canal. _____

2. Administering a drug directly into a vein is known as the _____.

3. The _____ is the administration of a drug through unbroken skin by an adhesive patch.

4. The intramuscular injection technique in which the skin and subcutaneous tissue are displaced laterally before inserting the needle is termed a _____.

5. Administering a drug beneath the tongue is called the _____.

Antimicrobial Drugs

antimicrobial agents

Antimicrobial agents are drugs that destroy microbes, prevent their multiplication or growth, or prevent their pathogenic action. Each class of antimicrobic is designed to act against a microbe by a specific mechanism. They are effective against bacteria and viruses.

antibiotics

Antibiotics are drugs that kill or inhibit the growth of bacteria. Antibiotics can be either bactericidal or bacteriostatic:

- **Bactericidal** drugs destroy bacteria.
- **Bacteriostatic** drugs hinder or arrest bacterial growth.

(The word part *-stat* refers to a "substance that keeps something from changing, flowing, or moving"; the word part *-cide* means "killer.") Notice the nuances in spelling: bacteri*o*static has a combining *o,* but bactericidal does not.

The proper administration of antibiotics requires that the organism be identified. However, this is often not done. In some cases, time does not permit thorough testing. Thus, physicians prescribe according to the clinical picture and experience. Prescribing an antibiotic for conditions that are not bacterial in origin (e.g., against viruses) or prescribing the wrong antibiotic causes unwarranted problems and leads to microbial resistance.

antiseptic

An **antiseptic** is a topical agent that prevents infection by inhibiting the growth of infectious agents. Antiseptics are used to inhibit the development of infection in cuts, scratches, or surgical incisions.

astringent

Another topically-applied agent, an **astringent**, shrinks blood vessels and draws skin tissue together. Astringents are used to absorb lesion secretions and lessen skin sensitivity.

broad-spectrum antibiotics

Broad-spectrum antibiotics offer benefit against both gram-positive (G^+) and gram-negative (G^-) bacteria. The Gram stain is a useful test for bacterial taxonomy and identification and is used to determine treatments. Bacteria are either gram-positive (taking up the purple stain) or gram-negative (taking up the red stain) (**Figure 19-4**). Broad-spectrum

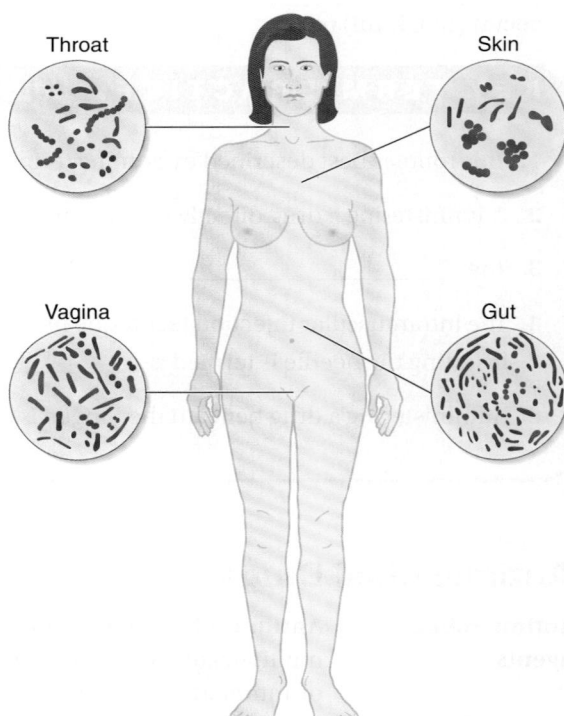

Figure 19-4 The typical bacteria seen in the microbe-laden sites of the body are shown in schematic fashion. Gram-positive bacteria are shown in purple, gram-negative bacteria are in red.

antibiotics are beneficial for a **superinfection**, a new infection in addition to one already present.

antimycobacterial drugs
Antimycobacterial drugs are effective against *Mycobacterium* species, which cause leprosy and tuberculosis. (Note the spelling of the term and avoid the temptation to write the nonsensical term "microbacterium" or the incorrectly spelled term "micobacterium.")

KEY TERM	Definition
antimicrobial (an-tee-migh-KROH-bee-ul) **agents**	drugs that destroy microbes, prevent their multiplication or growth, or prevent their pathogenic action
antibiotics (an-tee-bye-OT-icks)	drugs that kill or inhibit the growth of bacteria
bactericidal (back-teer-ih-SIGH-dul)	drug that destroys bacteria
bacteriostatic (back-teer-oh-STAT-ick)	drug that hinders or arrests bacterial growth
antiseptic (an-tih-SEP-tick)	topical agent that prevents infection by inhibiting the growth of infectious agents
astringent (uh-STRIN-jent)	topical agent that shrinks tissues
broad-spectrum antibiotics (an-tee-bye-OT-icks)	agents that are effective against both G$^+$ and G$^-$ bacteria
superinfection	a new infection in addition to one already present
antimycobacterial (an-tee-migh-koh-back-TEER-ee-ul) **drugs**	an agent effective against *Mycobacterium* species

KEY TERM PRACTICE: *Antimicrobial Drugs*

1. Drugs that destroy microbes, prevent their multiplication or growth, or prevent their pathogenic action are known collectively as _____.

2. Drugs that are aimed at both G$^+$ and G$^-$ organisms are called _____.

3. An _____ is a topical agent that shrinks tissues.

4. A drug that destroys bacteria is termed a _____ and is derived from the word part _____ for *bacteria* and the word part _____ for *killing*.

5. _____ are drugs that kill or inhibit the growth of bacteria.

Antiviral Drugs

antiviral drugs
Antiviral drugs react against viruses, which are minute particles that live as parasites in organisms. These drugs weaken, are antagonistic to, or destroy viruses. Drugs discussed in this section treat human immunodeficiency virus (HIV) and influenza.

HIV is a retrovirus that destroys the body's immune system. Acquired immunodeficiency syndrome (AIDS) is the disease that results from the absent or diminished immune response. HIV replicates using enzymes called reverse transcriptase and protease, which some drugs target.

- **Reverse transcriptase inhibitors (RTIs)** hamper an enzyme (reverse transcriptase) that the HIV virus uses to replicate, and for this reason serve as one method for targeting HIV for eradication.

- **Protease inhibitors** interfere with viral protein processing, preventing new viral particles from forming.

  Influenza (flu) is a viral illness that produces a fever, sore throat, runny nose, headache, dry cough, and muscle pain. The function of influenza drugs is to lessen the severity of the symptoms.

- **Neuraminidase inhibitors** block the release of the influenza virus from infected cells.

KEY TERM	Definition
antiviral (an-tee-VYE-rul) **drugs**	agents that act against viruses
reverse transcriptase (tran-SKRIP-tace) **inhibitors (RTIs)**	agents that block the enzyme reverse transcriptase to eradicate viruses that use it for replication
protease (PROH-tee-ace) **inhibitors**	agents that block the enzyme protease to eradicate viruses that use it for replication
neuraminidase (nur-uh-MIN-ih-daze) **inhibitors**	agents that block the release of influenza virus from infected cells

KEY TERM PRACTICE: *Antiviral Drugs*

1. Drugs acting against viruses are called _____.

2. _____ are agents that block the release of influenza virus from infected cells.

3. Agents that block the enzyme protease to eradicate viruses that use it for replication are known as

   _____.

4. Agents that block the enzyme reverse transcriptase to eradicate viruses that use it for replication are called

   _____.

Antifungal, Antiprotozoal, and Antihelminthic Drugs

antifungal drugs   **Antifungal drugs** suppress or destroy fungi. Fungal infections most commonly occur on the skin, hair, and nails and to a lesser extent in the mouth, gastrointestinal tract, and perianal region. A common fungal infection is athlete's foot (**Figure 19-5**).

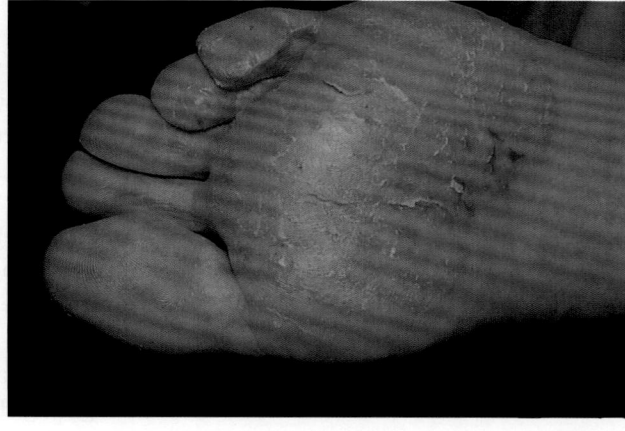

Figure 19-5 Athlete's foot skin lesions.

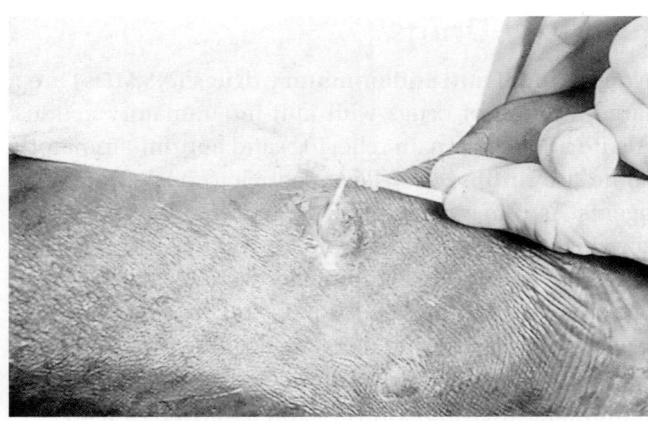

Figure 19-6 An adult female worm is removed by winding onto a stick. Gloves are not worn because this photo was taken in the field.

Protozoa are single-celled organisms, such as amoebae. **Antiprotozoal drugs** treat common protozoal infections, including African sleeping sickness (an infection transmitted by the tsetse fly), amebiasis (diarrhea), dysentery, giardiasis (diarrhea), trichomoniasis (genital infection), malaria, and toxoplasmosis.

Various parasitic worms such as flatworms, tapeworms, roundworms, or flukes are helminths (**Figure 19-6**). **Antihelminthic drugs** act against helminths.

KEY TERM	Definition
antifungal (an-tee-FUNG-gul) **drugs**	agents that suppress or destroy fungi
antiprotozoal (an-tee-proh-tuh-ZOH-ul) **drugs**	agents that are effective against protozoa infections
antihelminthic (an-tee-hel-MIN-thick) **drugs**	agents that target parasitic worms called helminths

KEY TERM PRACTICE: *Antifungal, Antiprotozoal, and Antihelminthic Drugs*

1. _____ are agents that suppress or destroy fungi.

2. Agents that act against protozoa are termed _____.

3. _____ target parasitic worms called helminths.

Cancer Drugs

Treatment of cancer generally involves the administration of several drugs used in combination to obtain synergistic effects. The goal of therapy is to eradicate cancer cells using **cytotoxic drugs**, which kill cells. Unfortunately, other cells in addition to cancer cells are killed, and numerous side effects occur with anticancer therapies. Cancer is discussed in the next chapter.

KEY TERM	Definition
cytotoxic (sigh-toh-TOCK-sick) **drugs**	agents that kill cells

KEY TERM PRACTICE: *Cancer Drugs*

1. The word part cyto- means _____, and the word part *toxi-* means _____; so _____ agents kill cells.

Nonsteroidal Anti-Inflammatory Drugs

nonsteroidal anti-inflammatory drugs (NSAIDs)

Nonsteroidal anti-inflammatory drugs (NSAIDs) are a large number of drugs with anti-inflammatory actions. All are **analgesic** (pain relieving) and anti-inflammatory; some are **antipyretic** (fever reducing) and antiplatelet agents. Aspirin is the classic example of an NSAID, and in the United States, approximately 80 billion aspirin tablets are taken yearly. Its components were used during the second millennium BCE for pain treatment, but aspirin was not developed into its recognizable form until 1897. Other examples of NSAIDs are acetaminophen (Tylenol), ibuprofen (Advil and Motrin), and naproxen (Aleve).

- **Aspirin** is a widely used analgesic, antipyretic, anti-inflammatory, and antiplatelet agent. The chemical name for aspirin is acetylsalicylic acid, and thus it is commonly abbreviated ASA. In 1981, English physician Sir John Vane won the Nobel Prize for medicine after discovering in 1971 that aspirin works by inhibiting prostaglandin synthesis.

- **Acetaminophen** has both analgesic and antipyretic properties, and its potency is similar to that of aspirin.

- **Ibuprofen** is used as an analgesic and anti-inflammatory agent.

- **Naproxen** is an anti-inflammatory commonly used to treat headaches and arthritis.

KEY TERM	Definition
nonsteroidal (non-sterr-OID-ul) **anti-inflammatory drugs (NSAIDs)**	large number of drugs with analgesic and anti-inflammatory actions
analgesic (an-al-JEE-zick)	pain reliever
antipyretic (an-tee-pye-RET-ick)	agent that reduces fever
aspirin	widely used analgesic, antipyretic, anti-inflammatory, and antiplatelet agent; also called acetylsalicylic acid (ASA); type of NSAID
acetaminophen (as-et-uh-MIH-noh-fen)	drug that relieves pain and reduces fever; type of NSAID
ibuprofen (eye-byoo-PROH-fen)	analgesic and anti-inflammatory agent; type of NSAID
naproxen (nuh-PROCKS-en)	anti-inflammatory commonly used to treat headaches and arthritis; type of NSAID

KEY TERM PRACTICE: *Nonsteroidal Anti-Inflammatory Drugs*

1. Acetylsalicylic acid is the chemical name for _____.

2. Name 3 common NSAIDS. _____

3. An _____ is an agent that reduces fever.

4. Agents that are not steroids that relieve pain and inflammation are called _____.

5. _____ is a drug that relieves pain and reduces fever.

Nervous System Drugs

Central nervous system (CNS) drugs affect the brain and spinal cord.

barbiturates	**Barbiturates** are CNS depressants. They are used for their tranquilizing (calming), hypnotic (causing sleep or drowsiness), and antiseizure effects. Barbiturates are used primarily to treat insomnia and epilepsy. Epilepsy is a chronic disorder in which the brain neurons discharge sporadically causing seizures. The seizure type determines the drug used**.**
benzodiazepines	**Benzodiazepines** are drugs with antianxiety, hypnotic, anticonvulsant, and skeletal muscle relaxant properties. They are used short term to treat anxiety disorders and insomnia.
anticonvulsants	Drugs that prevent or reduce the severity of convulsive seizures, such as epileptic events, are called **anticonvulsants.**
antidepressants	**Antidepressants** are drugs used to treat depression. Several are currently available: • **Selective serotonin reuptake inhibitors (SSRIs)** block the reuptake of the neurotransmitter serotonin, thereby allowing increased levels to remain in the circulation. The heightened amounts then positively affect mood. SSRIs are the first-line drugs used to treat depression. • **Serotonin-norepinephrine reuptake inhibitors (SNRIs)** are used to treat major depression and other mood disorders. The drugs inhibit the reuptake of serotonin and norepinephrine at the presynaptic neuron, causing increased levels to remain in circulation. • **Tricyclic antidepressants (TCAs)** are used to treat depression by blocking the reuptake of norepinephrine and serotonin. Thus, more norepinephrine and serotonin remain in circulation. • **Monoamine oxidase inhibitors (MAOIs)** increase the levels of norepinephrine and serotonin by inhibiting monoamine oxidase, the enzyme that breaks down these neurotransmitters.
psychotropic drugs	**Psychotropic drugs** are agents that can alter mental function, behavior, or experience and are used to treat psychiatric disorders: • Typical (first-generation) antipsychotics block dopamine receptors. • Atypical (second-generation) antipsychotics block dopamine and serotonin receptors. • Lithium carbonate is used to treat bipolar disorder, but its mechanism of action is unknown.
levodopa (L-dopa)	**Levodopa (L-dopa)** is a natural substance that is converted to the neurotransmitter, dopamine, in the brain after crossing the blood–brain barrier (BBB). Parkinson disease (PD) results from a loss of dopamine-containing neurons in the substantia nigra portion of the brain. Because dopamine cannot cross the BBB, it cannot be used to treat the disease, so instead a precursor such as levodopa is needed. A precursor is a substance that leads to another compound.

narcotics   **Narcotics** are drugs that dull the senses. In therapeutic doses, narcotics relieve pain and discomfort and produce sleep. In large doses, they cause stupor, coma, and convulsions.

Opiates act on specific CNS receptors to reduce pain perception. The opiates opium, morphine, and codeine are classified as narcotics.

- **Opium** is a brownish, gummy extract from the unripe seed pods of the opium poppy that contains highly addictive substances such as morphine and codeine.

- **Morphine** is used as a narcotic analgesic. Analgesics alleviate pain without loss of consciousness. Interestingly, in 1853, hypodermic needle syringes with a point fine enough to pierce the skin were invented—and their first use was for intravenous morphine injections.

- **Codeine** resembles morphine in its action, but it is weaker. Codeine is used as an analgesic, **antitussive** (cough suppressant), and **antidiarrheal** (diarrhea treatment).

KEY TERM	Definition
barbiturates (bar-BICH-ur-ates)	central nervous system depressants
benzodiazepines (ben-zoh-dye-AZ-uh-peenz)	drugs with antianxiety, hypnotic, anticonvulsant, and skeletal muscle relaxant properties
anticonvulsants (an-tee-kun-VUL-sunts)	drugs that prevent or reduce the severity of convulsive seizures
antidepressants (an-tee-de-PRES-unts)	drugs used to treat depression
selective serotonin (serr-oh-TOH-nin) **reuptake inhibitors (SSRIs)**	drugs that block the reuptake of serotonin, causing increased levels to remain in circulation
serotonin-norepinephrine reuptake inhibitors (SNRIs)	drugs that treat major depression and other mood disorders by inhibiting the reuptake of serotonin and norepinephrine at the presynaptic neuron, causing increased levels to remain in circulation
tricyclic antidepressants (TCAs) (try-SICK-lick an-tee-de-PRES-unts)	drugs used to treat depression by blocking the reuptake of norepinephrine and serotonin, causing increased levels to remain in circulation
monoamine oxidase (mon-oh-AM-een OCK-sih-dace) **inhibitors (MAOIs)**	drugs that increase the levels of norepinephrine and serotonin by inhibiting monoamine oxidase, the enzyme that breaks down these neurotransmitters
psychotropic (sigh-koh-TROP-ick) **drugs**	agents that can alter mental function, behavior, or experience and are used to treat psychiatric disorders
levodopa (lee-voh-DOH-puh) **(L-dopa)**	natural substance that is converted to the neurotransmitter dopamine in the brain after crossing the blood–brain barrier (BBB); it is used to treat Parkinson disease
narcotics	drugs that dull the senses
opiates	drugs that act on specific CNS receptors to reduce pain perception
opium	brownish, gummy extract from the unripe seed pods of the opium poppy that contains highly addictive substances such as morphine and codeine
morphine	narcotic analgesic
codeine (KOH-deen)	drug that acts as an analgesic, antitussive, and antidiarrheal
antitussive (an-tee-TUS-iv)	cough suppressant
antidiarrheal (an-tee-dye-uh-REE-ul)	drug that treats diarrhea

continued

continued from page 1058

KEY TERM PRACTICE: *Nervous System Drugs*

1. _____ are drugs that prevent or reduce the severity of convulsive seizures.

2. _____ are drugs that block the reuptake of serotonin, causing increased levels to remain in circulation.

3. Opium, morphine, and codeine belong to a class of drugs called _____.

4. The medical term for a cough suppressant is an _____.

5. A natural substance that is converted to the neurotransmitter dopamine in the brain and is used to treat Parkinson disease is _____.

Anesthetics

anesthetics   **Anesthetics** are drugs that reversibly depress neuronal function and cause insensitivity to pain. For example, a dentist may administer an anesthetic to "numb" your mouth prior to a tooth extraction. The first anesthetics were used in the 1840s, and the three used were all inhaled substances: chloroform, ether, and nitrous oxide. Today, anesthetics are given to patients before, during, and after surgery. The ideal anesthetic achieves several outcomes: rapid, pleasant induction and withdrawal from the drug, skeletal muscle relaxation, analgesia (conscious pain relief), and high potency.

The branch of medicine that deals with the study and use of anesthetic substances is **anesthesiology**. A doctor or other qualified person who administers anesthesia is known as an **anesthesiologist** or **anesthetist**. Physicians specializing in anesthesiology are generally called anesthesiologists, whereas nurses with specialized training in anesthesiology are known as **nurse anesthetists**. To anesthetize a person is to induce anesthesia.

Anesthetic agents are categorized as general (given by inhalation or intravenous injection), local (regional or topical anesthesia), and specific applications (spinal and epidural).

- **General anesthetics** produce drug-induced **anesthesia**, the absence of perception. There is a total loss of sensation and consciousness in the whole body. General anesthesia is often called "putting people under" or "putting people asleep" before a surgical procedure. The mechanism of action of general anesthetics remains mostly unknown. General anesthesia is induced through inhaled gases and IV routes.

- **Local anesthetics** typically cause loss of sensation at the site of administration by blocking nerve conduction.

- **Spinal anesthesia** involves injecting the drug into the subarachnoid space through a spinal needle (**Figure 19-7**). There is a loss of sensation in the region. This type of anesthesia is used for gynecological, obstetrical, orthopedic, and genitourinary surgeries.

- **Epidural anesthesia** involves injection of the anesthetic into the epidural space, usually the lumbar or caudal region, through a catheter (**Figure 19-8**). The drug is slowly absorbed into the cerebrospinal fluid and is commonly used for labor and delivery.

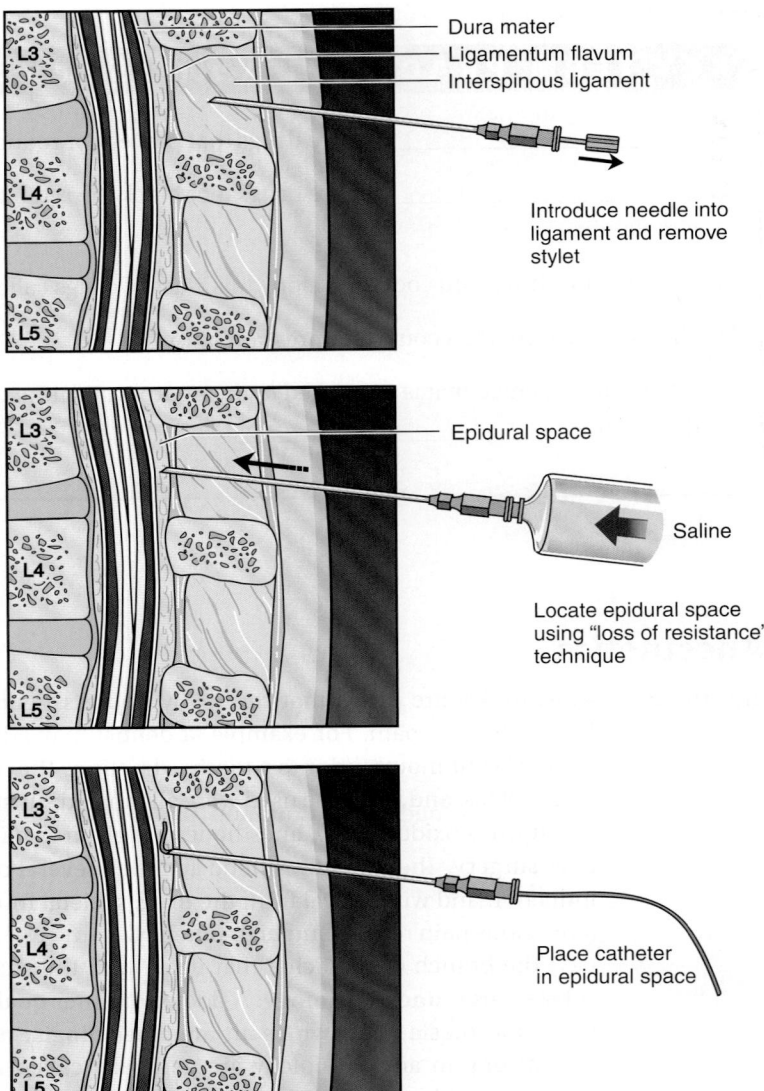

Figure 19-8 Epidural anesthesia.

Dura mater
Ligamentum flavum
Interspinous ligament

Introduce needle into ligament and remove stylet

Epidural space

Saline

Locate epidural space using "loss of resistance" technique

Place catheter in epidural space

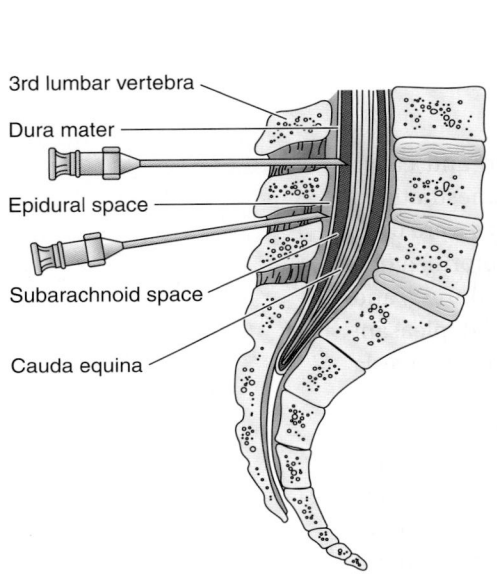

3rd lumbar vertebra
Dura mater
Epidural space
Subarachnoid space
Cauda equina

Figure 19-7 Spinal anesthesia.

KEY TERM	Definition
anesthetics (an-es-THET-icks)	drugs that reversibly depress neuronal function and cause insensitivity to pain
anesthesiology (an-es-THEEZ-ee-ol-uh-jee)	branch of medicine that deals with the study and use of anesthetic substances
anesthesiologist (an-es-theez-ee-OL-uh-jist)	physician specializing in anesthesiology who administers anesthesia
anesthetist (an-ES-the-tist)	health care professional who administers anesthetics
nurse anesthetists	nurses with specialized training in anesthesiology
general anesthetics (an-es-THET-icks)	drugs that produce loss of sensation in the whole body along with unconsciousness
anesthesia (an-es-THEEZH-uh)	complete loss of sensation

continued

continued from page 1060

KEY TERM	Definition
local anesthetics (an-es-THET-icks)	drugs that cause loss of sensation at the site of administration
spinal anesthesia	drug injection into the subarachnoid space through a spinal needle to induce anesthesia
epidural anesthesia	drug injection into the epidural space, usually the lumbar or caudal region, through a catheter to induce anesthesia

KEY TERM PRACTICE: *Anesthetics*

1. A complete loss of sensation is termed _____.

2. _____ are drugs that cause a loss of sensation at the site of administration.

3. The medical science dealing with anesthetics and anesthesia is known as _____.

4. A _____ is a nurse with specialized training in anesthesiology.

5. Drugs that reversibly depress neuronal function and cause insensitivity to pain are called _____.

Blood Drugs

Drugs used to treat blood disorders vary in what they do: Some prevent blood clotting and others dissolve already-formed clots. Common blood drug categories are anticoagulants, antiplatelet drugs, and thrombolytics.

anticoagulants   **Anticoagulants** are drugs that interfere with blood clotting by prolonging bleeding time. They are commonly called *blood thinners*. Examples of anticoagulant drugs are heparin, low-molecular-weight heparin (LMWH), and warfarin. Anticoagulants are used to prevent **thrombosis** (blood clot formation) in veins.

antiplatelet drugs   **Antiplatelet drugs** prevent the formation of blood clots by preventing platelets from sticking together. Recall from Chapter 10 that platelets are components of whole blood that function in clotting. Examples of antiplatelet drugs are aspirin and clopidogrel (Plavix). These drugs are used to prevent thrombosis in arteries.

thrombolytics   **Thrombolytics** are used to dissolve clots. They are used to treat deep vein thrombosis (DVT) and pulmonary embolism by clearing the blocked artery. Common thrombolytics are streptokinase and urokinase.

KEY TERM	Definition
anticoagulants (an-tee-koh-AG-yoo-lunts)	drugs that interfere with blood clotting by prolonging bleeding time; also called blood thinners
thrombosis (throm-BOH-sis)	blood clot formation
antiplatelet (an-tee-PLATE-let) **drugs**	prevent the formation of blood clots by preventing platelets from sticking together
thrombolytics (throm-boh-LIT-icks)	agents that dissolve blood clots

continued

continued from page 1061

KEY TERM PRACTICE: *Blood Drugs*

1. Drugs that dissolve already-formed blood clots are called _____.

2. _____, also called blood thinners, are drugs that interfere with blood clotting by prolonging bleeding time.

3. _____ prevent the formation of blood clots by preventing platelets from sticking together.

4. The term for blood clot formation is _____.

Cardiovascular System Drugs

Cardiovascular drugs treat coronary heart disease, heart failure, hypertension (high blood pressure), and arrhythmia (irregularity in the normal rhythm of heartbeat). The top 10 prescribed cardiovascular drugs are given in **Table 19-3**.

Coronary heart disease (CHD) occurs when the coronary circulation, which supplies the heart muscle itself with blood, fails. It is the most common disease of the heart and is responsible for many premature deaths. Drugs used to dilate coronary blood vessels in the treatment of CHD include nitrates, beta blockers, and calcium channel blockers. Many of these same drugs treat hypertension (high blood pressure).

nitrates   **Nitrates** are vasodilators (blood vessel relaxers). The most common nitrate is nitroglycerin. Usually administered sublingually, it is highly effective at treating angina (pain due to inadequate blood supply to the heart muscle).

beta blockers   **Beta blockers** (also called beta-adrenergic blockers) reduce the heart's oxygen demand by decreasing the heart rate. They do this by preventing

TABLE 19-3

TOP 10 PRESCRIBED CARDIOVASCULAR DRUGS

Generic	Trade Name	Use	Class
1. atorvastatin	Lipitor	Lowers cholesterol	Statin
2. amlodipine	Norvasc	Lowers blood pressure	Calcium channel blocker
3. lisinopril	Zestril	Lowers blood pressure	ACE inhibitor
4. digoxin	Lanoxin	Treats heart failure	Cardiac glycoside
5. simvastatin	Zocor	Lowers cholesterol	Statin
6. enalapril	Vasotec	Lowers blood pressure; treats heart failure	ACE inhibitor
7. warfarin sodium	Coumadin	Prevents blood clots	Anticoagulant
8. pravastatin	Pravachol	Lowers cholesterol	Statin
9. quinapril	Accupril	Lowers blood pressure; treats heart failure	ACE inhibitor
10. diltiazem	Cardizem	Lowers blood pressure; treats angina pectoris	Calcium channel blocker

sympathetic stimulation of the heart. Common beta blockers are atenolol and propranolol.

calcium channel blockers

Calcium channel blockers inhibit the movement of calcium ions through the cell membrane, causing vasodilation and relaxation of smooth muscle in the arterioles. (Calcium ions are necessary for the contraction of smooth muscle.) Common calcium channel blockers are amlodipine, diltiazem, and verapamil.

cardiac glycosides

Drugs used to treat heart failure are **inotropic agents,** which increase the force of cardiac muscle contraction. **Cardiac glycosides** are inotropic agents. Two commonly used cardiac glycosides are digitoxin and digoxin.

antihypertensive drugs

Medications used to lower blood pressure are termed **antihypertensive drugs**. The cause of 90% of hypertension cases is unknown. Common antihypertensive agents include diuretics, angiotensin-converting enzyme (ACE) inhibitors, angiotensin II receptor blockers, alpha blockers, calcium channel blockers, nitrates, and beta blockers.

- **Diuretics** increase urine output, thereby decreasing total fluid volume and blood pressure.
- **Angiotensin-converting enzyme (ACE) inhibitors** operate within the kidneys to block the synthesis of angiotensin II (AG II), which increases blood pressure. AG II cannot be synthesized because ACE inhibitors inhibit angiotensin-converting enzyme, the enzyme necessary for its synthesis. Common ACE inhibitors are lisinopril, enalapril, and quinapril.
- **Angiotensin II receptor blockers** interfere with the binding of AG II with its receptor. Blood pressure will not increase if the AG II signal is absent.
- **Alpha blockers** dilate arteries and veins to lower blood pressure.

antihyperlipidemics

Hyperlipidemia is elevated levels of lipids (fats) in the blood. It is characterized by increased levels of cholesterol and/or triglycerides that contain lipoproteins. The lipoproteins are characterized as low-density lipoprotein (LDL) and high-density lipoprotein (HDL). Patients with elevated LDLs and cholesterol levels are at increased risk for atherosclerosis, coronary heart disease, myocardial infarction, and hypertension. If the cholesterol and LDL levels cannot be decreased by diet and exercise, medication may be necessary. **Antihyperlipidemics** are lipid-lowering drugs. They act by either decreasing the production of lipoprotein carriers of cholesterol or increasing lipoprotein breakdown. **Statins** (HMG-CoA reductase inhibitors) are a group of antihyperlipidemics that lower cholesterol by inhibiting an enzyme that is essential for the production of cholesterol in the liver. Common statins are atorvastatin, simvastatin, and pravastatin.

KEY TERM	Definition
nitrates (NIGH-trates)	vasodilators (blood vessel relaxers)
beta blockers	drugs that reduce the heart's oxygen demand by decreasing the heart rate; also called beta-adrenergic blockers
calcium channel blockers	drugs that inhibit the movement of calcium ions through the cell membrane, causing vasodilation and relaxation of smooth muscle in the arterioles
inotropic (in-oh-TROP-ick) **agents**	drugs that increase the force of cardiac muscle contraction
cardiac glycosides (GLYE-koh-sides)	drugs that increase the force of cardiac muscle contraction
antihypertensive (an-tee-high-pur-TEN-siv) **drugs**	agents that lower blood pressure
diuretics (dye-yoo-RET-icks)	drugs that increase urine output
angiotensin-converting enzyme (ACE) inhibitors	drugs that lower blood pressure by blocking the synthesis of angiotensin II, which increases blood pressure
angiotensin II receptor blockers	drugs that interfere with the binding of angiotensin II with its receptor, thereby decreasing blood pressure
alpha blockers	drugs that dilate arteries and veins to lower blood pressure
hyperlipidemia (high-pur-lip-ih-DEE-mee-uh)	elevated levels of lipids (fats) in the blood
antihyperlipidemics (an-tee-high-pur-lip-ih-DEE-micks)	lipid-lowering drugs
statins (STAT-inz)	group of antihyperlipidemics that lower cholesterol by inhibiting an enzyme that is essential for the production of cholesterol in the liver; also called HMG-CoA reductase inhibitors

KEY TERM PRACTICE: *Cardiovascular System Drugs*

1. Drugs that increase the force of cardiac contraction are termed _____, derived from the word part _____, meaning *muscle fiber*.

2. _____ are a group of antihyperlipidemics that lower cholesterol by inhibiting an enzyme that is essential for the production of cholesterol in the liver.

3. Drugs that inhibit the movement of calcium ions through the cell membrane, causing vasodilation and relaxation of smooth muscle in the arterioles, are termed _____.

4. _____ is characterized by elevated levels of lipids (fats) in the blood.

5. Drugs that increase urine output are _____.

Respiratory System and Allergy Drugs

antihistamines   **Antihistamines** prevent, counteract, or diminish histamine's effects such as sneezing and itching. They block histamine, a mediator of inflammation and part of the allergic response. They also reduce acid secretion in the stomach by blocking cell receptors for histamine.

decongestants   **Decongestants** reduce or relieve nasal congestion and swelling.

bronchodilators   **Bronchodilators** dilate the bronchial tree (lung passages) and are used in aerosol sprays to treat asthma and chronic obstructive pulmonary disease (COPD).

expectorant   An agent that promotes secretion from the mucous membranes lining the air passages to be coughed up and out is termed an **expectorant**.

KEY TERM	Definition
antihistamines	drugs that block histamine to prevent allergic effects
decongestants	agents that reduce or relieve nasal congestion
bronchodilators (bronk-oh-dye-LAY-turz)	drugs that widen and relax the bronchial tree (lung passages)
expectorant (eck-SPECK-toh-runt)	a medicine that promotes mucus secretion to be coughed up and out

KEY TERM PRACTICE: *Respiratory System and Allergy Drugs*

1. _____ are drugs that block histamine.

2. A medicine that promotes mucus secretion to be coughed up and out is termed an _____.

3. _____ are agents that reduce or relieve nasal congestion.

4. Drugs that widen and relax the bronchial tree (lung passages) are known as _____.

Endocrine and Reproductive System Drugs

Drugs used to treat endocrine disorders replace hormones or impede hormonal action or secretion.

levothyroxine   A common disorder is hypothyroidism (low thyroid function.) **Levothyroxine** is a synthetic form of thyroxine (T_4) used to treat hypothyroidism.

hypoglycemic drugs   **Hypoglycemic drugs** are used to treat hyperglycemia (abnormally high levels of glucose in the blood). Most hypoglycemic drugs are called antidiabetic drugs because they are taken to treat diabetes mellitus. Diabetes mellitus is a disorder characterized by hyperglycemia, and **insulin** is the drug used to treat it (**Figure 19-9**). Insulin is a hormone secreted by the pancreas to lower blood glucose levels by facilitating

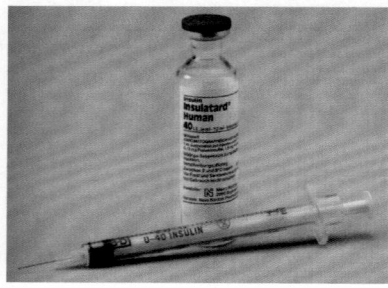

Figure 19-9 Vial of insulin with syringe.

glucose uptake in body cells. Injectable insulin has the same effect as the insulin the body produces naturally. *Oral antidiabetic drugs*, such as the sulfonylureas and biguanides, act to lower blood glucose levels.

adrenocortical hormones

Adrenocortical hormones are derived from the adrenal cortex and include glucocorticoids and mineralocorticoids. Glucocorticoids promote protein breakdown and glucose formation and have anti-inflammatory properties. Glucocorticoids are used to treat adrenal insufficiency, such as Addison disease. Mineralocorticoids are involved with sodium and water balance. They are used to treat adrenocortical deficiency.

testosterone

Testosterone is a steroid hormone that stimulates the development of secondary sexual characteristics. It is produced mainly in the male testes, but it is also produced in the ovaries (in females) and the adrenal cortex in both males and females. Synthetic testosterone is used to treat hypogonadism (decreased or absent hormone secretion in the testes) or to increase sperm production (**Figure 19-10**).

estrogen

Estrogen is a steroid hormone formed by the ovary, placenta, testes, and possibly the adrenal cortex. It stimulates the development of secondary sexual characteristics and has systemic effects. Estrogen is used therapeutically in treating menstrual disorders and problems related to menopause (**Figure 19-11**).

progesterone

Progesterone is an antiestrogenic hormone produced by the corpus luteum or placenta. It is used therapeutically to correct abnormalities of the menstrual cycles, as a contraceptive, and to maintain problematic pregnancy.

oxytocic agents

Drugs used to induce or stimulate labor are termed **oxytocic agents**. They are identical to naturally synthesized oxytocin. Oxytocic agents are also used to manage postpartum hemorrhage and to relieve painful breast engorgement (milk-filled mammary glands).

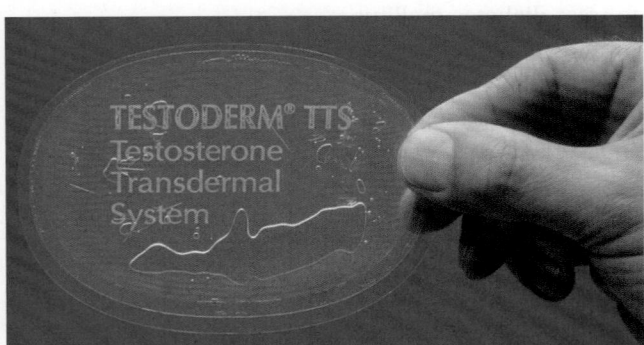

Figure 19-10 Transdermal testosterone patch.

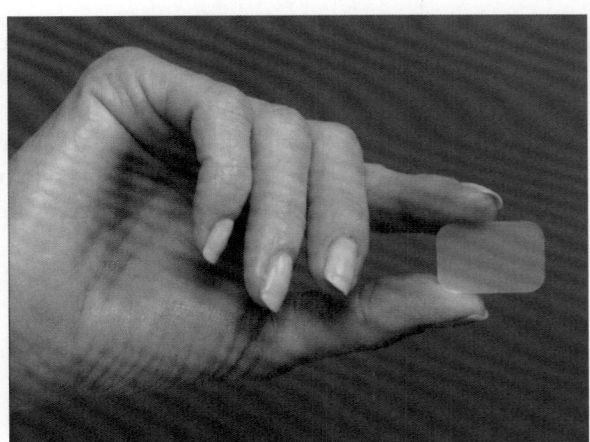

Figure 19-11 Skin patches impregnated with synthetic estrogen are an efficient means of administering hormone replacement therapy to women during and after menopause.

KEY TERM	Definition
levothyroxine (lev-oh-thigh-ROCK-seen)	synthetic form of thyroxine (T_4) used to treat hypothyroidism
hypoglycemic (high-poh-glye-SEE-mick) **drugs**	agents used to treat hyperglycemia
insulin	hormone and drug used to treat hyperglycemia
adrenocortical (a-dree-noh-KOR-ti-kul) **hormones**	glucocorticoids and mineralocorticoids from the adrenal cortex
testosterone (tes-TOS-teh-rohn)	steroid hormone that stimulates the development of secondary sexual characteristics
estrogen (es-TROH-jen)	steroid hormone formed by the ovary, placenta, testes, and possibly the adrenal cortex that stimulates the development of secondary sexual characteristics
progesterone (proh-JES-ter-ohn)	antiestrogenic hormone produced by the corpus luteum or placenta
oxytocic (ock-see-TOH-sick) **agents**	drugs used to induce or stimulate labor

KEY TERM PRACTICE: *Endocrine and Reproductive System Drugs*

1. Drugs used to induce or stimulate labor are termed _____.

2. The steroid hormone formed by the ovary, placenta, testes, and possibly the adrenal cortex that stimulates the development of secondary sexual characteristics is _____.

3. _____ is an antiestrogenic hormone produced by the corpus luteum or placenta.

4. Agents used to treat hyperglycemia are called _____.

5. The synthetic form of thyroxine (T_4) used to treat hypothyroidism is _____.

Gastrointestinal System Drugs

Drugs used for the gastrointestinal system treat ulcers, diarrhea, constipation, and vomiting. Ulcers are treated with antibiotics, antacids, H_2-receptor antagonists, proton pump inhibitors, and prostaglandins. Antibiotics are used to treat ulcers caused by bacteria. Diarrhea treatments are drugs that cause constipation, whereas constipation drugs are stimulants that increase motility and increase water and electrolytes in stools. Vomiting is treated by emetics (to induce vomiting) or antiemetics (to prevent vomiting).

antacid	An **antacid** is a drug that reduces or neutralizes hydrochloric acid (HCl) in the stomach to relieve symptoms of indigestion and reflux esophagitis (heartburn). As weak bases, the antacids combine with the HCl to neutralize it.
H$_2$ blockers	Histamine activates histamine (H_2) receptors to stimulate acid secretion. **H$_2$ blockers** reduce the secretion of gastric acid by blocking the H_2 receptors. A common H_2 blocker is cimetidine (Tagamet), which is used to treat gastroesophageal reflux disease (GERD).
proton pump inhibitors	To form hydrochloric acid, hydrogen ions (protons) are necessary. **Proton pump inhibitors** block the transport of hydrogen ions into the stomach and are thus useful in treating hyperacidity. They are used to heal stomach and duodenal ulcers and to relieve GERD symptoms.

prostaglandins	**Prostaglandins** stimulate motility in the intestinal tract. They also increase bicarbonate ion and mucus release and decrease acid secretion.
adsorbents	**Adsorbents** are antidiarrheals that act by coating the wall of the intestines and adsorbing the toxins that might be causing the diarrhea. These bulk-forming agents absorb water and soften feces.
laxatives	**Laxatives** promote bowel movement and defecation and are used to treat constipation or to evacuate the GI tract before surgery or radiographic examination. Bulk-forming laxatives include psyllium hydrophilic mucilloid (Metamucil) and methylcellulose (Citrucel), which add fiber to create bulk.
vomiting	**Vomiting** is the ejection of matter from the stomach through the esophagus and mouth. The vomiting reflex is controlled by the medulla oblongata. An **emetic** is an agent used to induce vomiting, especially in cases of poisoning. The emetic stimulates the vomiting center in the medulla oblongata. Ipecac syrup is a commonly used emetic. Agents that suppress vomiting are called **antiemetics**; their mechanism of action is not known. Antihistamines can be used as antiemetics. Drugs that prevent or alleviate nausea are termed **antinauseants**. The spice, ginger, is as effective as over-the-counter medicines for treating nausea, vomiting, morning sickness, and motion sickness.

KEY TERM	Definition
antacid	drug that reduces or neutralizes hydrochloric acid
H$_2$ blockers	drugs that reduce the secretion of gastric acid by blocking the H$_2$ receptors
proton pump inhibitors	drugs that block the transport of hydrogen ions into the stomach and are thus useful in treating hyperacidity
prostaglandins	hormones that stimulate motility in the intestinal tract, increase bicarbonate ion and mucus release, and decrease acid secretion
adsorbents	antidiarrheals that act by coating the wall of the intestines and adsorbing the toxins that might be causing the diarrhea
laxatives	drugs that relieve constipation or evacuate the bowel
vomiting	ejection of matter from the stomach through the esophagus and mouth
emetic (eh-MET-ick)	an agent that induces vomiting
antiemetics (an-tee-eh-MET-icks)	agents that prevent or relieve vomiting
antinauseants (an-tee-NAW-zee-unts)	drugs that prevent or alleviate nausea

KEY TERM PRACTICE: *Gastrointestinal System Drugs*

1. _____ are drugs that reduce or neutralize hydrochloric acid.

2. An agent that prevents vomiting is termed an _____.

3. _____ are drugs that prevent or alleviate nausea.

4. _____ are drugs that relieve constipation or evacuate the bowel.

5. Drugs that block the transport of hydrogen ions into the stomach and are thus useful in treating hyperacidity are called _____.

Immunosuppressive Drugs

| immunosuppressive drugs | **Immunosuppressive drugs** (immunosuppressants) inhibit the immune response to prevent rejection of transplanted organs or to treat autoimmune disorders. A common immunosuppressive drug is azathioprine, which is used to treat rheumatoid arthritis, polymyositis (autoimmune disease affecting the muscles), and multiple sclerosis. |

- **Cyclosporine** suppresses the body's immune system in order to prevent or inhibit tissue rejection after transplant surgery.
- A **monoclonal antibody (MAB, MoAb)** is a specific antibody produced by clone cells that reacts to a particular antigen. Monoclonal antibodies are used to prevent rejection of transplanted organs.

| corticosteroids | **Corticosteroids** are drugs used to reduce inflammation, control allergic disorders, and prevent tissue rejection. These synthetic drugs are identical to the natural corticosteroid hormones derived from the adrenal gland. |

| chrysotherapy | **Chrysotherapy** is the use of gold compounds in the treatment of disease, notably the autoimmune disease rheumatoid arthritis. |

KEY TERM	Definition
immunosuppressive (im-yoo-noh-suh-PRES-iv) **drugs**	agents that inhibit the immune response; also called immunosuppressants
cyclosporine (sigh-kloh-SPOR-een)	drug that suppresses the body's immune system in order to prevent or inhibit tissue rejection after transplant surgery
monoclonal antibody (MAB, MoAb) (mon-oh-KLOH-nul an-tuh-BOD-ee)	specific antibody produced by clone cells that reacts to a particular antigen
corticosteroids (kor-ti-koh-STEER-oidz)	drugs that are identical to hormones derived from the adrenal gland that are used to reduce inflammation, control allergic disorders, and prevent tissue rejection
chrysotherapy (kris-oh-THERR-uh-pee)	the use of gold compounds to treat disease

KEY TERM PRACTICE: *Immunosuppressive Drugs*

1. Drugs that inhibit the immune response are termed _____.

2. _____ suppresses the body's immune system in order to prevent or inhibit tissue rejection after transplant surgery.

3. The word part _____ refers to *gold*, and the use of gold compounds to treat disease is termed _____.

4. _____ are drugs that are identical to hormones derived from the adrenal gland that are used to reduce inflammation, control allergic disorders, and prevent tissue rejection.

5. _____ are specific antibodies produced by clone cells that react to a particular antigen.

LIFE SPAN

The effects of drugs vary considerably among fetuses, newborns, infants, children, adults, and older adults. Pharmacokinetics can also be quite different in a pregnant or lactating woman than in other women. Most drugs administered to a pregnant woman can cross the placenta and expose the embryo and fetus to their effects. Specific drugs are contraindicated during pregnancy due to their potential to cause birth defects. Drugs can also pass from mother to infant through breast milk. Furthermore, endocrine function during pregnancy may alter the effects of the drugs on the woman.

The first year of life marks the time in which the greatest drug variance can be found in a person. Unique factors in the newborn account for drug absorption variability. Gastric function, such as acid secretion and gastric emptying, fluctuates during the first few days of life and thus must be taken into consideration. Drug metabolism and excretion are also low in the newborn. The amount of drug remaining in the body changes as the infant develops.

The growing child presents further challenges because much of what is known about various drugs in children has been obtained through clinical experience and reporting, not by clinical tests (because of the ethical issues involved in exposing children to unknown health risks to advance science). The body of evidence is growing, and pediatric charts are available for drug dosages.

Regardless of a person's age, the mere process of growing older affects pharmacological reactions. Drug responses are affected by other medical disorders, the general health of the individual, compliance, and diet. There appears to be no age-associated decline in drug absorption. Drug distribution does change, however, as a result of reduced lean body mass and water composition and an increase in fat. Liver metabolism of drugs does not show a consistent decline to all agents.

The decline in kidney weight and hepatic blood flow in older adults ages 60 to 80 years affects drug pharmacokinetics. A high incidence of adverse drug reactions in the elderly occurs because these patients take an average of seven different prescriptions. Computer databanks are assisting in gathering critical information pertaining to drug interactions, pharmacokinetics, and pharmacodynamics throughout the life span.

COMMON Abbreviations

Abbreviation	Term
ACE inhibitors	angiotensin-converting enzyme inhibitors
ADR	adverse drug reaction
AG II	angiotensin II
AIDS	acquired immunodeficiency syndrome
ASA	acetylsalicylic acid (aspirin)
BBB	blood–brain barrier
CD	curative dose
CHD	coronary heart disease
CNS	central nervous system
COPD	chronic obstructive pulmonary disease
DEA	Drug Enforcement Agency
DVT	deep vein thrombosis
ED	effective dose

continued

continued from page 1070

Abbreviation	Term
FDA	Food and Drug Administration
FDCA	Food, Drug, and Cosmetic Act
G$^-$	gram-negative
G$^+$	gram-positive
GERD	gastroesophageal reflux disease
GI	gastrointestinal
HDL	high-density lipoprotein
HIV	human immunodeficiency virus
IM	intramuscular
IV	intravenous
LD	lethal dose
LDL	low-density lipoprotein
L-dopa	levodopa
LMWH	low-molecular-weight heparin
MAB	monoclonal antibody
MAOI	monoamine oxidase inhibitor
MoAb	monoclonal antibody
NPO	*non per os* (nothing by mouth)
NSAID	nonsteroidal anti-inflammatory drug
OTC	over-the-counter
PD	Parkinson disease
PDR	*Physicians' Desk Reference*
PM	polymyositis
POS	physician's order sheet
RPh	registered pharmacist
RSV	respiratory syncytial virus
RTI	reverse transcriptase inhibitor
Rx	prescription
SNRI	serotonin-norepinephrine reuptake inhibitor
SSRI	selective serotonin reuptake inhibitor
TCA	tricyclic antidepressant
USP	*United States Pharmacopeia*

COMMON ABBREVIATIONS EXERCISES

1. TCA is the abbreviation for _____.

2. SNRI is the abbreviation for _____.

3. The abbreviation for gastroesophageal reflux disease is _____.

4. The abbreviation for angiotensin-converting enzyme is _____.

5. USP stands for _____.

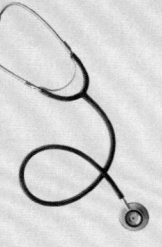

Case Study

Karen was working on a specific case with Dr. Wien, a rheumatologist, to best manage pharmacological treatment for a patient. Wendell Jensen, a 35-year-old woman, was diagnosed with polymyositis (PM) and mixed connective tissue disease. Raynaud phenomenon initially led her to seek medical care when she began noticing that her fingertips were dark and her hands were frequently cold. She has difficulty walking up stairs and raising her arms. Mrs. Jensen made an appointment because she was feeling extremely weak and tired and thought perhaps she had a respiratory infection. Mrs. Jensen currently takes medicines on a daily basis. Her pharmaceutical agents are as follows:

- methotrexate, 2.5 mg every day
- prednisone, 5 mg every other day
- diltiazem (Cardizem), 30 mg every day
- cimetidine (Tagamet), 400 mg bid
- azathioprine (Imuran), 50 mg every day

Case Study Questions

Select the best answer to each of the following questions.

1. **Polymyositis is an autoimmune disorder. Methotrexate, prednisone, and azathioprine are immunosuppressants. Immunosuppressants are best described as drugs that**
   _____.
   a. inhibit the immune response
   b. enhance the immune response
   c. alter cardiovascular function
   d. enhance tissue rejection

2. **Cardizem is classified as a calcium channel blocker. Calcium channel blockers**
   _____.
   a. are drugs that widen the arteries to slow the heart and treat heart conditions
   b. are diuretics
   c. are ACE inhibitors
   d. increase urinary output

3. **Cimetidine is used in the treatment of gastrointestinal conditions. This particular drug is an H_2 blocker, which**
   _____.
   a. increases histamine-induced acid release
   b. has no effect on acid
   c. blocks histamine-induced acid release
   d. treats diarrhea

4. **Cardizem, Imuran, and Tagamet are**
   _____.
   a. chemical names
   b. brand or trade names
   c. generic names
   d. formularies

5. **Cimetidine is prescribed at 400 mg bid. This means that Mrs. Jensen should take 400 mg**
   _____.
   a. once a day
   b. twice a day
   c. every other day
   d. every day

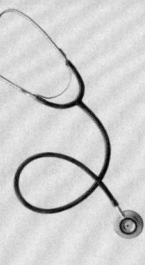

Real World Report

In the hospital, a physician's order sheet (POS), or chart order, is used. As an attending pharmacist, Karen relies on this document, which contains much of the same information as an outpatient prescription, but the duration of therapy or number of doses is often not listed. The POS contains the following information: patient's name, date of birth, name and strength of medication, dose, route and frequency of administration, date, time ordered, initials, and the physician's signature. Mrs. Jensen's report, which was received in the hospital pharmacy, follows:

CENTRAL HOSPITAL: PHYSICIAN'S ORDER SHEET

NAME: Wendell Jensen
DATE OF BIRTH: August 3, 1976
DATE: December 28, 2011

Time/Initials	Med, IV, Treatment	Dose	Route
1 1400/SKR	methotrexate	5 mg every day	oral
2 1400/SKR	prednisone	5 mg every other day	oral
3 1630/AMW	ampicillin	250 mg IV q6h 7 days	IV
4 1700/JBN	diltiazem (Cardizem)	30 mg every day	oral
5 1700/JBN	esomeprazole magnesium (Nexium)	40 mg qam	oral
6 1700/JBN	folic acid	1 mg every day pc	oral

Physician Signature:
Dr. Wien

Real World Report Questions

The following exercises review the medical terms used in the preceding medical report.

1. How often was each of the following drugs administered?

   a. drug 5 _____

   b. drug 6 _____

   c. drug 3 _____

2. Ampicillin was one of the prescribed drugs.

   a. How was it administered? _____

   b. How long was the drug to be given? _____

3. What are the trade names for the following drugs?

   a. drug 4 _____

   b. drug 5 _____

4. Identify the meaning of pc with respect to drug 6. _____

Review and Application

Multiple-Choice Questions

Select the best answer to each of the following questions.

1. The science and study of drugs is called _____.
   a. toxicology
   b. pharmacy
   c. apothecary
   d. pharmacology

2. The study of a drug's mechanism of action in the body is termed _____.
   a. pharmacodynamics
   b. pharmacology
   c. pharmacognosy
   d. toxicology

3. A natural or artificial substance other than food used to treat or prevent illness is a/an _____.
   a. drug
   b. toxin
   c. loading dose
   d. agonist

4. A _____ is a prescription medication or illegal drug.
   a. compliance
   b. controlled substance
   c. maintenance dose
   d. formulary

5. _____ is the ability of a drug to produce a desired result.
   a. Loading dose
   b. Lethal dose
   c. Efficacy
   d. Bioavailability

6. Which term means the amount of drug absorbed and obtainable for use at the target tissue? _____
   a. first-pass effect
   b. bioavailability
   c. antagonist
   d. therapeutic index

7. Drug metabolism in the liver is known as _____.
   a. first-pass effect
   b. first-pass metabolism
   c. bioavailability
   d. a and b

8. A _____ is a treatment plan for improving health.
   a. regimen
   b. compliance
   c. schedule
   d. formulary

9. A response to a drug that causes harm is termed a/an _____.
   a. adverse drug reaction
   b. standard
   c. formulary
   d. addiction

10. A reference book of medicinal preparations is known as a/an _____.
    a. palliative
    b. apothecary
    c. formulary
    d. regimen

11. The _____ is the national formulary of the United States.
    a. Drug Enforcement Agency (DEA)
    b. *U.S. Pharmacopeia (USP)*
    c. Food, Drug, and Cosmetic Act (FDCA)
    d. *Physicians' Desk Reference (PDR)*

12. Willingness to conform to treatment is termed _____.
    a. anesthetic
    b. diuretic
    c. agonist
    d. compliance

13. _____ are agents that directly affect bacteria.
    a. Antivirals
    b. Antibiotics
    c. Immunosuppressants
    d. Antifungals

14. Drugs effective against *Mycobacterium* species are termed _____.
    a. antivirals
    b. antihelminthics
    c. antimycobacterials
    d. antifungals

15. _____ is a drug that hinders bacterial growth, and a/an _____ destroys bacteria.
    a. Bactericidal; bacteriostatic
    b. Antibiotic; bacteriostatic
    c. Antimicrobial; antibiotic
    d. Bacteriostatic; bactericidal

16. Which class of drugs improves heart muscle contraction? _____

    a. cardiac glycosides   b. antihypertensives   c. calcium channel blockers   d. diuretics

17. While taking an antibiotic for a urinary tract infection, a patient comes down with a secondary respiratory infection. This is an example of a _____.

    a. superinfection   b. Gram stain   c. bactericide   d. contraindication

Word Parts Exercises

Using the following word parts, form a medical term for each definition. Each word part is used only once.

-cutaneous	-muscular
-dermal	pharmaco-
intra-	sub-
-lingual	sub-
-logy	trans-

18. study of drugs _____

19. across the skin _____

20. beneath the tongue _____

21. within the muscle _____

22. beneath the skin _____

Matching Exercises

Match the definition with its correct term.

_____ 23. effective dose

_____ 24. curative dose

_____ 25. lethal dose

_____ 26. loading dose

_____ 27. maintenance dose

a. amount of drug required to cure a disease or correct a deficiency
b. amount of drug that will produce the desired effects
c. amount of drug needed to maintain protection against exacerbation
d. amount of drug that will likely cause death
e. single, large dose of drug given at the onset of therapy

Match the definition or action with its drug type

_____ 28. inotropic

_____ 29. antihypertensive

_____ 30. diuretic

_____ 31. nitrate

_____ 32. antihyperlipidemic

a. drug that lowers blood pressure
b. drug that increases the force of cardiac contraction
c. drug that lowers lipid blood levels
d. vasodilator
e. drug that increases urine output

Match the term with its definition

_____ 33. contraindication

_____ 34. expectorant

_____ 35. pharmacist

_____ 36. dispensing

_____ 37. bronchodilator

a. one who practices pharmacy
b. preparing and distributing medicines
c. symptom or condition for which a treatment is inadvisable
d. drug that widens the respiratory passages
e. medicine that promotes mucus secretion to be coughed out

Match the definition with its correct term

_____ 38. enteral

_____ 39. cytotoxic drug

_____ 40. emetic

_____ 41. antipyretic

_____ 42. cyclosporine

a. drug that inhibits organ transplant rejection
b. agent that induces vomiting
c. agent that kills cells
d. drug route by way of the gastrointestinal tract
e. fever-reducing drug

Match the drug classification with its pharmacological agents.

_____ 43. blood drugs

_____ 44. cardiovascular drugs

_____ 45. lipid-lowering drugs

_____ 46. cancer drugs

_____ 47. endocrine system drugs

a. glucocorticoids, progesterone, estrogens
b. antiplatelet drugs, thrombolytics, anticoagulants
c. glycosides, diuretics, vasodilators, ACE inhibitors
d. lovastatin, atorvastatin, Zocor
e. cytotoxic agents

Match the pharmacological agent with its drug classification.

_____ 48. allergy and respiratory drugs

_____ 49. GI drugs

_____ 50. NSAIDs and analgesics

_____ 51. immunosuppressive drugs

_____ 52. reproductive drugs

a. aspirin, acetaminophen, ibuprofen
b. estrogen, testosterone, progesterone
c. cyclosporine, monoclonal antibodies
d. acid inhibitors, H_2 blockers
e. H_2 blockers, antihistamines

Definition

Define the following terms.

53. pharmacologist _____

54. pharmacotherapy _____

55. placebo _____

Provide a medical term for the following definitions

56. strength; dose required to bring about drug's maximum effect _____

57. science of the nature and effects of poisons, their detection, and treatments _____

58. drug that prevents the development of a disease _____

59. readiness to conform to a treatment _____

60. general term for a person who administers anesthetics _____

Alternate Terms

Give an alternate term for each of the following terms.

61. chemotherapy _____

62. blood thinners _____

63. first-pass effect _____

64. maintenance drug therapy _____

Spelling

Identify the correctly spelled term in each set.

65. _____	66. _____	67. _____	68. _____	69. _____
a. iatrogeneic	a. palliative	a. pharmicopeia	a. anesthetecs	a. analgesic
b. iatrogenic	b. paliative	b. pharmacopeea	b. anasthetics	b. anelgesic
c. itrogenic	c. pallative	c. pharmacopeia	c. enesthetics	c. analgesick
d. iatragenic	d. pallitive	d. pharmakopia	d. anesthetics	d. anallgesic

Unscramble

Unscramble the letters to form a medical term.

70. ticnoddai _____

71. exitvaal _____

72. senthazitee _____

73. acceffiy _____

74. aaoocghlmpry _____

Abbreviations

Provide the term for the abbreviations and then define the terms.

75. NPO = _____

76. NSAIDs = _____

77. ACE inhibitors = _____

78. bid = _____

79. p.c. = _____

Analogies

Provide a medical term to complete a meaningful analogy.

80. First-pass effect is to _____ as pharmaceutics are to _____.

81. Motrin is to _____ as _____ is to acetaminophen.

Short Answer

Answer the following questions.

82. A patient seeks medical attention for the common cold, which is caused by a virus. The physician prescribes the antibiotic amoxicillin. Is this an appropriate therapy? Explain. _____
_____

83. A friend has been taking spironolactone, a diuretic, for a period of 2 weeks and notices that she has been urinating more frequently than usual. Is this a normal or an abnormal response? Explain. _____
_____

84. Using common abbreviations for chart orders, write a prescription indicating 500 milligrams of aspirin to be used every 5 hours as needed. _____

Word Search

Find the medical terms hidden in the puzzle.

```
G  Q  S  N  K  Q  F  D  Y  E  Q  T  I  O  B
N  V  K  W  M  N  I  V  V  C  O  B  P  I  S
I  A  D  D  I  C  T  I  O  N  U  I  O  R  C
T  K  G  C  A  A  T  O  F  P  U  A  Y  E  I
I  L  S  T  U  A  H  H  R  M  V  D  R  G  T
M  O  N  H  I  T  J  O  X  A  O  S  M  I  Y
O  A  U  L  Q  K  F  D  I  R  V  O  K  M  L
V  L  L  X  E  E  X  L  E  F  L  R  Y  E  O
J  A  D  P  N  N  A  F  W  Z  F  B  B  N  B
P  K  E  M  A  B  I  I  I  U  C  E  L  H  M
C  O  D  E  I  N  E  H  V  F  P  N  L  Y  O
J  V  Y  L  X  I  M  O  P  S  H  T  X  Q  R
N  O  I  T  C  E  F  N  I  R  E  P  U  S  H
R  T  F  Z  F  Y  U  L  N  A  O  L  U  U  T
Y  S  C  I  T  O  C  R  A  N  V  M  T  E  Y
```

addiction
adsorbent
antacid
bioavailability
codeine
ibuprofen
morphine
narcotics
opium
palliative
regimen
superinfection
thrombolytics
vomiting

Vocabulary Review

Review the key terms from this chapter, study the spelling and pronunciation of each term, and write its definition in the space provided. Listen to the audio available for most terms at http://thepoint.lww.com/nath2e and pronounce each term for yourself. Then check the box when you feel confident that you know the definition and can pronounce the term correctly.

Key Term	Pronunciation	Definition
❏ **acetaminophen**	(as-et-uh-MIH-noh-fen)	_____
❏ **addiction**		_____
❏ **adrenocortical hormones**	(a-dree-noh-KOR-ti-kul)	_____
❏ **adsorbents**		_____
❏ **adverse drug reaction (ADR)**		_____
❏ **alpha-blockers**		_____
❏ **analgesic**	(an-al-JEE-zick)	_____
❏ **anesthesia**	(an-es-THEEZH-uh)	_____
❏ **anesthesiologist**	(an-es-theez-ee-OL-uh-jist)	_____
❏ **anesthesiology**	(an-es-THEEZ-ee-ol-uh-jee)	_____
❏ **anesthetics**	(an-es-THET-icks)	_____

Key Term	Pronunciation	Definition
❏ anesthetist	(an-ES-the-tist)	_____
❏ angiotensin-converting enzyme (ACE) inhibitors		_____
❏ angiotensin II receptor blockers		_____
❏ antacid		_____
❏ antibiotics	(an-tee-bye-OT-icks)	_____
❏ anticoagulants	(an-tee-koh-AG-yoo-lunts)	_____
❏ anticonvulsants	(an-tee-kun-VUL-sunts)	_____
❏ antidepressants	(an-tee-de-PRES-unts)	_____
❏ antidiarrheal	(an-tee-dye-uh-REE-ul)	_____
❏ antiemetics	(an-tee-eh-MET-icks)	_____
❏ antifungal	(an-tee-FUNG-gul) drugs	_____
❏ antihelminthic	(an-tee-hel-MIN-thick) drugs	_____
❏ antihistamines		_____
❏ antihyperlipidemics	(an-tee-high-pur-lip-ih-DEE-micks)	_____
❏ antihypertensive drugs	(an-tee-high-pur-TEN-siv)	_____
❏ antimicrobial agents	(an-tee-migh-KROH-bee-ul)	_____
❏ antimycobacterial drugs	(an-tee-migh-koh-back-TEER-ee-ul)	_____
❏ antinauseants	(an-tee-NAW-zee-unts)	_____
❏ antiplatelet drugs	(an-tee-PLATE-let)	_____
❏ antiprotozoal drugs	(an-tee-proh-tuh-ZOH-ul)	_____
❏ antipyretic	(an-tee-pye-RET-ick)	_____
❏ antiseptic	(an-tih-SEP-tick)	_____
❏ antitussive	(an-tee-TUS-iv)	_____
❏ antiviral drugs	(an-tee-VYE-rul)	_____
❏ aspirin		_____
❏ astringent	(uh-STRIN-jent)	_____
❏ bactericidal	(back-teer-ih-SIGH-dul)	_____
❏ bacteriostatic	(back-teer-oh-STAT-ick)	_____
❏ barbiturates	(bar-BICH-ur-ates)	_____
❏ benzodiazepines	(ben-zoh-dye-AZ-uh-peenz)	_____
❏ beta-blockers		_____
❏ bioavailability	(bye-oh-uh-vale-uh-BIL-ih-tee)	_____
❏ broad-spectrum antibiotics	(an-tee-bye-OT-icks)	_____
❏ bronchodilators	(bronk-oh-dye-LAY-turz)	_____
❏ buccal route	(BUCK-ul)	_____

Key Term	Pronunciation	Definition
❏ calcium channel blockers		_____
❏ cardiac glycosides	(GLYE-koh-sides)	_____
❏ chrysotherapy	(kris-oh-THERR-uh -pee)	_____
❏ codeine	(KOH-deen)	_____
❏ compliance		_____
❏ contraindication	(kon-truh-in-dih-KAY-shun)	_____
❏ controlled substance		_____
❏ corticosteroids	(kor-ti-koh-STEER-oidz)	_____
❏ curative dose (CD)	(KYUR-uh-tiv)	_____
❏ cyclosporine	(sigh-kloh-SPOR-een)	_____
❏ cytotoxic drugs	(sigh-toh-TOCK-sick)	_____
❏ decongestants		_____
❏ diuretics	(dye-yoo-RET-icks)	_____
❏ effective dose (ED)		_____
❏ efficacy	(EF-ih-kuh-see)	_____
❏ emetic	(eh-MET-ick)	_____
❏ enteral	(EN-tur-ul)	_____
❏ epidural anesthesia		_____
❏ estrogen	(es-TROH-jen)	_____
❏ expectorant	(eck-SPECK-toh-runt)	_____
❏ first-pass metabolism		_____
❏ formulary	(FOR-mew-lerr-ee)	_____
❏ general anesthetics	(an-es-THET-icks)	_____
❏ H_2 blockers		_____
❏ hyperlipidemia	(high-pur-lip-ih-DEE-mee-uh)	_____
❏ hypoglycemic drugs	(high-poh-glye-SEE-mick)	_____
❏ iatrogenic	(eye-at-roh-JEN-ick)	_____
❏ ibuprofen	(eye-byoo-PROH-fen)	_____
❏ immunosuppressive drugs	(im-yoo-noh-suh-PRES-iv)	_____
❏ inhalation route		_____
❏ inotropic agents	(in-oh-TROP-ick)	_____
❏ insulin		_____
❏ intradermal route	(in-truh-DUR-mul)	_____
❏ intramuscular route	(in-truh-MUS-kew-lur)	_____
❏ intravenous (IV) route		_____
❏ laxatives		_____
❏ lethal dose (LD)		_____
❏ levodopa (L-dopa)	(lee-voh-DOH-puh)	_____

Key Term	Pronunciation	Definition
❏ levothyroxine	(lev-oh-thigh-ROCK-seen)	_____
❏ loading dose		_____
❏ local anesthetics	(an-es-THET-icks)	_____
❏ maintenance dose		_____
❏ monoamine oxidase inhibitors (MAOIs)	(mon-oh-AM-een OCK-sih-dace)	_____
❏ monoclonal antibody (MAB, MoAb)	(mon-oh-KLOH-nul an-tuh-BOD-ee)	_____
❏ morphine		_____
❏ naproxen	(nuh-PROCKS-en)	_____
❏ narcotics		_____
❏ nasal route		_____
❏ nasogastric route		_____
❏ neuraminidase inhibitors	(nur-uh-MIN-ih-daze)	_____
❏ nitrates	(NIGH-trates)	_____
❏ nonsteroidal anti-inflammatory drugs (NSAIDs)	(non-sterr-OID-ul)	_____
❏ nurse anesthetists		_____
❏ opiates		_____
❏ opium		_____
❏ ophthalmic route	(off-THAL-mick)	_____
❏ oral route		_____
❏ otic route	(OH-tick)	_____
❏ oxytocic agents	(ock-see-TOH-sick)	_____
❏ palliative	(PAL-ee-uh-tiv)	_____
❏ parenteral	(puh-REN-tur-ul)	_____
❏ percutaneous administration	(pur-kew-TAY-nee-us)	_____
❏ pharmaceuticals	(far-muh-SUE-ti-kulz)	_____
❏ pharmaceutics	(far-muh-SUE-ticks)	_____
❏ pharmacist	(FAR-muh-sist)	_____
❏ pharmacodynamics	(far-muh-koh-dye-NAM-icks)	_____
❏ pharmacokinetics	(far-muh-koh-ki-NET-icks)	_____
❏ pharmacologist	(far-muh-KOL-uh-jist)	_____
❏ pharmacology	(far-muh-KOL-uh-jee)	_____
❏ pharmacotherapy	(far-muh-koh-THERR-uh-pee)	_____
❏ pharmacy	(FAR-muh-see)	_____
❏ placebo	(pluh-SEE-boh)	_____
❏ potency	(POH-tun-see)	_____
❏ potentiation	(poh-ten-shee-AY-shun)	_____

Key Term	Pronunciation	Definition
❑ prescription (Rx)		_____
❑ progesterone	(proh-JES-ter-ohn)	_____
❑ prophylactic	(proh-fih-LACK-tick)	_____
❑ prostaglandins		_____
❑ protease inhibitors	(PROH-tee-ace)	_____
❑ proton pump inhibitors		_____
❑ psychotropic drugs	(sigh-koh-TROP-ick)	_____
❑ rectal route	(RECK-tul)	_____
❑ regimen	(REJ-i-mun)	_____
❑ reverse transcriptase inhibitors (RTIs)	(tran-SKRIP-tace)	_____
❑ selective serotonin reuptake inhibitors (SSRIs)	(serr-oh-TOH-nin)	_____
❑ serotonin-norepinephrine reuptake inhibitors (SNRIs)		_____
❑ side effect		_____
❑ spinal anesthesia		_____
❑ statins	(STAT-inz)	_____
❑ subcutaneous route	(sub-kew-TAY-nee-us)	_____
❑ sublingual route	(sub-LING-gwul)	_____
❑ superinfection		_____
❑ testosterone	(tes-TOS-teh-rohn)	_____
❑ thrombolytics	(throm-boh-LIT-icks)	_____
❑ thrombosis	(throm-BOH-sis)	_____
❑ toxicology	(tock-si-KOL-uh-jee)	_____
❑ transdermal route	(trans-DUR-mul)	_____
❑ tricyclic antidepressants (TCAs)	(try-SICK-lick an-tee-de-PRES-unts)	_____
❑ vaginal route	(VAJ-i-nul)	_____
❑ vomiting		_____
❑ Z-tract injection		_____

Answers

Word Grouping Exercises

Definition	Word Part	Definition	Word Part
bacteri-, bacterio-	bacteria	place, topical, local	top-, topo-
drugs	pharmaco-	poison, toxin	tox-, toxi-, toxico-, toxo-
gold	chrys-, chryso-	rectum	rect-, recto-
muscle fiber	ino-	sensation, perception	esthesio-
pain	alge-, algesi-	substance that keeps something from changing, flowing, or moving	-stat
physicians, medicine, treatment	iatro-	substance that kills	-cide

Word Building Exercises

Word Part	Meaning	Common or Known Word	Example Medical Term
chrys-, chryso-	gold	chrysanthemum	chrysotherapy
alge-, algesi-	pain	analgesic	analgesia
bacteri-, bacterio-	bacteria	bacteria	bactericide
-cide	substance that kills	suicide	fungicide
esthesio-	sensation, perception	anesthesia	anesthesia
pharmaco-	drugs	pharmacy	pharmacology
rect-, recto-	rectum	rectum	rectal
-stat	substance that keeps something from changing, flowing, or moving	electrostatic	bacteriostatic
top-, topo-	place, topical, local	topical	topical
tox-, toxi-, toxico-, toxo-	poison, toxin	toxic	toxicology

Key Term Practice

Pharmacology Preview

1. prescription (Rx)
2. *pharmaco-*; study of; pharmacology
3. pharmaceuticals; pharmaceutics
4. pharmacy
5. Toxicology; *toxico-*

Basic Pharmacology Terms

1. lethal dose (LD)
2. Pharmacokinetics
3. Pharmacodynamics
4. efficacy
5. first-pass metabolism

Drug Reactions, Regulations, and References

1. Potentiation
2. palliative
3. iatrogenic; *iatro-*
4. addiction
5. formulary

Routes of Administration

1. otic route
2. intravenous (IV) route
3. transdermal route
4. Z-tract injection
5. sublingual route

Antimicrobial Drugs

1. antimicrobial agents
2. broad-spectrum antibiotics
3. astringent
4. bactericidal; bacteri-; -cide
5. Antibiotics

Antiviral Drugs

1. antiviral drugs
2. Neuraminidase inhibitors
3. protease inhibitors
4. reverse transcriptase inhibitors (RTIs)

Antifungal, Antiprotozoal, and Antihelminthic Drugs

1. Antifungal drugs
2. antiprotozoal drugs
3. Antihelminthic drugs

Cancer Drugs

1. cell, poison; cytotoxic

Nonsteroidal Anti-Inflammatory Drugs

1. aspirin
2. aspirin, acetaminophen, ibuprofen, and naproxen
3. antipyretic
4. nonsteroidal anti-inflammatory drugs (NSAIDs)
5. Acetaminophen

Nervous System Drugs

1. Anticonvulsants
2. Selective serotonin reuptake inhibitors (SSRIs)
3. narcotics
4. antitussive
5. levodopa (L-dopa)

Anesthetics

1. anesthesia
2. Local anesthetics
3. anesthesiology
4. nurse anesthetist
5. anesthetics

Blood Drugs

1. thrombolytics
2. Anticoagulants
3. Antiplatelet drugs
4. thrombosis

Cardiovascular System Drugs

1. inotropic agents; *ino-*
2. Statins
3. calcium channel blockers
4. Hyperlipidemia
5. diuretics

Respiratory System and Allergy Drugs

1. Antihistamines
2. expectorant
3. Decongestants
4. bronchodilators

Endocrine and Reproductive System Drugs

1. oxytocic agents
2. estrogen
3. Progesterone
4. hypoglycemic drugs
5. levothyroxine

Gastrointestinal System Drugs

1. Antacids
2. antiemetic
3. Antinauseants
4. Laxatives
5. proton pump inhibitors

Immunosuppressive Drugs

1. immunosuppressive drugs
2. Cyclosporine
3. *chryso-*; chrysotherapy
4. Corticosteroids
5. Monoclonal antibodies (MAB, MoAb)

Common Abbreviations Exercises

1. TCA = tricyclic antidepressant
2. SNRI = serotonin-norepinephrine reuptake inhibitor
3. gastroesophageal reflux disease = GERD
4. angiotensin-converting enzyme = ACE
5. USP = *United States Pharmacopeia*

Case Study

1. a is the correct answer.
   - b is incorrect because immunosuppressants do not enhance the immune system.
   - c is incorrect because immunosuppressants do not alter cardiac function.
   - d is incorrect because immunosuppressants do not enhance tissue rejection.
2. a is the correct answer.
   - b is incorrect because diuretics are not calcium channel blockers, although they are used in the treatment of some heart conditions.
   - c is incorrect because ACE inhibitors are not calcium channel blockers, although they are used in the treatment of some heart conditions.
   - d is incorrect because calcium channel blockers are not used to increase urinary output.
3. c is the correct answer.
   - a is incorrect because H_2 blockers reduce acid release.
   - b is incorrect because H_2 blockers reduce acid release.
   - d is incorrect because cimetidine is used to treat upper GI conditions, and diarrhea treatments target the lower GI tract, not the upper GI tract.
4. b is the correct answer.
   - a is incorrect because chemical names would indicate the drugs' chemical makeup.
   - c is incorrect because the generic names for these drugs are diltiazem, azathioprine, and cimetidine.
   - d is incorrect because formularies are reference books containing lists of pharmaceutical products with their descriptions and prescribing information.
5. b is the correct answer.
   - a, c, and d are incorrect by definition.

Real World Report

1. a. every morning; b. every day; c. every 6 h
2. a. intravenously (IV); b. every 6 h for 7 days
3. a. Cardizem; b. Nexium
4. after meals

Review and Application

1. d	6. b	11. b	16. a
2. a	7. d	12. d	17. a
3. a	8. a	13. b	18. pharmacology
4. b	9. a	14. c	19. transdermal
5. c	10. c	15. d	20. sublingual

21. intramuscular
22. subcutaneous
23. b
24. a
25. d
26. e
27. c
28. b
29. a
30. e
31. d
32. c
33. c
34. e
35. a
36. b
37. d
38. d
39. c
40. b
41. e
42. a
43. b
44. c
45. d
46. e
47. a
48. e
49. d
50. a
51. c
52. b

53. pharmacologist = person who studies pharmacology
54. pharmacotherapy = treatment of disease by drugs
55. placebo = substance with no medicinal ingredients, yet the person may derive therapeutic effects
56. potency
57. toxicology
58. prophylactic
59. compliance
60. anesthetist
61. pharmacotherapy
62. anticoagulants
63. first-pass metabolism
64. maintenance dose
65. b
66. a
67. c
68. d
69. a
70. addiction
71. laxative
72. anesthetize
73. efficacy
74. pharmacology
75. NPO = nothing by mouth, *non per os*; the patient is not to ingest any food or drink

76. NSAIDs = nonsteroidal anti-inflammatory drugs; large number of drugs with analgesic and anti-inflammatory actions
77. ACE inhibitors = angiotensin-converting enzyme inhibitors; drugs that lower blood pressure by blocking the synthesis of angiotensin II (AG II), which increases blood pressure
78. bid = twice per day, *bis in die*; the medication is to be taken twice per day
79. p.c. = after meals, *post cibum*; the medication is to be taken after meals
80. first-pass metabolism; pharmaceuticals
81. ibuprofen; Tylenol
82. This is an inappropriate prescription therapy because amoxicillin is an antibiotic and is effective only against bacterial infections. The physician should either prescribe an antiviral medication or nothing at all if the symptoms began more than 30 h earlier.
83. Spironolactone is a diuretic, which is an agent that causes increased urinary output. Thus, this is a normal response.
84. ASA 500 mg q5h prn

Word Search

```
G  Q  S  N  K  Q  F  D  Y  E  Q  T  I  O  B
N  V  K  W  M  N  I  V  V  C  O  B  P  I  S
I  A  D  D  I  C  T  I  O  N  U  I  O  R  C
T  K  G  C  A  A  T  O  F  P  U  A  Y  E  I
I  L  S  T  U  A  H  H  R  M  V  D  R  G  T
M  O  N  H  I  T  J  O  X  A  O  S  M  I  Y
O  A  U  L  Q  K  F  D  I  R  V  O  K  M  L
V  L  L  X  E  E  X  L  E  F  L  R  Y  E  O
J  A  D  P  N  N  A  F  W  Z  F  B  B  N  B
P  K  E  M  A  B  I  I  I  U  C  E  L  H  M
C  O  D  E  I  N  E  H  V  F  P  N  L  Y  O
J  V  Y  L  X  I  M  O  P  S  H  T  X  Q  R
N  O  I  T  C  E  F  N  I  R  E  P  U  S  H
R  T  F  Z  F  Y  U  L  N  A  O  L  U  U  T
Y  S  C  I  T  O  C  R  A  N  V  M  T  E  Y
```

addiction
adsorbent
antacid
bioavailability
codeine
ibuprofen
morphine
narcotics
opium
palliative
regimen
superinfection
thrombolytics
vomiting

Vocabulary Review

Key Term	Definition	Key Term	Definition
acetaminophen	drug that relieves pain and reduces fever; type of NSAID	anesthetist	health care professional who administers anesthetics
addiction	state of physiological or psychological dependence on a drug	angiotensin-converting enzyme (ACE) inhibitors	drugs that lower blood pressure by blocking the synthesis of angiotensin II, which increases blood pressure
adrenocortical hormones	glucocorticoids and mineralocorticoids from the adrenal cortex		
adsorbents	antidiarrheals that act by coating the wall of the intestines and adsorbing the toxins that might be causing the diarrhea	angiotensin II receptor blockers	drugs that interfere with the binding of angiotensin II with its receptor, thereby decreasing blood pressure
adverse drug reaction (ADR)	any response to a drug that causes harm when the drug is given at its normal dosage and usage	antacid	drug that reduces or neutralizes hydrochloric acid
alpha blockers	drugs that dilate arteries and veins to lower blood pressure	antibiotics	drugs that kill or inhibit the growth of bacteria
analgesic	pain reliever	anticoagulants	drugs that interfere with blood clotting by prolonging bleeding time; also called blood thinners
anesthesia	complete loss of sensation		
anesthesiologist	physician specializing in anesthesiology who administers anesthesia	anticonvulsants	drugs that prevent or reduce the severity of convulsive seizures
anesthesiology	branch of medicine that deals with the study and use of anesthetic substances	antidepressants	drugs used to treat depression
		antidiarrheal	drug that treats diarrhea
anesthetics	drugs that reversibly depress neuronal function and cause insensitivity to pain	antiemetics	agents that prevent or relieve vomiting
		antifungal drugs	agents that suppress or destroy fungi

Key Term	Definition
antihelminthic drugs	agents that target parasitic worms called helminths
antihistamines	drugs that block histamine to prevent allergic effects
antihyperlipidemics	lipid-lowering drugs
antihypertensive drugs	agents that lower blood pressure
antimicrobial agents	drugs that destroy microbes, prevent their multiplication or growth, or prevent their pathogenic action
antimycobacterial drugs	an agent effective against *Mycobacterium* species
antinauseants	drugs that prevent or alleviate nausea
antiplatelet drugs	prevent the formation of blood clots by preventing platelets from sticking together
antiprotozoal drugs	agents that are effective against protozoa infections
antipyretic	agent that reduces fever
antiseptic	topical agent that prevents infection by inhibiting the growth of infectious agents
antitussive	cough suppressant
antiviral drugs	agents that act against viruses
aspirin	widely used analgesic, antipyretic, anti-inflammatory, and antiplatelet agent; also called acetylsalicylic acid (ASA); type of NSAID
astringent	topical agent that shrinks tissues
bactericidal	drug that destroys bacteria
bacteriostatic	drug that hinders or arrests bacterial growth
barbiturates	central nervous system depressants
benzodiazepines	drugs with antianxiety, hypnotic, anticonvulsant, and skeletal muscle relaxant properties
beta blockers	drugs that reduce the heart's oxygen demand by decreasing the heart rate; also called beta-adrenergic blockers
bioavailability	degree to which a drug becomes available to target tissues after administration
broad-spectrum antibiotics	agents that are effective against both G^+ and G^- bacteria
bronchodilators	drugs that widen and relax the bronchial tree (lung passages)
buccal route	administering a drug between the gum and cheek
calcium channel blockers	drugs that inhibit the movement of calcium ions through the cell membrane, causing vasodilation and relaxation of smooth muscle in the arterioles
cardiac glycosides	drugs that increase the force of cardiac muscle contraction

Key Term	Definition
chrysotherapy	the use of gold compounds to treat disease
codeine	drug that acts as an analgesic, antitussive, and antidiarrheal
compliance	willingness to conform to treatment and/or a prescribed regimen
contraindication	any special symptom or circumstance that makes a particular treatment inadvisable
controlled substance	prescription medication or illegal drug
corticosteroids	drugs that are identical to hormones derived from the adrenal gland that are used to reduce inflammation, control allergic disorders, and prevent tissue rejection
curative dose (CD)	amount of drug required to cure disease or correct a deficiency
cyclosporine	drug that suppresses the body's immune system in order to prevent tissue rejection after transplant surgery
cytotoxic drugs	agents that kill cells
decongestants	agents that reduce or relieve nasal congestion
diuretics	drugs that increase urine output
effective dose (ED)	dose required to produce desired effects
efficacy	ability of a drug to produce a desired result
emetic	an agent that induces vomiting
enteral	drug route by way of the gastrointestinal tract
epidural anesthesia	drug injection into the epidural space, usually the lumbar or caudal region, through a catheter to induce anesthesia
estrogen	steroid hormone formed by the ovary, placenta, testes, and possibly the adrenal cortex that stimulates the development of secondary sexual characteristics
expectorant	a medicine that promotes mucus secretion to be coughed up and out
first-pass metabolism	breakdown of a drug in the liver before reaching the general circulation; also called the first-pass effect
formulary	detailed collection of formulas for medicines
general anesthetics	drugs that produce loss of sensation in the whole body along with unconsciousness
H_2 blockers	drugs that reduce the secretion of gastric acid by blocking the H_2 receptors
hyperlipidemia	elevated levels of lipids (fats) in the blood

Key Term	Definition	Key Term	Definition
hypoglycemic drugs	agents used to treat hyperglycemia	**nasal route**	dropping or spraying medications into the nose
iatrogenic	inadvertent, adverse response brought on unintentionally by the drug, treatment, or health care provider	**nasogastric route**	drug delivery through the nasal passages and into the stomach
ibuprofen	analgesic and anti-inflammatory agent; type of NSAID	**neuraminidase inhibitors**	agents that block the release of influenza virus from infected cells
immunosuppressive drugs	agents that inhibit the immune response; also called immunosuppressants	**nitrates**	vasodilators (blood vessel relaxers)
inhalation route	drug is inhaled and delivered directly to respiratory tissues	**nonsteroidal anti-inflammatory drugs (NSAIDs)**	large number of drugs with analgesic and anti-inflammatory actions
inotropic agents	drugs that increase the force of cardiac muscle contraction	**nurse anesthetists**	nurses with specialized training in anesthesiology
insulin	hormone and drug used to treat hyperglycemia	**opiates**	drugs that act on specific CNS receptors to reduce pain perception
intradermal route	administering a drug within the dermis	**opium**	brownish, gummy extract from the unripe seed pods of the opium poppy that contains highly addictive substances such as morphine and codeine
intramuscular route	administering a drug within a muscle		
intravenous (IV) route	administering a drug directly into a vein	**ophthalmic route**	administering drops or ointments directly into the eye
laxatives	drugs that relieve constipation or evacuate the bowel	**oral route**	administering a drug by mouth
		otic route	administering drops directly into the ear canal
lethal dose (LD)	amount of drug that will likely cause death	**oxytocic agents**	drugs used to induce or stimulate labor
levodopa (L-dopa)	natural substance that is converted to the neurotransmitter dopamine in the brain after crossing the blood–brain barrier (BBB); it is used to treat Parkinson disease	**palliative**	drug that relieves or soothes symptoms but does not cure a disorder
		parenteral administration	introduction of a drug outside the intestines, by intramuscular, subcutaneous, intravenous, or intradermal injection
levothyroxine	synthetic form of thyroxine (T_4) used to treat hypothyroidism	**percutaneous administration**	passage of drugs through unbroken skin
loading dose	single, large dose of a drug initially given to achieve the desired therapeutic level quicker than repeated small doses would	**pharmaceuticals**	medicinal drugs; also called pharmaceutics
		pharmaceutics	medicinal drugs; also called pharmaceuticals
local anesthetics	drugs that cause loss of sensation at the site of administration	**pharmacist**	person trained and licensed to dispense medicinal drugs and advise on their use
maintenance dose	the systemic dosage of medication required to maintain protection against exacerbation; also called maintenance drug therapy	**pharmacodynamics**	the study of a drug's mechanism of action in the body
		pharmacokinetics	pertains to the drug's absorption, distribution, metabolism, and elimination by the body
monoamine oxidase inhibitors (MAOIs)	drugs that increase the levels of norepinephrine and serotonin by inhibiting monoamine oxidase, the enzyme that breaks down these neurotransmitters	**pharmacologist**	person who studies pharmacology
		pharmacology	the science and study of drugs
monoclonal antibody (MAB, MoAb)	specific antibody produced by clone cells that reacts to a particular antigen	**pharmacotherapy**	use of drugs to treat disease; also called chemotherapy
		pharmacy	practice of preparing and dispensing drugs; it is also a drugstore
morphine	narcotic analgesic		
naproxen	anti-inflammatory commonly used to treat headaches and arthritis; type of NSAID	**placebo**	substance with no medicinal ingredients, yet the person may derive therapeutic effects
narcotics	drugs that dull the senses	**potency**	pharmacological strength of a drug measured by the amount needed to produce a certain effect

Key Term	Definition
potentiation	interaction between two or more drugs given together is greater than the sum of each acting separately
prescription (Rx)	written order by a medical practitioner that authorizes a patient to be provided medicine, treatment, or a medical device
progesterone	antiestrogenic hormone produced by the corpus luteum or placenta
prophylactic	drug that prevents the development of a disease
prostaglandins	hormones that stimulate motility in the intestinal tract, increase bicarbonate ion and mucus release, and decrease acid secretion
protease inhibitors	agents that block the enzyme protease to eradicate viruses that use it for replication
proton pump inhibitors	drugs that block the transport of hydrogen ions into the stomach and are thus useful in treating hyperacidity
psychotropic drugs	agents that can alter mental function, behavior, or experience and are used to treat psychiatric disorders
rectal route	administering a drug through the rectum
regimen	treatment plan directed at improving health
reverse transcriptase inhibitors (RTIs)	agents that block the enzyme reverse transcriptase to eradicate viruses that use it for replication
selective serotonin reuptake inhibitors (SSRIs)	drugs that block the reuptake of serotonin, causing increased levels to remain in circulation
serotonin-norepinephrine reuptake inhibitors (SNRIs)	drugs that treat major depression and other mood disorders by inhibiting the reuptake of serotonin and norepinephrine at the presynaptic neuron, causing increased levels to remain in circulation

Key Term	Definition
side effect	secondary, typically undesirable effect of a drug that is an expanded application of the drug's normal actions
spinal anesthesia	drug injection into the subarachnoid space through a spinal needle to induce anesthesia
statins	group of antihyperlipidemics that lower cholesterol by inhibiting an enzyme that is essential for the production of cholesterol in the liver; also called HMG-CoA reductase inhibitors
subcutaneous route	administering a drug beneath the epidermis and dermis into subcutaneous tissue using a hypodermic needle
sublingual route	administering a drug beneath the tongue
superinfection	a new infection in addition to one already present
testosterone	steroid hormone that stimulates the development of secondary sexual characteristics
thrombolytics	agents that dissolve blood clots
thrombosis	blood clot formation
toxicology	study of poisons, including their source, chemical composition, action on the body, and antidotes
transdermal route	administering a drug through unbroken skin by an adhesive patch
tricyclic antidepressants (TCAs)	drugs used to treat depression by blocking the reuptake of norepinephrine and serotonin, causing increased levels to remain in circulation
vaginal route	administering a drug into the vagina using a medicated suppository
vomiting	ejection of matter from the stomach through the esophagus and mouth
Z-tract injection	intramuscular technique in which the skin and subcutaneous tissue are displaced laterally before inserting the needle

CHAPTER 20

Oncology

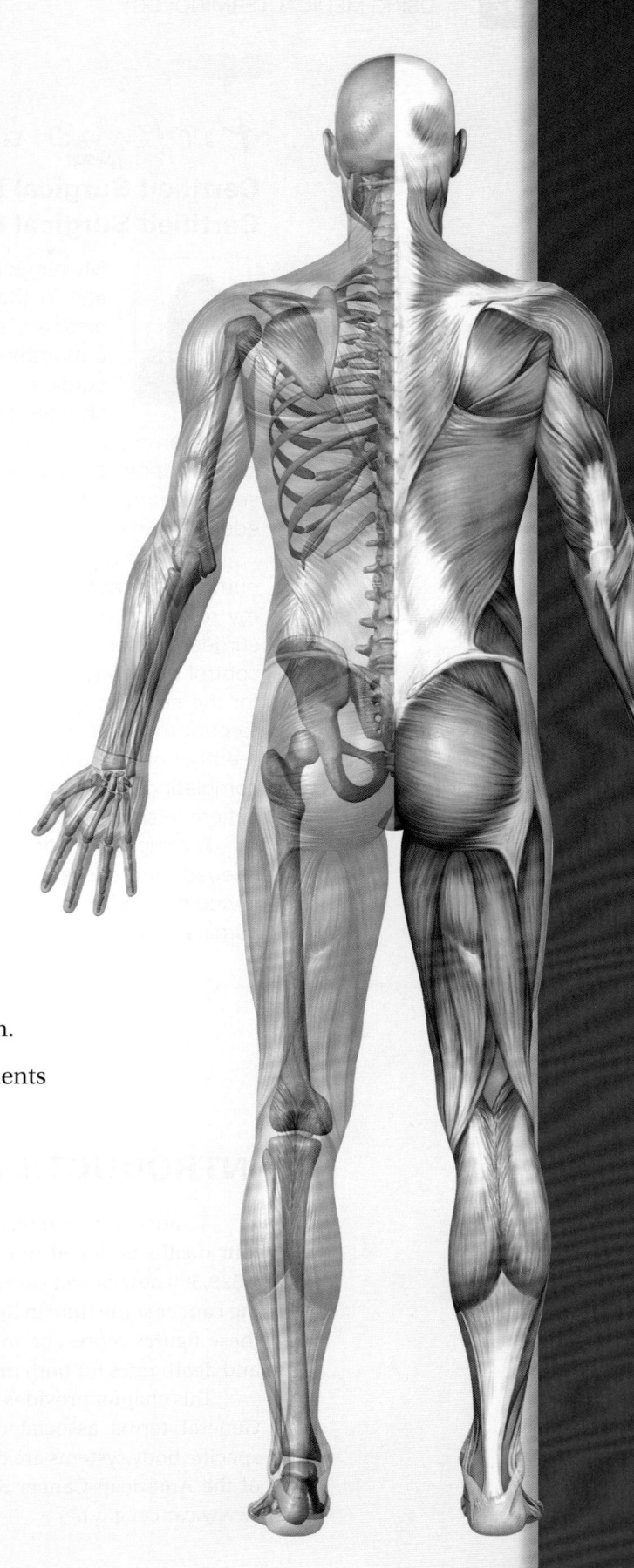

OBJECTIVES

After completing this chapter, you should be able to:

1. Define the meanings of word parts related to oncology.

2. List risk factors and causes of cancer.

3. Define terms associated with grading and staging of tumors.

4. Associate cancer types with their respective body system.

5. Become familiar with diagnostic procedures and treatments associated with cancer.

6. Identify key aspects of aging and cancer prevalence.

7. Define common abbreviations related to oncology.

8. Define terms used in medical reports involving cancer.

9. Correctly define, spell, and pronounce the chapter's medical terms.

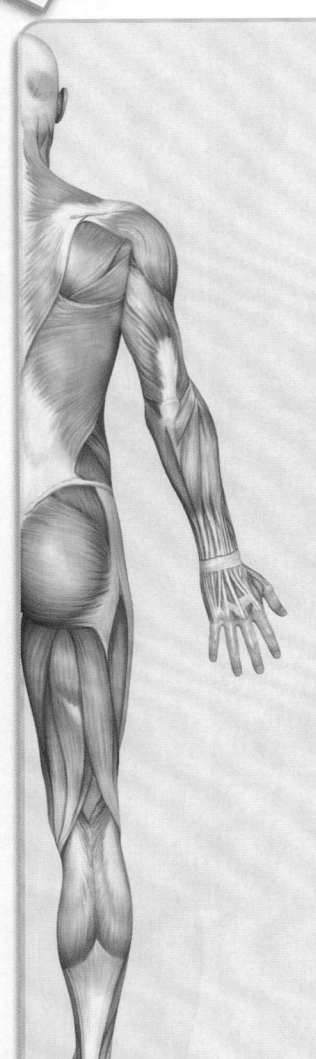

Professional Profile

Certified Surgical Technologist/ Certified Surgical First Assistant

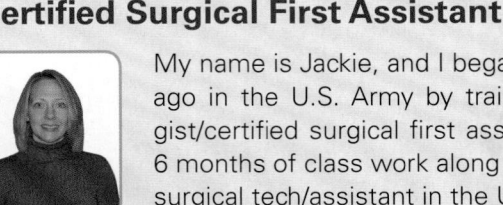

My name is Jackie, and I began my health care career almost 20 years ago in the U.S. Army by training to be a certified surgical technologist/certified surgical first assistant. My formal education began with 6 months of class work along with 8 months of on-the-job training as a surgical tech/assistant in the U.S. military, where I trained to be part of an Airborne Forward Surgical Team. After serving 5 years in the military and receiving an honorable discharge, I sat for the certification exam to practice as a civilian. Upon completion of my service, I continued my career in surgery and began to specialize more in general and vascular surgery. This led to the decision to further my education with an additional 4 years of training to become a registered nurse.

Many of our surgical cases are patients with cancer, and I have lost track of the number of lumpectomies and mastectomies we've done. While in the operating room, my role is to assist with surgical procedures under the supervision of the primary surgeon. As an integral member of the surgical team, I concentrate on aiding in the control of blood flow to prevent hemorrhage, providing exposure of the surgical site for the surgeon to better perform his job, and following the direction of the surgeon to perform additional technical functions critical to patient care. It is imperative as a member of this team to work in sync with the surgeon, anticipating his next move, and completing the surgical procedure as quickly and effectively as possible to decrease patient infection, complication, mortality, and morbidity rates.

A basic knowledge of medical terminology has provided me the solid foundation needed for a successful career in the field of surgery. Without this basic knowledge, it would be difficult for me to contribute successfully as a supportive member of the surgical team.

INTRODUCTION

*C*ancer is a leading public health issue worldwide. In the United States, one out of every four deaths is linked to cancer. The American Cancer Society estimated a total number of 1,529,560 new cancer cases in 2010 leading to 569,490 deaths. The chance of a woman developing cancer some time in her life is one in three. For men it is one in two. The good news is that these figures represent an overall decrease in both the incidence (frequency of occurrence) and death rates for both men and women during the past 16 years.

This chapter provides an overview of the field of cancer study formally known as *oncology*. General terms associated with cancer will be presented, and cancers associated with specific body systems are discussed. Further information can be found by visiting the websites of the American Cancer Society (www.cancer.org) and the National Cancer Institute (NCI) (www.cancer.gov).

MEDICAL TERM PARTS

Word Parts

Medical term prefixes, suffixes, and combining forms related to oncology are introduced in this section.

Word Part	Meaning
ana-	not
aden-, adeno-	gland
angi-, angio-	blood vessel
apo-	separated from or derived from
-atus	to change
carcin-, carcino-	cancer
chem-, chemo-	chemistry
chondro-	cartilage
cry-, cryo-	cold
cyt-, cyto-	cell
dys-	bad, difficult
-ectomy	removal of an anatomical structure
electro-	electricity
-emia	blood
fibr-, fibro-	fiber
-gen	precursor of
hyper-	excessive, above normal
hyster-, hystero-	uterus
leio-	smooth
leuk-, leuko-	white
lip-, lipo-	fatty
-logy	study of
lymph-, lympho-	lymph, colorless fluid
mast-, masto-	breast
melan-, melano-	black
mes-, meso-	middle, mesentery
meta-	change of position
myo-	muscle
myx-, myxo-	mucus
neo-	new, recent
neur-, neuri-, neuro-	nerve, nervous system
-oma	tumor or neoplasm
onco-	tumor
ost-, oste-, osteo-	bone
path-, -pathic, patho-, -pathy	disease
-plasia	formation
rhabd-, rhabdo-	rod, rod shaped
sarco-	muscle, flesh
tox-, toxi-, toxico-, toxo-	poison, toxin

Word Grouping Exercises

Using the *Medical Term Parts* table, identify the prefix, suffix, or combining form for each of the following definitions. The first one has been done as an example.

Definition	Word Part
new, recent	*neo-*
bad, difficult	
black	
blood	
blood vessel	
bone	
breast	
cancer	
cartilage	
cell	
change of position	
chemistry	
cold	
disease	
electricity	
excessive, above normal	
fatty	
fiber	
formation	
gland	
lymph	
middle, mesentery	
mucus	
muscle	
muscle, flesh	
nerve, nervous system	
new, recent	
not	
poison, toxin	
precursor of	
removal of an anatomical structure	
rod, rod shaped	
separated from or derived from	
smooth	
study of	
to change	
tumor	
tumor or neoplasm	
uterus	
white	

Word Building Exercises

Word parts introduced in the *Medical Term Parts* section are listed in the following table. For this exercise, first supply the meaning of each word part, then use the word part to build a word you already know. The word you list under *Common or Known Word* does not have to be a medical term; a commonly used word is fine. Be sure, however, that the word correctly reflects the intended meaning. The first one has been done as an example. Check your answers in a dictionary.

Word Part	Meaning	Common or Known Word	Example Medical Term
-emia	*blood*	*anemia*	leukemia
angi-, angio-			angiogenesis
carcin-, carcino-			carcinoma
chem-, chemo-			chemotherapy
cry-, cryo-			cryotherapy
-ectomy			hysterectomy
electro-			electrodessication
hyper-			hyperplasia
hyster-, hystero-			hysterectomy
leuk-, leuko-			leukemia
lip-, lipo-			lipoma
-logy			oncology
melan-, melano-			melanoma
neo-			neoplasm
onco-			oncogenes
tox-, toxi-, toxico-, toxo-			toxicology

ANATOMY AND PHYSIOLOGY

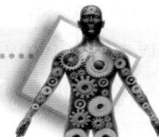

Cancer Preview

Cancer (CA) is a disease that results from uncontrolled division of abnormal body cells forming abnormal tissue called **neoplasms** or **tumors**. Neoplasms invade surrounding tissues, and spread or **metastasize,** by blood or lymph to new sites.

KEY TERM	Definition
cancer (KAN-ser) **(CA)**	disease resulting from uncontrolled division of abnormal body cells producing malignant tumors
neoplasms (NEE-oh-plaz-umz)	abnormal tissue formed from uncontrolled cellular division; also called tumors
tumors (TOO-merz)	abnormal tissue formed from uncontrolled cellular division; also called neoplasms
metastasize (meh-TAS-tuh-size)	to spread to other sites

KEY TERM PRACTICE: *Cancer Preview*

1. _____ means that the tumor has spread to other sites.

2. Abnormal tissue formed from uncontrolled cellular division is termed _____ or _____.

3. _____ is a disease resulting from uncontrolled division of abnormal body cells producing malignant tumors.

Causes of Cancer and Cancer Risk Factors

There are approximately 200 different types of cancer. Although a few forms are inherited, most are considered to be multifactorial. That is, many factors play a role in cancer development. **Carcinogens** are cancer-causing substances, such as tobacco or ultraviolet radiation. When studying cancer, we often discuss cases in terms of risk factors, morbidity, and mortality. It appears as if most cancers occur when several risk factors interact. A **risk factor** is something that increases the chance of developing a disease. Risk factors for cancer include age, genes, the immune system, viruses, bacteria, and the environment.

Statistics are reported using morbidity and mortality data. **Morbidity** is the presence of disease or illness. **Mortality** refers to the number of deaths. **Five-year survival rate** is the phrase used for estimating the prognosis of cancer. It describes the percentage of patients who are alive 5 years after their disease is diagnosed. The Surveillance, Epidemiology, and End Results (SEER) database calculates the 5-year survival rates. SEER is a resource maintained by the National Cancer Institute.

The American Cancer Society has listed seven warning signs and symptoms of cancer. The acronym for these is **CAUTION**. Although the list is not definitive, if an individual experiences a sign or symptom on the list, a health care professional should evaluate the person.

- **C**hange in bowel or bladder habits
- **A** sore that does not heal
- **U**nusual bleeding or discharge
- **T**hickening or lump in the breast, testicles, or elsewhere
- **I**ndigestion or difficulty swallowing
- **O**bvious change in the size, color, shape, or thickness of a wart, mole, or mouth sore
- **N**agging cough or hoarseness

In terms of genetic factors, **oncogenes** are genes that in certain circumstances can transform a normal cell into an abnormal tumor cell. This change in the chemistry of a gene is termed **mutation**. When a tumor invades the surrounding tissue it is said to be **malignant**. Tumors that are nonthreatening to survival or that are noncancerous are termed **benign**. Many times, abnormal cells undergo a programmed cell death known as **apoptosis**, but oncogenes have the ability to prevent apoptosis, allowing cancer cells to survive and reproduce. This rapid reproduction of cells is called **proliferation**.

The branch of medicine dealing with cancer is known as **oncology**. Physicians who specialize in the diagnosis and treatment of cancer are known as **oncologists**. There are several subspecialties within oncology, such as gynecological oncology, interventional oncology, medical oncology, pediatric oncology, radiation oncology, and surgical oncology.

KEY TERM	Definition
carcinogens (kar-SIN-oh-jinz)	cancer-causing substances
risk factors	variables associated with an increased chance of developing a disease
morbidity (mor-BID-i-tee)	a diseased state
mortality (mor-TA-lih-tee)	the number of deaths
five-year survival rate	the percentage of people who are alive 5 years after their initial cancer diagnosis
oncogenes (ON-koh-jeenz)	genes that can cause a cell to become malignant
mutation (myoo-TAY-shun)	structural change in a gene
malignant (muh-LIG-nunt)	tumor that invades surrounding tissue and may spread to other body parts; cancerous
benign (beh-NINE)	nonmalignant; noncancerous
apoptosis (a-pop-TOH-sis)	programmed cell death
proliferation (proh-lih-fuh-RAY-shun)	growth and rapid reproduction of similar cells
oncology (on-KOL-oh-jee)	branch of medicine that deals with the study and treatment of cancer
oncologists (on-KOL-oh-jists)	physicians specializing in cancer diagnosis and treatment

KEY TERM PRACTICE: *Causes of Cancer and Cancer Risk Factors*

1. When a tumor invades normal tissue it is termed _____.

2. A _____ is a cancer-causing substance.

3. Tumors that are noncancerous are termed _____.

4. _____ are genes that can cause a cell to become malignant.

5. _____ is the term for programmed cell death.

Staging and Grading of Neoplasms

Neoplasms are identified and described using staging and grading. Identifying the progression of cancer is known as **staging**. **Grading (G)** refers to determining the degree of a tumor's malignancy or tissue differentiation. It is done by determining the size and shape of the nucleus in the tumor cells and the percentage of tumor cells that are dividing. The grading system is used to classify cancer cells in terms of how abnormal they look and how dangerous they may be.

Body cells begin as **stem cells**, which are cells capable of giving rise to more cells of the same type. From these cells, other cells arise by **differentiation**, that is, the process of cells becoming different or distinct during their growth or development. Differentiated cells have a different character or function from the original cell line. Cell differentiation is one characteristic clinicians use in evaluating cancerous cells.

TNM staging			
T — primary tumor			
TX	primary tumor cannot be judged		
T0	no basis for primary tumor		
Tis	carcinoma/tumor in situ		
T1, T2, T3, T4 increasing sizes and/or extent of primary tumor invasion			
N — regional lymph nodes			
NX	regional lymph nodes cannot be judged		
N0	no regional lymph node metastases		
N1, N2, N3 increasing invasion of regional lymph nodes			
M — metastasis			
MX	existence of metastases cannot be judged		
M0	no metastases		
M1	metastases present		
	the category M1 can be subdivided as follows:		
	lung	PUL	marrow	MAR
	bone	OSS	rib	PLE
	liver	HEP	peritoneum	PER
	brain	BRA	skin	SKI
	lymph nodes	LYM	other organs	OTH
G — histopathologic differentiation grade (grading)			
GX	differentiation grade cannot be determined		
G1	well-differentiated		
G2	moderately differentiated		
G3	poorly differentiated		
G4	undifferentiated		

Figure 20-1 TNM staging.

To enable effective communication among clinicians worldwide, a standardized system of staging and grading has been developed. This staging standard is known as **TNM staging** (**Figure 20-1**). The system name is derived from **T** for **t**umor size and invasion, **N** for lymph **n**ode involvement, and **M** for **m**etastasis. To provide an example, a tumor classified T2N2M0 G1 has a better prognosis than a tumor classified as T3N3M1 G3.

Terms used to describe structural differentiation include anaplasia and hyperplasia (see below). **Anaplasia** refers to no differentiation, and a cancer that is poorly differentiated is called anaplastic. **Dedifferentiation** is a common synonym for anaplasia. Most malignant neoplasms are anaplastic, and when the cells infiltrate or destroy surrounding tissue the tumor is said to be **invasive**.

KEY TERM	Definition
staging	identifying the progression of cancer
grading (G)	determining the degree of tumor malignancy
stem cells	an undifferentiated cell from which specialized cells develop
differentiation (dih-fur-en-shee-AY-shun)	acquiring characteristics or functions different from that of the original cell
TNM staging	classification based on characteristics of the **t**umors, **n**odal involvement, and extent of **m**etastatic spread
anaplasia (an-uh-PLAY-zee-uh)	reversion of cells within a tumor to a simpler or less differentiated form; also called dedifferentiation
dedifferentiation (dee-dih-fur-en-shee-AY-shun)	reversion of cells within a tumor to a simpler or less differentiated form; also called anaplasia
invasive (in-VAY-siv)	growing aggressively, so as to infiltrate or destroy surrounding tissue

continued

continued from page 1098

KEY TERM PRACTICE: *Staging and Grading of Neoplasms*

1. The term that refers to no differentiation is _____; it is also called _____.

2. Identifying the progression of cancer is called _____.

3. Determining the degree of a tumor's malignancy is _____.

4. Specialized cells come from undifferentiated cells known as _____.

5. _____ is a classification system based on characteristics of tumors and includes nodal involvement and extent of metastatic spread.

Tissue Changes

Four types of tissue make up the human body: epithelial, connective, muscle, and nervous. All organs are composed of these tissue types, and cancers can be categorized by tissue type. **Pathologists**, physicians skilled in identifying the nature, origin, progress, and cause of disease, typically determine from which type of tissue a particular cancer is derived. They do this by studying tissue obtained from a living person in a procedure called a **biopsy**. In addition to determining anaplasia and differentiation, as previously discussed, pathologists examine the tissue for other characteristics.

For example, a pathologist might discover hyperplasia. **Hyperplasia** describes an increase in the number of normal cells, but hyperplastic tissue is not necessarily cancerous. Or, the tissue might exhibit **metaplasia**, the transformation of one kind of tissue into another undesirable type. Abnormal tissue development is termed **dysplasia**. Metaplasia and dysplasia are characteristic of tumor formation. A tumor composed of two or more kinds of tissue is termed a **mixed tumor** (**Figure 20-2**).

Epithelial tissue, also called the **epithelium**, is the avascular tissue that covers all free body surfaces (such as skin), lines body cavities and blood vessels, and forms glands. Common tumors associated with epithelial tissues are given in **Table 20-1**.

Connective tissue supports, binds, or separates other tissues and has cells embedded in an unstructured matrix, often with collagen or other fibers. It includes cartilage, adipose (fat), bone, and blood. Tumors associated with connective tissues are given in **Table 20-2**.

Muscle tissue is specialized for contraction. There are three types of muscle tissue: skeletal, smooth, and cardiac. Skeletal muscle attaches to bones and allows for movement. Smooth

---

TABLE 20-1   **EPITHELIAL TISSUE TUMORS**

Epithelial Tissue Tumor	Description
adenocarcinoma	cancer of glandular epithelium
angiosarcoma	cancer of blood vessel endothelial cells
carcinoma	any cancer of epithelial cell origin
mesothelioma	cancer of mesothelia cells, which line serous cavities (peritoneum, pleura, and pericardium)

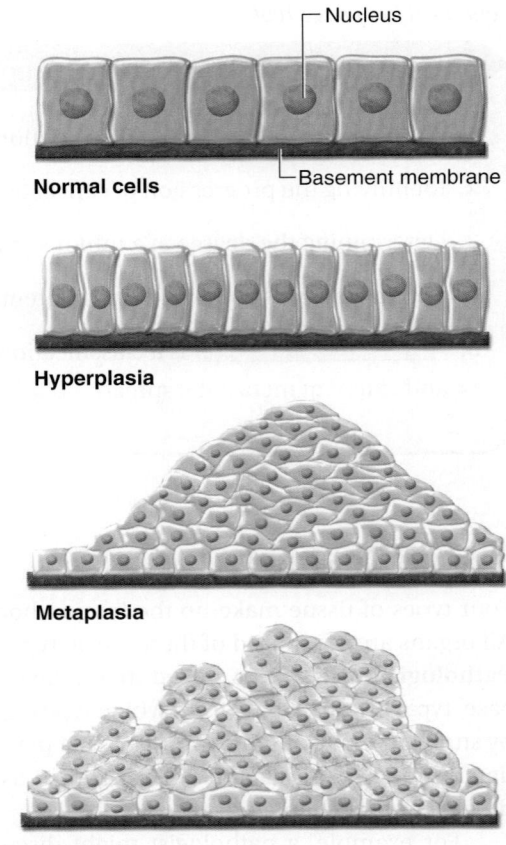

Nucleus

Normal cells — Basement membrane

Hyperplasia

Metaplasia

Dysplasia

Figure 20-2 Cellular changes. This figure compares normal cell growth with hyperplasia, metaplasia, and dysplasia.

muscle lines the walls of blood vessels and hollow organs. Cardiac muscle tissue is found only in the heart. Tumors associated with muscle tissues are given in **Table 20-3**.

Nervous tissue, also called *neural tissue*, is specialized for conducting electrical impulses. Two types of cells are found in neural tissue: neurons and neuroglia. **Neurons** transmit nerve impulses and are the basic functional units of the nervous system. The network of supporting tissue and fibers that nourish nerve cells in the brain and spinal cord consists of **neuroglia** or **glial cells**. **Table 20-4** lists tumors associated with neural tissue.

TABLE 20-2

CONNECTIVE TISSUE TUMORS

Connective Tissue Tumor	Description
chondroma	benign tumor of cartilage
chondrosarcoma	malignant tumor of cartilage
fibroma	benign tumor of fibrocartilage
leukemia	cancer of leukocytes (white blood cells)
lipoma	benign tumor of fatty tissue
liposarcoma	cancer of adipose tissue
lymphoma	malignant tumor of lymphatic tissue
myxoma	benign connective tissue tumor
osteoma	benign tumor of bone tissue
osteosarcoma	malignant bone tumor

T A B L E 20-3

MUSCLE TISSUE TUMORS

Muscle Tissue Tumor	Description
cardiac sarcoma	cancer of the heart
leiomyoma	benign tumor of smooth muscle tissue
leiomyosarcoma	cancer of smooth muscle tissue
myosarcoma	cancer of skeletal muscle tissue

KEY TERM	Definition
pathologists (puh-thol-OH-jists)	physicians skilled in identifying the nature, origin, progress, and cause of disease
biopsy (BYE-op-see)	process of removing tissue for diagnostic examination
hyperplasia (high-pur-PLAY-zee-uh)	abnormal growth (not necessarily cancerous) caused by excessive multiplication of cells
metaplasia (met-uh-PLAY-zhuh)	abnormal transformation from one tissue type into another tissue type
dysplasia (dis-PLAY-zhuh)	abnormal tissue development
mixed tumor	tumor made up of two or more types of tissue
epithelial tissue (ep-ih-THEE-lee-ul TISH-yoo)	tissue that forms a thin protective layer on exposed body surfaces and lines body cavities and blood vessels and forms glands; also called epithelium
epithelium (ep-ih-THEE-lee-um)	tissue that forms a thin protective layer on exposed body surfaces and lines body cavities and blood vessels and forms glands; also called epithelial tissue
connective tissue	supporting and binding tissue that has cells embedded in an unstructured matrix
muscle tissue	tissue that is specialized for contraction and includes skeletal muscle, smooth muscle, and cardiac muscle
nervous tissue	tissue that is specialized for conducting electrical impulses; also called neural tissue
neurons (NOOR-onz)	functional nerve cells of the nervous system that transmit nerve impulses
neuroglia (noor-OH-glee-uh)	supporting cells with metabolic functions found in the nervous system; also called glial cells
glial cells (GLEE-ul SELLS)	supporting cells with metabolic functions found in the nervous system; also called neuroglia

KEY TERM PRACTICE: *Tissue Changes*

1. The process of surgically obtaining a piece of tissue to be diagnostically examined is called a _____.

2. _____ are physicians who identify the nature, origin, progress, and cause of disease.

3. The abnormal transformation of one tissue into another tissue type is termed _____.

4. A tumor that is made up of two or more tissue types is a _____.

5. Abnormal tissue development is called _____.

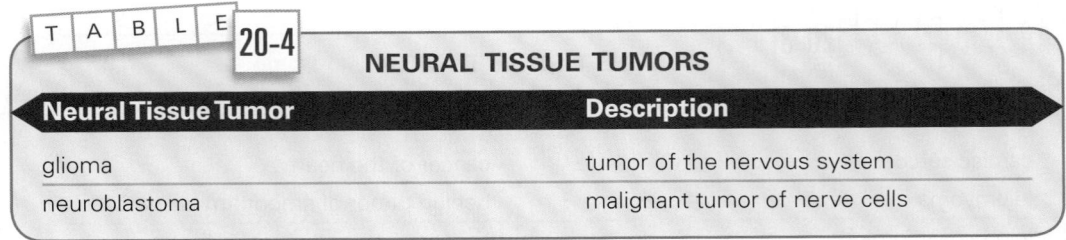

Neural Tissue Tumor	Description
glioma	tumor of the nervous system
neuroblastoma	malignant tumor of nerve cells

TABLE 20-4 NEURAL TISSUE TUMORS

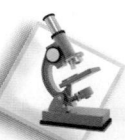

THE CLINICAL DIMENSION

Integumentary System Cancers

The integumentary system includes the skin, hair, nails, sweat glands, and oil glands. We will focus on the skin and skin cancer, the most common type of cancer. The National Cancer Institute estimated that in 2010 there were more than 1,000,000 new cases of skin cancer but fewer than 1,000 would die as a result of the disease. To read about other skin cancers not covered in this section, refer to Chapter 4, Integumentary System.

Repeated exposure to ultraviolet radiation is the greatest risk factor for developing skin cancer. The best prevention is to protect yourself from the sun by wearing long sleeves, avoiding midday sun exposure, using sunscreen lotions with a sun protection factor (SPF) of 15 or better, and avoiding tanning booths.

Most skin cancers can be detected by using the **ABCDEs of skin cancer**, a method used to examine moles, freckles, and skin spots by checking the **A**symmetry, **B**order, **C**olor, **D**iameter, and **E**levation of the skin area (**Figure 20-3**). Skin cancers are **a**symmetrical and have irregular **b**orders. The mole, freckle, or skin spot is abnormal if the **c**olor is not an even, uniform tone. A physician should examine any suspicious mole if the **d**iameter is larger than that of a pencil eraser (about 1/4 in.), regardless of color, border, or asymmetry. Cancers usually are **e**levated above the skin surface.

Skin cancers are diagnosed by one of four common types of skin biopsies: punch, incisional, excisional, and shave. With a **punch biopsy**, the doctor uses a sharp, hollow tool to remove a cylinder of tissue from an abnormal area (**Figure 20-4**). An **incisional biopsy** involves a removal of *part* of the growth, whereas an **excisional biopsy** involves the removal of the *entire* growth along with some surrounding tissue. A **shave biopsy** is the shearing off of abnormal growth layer by layer.

Skin cancer staging is based on tumor size, how deeply it has grown beneath the skin, and whether it has metastasized. If the cancer is located only in the superficial skin layer

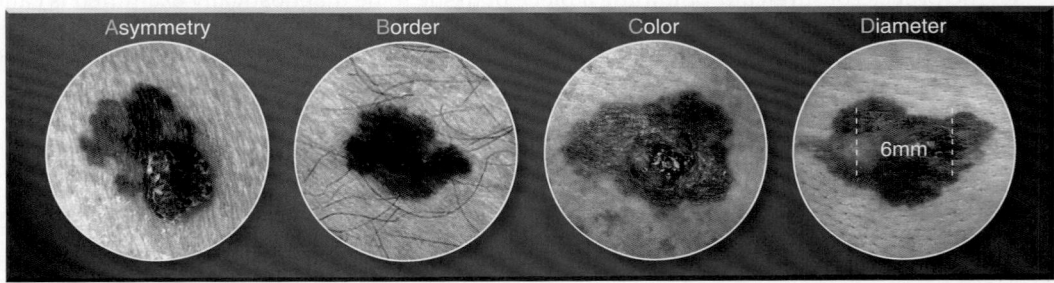

Figure 20-3 ABCDs of skin cancer.

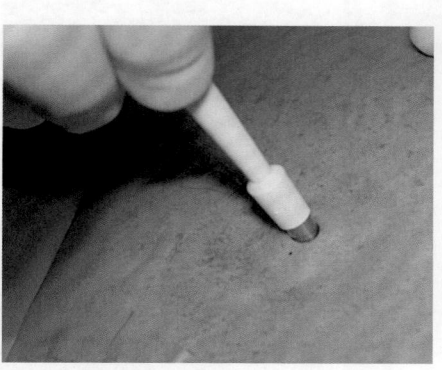

Figure 20-4 Punch biopsy.

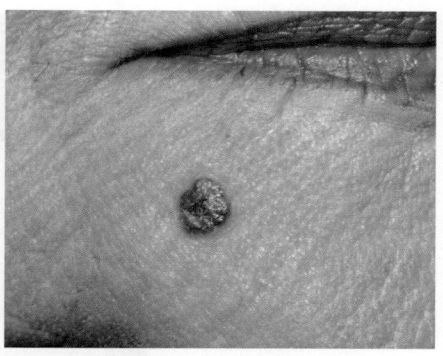

Figure 20-5 Basal cell carcinoma. Note the irregular surface.

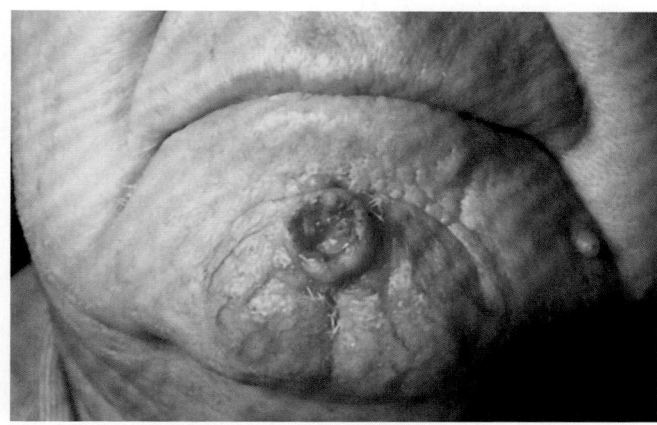

Figure 20-6 Squamous cell carcinoma on the chin.

(epithelium), it is termed **carcinoma in situ (CIS)**. *In situ* refers to the fact that the cancer does not extend beyond its origin. The stages of skin cancer are the following:

- Stage 0: The cancer is found in only the top layer of skin.
- Stage I: Growth is 2 cm (0.79 in.) wide or smaller.
- Stage II: Growth is greater than 2 cm (0.79 in.).
- Stage III: The cancer has spread to cartilage, muscle, bone, or nearby lymph nodes, but has not spread anywhere else.
- Stage IV: The cancer has metastasized throughout the body.

melanoma	**Melanoma** (malignant melanoma) is a type of skin cancer that forms in melanocytes. Melanocytes are the pigment-producing cells that cause our skin to darken when exposed to ultraviolet radiation. Although it is one of the less common types of skin cancer, it causes the majority of skin cancer-related deaths.
basal cell carcinoma	Cancer that forms in the deepest cells of the epidermis is termed **basal cell carcinoma** (Figure 20-5). This cancer is slow growing and invasive, but it usually does not metastasize. Basal cell carcinoma is commonly seen in the sun-damaged skin of the elderly.
squamous cell carcinoma	If the cancer forms in the flat cells that form the skin surface, it is called **squamous cell carcinoma** (Figure 20-6).

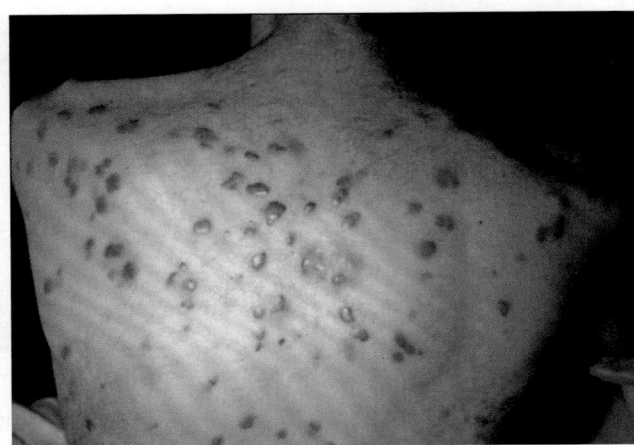

Figure 20-7 Kaposi sarcoma.

Kaposi sarcoma A malignant neoplasm that occurs in the skin and sometimes in the lymph nodes or organs is **Kaposi sarcoma**. It is characterized by purplish-red patches on the skin and is seen most commonly in men older than 60 years of age and in patients with AIDS (**Figure 20-7**). In patients with AIDS, it is an opportunistic disease associated with human herpes virus 8 infection. An **opportunistic disease** describes an infection that is not normally serious but can become pathogenic or life threatening when the person has a low level of immunity, as in patients with AIDS.

Treatment options for skin cancer include various types of surgery:

- In **excisional skin surgery**, the physician removes the growth and the skin surrounding the growth with a scalpel. The skin bordering the growth is termed the **margin**. Skin cells from the margin are examined under a microscope to be certain that all abnormal tissue has been removed.
- With **Mohs surgery**, a surgeon shaves away thin layers of the growth. Before shaving, the tissue is fixed in place with a zinc chloride paste. Each layer is microscopically examined, and the surgeon continues until no cancerous cells can be seen. The benefit of this surgery is that all the cancerous cells are removed, yet the least amount of healthy tissue is removed.
- **Electrodesiccation and curettage** is a relatively quick procedure in which an electrical current is passed through a sharp, spoon-like instrument called a curette. As the tissue is excised with the curette, the electric current controls bleeding and kills cancer cells in the region. Electrodesiccation and curettage is used to treat basal cell carcinoma.
- **Cryosurgery** uses extreme cold to treat early-stage skin cancer. Liquid nitrogen creates the extreme cold, which is applied directly to the site to destroy the diseased tissue.
- **Laser surgery** uses a focused beam of light to destroy cancer cells.
- **Skin grafts** are used to close openings in skin created by excisional surgery. With a skin graft, healthy skin is taken from one part of the body and used to replace lost or damaged skin in another location.

  Other treatments for skin cancer include the following:
- With **topical chemotherapy**, anticancer drugs are applied directly to the skin. Topical chemotherapy is usually used in cases where the skin cancer is too large for surgery.

- **Photodynamic therapy (PDT)** uses a chemical along with a laser to kill cancer cells. This treatment is used for cancers that are on the skin surface or close to the skin surface.
- **Radiation therapy (RTx)**, also called **radiotherapy**, uses high-energy x-rays directed at the cancer to kill cells. Radiation therapy is designed to target cells in a specific location and is given in one dose or in several doses over many weeks.

KEY TERM	Definition
ABCDEs of skin cancer	method used to examine skin area by checking the **a**symmetry, **b**order, **c**olor, **d**iameter, and **e**levation of a mole, freckle, or skin spot
punch biopsy (BYE-op-see)	method of removing a small cylinder of tissue using an instrument that pierces the skin
incisional biopsy (in-SIH-zhun-ul BYE-op-see)	removal of only a part of a growth by cutting into it
excisional biopsy (ek-SIH-zhun-ul BYE-op-see)	removal of entire growth by cutting it out
shave biopsy (BYE-op-see)	technique performed with a surgical blade or razor blade to shave off growths layer by layer
carcinoma in situ (CIS) (kar-sih-NOH-muh in SIGH-too)	cancer that is confined to the superficial skin layer (epithelium)
melanoma (mel-uh-NOH-muh)	malignant neoplasm derived from melanocytes
basal cell carcinoma (BAY-sul SELL kar-sih-NOH-muh)	slow-growing, invasive, nonmetastasizing neoplasm located in the epidermis
squamous cell carcinoma (SKWAY-mus SELL kar-sih-NOH-muh)	malignant neoplasm derived from squamous epithelium
Kaposi sarcoma (kuh-POH-zee sar-KOH-muh)	cancer of the skin and sometimes lymph nodes that causes purplish-red patches on the skin
opportunistic disease (op-or-too-NIS-tik dih-ZEEZ)	infection that results due to lowered resistance of the immune system
excisional skin surgery (ek-SIH-zhun-ul skin SUR-juh-ree)	scalpel removal of growth along with surrounding skin
margin	boundary or edge
Mohs surgery (MOZE SUR-juh-ree)	technique for removing skin tumors in which fixed sections of tissue are removed in thin layers and examined until all the tumor has been removed
electrodesiccation and curettage (ee-lek-troh-deh-sih-KAY-shun and KUE-ruh-tahzh)	destruction of tumor by electric current during tissue removal with a curette
cryosurgery (KRY-oh-sur-juh-ree)	using liquid nitrogen as a freezing agent to destroy tissue
laser surgery (LAY-zer SUR-juh-ree)	using an intense, narrow beam of light to remove tissue. It is an acronym coined from **l**ight **a**mplification by **s**timulated **e**mission of **r**adiation.
skin grafts	skin transplanted from one part of the body to another
topical chemotherapy (TAH-pih-kul KEE-moh-THERR-uh-pee)	anticancer drugs applied directly to the skin surface
photodynamic therapy (PDT) (foh-toh-dye-NAM-ick THERR-uh-pee)	a laser-assisted procedure in which the light beam and anticancer chemical are aimed at the tumor to destroy it
radiation therapy (RTx) (ray-dee-AY-shun THERR-uh-pee)	treatment with x-rays; also called radiotherapy
radiotherapy (ray-dee-oh-THERR-uh-pee)	treatment with x-rays; also called radiation therapy

continued

continued from page 1105

KEY TERM PRACTICE: *Integumentary System Cancers*

1. _____ is a malignant neoplasm derived from squamous epithelium.

2. _____ is a cancer of the connective tissue that is characterized by purplish-red patches on the skin.

3. The procedure of removing a small cylinder of tissue from the skin is called _____.

4. Cancer that is confined to the superficial skin layer is termed _____.

5. Using liquid nitrogen to freeze and destroy tissue is known as _____.

Skeletal System Cancers

Skeletal system cancers are commonly referred to as bone cancers. **Primary bone cancer** forms in the bone cells, but may also invade certain soft tissues. Types of primary bone cancers are osteosarcoma, Ewing sarcoma, and chondrosarcoma. When a cancer spreads to the bones from another body part, such as the breast, lung, or prostate gland, it is called **secondary bone cancer**. It was estimated that there would be 2,650 new cases of bone cancer in the United States in 2010 and 1,460 deaths from the disease. Chapter 5, Skeletal System: Bones and Joints, discusses other skeletal system cancers.

osteosarcoma   **Osteosarcoma**, the most common type of bone cancer, is a malignant bone tumor that usually begins in the bone-building cells called osteoblasts. It commonly affects teenagers and young adults and targets the ends of long bones (the epiphyses). In children and teenagers, it often develops in the knee joint. Osteosarcoma affects more males than females.

Ewing sarcoma   **Ewing sarcoma** is a group of cancers of the bone and soft tissue. Ewing sarcomas develop in the arms, chest, trunk, back, or head. There are three types of Ewing sarcoma: classic Ewing sarcoma, primitive neuroectodermal tumor (PNET), and Askin tumor (or PNET of the chest wall).

chondrosarcoma   **Chondrosarcoma** is a type of bone cancer that forms in cartilage, usually originating in the pelvis.

Risk factors for primary bone cancers include being a male teenager or having past treatment with radiation. Signs and symptoms of osteosarcoma include pain and swelling over a bone, joint pain, and bone fractures of unknown origin. Imaging tests (x-ray, CT scan, and MRI) are used to detect bone cancers, and biopsies are done to diagnose osteosarcoma.

Biopsy procedures include fine-needle aspiration, core biopsy, and incisional biopsy. Location and tumor size determine which biopsy method is used. The removal of tissue or fluid using a thin needle is called **fine-needle aspiration (FNA) biopsy**. The removal of tissue using a wide needle is called **core biopsy**. Incisional biopsy is used to remove part of a tissue sample that does not appear normal. Treatment options include chemotherapy and surgery.

KEY TERM	Definition
primary bone cancer	cancer that originates in bone cells
secondary bone cancer	cancer that originates in one part of the body and metastasizes to bones
osteosarcoma (os-tee-oh sar-KOH-muh)	cancer of the bone
Ewing sarcoma (YOO-ing sar-KOH-muh)	a type of cancer that forms in bone or soft tissue
chondrosarcoma (kon-droh-sar-KOH-muh)	a type of cancer that forms in cartilage
fine-needle aspiration (FNA) biopsy (NEE-dul as-pih-RAY-shun BYE-op-see)	removal of tissue or fluid with a thin needle for microscopic examination
core biopsy (BYE-op-see)	removal of a tissue sample with a wide needle for microscopic examination

KEY TERM PRACTICE: *Skeletal System Cancers*

1. Cancer that originates in bone cells is termed _____.

2. Cancer that originates in one tissue and metastasizes to bones is called _____.

3. _____ is the medical term for cancer of the bone.

4. A type of cancer that forms in cartilage is _____.

5. The use of a wide needle to remove a tissue sample is called a _____.

Muscular System Cancers

Soft tissue sarcomas are cancers that begin in muscle, fat, fibrous tissue, blood vessels, or other supporting body tissue. Soft tissue sarcomas are uncommon and in 2006, about 9,500 cases were diagnosed. In this section we turn our attention to cancers that affect muscle tissue.

myosarcoma	A general term for a malignant neoplasm derived from muscle tissue is **myosarcoma**.
rhabdomyosarcoma	Malignant cancer that forms specifically in skeletal muscle tissue is termed **rhabdomyosarcoma**. This type of cancer occurs more commonly in children than adults and is often referred to as *childhood rhabdomyosarcoma*. Risk factors include radiation or chemical exposure. Certain rare genetic disorders also increase the risk of childhood rhabdomyosarcoma.

Signs include a lump or mass that continues to enlarge. There is rarely any pain or swelling. Diagnosis is made by physical exam, bone scan, bone marrow aspiration with biopsy, x-rays, CT, MRI, and biopsy (Bx). During a **bone scan**, a small amount of radioactive material is injected into a vein and travels through the bloodstream where it eventually collects in bone tissue. A scanner then detects this radioactive dye and the resulting image that appears on a computer screen or film is evaluated for cancerous cells in the bone (**Figure 20-8**). During a **bone marrow aspiration and biopsy**, a hollow needle is inserted into the hipbone to collect bone marrow, blood, and a small piece of bone. Samples are taken from both hips and checked by a pathologist for cancerous cells (**Figure 20-9**). The usual treatment is surgical removal of the tumor. Radiation therapy and chemotherapy are also used.

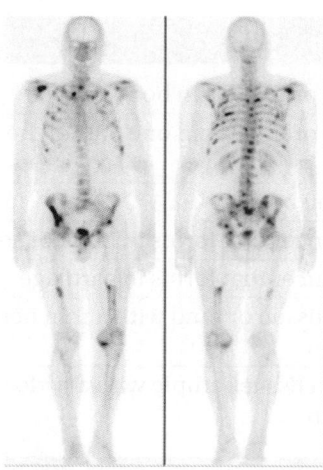

Figure 20-8 Bone scan of a 68-year-old male with lung cancer showing extensive metastases to the bones.

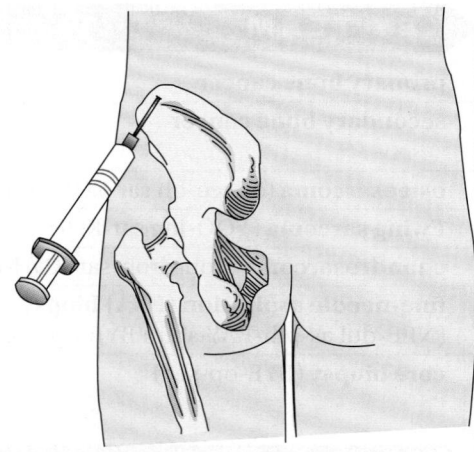

Figure 20-9 Bone marrow aspiration. Posterior view of pelvic region showing a common site for bone marrow aspiration and biopsy.

KEY TERM	Definition
myosarcoma (migh-oh-sar-KOH-muh)	malignant neoplasm derived from muscle tissue
rhabdomyosarcoma (rab-doh-my-oh-sar-KOH-muh)	malignant neoplasm derived from skeletal muscle tissue
bone scan	technique used to create images of bone by injecting the patient with radioactive dye that is taken up by bone tissue
bone marrow aspiration and biopsy (bone MAYR-oh as-pih-RAY-shun and BYE-op-see)	procedure in which a small sample of bone marrow and bone is removed for evaluation using a special needle that is pushed into the bone

KEY TERM PRACTICE: *Muscular System Cancers*

1. A malignant neoplasm derived from muscle tissue is called a _____.

2. The technique of injecting a patient with a dye that the bone absorbs and allowing for an image to be made is a _____.

3. A skeletal muscle malignant neoplasm is a _____.

4. The procedure in which a special needle is used to obtain a sample of a patient's bone and bone marrow is termed a _____.

Nervous System Cancers

The nervous system is an organized network of nerve tissue in the body. It includes the central nervous system, composed of the brain and spinal cord, and the peripheral nervous system, made up of the nerves that extend from the brain and spinal cord to the rest of the body. **Brain tumors** are defined as the growth of abnormal cells in the tissues of the brain. It was estimated that there would be 22,020 new cases of brain cancer in 2010 and in this same year, 13,140 would die as a result.

Primary brain tumors are named according to their location in the brain or the type of cells in which they begin. The most common types of adult brain tumors are astrocytomas, meningiomas, and oligodendrogliomas. Cancers of the nervous system are also discussed in Chapter 7, Nervous System.

astrocytoma	An **astrocytoma** is made up of star-shaped glial cells known as astrocytes. Astrocytomas often originate in the cerebrum or spinal cord.
meningioma	A **meningioma** is a slow-growing benign tumor that affects the meninges, the thin layers of tissue that cover and protect the brain and spinal cord. Meningiomas may cause serious damage by pressing on neural tissue.
oligodendroglioma	**Oligodendrogliomas** arise from oligodendrocytes, the cells that make the fatty covering on nerves. These rare, slow-growing tumors usually occur in the cerebrum and occur most commonly in middle-aged adults.

The most common types of neural tumors affecting children are medulloblastoma, grade I or grade II astrocytoma, ependymoma, brainstem glioma, and neuroblastoma.

medulloblastoma	A **medulloblastoma** is a rapidly growing malignant tumor that is usually located in the cerebellum and may be implanted on the surfaces of the brainstem and spinal cord. This type of cancer occurs most frequently in children.
grade I or **grade II astrocytoma**	In children, a **grade I** or **grade II astrocytoma** is a low-grade tumor that occurs anywhere in the brain. The most common type is **juvenile pilocytic astrocytoma**, a slow-growing tumor derived from glial cells in the brain and spinal cord.
ependymoma	An **ependymoma** arises from ependyma, which are cells that line the ventricles of the brain and the central canal of the spinal cord. It is commonly found in children and young adults.
brainstem glioma	**Brainstem gliomas** are found in the brainstem, the region where the brain is connected to the spinal cord. Gliomas may grow rapidly or slowly.
neuroblastoma	**Neuroblastomas** are malignant neoplasms of embryonic nerve cells called neuroblasts. These tumors occur frequently in infants and children and have widespread metastases to the liver, lungs, lymph nodes, brain, and skeleton.

Risk factors for developing brain cancer are difficult to identify. We do know that people exposed to ionizing radiation have an increased risk of developing brain tumors. However, research has failed to identify any links between cell phone use, previous head injury, and exposure to magnetic fields with the development of brain cancer.

The most common signs and symptoms of brain tumors are headache, memory loss, nausea, vomiting, muscle twitching, and numbness or tingling in the arms or legs. A complete neurological exam, accompanied by diagnostic tests (MRI, CT scan, and biopsy), is necessary to identify the underlying problem.

A **stereotactic biopsy**, a procedure that uses a computer and a three-dimensional scanning device to find a tumor site and guide the removal of tissue for microscopic examination, may be done. Treatment options include surgery (if the tumor is in a location that will not adversely affect other neural tissue), chemotherapy, and radiation therapy.

KEY TERM	Definition
brain tumor (TOO-mer)	abnormal growth of cells in the brain
astrocytoma (as-troh-sigh-TOH-muh)	tumor that begins in the brain (often the cerebrum) or spinal cord in small, star-shaped cells called astrocytes
meningioma (meh-nin-jee-OH-muh)	a slow-growing benign tumor that forms in the meninges
oligodendroglioma (oh-lih-goh-den-droh-glee-OH-muh)	a rare, slow-growing tumor that begins in oligodendrocytes
medulloblastoma (med-yoo-loh-blas-TOH-muh)	a malignant brain tumor that is usually located in the cerebellum and may be implanted on the surfaces of the brainstem and spinal cord
grade I or **grade II astrocytoma** (as-troh-sigh-TOH-muh)	a low-grade tumor affecting children that occurs anywhere in the brain
juvenile pilocytic astrocytoma (JOO-veh-nile pye-loh-SIH-tik as-troh-sye-TOH-muh)	tumor forming from glial cells that usually occurs in children and young adults
ependymoma (eh-pen-dih-MOH-muh)	a type of tumor that begins in the lining of the brain ventricles or spinal cord central canal
brainstem glioma (glee-OH-muh)	a tumor located in the brainstem, which is the part of the brain that connects to the spinal cord
neuroblastoma (noo-roh-blas-TOH-muh)	a malignant tumor of embryonic nerve cells (neuroblasts)
stereotactic biopsy (stayr-ee-oh-TAK-tik BYE-op-see)	removal of tumor using an apparatus that is attached to the head and is used to localize the precise location of the brain tumor using a computer

KEY TERM PRACTICE: *Nervous System Cancers*

1. An abnormal growth—either benign or malignant—of cells in the brain is called a _____.

2. A _____ is a malignant tumor of embryonic nerve cells.

3. A tumor that begins in the central nervous system in small, star-shaped cells is known as an _____.

4. A _____ is a malignant tumor that is usually located in the cerebellum and may be implanted on the surfaces of the brainstem and spinal cord.

5. A slow-growing tumor that forms in the meninges is a _____.

Endocrine System Cancers

The endocrine system is a system of glands that secrete hormones directly into the bloodstream. Important endocrine glands are the adrenal, thyroid, parathyroid, pituitary, and pancreas. Other endocrine system cancers are discussed in Chapter 9.

There are two adrenal glands, and one caps the superior part of each kidney. These glands make steroid hormones, epinephrine (adrenaline), and norepinephrine (noradrenaline) to control heart rate, blood pressure, and other body functions. A rare cancer that forms in the adrenal cortex, the outer surface of the gland, is called **adrenocortical carcinoma**. This rare cancer affects only 1 to 2 persons per 1 million and is treated by surgical removal.

pheochromocytoma   A **pheochromocytoma** is a tumor that forms in the medulla (center) of the adrenal gland and causes the gland to make too much epinephrine. Pheochromocytomas are usually benign but cause high blood pressure, pounding headaches, heart palpitations, facial flushing, nausea, and vomiting. These tumors are often hereditary.

thyroid cancer   The thyroid gland is a butterfly-shaped organ that is located at the base of the throat. Thyroid hormones regulate heart rate, blood pressure, body temperature, and weight. Cancer of this gland is termed **thyroid cancer** (**Figure 20-10**). It was estimated that there would be 44,670 new cases of thyroid cancer in 2010, and that 1,690 deaths would result.

parathyroid cancers   The parathyroid glands are four tiny glands embedded on the posterior surface of the thyroid glands. These glands secrete hormones to help the body maintain calcium balance. **Parathyroid cancers** are very rare tumors that affect only 0.015 per 100,000 people.

The pituitary gland is considered the body's "master gland" because it secretes hormones that affect many other glands and body functions. This gland is located in the center of the brain, and most pituitary tumors are benign.

KEY TERM	Definition
adrenocortical carcinoma (uh-dree-noh-KOR-tih-kul kar-sih-NOH-muh)	cancer of the adrenal cortex
pheochromocytoma (fee-oh-kroh-moh-sigh-TOH-muh)	tumor located in the adrenal medulla
thyroid cancer (THIGH-royd KAN-ser)	cancer that affects the thyroid gland
parathyroid cancers (pair-uh-THIGH-royd KAN-sers)	a rare cancer that forms in one or more of the parathyroid glands

KEY TERM PRACTICE: *Endocrine System Cancers*

1. Cancer of the adrenal cortex is termed _____.

2. _____ is a tumor in the adrenal medulla.

3. Any one of the four types of cancer affecting the thyroid gland is known as _____.

4. _____ is a rare type of cancer that forms in one or more of the parathyroid glands.

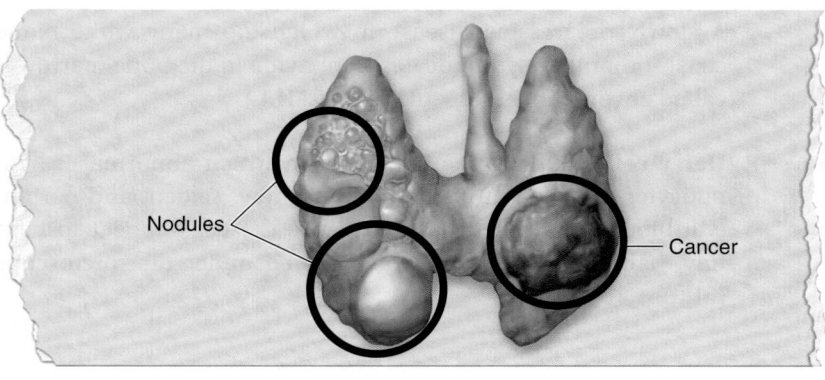

Nodules

Cancer

Figure 20-10 Thyroid cancer.

Blood Cancers

leukemia

Cancer that starts in blood-forming tissues is called **leukemia**. Leukemia was expected to affect 43,050 people in 2010, with death occurring in 21,840 of these new cases. There are numerous types of leukemia. See also the section on leukemia in Chapter 10, Blood.

Physical exam, complete blood cell count (CBC), peripheral smear, and bone marrow aspiration with biopsy, cytogenetic analysis, and immunophenotyping are used to confirm the diagnosis. A **peripheral blood smear** is a blood test that checks for the presence of **blast cells** (immature, undifferentiated blood cells), counts the number of white blood cells and platelets, and identifies the shape of blood cells. The test in which a sample of blood or bone marrow is viewed under the microscope to find out if malignant lymphocytes began as B lymphocytes or T lymphocytes is called **immunophenotyping**.

acute lymphoblastic leukemia (ALL) or **acute lymphocytic leukemia**

Acute lymphoblastic leukemia (ALL) is a fast-growing type of cancer (adult and childhood forms) in which the bone marrow makes too many lymphocytes. Lymphocytes are a type of white blood cell. It is also known as **acute lymphocytic leukemia**. Previous exposure to radiation or prior treatment with chemotherapy increases the risk of developing ALL. Signs and symptoms include fever, feeling tired, easy bruising or bleeding, and **petechiae** (flat, pinpoint spots under the skin caused by bleeding.)

acute myeloid leukemia (AML)

Acute myeloid leukemia (AML) is a type of fast-growing cancer (adult and childhood forms) in which the bone marrow makes abnormal myeloblasts, red blood cells, or platelets. Myeloblasts are a type of immature white blood cell. This is the most common type of acute leukemia and requires prompt treatment. Risk factors include smoking, previous chemotherapy treatment, and exposure to radiation. Signs, symptoms, and diagnostic tests are the same as for acute lymphoblastic leukemia.

chronic lymphocytic leukemia (CLL)

Chronic lymphocytic leukemia (CLL) is an **indolent** (slow-growing) cancer in which too many immature lymphocytes are found in the blood and bone marrow and/or in the lymph nodes.

chronic myeloid leukemia (CML)

A slowly progressing disease in which too many white blood cells—other than lymphocytes—are made in the bone marrow is called **chronic myeloid leukemia (CML)**.

hairy cell leukemia

Hairy cell leukemia is a leukemia in which abnormal B lymphocytes are present in the bone marrow, spleen, and peripheral blood. It is called hairy, because the cells appear to have tiny, hair-like projections when viewed under the microscope (**Figure 20-11**).

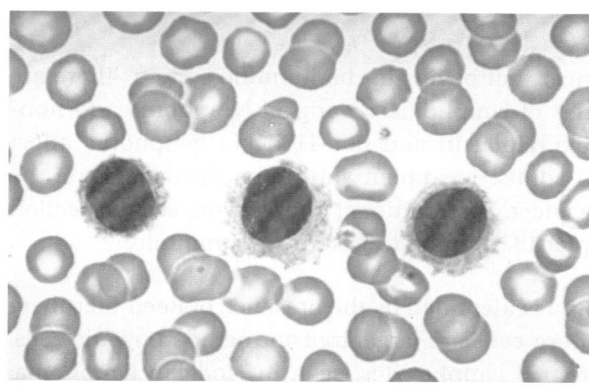

Figure 20-11 Blood smear showing hairy cell leukemia. Notice the fine cytoplasmic extensions that look like hair.

KEY TERM	Definition
leukemia (loo-KEE-mee-uh)	cancer that starts in blood-forming tissues
peripheral blood smear (peh-RIH-feh-rul)	procedure in which a sample of blood is viewed under a microscope to count different circulating blood cells and to see whether the cells look normal
blast cells	immature, undifferentiated blood cells
immunophenotyping (IM-yoo-noh-fee-noh-type-ing)	process used to identify cells and diagnose specific types of leukemia and lymphoma by comparing the cancer cells to normal immune cells
acute lymphoblastic leukemia (ALL) (uh-KYOOT lim-foh-BLAS-tik loo-KEE-mee-uh)	fast-growing type of blood cancer in which too many immature white blood cells appear in blood and bone marrow; also called acute lymphocytic leukemia
acute lymphocytic leukemia (ALL) (uh-KYOOT lim-foh-SIH-tik loo-KEE-mee-uh)	fast-growing type of blood cancer in which too many immature white blood cells appear in blood and bone marrow; also called acute lymphoblastic leukemia
petechiae (peh-TEH-kee-uh)	pinpoint, unraised, round red spots under the skin caused by bleeding
acute myeloid leukemia (AML) (uh-KYOOT MYE-eh-loyd loo-KEE-mee-uh)	fast-growing disease in which too many myeloblasts (immature white blood cells that are not lymphoblasts) are found in the bone marrow and blood
chronic lymphocytic leukemia (CLL) (KRAH-nik lim-foh-SIH-tik loo-KEE-mee-uh)	a slow-growing cancer in which too many immature lymphocytes are found in the blood and bone marrow and/or in the lymph nodes
indolent (IN-doe-lint)	describes a type of cancer that grows slowly
chronic myeloid leukemia (CML) (KRAH-nik MYE-eh-loyd loo-KEE-mee-uh)	a slowly progressing cancer in which too many white blood cells (not lymphocytes) are made in the bone marrow
hairy cell leukemia (HAYR-ee SELL loo-KEE-mee-uh)	a type of leukemia in which abnormal B lymphocytes are present in the bone marrow, spleen, and peripheral blood

KEY TERM PRACTICE: *Blood Cancers*

1. Immature, undifferentiated blood cells are called _____.

2. _____ is a fast-growing disease in which too many myeloblasts are found in the bone marrow and blood.

3. Pinpoint, round red spots that appear below the skin and are caused by bleeding are known as _____.

4. A cancer originating in blood-forming tissues is termed _____.

5. The process used to identify cells and diagnose types of leukemia and lymphoma by comparing cancer and normal cells is _____.

Immune System Cancers

lymphoma

Lymphoma is cancer that begins in the immune system. There are two basic categories of lymphomas: Hodgkin lymphoma and non-Hodgkin lymphoma. Hodgkin and non-Hodgkin lymphoma affect both children and adults. Treatment and prognosis depend on the stage and type of cancer. For additional information, see the section on tumors in Chapter 13, Lymphatic System and Immunity.

Hodgkin lymphoma

Hodgkin lymphoma is identified by the presence of Reed-Sternberg cells. **Reed-Sternberg cells** are large, transformed pathogenic cells, usually derived from B lymphocytes, seen in Hodgkin lymphoma. These cells increase in numbers as the disease advances. They are named for two researchers, Dorothy Reed Mendenhall and Carl Sternberg, who provided the first definitive microscopic description of Hodgkin lymphoma.

non-Hodgkin lymphoma

Non-Hodgkin lymphoma is any one of a diverse group of immune system cancers that are divided into **aggressive** (fast-growing) and indolent (slow-growing) types.

KEY TERM	Definition
lymphoma (lim-FOH-muh)	cancer that begins in immune system cells
Hodgkin lymphoma (HOJ-kin lim-FOH-muh)	cancer of the immune system marked by the presence of Reed-Sternberg cells
Reed-Sternberg cells	large, transformed pathogenic cells, usually derived from B lymphocytes, that appear in people with Hodgkin lymphoma
non-Hodgkin lymphoma (non-HOJ-kin lim-FOH-muh)	any of a large group of cancers of lymphocytes
aggressive	describes a tumor or disease that grows or spreads quickly

KEY TERM PRACTICE: *Immune System Cancers*

1. Reed-Sternberg cells are present in people with _____.

2. Cancer originating in the immune system is termed _____.

3. _____ is any of a diverse, large group of cancers of lymphocytes.

4. A tumor or disease that grows quickly is termed _____.

5. Large, transformed pathogenic cells that usually come from B lymphocytes and are typically found in cases of Hodgkin lymphoma are called _____.

Respiratory System Cancers

The respiratory system is made up of organs involved in breathing. These include the nose, pharynx, larynx, trachea, bronchi, and lungs. In this section we focus on lung cancers. Lung cancers usually form in the cells lining the air passages. The two main types of lung cancer are small cell lung cancer and non-small cell lung cancer, based on how they look under a microscope. The 2010 estimated number of new cases of lung cancer (both small cell and

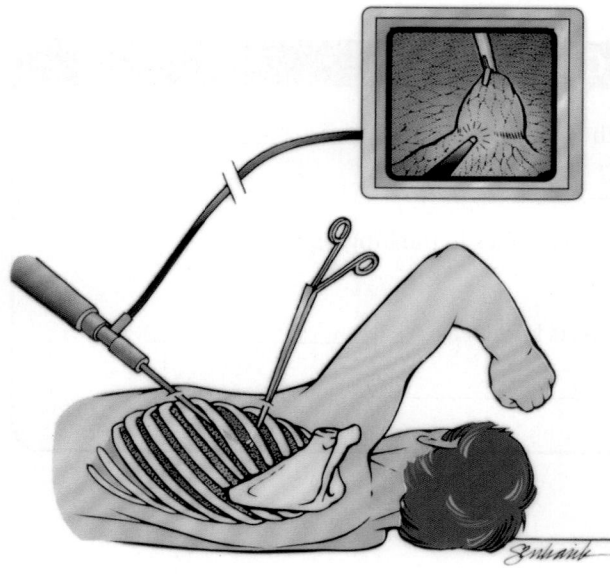

Figure 20-12 Thoracoscopy. Thoracoscopy uses fiberoptic instruments and a video camera for visualizing thoracic structures.

non-small cell) in the United States was 222,520. The number of deaths was expected to be 157,300. Cancer of the respiratory system is also discussed in Chapter 12.

The major risk factor for developing lung cancer is cigarette smoking. Signs and symptoms include persistent cough, chest pain, and shortness of breath. Physical exam, chest x-ray, CT scan, PET scan, and thoracoscopy diagnose it. **Thoracoscopy** is a surgical procedure in which an incision is made between two ribs and a thoracoscope is inserted into the chest to check for abnormal areas (**Figure 20-12**). For most patients, current treatments do not cure the cancer.

small cell lung cancer	**Small cell lung cancer** is a disease in which malignant cells form in lung tissues, and there are two types: small cell carcinoma (also called oat cell cancer) and combined small cell carcinoma. This is an aggressive form of cancer whose cells appear small and oval-shaped when viewed under a microscope.
non-small cell lung cancer	**Non-small cell lung cancer** is also characterized by metastatic cells in the lungs and is the most common kind of lung cancer. These cancers are grouped by the physical appearance of the cancerous cells. The main types of non-small cell lung cancer are squamous cell carcinoma, large cell carcinoma, and adenocarcinoma. Squamous cell carcinoma is cancer that begins in the thin, flat cells called squamous cells. Abnormal, large cells characterize **large cell carcinoma**. **Adenocarcinoma** is lung cancer that begins in the cells that line the alveoli (tiny air sacs where gas exchange takes place).

KEY TERM	Definition
thoracoscopy (thor-uh-KOS-koh-pee)	examination of the inside of the chest using a thoracoscope
small cell lung cancer (SELL lung KAN-ser)	aggressive cancer that forms in the lungs
non-small cell lung cancer (SELL lung KAN-ser)	group of lung cancers named for the kinds of cells found in the cancer and their appearance under the microscope
large cell carcinoma (SELL kar-sih-NOH-muh)	lung cancer in which the cells are large and look abnormal when viewed under a microscope
adenocarcinoma (a-den-oh-kar-sih-NOH-muh)	lung cancer that forms in the alveoli

continued

continued from page 1115

KEY TERM PRACTICE: *Respiratory System Cancers*

1. The procedure that uses a thoracoscope to examine the inside of the chest is called _____.

2. Lung cancer that forms in the alveoli is termed _____.

3. An aggressive cancer characterized by small, oval-shaped cells that originates in the lungs is

    _____.

4. A group of lung cancers named for the kinds and appearance of cells is known as _____.

5. Lung cancer characterized by large, abnormal-looking cells is _____.

Digestive System Cancers

Many cancers identified within the digestive system are discussed within the context of those specific body system chapters. Here, we briefly list the cancer types along with key statistics. Chapter 14 also discusses digestive system cancers.

The digestive system is made up of organs that take in food and turn it into nutrients that the body can use. Components of the digestive system include the mouth, salivary glands, esophagus, stomach, liver, pancreas, gallbladder, small and large intestines, and rectum. Digestive system cancers are varied and numerous. **Table 20-5** lists the various digestive system–related cancers and the estimated number of new cases and deaths for 2010.

colon cancer
Colon cancer is the most common type of cancer affecting the digestive system and forms in the longest section of the large intestine, known as the colon. The colon extends from the cecum to the rectum. Age and health history can affect the risk of developing colon cancer. For example, a history of polyps, ulcerative colitis, or Crohn disease increases the risk of developing colon cancer. Colon **polyps** are common growths that protrude from the tissue lining the colon. **Ulcerative colitis** is a chronic inflammation of the large intestine causing ulcers on the intestinal wall. It is marked by abdominal pain, cramps, and mucus in the bowel. **Crohn disease** is chronic inflammation of

TABLE 20-5 — **DIGESTIVE SYSTEM CANCERS**

Type	2010 Estimated New Cases	2010 Estimated Deaths
Anal	5,260	720
Colon and rectal	102,900 (colon) 39,670 (rectal)	51,370 for both combined
Esophageal	16,640	14,500
Gallbladder	9,760	3,320
Liver	24,120	18,910
Pancreatic	43,140	36,800
Small Intestine	6,980	1,100
Stomach	21,000	10,570

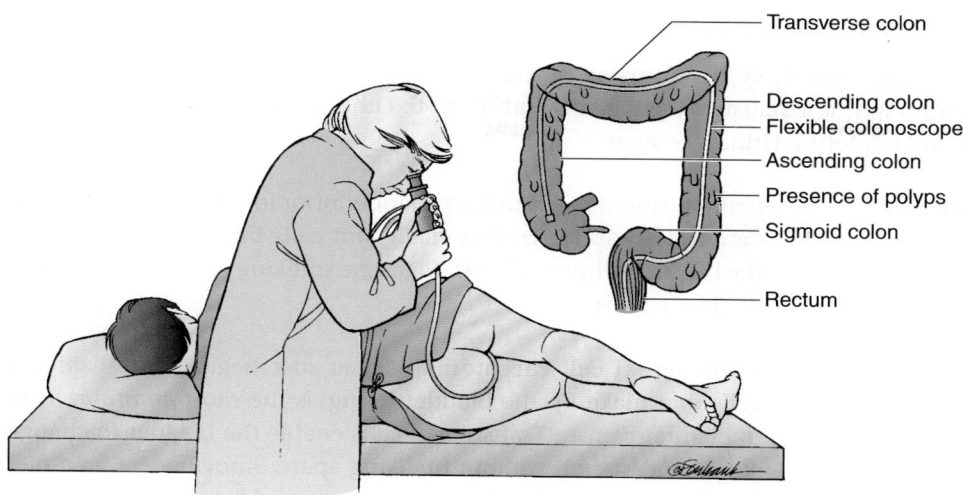

Transverse colon

Descending colon
Flexible colonoscope
Ascending colon
Presence of polyps
Sigmoid colon

Rectum

Figure 20-13 Colonoscopy. A flexible scope passes through the rectum and into the colon.

the gastrointestinal tract, usually of the lower portion. Scarring and thickening of the intestinal wall and obstruction mark it.

Signs of colon cancer include diarrhea or constipation, bloating, and vomiting. Tests that examine the rectum and large intestine, such as the fecal occult blood test and a colonoscopy, are used to detect and diagnose colon cancer. The **fecal occult blood test (FOBT)** checks for blood in the stool. With this test, small samples of stool are placed on special cards and tested for the presence of blood. A **colonoscopy** is a diagnostic procedure used to check for the presence of polyps, abnormal areas, or cancer. Using a colonoscope, a thin, tube-like instrument with a light and lens for viewing, the interior of the colon can be examined (**Figure 20-13**). The standard treatments are surgery, chemotherapy, and radiation therapy.

KEY TERM	Definition
colon cancer (KOH-lun KAN-ser)	cancer that forms in the tissues of the colon
polyps (PAH-lips)	growths that protrude from the tissue lining the colon
ulcerative colitis (UL-ser-uh-tiv koh-LIGH-tis)	chronic inflammation of the colon that produces ulcers in its lining
Crohn disease (KRONE dih-ZEEZ)	chronic inflammation of the gastrointestinal tract
fecal occult (FEE-kul uh-KULT) **blood test (FOBT)**	a test to check for blood in the stool
colonoscopy (koh-lun-OS-koh-pee)	examination of the inside of the colon using a colonoscope

KEY TERM PRACTICE: *Digestive System Cancers*

1. Growths extending out from the tissue lining the colon are called _____.

2. _____ is a chronic inflammation of the colon that produces ulcers.

3. _____ is a disease characterized by chronic inflammation of the lower gastrointestinal tract.

4. To determine whether there is blood in a patient's stool, a _____ test is performed.

5. The most common type of cancer that affects the digestive system is _____, which forms in the tissues of the colon.

Urinary System Cancers

The organs of the urinary system form, store, and eliminate urine. Common urinary system cancers and important statistics are given in **Table 20-6**. Other urinary system cancers are discussed in Chapter 15, Urinary System.

bladder cancer
Urine is stored in the urinary bladder prior to elimination. **Bladder cancer** is characterized by malignant cells that form in tissues of the bladder (**Figure 20-14**). Cigarette smoking is a leading cause of bladder cancer.

transitional cell carcinoma
Transitional cell carcinoma, cancer that begins in transitional cells that make up the bladder lining, is the most common form of bladder cancer. Transitional cells enable the bladder to change shape and stretch without breaking apart. Smoking, eating a diet high in fried meats and fat, and being an older male are risk factors for bladder cancer development. Signs and symptoms include **hematuria** (blood in the urine) and pain during urination. Tests that examine the urine (urinalysis) and bladder (IVP, biopsy, and cystoscopy) are used to detect and diagnose bladder cancer. In cystoscopy, a narrow tubular instrument is passed through the urethra to examine the interior of the urethra and urinary bladder. Treatment options include surgery, radiation therapy, chemotherapy, and biological therapy.

T A B L E 20-6

URINARY SYSTEM CANCERS

Type	2010 Estimated New Cases	2010 Estimated Deaths
Bladder	70,530	14,680
Kidney (renal cell carcinoma)	58,240	13,040

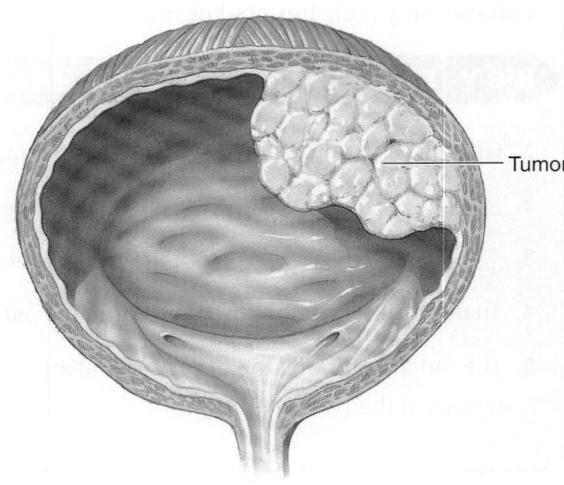

Tumor

Figure 20-14 Bladder cancer. Chemicals from tobacco are absorbed into the bloodstream and leave the body through the urine. These carcinogens are always in contact with the bladder, increasing the risk of cancer.

renal cell carcinoma
or **kidney cancer** or
renal adenocarcinoma

Renal cell carcinoma is a disease in which malignant cells form in the kidney tubules. Renal cell carcinoma is also called **kidney cancer** or **renal adenocarcinoma**. Cigarette smoking and long-term use of pain medications increase the risk of developing renal cell carcinoma. Signs include hematuria, weight loss for no known reason, and anemia.

Tests, such as urinalysis, intravenous pyelogram, and biopsy are used to detect kidney cancer. An **intravenous pyelogram (IVP)** is an x-ray image of the kidneys, ureter, and bladder after introduction of a dye, which illuminates the structures. Treatment options include surgery, radiation therapy, chemotherapy, biological therapy, and targeted therapy. Treatment to boost the ability of the person's immune system to fight cancer is called **biological therapy**. Agents used in biological therapy are **monoclonal antibodies** (special laboratory-made proteins that bind to tumor cells), growth factors, and vaccines.

KEY TERM	Definition
bladder cancer (BLA-der KAN-ser)	cancer that forms in tissues of the urinary bladder
transitional cell carcinoma (tran-ZIH-shuh-nul SELL kar-sih-NOH-muh)	cancer that forms in transitional cells lining the urinary bladder
hematuria (hee-muh-TOOR-ee-uh)	blood in the urine
renal cell carcinoma (REE-nul SELL kar-sih-NOH-muh)	most common type of urinary system cancer; also called kidney cancer and renal adenocarcinoma
kidney cancer (KID-nee KAN-ser)	most common type of urinary system cancer; also called renal cell carcinoma and renal adenocarcinoma
renal adenocarcinoma (REE-nul a-den-oh-kar-sih-NOH-muh)	most common type of urinary system cancer; also called renal cell carcinoma and kidney cancer
intravenous pyelogram (IVP) (in-truh-VEE-nus PYE-el-oh-gram)	an x-ray image of the kidneys, ureter, and bladder made after a substance that shows up on x-rays is injected into a blood vessel
biological therapy (bye-oh-LOJ-i-kul THAYR-uh-pee)	treatment to boost the ability of the immune system to fight cancer
monoclonal antibodies (mah-noh-KLOH-nul AN-tih-bah-dees)	proteins made in the laboratory that can bind to tumor cells

KEY TERM PRACTICE: *Urinary System Cancers*

1. Cancer that forms in transitional cells lining the urinary bladder is termed _____.

2. _____ is the medical term for blood in the urine.

3. The most common type of urinary system cancer that affects the kidneys is called _____; it is also called _____ or _____.

4. IVP is the abbreviation for _____.

5. A treatment intended to boost the immune system so it can fight cancer better is called _____.

Reproductive System Cancers

The reproductive system includes body organs and tissues used in the process of producing offspring. In this section, we focus on common cancers affecting males (prostate and testicular) and cancers affecting females (breast, ovarian, uterine, and cervical). Other cancers of the reproductive system are covered in Chapter 16, Reproductive Systems.

prostate cancer

Prostate cancer, a disease in which malignant cells form in the prostate, usually occurs in older men. The prostate is a chestnut-shaped gland that surrounds the male urethra and is located inferior to the bladder and anterior to the rectum. Structurally, it consists of 30 to 50 tubuloalveolar glands that secrete a milky fluid that is discharged during ejaculation. The National Cancer Institute predicted that there would be 217,730 new cases of prostate cancer in 2010, with 32,050 deaths as a result of the disease. Signs of prostate cancer include weak flow of urine or frequent urination.

Common tests used to detect prostate cancer include a digital rectal exam, prostate-specific antigen (PSA) test, and transrectal ultrasound. The procedure in which the prostate gland is felt through the wall of the rectum by inserting a lubricated, gloved finger into the rectum is called a **digital rectal exam (DRE)** (Figure 20-15). Prostate-specific antigen is a substance made in the prostate gland. The **prostate-specific antigen (PSA) test** measures the amount of PSA in the blood. Levels are increased in men who have prostate cancer. **Transrectal ultrasound** is a procedure in which a probe that sends out high-energy sound waves is inserted into the rectum to check the prostate. There are four types of standard treatment: watchful waiting, surgery, radiation therapy, and hormone therapy. In **watchful waiting**, the patient is closely monitored but not treated until symptoms appear or change.

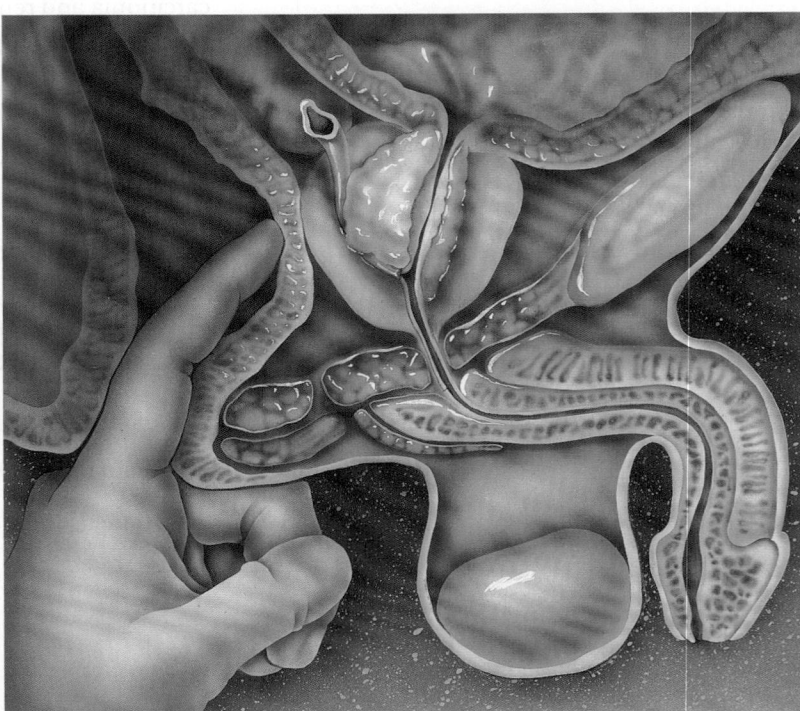

Figure 20-15 Digital rectal exam. A digital rectal exam is very useful in detecting early signs of prostatic enlargement.

testicular cancer
The testes are egg-shaped glands inside the scrotum that make sperm and male sex hormones. Malignant cells that form in one or both testes are termed **testicular cancer**. This form of cancer typically affects young or middle-aged men. There are two main types: seminomas and nonseminomas.

- **Seminomas**, cancers of the testes seen in young adult males, grow slowly and respond to radiation therapy. Seminomas may spread to the lungs, bones, liver, or brain.

- A group of testicular cancers that begin in the germ cells that give rise to sperm are called **nonseminomas**. Nonseminomas grow more quickly than seminomas.

The estimated new cases of testicular cancer in the United States in 2010 were 8,480 and the deaths were expected to number 350. Signs and symptoms include a lump or swelling in either testicle, a dull ache in the abdomen or groin, and pain or discomfort in the testicle or scrotum.

A **serum tumor marker test** is a procedure in which a sample of blood is examined to measure three **tumor markers** (substances released by malignant cells): alpha-fetoprotein (AFP), beta-human chorionic gonadotropin (β-hCG), and lactate dehydrogenase (LDH). It is used to confirm a diagnosis. Testicular cancer is treated by surgery, radiation therapy, and chemotherapy.

breast cancer
Breast cancer is a disease in which malignant cells form in the tissues of the breast. It usually forms in the ducts (tubes that transport milk to the nipple) and lobules (glands that produce milk). Breast cancer affects both men and women, but male breast cancer is rare. Cancer rates for breast, ovarian, uterine, and cervical cancers are shown in **Table 20-7**. Familial clustering of breast cancer has long been recognized. About 5% of all breast cancers are due to mutations in two genes: *BRCA1* and *BRCA2*. *BRCA1* and *BRCA2* are tumor suppressor genes located on chromosomes 17 and 13, respectively. These genes help repair damaged DNA. Individuals who are carriers of mutations in *BRCA1* and *BRCA2* have an increased risk of developing both breast and ovarian cancer. Risk factors for developing breast cancer include older age, menstruating at an early age, never having given birth, or hereditary (5% to 10% of all breast cancer cases). Early-stage breast cancer generally has no symptoms. Signs include breast tenderness, an abnormal lump felt when palpating breast tissue, discharge from the nipple, and breast tissue that appears different from any other area on either breast.

T A B L E 20-7

Type	FEMALE REPRODUCTIVE SYSTEM CANCERS	
	2010 Estimated New Cases	**2010 Estimated Deaths**
breast	207,090 (female)	39,840 (female)
	1,970 (male)	390 (male)
cervical	12,200	4,210
ovarian	21,880	13,850
uterine	43,470	7,950

Tests used to detect breast cancer include mammogram, ultrasound, biopsy, estrogen and progesterone receptor test, and MRI. A **mammogram** is an x-ray of the breast. The **estrogen and progesterone receptor test** is a lab test to determine if cancer cells have receptors for the hormones estrogen and progesterone. If the cancerous cells have estrogen or progesterone receptors, they may require estrogen or progesterone to grow. Once this is known, the clinician can determine whether or not hormone therapy may be used as an effective treatment.

Standard treatments are surgery, radiation therapy, chemotherapy, hormone therapy, and targeted therapy. Surgical options include:

- **Lumpectomy**: removal of the tumor and a small amount of normal tissue surrounding the tumor
- **Partial mastectomy**: removal of part of the cancerous breast and some normal tissue surrounding the tumor
- **Total mastectomy**: removal of the entire cancerous breast
- **Modified radical mastectomy**: removal of the entire cancerous breast, surrounding lymph nodes, lining over the chest muscles, and some chest wall muscles
- **Radical mastectomy**: removal of the cancerous breast, chest wall muscles under the breast, and all the lymph nodes under the arm. At one time, radical mastectomy was the standard treatment for breast cancer, but it is rarely used today. A radical mastectomy is only considered if the tumor has spread to chest muscles. A radical mastectomy is also called a **Halsted radical mastectomy**, named for Dr. William Halsted, who pioneered the procedure. When used within the context of medicine, *radical* means treatment by extreme or drastic measures as opposed to conservative measures, as in a lumpectomy.

In **targeted therapy** drugs such as monoclonal antibodies are used to attack specific cancer cells without harming normal tissue. There are fewer side effects associated with targeted therapy than with other forms of treatment.

IN THE NEWS: Cancer-Sniffing Canines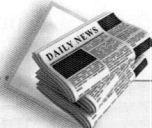

Cancer-sniffing dogs have shown promise in detecting cancer in humans. It appears as though dogs can smell cancerous proteins circulating in the bloodstream of people who have cancer. Research has demonstrated that specially trained dogs can detect lung cancer 99% of the time and breast cancer 88% of the time simply by smelling human exhaled breath. Researchers surmised that the canines are detecting metabolic waste from the tumor cells, which is chemically different from that of normal body cells.

The scenting ability of a dog's nose has detection thresholds as low as parts per trillion. Case reports appeared in the scientific literature as early as 1989, and recent studies have shown that dogs were able to detect melanoma and bladder cancer—all through the use of scent. Dogs correctly identified bladder cancer 41% of the time simply by sniffing the urine. Dr. Armand Cognetta of Tallahassee, Florida, is an expert in melanomas and trained dogs to detect melanoma. One particular dog, George, was able to detect melanoma 99% of the time, and was able to distinguish malignant melanoma from benign lesions. Although more research is needed, canines are showing great promise as a noninvasive technique for detecting some cancers.

ovarian cancer   The ovaries are a pair of female reproductive organs that function in egg cell production. **Ovarian cancer** occurs when malignant cells form in ovarian tissues. There are two types of ovarian cancer: ovarian epithelial carcinoma and malignant germ cell tumors. **Ovarian epithelial carcinoma** begins in the cells on the ovarian surface. Cancer that begins in egg cells is termed **malignant germ cell tumors**. Women with a familial history of ovarian cancer are at an increased risk of developing the disease.

Pelvic exam, ultrasound, and a CA-125 assay are used to detect ovarian cancer. CA-125 is a cancer antigen (tumor marker), and the **CA-125 assay** is a test that measures the level of CA-125 in the bloodstream. Elevated CA-125 levels are associated with ovarian cancer development. Treatments include surgery, radiation therapy, and chemotherapy.

uterine cancer   The uterus is a small, hollow, pear-shaped organ located in the pelvis. Cancer that forms in the tissues of the uterus is called **uterine cancer**. There are two types of uterine cancer: **endometrial cancer**, which begins in cells lining the uterus (endometrium), and **uterine sarcoma**, a rare cancer that begins in the myometrium (uterine muscle). Going further, there are two types of uterine sarcoma, **leiomyosarcoma** (cancer that begins in uterine smooth muscle cells) and **endometrial stromal sarcoma** (cancer that begins in connective tissue cells). Most uterine cancers begin in the cells that make and release mucus. Risk factors include taking the drug tamoxifen for breast cancer or taking estrogen alone without progesterone. Signs and symptoms are bleeding not related to menstruation, pain during sexual intercourse, and pain in the pelvic area.

Endometrial biopsy is used to detect endometrial cancer. Three types of standard treatment are used: surgery, radiation therapy, and hormone therapy. Surgical procedures include:

- **Total hysterectomy**: removal of the entire uterus and cervix
- **Total hysterectomy with salpingo-oophorectomy**: removal of uterus, cervix, uterine tube and ovary or removal of uterus, both uterine tubes, and ovaries
- **Radical hysterectomy**: removal of uterus, cervix, both uterine tubes, both ovaries, and a section of the vagina.

cervical cancer   The cervix is the organ connecting the uterus and vagina. **Cervical cancer** is a disease in which malignant cells form in the tissues of the cervix. It is usually slow growing and is detected by a **Pap test** (also called a **Pap smear**), a procedure in which cells are scraped from the cervix and viewed under a microscope to look for abnormalities. Nearly all cases of cervical cancer are caused by human papillomavirus (HPV) infection. There are usually no signs or symptoms but when present may include pelvic pain and unusual vaginal discharge. Cervical cancer is normally treated by **conization,** a procedure in which a cone-shaped tissue from the cervix is removed (**Figure 20-16**).

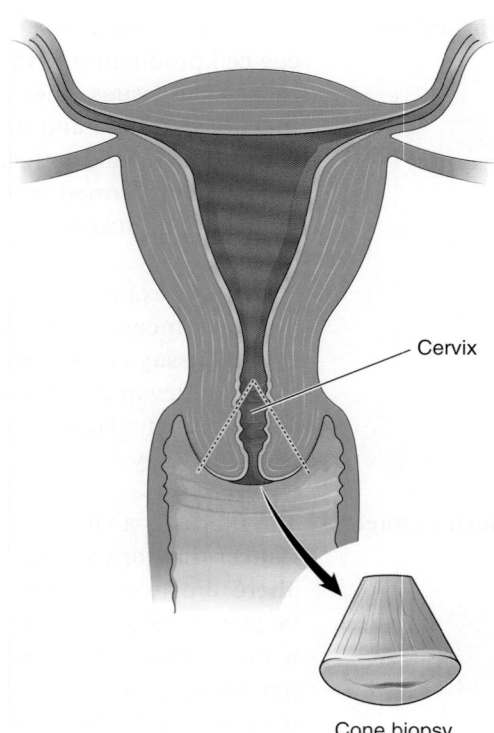

Cervix

Cone biopsy

Figure 20-16 Conization. Cone biopsy of the uterine cervix.

KEY TERM	Definition
prostate cancer (PROS-tayt KAN-ser)	cancer that forms in the tissues of the prostate gland
digital rectal exam (DRE) (DIH-jih-tul REK-tul)	an examination in which the health care provider inserts a lubricated, gloved finger into the rectum to feel for abnormalities
prostate-specific antigen (PSA) test (PROS-tayt-speh-SIH-fik AN-tih-jen)	a blood test that measures the level of prostate-specific antigen, a substance produced by the prostate; elevated levels of PSA may be a sign of cancer
transrectal ultrasound (tranz-REK-tul UL-truh-sound)	a procedure in which a probe that sends out high-energy sound waves is inserted into the rectum to look for abnormalities in the rectum and prostate
watchful waiting	closely watching a patient's condition but not giving treatment unless symptoms appear or change
testicular cancer	malignant cells that form in one or both testes
seminomas (seh-mih-NOH-muhz)	type of cancer of the testicles seen in young adult males that responds well to therapy
nonseminomas (non-seh-mih-NOH-muhz)	group of testicular cancers that begin in the germ cells that give rise to sperm
serum tumor marker (SEER-um TOO-mer MARK-er) **test**	a blood test that measures the amount of substances called tumor markers, which are released into the blood by tumor cells
tumor markers (TOO-mer MARK-erz)	substances released by malignant cells
breast cancer (BREST KAN-ser)	cancer that forms in breast tissue
mammogram (MAM-oh-gram)	an x-ray of the breast
estrogen and progesterone receptor (ES-truh-jin and proh-JES-ter-one ree-SEP-ter) **test**	a lab test to determine if cancer cells have estrogen and progesterone receptors

continued

continued from page 1124

KEY TERM	Definition
lumpectomy (lump-EK-toh-mee)	surgery to remove abnormal breast tissue and a small amount of normal tissue around it
partial mastectomy (PAR-shul ma-STEK-toh-mee)	removal of part of the cancerous breast and some normal tissue surrounding the tumor
total mastectomy (TOH-tul ma-STEK-toh-mee)	removal of the entire cancerous breast
modified radical mastectomy (mah-dih-FIDE RAD-ih-kul ma-STEK-toh-mee)	removal of the entire cancerous breast, surrounding lymph nodes, lining over the chest muscles, and some chest wall muscles
radical mastectomy (RAD-ih-kul ma-STEK-toh-mee)	removal of the entire cancerous breast, chest wall muscles under the breast, and all the lymph nodes under the arm; also called Halsted radical mastectomy
Halsted radical mastectomy (HAWL-sted RAD-ih-kul ma-STEK-toh-mee)	removal of the entire cancerous breast, chest wall muscles under the breast, and all the lymph nodes under the arm; also called radical mastectomy
targeted therapy (TAR-geh-ted THAYR-uh-pee)	treatment that uses drugs to attack specific cancer cells
ovarian cancer (oh-VAYR-ee-un KAN-ser)	cancer that forms in the tissues of the ovary
ovarian epithelial carcinoma (oh-VAYR-ee-un eh-pih-THEE-lee-ul kar-sih-NOH-muh)	cancer that occurs in the cells on the surface of the ovary
malignant germ cell tumors (muh-LIG-nunt)	cancer that begins in egg cells
CA-125 assay	test used to check the levels of the cancer antigen CA-125 in the blood
uterine cancer (YOO-teh-rin KAN-ser)	cancer that forms in the uterus
endometrial cancer (en-doh-MEE-tree-ul KAN-ser)	cancer that forms in the cells lining the uterus (endometrium)
uterine sarcoma (YOO-teh-rin sar-KOH-muh)	rare type of uterine cancer that forms in the uterine muscle (myometrium)
leiomyosarcoma (lye-oh-my-oh-sar-KOH-muh)	cancer that begins in uterine smooth muscle cells
endometrial stromal sarcoma (en-doh-MEE-tree-ul STROH-mul sar-KOH-muh)	cancer that begins in uterine connective tissue cells
total hysterectomy (TOH-tul his-teh-REK-toh-mee)	surgery to remove the entire uterus, including the cervix
total hysterectomy with salpingo-oophorectomy (TOH-tul his-teh-REK-toh-mee with sal-pin-goh-oh-oh-foh-REK-toh-mee)	surgery to remove the entire uterus, cervix, uterine tubes, and ovaries
radical hysterectomy (RAD-ih-kul his-teh-REK-toh-mee)	surgery to remove the uterus, cervix, uterine tubes, ovaries, and part of the vagina
cervical cancer (SER-vih-kul KAN-ser)	cancer that forms in tissues of the cervix
Pap test	procedure in which cells are scraped from the cervix for examination under a microscope; also called a Pap smear
Pap smear	procedure in which cells are scraped from the cervix for examination under a microscope; also called a Pap test
conization (ko-nih-ZAY-shun)	surgery to remove a cone-shaped piece of tissue from the cervix

continued

continued from page 1125

KEY TERM PRACTICE: *Reproductive System Cancers*

1. A slow-growing testicular cancer that develops in young male adults and responds to radiation therapy is termed a _____.

2. What test measures the presence of estrogen and progesterone receptors in breast cancer tissue?
_____

3. Removal of the entire cancerous breast is known as a _____.

4. Treatment that uses drugs to attack specific cancer cells is called _____.

5. Name two general types of uterine cancer. _____.

LIFE SPAN

The charge of the National Cancer Institute is to control cancer. The NCI is the U.S. government's principal agency for cancer research, and it provides accurate, up-to-date, comprehensive cancer information. Many individuals who develop cancer might be spared if information about how to prevent and detect the disease were made available to all and treatment protocols were adopted. In fact, lifestyle and environmental influences are responsible for the majority of cancer cases.

There are links between aging and cancer. As we age, there is greater risk, poorer prognosis, and poorer surgical outcomes related to cancer. A recent study found an association between leukocyte (white blood cell) telomere length and cancer. Telomeres are regions of DNA at the end of a chromosome that protect the start of the genetic coding sequence against shortening during successive replications. Telomere length gets shorter with each cell division, that is, with time and age. This study showed that the shorter the leukocyte telomere length, the greater the risk of cancer and death. The new rate of cancer incidence was independent of standard cancer risk factors.

Some research has shown that body fatness at young ages may be related to breast cancer risk throughout life. Obesity increases postmenopausal women's risk of developing colon cancer. Furthermore, obesity may increase the risk of postmenopausal women dying from colon cancer.

Cancer occurs in all ages, but growing older may be the greatest carcinogen after age 65. Sixty percent of new cancer cases and two-thirds of cancer deaths occur in persons 65 years and older. The good news is that the incidence of many cancers levels off after age 80.

COMMON Abbreviations

Abbreviation	Term
AFP	alpha-fetoprotein
ALL	acute lymphoblastic leukemia; acute lymphocytic leukemia
AML	acute myeloid leukemia
β-hCG	beta-human chorionic gonadotropin
Bx	biopsy
CA	cancer
CIS	carcinoma in situ
CLL	chronic lymphocytic leukemia
CML	chronic myeloid leukemia
DRE	digital rectal exam
FOBT	fecal occult blood test
G	grading
HPV	human papillomavirus
IVP	intravenous pyelogram
LDH	lactate dehydrogenase
M	metastasis
N	nodal involvement
NCI	National Cancer Institute
NHL	non-Hodgkin lymphoma
Pap test, Pap smear	Papanicolaou test, Papanicolaou smear
PDT	photodynamic therapy
PNET	primitive neuroectodermal tumor
PSA	prostate-specific antigen
RTx	radiation therapy
T	tumor
TNM	tumor, nodes, metastasis

COMMON ABBREVIATIONS EXERCISES

1. CML is the abbreviation for _____.

2. Write the abbreviation for primitive neuroectodermal tumor._____

3. Write the term for TNM._____

4. When discussing cancer, the abbreviation G refers to _____.

5. Write the term for CIS._____

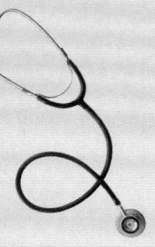

Case Study

Jackie works closely with a thoracic and vascular surgeon. As a team, they see patients routinely and discuss clinical care. Mrs. Eleanor presented in Jackie's office after being referred by her family physician. This patient is a 54-year-old female in good health, who is an active cyclist. During a routine self-breast exam, she discovered a lump in her right breast. She presented in her primary care physician's office with no other signs or symptoms beyond the lump in her right breast, which she estimated had been there approximately 1 month.

Her social history indicates that she is married with three teenage daughters. She is self-employed. With respect to alcohol use, she reports that she consumes about three alcoholic beverages per month.

The medical history indicates that she had her first menses at age 12. Her height is 5'9" and weight is 200 pounds. Blood pressure is 90/60. The last mammogram was 10 years ago.

A mammogram and ultrasound with guided biopsy were performed. The results showed two ill-defined shadowing areas in close proximity within the right upper-outer breast. The patient's pathology results show both invasive carcinoma and ductal carcinoma in situ. Surgical intervention was recommended.

Case Study Questions

1. What are common signs and symptoms of breast cancer?

_____

_____

_____

_____

2. Based on information provided in this chapter, which risk factor for breast cancer does Mrs. Eleanor exhibit?

_____

_____

_____

_____

3. Define mammogram.

_____

_____

_____

_____

4. Define invasive carcinoma.

_____

_____

_____

_____

5. Define ductal carcinoma in situ.

_____

_____

_____

_____

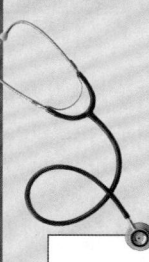

Real World Report

A lumpectomy was performed on Mrs. Eleanor and the pathology surgical report follows.

Pathological Diagnosis

Breast, right, core biopsy:
  Invasive ductal carcinoma, nuclear grade 2
  Ductal carcinoma in situ in association with tumor

Supplemental Report

Hormone receptor studies are performed on the right breast core biopsy specimen, showing invasive ductal carcinoma.
Estrogen receptor: 95% nuclear staining (positive)
Progesterone receptor: 70% nuclear staining (positive)
Scoring System:
  0% nuclear staining = negative
  1–5% nuclear staining = borderline positive
  >5% nuclear staining = positive

Real World Report Questions

The following exercises review the medical terms used in the preceding medical report.

1. Define core biopsy.

_____

_____

_____

_____

2. What is a grade 2 tumor?

_____

_____

_____

_____

3. Define the estrogen and progesterone receptor test.

_____

_____

_____

_____

Review and Application

Multiple-Choice Questions

Select the best answer to each of the following questions.

1. The ABCDEs of skin cancer are _____.
   a. Aggressive, Benign, Cancerous, Deadly, and Elongated
   b. Asymmetry, Border, Color, Diameter, and Elevation
   c. Apoptosis, Black, Caution, Differentiation, and Epithelium
   d. Acute, Basal, Cells, Deep, Excisional

2. This type of tissue forms a thin protective layer on exposed body surfaces and lines body cavities and blood vessels and forms glands. _____
   a. epidermal tissue
   b. subcutaneal tissue
   c. connective tissue
   d. epithelial tissue

3. _____ is the presence of disease or illness.
   a. Morbidity
   b. Five-year survival
   c. Proliferation
   d. Apoptosis

4. The main function of _____ is to support, bind, or separate other tissues.
   a. neuroglia
   b. muscles tissue
   c. nervous tissue
   d. connective tissue

5. Cancer that forms in the flat cells that form the skin surface is called _____.
   a. basal cell carcinoma
   b. melanoma
   c. squamous cell carcinoma
   d. basal cell sarcoma

6. The network of support tissue and fibers that nourishes nerve cells in the brain and spinal cord is referred to as _____.
   a. neurons
   b. glioma
   c. glial cells
   d. neuroblastoma

7. A/an _____ biopsy involves the removal of part of a growth, while a/an _____ biopsy involves the removal of an entire growth in addition to some surrounding tissue.
   a. punch; shave
   b. shave; punch
   c. incisional; excisional
   d. excisional; incisional

8. _____ is a therapy that uses a chemical along with a laser to kill cancer cells.
   a. Radiotherapy
   b. Topical chemotherapy
   c. Photodynamic therapy
   d. Radiation

9. Substances released by malignant cells are termed _____.
   a. carcinogens
   b. tumor markers
   c. dysplasia
   d. indolent

10. This type of tumor is found in the brainstem and may grow rapidly or slowly. _____
    a. brain cell glioma
    b. cardiac
    c. ependymoma
    d. brainstem glioma

11. _____ is characterized by too many immature lymphocytes in the blood, bone marrow, and/or lymph nodes. _____ is characterized by too many white blood cells being made in the bone marrow.
    a. Chronic lymphocytic leukemia; Chronic myeloid leukemia
    b. Chronic myeloid leukemia; Chronic lymphocytic leukemia
    c. Hairy cell leukemia; Acute myeloid leukemia
    d. Acute myeloid leukemia; Hairy cell leukemia

12. Special laboratory-made proteins that bind to tumor cells are called _____
    a. amino acids
    b. oncogenes
    c. monoclonal antibodies
    d. glucose

13. The levels of this substance, which is produced in the prostate gland, are higher in men who have prostate cancer. _____
    a. semen
    b. prostate-specific antigen
    c. serum
    d. sperm

14. In this treatment, treatment is withheld, and the patient is closely monitored until symptoms appear or change. _____

    a. watchful waiting   b. wishful waiting   c. targeted therapy   d. biological therapy

15. A/an _____ biopsy technique involves shearing off the abnormal growth in layers.

    a. punch   b. shave   c. excisional   d. incisional

16. In this procedure, healthy skin is taken from one part of the body and used to replace lost or damaged skin in another location. _____

    a. skin graft   b. topical chemotherapy   c. Mohs surgery   d. excisional skin surgery

17. This kind of biopsy uses a computer and a three-dimensional scanning device to find a tumor and guide the removal of tissue for microscopic examination. _____

    a. punch   b. incisional   c. core   d. stereotactic

18. A group of testicular cancers that begins in the germ cells that give rise to sperm are called _____.

    a. super seminomas   b. seminomas   c. nonseminomas   d. super nonseminomas

19. In this procedure, a sample of blood is examined to measure three tumor markers: alpha-fetoprotein, beta-human chorionic gonadotropin, and lactate dehydrogenase. _____

    a. prostate-specific antigen test   b. transrectal ultrasound   c. serum tumor marker test   d. mammogram

20. Which of the following is a surgical option to treat breast cancer? _____

    a. lumpectomy   b. hysterectomy   c. Mohs surgery   d. mammogram

21. The uterine sarcoma that begins in connective tissue cells is called _____.

    a. leiomyosarcoma   b. endometrial stromal sarcoma   c. myometrium   d. endometrial cancer

22. The type of ovarian cancer that begins in egg cells is _____, while the type of ovarian cancer that begins in cells on the ovarian surface is _____.

    a. ovarian epithelial carcinoma; benign germ cell tumor   b. benign germ cell tumor; malignant germ cell tumor   c. malignant germ cell tumor; ovarian epithelial carcinoma   d. ovarian endothelial carcinoma; ovarian epithelial carcinoma

23. The type of hysterectomy where the uterus, cervix, both uterine tubes, both ovaries, and a section of the vagina are removed is called _____.

    a. total hysterectomy   b. total hysterectomy with salpingo-oophorectomy   c. radical hysterectomy   d. partial hysterectomy

24. The most common type of astrocytoma in children is _____, a slow-growing tumor derived from glial cells in the brain and spinal cord.

    a. brain cell glioma   b. neuroblastoma   c. ependymoma   d. juvenile pilocytic astrocytoma

25. _____ is a lung cancer in which the cells are large and look abnormal when viewed under a microscope.

    a. Large cell carcinoma   b. Squamous cell carcinoma   c. Adenocarcinoma   d. Small cell lung cancer

Word Parts Exercises

Using the following word parts, form a medical term for each definition. Each word part is used only once.

melan- neo-   onco-   hyster-
-logy   -oma   -plasm -ectomy

26. the study of tumors _____

27. black tumors _____

28. new formation _____

29. removal of the uterus _____

Matching Exercises

Match the disorder with its description.

_____ 30. grade I or grade II astrocytoma

_____ 31. basal cell carcinoma

_____ 32. Ewing sarcoma

_____ 33. hairy cell leukemia

_____ 34. acute lymphocytic leukemia

a. fast-growing type of blood cancer in which too many immature white blood cells appear in blood and bone marrow
b. slow-growing, invasive, nonmetastasizing neoplasm located in the epidermis
c. a type of cancer that forms in bone or soft tissue
d. a low-grade tumor that occurs anywhere in the brain
e. a type of leukemia in which abnormal B lymphocytes are present in the bone marrow, spleen, and peripheral blood

Match the sign or symptom with its description.

_____ 35. hyperplasia

_____ 36. invasive

_____ 37. dedifferentiation

_____ 38. indolent

a. loss of structural differentiation; reversion to a simpler or less differentiated form
b. abnormal growth caused by excessive multiplication of cells
c. a type of cancer that grows slowly
d. growing aggressively

Match the clinical test with its description.

_____ 39. colonoscopy

_____ 40. transrectal ultrasound

_____ 41. CA-125

_____ 42. Pap smear

_____ 43. peripheral blood smear

a. test used to check the levels of cancer antigen in the blood
b. examination of the inside of the colon using a colonoscope
c. procedure in which cells are scraped from the cervix for examination under a microscope
d. procedure in which a sample of blood is viewed under a microscope to count different circulating blood cells and to see whether the cells look normal
e. procedure in which a probe that sends out high-energy sound waves is inserted into the rectum to look for abnormalities in the rectum and prostate

Match the treatment with its description.

_____ 44. laser surgery

_____ 45. electrodesiccation and curettage

_____ 46. conization

_____ 47. Halsted radical mastectomy

_____ 48. total hysterectomy with salpingo-oophorectomy

_____ 49. Mohs surgery

a. surgery to remove a cone-shaped piece of tissue from the cervix
b. destruction of tumor by electric current
c. removal of the entire cancerous breast, chest wall muscles under the breast, and all the lymph nodes under the arm
d. technique for removing skin tumors in which fixed sections of tissue are removed in thin layers and examined until all the tumor has been removed
e. surgery to remove the entire uterus, cervix, uterine tubes, and ovaries
f. surgery using a focused beam of light to destroy cancer cells

Definitions

Define the following terms.

50. five-year survival rate _____

51. mortality _____

52. oligodendroglioma _____

53. opportunistic disease _____

54. proliferation _____

Alternate Terms

Give an alternative term for each of the following terms.

55. nerve cell _____

56. glial cell _____

57. neural tissue _____

58. kidney cancer _____

Spelling

Identify the correctly spelled word in each set.

59. _____
   a. apendymoma
   b. epandymoma
   c. ependymoma
   d. ependimoma

60. _____
   a. apoptosis
   b. appoptosis
   c. ippoptosis
   d. apoptsis

61. _____
   a. liomyosarkoma
   b. leimyosarcoma
   c. leiomysarcoma
   d. leiomyosarcoma

62. _____
   a. oncolojist
   b. oncologist
   c. onclogist
   d. oncollogist

63. _____
   a. apithelium
   b. epithelium
   c. epitheliem
   d. eppithelium

Unscramble

Unscramble the letters to form a medical term.

64. nuatimot _____

67. ammmmorag _____

65. grinam _____

68. threapiodrady _____

66. stomur _____

Abbreviations

Provide the terms for the abbreviations and then define the terms.

69. ALL = _____

70. CA = _____

71. DRE = _____

72. Pap test = _____

73. RTx = _____

74. FNA biopsy = _____

Short Answer

Answer the following questions.

75. List five risk factors for cancer. _____

76. Describe the difference between a partial mastectomy, a modified radical mastectomy, and a radical mastectomy.

_____

77. Austin has skin cancer that covers his entire back. His wife believes excisional skin surgery is the best way to treat his cancer. Austin thinks that topical chemotherapy might be a better option. Who is right and why?

_____

Word Search

E	B	U	J	N	E	Q	K	L	B
Z	T	A	T	Y	R	I	A	A	R
I	U	A	Z	E	D	P	R	C	E
I	X	S	T	N	R	E	M	I	A
T	T	Y	E	S	D	I	T	V	S
J	Z	Y	I	D	O	T	N	R	T
E	J	B	A	F	A	R	C	E	B
R	N	L	J	M	B	X	P	C	Z
I	B	N	O	V	A	R	I	A	N
R	O	N	T	W	O	Z	F	C	B

bladder
breast
cervical
kidney
ovarian
prostate
uterine

Vocabulary Review

Review the key terms from this chapter, study the spelling and pronunciation of each term, and write its definition in the space provided. Listen to the audio available for most terms at http://thepoint.lww.com/nath2e and pronounce each term for yourself. Then check the box when you feel confident that you know the definition and can pronounce the term correctly.

Key Term	Pronunciation	Definition
☐ **ABCDEs of skin cancer**		_____
☐ **acute lymphoblastic leukemia**	(uh-KYOOT lim-foh-BLAS-tik loo-KEE-mee-uh)	_____
☐ **acute lymphocytic leukemia**	(uh-KYOOT lim-foh-SIH-tik loo-KEE-mee-uh)	_____
☐ **acute myeloid leukemia (AML)**	(uh-KYOOT MYE-eh-loyd loo-KEE-mee-uh)	_____
☐ **adenocarcinoma**	(a-den-oh-kar-sih-NOH-muh)	_____

Key Term	Pronunciation	Definition
❑ adrenocortical carcinoma	(uh-dree-noh-KOR-tih-kul kar-sih-NOH-muh)	_____
❑ aggressive		_____
❑ anaplasia	(an-uh-PLAY-zee-uh)	_____
❑ apoptosis	(a-pop-TOH-sis)	_____
❑ astrocytoma	(as-troh-sigh-TOH-muh)	_____
❑ basal cell carcinoma	(BAY-sul SELL kar-sih-NOH-muh)	_____
❑ benign	(beh-NINE)	_____
❑ biological therapy	(bye-oh-LOJ-i-kul THAYR-uh-pee)	_____
❑ biopsy	(BYE-op-see)	_____
❑ bladder cancer	(BLA-der KAN-ser)	_____
❑ blast cells		_____
❑ bone marrow aspiration and biopsy	(bone MAYR-oh as-pih-RAY-shun and BYE-op-see)	_____
❑ bone scan		_____
❑ brain tumor	(TOO-mer)	_____
❑ brainstem glioma	(glee-OH-muh)	_____
❑ breast cancer	(BREST KAN-ser)	_____
❑ CA-125 assay		_____
❑ cancer (CA)	(KAN-ser)	_____
❑ carcinogens	(kar-SIN-oh-jinz)	_____
❑ carcinoma in situ (CIS)	(kar-sih-NOH-muh in SIGH-too)	_____
❑ cervical cancer	(SER-vih-kul KAN-ser)	_____
❑ chondrosarcoma	(kon-droh-sar-KOH-muh)	_____
❑ chronic lymphocytic leukemia	(KRAH-nik lim-foh-SIH-tik loo-KEE-mee-uh)	_____
❑ chronic myeloid leukemia	(KRAH-nik MYE-eh-loyd loo-KEE-mee-uh)	_____
❑ colon cancer	(KOH-lun KAN-ser)	_____
❑ colonoscopy	(koh-lun-OS-koh-pee)	_____
❑ conization	(ko-nih-ZAY-shun)	_____
❑ connective tissue		_____
❑ core biopsy	(BYE-op-see)	_____
❑ Crohn disease	(KRONE dih-ZEEZ)	_____
❑ cryosurgery	(KRY-oh-sur-juh-ree)	_____
❑ dedifferentiation	(dee-dih-fur-en-shee-AY-shun)	_____
❑ differentiation	(dih-fur-en-shee-AY-shun)	_____
❑ digital rectal exam (DRE)	(DIH-jih-tul REK-tul)	_____
❑ dysplasia	(dis-PLAY-zhuh)	_____

Key Term	Pronunciation	Definition
❑ electrodesiccation and curettage	(ee-lek-troh-deh-sih-KAY-shun and KUE-ruh-tahzh)	_____
❑ endometrial cancer	(en-doh-MEE-tree-ul KAN-ser)	_____
❑ endometrial stromal sarcoma	(en-doh-MEE-tree-ul STROH-mul sar-KOH-muh)	_____
❑ ependymoma	(eh-pen-dih-MOH-muh)	_____
❑ epithelial tissue	(ep-ih-THEE-lee-ul TISH-yoo)	_____
❑ epithelium	(ep-ih-THEE-lee-um)	_____
❑ estrogen and progesterone receptor test	(ES-truh-jin and proh-JES-ter-one ree-SEP-ter)	_____
❑ Ewing sarcoma	(YOO-ing sar-KOH-muh)	_____
❑ excisional biopsy	(ek-SIH-zhun-ul BYE-op-see)	_____
❑ excisional skin surgery	(ek-SIH-zhun-ul skin SUR-juh-ree)	_____
❑ fecal occult blood test (FOBT)	(FEE-kul uh-KULT)	_____
❑ fine-needle aspiration (FNA) biopsy	(NEE-dul as-pih-RAY-shun BYE-op-see)	_____
❑ five-year survival rate		_____
❑ glial cells	(GLEE-ul SELLS)	_____
❑ grade I or grade II astrocytoma	(as-troh-sigh-TOH-muh)	_____
❑ grading		_____
❑ hairy cell leukemia	(HAYR-ee SELL loo-KEE-mee-uh)	_____
❑ Halsted radical mastectomy	(HAWL-sted RAD-ih-kul ma-STEK-toh-mee)	_____
❑ hematuria	(hee-muh-TOOR-ee-uh)	_____
❑ Hodgkin lymphoma	(HOJ-kin lim-FOH-muh)	_____
❑ hyperplasia	(high-pur-PLAY-zee-uh)	_____
❑ immunophenotyping	(IM-yoo-noh-fee-noh-type-ing)	_____
❑ incisional biopsy	(in-SIH-zhun-ul BYE-op-see)	_____
❑ indolent	(IN-doe-lint)	_____
❑ intravenous pyelogram (IVP)	(in-truh-VEE-nus PYE-el-oh-gram)	_____
❑ invasive	(in-VAY-siv)	_____
❑ juvenile pilocytic astrocytoma	(JOO-veh-nile pye-loh-SIH-tik as-troh-sye-TOH-muh)	_____
❑ Kaposi sarcoma	(kuh-POH-zee sar-KOH-muh)	_____
❑ kidney cancer	(KID-nee KAN-ser)	_____
❑ large cell carcinoma	(SELL kar-sih-NOH-muh)	_____
❑ laser surgery	(LAY-zer SUR-juh-ree)	_____

Key Term	Pronunciation	Definition
❏ leiomyosarcoma	(lye-oh-my-oh-sar-KOH-muh)	_____
❏ leukemia	(loo-KEE-mee-uh)	_____
❏ lumpectomy	(lump-EK-toh-mee)	_____
❏ lymphoma	(lim-FOH-muh)	_____
❏ malignant	(muh-LIG-nunt)	_____
❏ malignant germ cell tumors	(muh-LIG-nunt)	_____
❏ mammogram	(MAM-oh-gram)	_____
❏ margin		_____
❏ medulloblastoma	(med-yoo-loh-blas-TOH-muh)	_____
❏ melanoma	(mel-uh-NOH-muh)	_____
❏ meningioma	(meh-nin-jee-OH-muh)	_____
❏ metaplasia	(met-uh-PLAY-zhuh)	_____
❏ metastasize	(meh-TAS-tuh-size)	_____
❏ mixed tumor		_____
❏ modified radical mastectomy	(mah-dih-FIDE RAD-ih-kul ma-STEK-toh-mee)	_____
❏ Mohs surgery	(MOZE SUR-juh-ree)	_____
❏ monoclonal antibodies	(mah-noh-KLOH-nul AN-tih-bah-dees)	_____
❏ morbidity	(mor-BID-i-tee)	_____
❏ mortality	(mor-TA-lih-tee)	_____
❏ muscle tissue		_____
❏ mutation	(myoo-TAY-shun)	_____
❏ myosarcoma	(migh-oh-sar-KOH-muh)	_____
❏ neoplasms	(NEE-oh-plaz-umz)	_____
❏ nervous tissue		_____
❏ neuroblastoma	(noo-roh-blas-TOH-muh)	_____
❏ neuroglia	(noor-OH-glee-uh)	_____
❏ neurons	(NOOR-onz)	_____
❏ non-Hodgkin lymphoma	(non-HOJ-kin lim-FOH-muh)	_____
❏ nonseminomas	(non-seh-mih-NOH-muhz)	_____
❏ non-small cell lung cancer	(SELL lung KAN-ser)	_____
❏ oligodendroglioma	(oh-lih-goh-den-droh-glee-OH-muh)	_____
❏ oncogenes	(ON-koh-jeenz)	_____
❏ oncologists	(on-KOL-oh-jists)	_____
❏ oncology	(on-KOL-oh-jee)	_____
❏ opportunistic disease	(op-or-too-NIS-tik dih-ZEEZ)	_____
❏ osteosarcoma	(os-tee-oh sar-KOH-muh)	_____

Key Term	Pronunciation	Definition
❏ ovarian cancer	(oh-VAYR-ee-un KAN-ser)	
❏ ovarian epithelial carcinoma	(oh-VAYR-ee-un eh-pih-THEE-lee-ul kar-sih-NOH-muh)	
❏ Pap smear		
❏ Pap test		
❏ parathyroid cancers	(pair-uh-THIGH-royd KAN sers)	
❏ partial mastectomy	(PAR-shul ma-STEK-toh-mee)	
❏ pathologists	(puh-thol-OH-jists)	
❏ peripheral blood smear	(peh-RIH-feh-rul)	
❏ petechiae	(peh-TEH-kee-uh)	
❏ pheochromocytoma	(fee-oh-kroh-moh-sigh-TOH-muh)	
❏ photodynamic therapy (PDT)	(foh-toh-dye-NAM-ick THERR-uh-pee)	
❏ polyps	(PAH-lips)	
❏ primary bone cancer		
❏ proliferation	(proh-lih-fuh-RAY-shun)	
❏ prostate cancer	(PROS-tayt KAN ser)	
❏ prostate-specific antigen (PSA) test	(PROS-tayt-speh-SIH-fik AN-tih-jen)	
❏ punch biopsy	(BYE-op-see)	
❏ radiation therapy (RTx)	(ray-dee-AY-shun THERR-uh-pee)	
❏ radical hysterectomy	(RAD-ih-kul his-teh-REK-toh-mee)	
❏ radical mastectomy	(RAD-ih-kul ma-STEK-toh-mee)	
❏ radiotherapy	(ray-dee-oh-THERR-uh-pee)	
❏ Reed-Sternberg cells		
❏ renal adenocarcinoma	(REE-nul a-den-oh-kar-sih-NOH-muh)	
❏ renal cell carcinoma	(REE-nul SELL kar-sih-NOH-muh)	
❏ rhabdomyosarcoma	(rab-doh-my-oh-sar-KOH-muh)	
❏ risk factors		
❏ secondary bone cancer		
❏ seminomas	(seh-mih-NOH-muhz)	
❏ serum tumor marker test	(SEER-um TOO-mer MARK-er)	
❏ shave biopsy	(BYE-op-see)	
❏ skin grafts		
❏ small cell lung cancer	(SELL lung KAN-ser)	
❏ squamous cell carcinoma	(SKWAY-mus SELL kar-sih-NOH-muh)	
❏ staging		

Key Term	Pronunciation	Definition
❏ **stem cells**		_____
❏ **stereotactic biopsy**	(stayr-ee-oh-TAK-tik BYE-op-see)	_____
❏ **targeted therapy**	(TAR-geh-ted THAYR-uh-pee)	_____
❏ **thoracoscopy**	(thor-uh-KOS-koh-pee)	_____
❏ **thyroid cancer**	(THIGH-royd KAN-ser)	_____
❏ **TNM staging**		_____
❏ **topical chemotherapy**	(TAH-pih-kul KEE-moh-THERR-uh-pee)	_____
❏ **total hysterectomy**	(TOH-tul his-teh-REK-toh-mee)	_____
❏ **total hysterectomy with salpingo-oophorectomy**	(TOH-tul his-teh-REK-toh-mee with sal-pin-goh-oh-oh-foh-REK-toh-mee)	_____
❏ **total mastectomy**	(TOH-tul ma-STEK-toh-mee)	_____
❏ **transitional cell carcinoma**	(tran-ZIH-shuh-nul SELL kar-sih-NOH-muh)	_____
❏ **transrectal ultrasound**	(tranz-REK-tul UL-truh-sound)	_____
❏ **tumor markers**	(TOO-mer MARK-erz)	_____
❏ **tumors**	(TOO-merz)	_____
❏ **ulcerative colitis**	(UL-ser-uh-tiv koh-LIGH-tis)	_____
❏ **uterine cancer**	(YOO-teh-rin KAN-ser)	_____
❏ **uterine sarcoma**	(YOO-teh-rin sar-KOH-muh)	_____
❏ **watchful waiting**		_____

Answers

Word Grouping Exercises

Definition	Word Part	Definition	Word Part
new, recent	neo-	change of position	meta-
bad, difficult	dys-	chemistry	chem-, chemo-
black	melan-, melano-	cold	cry-, cryo-
blood	-emia	disease	path-, -pathic, patho-, -pathy
blood vessel	angi-, angio-	electricity	electro-
bone	ost-, oste-, osteo-	excessive, above normal	hyper-
breast	mast-, masto-	fatty	lip-, lipo-
cancer	carcin, carcino-	fiber	fibr-, fibro-
cartilage	chondro-	formation	-plasia
cell	cyt-, cyto-	gland	aden-, adeno-

Definition	Word Part	Definition	Word Part
lymph, colorless fluid	lymph-, lympho-	rod, rod shaped	rhabd-, rhabdo-
middle, mesentery	mes-, meso-	separated from or derived from	apo-
mucus	myx-, myxo-	smooth	leio-
muscle	myo-	study of	-logy
muscle, flesh	sarco-	to change	-atus
nerve, nervous system	neur-, neuri-, neuro-	tumor	onco-
new, recent	neo-	tumor or neoplasm	-oma
not	ana-	uterus	hyster-, hystero-
poison, toxin	tox-, toxi-, toxico-, toxo-	white	leuk-, leuko-
precursor of	-gen		
removal of an anatomical structure	-ectomy		

Word Building Exercises

Word Part	Meaning	Common or Known Word	Example Medical Term
-emia	blood	anemia	leukemia
angi-, angio-	blood vessel	angiogram	angiogenesis
carcin-, carcino-	cancer	carcinogen	carcinoma
chem-, chemo-	chemistry	chemical	chemotherapy
cry-, cryo-	cell	cryogenics	cryotherapy
-ectomy	removal of an anatomical structure	tonsillectomy	hysterectomy
electro-	electricity	electromagnet	electrodesiccation
hyper-	excessive, above normal	hypertension	hyperplasia
hyster-, hystero-	uterus	hysterectomy	hysterectomy
leuk-, leuko-	white	leukemia	leukemia
lip-, lipo-	fatty	liposuction	lipoma
-logy	study of	biology	oncology
melan-, melano-	black	melanoma	melanoma
neo-	new, recent	neo-Gothic	neoplasm
onco-	tumor	oncology	oncogenes
tox-, toxi-, toxico-, toxo-	poison, toxin	toxic	toxicology

Key Term Practice

Cancer Preview

1. Metastasize
2. neoplasms; tumors
3. Cancer

Causes of Cancer and Cancer Risk Factors

1. malignant
2. carcinogen
3. benign
4. Oncogenes
5. Apoptosis

Staging and Grading of Neoplasms

1. anaplasia; dedifferentiation
2. staging
3. grading
4. stem cells
5. TNM staging

Tissue Changes

1. biopsy
2. Pathologists
3. metaplasia
4. mixed tumor
5. dysplasia

Integumentary System Cancers

1. Squamous cell carcinoma
2. Kaposi sarcoma
3. punch biopsy
4. carcinoma in situ
5. cryosurgery

Skeletal System Cancers

1. primary bone cancer
2. secondary bone cancer
3. Osteosarcoma
4. chondrosarcoma
5. core biopsy

Muscular System Cancers

1. myosarcoma
2. bone scan
3. rhabdomyosarcoma
4. bone marrow aspiration and biopsy

Nervous System Cancers

1. brain tumor
2. neuroblastoma
3. astrocytoma
4. medulloblastoma
5. meningioma

Endocrine System Cancers

1. adrenocortical carcinoma
2. Pheochromocytoma
3. thyroid cancer
4. Parathyroid cancer

Blood Cancers

1. blast cells
2. Acute myeloid leukemia (AML)
3. petechiae
4. leukemia
5. immunophenotyping

Immune System Cancers

1. Hodgkin lymphoma
2. lymphoma
3. Non-Hodgkin lymphoma
4. aggressive
5. Reed-Sternberg cells

Respiratory System Cancers

1. thoracoscopy
2. adenocarcinoma
3. small cell lung cancer
4. non-small cell lung cancer
5. large cell carcinoma

Digestive System Cancers

1. polyps
2. Ulcerative colitis
3. Crohn disease
4. fecal occult blood
5. colon cancer

Urinary System Cancers

1. transitional cell carcinoma
2. Hematuria
3. renal cell carcinoma; kidney cancer; renal adenocarcinoma
4. intravenous pyelogram (IVP)
5. biological therapy

Reproductive System Cancers

1. seminoma
2. estrogen and progesterone receptor test
3. total mastectomy
4. targeted therapy
5. endometrial cancer and uterine sarcoma

Common Abbreviations Exercises

1. CML = chronic myeloid leukemia
2. primitive neuroectodermal tumor = PNET
3. TNM = tumor, nodes, metastasis
4. G = grading
5. CIS = carcinoma in situ

Case Study

1. Breast cancer usually has no symptoms in its early stages. Signs of breast cancer include an abnormal lump in the breast, breast tenderness, discharge from the nipple, and breast tissue that appears different from any other area on either breast.
2. Early onset of menses is a risk factor that Mrs. Eleanor exhibits.
3. A mammogram is an image obtained from x-ray examination of the breast.
4. Invasive carcinoma is a cancer that infiltrates and destroys surrounding tissue.
5. Ductal carcinoma in situ is cancer that is derived from the ducts in the breast and limited to the epithelium.

Real World Report

1. A core biopsy is removal of a sample of tissue with a wide needle for microscopic examination.
2. Tumors assigned a grade 2 (G2) rating are cancers that are moderately differentiated with cells that do not resemble normal cells. G2 cancers grow rapidly and spread quickly.
3. The estrogen and progesterone receptor test is a lab test used to determine if cancer cells have estrogen and progesterone receptors.

Review and Application

1. b	13. b	25. a	37. a
2. d	14. a	26. oncology	38. c
3. a	15. b	27. melanoma	39. b
4. d	16. a	28. neoplasm	40. e
5. c	17. d	29. hysterectomy	41. a
6. c	18. c	30. d	42. c
7. c	19. c	31. b	43. d
8. c	20. a	32. c	44. f
9. b	21. b	33. e	45. b
10. d	22. c	34. a	46. a
11. a	23. c	35. b	47. c
12. c	24. d	36. d	48. e

49. d
50. five-year survival rate = the percentage of patients who are alive 5 years after their disease is diagnosed
51. mortality = number of deaths
52. oligodendroglioma = a rare, slow-growing tumor that begins in oligodendrocytes

53. opportunistic disease = an infection that is not normally serious but can become life threatening when the person has a low level of immunity
54. proliferation = rapid reproduction of cells
55. neuron
56. neuroglia

57. nervous tissue
58. renal adenocarcinoma or renal cell carcinoma
59. c
60. a
61. d
62. b
63. b
64. mutation
65. margin
66. tumors
67. mammogram
68. radiotherapy
69. ALL = acute lymphoblastic leukemia; fast-growing type of blood cancer in which too many immature white blood cells appear in blood and bone marrow
70. CA = cancer; a disease resulting from uncontrolled division of abnormal body cells
71. DRE = digital rectal exam; internal examination of the rectum using gloved fingers
72. Pap test = Papanicolaou test; test used to detect cancer of the cervix or uterus, using cells collected from the cervix
73. RTx = radiation therapy; treatment of disease, especially cancer, using x-rays
74. FNA biopsy = fine-needle aspiration biopsy; removal of tissue or fluid with a thin needle for microscopic examination
75. Age, genes, the immune system, viruses, bacteria, and the environment are risk factors for cancer.
76. A partial mastectomy is the removal of part of a cancerous breast and some normal tissue surrounding the tumor. A modified radical mastectomy is the removal of an entire cancerous breast, surrounding lymph nodes, lining over the chest muscles, and some of the chest wall muscles. A radical mastectomy is the removal of an entire cancerous breast, chest wall muscles under the breast, and all the lymph nodes under the arm.
77. Austin is correct. Excisional skin surgery is a type of surgery using a scalpel to remove small growths and surrounding skin. Topical chemotherapy is used in cases like Austin's where the skin cancer is too large for surgery.

Word Search

E	+	U	+	+	+	+	K	L	B
+	T	+	T	+	+	I	+	A	R
+	+	A	+	E	D	+	R	C	E
I	+	+	T	N	R	E	+	I	A
T	+	+	E	S	D	I	+	V	S
+	+	Y	+	D	O	+	N	R	T
+	+	+	A	+	+	R	+	E	+
+	+	L	+	+	+	+	P	C	+
+	B	+	O	V	A	R	I	A	N
+	+	+	+	+	+	+	+	+	+

bladder
breast
cervical
kidney
ovarian
prostate
uterine

Vocabulary Review

Key Term	Definition	Key Term	Definition
ABCDEs of skin cancer	method used to examine skin area by checking the **a**symmetry, **b**order, **c**olor, **d**iameter, and **e**levation of a mole, freckle, or skin spot	**cancer**	disease resulting from uncontrolled division of abnormal body cells producing malignant tumors
acute lymphoblastic leukemia	fast-growing type of blood cancer in which too many immature white blood cells appear in blood and bone marrow; also called acute lymphocytic leukemia	**carcinogens**	cancer-causing substance
		carcinoma in situ (CIS)	cancer that is confined to the superficial skin layer (epithelium)
		cervical cancer	cancer that forms in tissues of the cervix
acute lymphocytic leukemia	fast-growing type of blood cancer in which too many immature white blood cells appear in blood and bone marrow; also called acute lymphoblastic leukemia	**chondro-sarcoma**	a type of cancer that forms in cartilage
		chronic lymphocytic leukemia	a slow-growing cancer in which too many immature lymphocytes are found in the blood and bone marrow and/or in the lymph nodes
acute myeloid leukemia	fast-growing disease in which too many myeloblasts (immature white blood cells that are not lymphoblasts) are found in the bone marrow and blood	**chronic myeloid leukemia**	a slowly progressing cancer in which too many white blood cells (not lympho-cytes) are made in the bone marrow
adeno-carcinoma	lung cancer that forms in the alveoli	**colon cancer**	cancer that forms in the tissues of the colon
adrenocortical carcinoma	cancer of the adrenal cortex	**colonoscopy**	examination of the inside of the colon using a colonoscope
aggressive	describes a tumor or disease that grows or spreads quickly	**conization**	surgery to remove a cone-shaped piece of tissue from the cervix
anaplasia	loss of structural differentiation; reversion to a simpler or less differenti-ated form; also called dedifferentiation	**connective tissue**	supporting and binding tissue that has cells embedded in an unstructured matrix
apoptosis	programmed cell death	**core biopsy**	removal of a tissue sample with a wide needle for microscopic examination
astrocytoma	tumor that begins in the brain or spinal cord in small, star-shaped cells called astrocytes	**Crohn disease**	chronic inflammation of the gastroint-estinal tract
basal cell carcinoma	slow-growing, invasive, nonmetastasizing neoplasm located in the epidermis	**cryosurgery**	using liquid nitrogen as a freezing agent to destroy tissue
benign	nonmalignant; noncancerous	**dedifferen-tiation**	loss of structural differentiation; rever-sion to a simpler or less differentiated form; also called anaplasia
biological therapy	treatment to boost the ability of the immune system to fight cancer		
biopsy	process of removing tissue for diagnostic examination	**differentiation**	acquiring characteristics or functions different from that of the original cell
bladder cancer	cancer that forms in tissues of the urinary bladder	**digital rectal exam (DRE)**	an examination in which the health care provider inserts a lubricated, gloved finger into the rectum to feel for abnormalities
blast cells	immature, undifferentiated blood cells		
bone marrow aspiration and biopsy	procedure in which a small sample of bone marrow and bone is removed for evaluation using a special needle that is pushed into the bone	**dysplasia**	abnormal tissue development
		electro-desiccation and curettage	destruction of tumor by electric current
bone scan	technique used to create images of bone by injecting the patient with radioactive dye that is taken up by bone tissue	**endometrial cancer**	cancer that forms in the cells lining the uterus (endometrium)
brain tumor	abnormal growth of cells in the brain	**endometrial stromal sarcoma**	cancer that begins in uterine connective tissue cells
brainstem glioma	a tumor located in the brainstem, which is the part of the brain that connects to the spinal cord	**ependymoma**	a type of tumor that begins in the lining of the brain ventricles or spinal cord central canal
breast cancer	cancer that forms in breast tissue		
CA-125 assay	test used to check the levels of cancer antigen in the blood		

Key Term	Definition	Key Term	Definition
epithelial tissue	tissue that forms a thin protective layer on exposed body surfaces and lines body cavities and blood vessels and forms glands; also called epithelium	**intravenous pyelogram (IVP)**	an x-ray image of the kidneys, ureter, and bladder made after a substance that shows up on x-rays is injected into a blood vessel
epithelium	tissue that forms a thin protective layer on exposed body surfaces and lines body cavities and blood vessels and forms glands; also called epithelial tissue	**invasive**	growing aggressively
		juvenile pilocytic astrocytoma	tumor forming from glial cells that usually occurs in children and young adults
estrogen and progesterone receptor test	a lab test to determine if cancer cells have estrogen and progesterone receptors	**Kaposi sarcoma**	cancer of connective tissue that causes purplish-red patches on the skin
Ewing sarcoma	a type of cancer that forms in bone or soft tissue	**kidney cancer**	most common type of urinary system cancer; also called renal cell carcinoma and renal adenocarcinoma
excisional biopsy	removal of entire growth by cutting it out	**large cell carcinoma**	lung cancer in which the cells are large and look abnormal when viewed under a microscope
excisional skin surgery	scalpel removal of growth along with surrounding skin	**laser surgery**	using an intense, narrow beam of light to remove tissue. It is an acronym coined from **l**ight **a**mplification by **s**timulated **e**mission of **r**adiation.
fecal occult blood test (FOBT)	a test to check for blood in the stool		
fine-needle aspiration (FNA) biopsy	removal of tissue or fluid with a thin needle for microscopic examination	**leiomyosarcoma**	cancer that begins in uterine smooth muscle cells
		leukemia	cancer that starts in blood-forming tissues
five-year survival rate	the percentage of people who are alive 5 years after their initial cancer diagnosis	**lumpectomy**	surgery to remove abnormal breast tissue and a small amount of normal tissue around it
glial cells	supporting cells with metabolic functions found in the nervous system; also called neuroglia	**lymphoma**	cancer that begins in immune system cells
grade I or **grade II astrocytoma**	a low-grade tumor that occurs anywhere in the brain	**malignant**	tumor that invades surrounding tissue and may spread to other body parts; cancerous
grading	determining the degree of tumor malignancy	**malignant germ cell tumors**	cancer that begins in egg cells
hairy cell leukemia	a rare type of leukemia in which abnormal B lymphocytes are present in the bone marrow, spleen, and peripheral blood	**mammogram**	an x-ray of the breast
		margin	boundary or edge
		medulloblastoma	a malignant brain tumor that is usually located in the cerebellum and may be implanted on the surfaces of the brainstem and spinal cord
Halsted radical mastectomy	removal of the entire cancerous breast, chest wall muscles under the breast, and all the lymph nodes under the arm; also called radical mastectomy	**melanoma**	malignant neoplasm derived from melanocytes
hematuria	blood in the urine	**meningioma**	a slow-growing tumor that forms in the meninges
Hodgkin lymphoma	cancer of the immune system marked by the presence of Reed-Sternberg cells	**metaplasia**	abnormal transformation from one tissue type into another tissue type
hyperplasia	abnormal growth caused by excessive multiplication of cells	**metastasize**	to spread to other sites
immunophenotyping	process used to identify cells and diagnose specific types of leukemia and lymphoma by comparing the cancer cells to normal immune cells	**mixed tumor**	tumor made up of two or more types of tissue
		modified radical mastectomy	removal of the entire cancerous breast, surrounding lymph nodes, lining over the chest muscles, and some chest wall muscles
incisional biopsy	removal of only a part of a growth by cutting into it	**Mohs surgery**	technique for removing skin tumors in which fixed sections of tissue are removed in thin layers and examined until all the tumor has been removed
indolent	describes a type of cancer that grows slowly		

Key Term	Definition	Key Term	Definition
monoclonal antibodies	proteins made in the laboratory that can bind to tumor cells	partial mastectomy	removal of part of the cancerous breast and some normal tissue surrounding the tumor
morbidity	a diseased state	pathologists	physicians skilled in identifying the nature, origin, progress, and cause of disease
mortality	death		
muscle tissue	tissue that is specialized for contraction and includes skeletal muscle, smooth muscle, and cardiac muscle	peripheral blood smear	procedure in which a sample of blood is viewed under a microscope to count different circulating blood cells and to see whether the cells look normal
mutation	structural change in a gene		
myosarcoma	malignant neoplasm derived from muscle	petechiae	pinpoint, unraised, round red spots under the skin caused by bleeding
neoplasms	abnormal tissue formed from uncontrolled cellular division; also called tumors	pheochromocy-toma	tumor located in the adrenal medulla
nervous tissue	tissue that is specialized for conducting electrical impulses; also called neural tissue	photodynamic therapy (PDT)	a laser-assisted procedure in which the light beam and anticancer chemical are aimed at the tumor to destroy it
neuroblastoma	a malignant tumor of embryonic nerve cells (neuroblasts)	polyps	growths that protrude from the tissue lining the colon
neuroglia	supporting cells with metabolic functions found in the nervous system; also called glial cells	primary bone cancer	cancer that originates in bone cells
neurons	functional nerve cells of the nervous system	proliferation	growth and reproduction of similar cells
		prostate cancer	cancer that forms in the tissues of the prostate gland
non-Hodgkin lymphoma	any of a large group of cancers of lymphocytes	prostate-specific antigen (PSA) test	a blood test that measures the level of prostate-specific antigen, a substance produced by the prostate; elevated levels of PSA may be a sign of cancer
nonseminomas	group of testicular cancers		
non-small cell lung cancer	group of lung cancers named for the kinds of cells found in the cancer and how the cells look under the microscope	punch biopsy	method of removing a small cylinder of tissue using an instrument that pierces the skin
oligodendro-glioma	a rare, slow-growing tumor that begins in oligodendrocytes	radiation therapy (RTx)	treatment with x-rays; also called radiotherapy
oncogenes	genes that can cause a cell to become malignant	radical hysterectomy	surgery to remove the uterus, cervix, uterine tubes, ovaries, and part of the vagina
oncologists	physicians specializing in cancer diagnosis and treatment		
oncology	branch of medicine that deals with the study and treatment of cancer	radical mastectomy	removal of the entire cancerous breast, chest wall muscles under the breast, and all the lymph nodes under the arm; also called Halsted radical mastectomy
opportunistic disease	pathology that results due to lowered resistance of the immune system		
osteosarcoma	cancer of the bone	radiotherapy	treatment with x-rays; also called radiation therapy
ovarian cancer	cancer that forms in the tissues of the ovary	Reed-Sternberg cells	large, transformed pathogenic cells, usually derived from B lymphocytes, that appear in people with Hodgkin lymphoma
ovarian epithe-lial carcinoma	cancer that occurs in the cells on the surface of the ovary		
Pap smear	procedure in which cells are scraped from the cervix for examination under a microscope; also called a Pap test	renal adenocarcinoma	most common type of urinary system cancer; also called renal cell carcinoma and kidney cancer
Pap test	procedure in which cells are scraped from the cervix for examination under a microscope; also called a Pap smear	renal cell carcinoma	most common type of urinary system cancer; also called kidney cancer and renal adenocarcinoma
parathyroid cancers	a rare cancer that forms in one or more of the parathyroid glands	rhabdomyosar-coma	malignant neoplasm derived from skeletal muscle tissue

Key Term	Definition	Key Term	Definition
risk factors	variables associated with an increased risk of disease	**TNM staging**	classification based on characteristics of the **t**umors, **n**odal involvement, and extent of **m**etastatic spread
secondary bone cancer	cancer that originates in one part of the body and metastasizes to bones	**topical chemotherapy**	anticancer drugs applied directly to the skin surface
seminomas	type of cancer of the testicles seen in young adult males that responds well to therapy	**total hysterectomy**	surgery to remove the entire uterus, including the cervix
serum tumor marker test	a blood test that measures the amount of substances called tumor markers, which are released into the blood by tumor cells	**total hysterectomy with salpingo-oophorectomy**	surgery to remove the entire uterus, cervix, uterine tubes, and ovaries
shave biopsy	technique performed with a surgical blade or razor blade to shave off growths layer by layer	**total mastectomy**	removal of the entire cancerous breast
skin grafts	skin transplanted from one part of the body to another	**transitional cell carcinoma**	cancer that forms in transitional cells lining the urinary bladder
small cell lung cancer	aggressive cancer that forms in the lungs	**transrectal ultrasound**	a procedure in which a probe that sends out high-energy sound waves is inserted into the rectum to look for abnormalities in the rectum and prostate
squamous cell carcinoma	malignant neoplasm derived from stratified squamous epithelium	**tumor markers**	substances released by malignant cells
staging	identifying the progression of cancer	**tumors**	abnormal tissue formed from uncontrolled cellular division; also called neoplasms
stem cells	an undifferentiated cell from which specialized cells develop		
stereotactic biopsy	removal of tumor using an apparatus that is attached to the head and is used to localize the precise location of the brain tumor	**ulcerative colitis**	chronic inflammation of the colon that produces ulcers in its lining
		uterine cancer	cancer that forms in the uterus
targeted therapy	treatment that uses drugs to attack specific cancer cells	**uterine sarcoma**	rare type of uterine cancer that forms in the uterine muscle (myometrium)
thoracoscopy	examination of the inside of the chest using a thoracoscope	**watchful waiting**	closely watching a patient's condition but not giving treatment unless symptoms appear or change
thyroid cancer	cancer that affects the thyroid gland		

CHAPTER 21

Gerontology

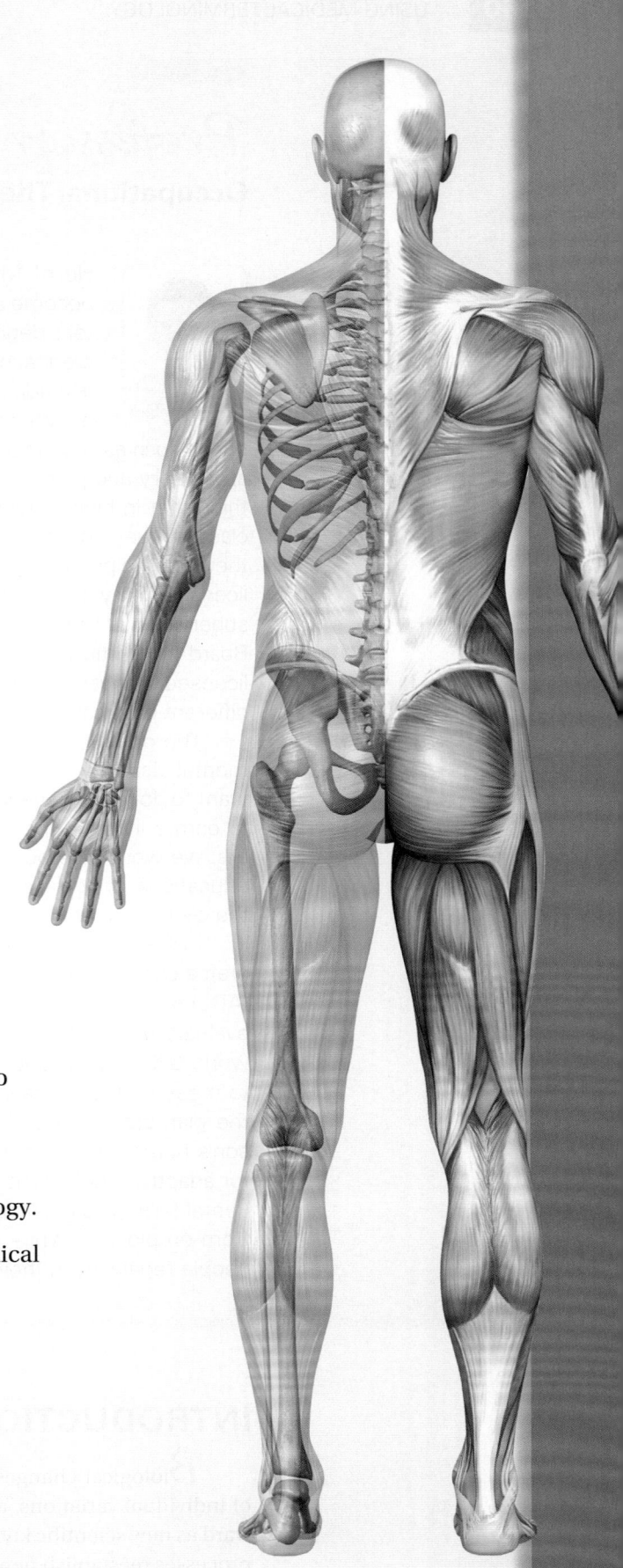

OBJECTIVES

After completing this chapter, you should be able to:

1. Define the meanings of word parts related to gerontology.

2. Name common age-related disorders affecting each body system.

3. Define common signs, symptoms, and treatments of various diseases related to aging.

4. Explain clinical tests and diagnostic procedures related to gerontology.

5. Define common abbreviations related to gerontology.

6. Define terms used in medical reports related to gerontology.

7. Correctly define, spell, and pronounce the chapter's medical terms.

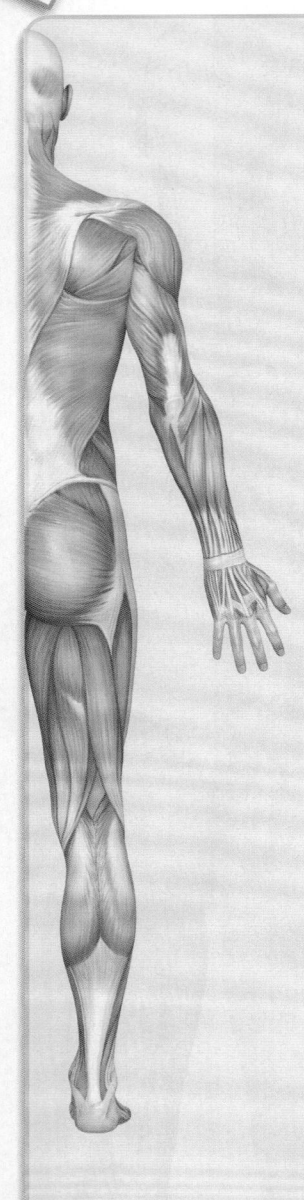

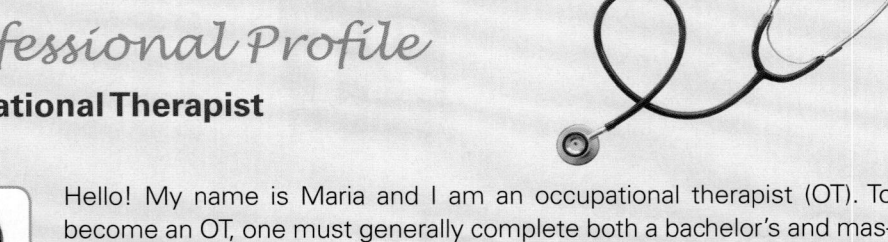

Professional Profile

Occupational Therapist

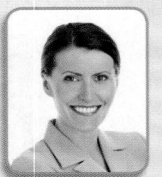

Hello! My name is Maria and I am an occupational therapist (OT). To become an OT, one must generally complete both a bachelor's and master's degree program that is accredited by an organization such as the Accreditation Council for Occupational Therapy Education (ACOTE), which accredits approximately 290 programs. My OT program coursework was heavily concentrated in chemistry, biology, anatomy, and behavioral sciences such as psychology, sociology, and anthropology in addition to occupational therapy theory and practical skills. Because this is a very rigorous program, it was a good thing that in high school I took biology, chemistry, physics, health, and social science classes. They not only provided me with a great foundation for success in college, but they also helped me get accepted into the occupational therapy program. To become licensed in my state, following graduation I had to work for 24 weeks under the direct supervision of licensed OTs and pass the occupational therapy board exam. The National Board for Certification in Occupational Therapy (NBCOT) gives this exam. Once I was licensed, I began working in a private OT practice helping clients of all ages with many different physical or mental problems to live rich and full lives.

The goal of my work is to help people who have experienced some physical or mental disability—whether permanent or temporary—to participate in the things they want to do in their everyday lives. Sometimes I work with clients to find ways for them to earn a living in their chosen field or to find a new line of work for them. For others, we work together to improve their quality of life and allow them to participate in educational or social activities of their choosing. For older people, I create a team with the client and their family to cope with the patient's physical and cognitive changes.

In every case, I make an individual evaluation and set goals for my patient and then draft a customized plan to improve the person's ability to perform activities of daily life (ADL) such as bathing, grooming, climbing stairs, walking, and dental hygiene. I also evaluate instrumental activities of daily life (IADL) such as cooking, shopping, housework, taking medications, and using transportation. Periodically I evaluate outcomes to measure if the goals we set for each client are being met or whether changes to the plan are needed. Evaluations often include a comprehensive report on the person's home, school, and workplace environments with necessary recommendations for adaptive equipment and training in its use or safety. My goals are to reduce accidental falls, give guidance and training to family or caregivers, and obtain cooperation from employers. While I do earn a good salary, the greater reward to me is helping people regain joy in their lives.

INTRODUCTION

*B*iological changes occur in the lifespan of the individual. There are many examples of individual variations, and the limits of a person's lifespan may be shifted forward or backward as new scientific knowledge and discoveries of cellular function and treatment of disease processes reestablish new guidelines. The aging phenomenon, termed *senescence*, begins with birth, as an inherent process, and is followed by infancy, childhood, adolescence, maturity, stabilization of the adult condition (at about age 25), and old age—leading eventually to death. Aging, however, varies with time, degree, physiology, and other factors affecting the individual and, thus, the process may change as we learn more about the course of development. As we find out more about the process, we will be able to alter some of the cellular changes, as well as repair or replace injured or aging tissues and organs.

Gerontology is the scientific study of aging and its effects. Several factors must be considered when studying the aging process. For example, environmental stress from one age period to another and the function, malfunction, and morphology of a single system are to be reviewed. The field recognizes the interrelated systems, such as the cardiovascular and respiratory systems. It is important to think about and assess the role of life history with all its specific biosocial complexities throughout the lifespan. The purpose of this chapter is to introduce you to the emerging study of aging and its terminology.

MEDICAL TERM PARTS

Word Parts

Medical term prefixes, suffixes, and combining forms related to gerontology are introduced in this section.

Word Part	Meaning
ankylo-	bent, crooked, stiff
arteri-, arterio-	artery
arthr-, arthro-	joint, articulation
centi-	hundred
derm-, derma-	skin
gero-, geront-, geronto-	old age
hyper-	above, over
hypo-	deficient, below normal
mort-	death
noct-	night
-ology	study of
-opia	vision
ost-, oste-, osteo-	bone
-penia	deficiency
phaco-	relating to the lens
phot-, photo-	light
presby-, presbyo-	old age
sarco-	muscle
scler-, sclero-	hard
spondyl-, spondylo-	vertebrae
xero-	dry

Word Grouping Exercises

Using the *Medical Term Parts* table, identify the prefix, suffix, or combining form for each of the following definitions. The first one has been done as an example.

Definition	Word Part
above, over	*hyper-*
artery	
bent, crooked, stiff	
bone	
death	
deficiency	
deficient, below normal	
dry	
hard	
hundred	
joint, articulation	
light	
muscle	
night	
old age	*A.*
	B.
relating to the lens	
skin	
study of	
vertebrae	
vision	

Word Building Exercises

Word parts introduced in the *Medical Term Parts* section are listed in the following table. For this exercise, first supply the meaning of each word part, then use the word part to build a word you already know. The word you list under *Common or Known Word* does not have to be a medical term; a commonly used word is fine. Be sure, however, that the word correctly reflects the intended meaning. The first one has been done as an example. Check your answers in a dictionary.

Word Part	Meaning	Common or Known Word	Example Medical Term
arteri-, arterio-	*artery*	*artery*	arterial
arthr-, arthro-			arthralgia
centi-			centimeter
derm-, derma-			dermatology

continued

continued from page 1152

Word Part	Meaning	Common or Known Word	Example Medical Term
gero-, geront-, geronto-			**gerontology**
hyper-			**hyperthermia**
hypo-			**hypoglycemia**
mort-			**mortality**
phot-, photo-			**photocoagulation**
scler-, sclero-			**arteriosclerosis**

FUNDAMENTALS

Aging

Aging is the process of growing old. It is characterized by irreversible changes in structure and function. For example, aging in the cardiovascular system is marked by the replacement of functional cells with fibrous connective tissue. **Gerontology** is the scientific study of the clinical, sociological, biological, and psychological aspects of aging, and a person who specializes in gerontology is known as a **gerontologist**. The branch of medicine concerned with the health care of the elderly (old people) is **geriatrics**. **Senescence** is the term used by biological gerontologists to describe the changes that occur as we age.

Terms closely associated with aging and senescence are longevity, lifespan, and life expectancy. **Longevity** refers to the duration of life beyond the norm for the species, whereas **lifespan** is the normal or average duration of life for members of a given species. The **life expectancy** is the average number of years a person born today can expect to live under current conditions. The latest census data (2010) indicate that life expectancy in the United States varies greatly by region and the average is 77.9 years. Japan has the highest overall life expectancy at 82.6 years, while Swaziland has the lowest at 39.6 years, which is 40% below the world average. The disparity can be attributed to access to health care and the high rates of HIV/AIDS. Worldwide, women tend to outlive men except in Zimbabwe, Lesotho, Swaziland, and Afghanistan.

The longest-lived documented person was Jeanne Calment of France (1875–1997), who died at 122 years and 164 days. At the writing of this text, the current oldest living person is Besse Cooper of the United State, born August 26, 1896 (115 years old). Such individuals, who live to be 100 years old or more, are called **centenarians**.

With respect to health, **morbidity** is the condition of being ill. The morbidity rate is the ratio of sick to well people in a community. **Mortality** refers to death, and the mortality rate is the total number of deaths in a year per 1,000 people. The Centers for Disease Control and Prevention (CDC) publishes a weekly digest, the *Morbidity and Mortality Weekly Report* (MMWR), that gives public health information, recommendations, and epidemiology data. **Epidemiology** is the branch of science that deals with the incidence, distribution, and possible control of diseases and other factors related to health.

As a person ages, the probability of dying doubles every 8 years. The leading cause of death among the elderly is heart disease. According to the CDC, the leading cause of death in the United States is heart disease. The top 10 causes of death in 2009 are listed in **Table 21-1**.

TABLE 21-1

LEADING CAUSES OF DEATH IN THE UNITED STATES, 2009

1. Heart disease
2. Cancer
3. Stroke (cerebrovascular diseases)
4. Chronic lower respiratory diseases
5. Accidents (unintentional injuries)
6. Alzheimer disease (AD)
7. Diabetes
8. Influenza and pneumonia
9. Nephritis, nephrotic syndrome, and nephrosis
10. Septicemia

Turning back the hands of time seems to be a quest for many, because antiaging products flood the market. How and why we age remains one of life's greatest mysteries; however, several theories help to explain aging. Some of these theories are biological, cellular, cognitive, and physiological. Regardless, one goal of all aging people is to retain physical functioning. **Activities of daily living (ADL)** are acts of basic care such as bathing, dressing, going to the bathroom, getting in or out of bed or a chair, walking, and eating. An expansion of the ADL is the **instrumental activities of daily living (IADL)**, which adds tasks to the ADL such as going shopping, preparing meals, managing money, using the telephone, and doing housework.

Another medical area involved with gerontology is occupational therapy. **Occupational therapy (OT)** is a form of therapy for individuals recuperating from physical or mental illness that encourages rehabilitation through the performance of activities required for daily life. An **occupational therapist (OT)** is a person trained to practice occupational therapy. Through the therapeutic use of self-care, work, and recreational activities, people increase independent function, enhance their development, and prevent disability. Occupational therapy may include adapting tasks or changing the living environment to achieve maximum independence and optimal quality of life.

Popular college courses with a gerontology focus include biology and physiology of aging, psychology of aging, social gerontology, and sociology of aging. The field is diverse, because aging encompasses biological and medical aspects as well as cultural, environmental, psychological, and social facets.

KEY TERM	Definition
aging	process of growing old
gerontology (jer-on-TOL-oh-jee)	scientific study of the clinical, sociological, biological, and psychological aspects of aging
gerontologist (jer-on-TOL-oh-jist)	person who specializes in gerontology
geriatrics (jer-ee-AT-riks)	branch of medicine concerned with the health care of the elderly
senescence (seh-NES-ens)	changes that occur with aging
longevity (lon-JEV-ih-tee)	duration of life beyond the norm for the species

continued

continued from page 1154

KEY TERM	Definition
lifespan	normal or average duration of life for members of a given species
life expectancy	average number of years a person born today can expect to live under current conditions
centenarians (sen-ten-AIR-ee-enz)	individuals who live to be 100 years old or more
morbidity (mor-BID-ih-tee)	condition of being ill
mortality (mor-TAL-ih-tee)	refers to death
epidemiology (ep-ih-dee-mee-OL-oh-jee)	branch of science that deals with the incidence, distribution, and possible control of diseases and other factors related to health
activities of daily living (ADL)	acts of basic care such as bathing, dressing, going to the bathroom, getting in or out of bed or a chair, walking, and eating
instrumental activities of daily living (IADL)	activities of daily living plus tasks such as shopping, preparing meals, managing money, using the telephone, and doing housework
occupational therapy (OT)	form of therapy for individuals recuperating from physical or mental illness that encourages rehabilitation through the performance of activities required for daily life
occupational therapist (OT)	person trained to practice occupational therapy

KEY TERM PRACTICE: *Aging*

1. _____ is the condition of being ill.

2. The scientific study of the clinical, sociological, biological, and psychological aspects of aging is termed _____ and is derived from the word part _____ for *old age* and the word part _____ for *study of.*

3. _____ is the branch of science that deals with the incidence, distribution, and possible control of diseases and other factors related to health.

4. Individuals who live to be 100 years old or more are termed _____, derived from the word part _____ for *hundred.*

5. The _____ is the average number of years a person born today can expect to live under current conditions.

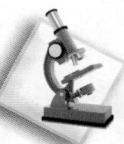

THE CLINICAL DIMENSION

Aging and the Integumentary System

The skin is constantly aging, but the most noticeable effects usually do not occur until after age 40. As the body ages, blood flow to the skin is diminished and the skin tends to thin out and become dry, a condition called xeroderma.

xeroderma   **Xeroderma** is excessive skin dryness (**Figure 21-1**).
In the elderly, the skin is more easily damaged than in younger people and repairs itself more slowly. In addition, the elastic fibers in the dermis

decrease in diameter and number, thicken and clump, resulting in a tendency for the skin to sag and wrinkle. At the cellular level, collagen fibers thicken and stiffen, break apart, and form shapeless, matted tangles. A loss of subcutaneous fat in the hypodermis, most often seen in the face, makes it thinner and results in sagging, wrinkled (permanent infolded) skin. Blood vessels in the dermis become thick walled and less permeable. Other changes are due to years of sun exposure.

photoaging Skin changes called **photoaging** are due to years of sun exposure and include mottled pigmentation, roughened texture, leatherlike appearance in severe cases, wrinkling, extreme furrowing and sagging, and a variety of skin outgrowths (**Figure 21-2**).

skin tag A skin outgrowth is called a **skin tag**, and it hangs from the surface by a thin stalk (**Figure 21-3**).

hypothermia A decrease in subcutaneous fat and a decline in the activity of skin glands result in dry, broken skin that has poor thermoregulatory ability and is susceptible to infection. The elderly are also more sensitive to cold because of the loss of insulating fat and diminished vascular circulation. **Hypothermia**, a body temperature lower than 98.6°F (37°C), as a result of the loss of subcutaneous fat and compromised thermoregulation, is common among the elderly.

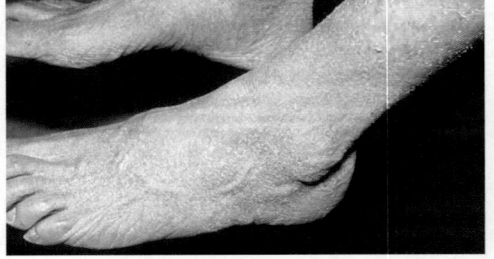

Figure 21-1 Dry skin tends to be most apparent on the hands and lower legs. This elderly patient's legs are dry and scaly.

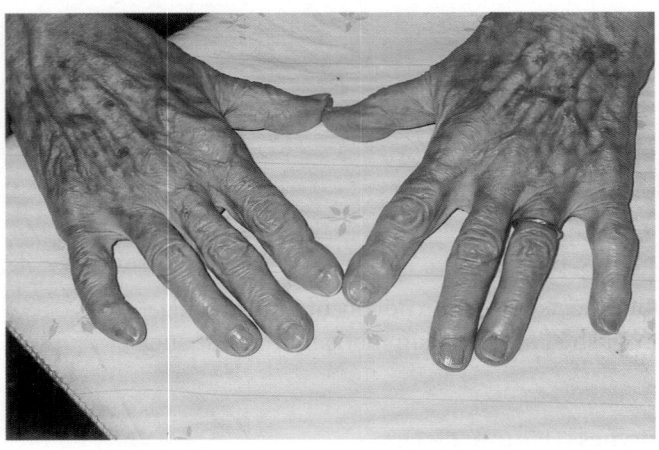

Figure 21-2 Hands with wrinkling, mottling, and overlapping folds common to aging skin.

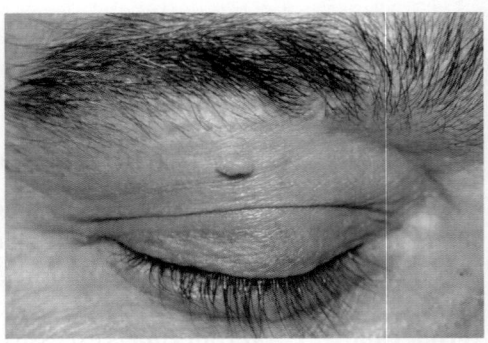

Figure 21-3 A solitary skin tag is present on the eyelid.

heatstroke   The inability to sweat in the elderly can lead to **heatstroke**, a severe and often fatal illness produced by exposure to excessively high temperatures.

The number of melanocytes (pigment-making cells) generally decreases in some areas. The decline in melanocyte activity makes the skin more sensitive to ultraviolet radiation, leading to disruption of cellular activity and subsequent skin cancer.

melanoma   **Melanoma**, a malignant cancer derived from melanocytes, becomes a concern in the elderly.

liver spots or   Melanocytes increase in some areas of skin to form age spots or pigment
senile lentigines   blotching called **liver spots** or **senile lentigines** (*lentigo* = singular), especially on the face and hands (**Figure 21-4**). **Senile** means relating to or characteristic of old age.

White or gray hairs also appear, and the skin takes on pallor (paleness) due to a decrease or lack of melanin production. Dendritic cells, which play a role in immunity, decrease in number in the skin by approximately 50%. So, the immune responsiveness of older skin also decreases. The 2011 Nobel Prize in Physiology or Medicine was awarded to Dr. Ralph M. Steinman for his discovery of the dendritic cell and its role in immunity. Sadly, he died of pancreatic cancer just 3 days prior to the October 3, 2011, award announcement. The prize is normally not awarded posthumously; however, the Nobel Committee decided that Dr. Steinman would be granted the award.

Aged skin heals poorly. Skin repair time is nearly double that of a younger person. Aged skin also becomes more susceptible to pathological conditions such as cancer and the following:

- **Senile pruritus**: itching associated with dryness of the skin in the elderly
- **Decubitus ulcers**: pressure sores that appear in areas of skin overlying bony projections
- **Shingles**: herpes zoster infection characterized by an eruption of vesicles on the skin following the course of a nerve (dermatome). Shingles is reactivation of the chickenpox virus in a nerve ganglion, resulting in inflammation, pain, and a rash of small blisters (**Figure 21-5**).

Furthermore, vitamin D_3 production declines about 75%, thereby increasing the necessity for receiving this important nutrient from the diet.

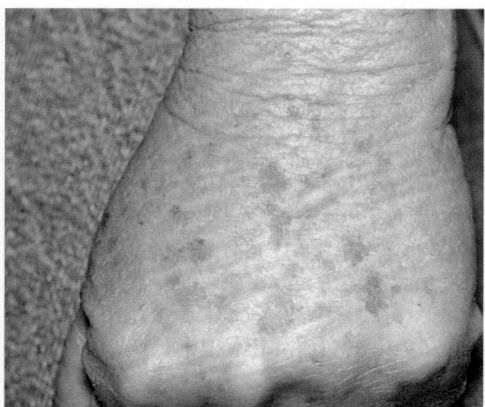

Figure 21-4 Lentigines are very common on aging skin.

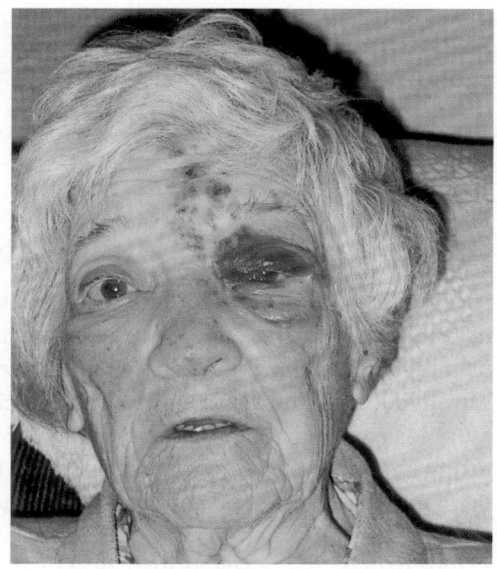

Figure 21-5 Herpes zoster (shingles).

As we age, hairs become finer and thinner. Although a general hair loss is characteristic of aging, females who go through menopause might develop more darkly pigmented, coarse facial hairs around the lips and on the chin as a result of changes in their androgen-to-estrogen ratio. There is also a decrease in the rate of nail growth.

KEY TERM	Definition
xeroderma (zeh-roh-DUR-muh)	excessive skin dryness
photoaging (foh-toh-AGE-ing)	skin wrinkling and damage due to years of sun exposure
skin tag	an outgrowth from the skin that hangs from the surface by a thin stalk
hypothermia (high-poh-THUR-mee-uh)	body temperature lower than 98.6°F (37°C)
heatstroke	severe and often fatal illness produced by exposure to excessively high temperatures
melanoma (mel-uh-NOH-muh)	malignant cancer derived from melanocytes
liver spots	age spots or pigment blotching on the skin due to increased melanin production; also called senile lentigines
senile lentigines (SEE-nile len-TIJ-ih-nez)	age spots or pigment blotching on the skin due to increased melanin production; also called liver spots
senile (SEE-nile)	relating to or characteristic of old age
senile pruritus (SEE-nile proo-RYE-tus)	itching associated with dryness of the skin in the elderly
decubitus ulcers (de-KYOO-bih-tus UL-surz)	pressure sores that appear in areas of skin overlying bony projections
shingles	herpes zoster infection characterized by an eruption of vesicles on the skin following the course of a nerve

KEY TERM PRACTICE: *Aging and the Integumentary System*

1. The term for "relating to or characteristic of old age" is _____.

2. Itching associated with dryness of the skin in the elderly is known as _____.

3. _____ is excessive skin dryness, and it is derived from the word part _____ for *dry* and the word part _____ for *skin*.

4. Pressure sores that appear in areas of skin overlying bony projections are called _____.

5. _____ is skin wrinkling and damage due to years of sun exposure.

Aging and the Skeletal System

Aging affects the skeletal system by decreasing bone mass and density and increasing porosity and erosion. One effect is the loss of calcium from the bones (*decalcification*). This loss usually begins after the age of 30, and in females, accelerates greatly at ages 40 to 45 due to estrogen loss. As much as 30% of bone calcium can be lost by the age of 70. In males, the calcium loss typically begins after the age of 60. In the jaw, tooth loss is a concern, and denture fitting becomes problematic because bone loss continues throughout life. The loss of calcium contributes to bone weakening and the condition called osteoporosis.

osteoporosis   **Osteoporosis**, a disease characterized by weak, very porous bones that break easily and heal slowly, is the most prevalent metabolic disorder of bone that develops in the elderly (**Figure 21-6**). Two types of osteoporosis exist: type I and type II.

Type I osteoporosis occurs after cessation of the menstrual cycle, and the term is used in reference to fractures as a result of spongy (trabecular) bone loss, primarily in the spine and wrist. Postmenopausal women are very susceptible to this condition, which is attributable to immobilization or inactivity, decreased estrogen levels, high steroid levels, poor diet, hormonal or other chemical imbalance in the blood, and other environmental conditions.

Measurement of bone mineral density is done by **dual energy x-ray absorptiometry (DEXA)**, which aims x-ray beams of differing energy levels at the bones (**Figure 21-7**). DEXA is used to evaluate osteoporosis.

There is no cure, as yet, but the condition can be prevented by good eating habits, regular exercise from youth through adulthood, and treatment with dietary calcium and estrogen. The drug alendronate (Fosamax) has been effective in managing osteoporosis and appears to work with hormones to block the activity of osteoclasts (cells associated with absorption and removal of bone).

Type II osteoporosis occurs later in life. It is marked by loss of dense (cortical) bone and represents loss of bone due to decreased action of osteoblasts (bone-building cells), decreased calcium absorption, and increased bone resorption as opposed to formation. Generally, the hips and less frequently, the proximal humeri, are involved.

Osteoporosis is a "pediatric problem with geriatric consequences." Central to the condition is calcium loss. It is the major cause of fractures in adults, and is characterized by chronic back pain, considerable loss of height, and teeth loss. It represents a disease of major public health significance; the United States spends in excess of $13 billion per year in medical expenses related to the disease. It is estimated that by 2025, the cost may be around $80 billion per year.

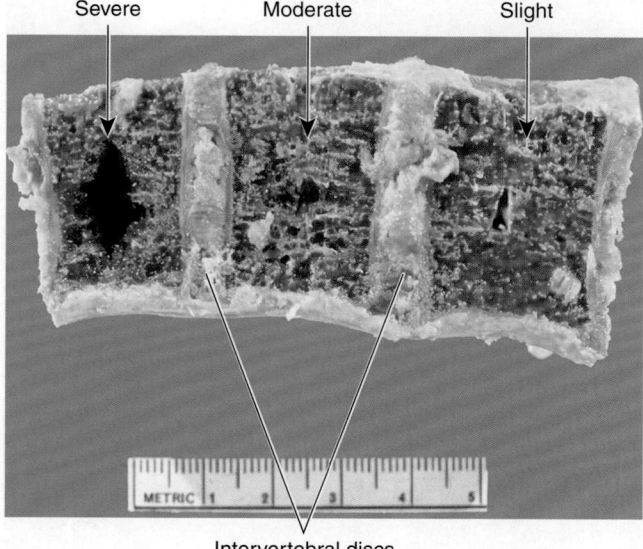

Severe   Moderate   Slight

Intervertebral discs

Figure 21-6 Osteoporosis of the spine. The degree of severity to which the vertebral bodies are affected decreases from left to right.

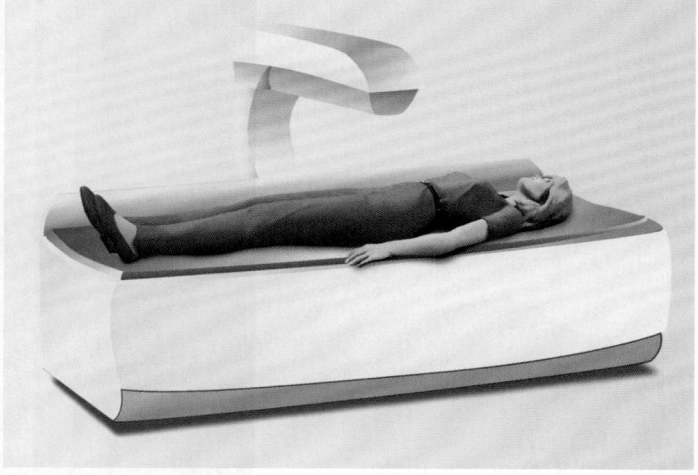

Figure 21-7 Bone mineral density test using DEXA.

kyphosis

A physical deformity related to osteoporosis is **kyphosis** (humpback), an abnormal concave curvature of the thoracic spine (**Figure 21-8**). Kyphosis causes the lower ribs to rest on the iliac crest and form a fibrous line of skin tissue. This also impairs proper chest cavity inflation. In postmenopausal women, this kyphosis is referred to as a **dowager hump** and is due to osteoporosis and compression fractures of vertebrae.

senile osteopenia

A bone condition characterized by decreased calcification or density of bone in the elderly is termed **senile osteopenia**. It results from inadequate osteoid synthesis. Osteoid is the newly formed bone matrix before calcification.

osteomalacia

Osteomalacia, bone softening and bending, is a condition resulting from vitamin D deficiency. The bones cannot calcify, and the weight of the body causes bowing of the leg bones, shortening of the spine, and flattening of the pelvic bones. It is sometime referred to as *adult rickets*.

Paget disease

Paget disease is a generalized skeletal disease of older people in which bone resorption and formation are both increased. There is irregular thickening and softening of the bones with bending of weight-bearing bones. This disease is rarely seen before the age of 50. Its cause is unknown.

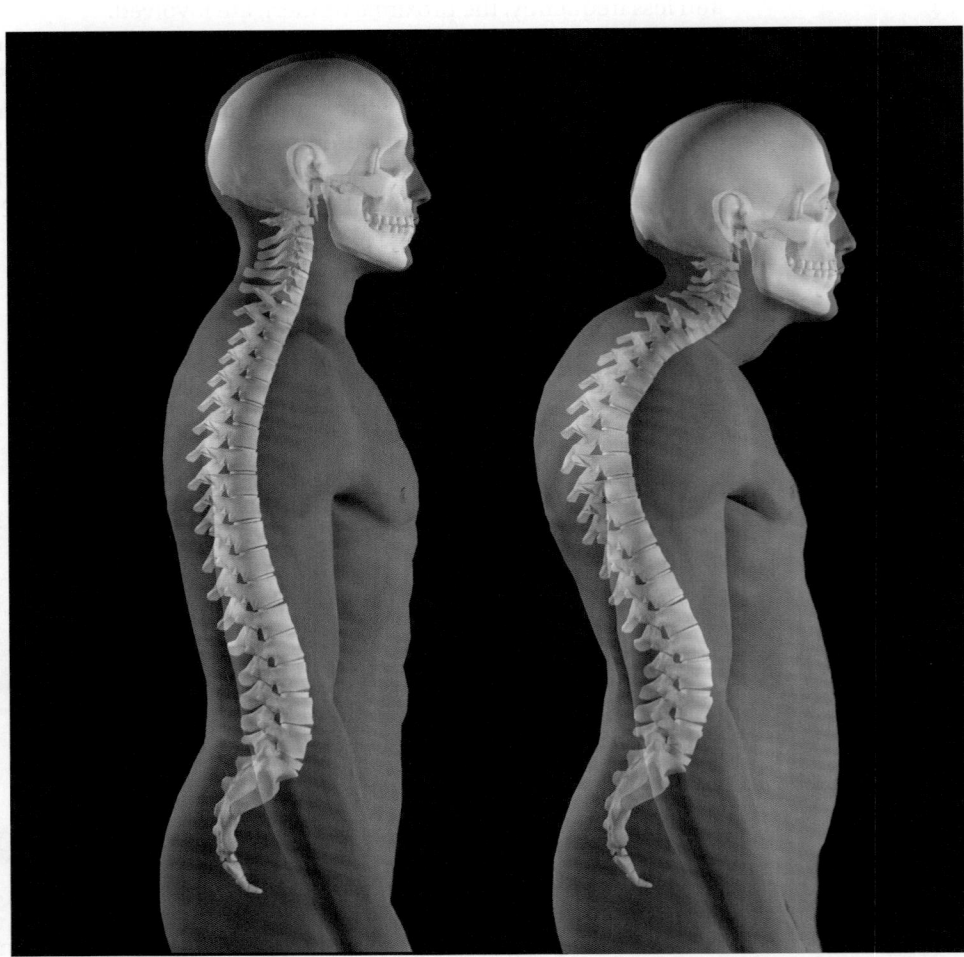

Figure 21-8 Kyphosis (right) versus normal spinal column (left).

Joints

As a result of aging, constant use, and trauma, joints (articulations) are subject to inflammation and a number of debilitating and degenerative diseases. Degenerative changes are also evident with aging articulations. The incidence of arthritis and rheumatism (a general term used to indicate diseases of muscles, bone, and joints) increases. Among the many disorders of joints, the most prevalent are arthritis, osteoarthritis, gouty arthritis, and bursitis.

arthritis

Arthritis is inflammation of a joint or chronic inflammation of the joints. Also known as degenerative arthritis, "wear-and-tear" arthritis, or degenerative joint disease (DJD), arthritis encompasses all rheumatic diseases affecting synovial joints. In essence, the joint is being worn out with use. Many forms of arthritis exist, and all involve inflammation, swelling, and pain of one or more joints. Its causes are unknown, but the chronic pain may be related to a deficiency or lack of endorphins (substances in the central nervous system that act as painkillers).

osteoarthritis

Osteoarthritis is characterized by erosion of the articular cartilage within a joint. It is the most common type of arthritis and results from a combination of aging, joint irritation, wear-and-tear, abrasion, excess body weight, some metabolic disorders, and a number of other factors. It affects a large proportion of the population over 60 years of age.

Although osteoarthritis is synonymous with aging and typically affects individuals age 60+, it is probably not a senescent change. It is a disease of articular cartilage as a result of a cartilage metabolism disorder. Genetic factors also affect the collagen formation in the cartilage. Osteophytes (bone spurs) form and can lead to bone fusion. With time, the articular cartilages soften and disintegrate gradually, leaving the articular surfaces roughened. The joints become painful and movement is restricted. The joints most likely involved are those used most often: the fingers, hips, knees, and lower parts of the vertebral column. As a disease process, it develops relatively slowly and many of its symptoms can be controlled by medications.

Continuous passive motion (CPM), a technique in which the joint is moved constantly through a variable range of motion to prevent stiffness and increase the range of motion, appears to encourage repair and improve circulation of the synovial fluid. A motorized passive motion device usually assists with the movement (**Figure 21-9**). Exercise, physical therapy, and anti-inflammatory drugs (such as aspirin) slow the progression. In severe cases, **arthroplasty** (joint replacement) may be necessary.

gouty arthritis

Gouty arthritis is a condition in which sodium urate crystals deposit in the joints of soft tissues and irritate the cartilage, causing inflammation and acute pain (**Figure 21-10**). It primarily occurs in males of any age. Treatment with various drugs seems to be effective.

bursitis

Bursitis is an acute or chronic inflammation of a bursa (a sac or pouch of synovial fluid found at friction areas in joints). It is usually caused by trauma, acute or chronic infection, or rheumatoid

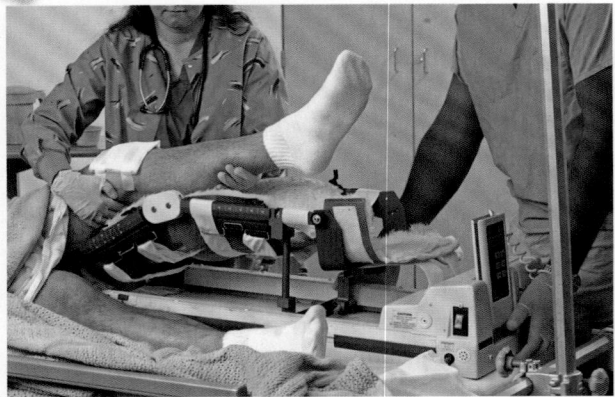

Figure 21-9 Continuous passive motion device. Support the affected extremity, elevate it to allow placement of the padded CPM device on the bed. Gently lower the leg onto the device.

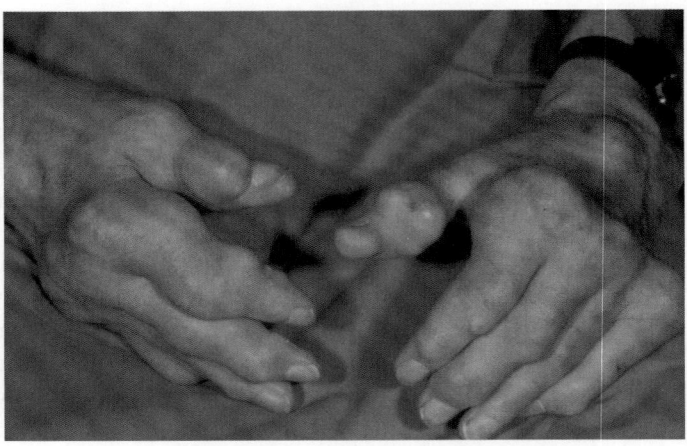

Figure 21-10 Gout affecting the finger joints.

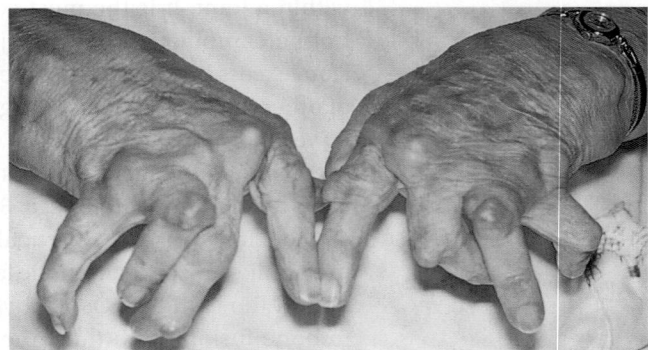

Figure 21-11 Characteristic joint deformities of the hands in long-standing rheumatoid arthritis.

arthritis. Repeated excessive friction can lead to bursitis and local inflammation with fluid accumulation. Signs and symptoms are pain, swelling, tenderness, and limitation of movement. Generally, it is treated with rest, but severe cases may need medication.

rheumatoid arthritis (RA)

Rheumatoid arthritis (RA) is an autoimmune disease in which the body attacks its own cartilage and joint linings. About 10% of RA patients developed the condition after age 60. It is the most painful and potentially crippling of the arthritic conditions. The synovial membrane of a joint becomes inflamed and grows thicker, to form a mass or *pannus*. This change is usually followed by damage to the articular cartilage of the joint and by invasion of fibrous tissue into the joint. These tissues interfere with joint movements and may become ossified in time, resulting in a fusion of the articulating bones (**Figure 21-11**). The mechanism for development of this disease is unknown, but may involve certain white blood cells that release substances that stimulate bone tissue destruction.

ankylosing spondylitis

Ankylosing spondylitis is arthritis of the spine that resembles rheumatoid arthritis. The disease is more common in males and may progress to fusion of vertebrae (**Figure 21-12**).

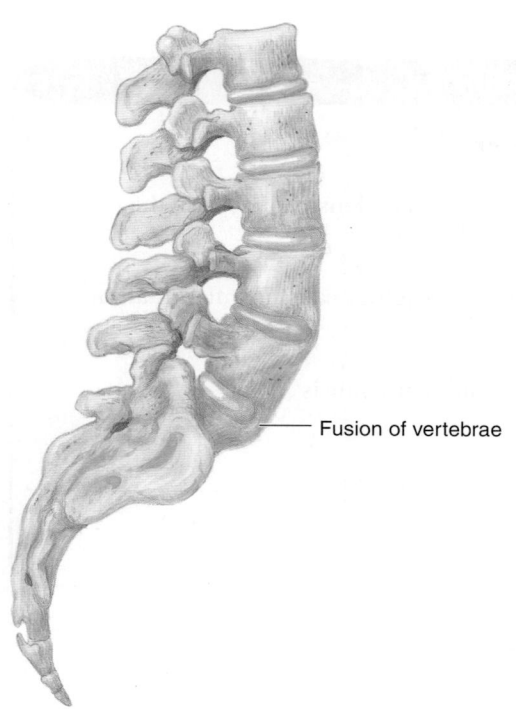

— Fusion of vertebrae

Figure 21-12 Fusion of vertebrae in ankylosing spondylitis.

KEY TERM	Definition
osteoporosis (os-tee-oh-puh-ROH-sis)	disease characterized by weak, very porous bones that break easily and heal slowly
dual energy x-ray absorptiometry (DEXA) (ab-sorp-tee-OM-eh-tree)	evaluative tool for osteoporosis that measures bone mineral density by aiming x-ray beams of differing energy levels at the bones
kyphosis (kigh-FOH-sis)	abnormal concave curvature of the thoracic spine; also called humpback
dowager hump	thoracic kyphosis in postmenopausal women due to osteoporosis and compression fractures of vertebrae
senile osteopenia (SEE-nile os-tee-oh-PEE-nee-uh)	bone condition characterized by decreased calcification or density of bone in the elderly
osteomalacia (os-tee-oh-muh-LAY-she-uh)	bone softening and bending as a result of a vitamin D deficiency; also called adult rickets
Paget (PAJ-et) **disease**	generalized skeletal disease of older people characterized by irregular thickening and softening of the bones with bending of weight-bearing bones
arthritis (ar-THRIGH-tis)	inflammation of a joint or chronic inflammation of the joints
osteoarthritis (os-tee-oh-ar-THRIGH-tis)	joint disease characterized by erosion of articular cartilage within a joint
continuous passive motion (CPM)	technique in which the joint is moved constantly through a variable range of motion to prevent stiffness and increase the range of motion
arthroplasty (AR-throh-plas-tee)	joint replacement
gouty arthritis (GOW-tee ar-THRIGH-tis)	condition in which sodium urate crystals deposit in the joints, causing inflammation and pain
bursitis (ber-SIGH-tis)	inflammation of a bursa
rheumatoid arthritis (RA) (ROO-muh-toid ar-THRIGH-tis)	autoimmune disease in which the body attacks its own cartilage and joint linings
ankylosing spondylitis (ang-kih-LOH-sing spon-dih-LIGH-tis)	arthritis of the spine that resembles rheumatoid arthritis and may progress to fusion of vertebral joints

continued

continued from page 1163

KEY TERM PRACTICE: *Aging and the Skeletal System*

1. Inflammation of a bursa is termed _____.

2. _____ is a bone condition characterized by decreased calcification or density of bone in the elderly.

3. _____ is a condition in which sodium urate crystals deposit in the joints, causing inflammation and pain.

4. The medical term for a hunchback or an abnormal concave curvature of the thoracic spine is _____.

5. The joint disease characterized by erosion of the articular cartilage within the joint is termed _____, which is derived from the word parts _____ for *bone* and _____ for *joint*.

Aging and the Muscular System

Although there is a general decrease in strength, endurance, and agility of skeletal muscle as we age, the extent of age-related changes varies considerably among individuals. This system is one in which the individual can actively slow down the aging changes.

fibrosis   As we age, skeletal muscle becomes less elastic because of **fibrosis**, the formation of fibrous connective tissue, which displaces skeletal muscle tissue.

    Changes in the muscular system are often related to alterations of body homeostasis. Due to the reduction in thermoregulatory ability, individuals are subject to overheating. Individuals age 65 and older cannot eliminate the heat produced from skeletal muscle activity as readily as younger people.

    Exercise tolerance decreases and overall repair and recovery rates decline. Muscle loss begins in the third decade of life, but it tends to go unnoticed for decades and seems to accelerate with time. The decline in muscle tissue has been linked to several factors, including hormones, satellite cells, and nerve cells. **Satellite cells**, believed to play a role in muscle repair and regeneration, are scattered throughout skeletal muscle. It appears that their performance dwindles with age.

    Nerve cells, too, play an important role. With age, nerve cells are lost, including those branching out from the spinal cord to muscles. Therefore, muscle performance is impeded.

flaccid muscles   **Flaccid muscles** are muscles with less-than-normal tone. They may result from damage or disease of the nerves supplying the muscle, or the result of disuse or inactivity (bedridden people or those with casts).

atrophy   Disuse leads to **atrophy**, or muscle wasting.

sarcopenia   It is important to include the term sarcopenia in the discussion of muscle aging. **Sarcopenia** is the loss of muscle and is generally associated with aging, but it is actually the result of deconditioning. Much of the muscle loss associated with aging is preventable and reversible. Moreover, muscle loss can contribute to loss of bone as well.

The consequences of sarcopenia are broad. One consequence is fatigue. Fatigue leads to decreased metabolic rate, reduced strength, and loss of bone. The loss of bone results because of the lack of muscular movement to stimulate bone-building activity. Through exercise, a person can reduce fatigue and muscle loss. Lastly, sarcopenia contributes to the decrease of lean-to-fat tissue ratios. This decrease is associated with decreased insulin sensitivity and subsequent development of type 2 diabetes.

KEY TERM	Definition
fibrosis (figh-BROH-sis)	formation of fibrous connective tissue, which displaces skeletal muscle tissue
satellite (SAT-eh-light) **cells**	cells scattered throughout muscle tissue that play a role in muscle repair and regeneration
flaccid (FLAH-sid) **muscles**	muscles with less-than-normal tone
atrophy (AT-roh-fee)	muscle wasting
sarcopenia (sar-koh-PEE-nee-uh)	loss of muscle as a result of deconditioning

KEY TERM PRACTICE: *Aging and the Muscular System*

1. _____ are muscles with less-than-normal tone.

2. The loss of muscle as a result of deconditioning is termed _____.

3. The medical term for muscle wasting is _____.

4. _____ is the formation of fibrous connective tissue, which displaces skeletal muscle tissue.

5. Cells scattered throughout muscle tissue that play a role in muscle repair and regeneration are known as

_____.

Aging and the Nervous System

In general, although the nervous system does "slow down" (apparent in a person's reaction time) and deteriorate with age, in most people, it functions very effectively throughout the lifespan. The actual extent of age-related changes within the brain is not known. An estimated 85% of people over age 65 lead relatively normal lives, but they exhibit noticeable changes in mental performance and in central nervous system (CNS) function. It has been estimated that perhaps the basic nerve cells of the nervous system are lost at the rate of about 100,000 neurons each day of our adult life. (The normal adult has about 10 to 12 billion neurons.) However, such claims are unfounded. Based on empirical studies, it is believed that relatively few neural cells are lost during the normal aging process. However, neurons are very sensitive and are susceptible to a variety of drugs or interruptions of vascular supply such as may result from strokes or other cardiovascular diseases. There is evidence, nevertheless, that the aging process alters neurotransmitters and that there is a decreased capacity for sending nerve impulses to and from the brain, so that processing of information is diminished.

Aging brings a reduction in brain size and weight. The weight of the brain decreases 7% to 11% from ages 20 to 96 years of age, with the greatest weight being at the age of 20. Blood flow to the brain decreases, as does the number of dendritic branches. The reduced blood flow also increases the chance of stroke.

stroke	A **stroke**, or brain attack, is a sudden impairment of blood circulation to the brain that lasts longer than 24 hours. An imprecise term for cerebral stroke is **cerebrovascular accident (CVA)**.

If the impairment resolves within 24 hours, it is called a **transient ischemic attack (TIA)**. Most TIAs last 15 to 20 minutes. Strokes, however, involve irreversible brain damage.

If the stroke affects the speech areas of the brain, aphasia may result. **Aphasia** is the partial or total inability to produce and understand speech, caused by brain injury.

About 600,000 people a year experience strokes in the United States, and one-fourth of strokes are fatal. It is estimated that strokes cost more than $40 billion annually.

The brains of elderly individuals have narrower gyri and wider sulci, and the subarachnoid space is larger. The aging in the brain impairs sensory perception and motor responses, which in turn have their effects on coordination, motivation, and ability and desire for many things, including exercise.

Aged brains show anatomical aberrations: accumulations of lipofuscin, neurofibrillary tangles, plaques, and amyloid. Lipofuscin is a granular pigment with no known function. Neurofibrillary tangles are masses of neurofibrils that form dense mats inside the neuron cell body and axon (see **Figure 18-5**). Amyloid is an unusual fibrillar protein, surrounded by abnormal dendrites and axons. Accumulations of amyloid form plaques. Evidence suggests that the accumulations appear in all aging brains, but when they are present in excess, they are associated with clinical abnormalities. |
organic brain syndrome	**Organic brain syndrome** is a collection of behavioral and psychological signs and symptoms including problems with attention, concentration, memory, confusion, anxiety, and depression. It is caused by transient or permanent brain dysfunction. This syndrome or disorder is a clinical consideration relative to an aging nervous system. Delirium and dementia fall under the classification of organic brain syndrome.
delirium	**Delirium** is an altered state of consciousness with confusion. It can develop at any age, but it is more likely in older adults. The causes are varied and include prescription drug use, infections (urinary bladder infections are common culprits), dehydration, electrolyte imbalance, heart attack, stroke, malnutrition (especially of the B vitamins), head trauma, hypothermia, chronic lung disease, and postoperative trauma. Generally, delirium is fairly brief, lasting hours to days, but rarely over a month. If the underlying cause is properly diagnosed, the outcome is good.
sundowner syndrome or **sundowning**	**Sundowner syndrome** or **sundowning** is the onset or exacerbation of delirium during the evening or night with improvement or disappearance during the day. People living in nursing homes who are already sensory deprived most often exhibit the behavior.

dementia

In **dementia**, an underlying structural brain disease causes a progressive loss of cognitive and intellectual functions. Most diagnoses of dementia are in older adults. Common types of dementia are vascular dementia (multi-infarct dementia), Huntington chorea, Parkinson disease (PD), and Alzheimer disease (AD).

vascular dementia or multi-infarct dementia

Vascular dementia, also known as **multi-infarct dementia,** is marked by a reduced blood flow to the brain. Risk factors include high blood pressure and diabetes. Multiple infarcts (areas of tissue that have died as a result of insufficient blood) over time result in decreased cognitive functions. Symptoms include dizziness, headaches, physical fatigue, and mental fatigue. The underlying problem is atherosclerosis (arterial plaque buildup). Onset of the disease occurs in a downward step-wise progression. Individuals may live for many years without being aware of the condition.

Huntington chorea

Huntington chorea is a hereditary neurodegenerative disorder characterized by irregular, spasmodic involuntary movements of the limbs or facial muscles and progressive dementia. Its onset is usually in the third or fourth decade.

Parkinson disease (PD)

Parkinson disease (PD) is a neurological syndrome usually resulting from deficiency of the neurotransmitter dopamine. Its cause is unknown, but it is common among the elderly. The environmental hypothesis suggests that the individual was exposed to any one of a number of possible neurotoxic agents that precipitated the onset of disease. Implicated agents include pesticides, fungicides, and anti sap stain agents found in lumber. The disease interferes with movement, and symptoms include slowed, monotonous speech pattern, reduced voice volume, masklike face that has no expression, and drooling from leaning forward and tongue weakness—not from oversalivating.

Brain changes seen in PD are varied. There is a loss of cells within the substantia nigra (midbrain). These cells secrete dopamine, so less dopamine is secreted. Dementia enters the picture in about 15% to 20% of the diagnosed cases. The older the individual is with initial onset, the more likely that dementia will result.

Treatment for PD has been pharmacological in nature. L-dopa has been the primary drug of choice. Dopamine itself cannot be used because it is unable to cross the blood–brain barrier, but the precursor molecule, L-dopa, has been used with success.

A newer treatment for Parkinson disease has focused on deep brain stimulation. With this procedure, bilateral wires are routed from the brain to positions just under the right and left clavicles where a pacemaker-like device alters electrical conductivity. This recent innovation is promising and appears to alleviate many physical manifestations of the disease.

Another treatment for PD is less glamorous: cigarette smoking. Smoking may alleviate symptoms of the disease due to the fact that it depletes the oxygen supply in the brain. Oxygen is necessary for free-radical damage, so if the supply is depleted, the disease may be thwarted.

Alzheimer disease (AD)

Alzheimer disease (AD) is a progressive degenerative disease of the brain (see **Figure 7-13**). It is the most common intellectual impairment in older adults; thus, it is the most common disorder. Over 4 million Americans are afflicted with the disease. Onset occurs over a wide age range, afflicting people anywhere between 40 and 100 years of age. The prevalence increases with age, and 20% of individuals over the age of 80 are afflicted with the condition. Symptoms unfold progressively with no abrupt changes, yet they do become more evident with time. AD is eventually fatal.

Epidemiological evidence shows that women on estrogen replacement therapy experience a decreased incidence and delayed progression of AD. Estrogen deficiency may be one of several factors that modify nerve injury and death. Humans evolved to survive merely long enough to procreate to carry on the species, but now that humans are living longer than their foraging ancestors, estrogen replacement therapy may be necessary.

Classic brain changes are obvious in AD: senile plaques, degenerated brain cells, and neurofibrillary tangles. The abnormal protein **beta amyloid** is at the core of the plaques. Both senile plaques and neurofibrillary tangles occur in all aged brains, but the extent of damage varies. The presence of these alterations is a hallmark of diagnosing the disease postmortem. Autopsies would provide valuable evidence, but they are limited.

KEY TERM	Definition
stroke	sudden impairment of blood circulation to the brain that lasts longer than 24 hours; also called brain attack
cerebrovascular accident (CVA) (se-ree-broh-VAS-kyoo-ler)	imprecise term for cerebral stroke
transient ischemic attack (TIA) (TRAN-see-ent is-KEE-mick)	sudden impairment of brain blood circulation that resolves within 24 hours
aphasia (uh-FAY-zhuh)	partial or total inability to produce and understand speech, caused by brain injury
organic brain syndrome	collection of behavioral and psychological signs and symptoms including problems with attention, concentration, memory, confusion, anxiety, and depression
delirium (de-LIR-ee-um)	altered state of consciousness with confusion
sundowner syndrome	the onset or exacerbation of delirium during the evening or night with improvement or disappearance during the day; also called sundowning
sundowning	the onset or exacerbation of delirium during the evening or night with improvement or disappearance during the day; also called sundowner syndrome
dementia (de-MEN-shuh)	underlying structural brain disease that causes a progressive loss of cognitive and intellectual functions
vascular dementia (vas-KYOO-lur de-MEN-shuh)	disorder marked by a reduced blood flow to the brain; also called multi-infarct dementia
multi-infarct dementia	disorder marked by a reduced blood flow to the brain; also called vascular dementia

continued

continued from page 1168

KEY TERM	Definition
Huntington chorea	hereditary neurodegenerative disorder characterized by irregular, spasmodic involuntary movements of the limbs or facial muscles and progressive dementia
Parkinson disease (PD)	neurological syndrome usually resulting from deficiency of the neurotransmitter dopamine
Alzheimer disease (AD) (ALTZ-high-mer)	progressive degenerative disease of the brain marked by senile plaques, degenerated brain cells, and neurofibrillary tangles
beta amyloid (BAY-tuh AM-ih-loyd)	abnormal protein at the core of the senile plaques of AD

KEY TERM PRACTICE: *Aging and the Nervous System*

1. Underlying structural brain disease that causes a progressive loss of cognitive and intellectual functions is termed _____.

2. _____ is a progressive degenerative disease of the brain marked by senile plaques, degenerated brain cells, and neurofibrillary tangles.

3. A neurological syndrome usually resulting from deficiency of the neurotransmitter dopamine is _____.

4. A disorder marked by a reduced blood flow to the brain is termed _____ or _____.

5. The onset or exacerbation of delirium during the evening or night with improvement or disappearance during the day is known as _____ or _____.

Aging and the Special Senses

Disease and degenerative conditions involving the special sense organs can alter vision or hearing in the elderly. Vision and hearing losses impact the quality of life and can lead to isolation and social withdrawal.

The lens of the eye is important to sight, and as we age, the lens yellows. The lens filters out cooler colors, thus the yellowing lens makes distinguishing them difficult. Warm colors (yellow, red, and orange) are still maintained.

presbyopia   **Presbyopia** is the inability of the aging eye to focus on near objects. The term literally means "old eye," and presbyopia is a senescent change. By age 65, 60% of men and 40% of females are affected. It basically involves the lens of the eye. Throughout the aging process, the lens becomes inflexible, gets locked in the distance position, and leads to farsightedness. Glasses (spectacles) can remedy the problem.

cataract   A **cataract** is an eye disease characterized by clouding of the lens (see **Figure 8-6**). Cataracts are the most common disability of older eyes. The condition happens uniformly with time, so it is a senescent change. Treatment involves surgical removal of the old lens and replacement with a new prescription lens.

    Phacoemulsification is a surgical technique that uses low-frequency ultrasonic needles to liquefy a cataract and remove it by suction through a small incision in the cornea. Phacoemulsification is the most widely used surgical procedure for the treatment of cataracts. There is no known preventive measure, although exposure to UV radiation seems to be important in developing cataracts. Vitamin C may slow the rate of development.

glaucoma

Glaucoma is increased fluid pressure in the eye that produces defects in the field of vision and eventual blindness. With this condition, a person sees halos around objects. It develops in middle age and is carried into old age, but is not considered normal senescence. The increased pressure in the eye can transfer to the optic nerve to cause irreparable damage. Treatments include medications to relieve pressure or surgery to allow fluid to escape.

age-related macular degeneration

Age-related macular degeneration usually affects older adults and is characterized by a loss of vision in the macula because of damage to the retina (see **Figure 8-15**). The macula is the center of the visual field that perceives fine detail and allows central focusing of an object. It is the leading cause of functional blindness in adults.

Two forms exist: wet and dry. The wet form is characterized by leaky blood vessels in retinal tissues, which lead to scar tissue formation. The dry form is characterized by mild atrophy. Causes and risk factors may be exposure to UV radiation, free-radical and oxidative damage, light eye color, and family history. Treatment involves laser therapy to destroy the vasculature.

diabetic retinopathy

The retinal changes occurring with diabetes mellitus characterized by leaky blood vessels and vessel overgrowth that causes scarring is termed **diabetic retinopathy** (see **Figure 8-13**). It is treated with laser therapy to cauterize the bleeding vessels. The use of a laser beam to treat retinal disorders in termed **photocoagulation**.

presbycusis

Presbycusis is hearing loss as a result of old age. The term literally means "old ear." Causes include senescence, exposure to noise, diseases, and genetics. It is characterized by a loss of hair cells within the organ of Corti, which functions in hearing. Individuals with the condition lose sounds in the higher frequencies first. People living in less developed areas do not develop it at the rate that people living in industrialized regions do. Prevention is aimed at reducing noise exposure. Current treatments include **hearing aids**, electronic devices for amplifying sound to the ear (**Figure 21-13**).

deafness

Deafness is the inability to hear.

- *Conduction deafness* is caused by impairment of the external and middle ear mechanisms for transmitting sounds to the cochlea.
- *Sensorineural deafness* is caused by impairment of the cochlea or cochlear branch of vestibulocochlear nerve (cranial nerve VIII).

Age-related deafness may be due to reduced blood supply to the ears, otosclerosis, atherosclerosis, repeated exposure to loud sounds, certain drugs, impacted cerumen (earwax), thickening of the eardrum, and stiffening of joints between ossicles.

Hearing aids substitute for hair cells, but they are quite expensive and expectations have not been met because they are a poor replacement for hair cells. Compliance rate is not high due to many reasons: stigma, pain, and the amplification of background noise.

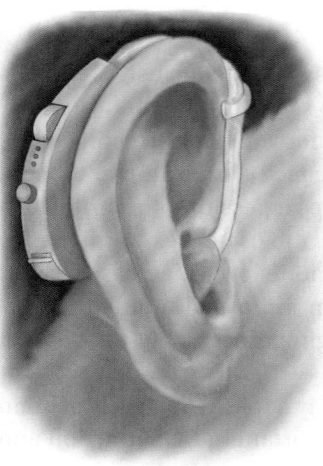
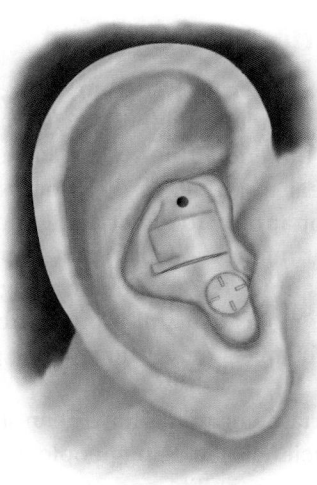
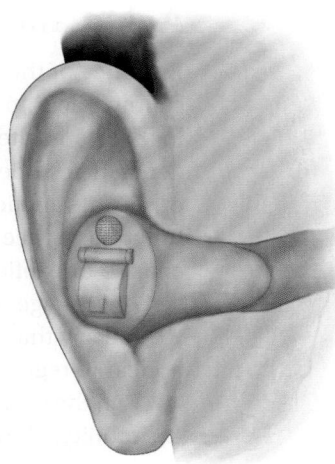

Behind the ear
(moderate to severe loss)

In the ear
(mild to severe loss)

In the canal
(mild to moderate loss)

Figure 21-13 Several types of hearing aids.

KEY TERM	Definition
presbyopia (prez-bee-OH-pee-uh)	inability of the aging eye to focus on near objects
cataract (KAT-uh-rakt)	eye disease characterized by clouding of the lens
phacoemulsification (fak-oh-ee-mul-sih-fi-KAY-shun)	surgical technique that uses low-frequency ultrasonic needles to liquefy a cataract and remove it by suction through a small incision in the cornea
glaucoma (glaw-KOH-muh)	increased fluid pressure in the eye that produces defects in the field of vision and eventual blindness
age-related macular (MACK-yoo-lur) **degeneration**	eye disorder affecting older adults characterized by a loss of vision in the macula (center of the visual field) because of damage to the retina
diabetic retinopathy (dye-uh-BET-ick ret-ih-NOP-uh-thee)	retinal changes occurring with diabetes mellitus characterized by leaky blood vessels and vessel overgrowth that causes scarring
photocoagulation (foh-toh-koh-ag-yoo-LAY-shun)	the use of a laser beam to treat retinal disorders
presbycusis (prez-bee-KYOO-sis)	hearing loss as a result of old age
hearing aids	electronic devices for amplifying sound to the ear
deafness	inability to hear; two forms are conduction deafness and sensorineural deafness

KEY TERM PRACTICE: *Aging and the Special Senses*

1. _____ is hearing loss as a result of old age.

2. Increased fluid pressure in the eye that produces defects in the field of vision and eventual blindness is known as _____.

3. An eye disease characterized by clouding of the lens is called a _____.

4. Electronic devices for amplifying sound to the ear are _____.

5. _____ is the use of a laser beam to treat retinal disorders.

Aging and the Endocrine System

Evidence of the role of the endocrine system in the aging process is not conclusive, and it is still not clear to what extent endocrine deficiencies may exert a secondary influence on aging. Various alterations of the endocrine system have been witnessed, but correcting these deficiencies does not appear to influence the process of senescence. For example, the loss of sexual function does not appear to affect aging, nor does the regression of reproductive function reduce physical or intellectual efficiency. Furthermore, the use of sex hormones to change the deficiency does not prevent or delay aging. Sex hormone levels decrease in both sexes with age, but elderly males can still produce active sperm in normal numbers. Thus, we can say that hormonal changes may influence the general aging process, but they do not appear to regulate it.

On the other hand, certain hormones have been shown to play a role in the levels of brain excitability. Hormonal deficiencies in aging people would be important in CNS function and are probably related to mood, irritability, and depression, which are marked in the older population. In addition, hyperfunction of an endocrine organ can produce abnormally high blood levels of hormones. Increased levels of norepinephrine and epinephrine from the adrenal cortex can raise blood pressure. Infections and circulatory disturbances, particularly of the adrenal gland, are a common consequence of the wear-and-tear of everyday life and affect the aging process and homeostasis of the organism.

Regarding thyroid function, hypothyroidism and myxedema are seen in aging adults.

hypothyroidism	**Hypothyroidism** is a deficiency of thyroid hormones, leading to a slow metabolic rate. There is also a tendency to gain weight, tiredness, and sometimes myxedema.
myxedema	**Myxedema** is extreme hypothyroidism in adults, characterized by dry swelling of the skin and subcutaneous tissues (**Figure 21-14**). It is treated with thyroid hormone replacement.
hyperthyroidism or **thyrotoxicosis**	**Hyperthyroidism** or **thyrotoxicosis** is excessive thyroid hormone production. About 25% to 30% of thyrotoxicosis cases occur in people over age 65. The excess thyroid hormones stress the heart, and treatment options include surgical removal of the thyroid gland or antithyroid drugs.
hyponatremia	**Hyponatremia**, an abnormally low concentration of sodium ions in the blood, is one of the most serious and least recognized disorders in

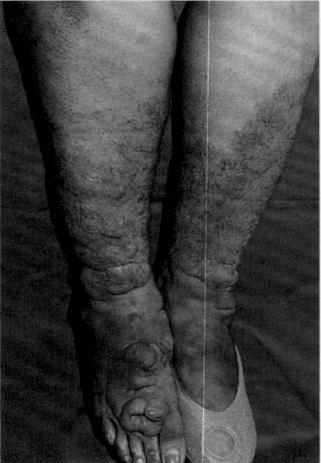

Figure 21-14 Myxedema affecting tibial region of leg.

the elderly. It is associated with oversecretion of antidiuretic hormone (ADH) from the posterior pituitary gland. ADH regulates sodium and water balance in the body.

water intoxication   **Water intoxication** is a metabolic brain disorder that results from severe overhydration. Oversecretion of ADH leads to water intoxication by causing water retention in the body.

KEY TERM	Definition
hypothyroidism (high-poh-THIGH-royd-izm)	deficiency of thyroid hormones
myxedema (micks-eh-DEE-muh)	extreme hypothyroidism in adults characterized by dry swelling of the skin and subcutaneous tissues
hyperthyroidism (high-pur-THIGH-royd-izm)	excessive thyroid hormone production; also called thyrotoxicosis
thyrotoxicosis (thigh-roh-tok-sih-KOH-sis)	excessive thyroid hormone production; also called hyperthyroidism
hyponatremia (high-poh-nay-TREE-mee-uh)	abnormally low concentration of sodium ions in the blood
water intoxication	metabolic brain disorder that results from severe overhydration

KEY TERM PRACTICE: *Aging and the Endocrine System*

1. _____ is an abnormally low concentration of sodium ions in the blood; it is derived from the word part _____, which means *below normal.*

2. An extreme hypothyroidism in adults characterized by dry swelling of the skin and subcutaneous tissues is termed _____.

3. Excessive thyroid hormone production is known as _____ or _____.

4. A metabolic brain disorder that results from severe overhydration is called _____.

5. _____ is a deficiency of thyroid hormones.

Aging and the Cardiovascular System

The leading cause of death in the elderly is cardiovascular senescence. A person becomes susceptible to life-threatening diseases as the heart and blood vessels age. The most common age-related change in the cardiovascular system is a general stiffening of the cardiovascular structures.

Changes in vessels that supply the brain tissue may lead to undernourishment of nerve cells and their malfunction or death. By age 80, renal blood flow is 50% less and brain blood flow 20% less than that of a 30-year-old. In addition, there is a progressive reduction in heart muscle fiber size and strength. The result of these changes is a decrease in the cardiac output at a given level of energy or pressure, and a depression in maximum heart rate. Consequently, the heart must work harder as we age in order to maintain an adequate supply of oxygen to the tissues throughout the body.

The heart generally shrinks with age and accumulates fat along its coronary vessels. The inner lining of the heart (endocardium) thickens by 25% from the age of 10 to 80. The heart valves also change and gradually become thickened, rigid, and even distorted by sclerosis. As we age, the heart reacts poorly to stress and cannot use oxygen as well. In addition, the average blood flow through the heart vessels is about 35% lower at age 60 than it is at age 30.

coronary artery disease (CAD)	**Coronary artery disease (CAD)** is the narrowing of the lumen of one or more coronary arteries. It is the leading cause of death in the United States. Because the heart muscle receives an inadequate supply of blood, it is unable to effectively pump the blood around the body. It can cause myocardial infarction.
myocardial infarction (MI)	**Myocardial infarction (MI)**, or heart attack, refers to the death of an area of the heart tissue due to interrupted blood supply. An embolus (blood clot) in a coronary artery prevents blood from flowing, and the tissue beyond the blockage dies. **Angina pectoris**, severe chest pain that radiates from the heart to the shoulder (usually the left) and down the arm, is a symptom of myocardial infarction.
arteriosclerosis	**Arteriosclerosis** is hardening of the arteries. One type of arteriosclerosis is atherosclerosis.
atherosclerosis	**Atherosclerosis** is a pathological condition in which fatty substances, especially cholesterol and triglycerides, are deposited in the arterial walls (see **Figure 11-21**). These deposits calcify and interfere with normal blood flow and may produce clots or plaques inside the vessels. The plaques build up on the walls of the blood vessels, thereby narrowing the lumen of the vessel. Clots can break off and send emboli into the cardiovascular system. Atherosclerosis is seen in most middle-aged and elderly people. It contributes to stroke, renal failure, coronary artery disease, and hypertension.
hypertension	**Hypertension** (high blood pressure) is the most common disease of the heart and blood vessels. It affects about 20% of American adults at some time in their lives. The definition of the term *hypertensive* varies with the age of the person. Normal blood pressure for young adults is less than 120/80 and a reading over 140/90 is cause for concern and treatment. The top number is the *systolic pressure*, the pressure when the heart beats and sends blood into the arteries. The bottom number is the *diastolic pressure*, the pressure in arteries when the heart relaxes.
	Hypertension leaves a person at risk for damage to the cardiovascular system itself and at an increased risk for strokes. However, since the heart muscle and vessels are less efficient as someone ages, health professionals recognize that the blood pressure necessary to satisfactorily perfuse the cells gradually rises as the person ages. To clarify, if the blood pressure is not high enough to adequately oxygenate the brain cells, the person may become dizzy when he or she stands up and be at risk for falls. Therefore, the level of blood pressure that is classified as necessitating treatment may rise as the person ages. As yet, medical science cannot cure hypertension, but it can usually be controlled through the combination of a low-salt diet, weight loss, smoking cessation, moderate alcohol consumption, exercise, and antihypertensive medications.
aneurysm	An **aneurysm** is a thin, weakened section of the wall of an artery that bulges outward, forming a balloon-like sac of the blood vessel (see

Figure 11-31). A common cause is atherosclerosis. If untreated, it may result in interrupted blood flow, pressure on surrounding structures, massive hemorrhage, stroke, severe pain, and even death (depending on the vessel involved).

congestive heart failure (CHF)

In **congestive heart failure (CHF)**, the heart muscle is unable to pump sufficient quantities of blood fast enough to satisfy the oxygen demands of the tissues and to maintain adequate pressure for the venous system. The sympathetic nervous system compensates for the failing heart by increasing the heart rate and increasing the venous return (amount of blood returning to the heart by the veins), which contributes to the congestion in the lungs and other tissues. It is characterized by peripheral and pulmonary edema.

claudication

Claudication is lameness, limping, tension, and pain caused by defective circulation of the blood in the vessels of the limbs. It is seen in occlusive arterial disease or in congestive heart failure.

deep vein thrombosis (DVT)

Deep vein thrombosis (DVT) is the presence of a blood clot (thrombus) in a vein, usually in deep veins of the lower extremity. It can lead to a **pulmonary embolism**, a clot in a pulmonary artery.

varicose veins

Varicose veins are dilated and twisted veins caused by incompetent or ineffective valves (**Figure 21-15**). The function of the venous valves is to counteract the forces of gravity by preventing backflow, thereby assisting blood return to the heart to be reoxygenated. Varicose veins develop as the result of the extra pressure put on the blood vessel walls from the slow-moving blood. The venous walls lose their elasticity and become flabby and stretched. Varicose veins can be due to heredity, pressure from prolonged standing, pregnancy, and aging.

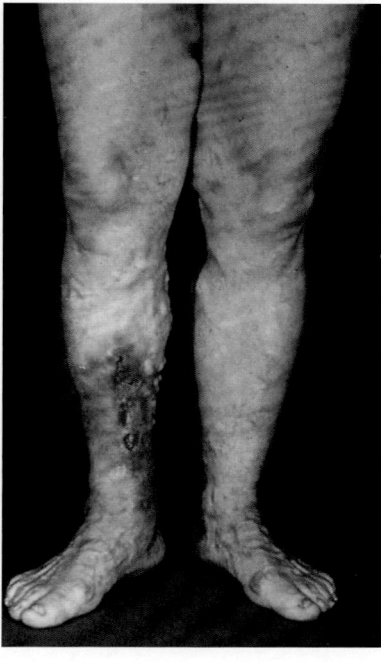

Figure 21-15 Varicose veins in the legs.

restless legs syndrome (RLS)	**Restless legs syndrome (RLS)** is an uneasiness, twitching, or restlessness that occurs in the legs after going to bed. It may be caused by inadequate circulation or as a side effect of antipsychotic and neuroleptic medications. Restless legs syndrome may be relieved temporarily by walking about.

KEY TERM	Definition
coronary artery (KOR-uh-nair-ee AR-ter-ee) **disease (CAD)**	narrowing of the lumen of one or more coronary arteries
myocardial infarction (MI) (migh-oh-KAR-dee-ul in-FARK-shun)	death of an area of the heart tissue due to interrupted blood supply; also called heart attack
angina pectoris (an-JYE-nuh PECK-toh-ris)	severe chest pain that radiates from the heart to the shoulder (usually the left) and down the arm
arteriosclerosis (ar-TEER-ee-oh-skler-oh-sis)	hardening of the arteries
atherosclerosis (ATH-er-oh-skler-oh-sis)	pathological condition in which fatty substances, especially cholesterol and triglycerides, are deposited in the arterial walls causing hardening of the arteries
hypertension (high-per-TEN-shun)	high blood pressure
aneurysm (AN-yoo-riz-um)	thin, weakened section of the wall of an artery that bulges outward, forming a balloon-like sac of the blood vessel
congestive heart failure (CHF)	inadequacy of the heart to pump blood and maintain systemic circulation
claudication (klaw-di-KAY-shun)	lameness, limping, tension, and pain caused by defective circulation of the blood in the vessels of the limbs
deep vein thrombosis (throm-BOH-sis) **(DVT)**	presence of a blood clot (thrombus) in a vein, usually in deep veins of the lower extremity
pulmonary embolism (pul-muh-NAIR-ee em-BOH-liz-um)	clot in a pulmonary artery
varicose (VAIR-ih-kose) **veins**	dilated and twisted veins caused by incompetent or ineffective valves
restless legs syndrome (RLS)	an uneasiness, twitching, or restlessness that occurs in the legs after going to bed

KEY TERM PRACTICE: *Aging and the Cardiovascular System*

1. _____ describes lameness, limping, tension, and pain caused by defective circulation of the blood in the vessels of the limbs.

2. An uneasiness, twitching, or restlessness that occurs in the legs after going to bed is termed _____.

3. Severe chest pain that radiates from the heart to the shoulder (usually the left) and down the arm is known as _____.

4. _____ is characterized by narrowing of the lumen of one or more coronary arteries.

5. A pathological condition in which fatty substances, especially cholesterol and triglycerides, are deposited in the arterial walls causing hardening of the arteries is termed _____.

Aging and the Respiratory System

As we age, changes in the respiratory system adversely affect the ability to breathe deeply. For example, the chest wall musculature weakens, skeletal changes affect posture, and the exchange of oxygen and carbon dioxide becomes less efficient. Arthritic changes in the rib cage restrict chest movements and alter breathing. Diminished chest wall mobility (rigidity) affects the vital capacity of the lungs. *Vital capacity* is the greatest amount of air that can be exhaled from the lungs after a maximum inhalation. In fact, this capacity can decrease to 35% by the age of 70 years. Decreased flexibility at the costal cartilages leads to stiffening. The lungs also experience reduced compliance (the ease with which the lungs expand and contract) due to stiffening of the thoracic cage.

There is also a reduced ability to clear the airways by coughing, making the elderly more susceptible to respiratory infections. Pneumonia and influenza must be considered when dealing with an aging population. Tuberculosis (TB) is also a possibility.

Because the respiratory and cardiovascular systems operate together, a disease or damage to one system greatly affects the other.

right ventricular hypertrophy or **cor pulmonale**	**Right ventricular hypertrophy**, also called **cor pulmonale**, is an abnormal enlargement of the right side of the heart in response to lung disease. Recall from the cardiovascular system that the right atrium and right ventricle receive the venous blood and pump it to the lungs to be oxygenated. If a significant number of alveoli are destroyed as a result of lung disease, blood backs up in the right ventricle. The right ventricle compensates for the strain by enlarging (hypertrophy). Acute cor pulmonale is characterized by dilation and failure of the right side of the heart due to pulmonary embolism (blood clot in a pulmonary artery).
pulmonary edema	**Pulmonary edema** is swelling of the lungs that is caused by mitral stenosis (narrowing of the opening of the mitral valve) or left ventricular failure. Left ventricular failure (left-sided heart failure) is the inability of the left heart to maintain its circulatory load. This leads to an increase in the pulmonary circulation and eventually pulmonary edema.
chronic obstructive pulmonary disease (COPD)	**Chronic obstructive pulmonary disease (COPD)** is a general term used to describe lung disorders that result in respiratory failure because the respiratory system cannot supply enough oxygen to maintain metabolism or eliminate carbon dioxide to prevent acidosis. It is relatively common in the elderly, especially those who have smoked. Emphysema (characterized by deterioration of the lungs' alveoli leading to the loss of their elasticity) and chronic bronchitis (inflammation of the bronchial tree) are types of COPD. In general, the disease is characterized by airway obstruction, which may lead to a chronic productive cough. Wheezing may also be present, as is labored breathing. There is no cure for COPD, but medical treatment and general physical conditioning with an emphasis on aerobic exercises can be very useful in making breathing easier.
emphysema	**Emphysema** is an anatomical alteration of the lung with abnormal enlargement of air sacs and eventual destruction of air sac walls. It

results from breathing under bronchitis conditions. The alveoli become hyperinflated and their appearance becomes balloon-like, rather than the characteristic grapelike appearance (see **Figure 12-19**). With 400 million alveoli in both lungs, representing 30% of the surface area of the entire body, this alteration becomes physiologically significant. The chief symptom is shortness of breath (dyspnea). Emphysema is not a senescent change, but it is one of the ten leading causes of death in the United States.

chronic bronchitis

Chronic bronchitis is a condition of the bronchial tree characterized by excessive mucus production and a persistent cough over a long period of time (see **Figure 12-18**). Chronic inflammation of the bronchial tree initiates a problem with subsequent destruction of airways. Cigarette smoke (firsthand or secondhand) is the number one cause. It chronically insults the respiratory tract, resulting in hypertrophy of the airways.

pneumonia

Pneumonia is inflammation of the lung with most cases caused by bacterial or viral infection (see **Figure 12-23**). Pneumonia is the eighth leading cause of death in older persons; 90% of deaths occur in persons older than age 65. Pneumococcal pneumonia disease requires hospitalization and accounts for 40,000 deaths annually. The U.S. government has adopted the World Health Organization's goal of aiming to vaccinate over 60% of the elderly population for pneumonia.

influenza

Influenza is an acute infectious respiratory disease caused by influenza viruses. Over $1 billion per year is spent in hospital costs in the treatment of influenza. Influenza vaccines are available.

tuberculosis (TB)

Tuberculosis (TB) is an infection of the lungs caused by *Mycobacterium tuberculosis* (see **Figure 12-24**). Although not the problem it once was, TB still occurs. In fact, 60% of cases occur in patients over 45 years of age. TB is usually treated without hospitalization. A cure rate of almost 100% can be achieved if the disease is diagnosed and treatment with antituberculosis medications is started early. Fever, weight loss, **anorexia** (poor appetite), and coughing up blood are signs that TB may be present.

lung cancer

Lung cancer is a common fatal malignancy in the elderly. Cancerous cells replace the bronchial epithelial cells (see **Figure 12-25**). The most important cause of lung cancer is smoking. The disease is also associated with long-term exposure to certain pollutants such as asbestos and uranium. Treatment is surgical if the tumor is small and if the disease has not spread too far. Radiation therapy can be combined with surgery, and in some select cases, chemotherapy (drug therapy) can be used. Persistent cough, which is sometimes bloody, and an increasing shortness of breath should alert one that cancer may be present or at least that it must be ruled out. Not smoking is the best prevention.

KEY TERM	Definition
right ventricular hypertrophy (ven-TRIK-yoo-lur high-PUR-troh-fee)	abnormal enlargement of the right side of the heart in response to lung disease; also called cor pulmonale
cor pulmonale (KOR pool-muh-NAL-ee)	abnormal enlargement of the right side of the heart in response to lung disease; also called right ventricular hypertrophy
pulmonary edema (pul-moh-NAIR-ee e-DEE-muh)	swelling of the lungs that is caused by mitral stenosis (narrowing of the opening of the mitral valve) or left ventricular failure
chronic obstructive pulmonary disease (COPD)	general term for lung disorders that result in respiratory failure
emphysema (em-fih-SEE-muh)	anatomical alteration of the lung with abnormal enlargement of air sacs and eventual destruction of air sac walls
chronic bronchitis (brong-KIGH-tis)	condition of the bronchial tree characterized by excessive mucus production and a persistent cough over a long period of time
pneumonia (new-MOH-nee-uh)	inflammation of the lung with most cases caused by bacterial or viral infection
influenza (in-floo-EN-zuh)	acute infectious respiratory disease caused by influenza viruses
tuberculosis (too-ber-kyoo-LOH-sis) **(TB)**	infection of the lung caused by *Mycobacterium tuberculosis*
anorexia (an-oh-REK-see-uh)	poor appetite
lung cancer	fatal malignancy in which cancerous cells replace the bronchial epithelial cells

KEY TERM PRACTICE: *Aging and the Respiratory System*

1. _____ is an infection of the lung caused by *Mycobacterium tuberculosis*.

2. Anatomical alteration of the lung with abnormal enlargement of air sacs and eventual destruction of air sac walls is known as _____.

3. A fatal malignancy in which cancerous cells replace the bronchial epithelial cells is called _____.

4. The medical term for swelling of the lungs that is caused by mitral stenosis (narrowing of the opening of the mitral valve) or left ventricular failure is _____.

5. Abnormal enlargement of the right side of the heart in response to lung disease is termed _____ or _____.

Aging and the Lymphatic System and Immunity

Immunologic responses remain indispensable for good health in the adult and older years. A decline in the body's immunologic "watchfulness and control" (surveillance) has been linked not only to an increase in autoimmune diseases and infections with advancing years, but also to the occurrence of diseases such as cancer and other malignancies. To what extent these specific age-related changes are the cause or consequence of the aging process is still not fully understood, since aging entails numerous and complex interactions at a number of levels.

With aging, there is also a decrease in the production of special lymphocytes that attach to and destroy antigens and an overall decrease in the production of antibodies that destroy antigens. Moreover, T lymphocytes (T cells) become less responsive to antigens. **T lymphocytes** are types of white blood cells essential for various aspects of immunity. The magnitude or degree of the immune responses appears to decline with age, as is seen in the decreased response to vaccines. It has long been noted that susceptibility to infectious disease is greater in the two extremes of life, the very young and the very old, and that resistance to a number of environmental factors progressively declines with age.

autoimmune diseases   **Autoimmune diseases** are diseases that result when the body does not recognize its own tissue (self) antigens and produces antibodies against them. Several human autoimmune diseases are lupus, hemolytic and pernicious anemias, and multiple sclerosis.

KEY TERM	Definition
T lymphocytes (lim-FOH-sights)	types of white blood cells essential for various aspects of immunity
autoimmune (aw-toh-ih-MYOON) **diseases**	disorders in which the body does not recognize its own tissue (self) antigens and produces antibodies against them

KEY TERM PRACTICE: *Aging and the Lymphatic System and Immunity*

1. Disorders in which the body does not recognize its own tissue (self) antigens and produces antibodies against them are termed _____.

2. _____ are types of white blood cells essential for various aspects of immunity.

Aging and the Digestive System

General alterations of the digestive system are varied. The cumulative or "wear-and-tear" damage of aging affects the lumen to a great extent. Additionally, there is a decline in epithelial stem cell divisions. Therefore, the walls of the gastrointestinal (GI) tract cannot undergo repair processes as rapidly. Changes associated with aging of the digestive system usually include decreased motility within the digestive organs, decreased secretion, loss of tone and strength of the muscular tissue and its supporting structures, alterations in the neurosecretory feedback mechanism regarding enzyme and hormone release, and a decreased response to pain and internal sensations. Smooth muscle tone also decreases. This is significant because the bulk of the digestive tract is composed of involuntary smooth muscle.

Other age-related changes include an increase in certain pathologies of the system, namely, duodenal ulcers, stomach cancer, malabsorption, maldigestion, and appendicitis. The terminal portion of the system is not necessarily spared from changes as the system ages, resulting in more constipation, cancer of the colon or rectum, hemorrhoids, and diverticular disease of the colon.

Taste buds also atrophy, resulting in loss of taste. We have 70% fewer taste buds at age 70 than at age 30. Saliva production diminishes as we age and contributes to dry mouth.

dry mouth   **Dry mouth** is a condition of diminished saliva production. Saliva protects the tissues of the mouth and aids the sense of taste. Dry mouth also results from mouth breathing and medications. Simple remedies such as increased fluid intake, wetting agents, and saliva stimulants (citrus fruits) can alleviate the condition temporarily.

oral cancer   **Oral cancer** (cancer of the mouth) peaks in the seventh decade of life and is frequently related to smoking and alcohol consumption.

Professional inspection of the oral cavity and evaluation of lumps in the head and neck area should be a part of a person's routine health habits.

stomach cancer   The incidence of **stomach cancer** (cancer of the stomach) increases with age and affects men more than women. Symptoms such as unexplained weight loss, change in bowel habits, and difficulty swallowing need to be evaluated by health care professionals.

colorectal cancer   The incidence of **colorectal cancer** (cancer of the colon and rectum) increases with age, in those with a family history of GI cancer, and in those with diets low in dietary fiber. Changes in bowel habits, mucus discharge, and rectal bleeding are signs that need to be evaluated. Special screening tests are available to identify the presence of hidden or occult blood in the rectum.

pancreatic cancer   **Pancreatic cancer** (cancer of the pancreas) is generally a disease of those over age 50 and is very difficult to diagnose during the early stages of the pathology. Weight loss, upper abdominal distress, and progressive yellowing of the skin (jaundice) may occur. Treatment is usually palliative and concentrates on symptom management.

constipation   **Constipation** refers to infrequent or difficult bowel movements due to decreased motility of the intestines, which allows the feces to remain in the colon longer than usual. Since water is reabsorbed into the circulation from the large intestine at a constant rate, a longer transit time may result in hard, dry feces. It is not an inevitable outcome of aging. Constipation can be alleviated by increasing fluids and fiber in the diet, by increasing physical exercise, by careful medication selection, and, if necessary, by using laxatives, stool softeners, or enemas. An **enema** is the rectal insertion of a liquid for clearing out the bowel as a treatment for constipation (**Figure 21-16**).

diarrhea   **Diarrhea**, frequent and excessive watery bowel movements, in the elderly can lead rather quickly to serious problems with fluid balance. Frequent causes of diarrhea in the elderly are bacterial and viral infections, too much fruit, and milk intolerance. Prompt

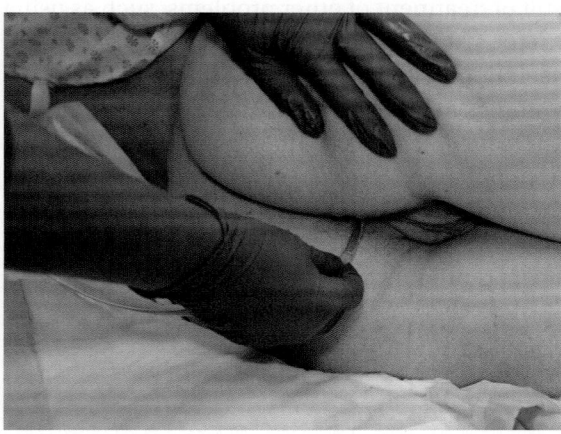

Figure 21-16 Enema administration. Advance the tube 2 to 4 inches (5 to 10 cm), aiming it toward the umbilicus. Avoid forcing the tube to prevent rectal wall trauma. If it does not advance easily, allow a little solution to flow in to relax the inner sphincter enough to allow passage.

action to alleviate the condition is necessary because diarrhea can easily lead to dehydration and electrolyte imbalances. Over-the-counter medications can assist with temporary management; however, removal of the causative factors is the most effective long-term management.

diverticulitis

Diverticulitis is inflammation of the diverticula with abdominal pain. Diverticula are pouches that develop in the wall of the colon where the muscular layer (muscularis) has become weak (diverticulosis; see **Figure 14-27**). Diverticulitis will cause numerous GI symptoms such as diarrhea, pain, and/or constipation. Treatment is symptomatic for the specific episode, followed by long-term change to a diet high in fiber.

periodontal disease

Periodontal disease is a collective term for a variety of oral conditions that are characterized by inflammation and degeneration of the gums (gingivae), alveolar bone, cementum, and periodontal ligament. It frequently results in soft tissue degeneration, alveolar bone resorption, gum recession, and even tooth loss. Signs are usually inflammation and enlargement of soft tissue and bleeding gums. The major causes of this disease are poor oral hygiene, vitamin C deficiency, local irritation of teeth and gums (bacteria, impacted food, cigarette smoke, poor bite, and poor dentures resulting in a poor bite), infections, mouth breathing, and medications. The most effective treatment for periodontal disease is regular removal of plaque and other debris from the tooth surfaces and gum areas.

hiatal hernia

Hiatal hernia is a weakening around the diaphragmatic opening for the esophagus that allows the stomach to move up into the chest cavity (see **Figure 14-25**). Although many hiatal hernias are asymptomatic, many people experience severe problems related to the condition. The hernia allows reflux or regurgitation of gastric juices into the lower esophagus, causing heartburn, ulceration, and/or stricture of the lower esophagus. Medical treatment focuses on the use of antacids, keeping the abdominal pressure low, and weight control. Elevating the head of the bed 4 to 6 inches and eating small, frequent meals can diminish reflux.

peptic ulcers

Peptic ulcers, sores in the stomach or duodenum, occur in the older adult primarily as a result of treatment of other problems, such as using large amounts of aspirin for arthritis management (see **Figure 14-16**). It can be due to hyposecretion of mucus, which normally protects the stomach and duodenal linings from acid, or an inadequate secretion of bicarbonate ions in pancreatic juices that buffer gastric acid. Five percent to 10% of the U.S. population develops peptic ulcers. Treatment usually is limited to removing the offending agents (caffeine or alcohol), using antacids (Tums, Maalox), and using certain drugs to eliminate the bacterial-caused ulcers (antibiotics) or medications to reduce acid secretion.

KEY TERM	Definition
dry mouth	condition of diminished saliva production
oral cancer	cancer of the mouth
stomach cancer	cancer of the stomach
colorectal cancer	cancer of the colon and rectum
pancreatic cancer	cancer of the pancreas
constipation (kon-stih-PAY-shun)	condition in which bowel movements are infrequent
enema (EN-eh-muh)	rectal insertion of a liquid for clearing out the bowel as a treatment for constipation
diarrhea (dye-uh-REE-uh)	frequent and excessive watery bowel movements
diverticulitis (dye-ver-tick-yoo-LYE-tis)	inflammation of the diverticula with abdominal pain
periodontal (per-ee-oh-DON-tul) **disease**	collective term for a variety of oral conditions
hiatal hernia (high-AYE-tul HER-nee-uh)	weakening around the diaphragmatic opening for the esophagus that allows the stomach to move up into the chest cavity
peptic ulcers (PEP-tik UL-serz)	sores in the stomach or duodenum lining

KEY TERM PRACTICE: *Aging and the Digestive System*

1. _____ is characterized by frequent and excessive bowel movements.

2. The collective term for a variety of oral conditions is _____.

3. The condition in which bowel movements are infrequent is termed _____.

4. _____ is a condition of diminished saliva production.

5. Sores in the stomach or duodenum lining are known as _____.

Aging and the Urinary System

Kidney function decreases with aging. Nephron numbers decline 30% to 40% between 25 and 85 years of age. By the age of 70, the filtering mechanism of the kidney is about half of what it was at the age of 40. This is due to decreased numbers of glomeruli, reductions in renal blood flow, and alterations in pH. With age there is also a diminished sensitivity to antidiuretic hormone (ADH). This leads to increased excretion of sodium in the urine.

Because fluid balance implies electrolyte balance, it is important to discuss the aging acid/base balance system with the urinary system. (Electrolytes are minerals important for body functions.) With age, the water content in the entire body decreases. Between the ages of 40 and 60, fluid accounts for nearly 55% of the total body content for males and 47% for females. After age 60, those numbers diminish to 50% for males and 45% for females. During this time, more water is lost in the urine. Other systems also influence fluid and electrolyte balance. A loss of vital capacity in the respiratory system can increase the risk of acidosis. The loss of mineral content in muscles affects fluid balance. Thus, exercise and proper nutrition are essential.

Two major problems associated with aging of the urinary system are urinary incontinence and urinary tract infections. Other common pathologies seen with aging are urinary retention and nocturia.

urinary incontinence   **Urinary incontinence** is the inability to control urination. It has been estimated that more that 20% of admissions to geriatric units were prompted by urinary incontinence. The condition is not well understood, but research suggests that the micturition (urination) reflex may be altered with age. This may be due to a loss of sphincter muscle tone. Men and women are encouraged to perform Kegel exercises that strengthen pelvic floor muscles.

urinary tract infections (UTIs)	**Urinary tract infections (UTIs)** are microbial (usually bacteria) infections in any part of the urinary tract. Acute UTI is more common in females (due to the shorter urethra) than in males and is usually caused by bacteria. It can result in **dysuria** (painful urination), urinary urgency and frequency, back pain, cloudy urine, chills, fever, nausea, vomiting, and urethral discharge. It is treated with antibiotics if the cause is bacterial.
urinary retention	**Urinary retention** is the inability to urinate. In men, it is commonly associated with prostate enlargement, which interferes with urine flow in the urethra. In females, **fecal impaction** (hardened feces in the colon or rectum) and urinary tract obstruction are common causes.
nocturia	**Nocturia** is the need to get up from sleep during the night to urinate. Nearly two-thirds of the elderly population awakens to urinate two to three times per night. Its cause may be too much fluid intake too soon before sleeping, urinary infection, renal disease, or prostate enlargement.
renal calculi	**Renal calculi** (kidney stones) are crystals of salts in the urine that can solidify into insoluble stones (see **Figure 15-7**). Interestingly, they are seen in 30- to 60-year-olds, but on autopsy, they are found in high numbers in 50- to 70-year-olds. They can be formed in any part of the urinary system and can cause pain, hematuria (blood in the urine), and pyuria (pus in the urine). They can be removed by surgery and by shock waves using the ultrasound waves of a lithotriptor (see **Figure 15-8**).

KEY TERM	Definition
urinary incontinence (in-KON-ti-nens)	the inability to control urination
urinary tract infections (UTIs)	microbial (usually bacteria) infections in any part of the urinary tract
dysuria (dis-YOO-ree-uh)	painful urination
urinary retention	the inability to urinate
fecal impaction (FEE-kul im-PAK-shun)	hardened feces in the colon or rectum
nocturia (nokt-YOO-ree-uh)	the need to get up from sleep during the night to urinate
renal calculi (ree-nul KAL-kyoo-lye)	kidney stones

KEY TERM PRACTICE: *Aging and the Urinary System*

1. _____ is the need to get up from sleep during the night to urinate.

2. The medical term for kidney stones is _____.

3. The inability to control urination is called _____.

4. The inability to urinate is termed _____.

5. _____ is the term for painful urination.

Aging and the Reproductive System

There are few age-specific disorders associated with the reproductive system even though there are major age-specific physical changes in function and structure. It appears as though the aging changes in the system in both males and females are more important psychologically than pathologically. The relationship between the end of reproductive function and aging of the entire body has been widely studied. There is generally a decline in the production of sex hormones and a loss of sexual vigor in both the male and female, but no facts establish that the loss of sexual function represents a primary cause of aging. Furthermore, there are no treatments available that can permanently restore the sexual vigor of youth—no true "fountain of youth."

Cultural sex roles may also play an important part. With aging, the decrease in testosterone production (at about age 55) produces less muscle strength, fewer viable sperm, and a decreased sexual drive. There is also a decreased sensitivity of the genitalia, which may affect sexual responsiveness. Nevertheless, abundant sperm are present even in old age.

Most age-dependent pathologies of the reproductive systems do not affect general health, except for prostate gland problems, which can be very serious. Healthy males maintain the ability to ejaculate throughout old age, but there is a reduction in the force of ejaculation, volume of the ejaculate, and quality of the seminal fluid (semen).

Female alterations include a gradual aging and the cessation of reproductive function. This is related to changes in the ovaries. These changes are responsible for many endocrine imbalances characteristic of menopause and postmenopause, and are reflected in the metabolic, cardiovascular, and nervous systems. The typical age for menopause is 45 to 55 years. During this time, GnRH, FSH, and LH levels rise, while estrogen and progesterone levels decline. Many women experience a number of postmenopausal phenomena, including hot flashes, excessive sweating, headache, hair loss, muscular pains, vaginal dryness, insomnia, depression, weight gain, and psychiatric changes or mood swings. Sexual desire, however, does not necessarily show a similar decline since it may receive support from adrenal gland hormone secretions.

In females, the reproductive system does have a time-limited period of fertility between menarche (onset of menstruation) and menopause (permanent cessation of menstruation). The system shows an age-dependent decline in fertility, possibly due to less frequent ovulation and declining ability of the uterus and uterine tubes to support the passage and development of the young embryo and fetus.

Other pathological events are also evident. Due to lower levels of estrogen, osteoporosis is common in aging females. Uterine cancer appears to reach its peak at age 65 in females, whereas cervical cancer is more common in younger females. Breast cancer is the second leading cause of death in females between the ages of 40 and 60 (lung cancer has become the number one cause in this female age group).

It has generally been established that the frequency of sexual intercourse decreases with age, even though effective sexual response can be maintained into advanced years. It has also been shown that regular physical activity contributes not only to the health and adequacy of a specific response, but also to the general health of the whole body. In women of advanced age (postmenopausal), all phases of sexual response associated with intercourse are fully attainable, yet there is a loss of sex steroids, which may result in a decline in the intensity and duration of the response.

In the same way, reaction patterns of erection and ejaculation in the male in advancing age are also slowed. The erect penis angle between the abdominal wall and the shaft of the penis is 90° in the elderly, whereas it is 45° in young men (**Figure 21-17**).

benign prostatic hyperplasia (BPH)	**Benign prostatic hyperplasia (BPH)** is progressive enlargement of the prostate gland that begins around the fifth decade. It typically increases anywhere from two to four times normal, occurs in about one-third of all males over the age of 60, and is often of unknown origin. It is characterized by hesitancy in urination, posturination dribbling,

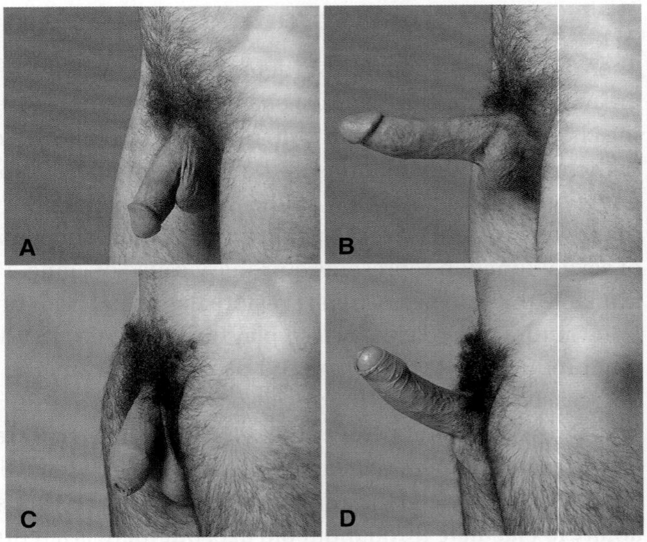

Figure 21-17 Photographs of two penises in the nonerect state (**A** and **C**) and the erect state (**B** and **D**). Part **B** shows the 90° angle of an erect penis, while **D** shows the 45° of an erect penis.

decreased force of the urinary stream, and the general sensation of incomplete emptying of the bladder. It does not progress to prostate cancer. It can usually be detected by **digital rectal examination (DRE)**, a manual examination done with a gloved hand to check anatomical structures by palpating them through the rectum (see **Figure 16-17**).

prostatitis   **Prostatitis** is an inflammation of the prostate gland. Acute and chronic infections of the prostate gland are relatively common in postpubescent males and are associated with urethral inflammation. Acute prostatitis is common in sexually active young men by infection from bacteria. The gland becomes swollen and tender, urination is painful, and in some cases pus drips from the penis. Treatment is generally antibiotic therapy, increased fluid intake, and bed rest. Chronic prostatitis is a very common chronic infection in men of middle and later years. It often produces no symptoms, but the gland may feel enlarged, soft, and tender. If bacterial in origin, it is treated with long-term antibiotics, but it may prove difficult to treat if the inflammation is autoimmune in nature. The prostate is believed to harbor infectious organisms responsible for some allergic conditions such as arthritis, inflammation of the nerves (neuritis), muscles (myositis), and iris (iritis).

prostate cancer   Tumors of the male reproductive system usually involve the prostate gland. **Prostate cancer** is the second leading cause of death from cancer in men in the United States and amounts to about 30,000 deaths per year. Its incidence has been related to age, occupation, geography, and ethnic origin. There is a blood test for prostate-specific antigen (PSA), which is an enzyme produced by prostate epithelial cells. PSA levels increase with an enlarged prostate gland and may indicate prostate cancer. Both benign and malignant growths are common in elderly men. Both press on the urethra making urination painful and difficult. In advanced stages, the patient usually dies from metastases to the spinal column and brain.

Treatments vary, depending on the age of the patient. Some cases require surgical removal, or **prostatectomy**. Two common prostate removal procedures are suprapubic prostatectomy and transurethral resection of the prostate. With **suprapubic prostatectomy**, the prostate gland is removed through an incision in the abdominal wall just above the pubic bone.

With **transurethral resection of the prostate (TURP)** the prostate gland is removed using an endoscope through the urethra (see **Figure 16-18**).

inguinal hernia   The inguinal or groin area represents a weak area in the abdominal wall. It is a frequent site of **inguinal hernia**, a rupture or separation of a portion of the abdominal wall resulting in the protrusion of a part of an organ. With age, the abdominal wall musculature becomes weaker. Exercise can help strengthen the wall. Inguinal hernias occur much less frequently in females.

Two general types of hernias are usually described: indirect and direct. An indirect hernia occurs when part of the small intestine protrudes down into the scrotum. A direct hernia occurs when part of the small intestine protrudes into the posterior wall of the inguinal canal and produces a localized "bulging" in the wall of the inguinal canal.

atrophic vaginitis   Inflammation of the vagina due to thinning and atrophy of the vaginal epithelium is termed **atrophic vaginitis**. It results from diminished estrogen secretion and commonly occurs in postmenopausal women. Symptoms include vaginal soreness, itching, and **dyspareunia** (pain during sexual intercourse). Treatments are estrogen replacement therapy, vaginal creams, and lubricants.

KEY TERM	Definition
benign prostatic hyperplasia (BPH) (beh-NINE pros-TAT-ik high-per-PLAY-zhe-uh)	progressive enlargement of the prostate gland that begins around the fifth decade
digital rectal examination (DRE)	manual examination done with a gloved hand to check anatomical structures by palpating them through the rectum
prostatitis (pros-tuh-TYE-tis)	inflammation of the prostate gland
prostate cancer	cancer of the prostate gland
prostatectomy (pros-tuh-TEK-toh-mee)	surgical removal of the prostate gland
suprapubic prostatectomy (soo-pruh-PYOO-bik pros-tuh-TEK-toh-mee)	removal of the prostate gland through an incision in the abdominal wall just above the pubic bone
transurethral (trans-yoo-REE-thrul) **resection of the prostate (TURP)**	endoscopic prostate gland removal through the urethra
inguinal hernia (ING-gwi-nul HER-nee-uh)	rupture or separation of a portion of the abdominal wall resulting in the protrusion of a part of an organ
atrophic vaginitis (a-TROH-fik vaj-ih-NIGH-tis)	inflammation of the vagina due to thinning and atrophy of the vaginal epithelium
dyspareunia (dis-pa-ROO-nee-uh)	pain during sexual intercourse

KEY TERM PRACTICE: *Aging and the Reproductive System*

1. Pain during sexual intercourse is termed _____.

2. _____ is inflammation of the vagina due to thinning and atrophy of the vaginal epithelium.

3. The medical term for prostate gland inflammation is _____.

4. Progressive enlargement of the prostate gland that begins around the fifth decade is called _____.

5. An _____ is a rupture or separation of a portion of the abdominal wall resulting in the protrusion of a part of an organ.

Pharmacology and Older Adults

Older adults as patients generally suffer from **comorbidity**, the coexistence of two or more disease processes. The involvement of multiple organ system deficiency (MOSD) has implications in terms of arriving at a single diagnosis because symptoms of the disease are frequently shared. There is also an alteration of classic symptoms and presentation of disease, increased likelihood of mental complications, as well as a greater possibility of physical complications in the elderly population.

The older adult also experiences **polypharmacy**, the administration of multiple drugs at the same time. The use of prescription and over-the-counter medications necessitates caution. There is polypharmacy due to comorbidity, and older patients are at increased risk for negative health outcomes and serious drug reactions. It has been proposed that **iatrogenic disease** (medically induced unfavorable response) is probably the most common preventable condition in older individuals, and most reactions are related to prescription drug use.

With the widespread use of antibiotics to treat most ailments, at all ages, a word of caution is very important, especially in the treatment of the elderly. Incomplete absorption of broad-spectrum antibiotics such as ampicillin and tetracycline affect the large intestinal flora and may lead to overgrowth of *Proteus*, *Pseudomonas*, and *Staphylococci* organisms. The overgrowth may result in severe nausea, indigestion, abdominal pain, flatulence, diarrhea, and even fecal incontinence. In addition, severe itching may accompany dermatitis of the anus and vulva, which can be very severe and prolonged.

Absorption of drugs in older adults is not usually compromised. However, the metabolism of drugs is complex and some drugs remain in circulation longer as a result of decreased kidney function.

KEY TERM	Definition
comorbidity (koh-mor-BID-ih-tee)	the coexistence of two or more disease processes
polypharmacy (pol-ee-FAR-muh-see)	the administration of multiple drugs at the same time
iatrogenic (eye-at-roh-JEN-ik) **disease**	medically induced unfavorable response

KEY TERM PRACTICE: *Pharmacology and Older Adults*

1. The coexistence of two or more disease processes is termed _____.

2. An _____ is a medically induced unfavorable response.

3. The administration of multiple drugs at the same time is known as _____.

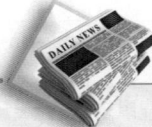

IN THE NEWS: Long-Lived Okinawans

Is the Japanese island of Okinawa the modern Shangri-La? Amazingly, the native people of Okinawa are the longest-lived people on earth. What is their secret? Well, they do have a cultural practice called *hara hachi bu*, which is defined as "eating until you are 80% full." It is likely that this calorie restriction along with lots of fruits and vegetables results in less damage to their bodies from free radicals. Carefully collected statistics show that Okinawa has more people over 100 years of age proportionately than any other place on earth. They have the lowest death rate from cancer, heart disease, and stroke—the top three killer diseases in the United States. Furthermore, they have the highest life expectancy for males and females over age 65, and females in Okinawa have the highest life expectancy of all age groups in the world, living to be 86.

continued

continued from page 1188

IN THE NEWS: Long-Lived Okinawans

These statistics probably reflect the Okinawans' good diet, emphasis on lots of physical activity throughout life, moderate alcohol use, little or no tobacco use, and an overall positive attitude that reduces stress. The Okinawans clearly demonstrate that living a healthy lifestyle will help us live longer and with less disease. We all can achieve these benefits with changes to our lifestyles, and it is never too late to start.

COMMON Abbreviations

Abbreviation	Term
ACOTE	Accreditation Council for Occupational Therapy Education
AD	Alzheimer disease
ADL	activities of daily living
BPH	benign prostatic hyperplasia
CAD	coronary artery disease
CDC	Centers for Disease Control and Prevention
CHF	congestive heart failure
CNS	central nervous system
CPM	continuous passive motion
CVA	cerebrovascular accident
DEXA	dual energy x-ray absorptiometry
DJD	degenerative joint disease
DRE	digital rectal examination
DVT	deep vein thrombosis
IADL	instrumental activities of daily living
MI	myocardial infarction
MMWR	*Morbidity and Mortality Weekly Report*
MOSD	multiple organ system deficiency
NBOT	National Board for Certification in Occupational Therapy
OT	occupational therapist; occupational therapy
PD	Parkinson disease
PT	physical therapist; physical therapy
RA	rheumatoid arthritis
RLS	restless legs syndrome
TB	tuberculosis
TIA	transient ischemic attack
TURP	transurethral resection of the prostate
UTI	urinary tract infection

continued

continued from page 1189

COMMON ABBREVIATIONS EXERCISES

1. IADL is the abbreviation for _____.

2. RLS is the abbreviation for _____.

3. The abbreviation for tuberculosis is _____.

4. CHF is the abbreviation for _____.

5. The abbreviation for transient is chemic attack is _____.

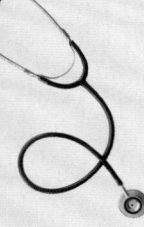

Case Study

Mr. Michael James is a 75-year-old married man afflicted with osteoarthritis of the right hip. After 2 years of physical therapy and a regular regimen of continuous passive motion (CPM), his hip was not improving. X-rays taken once per year revealed progressive degenerative joint disease, and a total hip replacement was recommended. Preadmission testing demonstrated nothing remarkable. Mr. James has slight presbycusis in his left ear and does have presbyopia of both eyes. A total hip arthroplasty was scheduled for October 31, 2011.

DOB: February 25, 1936
BP: 140/85
Height: 6'1"
Weight: 226 lbs/102.5 kg
Consults: PT and OT

Case Study Questions

1. **Identify and define the medical conditions that are affecting Mr. James.**

   _____

   _____

2. **Describe CPM.** _____

   _____

3. **What is an arthroplasty?** _____

   _____

4. **What do PT and OT mean?** _____

   _____

   _____

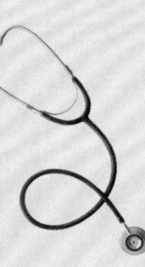

Real World Report

Client Name: Mr. Michael James

Date: November 3, 2011

Assessment: Postsurgery right hip replacement

An occupational therapy interview was conducted with the following findings.

HOME ENVIRONMENT

Two-storey home environment is acceptable. Wide passageways between bedroom, bathroom, living room, and kitchen are assured and will accommodate client and walker. There is no full bath facility on the first floor; however, the client has been taught how to go up and down stairs safely by the physical therapist (PT). The client could use the half-bath on the first floor for a sponge bath. PT taught client how to use his walker. Additionally, a single bed has been brought in for use on the first floor if needed. Client has been taught how to get into and out of bed.

Client has been taught how to get into and out of a chair. Patient has a proper chair with armrests. Household has been modified to accommodate client and his walker. Area rugs have been removed. All pathways have been cleared of potential obstacles to allow client to move about safely with his walker. Three large pet dogs will be confined until client is settled at home.

Food preparation and dressing require assistance from his spouse. Phones are within reach. Medications and palliative items are on hand and accessible by patient. Walk-in shower has had hand-grips and a seat added.

Arrangements have been made with a lawn service to perform any necessary yard work and snow/ice removal.

AUTOMOBILE TRANSPORT

PT taught client how to transfer into and out of an automobile. Client can be driven the short distance to his physical therapy sessions. No drives longer than 1 hour are allowed without physician's approval.

ASSISTANCE

Spouse or another person will be available to assist client at all times.

WORK ENVIRONMENT

Client is retired.

continued

continued from page 1191

ACTIVITIES OF DAILY LIVING (ADL)

ADL FUNCTION	Independent	Needs Help	Dependent	Cannot Do
Bathing	X			
Dressing		X		
Grooming	X			
Mouth care	X			
Toileting		X		
Transferring bed/chair	X			
Walking	X			
Climbing stairs		X		
Eating	X			

INSTRUMENTAL ACTIVITIES OF DAILY LIVING (IADL)

IADL Function	Independent	Needs Help	Dependent	Cannot Do
Shopping				X
Cooking				X
Managing medications		X		
Using the phone	X			
Doing housework				X
Doing laundry				X
Driving or public transportation				X
Managing finances		X		
Signature	Maria Wagner, OT		November 3, 2011	

Real World Report Questions

Answer the following questions related to the preceding medical report.

1. **Identify the health care workers involved with this case.** _____

2. **What was the reason for the OT consult?** _____

3. **What ADL can Mr. James do by himself?** _____

4. **For which IADL will Mr. James require assistance?** _____

5. **What are Mr. James's restrictions for driving?** _____

Review and Application

Multiple-Choice Questions

Select the best answer to each of the following questions.

1. The process of growing old is _____.
   a. senescence   b. senility   c. aging   d. longevity

2. Changes in the skin such as mottled pigmentation, roughened texture, and wrinkling, which result from years of sun exposure, are generally termed _____.
   a. aging   b. photoaging   c. photocoagulation   d. skin cancer

3. The progressive degenerative disease of the brain marked by senile plaques, degenerated brain cells, and neurofibrillary tangles is termed _____.
   a. ankylosing spondylitis   b. beta amyloid disease   c. Alzheimer disease   d. Paget disease

4. The joint disease characterized by erosion of the articular cartilage within the joint is termed _____.
   a. osteoporosis   b. osteoarthritis   c. atherosclerosis   d. prostatitis

5. Renal calculi are commonly called _____.
   a. aneurysms   b. abnormal proteins   c. cataracts   d. kidney stones

6. The condition of painful urination is termed _____.
   a. dysuria   b. hysuria   c. hernia   d. hyponatremia

7. When weakening around the diaphragmatic opening for the esophagus allows the stomach to move up into the chest cavity, the condition is termed a/an _____.
   a. myxedema   b. hyponatremia   c. inguinal hernia   d. hiatal hernia

8. The collective term for a variety of oral conditions is _____.
   a. polypharmacy   b. senile osteopenia   c. periodontal disease   d. iatrogenic disease

9. Severe chest pain that radiates from the heart to the shoulder, usually the left, and then down the arm is called _____.
   a. angina pectoris   b. angina femoris   c. ankylosing angina   d. beta amyloid angina

10. Increased fluid pressure in the eye that produces defects in the field of vision and eventually leads to blindness is termed _____.
    a. aphasia   b. emphysema   c. glaucoma   d. melanoma

Word Parts Exercises

Using the following word parts, form a medical term for each definition. Each word part is used only once.

arterio-	arth-	geront-
hypo-	-ologist	-opia
osteo-	-porosis	presby-
-ritis	-sclerosis	-thermia

11. hardening of the arteries _____

12. inflammation of the joints _____

13. person who specializes in gerontology _____

14. low body temperature _____

15. disease of porous, weak bones _____

16. inability of aging eye to focus on near objects _____

Matching Exercises

Match the disorder with its description.

_____ 17. age-related macular degeneration

_____ 18. Huntington chorea

_____ 19. organic brain syndrome

_____ 20. Paget disease

_____ 21. shingles

a. collection of behavioral and psychological problems
b. herpes zoster infection following the course of a nerve
c. generalized skeletal disease of older people
d. hereditary neurodegenerative disorder with spasmodic movements and progressive dementia
e. eye disorder affecting older persons characterized by a loss of vision in the macula

Match the disorder with its description.

_____ 22. acute infectious respiratory disease caused by influenza viruses

_____ 23. arthritis of the spine that may progress to fusion of vertebral joints

_____ 24. condition in which sodium urate crystals deposit in the joints

_____ 25. autoimmune disease in which the body attacks its own cartilage and joint linings

_____ 26. cancer of the prostate gland

a. ankylosing spondylitis
b. gouty arthritis
c. influenza
d. prostate cancer
e. rheumatoid arthritis

Match the sign or symptom with its description.

_____ 27. fecal impaction

_____ 28. heatstroke

_____ 29. hypertension

_____ 30. nocturia

_____ 31. urinary incontinence

a. high blood pressure
b. the inability to control urination
c. hardened feces in the colon or rectum
d. the need to get up from sleep during the night to urinate
e. severe and often fatal illness produced by exposure to excessively high temperatures

Match the clinical test or diagnostic procedure with its description.

_____ 32. digital rectal examination

_____ 33. dual energy x-ray absorptiometry

a. manual examination done with a gloved hand to check anatomical structure by palpation
b. evaluative tool for osteoporosis that measures bone mineral density

Match the treatment with its description.

_____ 34. technique in which the joint is moved constantly through a variable range of motion

_____ 35. surgical technique that uses low-frequency ultrasonic needles to liquefy a cataract and remove it

_____ 36. removal of the prostate gland through an incision in the abdominal wall

_____ 37. endoscopic prostate gland removal through the urethra

_____ 38. surgical removal of the prostate gland

a. prostatectomy
b. continuous passive motion
c. suprapubic prostatectomy
d. phacoemulsification
e. transurethral resection of the prostate

Definitions

Define the following terms.

39. delirium _____

40. geriatrics _____

41. lifespan _____

42. longevity _____

43. mortality _____

44. senescence _____

45. senile _____

Provide a medical term for the following definitions.

46. the inability to hear _____

47. person trained to practice occupational therapy _____

48. form of therapy for individuals recuperating from physical or mental illness that encourages rehabilitation through the performance of activities required for daily life _____

49. an outgrowth from the skin that hangs from the surface by a thin stalk _____

50. the inability to urinate _____

Alternate Terms

Give an alternate term for each of the following terms.

51. thyrotoxicosis _____

52. humpback _____

53. senile lentigines _____

54. multi-infarct dementia _____

55. myocardial infarction _____

56. adult rickets _____

Spelling

Identify the correctly spelled term in each set.

57. _____
   a. aneurysm
   b. anyeurism
   c. eneurism
   d. enyeurism

58. _____
   a. newmonia
   b. neumonia
   c. pneumonia
   d. pnumonia

59. _____
   a. diarhea
   b. diarria
   c. diarrhia
   d. diarrhea

60. _____
   a. emphysema
   b. emphesema
   c. emphesima
   d. emfysema

61. _____
   a. melonoma
   b. melanoma
   c. melonomma
   d. melinomma

Unscramble

Unscramble the letters to form a medical term.

62. sapahai _____

63. amene _____

64. kroset _____

65. xeroania _____

66. phortay _____

Abbreviations

Provide the term for the abbreviations and then define the terms.

67. CVA = _____

68. COPD = _____

69. CHF = _____

70. DVT = _____

71. TIA = _____

72. UTI = _____

Analogies

Provide a medical term to complete a meaningful analogy.

73. An aneurysm is to an artery as a deep thrombosis is to a _____.

74. A heart attack is to a _____ as a brain attack is to a _____.

75. Osteopenia is to bone as _____ is to muscle.

Short Answer

Answer the following questions.

76. Differentiate between activities of daily living and instrumental activities of daily living.

_____

_____

77. Briefly discuss the retinal changes due to diabetic retinopathy and how they are treated.

_____

_____

Word Search

Find the medical terms hidden in the puzzle.

```
D  G  P  K  G  U  C  C  U  Q  K  A  I  G  A  C
E  N  H  S  K  H  C  A  J  Y  M  S  E  I  N  O
M  I  O  U  N  T  T  O  T  R  Q  R  M  H  O  M
E  N  T  F  E  A  J  V  E  A  O  E  Y  Q  I  O
N  W  O  D  B  F  I  D  F  N  R  P  J  J  T  R
T  O  C  G  K  J  O  R  T  T  O  A  J  W  A  B
I  D  O  E  K  R  F  O  A  T  M  C  C  O  C  I
A  N  A  E  E  K  L  N  H  N  D  M  T  T  I  D
M  U  G  X  H  O  O  Y  A  M  E  Y  C  R  D  I
E  S  U  J  G  P  R  Z  D  C  S  T  I  I  U  T
D  H  L  Y  Y  O  C  N  V  N  F  X  N  X  A  Y
E  Y  A  H  I  B  U  R  S  I  T  I  S  E  L  H
X  Z  T  D  S  I  S  O  R  B  I  F  Y  F  C  V
Y  O  I  T  U  B  E  R  C  U  L  O  S  I  S  T
M  S  O  Y  T  S  A  L  P  O  R  H  T  R  A  O
M  Q  N  S  I  T  I  T  A  T  S  O  R  P  Q  F
```

arthroplasty
bursitis
cataract
centenarians
claudication
comorbidity
dementia
fibrosis
gerontology
hyponatremia
hypothyroidism
myxedema
photocoagulation
prostatitis
sundowning
tuberculosis
xeroderma

Vocabulary Review

Review the key terms from this chapter, study the spelling and pronunciation of each term, and write its definition in the space provided. Listen to the audio available for most terms at http://thepoint.lww.com/nath2e and pronounce each term for yourself. Then check the box when you feel confident that you know the definition and can pronounce the term correctly.

Key Term	Pronunciation	Definition
❏ activities of daily living (ADL)		_____
❏ age-related macular degeneration	(MACK-yoo-lur)	_____
❏ aging		_____
❏ Alzheimer disease (AD)	(ALTZ-high-mer)	_____
❏ aneurysm	(AN-yoo-riz-um)	_____
❏ angina pectoris	(an-JYE-nuh PECK-toh-ris)	_____
❏ ankylosing spondylitis	(ang-kih-LOH-sing spon-dih-LIGH-tis)	_____
❏ anorexia	(an-oh-REK-see-uh)	_____
❏ aphasia	(uh-FAY-zhuh)	_____

Key Term	Pronunciation	Definition
❏ arteriosclerosis	(ar-TEER-ee-oh-skler-oh-sis)	_____
❏ arthritis	(ar-THRIGH-tis)	_____
❏ arthroplasty	(AR-throh-plas-tee)	_____
❏ atherosclerosis	(ATH-er-oh-skler-oh-sis)	_____
❏ atrophic vaginitis	(a-TROH-fik vaj-ih-NIGH-tis)	_____
❏ atrophy	(AT-roh-fee)	_____
❏ autoimmune diseases	(aw-toh-ih-MYOON)	_____
❏ benign prostatic hyperplasia (BPH)	(beh-NINE pros-TAT-ik high-per-PLAY-zhe-uh)	_____
❏ beta amyloid	(BAY-tuh AM-ih-loyd)	_____
❏ bursitis	(ber-SIGH-tis)	_____
❏ cataract	(KAT-uh-rakt)	_____
❏ centenarians	(sen-ten-AIR-ee-enz)	_____
❏ cerebrovascular accident (CVA)	(se-ree-broh-VAS-kyoo-ler)	_____
❏ chronic bronchitis	(brong-KIGH-tis)	_____
❏ chronic obstructive pulmonary disease (COPD)		_____
❏ claudication	(klaw-di-KAY-shun)	_____
❏ colorectal cancer		_____
❏ comorbidity	(koh-mor-BID-ih-tee)	_____
❏ congestive heart failure (CHF)		_____
❏ constipation	(kon-stih-PAY-shun)	_____
❏ continuous passive motion (CPM)		_____
❏ cor pulmonale	(KOR pool-muh-NAL-ee)	_____
❏ coronary artery disease (CAD)	(KOR-uh-nair-ee AR-ter-ee)	_____
❏ deafness		_____
❏ decubitus ulcers	(de-KYOO-bih-tus UL-surz)	_____
❏ deep vein thrombosis (DVT)	(throm-BOH-sis)	_____
❏ delirium	(de-LIR-ee-um)	_____
❏ dementia	(de-MEN-shuh)	_____
❏ diabetic retinopathy	(dye-uh-BET-ick ret-ih-NOP-uh-thee)	_____
❏ diarrhea	(dye-uh-REE-uh)	_____
❏ digital rectal examination (DRE)		_____

Key Term	Pronunciation	Definition
❑ diverticulitis	(dye-ver-tick-yoo-LYE-tis)	_____
❑ dry mouth		_____
❑ dual energy x-ray absorptiometry (DEXA)	(ab-sorp-tee-OM-eh-tree)	_____
❑ dyspareunia	(dis-pa-ROO-nee-uh)	_____
❑ dysuria	(dis-YOO-ree-uh)	_____
❑ emphysema	(em-fih-SEE-muh)	_____
❑ enema	(EN-eh-muh)	_____
❑ epidemiology	(ep-ih-dee-mee-OL-oh-jee)	_____
❑ fecal impaction	(FEE-kul im-PAK-shun)	_____
❑ fibrosis	(figh-BROH-sis)	_____
❑ flaccid muscles	(FLAH-sid)	_____
❑ geriatrics	(jer-ee-AT-riks)	_____
❑ gerontologist	(jer-on-TOL-oh-jist)	_____
❑ gerontology	(jer-on-TOL-oh-jee)	_____
❑ glaucoma	(glaw-KOH-muh)	_____
❑ gouty arthritis	(GOW-tee ar-THRIGH-tis)	_____
❑ hearing aids		_____
❑ heatstroke		_____
❑ hiatal hernia	(high-AYE-tul HER-nee-uh)	_____
❑ Huntington chorea		_____
❑ hypertension	(high-per-TEN-shun)	_____
❑ hyperthyroidism	(high-pur-THIGH-royd-izm)	_____
❑ hyponatremia	(high-poh-nay-TREE-mee-uh)	_____
❑ hypothermia	(high-poh-THUR-mee-uh)	_____
❑ hypothyroidism	(high-poh-THIGH-royd-izm)	_____
❑ iatrogenic disease	(eye-at-roh-JEN-ik)	_____
❑ influenza	(in-floo-EN-zuh)	_____
❑ inguinal hernia	(ING-gwi-nul HER-nee-uh)	_____
❑ instrumental activities of daily living (IADL)		_____
❑ kyphosis	(kigh-FOH-sis)	_____
❑ life expectancy		_____
❑ lifespan		_____
❑ liver spots		_____
❑ longevity	(lon-JEV-ih-tee)	_____
❑ lung cancer		_____
❑ melanoma	(mel-uh-NOH-muh)	_____
❑ morbidity	(mor-BID-ih-tee)	_____

Key Term	Pronunciation	Definition
❏ mortality	(mor-TAL-ih-tee)	_____
❏ multi-infarct dementia		_____
❏ myocardial infarction (MI)	(migh-oh-KAR-dee-ul in-FARK-shun)	_____
❏ myxedema	(micks-eh-DEE-muh)	_____
❏ nocturia	(nokt-YOO-ree-uh)	_____
❏ occupational therapist (OT)		_____
❏ occupational therapy (OT)		_____
❏ oral cancer		_____
❏ organic brain syndrome		_____
❏ osteoarthritis	(os-tee-oh-ar-THRIGH-tis)	_____
❏ osteomalacia	(os-tee-oh-muh-LAY-she-uh)	_____
❏ osteoporosis	(os-tee-oh-puh-RO-sis)	_____
❏ Paget disease	(PAJ-et)	_____
❏ pancreatic cancer		_____
❏ Parkinson disease (PD)		_____
❏ peptic ulcers	(PEP-tik UL-serz)	_____
❏ periodontal disease	(per-ee-oh-DON-tul)	_____
❏ phacoemulsification	(fak-oh-ee-mul-sih-fi-KAY-shun)	_____
❏ photoaging	(foh-toh-AGE-ing)	_____
❏ photocoagulation	(foh-toh-koh-ag-yoo-LAY-shun)	_____
❏ pneumonia	(new-MOH-nee-uh)	_____
❏ polypharmacy	(pol-ee-FAR-muh-see)	_____
❏ presbycusis	(prez-bee-KYOO-sis)	_____
❏ presbyopia	(prez-bee-OH-pee-uh)	_____
❏ prostate cancer		_____
❏ prostatectomy	(pros-tuh-TEK-toh-mee)	_____
❏ prostatitis	(pros-tuh-TYE-tis)	_____
❏ pulmonary edema	(pul-moh-NAIR-ee e-DEE-muh)	_____
❏ pulmonary embolism	(pul-muh-NAIR-ee em-BO-liz-um)	_____
❏ renal calculi	(ree-nul KAL-kyoo-lye)	_____
❏ restless legs syndrome (RLS)		_____
❏ rheumatoid arthritis (RA)	(ROO-muh-toid ar-THRIGH-tis)	_____
❏ right ventricular hypertrophy	(ven-TRIK-yoo-lur high-PUR-troh-fee)	_____
❏ sarcopenia	(sar-koh-PEE-nee-uh)	_____

Key Term	Pronunciation	Definition
❏ satellite cells	(SAT-eh-light)	_____
❏ senescence	(seh-NES-ens)	_____
❏ senile	(SE-nile)	_____
❏ senile lentigines	(SEE-nile len-TIJ-ih-nez)	_____
❏ senile osteopenia	(SEE-nile os-tee-oh-PEE-nee-uh)	_____
❏ senile pruritus	(SEE-nile proo-RYE-tus)	_____
❏ shingles		_____
❏ skin tag		_____
❏ stomach cancer		_____
❏ stroke		_____
❏ sundowner syndrome		_____
❏ sundowning		_____
❏ suprapubic prostatectomy	(soo-pruh-PYOO-bik pros-tuh-TEK-toh-mee)	_____
❏ T lymphocytes	(lim-FOH-sights)	_____
❏ thyrotoxicosis	(thigh-roh-tok-sih-KOH-sis)	_____
❏ transient ischemic attack (TIA)	(TRAN-see-ent is-KEE-mick)	_____
❏ transurethral resection of the prostate (TURP)	(trans-yoo-REE-thrul)	_____
❏ tuberculosis (TB)	(too-ber-kyoo-LOH-sis)	_____
❏ urinary incontinence	(in-KON-ti-nens)	_____
❏ urinary retention		_____
❏ urinary tract infections (UTIs)		_____
❏ varicose veins	(VAIR-ih-kose)	_____
❏ vascular dementia	(vas-KYOO-lur de-MEN-shuh)	_____
❏ water intoxication		_____
❏ xeroderma	(zeh-roh-DUR-muh)	_____

Answers

Word Grouping Exercises

Definition	Word Part	Definition	Word Part
above, over	hyper-	joint, articulation	arthr-, arthro-
artery	arteri-, arterio-	light	phot-, photo-
bent, crooked, stiff	ankylo-	muscle	sarco-
bone	ost-, oste-, osteo-	night	noct-
death	mort-	old age	A. gero-, geront-, geronto- B. presby-, presbyo-
deficiency	-penia	relating to the lens	phaco-
deficient, below normal	hypo-	skin	derm-, derma-
dry	xero-	study of	-ology
hard	scler-, sclero-	vertebrae	spondyl-, spondylo-
hundred	centi-	vision	-opia

Word Building Exercises

Word Part	Meaning	Common or Known Word	Example Medical Term
arteri-, arterio-	artery	artery	arterial
arthr-, arthro-	joint, articulation	arthritis	arthralgia
centi-	hundred	centimeter	centimeter
derm-, derma-	skin	dermatologist	dermatology
gero-, geront-, geronto-	old age	gerontologist	gerontology
hyper-	above, over	hyperactive	hyperthermia
hypo-	deficient, below normal	hypoallergenic	hypoglycemia
mort-	death	mortal	mortality
phot-, photo-	light	photograph	photocoagulation
scler-, sclero-	hard	sclera	arteriosclerosis

Key Term Practice

Aging

1. Morbidity
2. gerontology; *geront-*; *-ology*
3. Epidemiology
4. centenarians; *centi-*
5. life expectancy

Aging and the Integumentary System

1. senile
2. senile pruritus
3. Xeroderma; *xero-*; *derma-*
4. decubitus ulcers
5. Photoaging

Aging and the Skeletal System

1. bursitis
2. Senile osteopenia
3. Gouty arthritis
4. kyphosis
5. osteoarthritis; *osteo-, arthr-*

Aging and the Muscular System

1. Flaccid muscles
2. sarcopenia
3. atrophy
4. Fibrosis
5. satellite cells

Aging and the Nervous System

1. dementia
2. Alzheimer disease (AD)
3. Parkinson disease (PD)
4. vascular dementia; multi-infarct dementia
5. sundowner syndrome; sundowning

Aging and the Special Senses

1. Presbycusis
2. glaucoma
3. cataract
4. hearing aids
5. Photocoagulation

Aging and the Endocrine System

1. Hyponatremia; *hypo-*
2. myxedema
3. hyperthyroidism; thyrotoxicosis
4. water intoxication
5. Hypothyroidism

Aging and the Cardiovascular System

1. Claudication
2. restless legs syndrome (RLS)
3. angina pectoris
4. Coronary artery disease (CAD)
5. atherosclerosis

Aging and the Respiratory System

1. Tuberculosis
2. emphysema
3. lung cancer
4. pulmonary edema
5. right ventricular hypertrophy; cor pulmonale

Aging and the Lymphatic System and Immunity

1. autoimmune diseases
2. T lymphocytes

Aging and the Digestive System

1. Diarrhea
2. periodontal disease
3. constipation
4. Dry mouth
5. peptic ulcers

Aging and the Urinary System

1. Nocturia
2. renal calculi
3. urinary incontinence
4. urinary retention
5. Dysuria

Aging and the Reproductive System

1. dyspareunia
2. Atrophic vaginitis
3. prostatitis
4. benign prostatic hyperplasia (BPH)
5. inguinal hernia

Pharmacology and Older Adults

1. comorbidity
2. iatrogenic disease
3. polypharmacy

Common Abbreviations Exercises

1. IADL = instrumental activities of daily living
2. RLS = restless legs syndrome
3. tuberculosis = TB
4. CHF = congestive heart failure
5. transient ischemic attack = TIA

Case Study

1. Mr. James has the following disorders:
   - a. osteoarthritis of the right hip = joint disease characterized by erosion of articular cartilage within a joint; this is a progressive degenerative joint disease
   - b. presbycusis of the left ear = hearing loss as a result of old age in the left ear
   - c. presbyopia = inability of the aging eyes to focus on near objects
   - d. slight hypertension, or high blood pressure
2. CPM is the abbreviation for continuous passive motion, a technique in which the joint is moved constantly through a variable range of motion to prevent stiffness and to increase the range of motion.
3. Arthroplasty is the medical term for a joint replacement.
4. PT is the abbreviation for physical therapy or physical therapist and OT is the abbreviation for occupational therapy or occupational therapist.

Real World Report Questions

1. The health care workers involved with this case are a physician, physical therapist (PT), and occupational therapist (OT).
2. Mr. James has just had hip replacement surgery and is getting ready to go home, so he needs to be assessed and evaluated.
3. Mr. James can bathe, groom, perform mouth care, do bed and chair transfers, walk, and eat independently.
4. Mr. James requires assistance for the following IADL: shopping, cooking, managing medications, doing housework, doing laundry, driving or using public transportation, and managing finances.
5. Mr. James cannot drive, but he may be driven distances of short duration (less than 1 hour).

Review and Application

1. c	10. c	19. a.	28. e.
2. b	11. arteriosclerosis	20. c.	29. a.
3. c	12. arthritis	21. b.	30. d.
4. b	13. gerontologist	22. c.	31. b.
5. d	14. hypothermia	23. a.	32. a.
6. a	15. osteoporosis	24. b.	33. b.
7. d	16. presbyopia	25. e.	34. b.
8. c	17. e.	26. d.	35. d.
9. a	18. d.	27. c.	36. c.

37. e.
38. a.
39. delirium = altered state of consciousness with confusion
40. geriatrics = the branch of medicine concerned with the health care of the elderly
41. lifespan = normal or average duration of life for members of a given species
42. longevity = duration of life beyond the norm for the species
43. mortality = refers to death
44. senescence = changes that occur with aging
45. senile = relating to or characteristic of old age
46. deafness
47. occupational therapist
48. occupational therapy
49. skin tag
50. urinary retention
51. hyperthyroidism
52. kyphosis
53. liver spots
54. vascular dementia
55. heart attack
56. osteomalacia
57. a.
58. c.
59. d.
60. a.
61. b.
62. aphasia
63. enema
64. stroke

65. anorexia
66. atrophy
67. CVA = cerebrovascular accident; imprecise term for cerebral stroke
68. COPD = chronic obstructive pulmonary disease; general term for lung disorders that result in respiratory failure
69. CHF = congestive heart failure; inadequacy of the heart to pump blood and maintain systemic circulation
70. DVT = deep vein thrombosis; presence of a blood clot (thrombus) in a vein, usually in deep veins of the lower extremity
71. TIA = transient ischemic attack; sudden impairment of brain blood circulation that resolves within 24 hours
72. UTI = urinary tract infection; microbial (usually bacteria) infection in any part of the urinary tract
73. vein
74. myocardial infarction; stroke
75. sarcopenia
76. Activities of daily living are acts of basic care such as bathing, dressing, going to the bathroom, walking, and eating. Instrumental activities of daily living are activities of daily living plus tasks such as shopping, preparing meals, managing money, using the telephone, and doing housework.
77. Retinal changes occurring with diabetes mellitus are mainly characterized by leaky blood vessels and vessel overgrowth, causing scarring of the retina and severe problems with vision. Laser beams are used to cauterize the leaky blood vessels.

Word Search

```
D  G  P  K  G  U  C  C  U  Q  K  A  I  G  A  C
E  N  H  S  K  H  C  A  J  Y  M  S  E  I  N  O
M  I  O  U  N  T  T  O  T  R  Q  R  M  H  O  M
E  N  T  F  E  A  J  V  E  A  O  E  Y  Q  I  O
N  W  O  D  B  F  I  D  F  N  R  P  J  J  T  R
T  O  C  G  K  J  O  R  T  T  O  A  J  W  A  B
I  D  O  E  K  R  F  O  A  T  M  C  C  O  C  I
A  N  A  E  E  K  L  N  H  N  D  M  T  T  I  D
M  U  G  X  H  O  O  Y  A  M  E  Y  C  R  D  I
E  S  U  J  G  P  R  Z  D  C  S  T  I  I  U  T
D  H  L  Y  Y  O  C  N  V  N  F  X  N  X  A  Y
E  Y  A  H  I  B  U  R  S  I  T  I  S  E  L  H
X  Z  T  D  S  I  S  O  R  B  I  F  Y  F  C  V
Y  O  I  T  U  B  E  R  C  U  L  O  S  I  S  T
M  S  O  Y  T  S  A  L  P  O  R  H  T  R  A  O
M  Q  N  S  I  T  I  T  A  T  S  O  R  P  Q  F
```

arthroplasty
bursitis
cataract
centenarians
claudication
comorbidity
dementia
fibrosis
gerontology
hyponatremia
hypothyroidism
myxedema
photocoagulation
prostatitis
sundowning
tuberculosis
xeroderma

Vocabulary Review

Key Term	Definition	Key Term	Definition
activities of daily living (ADL)	acts of basic care such as bathing, dressing, going to the bathroom, getting in or out of bed or a chair, walking, and eating	**anorexia**	poor appetite
		aphasia	partial or total inability to produce and understand speech, caused by brain injury
age-related macular degeneration	eye disorder affecting older adults characterized by a loss of vision in the macula (center of the visual field) because of damage to the retina	**arteriosclerosis**	hardening of the arteries
		arthritis	inflammation of a joint or chronic inflammation of the joints
aging	process of growing old	**arthroplasty**	joint replacement
Alzheimer disease (AD)	progressive degenerative disease of the brain marked by senile plaques, degenerated brain cells, and neurofibrillary tangles	**atherosclerosis**	pathological condition in which fatty substances, especially cholesterol and triglycerides, are deposited in the arterial walls causing hardening of the arteries
aneurysm	thin, weakened section of the wall of an artery that bulges outward, forming a balloon-like sac of the blood vessel	**atrophic vaginitis**	inflammation of the vagina due to thinning and atrophy of the vaginal epithelium
angina pectoris	severe chest pain that radiates from the heart to the shoulder (usually the left) and down the arm	**atrophy**	muscle wasting
		autoimmune diseases	disorders in which the body does not recognize its own tissue (self) antigens and produces antibodies against them
ankylosing spondylitis	arthritis of the spine that resembles rheumatoid arthritis and may progress to fusion of vertebral joints		

Key Term	Definition	Key Term	Definition
benign prostatic hyperplasia (BPH)	progressive enlargement of the prostate gland that begins around the fifth decade	**diarrhea**	frequent and excessive watery bowel movements
beta amyloid	abnormal protein at the core of the senile plaques of Alzheimer disease	**digital rectal examination (DRE)**	manual examination done with a gloved hand to check anatomical structures by palpating them through the rectum
bursitis	inflammation of a bursa	**diverticulitis**	inflammation of the diverticula with abdominal pain
cataract	eye disease characterized by clouding of the lens	**dry mouth**	condition of diminished saliva production
centenarians	individuals who live to be 100 years old or more	**dual energy x-ray absorptiometry (DEXA)**	evaluative tool for osteoporosis that measures bone mineral density by aiming x-ray beams of differing energy levels at the bones
cerebrovascular accident (CVA)	imprecise term for cerebral stroke		
chronic bronchitis	condition of the bronchial tree characterized by excessive mucus production and a persistent cough over a long period of time	**dyspareunia**	pain during sexual intercourse
		dysuria	painful urination
		emphysema	anatomical alteration of the lung with abnormal enlargement of air sacs and eventual destruction of air sac walls
chronic obstructive pulmonary disease (COPD)	general term for lung disorders that result in respiratory failure	**enema**	rectal insertion of a liquid for clearing out the bowel as a treatment for constipation
claudication	lameness, limping, tension, and pain caused by defective circulation of the blood in the vessels of the limbs	**epidemiology**	branch of science that deals with the incidence, distribution, and possible control of diseases and other factors related to health
colorectal cancer	cancer of the colon and rectum		
		fecal impaction	hardened feces in the colon or rectum
comorbidity	the coexistence of two or more disease processes	**fibrosis**	formation of fibrous connective tissue, which displaces skeletal muscle tissue
congestive heart failure (CHF)	inadequacy of the heart to pump blood and maintain systemic circulation	**flaccid muscles**	muscles with less-than-normal tone
		geriatrics	branch of medicine concerned with the health care of the elderly
constipation	condition in which bowel movements are infrequent	**gerontologist**	person who specializes in gerontology
continuous passive motion (CPM)	technique in which the joint is moved constantly through a variable range of motion to prevent stiffness and increase the range of motion	**gerontology**	scientific study of the clinical, sociological, biological, and psychological aspects of aging
		glaucoma	increased fluid pressure in the eye that produces defects in the field of vision and eventual blindness
cor pulmonale	abnormal enlargement of the right side of the heart in response to lung disease; also called right ventricular hypertrophy		
		gouty arthritis	condition in which sodium urate crystals deposit in the joints, causing inflammation and pain
coronary artery disease (CAD)	narrowing of the lumen of one or more coronary arteries		
deafness	inability to hear; two forms are conduction deafness and sensorineural deafness	**hearing aids**	electronic devices for amplifying sound to the ear
decubitus ulcers	pressure sores that appear in areas of skin overlying bony projections	**heatstroke**	severe and often fatal illness produced by exposure to excessively high temperatures
deep vein thrombosis (DVT)	presence of a blood clot (thrombus) in a vein, usually in deep veins of the lower extremity	**hiatal hernia**	weakening around the diaphragmatic opening for the esophagus that allows the stomach to move up into the chest cavity
delirium	altered state of consciousness with confusion		
dementia	underlying structural brain disease that causes a progressive loss of cognitive and intellectual functions	**Huntington chorea**	hereditary neurodegenerative disorder characterized by irregular, spasmodic involuntary movements of the limbs or facial muscles and progressive dementia
diabetic retinopathy	retinal changes occurring with diabetes mellitus characterized by leaky blood vessels and vessel overgrowth that causes scarring		
		hypertension	high blood pressure

Key Term	Definition
hyperthyroidism	excessive thyroid hormone production; also called thyrotoxicosis
hyponatremia	abnormally low concentration of sodium ions in the blood
hypothermia	body temperature lower than 98.6°F (37°C)
hypothyroidism	deficiency of thyroid hormones
iatrogenic disease	medically induced unfavorable response
influenza	acute infectious respiratory disease caused by influenza viruses
inguinal hernia	rupture or separation of a portion of the abdominal wall resulting in the protrusion of a part of an organ
instrumental activities of daily living (IADL)	activities of daily living plus tasks such as shopping, preparing meals, managing money, using the telephone, and doing housework
kyphosis	abnormal concave curvature of the thoracic spine; also called humpback
life expectancy	average number of years a person born today can expect to live under current conditions
lifespan	normal or average duration of life for members of a given species
liver spots	age spots or pigment blotching on the skin due to increased melanin production; also called senile lentigines
longevity	duration of life beyond the norm for the species
lung cancer	fatal malignancy in which cancerous cells replace the bronchial epithelial cells
melanoma	malignant cancer derived from melanocytes
morbidity	condition of being ill
mortality	refers to death
multi-infarct dementia	disorder marked by a reduced blood flow to the brain; also called vascular dementia
myocardial infarction (MI)	death of an area of the heart tissue due to interrupted blood supply; also called heart attack
myxedema	extreme hypothyroidism in adults characterized by dry swelling of the skin and subcutaneous tissues
nocturia	the need to get up from sleep during the night to urinate
occupational therapist (OT)	person trained to practice occupational therapy
occupational therapy (OT)	form of therapy for individuals recuperating from physical or mental illness that encourages rehabilitation through the performance of activities required for daily life
oral cancer	cancer of the mouth

Key Term	Definition
organic brain syndrome	collection of behavioral and psychological signs and symptoms including problems with attention, concentration, memory, confusion, anxiety, and depression
osteoarthritis	joint disease characterized by erosion of articular cartilage within a joint
osteomalacia	bone softening and bending as a result of a vitamin D deficiency; also called adult rickets
osteoporosis	disease characterized by weak, very porous bones that break easily and heal slowly
Paget disease	generalized skeletal disease of older people characterized by irregular thickening and softening of the bones with bending of weight-bearing bones
pancreatic cancer	cancer of the pancreas
Parkinson disease (PD)	neurological syndrome usually resulting from deficiency of the neurotransmitter dopamine
peptic ulcers	sores in the stomach or duodenum lining
periodontal disease	collective term for a variety of oral conditions
phacoemulsification	surgical technique that uses low-frequency ultrasonic needles to liquefy a cataract and remove it by suction through a small incision in the cornea
photoaging	skin wrinkling and damage due to years of sun exposure
photocoagulation	the use of a laser beam to treat retinal disorders
pneumonia	inflammation of the lung with most cases caused by bacterial or viral infection
polypharmacy	the administration of multiple drugs at the same time
presbycusis	hearing loss as a result of old age
presbyopia	inability of the aging eye to focus on near objects
prostate cancer	cancer of the prostate gland
prostatectomy	surgical removal of the prostate gland
prostatitis	inflammation of the prostate gland
pulmonary edema	swelling of the lungs that is caused by mitral stenosis (narrowing of the opening of the mitral valve) or left ventricular failure
pulmonary embolism	clot in a pulmonary artery
renal calculi	kidney stones
restless legs syndrome (RLS)	an uneasiness, twitching, or restlessness that occurs in the legs after going to bed

Key Term	Definition	Key Term	Definition
rheumatoid arthritis (RA)	autoimmune disease in which the body attacks its own cartilage and joint linings	sundowning	the onset or exacerbation of delirium during the evening or night with improvement or disappearance during the day; also called sundowner syndrome
right ventricular hypertrophy	abnormal enlargement of the right side of the heart in response to lung disease; also called cor pulmonale	suprapubic prostatectomy	removal of the prostate gland through an incision in the abdominal wall just above the pubic bone
sarcopenia	loss of muscle as a result of deconditioning	T lymphocytes	types of white blood cells essential for various aspects of immunity
satellite cells	cells scattered throughout muscle tissue that play a role in muscle repair and regeneration	thyrotoxicosis	excessive thyroid hormone production; also called hyperthyroidism
senescence	changes that occur with aging	transient ischemic attack (TIA)	sudden impairment of brain blood circulation that resolves within 24 hours
senile	relating to or characteristic of old age		
senile lentigines	age spots or pigment blotching on the skin due to increased melanin production; also called liver spots	transurethral resection of the prostate (TURP)	endoscopic prostate gland removal through the urethra
senile osteopenia	bone condition characterized by decreased calcification or density of bone in the elderly	tuberculosis (TB)	infection of the lung caused by *Mycobacterium tuberculosis*
senile pruritus	itching associated with dryness of the skin in the elderly	urinary incontinence	the inability to control urination
shingles	herpes zoster infection characterized by an eruption of vesicles on the skin following the course of a nerve	urinary retention	the inability to urinate
skin tag	an outgrowth from the skin that hangs from the surface by a thin stalk	urinary tract infections (UTIs)	microbial (usually bacteria) infections in any part of the urinary tract
stomach cancer	cancer of the stomach	varicose veins	dilated and twisted veins caused by incompetent or ineffective valves
stroke	sudden impairment of blood circulation to the brain that lasts longer than 24 hours; also called brain attack	vascular dementia	disorder marked by a reduced blood flow to the brain; also called multi-infarct dementia
sundowner syndrome	the onset or exacerbation of delirium during the evening or night with improvement or disappearance during the day; also called sundowning	water intoxication	metabolic brain disorder that results from severe overhydration
		xeroderma	excessive skin dryness

Index

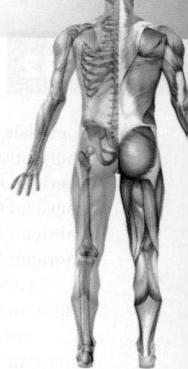

Page numbers followed by *f* and *t* indicate figures (illustrations) and tables, respectively.
Page numbers in **purple** where a key term is defined in a Key Term table.

A

A. *See* Anterior (A)
A$_{1c}$ test. *See* Glycosylated hemoglobin (A$_{1c}$) test
AA. *See* Alcoholics Anonymous (AA); Associate of arts (AA)
AAP. *See* American Academy of Pediatrics (AAP)
Ab. *See* Antibody(ies) (Ab)
ABCD. *See* Asymmetry, border, color, diameter (ABCD)
ABCDEs of skin cancer, **1105**
Abdominal cavity, **57**
Abdominal hernia, 725
Abdominal region, 63*f*, 64*t*
Abdominopelvic cavity, **57**
Abdominopelvic quadrants, 59, 60*f*
Abdominopelvic region(s), 59–61
Abducens nerve (CN VI), 330, 330*f*
Abduction, **246**
Abductors, **299**
ABGs. *See* Arterial blood gases (ABGs)
Abortion, **912**
spontaneous, 909
Abrasion, **162**
Abruptio placentae, **923**
Abscess(es), **170**, 237, 710
Absorption, **698**
Abstinence, **868**
Abulia, **995**
Accessory nerve (CN XI), 329, 330*f*
Accommodation, **372**
Accreditation Council for Occupational Therapy Education (ACOTE), 1150
ACE inhibitors. *See* Angiotensin-converting enzyme (ACE) inhibitors
Acetabulum, **229**
Acetaminophen, **1056**
Acetylsalicylic acid (ASA), 250, 537
Acid-fast bacilli (AFB), 605
Acid-fast stain, 605
Acidemia, 608, **610**
ACL. *See* Anterior cruciate ligament (ACL)
ACLS. *See* Advanced cardiac life support (ACLS)
Acne, **162**
ACOTE. *See* Accreditation Council for Occupational Therapy Education (ACOTE)
Acquired immunodeficiency syndrome (AIDS), **658**, 863, 1053
Acromegaly, **434**
Acromial region, 63*f*, 64*t*
Acromion process, 219*t*
Acrosome, **829**, 903
ACTH. *See* Adrenocorticotropic hormone (ACTH)
Actinic keratosis, 168
Active immunity, **648**

Activities of daily living (ADLs), 299, **1155**
Acute asthma, 655
Acute bronchitis, 597
Acute lymphoblastic leukemia (ALL), 486, **1113**
Acute lymphocytic leukemia (ALL), **1113**
Acute lymphocytic/lymphoid leukemia (ALL), **1113**. *See* Acute lymphoblastic leukemia (ALL)
Acute myeloid leukemia (AML), 486, **1113**
Acute renal failure (ARF), 780
Acute rhinitis, 601
A.D. *See* Right ear (*auris dextra,* A.D.)
AD. *See* Alzheimer disease (AD)
ADA. *See* American Dietetic Association (ADA)
Adaptive immunity, **648**
Addiction, 992, **1047**
Addison disease, **428**
Adduction, **246**
Adductors, **299**
Adenocarcinoma, **1115**
Adenohypophysis, **416**
Adenoid, 579, **646**
Adenosine triphosphate (ATP), **49**
ADH. *See* Antidiuretic hormone (ADH)
Adhesions, 727, 729
Adhesive capsulitis, 255
Adipose tissue, **153**
ADLs. *See* Activities of daily living (ADLs)
Adnexa, **849**
Adolescence, **917**
Adrenal cortex, **421**
Adrenal glands, **421**
disorders of, 425–428
Adrenal medulla, **421**
Adrenaline, **421**
Adrenocortical carcinoma, **1111**
Adrenocortical hormones, **1067**
Adrenocorticotropic hormone (ACTH), **416**
Adsorbents, **1068**
Adult respiratory distress syndrome (ARDS), **610**
Adult rickets, 1160
Adulthood, **917**
Advanced cardiac life support (ACLS), 508
Adverse drug reaction (ADR), **1047**
AFB. *See* Acid-fast bacilli (AFB)
Affect, **977**
AFP. *See* α-fetoprotein (AFP)
African sleeping sickness, 1055
Afterbirth, 909
Ag. *See* Antigen (Ag)
Age-related deafness, 1170
Age-related macular degeneration (AMD), 385, **1171**
dry form, 1170
wet form, 1170
Age spots, 183

Agglutination, **471**
Agglutinin, **471**
Agglutinogen, **471**
Aggressive, **1114**
Aging, 71, 948, **1154**
and cardiovascular function, 548
and cardiovascular system, 1173–1176
and digestive system, 734, 1180–1183
and endocrine system, 1172–1173
and immunity, 665
and integumentary system, 1155–1158
and lymphatic system and immunity, 1179–1180
and muscular system, 1164–1165
and nervous system, 1165–1169
and reproductive system, 870, 1185–1187
and respiratory system, 612, 1177–1179
and skeletal system, 1158–1164
and skin, 183
and special senses, 1169–1171
and urinary system, 791, 1183–1184
Agranulocytes, **465**
AHF. *See* Antihemophilic factor (AHF)
AIDS. *See* Acquired immunodeficiency syndrome (AIDS)
AIDS-related complex, **658**
Albinism, **156**, 925
Albumin, **462**
Albuminuria, **775**
Alcohol abuse, **991**
Alcoholics Anonymous (AA), 992
Alcoholism, **992**
Aldosterone, **421**, 771
Aliment, **690**
Alimentary canal, **691**
ALL. *See* Acute lymphocytic/lymphoid leukemia (ALL)
Allantois, **905**
Allergic rhinitis, 601, **655**
Allergy, **655**
drugs, 1064–1065
Allograft, **664**
Alogia, **995**
Alopecia, **164**
Alpha blockers, **1064**
α-fetoprotein serum test, **928**
α$_1$-Antiprotease deficiency, 596
α$_1$-Antitrypsin deficiency, 596
ALS. *See* Amyotrophic lateral sclerosis (ALS)
Altitude sickness, **610**
Alveolar ducts, 582*f*
Alveolar sacs, 582*f*
Alveoli, **583**
Alzheimer disease (AD), 339, **990**, **1169**
Amblyopia, **379**
AMD. *See* Age-related macular degeneration (AMD)

Amebiasis, 1055
American Academy of Pediatrics (AAP), 942
American Cancer Society, 850
American College of Surgeons, 71
American Dietetic Association (ADA), 686
American Massage Therapy Association
  (AMTA), 638
American Registry of Diagnostic Medical
  Sonographers (ARDMS), 898
American Society for Clinical Pathology
  (ASCP), 146
Amino acids, 705
Amnesia, 336, 990
  dissociative, 1005
Amniocentesis, 928
Amnion, 905
Amnionic, definition of, 903
Amphetamine(s), 986
Amphetamine-dextroamphetamine
  (Adderall), 986
AMTA. *See* American Massage Therapy
  Association (AMTA)
Amylase, 698
  salivary, 692
  serum, 717
  urine, 717
Amyloid, 1166
Amyotrophic lateral sclerosis (ALS), 345
Amyotrophy, 342
AN. *See* Anorexia nervosa (AN)
Anabolism, 701
Anal canal, 704
Anal sphincters, 703, 703*f*
Analgesics, 177, 341, 1056
Anaphylactic shock, 654
Anaphylaxis, 655
Anaplasia, 1098
Anatomic plane(s), 61–62
Anatomic position, 57
Anatomic terms, 63, 64–65*t*
  medical term parts used in, 42–46
  for superficial landmarks, 63, 63*f*
Anatomy, 47
Androgens, 421
Anemia, 474
  aplastic, 472
  hemolytic, 472
  hemorrhagic, 472
  iron-deficiency, 473
  nutritional, 473
  pernicious, 473–474
  sickle cell, 473, 473*f*, 474
Anencephaly, 937
Anesthesia, 1060
Anesthesiologist, 1060
Anesthesiology, 1060
Anesthetics, 1060
Anesthetist, 1060
Anesthetize, 1059
Aneurysm, 546, 1176
  dissecting, 544, 544*f*, 547
  false, 545, 547
  fusiform, 544, 544*f*, 547
  saccular, 544, 544*f*, 546
Angina pectoris, 532, 1176
Angiocardiography, 111
Angiogenesis, 520
Angiogram, 532

Angiography, 111
  cerebral, 336, 337
  computed tomographic, 103
  digital subtraction (DSA), 110
  fluorescein, 382, 385, 394–395
  magnetic resonance (MRA), 107
Angioplasty, 532
Angiotensin-converting enzyme (ACE)
  inhibitors, 537, 1064
Angiotensin II receptor blockers, 1064
Anhedonia, 995
Ankle, 228*f*
  bones of, 227
  disorders of, 252–254
Ankylosing spondylitis, 251, 1163
Ankylosis, 251
Anorexia, 718, 1179
Anorexia nervosa (AN), 721, 1010
ANS. *See* Autonomic nervous system (ANS)
Antacid, 712, 1068
Antagonist, 1053
Antebrachial, 63*f*, 64*t*
Antecubital, 63*f*, 64*t*
Anterior (A), 57
Anterior chamber, of eye, 370, 370*f*
Anterior cruciate ligament (ACL), 252, 305
Anterior pituitary gland, 418
Anteroposterior (AP), 57
Anthracosis, 600
Antibiotic(s), 712, 1053, 1067
  broad-spectrum, 1052–1053
Antibody(ies) (Ab), 471, 643, 649, 651, 651*f*, 665
Antibody-mediated immunity, 648
Antibody titer, 665
Anticholinergics, 335, 729
Anticoagulant, 335, 466, 470, 1061
Anticonvulsants, 1058
Antidepressants, 997, 1058
Antidiarrheal, 1058
Antidiuretic hormone (ADH), 417, 771
  deficiency of, 432
Antiemetics, 336, 1068
Antiestrogenic hormone, 1066
Antifungal drugs, 1055
Antigen (Ag), 471, 643
Antihelminthic drugs, 1055
Antihemophilic factor (AHF), 477
Antihistamines, 655, 1065
Antihyperlipidemics, 1064
Antihypertensive drugs, 1064
Antimicrobial agents, 1053
Antimycobacterial drugs, 1053
Antinauseants, 1068
Antineoplastic drugs, 486
Antiplatelet, 1061
Antiprotozoal drugs, 1055
Antipsychotic drugs, 995
  atypical, 1057
  typical, 1057
Antipyretic agent, 1056
Antiseptic agent, 1053
Antisocial personality disorder, 1013
Antitussive, 1058
Antiviral drugs, 1054
Anuria, 781
Anus, 704
Anxiety, 987
  disorders, 1001

Anxiolytic, 1001
Aorta, 514, 520
Aortic coarctation, 529
Aortic semilunar valve (ASLV), 512, 513*f*
Aortic valve, 514
Aortography, 111
Aortoplasty, 529
Apathy, 990
Apex, 513, 584
Apgar score, 913
Aphasia, 1168
Aphonia, 605
Aphtha, 710
Apical heartbeat, 513
Aplastic anemia, 474
Apnea, 589
  sleep, 589, 609, 1011, 1012
  reflex, 589
Aponeurosis, 291
Apoptosis, 348, 1097
Appendicitis, 713
Appendicular, 57
Appendix, 704
Apperception, 982
Aquaphobia, 999
Aqueous humor, 373
Arachnoid mater, 332
Arachnophobia, 999*t*
ARDMS. *See* American Registry of Diagnostic
  Medical Sonographers (ARDMS)
ARDS. *See* Adult respiratory distress
  syndrome (ARDS)
Areola, 833
ARF. *See* Acute renal failure (ARF)
Argus II system, 379
Arousal, 839
Arrector pili muscles, 156
Arrhythmia, 422, 541, 1062
Arterial blood gases (ABGs), 610, 939
Arterial catheter placement
  nonselective, 104, 106
  selective, 104, 106
Arteries, 518
Arteriography, 111
Arterioles, 518
Arteriosclerosis, 531, 1176
Arteriovenous (AV) fistula, 546
Artery(ies), 508, 514, 518
  disorders of, 543–547
Arthralgia, 473
Arthritis, 249, 1163. *See also* Lyme arthritis;
  Rheumatoid arthritis (RA)
Arthrocentesis, 249
Arthrography, 102, 254
Arthroplasty, 254, 1163
Arthroscope, 254
Arthroscopy, 254
Articular, 214
Articular cartilage, 214, 243
Articulation, 241
  autoimmune disease and, 249–251
  classification of, 241–244
  injury to, case study, 260
  movements, 244–246, 245*f*
  structures of, 240
  trauma to, 256–257
Artificial pacemaker, 536
A.S. *See* Left ear (*auris sinistra*, A.S.)

ASA. *See* Acetylsalicylic acid (ASA); Aspirin
Asbestosis, **600**
Ascending colon, **704**
Ascites, 852
Ascorbic acid, 215
ASCP. *See* American Society for Clinical Pathology (ASCP)
ASD. *See* Atrial septal defect (ASD)
ASLV. *See* Aortic semilunar valve (ASLV)
Aspartate aminotransferase (AST) test, 534
Asperger disorder, **987**
Asphyxia, **589**
Aspiration pneumonia, **605**
Aspirin, 250, 341, 537–538, 929, **1056**
Assessment, 5
AST. *See* Aspartate aminotransferase (AST)
Asthma, 597–599, **598**, **655**, 1065
    acute, 654
    bronchial, 597
    exercise-induced, 598
    extrinsic, 654, 655
    intrinsic, 654, 655
Astigmatism, **382**
Astringent, **1053**
Astrocytes, 324
Astrocytoma, **340**, **1110**
Asymmetry, border, color, diameter (ABCD), 167
Asymmetry, border, color, diameter, and elevation (ABCDE) method, of skin cancer, 1102, 1102*f*
Atherectomy, **531**
Atheroma, **106**
Atherosclerosis, **531**, 547, **1176**
Athlete's foot, 175
Athletic trainer, professional profile, 208
Atlas, 219*t*, 223
Atomizer, **592**
Atopic dermatitis, **174**
Atopic eczema, **175**
Atopy, **175**
ATP. *See* Adenosine triphosphate (ATP)
Atria, **513**
Atrial natriuretic peptide (ANP), **425**
Atrial septal defect (ASD), **529**, **933**
Atrioventricular (AV) bundle, **523**
Atrioventricular (AV) node, **523**
Atrioventricular (AV) valves, **513**
Atrium, 511, 512*f*, 519*f*
Atrophic vaginitis, **1187**
Atrophy, **216**, **291**, **1165**
Attention deficit disorder (ADD), **987**
Attention deficit hyperactivity disorder (ADHD), **987**
Attenuated vaccine, 651
Atypical antipsychotics, 1057
A.U. *See* Each ear (*auris uterque*, A.U.)
Audiogram, **388**
Audiometry, **388**
Auditory ossicles, **375**
Auditory tube, **375**
Aura, **336**
Auricle, **375**
Auscultation, **68**, **589**
Autism, **987**
Autograft, **664**
Autoimmune diseases, **653**, **1180**
Autoimmune disorder, **165**

Autologous transfusion, **474**
Automaticity, 522
Autonomic nervous system (ANS), **323**
AV. *See* Arteriovenous (AV); Atrioventricular (AV)
Axial, **57**
Axillary, 63*f*, 64*t*
Axis, 223
Axon, **325**
Azathioprine (AZT), **663**
Azotemia, 779
AZT. *See* Azathioprine (AZT)

B

B cells (B lymphocytes), **466**, **650**, 665
Bacteria
    gram-negative, 608, 1052, 1052*f*
    gram-positive, 1052, 1052*f*
Bactericidal drugs, **1053**
Bacteriostatic drugs, **1053**
Bacteriuria, **775**
Baldness, 163
Ball-and-socket joint, **244**
Barbiturates, **1058**
Barium enema (BE), **109**, 727, **732**
Barium sulfate (BaSO$_4$), **109**, 721
Barium swallow, **109**, **723**
Barrel chest, 597
Bartholin glands, 831
Basal cell carcinoma, **169**, **1105**
    case study, 185–186
Basal, definition of, 705
Basal ganglia, 340
Basal metabolic rate (BMR), **705**
Base, **584**
BaSO$_4$. *See* Barium sulfate (BaSO$_4$)
Basophils, **466**
BBB. *See* Blood–brain barrier (BBB)
BC. *See* Birth control (BC)
BCP. *See* Birth control pills (BCPs)
BE. *See* Barium enema (BE)
Bedsore. *See* Decubitus ulcers
Bedwetting, 789
Behavior therapy, **987**
Bell palsy, **342**
Benign prostatic hyperplasia (BPH), **845**, **1187**
Benign tumors, **167**, **1097**
Benzodiazepines, **1058**
Berylliosis, **600**
Beta-adrenergic blocker, **537**, **1064**
Beta amyloid, **1169**
Bicarbonate ion (HCO$_3^-$), 609
Bicuspid valve, **513**
Bicuspids (teeth), **695**
Bilateral salpingo-oophorectomy (BSO), 847
Bile, **702**, 714
Bilirubin pigment, **464**
Binding site, 415
Binge-purge syndrome, 719
Bioavailability, **1045**
Biofeedback, **1001**
Biological naming system, 11
Biological therapy, **1119**
Biopsy, 104–106, 164, **165**, **1101**, 1108
    bone marrow aspiration, 476, 477, 477*f*
    chorionic villus biopsy (CVB), 925, 926*f*, 928
    lung, 595, 597
    muscle, 300, 301
    needle aspiration, 436

    percutaneous needle, 104, 106
    transcatheter, 104, 106
Biot respirations, **590**
Bipolar disorder, **997**
Birth control (BC) methods, 864–869
Birth control implant, **868**
Birth control injection, **868**
Birth control patch, **868**
Birth control pills (BCPs), **868**
Birthmarks, 154–155
Bladder, 766*f*, 769–770, 770*f*
    cancer, **1119**
    neurogenic, 789
Bladder catheterization, **790**
Bladder neck obstruction (BNO), **790**
Bladder stones, **790**
Blast cells, **1113**
Blastocyst, **903**
Bleeding time, **477**
Blepharitis, **387**
Blepharoptosis, **387**
Blood, 215–216, 455–506
    across lifespan, 486–487
    cancers, 1112–1113, 1113*f*
    components of, 462*f*
    pathology of, 472
    sample, 460*f*
    types, 470–472, 471*f*
Blood cells, development of, 461*f*
Blood chemistry, case study, 488–489
Blood clotting, 468–470
Blood doping, 480
Blood drugs, 1061–1062
Blood pH, 460, 584
Blood pressure (BP), **524**, 547
Blood tests, **428**
Blood thinners, 1061
Blood urea nitrogen (BUN), **779**
Blood vessels, 514–518
    radiography of, 110–111
    thrombus in, 469*f*
Blood–brain barrier (BBB), 324, 1057
Blumberg sign, 713
BM. *See* Bowel movement (BM)
BMI. *See* Body mass index (BMI)
BMR. *See* Basal metabolic rate (BMR)
BMT. *See* Bone marrow transplant (BMT)
BNO. *See* Bladder neck obstruction (BNO)
Body
    human, structural organizational levels of, 48*f*
    of penis, 825–827
    of stomach, 697
    of uterus, 830–831
Body cavity(ies), 55–57, 56*f*
    anterior, 55–56, 56*f*, 57
    posterior, 55–57
Body dysmorphic disorder, **1003**
Body mass index (BMI), 716
Boil, 170
Bolus, **693**
Bone(s), 208
    anatomy of, 211–214
    cancellous, 213
    classification of, 211
    compact, 213*f*, 214
    congenital disorders of, 930–931
    flat, 211, 212*f*, 214

Bone(s) (*continued*)
  genetic diseases of, 232–233
  irregular, 211, 212*f*, 214
  long, 211, 212*f*, 214
  round, 211
  short, 211, 212*f*, 214
  spongy, 213, 213*f*
  surface markings of, 216, 217–218*t*, 217*f*
Bone density scan, 115
Bone formation, 214–216
Bone marrow, 208
Bone marrow aspiration and biopsy, **1108**
Bone marrow aspiration biopsy, **477**
Bone marrow transplant (BMT), **486**, **664**
Bone mass, 257
Bone remodeling, **216**
Bone scan, **123**, **1108**
Bony labyrinth, **375**
Borborygmi, **699**
Borderline personality disorder, **1013**
Botox, 292
Botulism, 292
Bowel movement (BM), 704
Bowman capsule, 767
BP. *See* Blood pressure (BP)
BPD. *See* Bronchopulmonary dysplasia (BPD)
BPH. *See* Benign prostatic hyperplasia (BPH)
Brachial plexus, 326, 326*f*
Brachial region, 63*f*, 64*t*
Brachytherapy, **119**
Bradycardia, **536**, 719
Bradypnea, **589**
Brain, 320*f*, 328–332, 329–330*f*, 975
  disorders of
    general, 333–337
    pediatric, 340–341
    neoplasms of, 340
Brain contusion, **336**
Brain tumor, **1110**
Brainstem, **331**
Brainstem glioma, **1110**
Braxton Hicks contractions, **908**
Breast bone, 224
Breast cancer, **852**, **1124**
Breast self-examinations (BSEs), 850
Breathing, 584
  altered, 588–590
Breech, **912**
Brittle bone disease. *See* Osteogenesis
    imperfecta (OI)
Broad-spectrum antibiotics, **1053**
Bronchi, **582**
Bronchial asthma, **598**
Bronchial tree, **577**, 581–583, 582*f*, 584*f*
Bronchiectasis, **597**
Bronchioles, **582**
Bronchitis, **597**
Bronchodilators, **597**, 655, **1065**
Bronchopulmonary dysplasia (BPD), **940**
Bronchoscope, **597**
Bronchoscopy, **597**
Bronchospasm, **598**
Brudzinski sign, 347
Bruit, **546**
Bruxism, **710**
BSEs. *See* Breast self-examinations (BSEs)
BSO. *See* Bilateral salpingo-oophorectomy (BSO)
Buccal region, 63*f*, 64*t*

Buccal route, **1051**
Bulbourethral glands, 3, 3*f*, **825**
Bulimia, **721**
Bulimia nervosa, **1010**
Bullae, **162**
Bull's-eye rash, 248*f*
BUN. *See* Blood urea nitrogen (BUN)
Bundle branches, right and left, 522,
    522*f*, 523
Bundle of His, 522, 522*f*
Bunion, **253**
Bunionectomy, **253**
Burkitt lymphoma, **663**
Burn(s), **163**
  classification of, 162, 163*f*
  first-degree, 162, 163*f*
  second-degree, 162, 163*f*
  third-degree, 162, 163*f*
Bursae, **244**
Bursitis, **257**, **1163**
Bx. *See* Biopsy
Bypass surgery, **537**
  coronary artery bypass graft (CABG), 531, 532

C

C. *See* Carbon (C)
C-section. *See* Cesarean section
C&S studies. *See* Culture and sensitivity (C&S)
    studies
C_1. *See* Atlas
C_1–C_7. *See* Cervical vertebrae (C_1–C_7)
C_2. *See* Axis
$C_6H_{12}O_6$. *See* Glucose
CA. *See* Cancer
CA-125 assay test, **1125**
  across lifespan, 1126
  blood, 1112–1113, 1113*f*
  risk factors, 1096
CAAHEP. *See* Commission on Accreditation
    of Allied Health Education Programs
    (CAAHEP)
CABG. *See* Coronary artery bypass graft (CABG)
    surgery
CAD. *See* Coronary artery disease (CAD)
Calcaneal, 63*f*, 65*t*
Calcaneus, **229**
Calcification, 247
Calcitonin (CT), 235, **419**
Calcitriol, **425**
Calcium (Ca^{2+}), **216**
Calcium channel blocker, **537**, **1064**
Calculi, 714
Callus, **171**
Calorie (cal), **705**
Calyces, **769**
Cancellous bone, 213
Cancer (CA), **167**, 1092, 1095–1096
  across lifespan, 1126
  blood, 1112–1113, 1113*f*
  causes and risk factors, 1096–1097
  digestive system, 1116–1117, 1116*t*, 1117*f*
  drugs, 1055
  endocrine system, 1110–1111, 1111*f*
  five-year survival rate, 1097
  immune system, 1114
  integumentary system, 1102–1106, 1102*f*,
    1103*f*, 1104*f*
  muscular system, 1107–1108, 1108*f*

nervous system, 1108–1110
reproductive system, 1120–1126, 1120*f*,
    1121*t*, 1124*f*
respiratory system, 1114–1116, 1115*f*
skeletal system, 1106–1107
urinary system cancers, 1118*t*, 1118–1119, 1118*f*
Candida albicans, 709
Candidiasis, **858**
Canine (teeth), 694*f*
Capacitation, **829**
CAPD. *See* Continuous ambulatory peritoneal
    dialysis (CAPD)
Capillaries, 508, **518**
  vascular and lymphatic, relationship of,
    644, 644*f*
Capitate, 225*f*
Capsule, of lymph node, 644, 644*f*
Carbohydrates (CHO), **705**
Carbon (C), 120, 705
Carbon dioxide (CO_2), 463, 572, 589
Carbon monoxide (CO) poisoning, **611**
Carbuncle, **170**
Carcinogens, **1097**
Carcinoma in situ (CIS), **1105**
Carcinomas, **169**
Cardia, **697**
Cardiac arrest, **536**
Cardiac catheterization, **106**, 531
Cardiac conducting system, **523**
Cardiac cycle, **523**
Cardiac enzyme test, **537**
Cardiac glycosides, **1064**
Cardiac muscle, **291**
Cardiac tamponade, **536**
Cardiac wall, 511*f*
Cardiomegaly, 534
Cardiomyopathy, **536**
Cardiopulmonary resuscitation (CPR),
    208, **536**
Cardiovascular (CV) system, **53**, 507–569
  across lifespan, 547–548
  aging and, 1173–1176
  disorders of, affecting lungs, 590–592
  drugs for, 1062–1064, 1062*t*
  pathology of, 525
Cardiovascular intensive care unit (CVICU),
    registered nurse professional
    profile, 508
Carpal bones, **226**
Carpal region, 63*f*, 64*t*
Carpal tunnel syndrome, **255**
Cartilage, **214**, 240
Cartilaginous joints, **244**
Case study, 1128
  anatomy and physiology, 73–75
  basal cell carcinoma, 185–186
  blood chemistry, 488–489
  cardiovascular disorder, 550
  chronic obstructive pulmonary disease, 614
  digestive disorder, 736–737
  endocrine disorder, 439
  eye examination, 350, 393–394
  gerontology, 1190
  hyperthyroidism, 439
  joint injury, 260
  lymphatic disorder, 667
  mental health, 1016
  muscular injury, 305–306

neurological examination, 350
oncology, 1128
pharmacology, 1072
polymyositis, 1072
pregnancy, 950
radiology, 126
renal failure, 736–737
reproductive disorder, 873
skeletal injury, 260
urinary disorder, 792–794
Castration, 843
CAT. *See* Computed axial tomography (CAT);
    Computer-assisted tomography (CAT);
    Computerized axial tomography (CAT)
Catabolism, 701
Catalysts, **698**
Cataract, 379, **1171**
Catatonic-type schizophrenia, **994**
Catheter, 531
    arterial, placement
      nonselective, 104, 106
      selective, 104, 106
    venous, placement
      nonselective, 104, 106
      selective, 104, 106
Catheterization, 104–106
    cardiac, 105, 106, 530, 531
    endoscopic, 105, 106
Cat's cry syndrome, 926
Cauda equina, 328
Caudal, **59**
Causalgia, 162
CAUTION, cancer, 1096
Cavities. *See* Dental caries
CBC. *See* Complete blood (cell) count (CBC)
CBD. *See* Common bile duct (CBD)
CBT. *See* Cognitive-behavioral therapy (CBT)
CC. *See* Chief complaint (CC)
CCK. *See* Cholecystokinin (CCK)
CCPD. *See* Continuous cycling peritoneal
    dialysis (CCPD)
CD. *See* Curative dose (CD)
CDC. *See* Centers for Disease Control (CDC)
CDR. *See* Commission on Dietetic
    Registration (CDR)
Cecum, **704**
Celiac disease, **726**
Celiac sprue, 726
Cell body, **325**
Cell-mediated immunity, **648**
Cell membrane, **50**
Cells, **50**
    differentiation, 1097
Cellulitis, **177**
Cellulose, 705
Cementum, **695**
Centenarians, **1155**
Centers for Disease Control (CDC), 716, 942
Central canal, **328**
Central nervous system (CNS), **323**, 975
    drugs affecting, 1057–1059
    infectious diseases of, 345–348
Cephalalgia, **336**
Cephalic region, **59**
Cerebellum, **331**
Cerebral angiography, **337**
Cerebral cortex, **331**
Cerebral hemispheres, **331**

Cerebral palsy (CP), **341**, **937**
Cerebral seizures, 337
Cerebrospinal fluid (CSF), **328**, 935
Cerebrovascular accident (CVA), **337**, 537, **1168**
Cerebrum, **331**
Certified nurse midwife (CNM), 816
Certified respiratory therapist (CRT), 572
Certified surgical technologist/first assistant,
    professional profile, 1092
Cerumen, 373
Ceruminous glands, **158**, 375
Cervical cancer, 852, **1125**
Cervical cap, **869**
Cervical plexus, 326, 326*f*
Cervical region, 63*f*, 64*t*
Cervical vertebrae (C₁–C₇), **224**
Cervix, **831**
    incompetent, 909, 912
Cesarean section (C-section), **913**
CF. *See* Cystic fibrosis (CF)
Chadwick sign, **908**
Chalazion, **387**
Chancres, **863**
Chancroid, **863**
CHD. *See* Congenital hip dysplasia (CHD)
Cheilectomy, **249**
Chemical digestion, **691**, **697**
Chemical sterility, 857
Chemotherapy, **70**, **486**
Chest pain, 530
Chest x-ray, **113**
Cheyne–Stokes respiration, 590
CHF. *See* Congestive heart failure (CHF)
Chickenpox, 179, 179*f*, **947**
Chief complaint (CC), 4
Child health, 897–970
Childhood, **917**
    infectious diseases of, 941–947
    rhabdomyosarcoma, 1107
Chlamydia, **863**
Chloasma, **182**, 908
CHO. *See* Carbohydrates (CHO)
chol. *See* Cholesterol
Cholangiogram, **715**
Cholangiography, 106, 109
Cholecystectomy, **715**
Cholecystitis, **715**
Cholecystogram, **715**
Cholecystography, **109**
Cholecystokinin (CCK), **702**
Cholelithiasis, **715**
Cholesteatoma, **389**
Cholesterol, 467–468, 548
Cholinergics, 725
Chondrosarcoma, **1107**
Chordae tendineae, **514**
Chorea, **339**
Chorioangioma, **923**
Choriocarcinoma, **923**
Chorion membrane, **905**
Chorionic villi, **905**
Chorionic villus biopsy (CVB), **928**
Chorionic villus sampling (CVS), **928**
Choroid, **372**
Choroid plexus, 329
Chromosome, **50**, **919**
Chronic bronchitis, 597, **1179**
Chronic inflammation, **1178**

Chronic lymphocytic leukemia (CLL), 486, **1113**
Chronic myeloid leukemia (CML), 486, **1113**
Chronic obstructive pulmonary disease (COPD),
    534, 597, 612, 1065, **1179**
    case study, 614
Chronic renal failure (CRF), 736, 780
Chrysotherapy, **1069**
Chyle, 642
Chyme, **698**, 721
Ciliary body, 372
Cinefluoroscopy, **102**
Cineradiography, **102**
Circadian cycle, 423*f*
Circadian rhythm, **424**
Circumcision, **826**
Circumduction, **246**
Circumflex artery, **520**
Cirrhosis, 722, **734**
CIS. *See* Carcinoma in situ (CIS)
CK test. *See* Creatine kinase (CK) test
Claudication, **1176**
Clavicles, **226**
Clavus, **171**
Clean-catch urine specimen, **785**
Clearance test, 779
Cleft lip, **931**
Cleft palate, **931**
Climax, **839**
Clinical psychologist, professional profile, 972
Clitoris, **832**
CLL. *See* Chronic lymphocytic leukemia (CLL)
Closed reduction, **232**
Clotting factor VIII, 475
Clotting factors, 469
Clubbing of fingers, **593**
Clubfoot, 234, **931**
CML. *See* Chronic myeloid leukemia (CML)
CMV. *See* Cytomegalovirus (CMV)
CNM. *See* Certified nurse midwife (CNM)
CNs. *See* Cranial nerves
CNS. *See* Central nervous system
CO. *See* Carbon monoxide (CO)
CO₂. *See* Carbon dioxide (CO₂)
Coagulation, 456, 470, 475–478
Coarctation of aorta, 525–526, 529, **933**
Coccyx, **224**
Cochlea, **375**
Codeine, **1058**
Coding, 95
Cognition, **976**
Cognitive-behavioral therapy (CBT), **987**
Coitus, **826**
Cold sores, **710**
Colic, **715**
Colitis, **732**
Collagen, **153**
Colles fracture, 231*t*
Colon cancer, 704, **1117**
    disorders of, 730–732
      polyps, 1116
      spastic, 730, 732
Colonoscopy, 732, **1117**
Colorectal cancer, 732, **1183**
Colostomy, 732, **936**
Colostrum, **833**, 914
Colpoplasty, **856**
Colporrhaphy, **856**
Coma, **336**

Combining forms, 13
Combining vowels, 10
Comedo, 158
Comminuted fracture, 231*f*, 231*t*
Commission on Accreditation of Allied
    Health Education Programs
    (CAAHEP), 2, 146
Commission on Dietetic Registration (CDR), 686
Commissurotomy, 543
Common bile duct (CBD), 702
Common diseases and ICD-9 codes, 7, 8*t*
Common hepatic duct, 702
Comorbidity, 1188
Compact bone, 214
Complement system, 647
Complete blood (cell) count (CBC), 464, 539
Complete fracture, 231*t*
Compliance, 1047
Compound (open) fracture, 231*f*, 231*t*
Compression fracture, 231*t*
Computed axial tomography (CAT), 103
Computed tomographic angiography, 104
Computed tomography (CT), 68, 104, 336, 427
Computer-assisted tomography (CAT), 103
Computerized axial tomography (CAT), 103
Concomitant, definition of, 546
Concussion, 336
Condoms, 864, 865–866
Conducting airway, 583
Conduction deafness, 388, 1170
Conduction myofibers, 523
Condyle, 218*t*
Cones, 373
Congenital, 905
    heart defects, 525–529
    syndromes, 925–928
Congenital articular disorders, 257–258
Congenital blood and cardiac disorders,
    932–933
Congenital hip dysplasia (CHD), 930, 931*f*
Congenital megacolon, 937
Congenital neuromuscular system disorders,
    934–937
Congestive heart failure (CHF), **536**, **1176**
Coniosis, 599
Conization, **825**, **1125**
Conjunctiva, 372
Conjunctivitis, 379
Connective tissue, 50, **1101**
Consciousness, 977
Constipation, **713**, **1183**
Contact dermatitis, 174
Continuous ambulatory peritoneal dialysis
    (CAPD), 782
Continuous cycling peritoneal dialysis
    (CCPD), 782
Continuous passive motion (CPM), **1163**, 1190
Continuous positive airway pressure (CPAP),
    610, **1012**
Contraception, **868**
Contractions, **912**
    Braxton Hicks, 908
Contraindication, **1047**
Contrast medium, **99**
Contrast studies, 108
Controlled substance, **1047**
Contusion, **162**, 334
Conversion disorder, **1003**

Convolutions, of brain, 329*f*
COPD. *See* Chronic obstructive pulmonary
    disease (COPD)
Copper T-380A IUD, 867*f*
Cor pulmonale, **539**, **1179**
Core biopsy, **1107**
Corn, 171
Cornea, 372
Coronal plane, 62
Coronal suture, 220*f*
Coronary artery
    left, 520, 521*f*
    right, 520, 521*f*
Coronary artery bypass graft (CABG)
    surgery, **532**
Coronary artery disease (CAD), **531**, **1176**
Coronary circulation, **520**
Coronary heart disease (CHD), 1062
Coronary sinus, 520, 521
Coronary vein(s), 521*f*
Corpora cavernosa, **826**
Corpus callosum, 331
Corpus luteum, 834
Corpus spongiosum, **826**
Correct-site/wrong-procedure surgery, 71
Cortex
    of lymph node, 644, 644*f*
    renal, 767, 768*f*
Corticosteroids, 251, 341–342, **663**, **1069**
Cortisol, **421**
Coryza, **602**
Costal region, 63*f*, 64*t*
Cot death, 609
Cough, 585, 595
    productive, 595
Counseling, **978**
Counselors, **978**
Cowper glands, 3, 3*f*, 823
Coxal region, 63*f*, 64*t*
    bones, 226
CP. *See* Cerebral palsy (CP)
CPAP. *See* Continuous positive airway
    pressure (CPAP)
CPK test. *See* Creatine phosphokinase
    (CPK) test
CPM. *See* Continuous passive motion (CPM)
CPR. *See* Cardiopulmonary resuscitation
    (CPR)
*CPT. See Current Procedural Terminology
    (CPT)*
Cradle cap, **174**
Cranial nerves, **332**
    disorders of, 341–342
Cranial region, 59, 63*f*, 64*t*
    bones, 216, 217*f*
Craniostenosis, **237**
Cranium, **221**
Creatine kinase (CK) test, 535
Creatine phosphokinase (CPK) test, 300
Creatinine clearance test, **780**
Cremaster muscle, 824
Crepitus, **232**
Crest surface marking, 217*t*
CRF. *See* Chronic renal failure (CRF)
Cri-du-chat syndrome, **928**
Crib death, 609
Crohn disease, **729**, **1117**
Cross-eyes, 378

Crown of tooth, **695**
CRT. *See* Certified respiratory therapist (CRT)
Crusts, 169
Cryosurgery, 168, 729, 852, 1105
Cryotherapy, 385
Cryptorchidism, **843**
CSF. *See* Cerebrospinal fluid (CSF)
CT. *See* Calcitonin (CT); Computed tomography
    (CT); Cytotechnologist (CT)
CT pelvimetry, 104
Cubital region, 63*f*, 65*t*
Cuboid, 228*f*
Culture and sensitivity (C&S) studies, **605**
Cuneiform bones, 228*f*
Curative dose (CD), **1044**
Curettage, 168. *See also* Dilation and curettage
    (D&C)
Current Procedural Terminology (CPT), 8
Cushing disease, **428**
Cuspids (of teeth), **695**
Cutaneous, 151
Cutaneous papillomas, 167
Cuticle, 159
CV. *See* Cardiovascular (CV)
CVA. *See* Cerebrovascular accident (CVA)
CVB. *See* Chorionic villus biopsy (CVB)
CVICU. *See* Cardiovascular intensive care
    unit (CVICU)
CVS. *See* Chorionic villus sampling (CVS)
Cyanosis, 156, 482, 546, 572, **592**, 932
Cyclophosphamide, 663
Cyclosporine, 663, 1069
Cyclothymic disorder, **998**
Cystic duct, **702**
Cystic fibrosis (CF), **593**, **718**, **925**
Cystitis, **786**
Cystocele, **856**
Cystography, 114
Cystoscope, 788
Cystoscopy, 788*f*
Cytology, 47
Cytomegalovirus (CMV), **904**
Cytoplasm, 49, 49*f*
Cytotechnologist (CT), professional profile, 146
Cytotoxic drugs, 663, **1055**
Cytotoxic T (T_c) cells, **650**

D

D&C. *See* Dilation and curettage (D&C)
DA. *See* Dopamine (DA)
Dartos muscle, 824
DEA. *See* Drug Enforcement Agency (DEA)
Deafness, **388**, **1171**
Débridement, 172
Deciduous, definition of, 693
Deciduous teeth, **695**
Decongestant, **601**, **655**, **1065**
Decubitus ulcers, **172**, 1158
Dedifferentiation, **1098**
Deep, **59**
Deep vein thrombosis (DVT), **547**, 1061, **1176**
Deer ticks, 258, 258*f*
Defecation, **704**
Defibrillation, **536**
Degenerative arthritis, 1161
Degenerative joint disease (DJD), 248
Deglutition, **693**
Dehydration, 791

Dehydroepiandrosterone (DHEA), 422
Delirium, 338, **990**, **1168**
Delirium tremens (DT), **992**
Delivery, 909–913
Delta-5 androstenediol, 422
Delusion, **990**
Dementia, 339, 990, 1168
Dendrites, **325**
Dendritic cells, 1157
Densitometer, **115**, **238**
Densitometry, **115**
Dental caries, **710**
Dentin, **695**
Deoxyribonucleic acid (DNA), 49
Depo-Provera, 865, 868
Depression, **990**, 1014
Dermal puncture, 456
Dermatitis, **174**
    types of, 173–174
Dermatologist, **151**
Dermatology, **151**
Dermatome, **180**, **328**
Dermatomyositis, **165**, 300
Dermatophyte, **176**
Dermatophytoses, **176**
Dermis, **153**
DES. *See* Diethylstilbestrol (DES)
Descending colon, **704**
Desensitization, **655**
Detached retina, **385**
Detrusor muscle, **770**
Detumescence, **839**
Development, 71, 897–970
    across lifespan, 947–948
    nongenetic syndromes affecting, 928–929
Developmental hip dysplasia, **931**
Developmental stages, 916–917
DEXA. *See* Dual energy x-ray absorptiometry (DEXA)
Dextroamphetamine (Dexedrine), **986**
DHEA. *See* Dehydroepiandrosterone (DHEA)
DHT. *See* Dihydrotestosterone (DHT)
Diabetes insipidus, **434**, **783**
Diabetes mellitus (DM), **430**, 716, **783**
Diabetic retinopathy, **385**, **1171**
Diagnostic and Statistical Manual of Mental Disorders, Fourth Edition, Text Revision (DSM-IV-TR), 973, 979–981
Diagnostic imaging, 100, 101
Diagnostic medical sonographer, professional profile, 898
Diagnostic procedures, 66–68
Diagnostic radiology, **101**
    procedures, 101*b*
Diagnostic ultrasound, **98**. *See also* Ultrasound, diagnostic
Dialysis, 736, **782**. *See also* Hemodialysis; Peritoneal dialysis (PD)
Dialysis nurse, professional profile, 762
Diaphoresis, **537**, 717
Diaphragm (muscle), **57**, **585**, **869**
Diaphragm (contraceptive), 867–868
Diaphysis, **214**
Diarrhea, 703, 713, **1183**
Diastole, **523**
Diastolic blood pressure, **524**
DIC. *See* Disseminated intravascular coagulation (DIC)

Diencephalon, **331**
Diethylstilbestrol (DES), 852
Dietitian, 686
Differential white blood count, **466**
Differentiation, **1098**
Digestion, **691**
Digestive system, **53**, 685–760
    across lifespan, 734
    aging and, 1180–1183
    anatomy of, 690–706
    cancers, 1116–1117, 1116*t*, 1117*f*
    radiography of, 108
    structures of, 691*f*
Digestive tract, 690, 692
Digital rectal examination (DRE), **845**, **1124**, **1187**
Digital region, 63*f*, 65*t*
Digital subtraction angiography (DSA), **111**
Digitalis, **536**
Dihydrotestosterone (DHT), **870**
Dilation and curettage (D&C), **849**, **923**
Diphtheria, **946**
Diphtheria, tetanus, pertussis (DTP) vaccine, 941*t*, 942*t*
Diploid, **829**
Directional terms, 58–59, 58*f*
Diskography, **102**
Dislocation, **257**
Disorders, 68–69
Disorganized-type schizophrenia, **994**
Dispensing, **1040**
Dissecting aneurysm, **547**
Disseminated intravascular coagulation (DIC), **477**
Dissociative amnesia, **1006**
Dissociative disorders, **1006**
Dissociative fugue, **1006**
Dissociative identity disorder, **1006**
Distal, **59**
Distal convoluted tubule, 768, 768*f*
Distend, **697**
Diuresis, 779, **1064**
Diuretics, **536**
Diverticulitis, **729**, **1183**
Diverticulosis, **729**
Diverticulum, **729**
Diving reflex, **586**
Dizygotic twins, **915**
DJD. *See* Degenerative joint disease (DJD)
DM. *See* Dermatomyositis; Diabetes mellitus (DM)
DMD. *See* Duchenne muscular dystrophy (DMD)
DNA. *See* Deoxyribonucleic acid (DNA)
Dominant genes, 917–918
Dopamine (DA), 335, **975**
Doppler echocardiography, **117**
Doppler effect, 116–118
Doppler ultrasonography, **117**, **547**
Doppler ultrasound
    2D, 552
    M-Mode, 552
    TM-Mode, 552
Dorsal region, **59**, 63*f*, 65*t*
Dorsiflexion, **246**
Dosimetry, **119**
Dowager hump, **1163**
Down syndrome, **928**, **984**
DRE. *See* Digital rectal examination (DRE)

Drug Enforcement Agency (DEA), **1047**
Drug reactions, 1045–1048
Drug references, **1047**
Drug regulations, 1045–1046
Drug schedules, 1046, 1046*t*
Drugs, **1044**
    routes of administration, 1048–1051
Dry form of age-related macular degeneration, **1170**
Dry mouth, **1183**
DSA. *See* Digital subtraction angiography (DSA)
DSM-IV-TR. See Diagnostic and Statistical Manual of Mental Disorders, Fourth Edition, Text Revision
DT. *See* Delirium tremens (DT)
DTP vaccine. *See* Diphtheria, tetanus, pertussis (DTP) vaccine
Dual energy x-ray absorptiometry (DEXA), **1163**
Duchenne muscular dystrophy (DMD), 300, **937**
Duct(s)
    alveolar, 582*f*
    common bile, 701, 701*f*, 702
    common hepatic, 701, 701*f*, 702
    cystic, 701, 701*f*, 702
    ejaculatory, 825, 826*f*
    lactiferous, 833, 833*f*
    lymphatic, 642*f*, 644, 645*f*
    pancreatic, 700, 700*f*
    paramesonephric, **870**
    right lymphatic, 642*f*, 644, 645, 645*f*
    thoracic, 642*f*, 644, 645, 645*f*
Ductography, **112**
Ductus arteriosus, **547**
Ductus deferens, **825**, 868*f*
Ductus venosus, **547**
Duodenal ulcer, **712**
Duodenography, **109**
Duodenum, **699**
Dura mater, **332**
Dyscrasia, **474**
Dysentery, **1055**
Dysmenorrhea, **849**
Dysmorphophobia, **1003**
Dyspareunia, **863**, **1187**
Dyspepsia, **732**
Dysphagia, **602**, **723**
Dysphasia, **337**, 721
Dysphonia, **602**
Dysphoria, **1001**
Dysplasia, **1101**
Dyspnea, **529**, **589**, 932
Dysrhythmia, **541**
Dyssomnias, **1012**
Dysthymic disorder, **997**
Dysuria, **785**, **1184**

E

E. *See* Epinephrine (E)
Each ear (*auris uterque*, A.U.), **375**
Each eye (*oculus uterque*, O.U.), **370**
Ear(s), 373–376
    anatomy of, 373
Eardrum, **373**
Earwax, **373**
Eating disorders, 718–721, 1009–1010
EBV. *See* Epstein-Barr virus (EBV)

EC. *See* Emergency contraception (EC)
Ecchymosis, **182**, **477**
ECG. *See* Electrocardiogram (ECG, EKG)
Echocardiogram, **529**
    of popliteal artery, 117*f*
Echocardiography, **117**
Echography, **117**
Echolalia, **987**
Eclampsia, **923**
ECT. *See* Electroconvulsive therapy (ECT)
Ectoderm, 70, **183**, 903
Ectopic, definition of, 847
Ectopic pregnancy, **923**
ED. *See* Effective dose (ED) or erectile
    dysfunction (ED)
Edema, **162**, **249**
    pulmonary, 539, 608
Edwards syndrome, **928**
EEG. *See* Electroencephalogram (EEG); Electro-
    encephalograph (EEG); Electroencepha-
    lography (EEG)
Effacement, **912**
Effective dose (ED), **1044**
Efferent, definition of, 644
Efficacy, **1044**
Effusion, **538**
Ejaculation, 824, **839**
Ejaculatory duct, **825**
EKG. *See* Electrocardiogram (ECG, EKG)
Elbow, 225*f*, 243
Electrocardiogram (ECG, EKG), **529**
Electrocoagulation, **852**
Electroconvulsive therapy (ECT), **997**
Electrodesiccation and curettage, **1105**
Electroencephalogram (EEG), **333**
Electroencephalograph (EEG), **333**
Electroencephalography (EEG), **336**
Electrolytes, **704**, 771
Electromyogram (EMG), **301**
Electromyography (EMG), **115**, **301**, 342
Electronystagmography (ENG), **391**
Elephantiasis, **162**, **659**
Emaciation, **721**
Embolism, **470**
    pulmonary, 592, 1061
Embolus, **470**
Embryo, 822, **902**
Embryology, **47**
Emergency contraception (EC), 868
Emesis, **698**
Emetic agent, **1068**
EMG. *See* Electromyogram (EMG); Electromyo-
    graphy (EMG)
Emission, **839**
Emphysema, **597**, 1179
Enamel, **695**
Encephalitis, **348**
End-stage renal disease (ESRD), 736, **781**
Endarterectomy, **531**
Endocarditis, **541**
Endocardium, **513**
Endocrine system, **53**, **416**
    across lifespan, 431
    aging and, 1172–1173
    anatomy of, 415–425, 417*f*
    cancers, 1110–1111, 1111*f*
    drugs affecting, 1067
    pathology of, 425

Endoderm, 70, 903
Endolymph, 374
Endometrial cancer, **853**, 1125
Endometrial stromal sarcoma, **1125**
Endometriosis, **849**
Endometrium, **831**
Endoscope, **723**
Endoscopic catheterization, **106**
Endothelium, 515*f*
Endotracheal tube, **592**
Enema, **1183**
ENG. *See* Electronystagmography (ENG)
Enteral, **1051**
Enuresis, **790**
Environmental hypothesis, 1167
Enzymes, **691**, 697
Eosinophils, **466**
Ependymal cells, 324
Ependymoma, **340**, 1110
Epicardium, **513**
Epicondyle projection, 217*t*
Epidemic parotitis, 944
Epidemiology, **69**, 1155
Epidermis, **153**, 183
Epididymis, **825**
Epididymitis, **843**
Epidural, 332
Epidural anesthesia, **1061**
Epigastric region, **61**
Epiglottis, **581**
Epilepsy, **337**, 1057
Epinephrine (E), **421**, 427, 975
Epiphyseal line, **216**
Epiphyseal plate, **216**
Epiphysis, **214**
Episiotomy, **913**
Epispadias, **787**, **843**
Epithelial tissue, **50**, 1101
Epithelium, **50**, 1101
EPO. *See* Erythropoietin (EPO)
Epoetin, **480**
Epogen, **480**
Eponychium, **159**
Eponyms, **8**
Epstein-Barr virus (EBV), 479, 658
Equilibrium, 322, 369, 375
    dynamic, 375
    static, 375
Equinovarus, **234**
Erectile dysfunction (ED), **843**
Erection, **826**, 838
ERP. *See* Exposure and response
    prevention (ERP)
ERT. *See* Estrogen-replacement therapy (ERT)
Eructation, **697**
ERV. *See* Expiratory reserve volume (ERV)
Erythema, **165**
Erythroblastosis fetalis, **484**, **933**
Erythroblasts, **484**
Erythrocyte sedimentation rate (ESR), **539**
Erythrocytes/red blood cells (RBCs), 460,
    462*f*, 464
Erythrocytosis, **464**
Erythropenia, **464**
Erythropoiesis, **464**
Erythropoietin (EPO), 464, 480, **771**
Esophageal hiatus, **696**
Esophageal varices, **723**

Esophagus, 579, 690, 691*f*, **696**
Esotropia, 378
ESR. *See* Erythrocyte sedimentation rate (ESR)
ESRD. *See* End-stage renal disease (ESRD)
Estimated date of confinement (EDC), 950
Estrogen, 425, 834, 904, 1067
    deficiency, 1168
    and progesterone receptor test, 1122, **1124**
Estrogen-replacement therapy (ERT), 237,
    238, 851
ESWL. *See* Extracorporeal shock wave lithotripsy
    (ESWL)
Ethmoid bone, 216, 219*f*, **221**
Ethmoidal sinus(es), 578
Etiology, **69**
Etymology, **13**
Euphoria, **998**
Eupnea, **585**
Eversion, **246**
Ewing sarcoma, **238**, 1107
Exchange transfusion, **474**
Excisional biopsy, **1105**
Excisional skin surgery, **1105**
Excretion, 416, 767
Exercise-induced asthma, **598**
Exercise stress test, **531**
Exfoliation, **162**
Exhalation, **585**
Exhibitionism, **1008**
Exophthalmos, **436**
Expectorant, **1065**
Expectorated, **593**
Expiratory reserve volume (ERV), **587**
Exposure and response prevention (ERP), **1001**
Extension, **246**
Extensors, **299**
External acoustic meatus, **375**
External anal sphincter, 703, 703*f*
External ear, **375**
    disorders of, 387
External fixation, **232**
External urethral orifice, **770**
Extracapsular extraction, 377
Extracorporeal shock wave lithotripsy (ESWL),
    716, 777
Extraction, of tooth, 707
Extraembryonic membranes, 903
Extrinsic asthma, **655**
Exudate, 169, **605**
Exudative eruptions, **175**
Eye(s), 369–373
    disorders of, 376–379
    examination, case study, 393–394
    structures of, 370*f*
Eyelid(s), 369
    disorders of, 387

F

Facet, 218*t*
Facial nerve (CN VII), 329, 330, 330*f*
    and Bell palsy, 341–342
Facial region, 63*f*, 64*t*
    bones, 216, 220*f*
Factitious disorder(s), **1004**
Factitious illness by proxy, **1001**
Falciform ligament, 701
Fallopian tubes, 830
False aneurysm, **547**

False ribs, **226**
False vocal cords, 581, 581*f*
Family history (FH), 5
Farsightedness, 380
FAS. *See* Fetal alcohol syndrome (FAS)
Fascia, 173, **291**, 317
FDA. *See* Food and Drug Administration (FDA)
FDCA. *See* Food, Drug, and Cosmetic Act (FDCA)
Fecal impaction, **1184**
Fecal incontinence, **713**
Fecal occult blood test (FOBT), **732**, **1117**
Feces, **704**
Female
    external genitalia of, 822
    pelvic disorders of, 846–849
    pelvis of, 226, 227*f*
    reproductive hormones of, 834
    reproductive system of, 822–823, 822*f*
    benign tumors of, 853–854
    cancer of, 850–853
    hernias in, 855
    inflammatory disorders of, 846–849
Female condom, **869**
Female sponge, 866, **869**
Femoral region, 63*f*, 65*t*
Femur, **229**, 248*f*
Fertility awareness–based method (FAM), **869**
Fertility, male, **829**
Fertilization, **902**, 903
    artificial, 914–915
Fetal alcohol syndrome (FAS), **929**
Fetal heart rate (FHR), 950
Fetal hemoglobin (HbF), 486
Fetishism, **1008**
Fetus, 46, 822, **902**
Fetus in fetu, 915–916
Fever blisters. *See* Cold sores
FH. *See* Family history (FH)
FHR. *See* Fetal heart rate (FHR)
Fibrillation, **536**
Fibrin, **470**
Fibrinogen, **462**
Fibrocystic breast changes, **854**
Fibromyalgia, **301**
Fibrosis, 251, **301**, **1165**
Fibrositis, **301**
Fibrous joints, **244**
Fibula, **229**, 243*f*
Filtration, **767**
Fimbriae, **831**
Fine-needle aspiration (FNA) biopsy, **1107**
Fingernails. *See* Nails
First-degree burn, **163**
First-pass metabolism, **1045**
Fissures, **176**, 218*t*, 331
Fistula, **782**
Five-year survival rate, **1097**
Fixation, **232**
Flacid muscles, **1165**
Flagellum, **829**
Flail chest, **611**
Flashes, **385**
Flat bones, **214**
Flatulence, **713**
Flexion, **246**
Flexors, 292, **299**, 317
Flexure, **704**
Floaters, 353, **385**

Floating ribs, **226**
Flu, 604
Fluorescein angiography, **385**
FNA. *See* Fine-needle aspiration (FNA) biopsy
Folate deficiency, 473
Foley catheter, 789, 790, 790*f*
Follicle, **156**, 835
    disorders of, 177–178
Follicle-stimulating hormone (FSH), 416, **827**, 834, 916
Folliculitis, **178**
Fontanelles, **221**, 236
Food and Drug Administration (FDA), 1046
Food, Drug, and Cosmetic Act (FDCA), 1046
Foot disorders, 234–235, 252–254
Foramen, 218*t*
Foramen ovale, 547
Foreskin, 826
Formulary, **1047**
Fossa, 218*t*
Fovea centralis, **373**
Fowler position, 539, 607
Fracture (Fx), **232**
    skull, 334
    types of, 231*t*
Free edge (nail), **159**
Fremitus, **529**
Frequency, **790**
Friction rub, 540
Frontal bone, **221**
Frontal plane, **62**
Frontal region, 63*f*, 64*t*
    bone, 216, 219*f*, 220*f*, 221, 221*f*
Frontal sinus(es), 578, 578*f*
Frotteurism, **1008**
FSH. *See* Follicle-stimulating hormone (FSH)
Fugue, **1006**
Fundus, **697**, 831
Fungus (pl. fungi), skin disease caused by, 175
Furuncles, **170**
Fusiform aneurysm, **547**
Fx. *See* Fracture(s) (Fx)

G

G⁻. *See* Gram-negative
G⁺. *See* Gram-positive
⁶⁷Ga. *See* Gallium-67 (⁶⁷Ga)
GABA. *See* γ-aminobutyric acid (GABA)
GAD. *See* Generalized anxiety disorder (GAD)
Galactography, **112**
Gallbladder, 690, 691*f*, 702
    disorders of, 714–716, 714*f*
Gallium-67 (⁶⁷Ga), 120
Gallium scan, **123**
Gallstones, **715**
Gametes, **820**, 903
γ-aminobutyric acid (GABA), 975
γ-glutamyltransferase (GGT), 992
Ganglion, **255**
Ganglionectomy, 255
Gangrene, **172**
Gas exchange, respiratory, 572, 573*f*, 585, 586
Gastric, definition of, 697
Gastric ulcer, **712**
Gastrin, 711
Gastroenteritis, **726**
Gastroesophageal disorders, 721–723
Gastroesophageal reflex disease (GERD), **723**, 1067

Gastrointestinal (GI) system, 1180. *See also* Digestive system
    drugs affecting, 1067–1068
GDM. *See* Gestational diabetes mellitus (GDM)
Gender identity disorder, **1008**
General anesthetics, **1060**
Generalized anxiety disorder (GAD), **1001**
Generalized tonic-clonic seizure, 337
Generic name, definition of, 1043
Genes, **50**, 919
Genetic disorder, 924–925
Genital herpes, **863**
Genital human papillomavirus (HPV) infection, **863**
Genital region, 63*f*, 64*t*
Genital warts, 861*f*
Genitourinary system, 763
Genus name, 11
GERD. *See* Gastroesophageal reflex disease (GERD)
Geriatrics, **1154**
Germ layers, 70, 183
German measles, 945, 947. *See also* Rubella
Germinal centers, 645
Gerontologist, **1154**
Gerontology, 1149–1209, **1154**
    aging, 1153–1155
    and cardiovascular system, 1173–1176
    and digestive system, 1180–1183
    and endocrine system, 1172–1173
    and integumentary system, 1155–1158
    and lymphatic system and immunity, 1179–1180
    and muscular system, 1164–1165
    and nervous system, 1165–1169
    and reproductive system, 1185–1187
    and respiratory system, 1177–1179
    and skeletal system, 1158–1164
    and special senses, 1169–1171
    and urinary system, 1183–1184
    pharmacology and older adults, 1188
Gestation, **902**, 903–906
Gestational age, **908**
Gestational diabetes mellitus (GDM), **430**, 923
GFR. *See* Glomerular filtration rate (GFR)
GGT. *See* γ-glutamyltransferase (GGT)
GH. *See* Growth hormone (GH) targets
GI. *See* Gastrointestinal (GI)
Giantism. *See* Gigantism
Giardiasis, **1055**
Gigantism, **434**
Gingiva, **695**
Gingivitis, **710**
Gland, **416**
    of integumentary system, 157–158
    disorders of, 177–178
Glans penis, **826**
Glasgow Coma Scale (GCS), **336**
Glaucoma, 379, **1171**
Glenoid cavity, 219*t*
Glial cells, 324, 996, **1101**
Glioma, **340**
Globulin, **462**
Glomerular capsule, **769**
Glomerular disorders, 778–780
Glomerular filtration rate (GFR), **780**

Glomerulonephritis, **779**
Glomerulosclerosis, **784**
Glomerulus, **769**
Glossopharyngeal nerve (CN IX), 330, 330*f*
Glottis, **581**
Glucagon, **420**, 700
Glucocorticoids, 1066
Gluconeogenesis, **702**
Glucose, 701
Glucose tolerance test (GTT), **430**
Glucosuria, **775**
Gluteal region, 63*f*, 65*t*
Gluten, 726
Glycogen, 420
Glycogenesis, **702**
Glycogenolysis, **702**
Glycosuria, 426, 775, 783
Glycosylated hemoglobin (A$_{1c}$) test, **430**
GnRH. *See* Gonadotropin-releasing
hormone (GnRH)
Goiter, **436**
Gonad(s), 425, **820**
Gonadotropin-releasing hormone
(GnRH), 916
Goniometer, 256
Gonorrhea, **863**
Goodell sign, **908**
Goodenough-Harris drawing test, **983**
Gout, **249**
Gouty arthritis, 249, **1163**
Grade I or grade II astrocytoma, **1110**
Grading (G), **1098**
Graft versus host disease (GVHD), **664**
Grafts, **664**
Gram-negative (G⁻), 608, 1052, 1052*f*
Gram-positive (G⁺), 1052, 1052*f*
Gram stain, **849**
Granulocytes, 465
Graves disease, **436**
Gray matter, **328**
Greater sciatic notch, 219*t*
Greater trochanter, 219*t*
Greater vestibular glands, **832**
Greenstick fracture, 231*f*, 231*t*
Gross anatomy, **47**
Growth hormone (GH) targets, 416
Growth plate, 215
GTT. *See* Glucose tolerance test (GTT)
Gubernaculum testis, 823
Guillain-Barré syndrome, **348**
Gumma, **863**
Gustation, 322, 330–331
Guthrie test, **925**
GVH. *See* Graft versus host disease (GVHD)
GYN. *See* Gynecology (GYN)
Gynecology (GYN), **908**
Gynecomastia, 422, 927
Gyri (sing. gyrus), 328, **331**

H

H. *See* Hydrogen (H)
H&P form. *See* History and physical (H&P) form
H$_2$. *See* Histamine (H$_2$)
H$_2$ blockers, **1068**
Haemophilus influenzae type b, 941, **946**
Hair, **151**, 156–157
disorders of, 177–178
loss of, 164

Hair cells, 375
Hairy cell leukemia, **1113**
Half-life (T$_{1/2}$), 99
Halitosis, **710**
Hallucinations, 976, **990**
Hallux, 64*t*, 247, 252
Hallux valgus, **253**
Haloperidol (Haldol), 987
Halsted radical mastectomy, **1125**
Hamate bone, 225, 225*f*
Hand(s)
bones of, 225*f*
disorders of, 234–235
Haploid, **829**
Hashimoto thyroiditis, **436**
HAV. *See* Hepatitis A virus (HAV)
Hay fever, **655**
HbO$_2$. *See* Oxyhemoglobin (HbO$_2$)
HBV. *See* Hepatitis B virus (HBV)
hCG. *See* Human chorionic gonadotropin
(hCG)
HCl. *See* Hydrochloric acid (HCl)
HCO$_3^-$. *See* Bicarbonate ion (HCO$_3^-$)
Hct. *See* Hematocrit (Hct)
HCV. *See* Hepatitis C virus (HCV)
HD. *See* Hodgkin disease (HD)
HDL. *See* High-density lipoprotein (HDL)
HDN. *See* Hemolytic disease of the newborn
(HDN)
HDV. *See* Hepatitis D virus (HDV)
Head, eyes, ears, nose, and throat (HEENT), 5
Head, of bone, 218*t*
Headache, 333
Health Insurance Portability & Accountability
Act (HIPAA), **8**
Hearing, 322, 373–376
receptors, 374
Hearing aids, **1171**
Heart, 54*f*, **513**.
anatomy of, 511–514, 512*f*
blood flow through, 518–520, 519*f*
congenital defects of, 525–529
disorders of, 532–537
associated with lungs, 538–539
inflammation, 539–541
radiography of, 110–111
size of, 511
Heart attack, 535
Heart block, **536**
Heart sounds, 524
Heartburn, **712**
Heart–lung machine, **529**
Heatstroke, **1158**
HEENT. *See* Head, eyes, ears, nose, and
throat (HEENT)
Hegar sign, **908**
Helicobacter pylori, 711
Helminths, 1055
Helper T (T$_H$) cells, **650**
Hemangioma, **167**
Hemarthrosis, **477**
Hematochezia, **729**
Hematocrit (Hct), 462, 464
Hematology, **462**
Hematoma, **477**
Hematopoiesis, 462, 646
Hematuria, 775, 778, 1119
Heme, 464

Hemibody radiation, **119**
Hemiparesis, **337**
Hemochromatosis, **482**
Hemocytoblasts, 460
Hemodialysis, 686, 736, 738, 782
Hemodialyzer, **782**
Hemoglobin (Hg, Hgb), 213, 464, 611
fetal (Hb F), 486
glycosylated (A$_{1c}$), 425, 429
Hemoglobin count, **464**
Hemoglobin S (HbS), 473
Hemolysis, 472
Hemolytic anemia, **474**
Hemolytic disease of the newborn (HDN),
484, 932
Hemolytic uremic syndrome (HUS), 781
Hemophilia, 477, 486
Hemopoiesis, 208, **462**
Hemoptysis, 539, 597
Hemorrhage, **470**
Hemorrhagic anemia, **474**
Hemorrhoid(s), 728–729
Hemorrhoidectomy, **729**
Hemosiderin, 478
Hemostasis, 470
Hemothorax, **607**
Heparin, 466, 470
Hepatic portal vein, **702**
Hepatitis, **734**
infectious, 733
serum, 733
Hepatitis A virus (HAV), 733, 947
vaccine, 941*t*, 942*t*
Hepatitis B virus (HBV), 733, 946
vaccine, 941*t*, 942*t*, 946
Hepatitis C virus (HCV), 733
Hepatitis D virus (HDV), 733
Hepatitis E virus (HEV), 733
Hepatitis G virus (HGV), 733
Hepatocytes, **702**
Hepatomegaly, 422, 538, 602
Hernia(s), **303**
abdominal, 725
hiatal, 721, 725
inguinal, 303, 725
reducible, 725
reproductive, 856
strangulated, 725
umbilical, 303
Herniated disc, **257**
Herniorrhaphy, **725**
Herpes simplex virus 1 (HSV1), 708–709
Herpes simplex virus type II (HSV-II), 860
Herpes zoster, **180**, 1157, 1157*f*
Hertz (Hz), 116
HEV. *See* Hepatitis E virus (HEV)
HGV. *See* Hepatitis G virus (HGV)
Hiatal hernia, **725**, **1183**
Hiatus, 695
Hiccupping, **585**
Hidrosis, **158**
High-density lipoprotein (HDL), **468**
Hilum, 584, 769
Hinge joints, 244
Hip(s)
bones, 226
congenital dysplasia (CHD), 930, 931*f*
joint, 228*f*

HIPAA. *See* Health Insurance Portability & Accountability Act (HIPAA)
Hirschsprung disease, 936, 937
Hirsutism, **178**, **428**
Histamine (H₂), **466**, 653, 1064
Histology, **47**
Histoplasmosis, **605**
History (Hx), medical, 4–8
History and physical (H&P) form, 5, 6*f*
Histrionic personality disorder, **1013**
HIV. *See* Human immunodeficiency virus (HIV)
Hives, 174
HLA. *See* Human leukocyte antigen (HLA)
HMD. *See* Hyaline membrane disease (HMD)
Hobnail liver, 732
Hodgkin disease (HD), **662**
Hodgkin lymphoma, **1114**
Holandric inheritance, **919**
Holter monitor, **532**
Homeostasis, 42, 415
Hordeolum, **387**
Horizontal plane, **62**
Hormone replacement therapy (HRT), **238**, **428**, **838**
Hormones, 416, 771
hPL test. *See* Human placental lactogen (hPL) test
HPV. *See* Human papillomavirus (HPV)
HRT. *See* Hormone replacement therapy (HRT)
HSV-II. *See* Herpes simplex virus type II (HSV-II)
HSV1. *See* Herpes simplex virus 1 (HSV1)
Human body systems, 50–53
Human chorionic gonadotropin (HCG), **906**
  in maternal serum or urine, 904
Human immunodeficiency virus (HIV), **658**, 859, 1053
Human leukocyte antigen (HLA), 664
Human papillomavirus (HPV), 850–851, **947**
Human placental lactogen (hPL) test, 429, **906**
Humerus, **226**
Humor(s), 370
Huntington chorea, 339, **1169**
Huntington disease (HD). *See* Huntington chorea
HUS. *See* Hemolytic uremic syndrome (HUS)
Hx. *See* History (Hx)
Hyaline membrane disease (HMD), **610**
  of newborn, 939
Hydatidiform mole, **923**
Hydrocele, **843**
Hydrocephalus, 345, **937**
Hydrochloric acid (HCl), **697**
Hydrocortisone, 421
Hydrogen (H), 705
Hydronephrosis, **777**
Hydroxycorticosteroid urine test, 426
Hymen, **831**
Hyoid bone, **222**
Hypercalcemia, **431**
Hypercapnia, **610**
Hyperextension, 246
Hyperglycemia, **430**, 717, 783
Hyperlipidemia, **1064**
Hyperopia (H), **382**
Hyperparathyroidism, **431**
Hyperplasia, **178**, **1101**
Hyperpnea, **589**

Hyperpyrexia, **119**
Hypersensitivity, **655**
  disorders, 653–655
Hypertension, 537, 1062, **1176**
  malignant, 535
  primary (essential), 534
  renal, 783, 784
  secondary, 535
Hyperthermia, **119**
Hyperthyroidism, **436**, **1173**
  case study, 439
Hypertrichosis, **178**
Hypertrophy, 216, 291
Hyperuricemia, **781**
Hyperventilation, **589**
Hypnosis, **1001**
Hypoalbuminemia, **779**
Hypocalcemia, 431
Hypochondria, **1003**
Hypochondriac region(s)
  left, 60, 60*f*
  right, 60, 60*f*
Hypochondriasis, **1003**
Hypochromic, definition of, 473
Hypodermis, 153, 183
Hypogastric region, **61**
Hypoglossal nerve (CN XII), 330*f*
Hypoglycemia, 334, **430**
Hypoglycemic drugs, **1067**
Hypogonadism, **927**
Hyponatremia, **1173**
Hypoparathyroidism, **431**
Hypophysis, 416
Hyposensitization, **655**
Hypospadias, **787**, **843**
Hypotension, **719**
Hypothalamus, **331**, **418**
Hypothermia, 719, **1158**
  and diving reflex, 586
Hypothyroidism, **436**, **1173**
  infantile, 434–435
Hypoventilation, **589**
Hypoxemia, **610**
Hypoxia, **593**, 933
Hysterectomy, **849**
Hysteria, **1003**
Hysterosalpingography, **112**
Hz. *See* Hertz (Hz)

I

¹³¹I. *See* Iodine-131 (¹³¹I)
I&D. *See* Incision and drainage (I&D)
Iatrogenic, definition of, **1047**
Iatrogenic disease, **1188**
IBD. *See* Inflammatory bowel disease (IBD)
IBS. *See* Irritable bowel syndrome (IBS)
Ibuprofen, **1056**
IC. *See* Interstitial cystitis (IC)
ICD. See International Classification of Diseases (ICD)
ICD-9-CM. *See* International Statistical Classification of Diseases and Related Health Problems, Ninth Edition, Clinical Modification (ICD-9-CM)
Ichthyosis, **162**
ICP. *See* Intracranial pressure (ICP)
ICSH (interstitial cell-stimulating hormone). *See* Luteinizing hormone (LH)

Idiopathic disease, **69**
  definition of, 174
IEP. *See* Individual educational plan (IEP)
IFNs. *See* Interferons (IFNs)
Ig. *See* Immunoglobulin(s) (Ig)
Ileocecal valve, **704**
Ileum, **699**, **702**
  vs. ilium, 9, 9*f*
Ileus, **729**
Iliac crest, 228*f*
Ilium, **229**
  vs. ileum, 9, 9*f*
IM. *See* Infectious mononucleosis (IM); Intramuscular (IM) route
Immune activation, 651
Immune system. *See* Lymphatic/immune system
Immune system cancers, **1114**
Immunity, **466**, **643**
  nonspecific, 643
  specific, 643
Immunizations, **946**
Immunodeficiency disorders, 656–658
Immunoglobulin(s) (Ig), 643, **652**
Immunologic surveillance, 647
Immunophenotyping, **1113**
Immunosuppressant, **729**
Immunosuppressive drugs, **1069**
Immunotherapy, **658**
Imp. *See* Impression (Imp)
Impetigo, **180**
Implantation, **903**
Impotence, **843**
Impression (IMP), 5
In utero, 902
In vitro fertilization (IVF), **915**
Incision and drainage (I&D), **170**
Incisional biopsy, **1105**
Incisors, **695**
Incompetent cervix, **912**
Incontinence, **790**
  fecal, 712, 713
  urinary, 789
Incubation, **947**
Incus, **375**
Index case, **69**
Individual educational plan (IEP), **985**
Indolent, **1113**
Infancy, **917**
Infant respiratory distress syndrome (IRDS), **610**, **940**
Infantile hypothyroidism, **436**
Infection, **648**, 658–660
  opportunistic, 656, 658
  of reproductive system, 857–858
Infectious disease(s)
  of central nervous system, 345–348
  of childhood, 941–947
  of skin, 179–181
Infectious mononucleosis (IM), **482**, **659**
Inferior, definition of, 59
Inferior nasal conchae, **221**
Inferior vena cava, **520**
Infertility, **857**
Inflammatory bowel disease (IBD), **729**
Influenza, **605**, **947**, **1179**
  deaths caused by, 612
  vaccine, 941*t*, 942*t*

Infundibulum, of uterine tube, **831**
Ingestion, 693
Inguinal hernia, **725, 1187**
Inguinal region(s), 63*f*, 64*t*
    left, 60*f*, 61
    right, 60*f*, 61
INH. *See* Isoniazid
Inhalation route, **585, 1051**
Inheritance, **919**
Inhibin, **834**
Innate immunity, **648**
Inotropic agents, **1064**
Insertion, muscle, **291**
Inspiration, **584**
Inspiratory reserve volume (IRV), **587**
Instrumental activities of daily living
    (IADL), **1155**
Insulin, 420, 429, 700, **1067**
Integument, 146, 149
Integumentary system, 50, 51*f*, 52*t*, 53,
    145–206, 151
    across lifespan, 183
    aging and, 1155–1158
    medical term parts in, 147–149
    pathology of, 160
Integumentary system cancers, 1102–1106,
    1102*f*, 1103*f*, 1104*f*
Intelligence quotient (IQ), **983**
Interferons (IFNs), **648**
Intermittent peritoneal dialysis
    (IPD), **782**
Internal anal sphincter, 703, 703*f*
Internal ear, **375**
    disorders of, 390–391
Internal fixation, **232**
International Classification of
    Diseases (ICD), 8
International Statistical Classification of
    Diseases and Related Health Problems,
    Ninth Edition, Clinical Modification
    (ICD-9-CM), 973
Interstitial brachytherapy, **119**
Interstitial cells, **821**
Interstitial cystitis (IC), **790**
Interstitial, definition of, **641**
Interventional radiology, **101**
Intervertebral disc, **244**
Intracranial pressure (ICP), **344**
Intradermal route, **1051**
Intradermal test, **655**
Intramuscular (IM) route, **1051**
Intraocular gas bubble, **385**
Intraocular lens (IOL), **377**
Intraocular pressure (IOP), 377–378
Intraoperative cone irradiation, **119**
Intrauterine device (IUD), **869**
Intravenous (IV) route, **1051**
Intravenous pyelogram (IVP), **114, 777**
Intravenous urogram (IVU), **777**
Intrinsic asthma, **655**
Intrinsic factor, **698**
Invasive tumor, **1098**
Inversion, **246**
Iodine 131 (^{131}I), **434**
Iodine, 419, 435
IOL. *See* Intraocular lens (IOL)
IOP. *See* Intraocular pressure (IOP)
IPD. *See* Intermittent peritoneal dialysis (IPD)

IQ. *See* Intelligence quotient (IQ)
IRDS. *See* Infant respiratory distress
    syndrome (IRDS)
Iris, **372**
Iron-deficiency anemia, **473**
Irradiation, **119**
    intraoperative cone, 118, 119
    total body, 118, 119
Irregular bones, **214**
Irritable bowel syndrome (IBS), **732**
IRV. *See* Inspiratory reserve volume (IRV)
Ischemia, **532**
Ischium, **229**
Islets of Langerhans, **420**
Isoniazid, **605**
Itching, **173**
IUD. *See* Intrauterine device (IUD)
IV. *See* Intravenous (IV) route
IVP. *See* Intravenous pyelogram (IVP)
IVU. *See* Intravenous urogram (IVU)

J

Jaundice, **156, 474**
JCAHO. *See* Joint Commission on
    Accreditation of Healthcare
    Organizations (JCAHO)
Jejunum, **699**
Joint(s), 238, **241**. *See also* Articulation(s)
    across lifespan, 257–258
    movements, 244–246, 245*f*
Joint capsule, **244**
Joint Commission on Accreditation of Health-
    care Organizations (JCAHO), 71
Joint Commissionís Universal Protocol, 71
Juvenile pilocytic astrocytoma, **1110**
Juxtaglomerular cells, **771**

K

K$^+$. *See* Potassium (K$^+$)
Kaposi sarcoma (KS), **169, 663, 1105**
Karyotype, 917, 918*f*
Kegel exercises, **790, 856**
Keloid, **168**
Keratin, **151**
Keratinization, 153, 156
Keratitis, **379**
Keratometer, **380**
Keratosis (pl. keratoses)
    actinic, 167, 168
    seborrheic, 166, 168
Kidney, 766, 767–769, 777*f*
    cancer of, 787–789, 1118*t*, 1119
    development of, 790–791
    disorders of, 775–778
    inherited and congenital disorders, 786–787
    function, disorders of, 780–781
    intravenous pyelogram of, 113*f*
    physiology of, 771–772
Kidney stones. *See* Renal calculi
Kidney transplant, **782**
Kidney, ureter, bladder (KUB) radiographic
    studies, 776, 777
Killed vaccines, **651**
Klinefelter syndrome, **928**
Knee, 228*f*
    disorders of, 252, 253–254
Koplik spots, **947**
KS. *See* Kaposi sarcoma (KS)

KUB radiographic study, **777**
Kussmaul respirations, **590**
Kwashiorkor, **721**
Kyphosis, 230, **1163**

L

L. *See* Lumbar (L)
L-dopa. *See* Levodopa (L-dopa)
L&W. *See* Living and well (L&W)
L$_1$–L$_5$. *See* Lumbar vertebrae
Labia majora (sing. labium majus), **832**
Labia minora (sing. labium minus), **832**
Labial cancer, **853**
Labor, **908**, 909–913
    stages of, 909, 910*f*
Labyrinthitis, **391**
Lacrimal bones, **222**
Lacrimal glands, **372**
Lacrimation, **602**
Lactation, **833, 914**
Lacteals, **643**
Lactic dehydrogenase (LDH) test, **535**
Lactiferous ducts, 833, 833*f*
Lactiferous sinuses, 833, 833*f*
Lamina, **224**
Language, 9–11
Lanugo, **183**
Laparoscope, **716**
Laparoscopy, **849**
Large cell carcinoma, **1115**
Large intestine, 690, 691*f*, **704**
    disorders of, 727–729
Laryngitis, **605**
Laryngography, **113**
Laryngopharynx, **579**
Laryngoscope, **605**
Laryngoscopy, **605**
Larynx, 577, 580–581, 582*f*
Laser ablation, **852**
Laser-assisted in situ keratomileusis (LASIK).
    See LASIK
Laser photocoagulation, **385**
Laser surgery, **1105**
LASIK surgery, **382**
Last menstrual period (LMP), 907, 950
lat. *See* Lateral
Lateral, definition of, 58*f*, 59
Lateral meniscus, 243*f*
Latex allergy, **655**
Laxatives, **1068**
LD. *See* Learning disorder (LD); Lethal dose
    (LD); Licensed dietitian (LD)
LDH test. *See* Lactic dehydrogenase
    (LDH) test
LDLs. *See* Low-density lipoproteins (LDLs)
Learning disorder (LD), **987**
Left atrioventricular (AV) valve, **513**
Left coronary artery, **520**
Left ear (*auris sinistra*, A.S.), **375**
Left eye (*oculus sinister*, O.S.), **371**
Left hypochondriac region, **61**
Left inguinal region, **61**
Left lower quadrant (LLQ), **61**
Left lumbar region, **61**
Left upper quadrant (LUQ), **61**
Legionellosis, **605**
Legionnaires' disease, **605**
Leiomyomas, 853, 854

Leiomyosarcoma, 1125
Lens, ocular, 372
Leptin, 425
LES. *See* Lower esophageal sphincter (LES)
Lesions, 156, 987
Lesser vestibular glands, 832
Lethal dose (LD), 1044
Leukopoiesis, 466
Leukemia, 486, 1113
    acute lymphoblastic leukemia (ALL), 485, 486
    acute lymphocytic leukemia (ALL), 485
    acute myeloid leukemia (AML), 485, 486
    chronic lymphocytic leukemia (CLL), 485, 486
    chronic myeloid leukemia (CML), 485, 486
Leukocytes, 460, 462*f*, 465–467, 466
    agranular, 466
    granular, 466
Leukocytosis, 482
Leukoderma, 182
Leukopenia, 482
Leukopoiesis, 465, 466
Level of consciousness (LOC), 334
Levodopa (L-dopa), 335, 1058
Levothyroxine, 434, 1067
LH. *See* Luteinizing hormone (LH)
Libido, 870
Lice, 180
Licensed dietitian (LD), 686
Licensed independent social worker (LISW), 978
Licensed practical nurse (LPN), 412
Licensed social worker (LSW), 978
Life expectancy, 70–71, 902, 1155
Lifespan, 70–71, 902, 1155
    and blood, 486–487
    and cancer, 1126
    and cardiovascular system, 547–548
    and development, 947–948
    and digestive system, 734
    and endocrine system, 431
    and integumentary system, 183
    and joints, 257–258
    and lymphatic/immune system, 665
    and mental disorders, 1014
    and muscular system, 304
    and nervous system, 348
    and pharmacologic effects, 1070
    and radiology, 124
    and reproductive system, 870
    and respiratory system, 612
    and skeletal system, 257–258
    and special senses, 391
    and urinary system, 790–791
Ligaments, 241
Ligation, 729
Lightening, 912
Linea nigra, 908
Lipase, 698
    serum, 717
Lipids, 705, 1063
Lipocytes, 153
Lipoma, 168
Lipoproteins, 467–468, 468
    classification of, 468*f*
Lipping, 948

LISW. *See* Licensed independent social worker
Lithium carbonate, 998, 1057
Lithotripsy, 777
Liver, 690, 691*f*, 701–702, 702. *See also* Hepatic
    disorders of, 732–734
    hobnail, 732
    spots, 1158
Living and well (L&W), 5
LLQ. *See* Left lower quadrant (LLQ)
LMP. *See* Last menstrual period (LMP)
Loading dose, 1044
Lobar pneumonia, 605
Lobectomy, 436, 606
Lobules, of liver, 702
LOC. *See* Level of consciousness (LOC)
Local anesthetics, 1061
Lockjaw, 943
Long bones, 214
Longevity, 1154
Lordosis, 230
Louse (pl. lice), 180
Low birth weight, 937
Low-density lipoproteins (LDLs), 468, 530
Lower esophageal sphincter (LES), 696
Lower respiratory tract, 576, 577*f*
    disorders of, 602–605
LPN. *See* Licensed practical nurse (LPN)
LSW. *See* Licensed social worker
Lumbar (L), 63*f*, 65*t*
Lumbar puncture, 348
Lumbar region(s)
    left, 61
    right, 61
Lumbar vertebrae (L$_1$–L$_5$), 224
Lumen, arterial, 531
Lumpectomy, 1125
Lunar month, 907
Lunate (bone), 225*f*
Lung(s), 577, 583–584
    biopsy, 597
    cancer, 606, 1179
    capacities, 586, 587*t*
    cardiovascular disorders affecting, 590–592
    heart disorders associated with, 538–539
    volumes, 586, 587*t*
Lung biopsy, 597
Lung cancer, 606, 1179
Lunula, 159
Lupus *See* Systemic lupus erythematosus (SLE)
LUQ. *See* Left upper quadrant (LUQ)
Luteinizing hormone (LH), 416, 827, 834, 916
Luxation, 257
Lyme arthritis, 249, 258
Lyme disease, 247, 248*f*
Lymph, 643
Lymph channels and nodes, radiography of, 110–111
Lymph node(s), 641, 643, 644
Lymph nodules, 645
Lymphadenopathy, 658
Lymphangiography, 663
Lymphangitis, 659
Lymphatic system, 53
Lymphatic vessels, 641, 642*f*

Lymphatic/immune system, 51*f*, 52, 52*t*, 53, 637–684, 642*f*, 643
    across lifespan, 665
    aging and, 1179–1180
    anatomy of, 641–652
    overview of, 641, 642*f*
    physiology of, 641–652
    tumors of, 661–663
Lymphedema, 659
Lymphocytes, 466, 642, 643
Lymphography, 111
Lymphomas, 662, 1114
Lysosome, 465
Lysozyme, 372

M

M. *See* Myopia
M-Mode Doppler ultrasonography, 552
MAB, MoAb. *See* Monoclonal antibody (MAB, MoAb)
Macrophages, 466
Macula, 373
Macular degeneration, 385
Macule(s), 180, 945
Magnetic resonance angiography (MRA), 107
Magnetic resonance imaging (MRI), 68, 107, 333, 427, 590
Magnetic resonance spectroscopy, 107
Maintenance dose, 1045
Major depressive disorder, 997
Major histocompatibility complex (MHC), 664
Malaise, 249, 258, 599
Malaria, 1055
Male
    pelvis of, 226, 227*f*
    reproductive hormones of, 827
    reproductive system of, 820–821, 821*f*
    testes and accessory glands of, 823–825
Male condoms, 869
Malignant, 167, 1097
    definition of, 166, 167
    germ cell tumors, 1123, 1125
    hypertension, 535
    melanoma, 168
Malignant germ cell tumors, 1125
Malignant melanoma, 169
Malleus, 375
Malnutrition, 718
Malocclusion, 710
Mammary galactography. *See* Ductography
Mammary glands, 822, 833–834
Mammogram, 1124
Mammography, 112, 852
Mandible, 222
Mania, 996
Mantoux test, 605
Manual region, 63*f*, 65*t*
MAOIs. *See* Monoamine oxidase inhibitors (MAOIs)
Marasmus, 721
Marfan syndrome, 233
Margin, 1105
Mask of pregnancy. *See* Chloasma
Massage therapist (MT), professional profile, 638
Massage therapy, 667
Mastectomy, 852

Mastication, 693
Mastoid process, 216, 217*t*
Mastoidectomy, 389
Mastoiditis, **389**
Masturbate, **1008**
Maxillary bones, **221**
Maxillary sinus(es), 578, 578*f*
McBurney point, 713
μCi. *See* Microcurie (μCi)
MCL. *See* Medial collateral ligament (MCL)
MDs. *See* Muscular dystrophies (MDs)
Measles, **947**
Measles, mumps, rubella (MMR) vaccine, 941*t*,
    942*t*, 947. *See also* Rubeola
Meatus, 218*t*
Mechanical digestion, **691**
Mechanical ventilator, **610**
Mechlorethamine, Oncovin, prednisone,
    and procarbazine (MOPP), 661
Meconium, **914**
Medial collateral ligament (MCL), 305
Medial, definition of, 59
Mediastinum, **57**
Medical assistant, 2
Medical record, 4–8
Medical terminology, careers requiring
    knowledge of, 3, 4*b*
Medulla
    of lymph node, 644, 644*f*
    renal, 767, 768*f*, 769
Medulla oblongata, **332**
Medullary cavity, **214**
Medulloblastoma, **1110**
Megacolon, 936
Meibomian glands, 386
Meiosis, **828**
Melanin, **151**, 154
Melanocyte-stimulating hormone (MSH), 417
Melanocytes, **151**, 154, 183
Melanoma, **168**, **1105**, **1158**
Melatonin, **424**
Melena, **729**
Membrane(s), **55**
    pericardial, 55
    peritoneal, 55
    pleural, 55
    serous, 55
Membranous labyrinth, **375**
Memory B cells, **650**
Memory T cells, **650**
Menarche, **838**
Ménière disease, **391**
Meningeal spaces, 329
Meninges (sing. meninx), **332**
Meningioma, **1110**
Meningitis, **348**
Meningocele, **345**, **937**
Meningococcal meningitis, **947**
Meniscus (pl. menisci), **244**
    torn, 252–253
Menopause, **838**
Menses, **838**
Menstrual cycle, **838**
Menstruation, **838**
Mental (chin), 63*f*, 64*t*
Mental health, 971–1036
    case study, 1016
    disorders, across lifespan, 1014

usually first diagnosed in infancy, childhood,
    or adolescence, 984–988
Mental health professionals, 977–979
Mental retardation, **987**
Mesentery, **55**
Mesoderm, 70, 183, 486, 903
Mesonephric ducts, 870
Mesothelioma, **606**
Metabolic disorders, 718–721
Metabolism, 43, 49, **702**
Metacarpal bones, **226**
Metaphysis, **214**
Metaplasia, **1101**
Metastasis, 606
Metastasize, 1095, 1096
Metatarsal bones, **229**
Metatarsophalangeal (MTP) joint(s), 252
Methylphenidate (Ritalin), 986
MHC. *See* Major histocompatibility complex
    (MHC)
MI. *See* Myocardial infarction (MI)
Microcurie (μCi), 434
Microglia, 324
Microvilli, intestinal, **699**
Micturition, **766**
Midbrain, **332**
Middle ear, **375**
    disorders of, 389–390
Midsagittal plane, **62**
Midwife, professional profile, 816
Migraine, **336**
Milia, 183
Millimeters of mercury (mm Hg), 523
Mind, **976**
Mineralocorticoids, 1066
Minerals, **705**
Minnesota multiphasic personality inventory
    (MMPI), **983**
Mirena IUD, 866
MIS. *See* Müllerian-inhibiting substance
    (MIS)
Miscarriage, 909
Mite(s), 180
Mitochondria, **50**, 463
Mitosis, 828
Mitral stenosis, 543
Mitral valve, **514**
Mitral valve prolapse (MVP), **543**
Mixed tumor, 1101
mm Hg. *See* Millimeters of mercury
    (mm Hg)
MMPI. *See* Minnesota Multiphasic Personality
    Inventory (MMPI)
MMR. *See* Measles, mumps, rubella (MMR)
Modafinil (Provigil), 1011
Modified radical mastectomy, 1125
Modified respiratory movements, 585
Mohs surgery, **169**, **1105**
Molar (tooth), **695**
Molar pregnancy, 920
Moles, 166
Monoamine oxidase inhibitors (MAOIs),
    996, 1058
Monoclonal antibodies (MAB, MoAb), **658**,
    1069, 1119
Monocytes, **466**
Monosomy, 927
Monozygotic twins, **915**

Mons pubis, 832
Mood disorders, 995–998, **997**
MOPP. *See* Mechlorethamine, Oncovin,
    prednisone, and procarbazine (MOPP)
Morbidity, **1097**, **1155**
Morning-after pill, **869**
Morphine, **1058**
Morphology, 47, 146, 211, 856
Mortality, **1097**, **1155**
MOSD. *See* Multiple organ system deficiency
    (MOSD)
Mountain sickness, **610**
Mouth, 692–693, 692*f*
MRA. *See* Magnetic resonance angiography
    (MRA)
MRI. *See* Magnetic resonance imaging (MRI)
MS. *See* Multiple sclerosis (MS)
MSH. *See* Melanocyte-stimulating
    hormone (MSH)
MT. *See* Massage therapist (MT)
MTP. *See* Metatarsophalangeal (MTP)
Mucolytics, 590
Mucopurulent, definition of, 595, 597
Mucous cells, 697
Müllerian ducts, 870
Müllerian-inhibiting substance (MIS), 870
Multi-infarct dementia, **1168**
Multiaxial classification, **981**
Multiple births, 914–915
Multiple myeloma, **482**
Multiple organ system deficiency (MOSD), **1188**
Multiple sclerosis (MS), **345**
Mumps, **947**
Munchausen syndrome, **1004**
Munchausen syndrome by proxy, **1004**
Murmur, 932
    cardiac, 541
    vascular, 544, 546
Muscle(s)
    of arm and forearm, 295*t*, 295*f*
    biopsy of, 300, 301
    contraction, 291
    of face, head and neck, 293*t*, 293*f*
    movement, 291–292
    names of, 292, 293*t*, 294*t*, 295*t*, 296*t*, 299
    of thigh and leg, 296*t*, 297–298*f*
    of trunk, 294*t*, 294*f*
Muscle biopsy, **301**
Muscle cells, **289**
Muscle fibers, **289**
Muscle tissue, **289**, **1101**
    tumors, 1099–1100, 1099*t*, 1101, 1101*t*
Muscular dystrophies (MDs), **301**
Muscular system, **53**, 285–318
    across lifespan, 304
    aging and, 1164–1165
    cancers, 1107–1108, 1108*f*
    case study, 305–306
    trauma to, 301–303
Muscular tissue, **50**
Musculoskeletal, definition of, 286
Mutation(s), **919**, **1097**
MVP. *See* Mitral valve prolapse (MVP)
Myalgia, 301
Mycobacterium tuberculosis, 1178
Myelin, **325**
Myelography, **109**
Myocardial infarction (MI), **537**, **1176**

Myocarditis, 541
Myocardium, 513
Myometrium, 830, 830*f*
Myopathy, **301**
Myopia (M), **382**
Myosarcoma, **1108**
Myositis, **301**
Myringotomy, **389**
Myxedema, **436, 1173**

N

Na⁺. *See* Sodium ion (Na⁺)
NAD. *See* No acute distress (NAD)
Nägele's rule, **908**
Nail bed, **159**
Nail body, **159**
Nail root, **159**
Nails, **151,** 158–160
    disorders of, 181
    free edge of, 158, 159, 159*f*
    structures of, 158, 159*f*
Naming system, biologic, 11
Naproxen, **1056**
Narcissistic personality disorder, **1013**
Narcolepsy, **1012**
Narcotics, **1058**
Nares, **579**
Nasal bones, **221**
Nasal cannula, **592**
Nasal catarrh, **601**
Nasal cavity, 57, 577, 578–579, 578*f*
Nasal polyp, **601**
Nasal region, 63*f*, 64*t*
Nasal route, **1051**
Nasal septum, **579**
Nasal speculum, **601**
Nasogastric (NG) tube, **718**
Nasogastric route, **1051**
Nasopharynx, **579**
National Board for Respiratory Care
    (NBRC), 572
National Center for Health Statistics
    (NCHS), 716
National Certification Examination for
    Therapeutic Massage and Bodywork
    (NCETMB), 638
National Collegiate Athletic Association
    (NCAA), 422
National Council Licensure Examination
    (NCLEX), 508
National Health and Nutrition Examination
    Survey (NHANES), 716
Natriuresis, 424
Natural killer (NK) cells, 641
Nausea, **713**
Navicular (bone), 228, 228*f*
NBRC. *See* National Board for Respiratory Care
    (NBRC)
NCAA. *See* National Collegiate Athletic Associa-
    tion (NCAA)
NCETMB. *See* National Certification Examination
    for Therapeutic Massage and Bodywork
    (NCETMB)
NCHS. *See* National Center for Health Statistics
    (NCHS)
NCLEX. *See* National Council Licensure
    Examination (NCLEX)
NE. *See* Norepinephrine (NE)

Nearsightedness, 382
Nebulizer, **592**
NEC. *See* Necrotizing enterocolitis (NEC)
Neck (of tooth), **695**
Necrosis, **172**
Necrotizing enterocolitis (NEC), **940**
Necrotizing fasciitis, 173
Necrotizing ulcerative gingivitis, **710**
Needle aspiration biopsy, 436
Neonatal respiratory distress syndrome
    (NRDS), **610**
Neonate, 902, **917**
Neoplasms, 1095, 1096. *See also* Tumor(s)
    staging and grading of, 1097–1099, 1098*f*
Neovascularization, 384
Nephrectomy, **788**
Nephritis, **777**
Nephron loop, 768
Nephrons, **769**
Nephropathy, **783**
Nephroptosis, **777**
Nephrotic syndrome, **779**
Nerve cells, 324
Nervous system, **53,** 320, 366
    across lifespan, 348
    aging and, 1165–1169
    anatomy of, 322–323, 369–376
    cancers, 1108–1110
    radiography of, 109
Nervous tissue, 50, **1101**
Neural tissue, 1100
Neuraminidase inhibitors, **1054**
Neuroblastoma, **1110**
Neuroendocrine system, 412
Neurogenic bladder, **790**
Neuroglia, 325, **1101**
Neurohypophysis, 416
Neurological examination, case study, 350
Neurologists, 332
Neuromuscular system, congenital disorders
    of, 934–937
Neurons, 325, 977, **1101**
Neuropathy, 488
Neurosis, **977**
Neurosurgeons, 332
Neurotransmitters, 325, **977**
Neutropenia, **482**
Neutrophils, **466**
Nevi, **156**
NG. *See* Nasogastric (NG)
NHANES. *See* National Health and Nutrition
    Examination Survey (NHANES)
NHL. *See* Non-Hodgkin lymphoma (NHL)
Nipple, 833, 833*f*
Nitrates, **1064**
Nitroglycerin, **537**
NK cells. *See* Natural killer (NK) cells
NKA. *See* No known allergies (NKA)
NKDA. *See* No known drug allergies (NKDA)
NMR. *See* Nuclear magnetic resonance (NMR)
No acute distress (NAD), 5
No known allergies (NKA), 5
No known drug allergies (NKDA), 5
Nocturia, **1184**
Node, 522
Nodules, **162**
Nomenclature, **8, 973**
    standard, 3

Non-Hodgkin lymphoma (NHL), **663, 1114**
Non per os (NPO), 940, 1049
Non-small cell lung cancer, **1115**
Nondisjunction, 927
Nongenetic syndromes, 928–929
Nonrespiratory air movements, 585
Nonselective arterial catheter placement, **106**
Nonselective venous, **106**
Nonseminomas, **1124**
Nonspecific immunity, **643**
Nonsteroidal anti-inflammatory drugs
    (NSAIDs), 251, 300, 540, 711, **1056**
Noradrenaline, 421
Norepinephrine (NE), **421,** 975
Nose, 330, 330*f*, 576, 577*f*, 578–579
Nostrils, 578, 578*f*
NPO. *See* Non per os (NPO)
NRDS. *See* Neonatal respiratory distress
    syndrome (NRDS)
NSAIDs. *See* Nonsteroidal anti-inflammatory
    drugs (NSAIDs)
Nuchal rigidity, **348**
Nuclear magnetic resonance (NMR), 107
Nuclear medicine, **98,** 120–123
    medical term parts used in, 95
    procedures in, 120–123
Nuclear scan studies, **123**
Nucleus, **50**
Nulliparous, **849**
Nurse anesthetists, **1060**
Nutrients, **705**
Nutrition, 687, **705**
Nutrition strategies, 70
Nutritional anemia, **474**
Nutritional disorders, 718–721
Nystagmus, **385**

O

O₂. *See* Oxygen (O₂)
OB. *See* Obstetrician (OB); Obstetrics (OB)
Obesity, 715, 716–717, 1009
Obsessive–compulsive disorder (OCD), **1001**
Obsessive–compulsive personality disorder
    (OCPD), 1000
Obstetric forceps, **913**
Obstetrician (OB), **908**
Obstetrics (OB), **908**
Obturator foramen, **229**
Occipital bone, **221**
Occipital region, 63*f*, 65*t*
Occult, **732**
Occult blood, 731
Occulta, **936**
Occupational history (OH), 5
Occupational therapist (OT), 1150, **1155**
Occupational therapy (OT), 299, 984, **1155**
OCD. *See* Obsessive–compulsive disorder (OCD)
OCDP. *See* Obsessive–compulsive personality
    disorder (OCPD)
OCPs. *See* Oral contraceptive pills (OCPs)
OCTs. *See* Oral contraceptives (OCTs)
Oculomotor nerve (CN III), 330*f*
O.D. *See* Right eye (*oculus dexter,* O.D.)
OH. *See* Occupational history (OH)
OI. *See* Osteogenesis imperfecta (OI)
Okinawans, 1188–1189
Olecranal region, 63*f*, 65*t*
Olfaction, 322

Olfactory nerve (CN I), 330*f*
Oligodendrocytes, 324
Oligodendroglioma, 340, **1110**
Oligospermia, 857
Oliguria, 779
Oncogenes, **1097**
Oncologists, **1097**
Oncology, 1091–1147, **1097**
Onychia, **181**
Onychomycosis, **181**
Onychophagia, **159**
Oocyte, **820**, 830
Oogenesis, 835
Oogonium, 835
Open reduction, 232
Ophthalmic route, 1051
Ophthalmoscope, 379
Opiates, 991, **1058**
Opium, **1058**
Opportunistic disease, **1105**
Opportunistic infection, 658
Optic disc, 373
Optic nerves (CN II), 330*f*, 373
Optometric assistant, professional profile, 366
Oral cancer, **1183**
Oral cavity, 57, 690, 692–693, 692*f*
  disorders of, 707–710
Oral contraceptive pills (OCPs), 865
Oral contraceptives (OCTs), **869**
Oral leukoplakia, **710**
Oral region, 63*f*, 64*t*
Oral route, 1051
Orbital region, 63*f*, 64*t*
Orchiectomy, **843**
Orchiopexy, **843**
Orchitis, **843**
Organ of Corti, 374
Organ system, **50**
Organelles, **50**
Organic brain disease, 977
Organic brain syndrome, 1168
Organism, **47**
Orgasm, **839**
Origin, 291
Oropharynx, **579**
Orthodontics, **710**
Orthopnea, **539**
Orthoptic training, 378
Ortolani sign, 931*f*
O.S. *See* Left eye (*oculus sinister,* O.S.)
Osmolarity, 775
Osmotic pressure, 462
Ossification, 216
Osteitis deformans, 237
Osteoarthritis, **249**, 1163
Osteoblasts, 216, 1106
Osteochondroma, 238
Osteoclastic activity, 257
Osteoclasts, 216
Osteocytes, 216
Osteogenesis imperfecta (OI), **232**
Osteogenic sarcoma, 238
Osteoid, 1160
Osteomalacia, **235**, 1163
Osteomyelitis, **237**
Osteophytes, **249**
Osteoporosis, **238**, 1163
Osteosarcoma, 238, **1107**

OT. *See* Occupational therapy
OTC. *See* Over-the-counter (OTC)
Otic region, 63*f*, 64*t*
Otic route, 1051
Otitis externa, **388**
Otitis media, **389**, 604
Otosclerosis, **391**
Otoscope, 388, 389*f*
Otoscopy, **389**
O.U. *See* Each eye (*oculus uterque,* O.U.)
Ova (sing. ovum), 830, 901
Oval window, 375
Ovarian cancer, 853, **1125**
Ovarian cysts, 849
Ovarian epithelial carcinoma, **1125**
Ovaries, 415*f*, **822**, 846, 901
Over-the-counter (OTC), **1041**
Overweight, 716
Oviducts, 822, 830
Ovulation, **831**, 836
Ovum, 831, 903
OXT. *See* Oxytocin (OXT)
Oxycodone (OxyContin), 991
Oxygen (O$_2$), 463, 572, 582, 705
Oxygen tent, 592
Oxygen therapy, 592
Oxyhemoglobin (HbO$_2$), **464**
Oxytocic agents, **1067**
Oxytocin (OXT), 417, **833**, 909

P

P. *See* Plan (P); Posterior (P)
P wave, **529**
Pacemaker
  artificial, 533, 533*f*, 536
  cardiac, 522
Pachyderma, **162**
Packed cell volume (PCV), **462**
Paget disease, 237, **1163**
Pain disorder, **1003**
Palatine bones, 221
Palatine tonsils, **579**
Palatine torus, 692
Palatopharyngoplasty, 1011
Palliative, **180**, 1047
Pallor, 546
Palmar region, 63*f*, 64*t*
Palpable, definition of, 166
Palpation, **68**
Palpebrae, 372
Palpitation, 536
Palsy, 340
Pancreas, 415, 415*f*, 419–420, **420**, 691*f*, **700**
  disorders of, 428–430, 718
Pancreatic duct, **700**, 1183
Pancreatic islets, 420
Pancreatic juice, **700**
Pancreatitis, **718**
Panic disorder, **1001**
Pap smear, 850, 851*f*, **1125**
Pap test, **852**, 1125
Papillae, **693**, 769
Papillary muscles, 514
Papilloma(s), cutaneous, 166, 167
Papule, 156, 160*f*, 945
Paradoxical respiration, **611**
ParaGard, 866
Paramesonephric ducts, 870

Paranasal sinuses, 218*t*, 221, 221*f*, 578–579, **579**
Paranoid personality disorder, **1013**
Paranoid-type schizophrenia, **994**
Paraphilias, **1008**
Parasomnias, **1012**
Parasympathetic nervous system, **323**
Parathyroid cancers, **1111**
Parathyroid glands, 418–419
  disorders of, 430–432
Parathyroid hormone (PTH), **419**
Parathyroidectomy, **431**
Parenteral administration, 1051
Parenteral route, 1049, 1051
Paresis, **337**
Parietal, 55
Parietal bones, **221**
Parietal pleura, **584**
Parkinson disease (PD), 337, 1057, **1169**
  symptoms of, 338
Parotid glands, **693**
Paroxysmal sleep, 1011
Partial (incomplete) fracture, 231*t*
Partial mastectomy, **1125**
Partial thromboplastin time (PTT), **477**
Parturition, **908**
Passive immunity, **648**
Patch test, **655**
Patella, 211, **229**, 243*f*
Patellar region, 63*f*, 64*t*
Patellar tendon, 243*f*
Patent, definition of, 526
Patent ductus arteriosus (PDA), **529**, 933
Pathogenesis, **69**
Pathogens, **643**
Pathologist, 47, **1101**
Pathology, 47, 146
  of blood, 472
  cardiovascular system, 525
  endocrine system, 425
  integumentary system, 160
  lymphatic/immune system, 652
  reproductive system, 839–864
  skeletal system, 229
Pathophysiology, **69**
PC. *See* Professional counselor (PC)
PCC. *See* Professional clinical counselor (PCC)
PCV. *See* Packed cell volume (PCV)
PD. *See* Parkinson disease (PD); Peritoneal
  dialysis (PD); Postural drainage (PD);
  Pupil distance (PD)
PDA. *See* Patent ductus arteriosus (PDA)
PDR. See Physicians' Desk Reference (PDR)
PDT. *See* Photodynamic therapy (PDT)
PE. *See* Physical examination (PE, Px)
Peak expiratory flow (PEF) test, **593**
Pectoral region, 64*t*
Pectoral girdle, **224**, 225*f*
Pedal region, 63*f*, 64*t*
Pediatrician, **913**
Pediatrics, **913**
Pedicles, 219*t*, 224
Pediculosis, **181**
Pediculosis capitis, **181**
Pedophilia, **1008**
PEEP. *See* Positive end-expiratory pressure (PEEP)
PEF test. *See* Peak expiratory flow (PEF) test
Pelvic cavity, 57, 63*f*, 64*t*
Pelvic examination, 849

Pelvic girdle, 226
Pelvic inflammatory disease (PID), **849**
Pelvimetry, **913**
Pelvis, 64*t*
    female, 226, 227*f*
    male, 226, 227*f*
    renal, 767, 768*f*, 769
PEM. *See* Protein-energy malnutrition (PEM)
Pemphigus, 162
Penis, 821, 825–827, 826*f*
    anatomy of, 826*f*
    disorders of, 839–846
Pepsin, 698
Peptic ulcers, 712, **1183**
Per os, 1049
Percussion, 68, **589**, 593
Percutaneous administration, **1051**
Percutaneous needle biopsy, **106**
Percutaneous transhepatic cholangiography
    (PCT, PTHC), **106**
Percutaneous transhepatic portography, 106
Percutaneous transluminal angioplasty
    (PTA), **106**
Percutaneous transluminal coronary angio-
    plasty (PTCA), **532**
Perennial allergic rhinitis, **655**
Pericardial fluid, 54*f*
Pericardial membranes, **55**
Pericardiocentesis, **536**
Pericarditis, **541**
Pericardium, 511*f*, **513**
    parietal, 54*f*
    visceral, 54*f*
Perilymph, 374
Perimenopause, **838**
Perimetrium, 830, 830*f*
Perineal region, 63*f*, 65*t*
Perineum, **823**
    female, 832*f*
Periodontal disease, 710, **1183**
Periodontal ligament, 694
Periosteum, **214**
Peripheral, **59**
Peripheral blood smear, **1113**
Peripheral nervous system (PNS), **323**
Peripheral vascular disease (PVD), **546**
Peristalsis, **291**, **318**, **691**, **770**
    in uterine tube, 830
Peritoneal cavity, 54*f*
Peritoneal dialysis (PD), **782**
    continuous ambulatory (CAPD), 782
    continuous cycling (CCPD), 782
    intermittent (IPD), 782
Peritoneal fluid, 54*f*
Peritoneal membranes, **55**
Peritoneum, **55**, **697**
    parietal, 54*f*
    visceral, 54*f*, 57
Peritonitis, **729**
Permanent teeth, **695**
Pernicious anemia, **474**
PERRLA. *See* Pupils equal, round, and reactive
    to light and accommodation (PERRLA)
Personality disorders, **1013**
Pertussis, **946**
Pervasive developmental disorders, **987**
Pessary, **1050**
PET. *See* Positron emission tomography (PET)

Petechiae, 162, 475, **1113**
PFT. *See* Pulmonary function test (PFT)
pH, of blood, 460, 584
Phacoemulsification, **1171**
Phagocytes, **648**
Phagocytosis, **646**
Phalangeal region, 63*f*, 65*t*
Phalanges, **226**
Pharmaceuticals, **1043**
Pharmaceutics, **1043**
Pharmacist, **1043**
Pharmacodynamics, **1044**
Pharmacognosy, **1040**
Pharmacokinetics, **1044**
Pharmacologist, **1043**
Pharmacology, 1037–1090, **1043**
    across lifespan, 1070
Pharmacopeia, **1047**
Pharmacotherapy, **1043**
Pharmacy, **1043**
Pharyngeal tonsil, **579**
Pharyngitis, **602**
Pharynx, 577, 579–580, 693
Phenylketonuria (PKU), 721, 919, **925**
Pheochromocytoma, **428**, **1111**
Phimosis, **787**
Phlebitis, **547**
Phlebography, 110
Phlebotomist, professional profile, 456
Phlebotomy, 456, **482**
Phlegm, **593**
Phobias, **1001**
Phonocardiography, **115**
Phosphate, **419**
Photoaging, **1158**
Photocoagulation, **1171**
Photodynamic therapy (PDT), **1105**
Photophobia, **336**
Photoreceptors, **370**
Physical examination (PE, Px), 5
Physical rehabilitation, **70**
Physical therapist (PT), professional profile, 286
Physical therapy (PT), 299, 307–308, 984
Physical therapy assistant (PTA), 286
Physicians' Desk Reference (PDR), **1047**
Physicians' order sheet (POS), **1073**
Physiology, 42, **47**
    terminology for, medical term parts used
    in, 42–46
Pia mater, **332**
Pica, **987**
PID. *See* Pelvic inflammatory disease (PID)
Pigment disorders, 182
Piles, 728
Pill, the, 865
Pilocytic astrocytoma, 1109
Pineal gland, 415, 415*f*, **423–424**, **424**
Pitocin, 909
Pituitary dwarfism, **434**
Pituitary gland, 415, 415*f*, **416–418**, **418**
    disorders of, 432–434
PKU. *See* Phenylketonuria (PKU)
Placebo, **1047**
Placenta, **902**
    delivery of, 909, 910*f*
Placenta formation, 903–906
Placenta previa, **923**
Plan (P), 5

Planes, **62**
Plantar flexion, **246**
Plantar region, 63*f*, 64*t*
Plantar wart, **181**
Plaque, **531**, **710**
    atherosclerotic, 544
    dental, 707, 710
    on skin, 165
Plasma, **462**
Plasma cells, **650**
Plasma electrolytes, 460
Plasma prothrombin time (PT; protime), **477**
Plasma test, 425
Plasmapheresis, **482**
Platelet(s), 462*f*, **467**, 467*f. See also* Thrombocytes
    disorders of, 475–478
    phase, 469
Plethysmography, **616**
Pleura
    parietal, 54*f*
    visceral, 54*f*
Pleural cavity, 56*f*
Pleural fluid, 54*f*
Pleural membranes, **55**
Plexus, **328**
Plural forms, rules for, 13, 13*t*
Pluripotential hemopoietic stem cell
    (PHSC), **462**
PM. *See* Polymyositis (PM)
PMDD. *See* Premenstrual dysphoric disorder
    (PMDD)
PMS. *See* Premenstrual syndrome (PMS)
Pneumococcal pneumonia disease, 1178
Pneumococcal vaccine, 941*t*, 942*t*
Pneumoconiosis, **600**
Pneumocystis carinii, 656
Pneumocystis jiroveci, 656
Pneumonia, **605**, 946, 1179
    aspiration, 603, 605
    deaths caused by, 612
    lobar, 603, 603*f*, 605
    respiratory syncytial virus (RSV), 603, 605
Pneumothorax, **607**
PNI. *See* Psychoneuroimmunology (PNI)
PNS. *See* Peripheral nervous system (PNS)
Poisoning, respiratory system in, 610–611
Polio, **947**
    vaccine, 941*t*, 942*t*
Poliomyelitis, **348**
Pollex, 64*t*
Polycystic kidney disease, **787**
Polycythemia, **482**
Polycythemia vera, **482**
Polydactyly, **235**
Polydipsia, 428, 432, 783, 919
Polymyositis (PM), **301**, 1072
    case study, 1072
Polyp(s), **1117**
    intestinal, 731
Polyphagia, 428, 920
Polypharmacy, **1188**
Polysomnography, **1012**
Polyuria, 428, 432, 783, 919
Pons, **332**
Popliteal artery, echocardiogram of, 117*f*
Popliteal bursa, 243*f*
Popliteal region, 63*f*, 65*t*
Pores, **158**

Port wine stain, 156
POS. *See* Physician's order sheet (POS)
Positive end-expiratory pressure (PEEP), 610
Positron emission tomography (PET), 68, 123
Post partum, 908
Post-polio syndrome (PPS), 347
Post-traumatic stress disorder (PTSD), 1001
Posterior (P), 57, 58, 58*f*
Posterior chamber, of eye, 370, 370*f*
Posterior pituitary gland, 418
Postpartum, 908
Postprandial, 430
    definition of, 429, 920
    glucose test, 429
Postural drainage (PD), 593
    positions, 594
Potassium (K⁺), 421
Potency, 1044
Potentiation, 1047
PPS. *See* Post-polio syndrome (PPS)
Pr. *See* Presbyopia
Preadmission testing, 1190
Precocious puberty, 434
Precursor, 422, 1057
Predonation, 472
Preeclampsia, 923
Preemies, 937
Prefixes, 9, 13
    common (list of), 14–15
    related to measurement, 21
    related to number and size, 19
Pregnancy, 897–970, 908
Premalignant, 167
Premature birth, 923
Premature infant, 937–940
Premenstrual dysphoric disorder (PMDD), 849
Premenstrual syndrome (PMS), 849
Premolar, 694*f*
Prepuce, 826
Presbycusis, 388, 1171
Presbyopia (Pr), 382, 1171
Prescription (Rx), 1043
    abbreviations used in, 1041–1042*t*
    sample, 1041*f*
Prevertebral tissue, 262
Prick test, 655
Primary bone cancer, 1107
Primary bronchi, 581, 582*f*
Primary insomnia, 1012
Primary malnutrition, 721
Primary oocyte, 835, 835*f*
Primary response, 652
PRL. *See* Prolactin (PRL)
Process projection, 217*t*
Procreation, 820
Procrit, 480
Proctocele, 856
Productive cough, 595
Professional clinical counselor (PCC), 978
Professional counselor (PC), 978
Professional profile
    athletic trainer, 208
    certified surgical first assistant, 1092
    certified surgical technologist, 1092
    clinical psychologist, 972
    cytotechnologist, 146
    diagnostic medical sonographer, 898
    dialysis nurse, 762

massage therapist, 638
medical assistant, 2
midwife, 816
optometric assistant, 366
phlebotomist, 456
physical therapist, 286
registered dietitian, 686
registered nurse in cardiovascular intensive
    care unit, 508
registered pharmacist, 1038
respiratory therapist, 572
Progesterone, 425, 834, 1067
Progress notes, 5, 8
Prolactin (PRL), 417, 833, 913
Prolapse, 542
Proliferation, 1097
Proliferative phase, 838
Pronation, 246
Prone, 57
Pronunciation key, 11, 11–12*t*
Prophylactic drug, 540, 1047
Prostaglandins, 1068
Prostate, 821
    cancer of, 845, 1124, 1187
    disorders of, 843–846
Prostatectomy, 846, 1187
Prostate-specific antigen (PSA) test, 845,
    1124, 1186
Prostatitis, 845, 1187
Protease inhibitors, 1054
Protein, 705
Protein-energy malnutrition (PEM), 719
Proteinuria, 775
Prothrombin, 469, 470
Protime. *See* Plasma prothrombin time (PT)
Proton pump inhibitors, 712, 1068
Protozoa, 1055
Protriptyline, 996, 1011
Proximal, 59
Proximal convoluted tubule, 768, 768*f*, 771
Pruritus, 174
PSA test. *See* Prostate-specific antigen (PSA) test
Psoriasis, 165
Psyche, 976
Psychiatrists, 978
Psychiatry, 978
Psychoanalysts, 978
Psychological therapy, 70
Psychologists, 979
Psychology, 978
Psychoneuroimmunology (PNI), 648
Psychosis, 977
Psychosomatic disorder, 1003
Psychotherapy, 978
Psychotic disorder, 976
Psychotropic drugs, 1058
PT. *See* Physical therapist (PT); Physical therapy
    (PT); Prothrombin time (PT)
PTA. *See* Percutaneous transluminal angioplasty
    (PTA); Physical therapy
    assistant (PTA)
PTC. *See* Percutaneous transhepatic
    cholangiography (PTHC, PTC)
PTCA. *See* Percutaneous transluminal coronary
    angioplasty (PTCA)
PTH. *See* Parathyroid hormone (PTH)
PTHC. *See* Percutaneous transhepatic
    cholangiography (PTHC, PTC)

PTSD. *See* Post-traumatic stress disorder (PTSD)
PTT. *See* Partial thromboplastin time (PTT)
Ptyalography, 109
Puberty, 870, 917
    precocious, 433
Pubic region, 63*f*
Pubis, 229
Pulmonary artery(ies), 519, 519*f*
    right and left, 519, 520
Pulmonary circuit, 520
Pulmonary edema, 539, 610, 1179
Pulmonary embolism, 592, 1176
Pulmonary function test (PFT), 587
Pulmonary semilunar valve (PSLV), 513*f*, 514
Pulmonary valve, 514
Pulmonary vein(s), 519, 519*f*
    right and left, 519, 520
Pulmonary ventilation, 585
Pulmonary volumes and capacities, 587*t*
Pulp (of tooth), 695
Pulse, 524
Pulse oximeter, 593
Pulse oximetry, 593
Punch biopsy, 1105
Pupil, 372
Pupil distance (PD), 366
Pupils equal, round, and reactive to light and
    accommodation (PERRLA), 5
Purkinje fibers, 523
Purpura, 162, 477
Pustules, 162
PVD. *See* Peripheral vascular disease (PVD)
Px. *See* Physical examination (PE, Px)
Pyelitis, 777
Pyelogram, 114
Pyelography, 114
Pyelonephritis, 785
Pyloric sphincter, 698
Pylorus, 697
Pyramids, renal, 767, 768*f*, 769
Pyrosis, 712
Pyuria, 775

Q

QRS complex, 529
Quadrants, 61
    abdominopelvic, 60*f*, 61
Quickening, 908

R

RA. *See* Rheumatoid arthritis (RA)
Radial keratotomy, 382
Radiation oncology, 98, 118–119
Radiation therapy (RTx), 70, 663, 1105, 1178
Radical hysterectomy, 1125
Radical mastectomy, 1125
Radioactive, 99
Radioactive iodine uptake (RIU) test,
    123, 436
Radiographs, 99
Radiography, 68, 102
    of blood vessels, 110–111
    conventional, 66
    of digestive system, 108
    of heart, 110–111
    of lymph channels and nodes, 110–111
    in motion, 102
    of nervous system, 109

percutaneous procedures, 104–106
of reproductive system, 111–112
of respiratory system, 113
technique, 99*f*
of urinary system, 113–114
Radioimmunoassay (RIA), **123**, **431**
Radioiodine, 434
ablation, 436
Radiologist, **98**
Radiology, **98**
abbreviations used in, 125
basic terms in, 98–99
diagnostic, 100, 101
interventional, 100, 101
lifespan and, 124
medical term parts used in, 95
Radionuclide, **100**
scan, 534, 536
Radionuclide ejection fraction, **123**
Radionuclide seeds, **119**
Radiopaque, **99**
Radiopharmaceutical, **123**
Radiosensitizers, 852
Radiotherapy, **119**, **663**, **1105**
Radiotracer, **100**
Radius, **226**
Rales, **592**
Ramus, projection, 217*t*
Range of motion (ROM), 248, 256, 305–306
Raphe, **821**
Rapid eye movement (REM), 1010
Raynaud phenomenon, **547**
RBCs. *See* Red blood cells (RBCs)
RD. *See* Registered dietitian (RD)
Reabsorption, **767**
Real world report
anatomy and physiology, 74–75
basal cell carcinoma, 186–187
blood chemistry and immunology, 489–490
cardiovascular disorder, 551
chronic obstructive pulmonary disease, 615–616
fluorescein angiography, 394–395
gerontology, 1191–1192
hemodialysis, 738
joint disorder, 261–262
lymphatic disorder, 668
multiaxial assessment, 1017–1018
pathological diagnosis, 1129
physical therapy, 307–308
physician's order sheet, 1073
pregnancy, 951
radiology, 127
reproductive disorder, 874
skeletal imaging, 261–262
urinary disorder, 794–795
whole-body thyroid scan, 440
Reality testing, 976
Rebound pain, **713**
Recessive gene, 918
Rectal route, **1051**
Rectocele, **856**
Rectum, **704**
Red blood cell count, **464**
Red blood cells (RBCs)/erythrocytes, 460, 462*f*, 463–464
Red bone marrow, **214**
Reducible hernia, **725**

Reduction, **232**
closed, 231–232
open, 232
Reed-Sternberg cells, 661, **1114**
Reflex apnea, **589**
Reflex response, **68**
Refraction, **372**
Refractive problems, 380
Regimen, **1047**
Region(s), **61**
abdominopelvic, 60–61, 60*f*
Regional enteritis, **729**
Registered dietitian (RD), professional profile, 686
Registered nurse (RN), 412, 508, 816
in cardiovascular intensive care unit, professional profile, 508
Registered pharmacist (RPh), professional profile, 1038
Registered respiratory therapist (RRT), 572
Regurgitation, **712**
Relaxin, **834**, **906**
Releasing hormones, 416
REM. *See* Rapid eye movement
Renal adenocarcinoma, **788**, **1119**
Renal arteries, **769**
Renal calculi, 777, **1184**
Renal cell carcinoma, 787, **1119**
Renal corpuscle, **769**
Renal cortex, **769**
Renal failure, **781**
acute, 780
chronic, 736, 780
end-stage, 780, 781
Renal hypertension, **784**
Renal medulla, **769**
Renal pelvis, **769**
Renal pyramids, **769**
Renal tubule, **769**
ascending limb of, 768
descending limb of, 768
Renal veins, **769**
Renin, **771**
vs. rennin, 11
Reproduction, **820**
Reproductive system, 53, 815–896
across lifespan, 870
aging and, 1185–1187
anatomy of, 820–839
cancers, 1120–1126, 1120*f*, 1121*t*, 1124*f*
infections of, 857–858
pathology of, 839–864
radiography of, 111–112
structures of, 821*f*, 822*f*
Resectoscope, **846**
Residual-type schizophrenia, **995**
Residual volume (RV), **587**
Resistance, **648**
Respiration, **585**
Respiratory acidosis, **608**
Respiratory airway, **583**
Respiratory alkalosis, **608**
Respiratory bronchioles, 582*f*
Respiratory failure, **610**
Respiratory syncytial virus (RSV)
pneumonia, **605**
Respiratory syndromes, 608–610
Respiratory system, 53, 571–636

across lifespan, 612
aging and, 1177–1179
anatomy of, 576–588
cancers, 1114–1116, 1115*f*
drugs affecting, 1064–1065
function of, 572, 573*f*, 584–585
radiography of, 113
structures of, 577, 577*f*
Respiratory therapist (RT), professional profile, 572
Restless legs syndrome (RLS), **1176**
Resuscitation bag, **592**
Reticulocyte, **464**
Retina, **373**
detached, 382–383, 385
disorders of, 382–385
Retinopathy, **385**
diabetic, **385**
Retinopathy of prematurity (ROP), 938, **940**
Retrograde pyelography (RP), **114**
Retrovirus, 656
Reverse transcriptase (RT), 656
Reverse transcriptase inhibitors (RTIs), **1054**
Review of systems (ROS), 5
Reye syndrome, **341**, **929**
Rh factor. *See* Rhesus (Rh) factor
Rhabdomyosarcoma, **1108**
RHD. *See* Rheumatic heart disease (RHD)
Rhesus (Rh) factor, 471, 482–483
Rheumatic heart disease (RHD), **543**
Rheumatism, **251**
Rheumatoid arthritis (RA), **251**, 652, **1163**
Rhinitis, 601
acute, 600–601
allergic, 600, 653, 655
perennial allergic, 653, 655
Rhinophyma, **178**
Rhinoviruses, **601**
Rhodopsin, **373**
RhoGAM, 483
Rhonchus, **598**
RIA. *See* Radioimmunoassay (RIA)
Rib(s), 224, 225*f*
false, 224
true, 224
vertebral, 224
Ribonucleic acid (RNA), 49
Ribosomes, **50**
Rickets, **235**
Rifampin, 605
Right and left bundle branches, **523**
Right and left pulmonary arteries, **520**
Right and left pulmonary veins, **520**
Right atrioventricular (AV) valve, **513**
Right coronary artery, **520**
Right ear (*auris dextra,* A.D.), 375
Right eye (*oculus dexter,* O.D.), 371
Right hypochondriac region, **61**
Right inguinal region, **61**
Right lower quadrant (RLQ), **61**
Right lumbar region, **61**
Right lymphatic duct, **645**
Right upper quadrant (RUQ), **61**
Right ventricular hypertrophy, **1179**
Ringworm, 175, 176*f*
Risk factors, **1097**
RIU test. *See* Radioactive iodine uptake (RIU) test

RLQ. *See* Right lower quadrant (RLQ)
RLS. *See* Restless legs syndrome (RLS)
RN. *See* Registered nurse (RN)
RNA. *See* Ribonucleic acid (RNA)
R/O. *See* Rule out (R/O)
Rods, **373**
Roentgen rays, 98
ROM. *See* Range of motion (ROM)
Root(s), **156**, **695**
    of hair, 156, 157*f*
    of penis, 825
    of teeth, 694*f*, 695
Root canal, **695**
    procedure, 708
    structure, 694*f*, 695
ROP. *See* Retinopathy of prematurity (ROP)
Rorschach test, 983, **994**
ROS. *See* Review of systems (ROS)
Rosacea, **178**
Rotation, **246**
Rotator cuff injury, **303**
Rotavirus, **946**
Round bones, 211
Routes of administration, 1048–1051
Rovsing sign, 713
RP. *See* Retrograde pyelography (RP)
RPh. *See* Registered pharmacist (RPh)
RRT. *See* Registered respiratory therapist (RRT)
RSV. *See* Respiratory syncytial virus (RSV)
RT. *See* Respiratory therapist (RT); Reverse
    transcriptase (RT)
RTIs. *See* Reverse transcriptase inhibitors (RTIs)
RTx. *See* Radiation therapy (RTx)
Rubella, **180**, **947**
Rubeola, 943–944
Rubor, 546
Rugae, **698**, 769
    of bladder, 770*f*
    gastric, 696*f*, 697
Rule out (R/O), 5, 711
Ruptured bladder, **790**
RUQ. *See* Right upper quadrant (RUQ)
RV. *See* Residual volume (RV)

S

S&S. *See* Signs and symptoms (S&S)
SA. *See* Sinoatrial (SA)
Saccular aneurysm, **546**
Sacral region, 63*f*, 65*t*
Sacrum, **224**
SAD. *See* Seasonal affective disorder (SAD)
Sagittal plane, **62**
Salivary amylase, 692
Salivary glands, **693**
Salpingo-oophorectomy, **849**
Sarcopenia, **1165**
Satellite cells, 304, 324, **1165**
Scabies, **181**
Scales, **983**
Scaphoid, 225*f*
Scapulae, **226**
Scar, **163**
Schedule drugs, 1046*t*
Schilling test, 123, **474**
Schizoid personality disorder, **1013**
Schizophrenia, **994**
    catatonic-type, 992, 994
    disorganized-type, 993, 994

    paranoid-type, 993, 994
    residual-type, 993, 995
    undifferentiated-type, 993, 995
Schwann cells, 324
Sciatica, **345**
SCID. *See* Severe combined immunodeficiency
    (SCID)
Scintigram, **662**
Scintigraphy, 123, **662**
Scintiscan, **662**
Sclera, **372**
Scleral buckle, **385**
Scleroderma, **165**
Sclerosis (ALS), **345**
Scoliosis, **230**
Scrotal swelling, 779*f*
Scrotum, **821**
Scurvy, **235**
Seasonal affective disorder
    (SAD), **998**
Sebaceous cysts, **167**
Sebaceous glands, **151**, 157
Seborrhea, **178**
Seborrheic dermatitis, **174**
Seborrheic keratosis, **168**
Sebum, **151**
Second-degree burn, **163**
Secondary bone cancer, **1107**
Secondary bronchi, 582*f*
Secondary malnutrition, **721**
Secondary oocyte, **831**, 835, 835*f*
Secondary response, **652**
Secondary sexual characteristics, **827**
Secretion, 416, 767
Secretory phase, **838**
SEER. *See* Surveillance, Epidemiology, and End
    Results (SEER)
Segmentation, **699**
Seizures
    cerebral, 335, 337
    generalized tonic–clonic, 335, 337
Selective arterial catheter placement, **106**
Selective serotonin reuptake inhibitors (SSRIs),
    996, **1058**
Selective venous, **106**
Self vs. nonself, **639**
Semen, 823–824, **825**
    analysis, 856, **857**
Semi-Fowler position, **607**
Semicircular canals, **375**
Semilunar (SL) valves, **513**
Seminal glands, **825**
Seminiferous tubules, **821**, 823, 824
Seminomas, **1124**
Senescence, 917, 1150–1151, **1154**
Senile, **1158**
Senile lentigines, **1158**
Senile osteopenia, **1163**
Senile pruritus, **1158**
Sensitization, **655**
Sensorineural deafness, **388**, 1170
Sensory function, **323**
Septicemia, 477, **848**
Septum, nasal, 578
Sequela (pl. sequelae), 342, **543**
Serosa, **55**
Serotonergic blockade, 994
Serotonin, **466**, 975

Serotonin-norepinephrine reuptake inhibitors
    (SNRIs), **1058**
Serous membranes, **55**
Serum, **462**
    test, 425
Serum amylase, **717**
Serum gastrin test, **712**
Serum glutamic-oxaloacetic transaminase
    (SGOT) test, 534
Serum lipase, **717**
Serum tumor marker, **1124**
Serum α-fetoprotein (AFP) test, 925, 928
Sesamoid bones, **214**
17-Ketosteroids (17-KS) test, 426
Severe combined immunodeficiency (SCID),
    658, 925
Severed tendon, **303**
Severity and course specifiers, **981**
Sex chromosomes, **919**
Sex-determining region of Y chromosome (SRY),
    870
Sex hormones, **421**
Sex-linked inheritance, **919**
Sex-linked traits, 918
Sexual and gender-identity disorders,
    1006–1009
Sexual dysfunction, **1008**
Sexual intercourse, 838–839
Sexual masochism, **1008**
Sexual sadism, **1008**
Sexually transmitted diseases (STDs),
    858–863
Sexually transmitted infections, 858
SGA. *See* Small for gestational age (SGA)
SGOT. *See* Serum glutamic-oxaloacetic
    transaminase (SGOT)
SH. *See* Social history (SH)
Shaft (of hair), **156**
    of penis, **825**
Shave biopsy, **1105**
Shin splints, **303**
Shingles, **180**, **1158**
Shock, **541**
    anaphylactic, **654**
    cardiogenic, 541
    hypovolemic, 541
    septic, 541
Short bones, **214**
Shoulder, 225*f*
    disorders of, 254–255
Shunt, **102**
Shuntogram, **102**
Sialography, **109**
Sickle cell anemia, **474**
Side effect, **1047**
SIDS. *See* Sudden infant death syndrome (SIDS)
Sigmoid colon, **704**
Sigmoidoscopy, **732**
Signs, 8, **66**
Signs and symptoms (S&S), 66
Silicosis, **600**
Simian line, 926, 927
Simple (closed) fracture, 231*f*, 231*t*
Sinoatrial (SA) node, **523**
Sinus(es), **222**, 579
    coronary, 520
    ethmoidal, 578, 578*f*
    frontal, 578, 578*f*

lactiferous, 833, 833*f*
maxillary, 578, 578*f*
paranasal, 218*t*, 221, 221*f*, 222, 577, 578–579, 578*f*
sphenoidal, 578, 578*f*
Sinusitis, **602**
Sjögren syndrome, **653**
Skeletal muscle, **291**, **318**
names of, 292, 293*t*, 294*t*, 295*t*, 296*t*, 299
Skeletal system, 51*f*, 52*t*, 53, 207–238
across lifespan, 257–258
aging and, 1158–1164
cancers, 1106–1107
injury to, case study, 260
pathology of, 229
structures of, 211
Skeletal traction, **232**
Skin, 146
anatomy of, 151–153, 152*f*
autoimmune disorders and, 164–165
cancer, ABCDE method of, 1102, 1102*f*, 1105
cancerous tumors of, 168–169
color of, 155
disorders affecting, 182
word parts pertaining to, 155, 155*t*
cracks in, 175
infectious diseases of, 179–181
layers of, 151–153
as membrane, 149
noncancerous tumors of, 166–168
as organ, 149
pathology of, 160
thick, 151
Skin conditions, 160–162
Skin grafts, **1105**
Skin lesions, in athlete's foot, 1054*f*
Skin tags, 166, **1158**. *See also* Cutaneous papillomas
Skin test, 654
Skull, 211, 219, 220*f*
fracture(s), 334
SL. *See* Semilunar (SL)
SLE. *See* Systemic lupus erythematosus (SLE)
Sleep apnea, **589**, **1012**
Sleep disorders, 1010–1012
Slit lamp, **379**
Small cell lung cancer, **1115**
Small for gestational age (SGA), 928, **940**
Small intestine, 690, 691*f*, 698–699
disorders of, 726–727
Smoking cessation, benefits of, 548
Smooth muscle, **291**, **318**
Sneezing, 585
SNRIs. *See* Serotonin-norepinephrine reuptake inhibitors (SNRIs)
SOAP notes, **8**
Social history (SH), 5
Social workers, **979**
Sodium ion (Na$^+$), 421
Soft palate, 1011
Soluble, definition of, 469
Somatic nervous system (SNS), **323**
Somatization disorder, **1003**
Somatoform disorder, 1001–1003
Sonography, **117**, **898**
Sore throat, 601

sp. gr. *See* Specific gravity (sp. gr.)
Spasm, 292, 468–469
Spastic colon, 732
Special senses, **323**, **369**
across lifespan, 391
aging and, 1169–1171
Species name, 11
Specific gravity (sp. gr.), **775**
Specific immunity, **643**
Spectroscopy, 107
Spectrum, 107
Sperm, **820**
regions of, 828, 829*f*
Spermatic cord, **825**
Spermatids, 828, 828*f*
Spermatogenesis, **821**, 828, 828*f*
Spermatogonium, **829**
Spermatozoa (sperm), 820, 828–829
Spermicide, **869**
Spermiogenesis, **829**
Sphenoid bone, 216, **221**
Sphenoidal sinus(es), 578, 578*f*
Sphincter, **770**
Sphygmomanometer, **524**
Spina bifida, **345**, **937**
Spina bifida cystica, **345**
Spina bifida occulta, **345**
Spinal anesthesia, **1061**
Spinal cord, 322, 323*f*, 325–328, 326*f*
disorders of, 342–345
Spinal nerve(s), 325–328, 326*f*
disorders of, 342–345
Spine, curvature of, 223*f*, 230
abnormal, 229–230
Spinous process, **224**
Spiral fracture, 231*f*, 231*t*
Spiral organ, **375**
Spirometer, **587**
Spleen, **643**, 646, 646*f*, 691*f*
imaging, 120, 123
Splenomegaly, 473, 602, **662**
Splenoportography, **109**
Split personality, 993
Sponge, **869**
Spongy bone, **214**
Spontaneous abortion, 909
Sprain, 254, 302–303
Sputum, 593
studies, 603, **605**
Squamous cell carcinoma, 169, **1105**
Squamous epithelium, simple, 53
SRY. *See* Sex-determining region of Y chromosome (SRY)
SSRIs. *See* Selective serotonin reuptake inhibitors (SSRIs)
Staging, **1098**
Stanford-binet intelligence scale, **983**
Stapedectomy, **391**
Stapes, **375**
Starch, 705
Statins, **1064**
Status asthmaticus, **655**
STDs. *See* Sexually transmitted diseases (STDs)
Steatorrhea, **726**
Stem cell transplant, **486**
Stem cells, 460, **1098**
Stereotactic biopsy, **1110**
Sterility, **857**

Sterilization, **869**
Sternal region, 63*f*
Sternberg-Reed cells, 661
Sternum, 224, 225*f*
Stethoscope, 68, **524**
Stillbirth, **923**
Stomach, 690, 691*f*, 696–697
cancer, **1183**
Strabismus, **379**, 928, 929*f*
Strain, **303**
Strangulated hernia, **725**
Strata, **153**
Strawberry hemangioma, 142, **156**
Streptococcus pyogenes, 173
Streptokinase, **477**
Stress fracture, 231*t*
Striae, **153**
Striae gravidarum, **908**
Striated muscle, 289, 289*f*
Stroke, 337, 535, **1168**
Stuttering, **987**
Styloid process, 216
Sub-unit vaccines, 651
Subarachnoid space, **332**
Subcutaneous (SC)
abbreviations for, 152
definition of, 152
route, **1051**
tissue, 152, 152*f*
Subcutaneous layer, **153**
Subdural space, **332**
Sublingual glands, **693**
Sublingual route, **1051**
Subluxation, **257**
Submandibular glands, **693**
Substance abuse, 991–992
Sudden infant death syndrome (SIDS), **610**
Sudoriferous glands, 151, 157
Suffixes, 9, **13**
medical term parts used as, 22–24, 24*t*
Sugar(s), 705
Sulci (sing. sulcus), 218*t*, 331
cerebral, 328, 331
Sundowner syndrome, **1168**
Sundowning, **1168**
Superficial, definition of, **59**
Superinfection, **1053**
Superior, **59**
Superior vena cava, **520**
Supination, **246**
Supine position, 57
Suppressor T (T$_s$) cells, **650**
Suprapatellar bursa, 243*f*
Suprapubic prostatectomy, **1187**
Surfactant, **584**, 612, 939
Surgery, **70**
wrong-site, 71–72
Surveillance, Epidemiology, and End Results (SEER), 1096
Susceptibility, 639, **648**
Sutural bones, **214**
Sutures(s), 212*f*, 219, 220*f*, **244**
Swallowing, 693
"Swan-neck" deformity, 250
Sweat glands, 151, 157
Sx. *See* Symptom(s) (Sx)
Sympathetic nervous system, **323**, 1175

Symphysis, 244
Symphysis pubis, 228*f*, 244
Symptoms(s) (Sx), 5, 8, 66
Synapses, 325, 975
Syncope, 537, **932**
Syndactyly, 235
Syndrome, 925
Syngraft, 664
Synovial cavity, 242*f*, 243
Synovial joints, 242–243, **244**
Synovial membrane, 242*f*, 243
Synovitis, **251**
Synthroid. *See* Levothyroxine
Syphilis, 859*t*, **863**
Syphiloma, **863**
Systemic circuit, **520**
Systemic lupus erythematosus (SLE), **165**, 165*f*
    251, 422, 652
Systole, **523**, 524
Systolic blood pressure, **524**

T

T. *See* Thoracic (T)
T cells (T lymphocytes), 642, 644, 646, **650**, 665,
    1179, **1180**
    cytotoxic, 649, 650
    helper, 649, 650
    memory T_c, 649, 650
    suppressor, 649, 650
T wave, **529**
$T_{1/2}$. *See* Half-life ($T_{1/2}$)
T_1–T_{12}. *See* Thoracic vertebrae
T_3. *See* Triiodothyronine (T_3)
T_4. *See* Thyroxine (T_4)
Tachycardia, **536**, 717
Tachypnea, **589**
Talipes, 235, **931**
Talipes equinovarus, **235**, **931**
Talus, **229**
Tamoxifen, 850
Tardive dyskinesia (TD), 992–995
Target cell, **416**
Targeted therapy, **1125**
Tarsal glands, 386
Tarsal region, 63*f*, 64*t*, **229**
    bones, 227, 228*f*, 229
TAT. *See* Thematic apperception test (TAT)
Tay–Sachs disease, **925**
TB. *See* Tuberculosis (TB)
^{99}Tc. *See* Technetium-99 (^{99}Tc)
T_c cells. *See* Cytotoxic T cells
TCAs. *See* Tricyclic antidepressants (TCAs)
TD. *See* Tardive dyskinesia (TD)
Technetium-99 (^{99}Tc), 120
Teeth, 690, 693–695, 694*f*, 734
    discolored, 707
    disorders of, 707
Teletherapy, **119**
Temporal bones, **221**
Temporomandibular joint (TMJ) syndrome,
    250, **710**
Tendinitis, **303**
Tendon(s), 241, 289, **291**
    severed, 302, 303
Tenoplasty, **303**
Tension headache, 333
Teratogens, **905**
Teratology, **906**

Teratoma, **916**
Terminal bronchioles, **582**
Terminologia Anatomica, **8**
Tertiary bronchi, 582*f*
Testes, 415*f*, **821**, 828
    disorders of, 839–843
Testicles, **821**
Testicular cancer, **843**, **1124**
Testicular self-examinations (TSEs), 842
Testicular torsion, **843**
Testosterone, **425**, **827**, **1067**
Tetanus, **946**
Tetanus immunoglobulin (TIG), 943
Tetany, 431
Tetracycline, 707
Tetraiodothyronine, 419. *See also* Thyroxine (T_4)
Tetralogy, **932**
Tetralogy of Fallot, **529**, 932–933
T_H cells. *See* Helper T cells
Thalamus, **331**
Thalassemia, **474**
Thallium (Tl) scan, **123**, 532
Thallium-201 (^{201}Tl), 120
Thematic apperception test (TAT), **983**, 994
Theophylline, **939**
Therapy vest, **593**
Thiamin deficiency, 473
Third-degree burn, **163**
Thoracentesis, **607**
Thoracic (T) region, 63*f*, 64*t*
Thoracic cage, 224, 225*f*
Thoracic cavity, **57**
Thoracic duct, **645**
Thoracic vertebrae (T_1–T_{12}), **224**
Thoracoscopy, **1115**
Thready, definition of, 533
Three-dimensional shape, of red blood cells, 463*f*
Thrill, **529**, 932
Throat, **579**
Thrombin, **470**
Thrombocytes/platelets, **467**
Thrombocytopenia, **477**
Thrombolytic drugs, 477, 535, **1061**
Thrombophlebitis, **547**
Thrombosis, 469, 476, **1061**
Thromboxane, 476
Thrombus, in blood vessel, 469, 469*f*, **470**
Thrush, **710**
Thymosins, **424**
Thymus, 415, 415*f*, **424**, 643, 646, 665
Thyroid cancer, **436**, **1111**
Thyroid function tests, 436
Thyroid gland, 415, 415*f*, 418–419
    disorders of, 434–437
Thyroid imaging, **123**
Thyroid scan, 439
Thyroid-stimulating hormone (TSH), **416**, 417
Thyroid storm, **436**
Thyroidectomy, **436**
Thyrotoxic crisis, 436
Thyrotoxicosis, **436**, **1173**
Thyroxine (T_4), **419**
TIA. *See* Transient ischemic attack (TIA)
Tibia, **229**, 243*f*
Tibial region, 63*f*, 64*t*
Tic disorders, **987**
Tic douloureux, **342**
Tidal volume (TV), **587**

TIG. *See* Tetanus immunoglobulin (TIG)
Tinea, **176**
Tinea capitis, **176**
Tinea corporis, **176**
Tinea pedis, **176**
Tinea unguium, **176**
Tinel sign, 254–255
Tinnitus, **391**
Tissue, **50**
Tissue changes, 1099–1102, 1100*f*, 1100*t*,
    1101*t*, 1102*t*
Tissue plasminogen activator, **337**
Tissue plasminogen activator (TPA, tPA),
    336, **337**, 470
Tissue rejection, **664**
TJR. *See* Total joint replacement (TJR)
^{201}Tl. *See* Thallium-201 (^{201}Tl)
TLC. *See* Total lung capacity (TLC)
TM-Mode Doppler ultrasonography, 552
TMJ. *See* Temporomandibular joint (TMJ)
TMS. *See* Transcranial magnetic stimulation
    (TMS)
TNM staging, **1098**
Toenails. *See* Nails
Tomography, **104**
Tongue, 690, 692
Tonometry, **379**
Tonsillectomy, **659**
Tonsillitis, **659**
Tonsils, 643, 646, 646*f*
    pharyngeal, 579, 580*f*
Topical chemotherapy, **1105**
TORCH series, **906**
Torn meniscus, 254
Tortuous, definition of, 547
Total body irradiation, 119
Total hysterectomy with salpingo-
    oophorectomy, **1125**
Total joint replacement (TJR), 248
Total lung capacity (TLC), **587**
Total mastectomy, **1125**
Tourette disorder, **987**
Toxemia of pregnancy, **923**
Toxic shock syndrome (TSS), **858**
Toxicology, **1043**
Toxins, 456
Toxoid vaccines, 651
Toxoplasmosis, 1055
TPA, tPA. *See* Tissue plasminogen activator
    (TPA, tPA)
TPI test. *See* *Treponema pallidum* immobiliza-
    tion (TPI) test
Trabeculae, **214**
Trachea, 577, 581–583, 582*f*
Tracheostomy tube, **592**
TRAM flap. *See* Transverse rectus abdominis
    myocutaneous (TRAM) flap
Transcatheter biopsy, **106**
Transcranial magnetic stimulation (TMS), **997**
Transdermal route, **1051**
Transesophageal echocardiography, **536**
Transfusion, **471**
Transient, definition of, 335
Transient ischemic attack (TIA), 337, 537, **1168**
Transitional cell carcinoma, **1119**
Transitional epithelial tissue, 769
Transluminal atherectomy, **106**
Transplants, 663–664

Transposition of great arteries, **933**
Transrectal ultrasound, **1124**
Transsexualism, **1008**
Transurethral resection (TUR), **846**
Transurethral resection of the prostate (TURP), 845, 845*f*, **1187**
Transvaginal sonography, **853**
Transverse colon, **704**
Transverse fracture, 231*f*, 231*t*
Transverse plane, **62**
Transverse processes, 219*t*, **224**
Transverse rectus abdominis myocutaneous (TRAM) flap, **852**
Transvetic fetishism, **1008**
Trapezium, 225*f*
Trapezoid, 225*f*
Trauma. *See also* Post-traumatic stress disorder (PTSD)
    to joints, 265–266
    muscular, 301–303
    respiratory system in, 610–611
Traveler's diarrhea, 725–726
Treatment(s), 69
Treponema pallidum immobilization (TPI) test, 862
Trichomoniasis, **863**, 1055
Tricuspid valve, **513**, 519, 519*f*
Tricyclic antidepressants (TCAs), 996, **1058**
Trigeminal nerve (CN V), 330*f*
    disorder of, 342
Trigeminal neuralgia, **342**
Trigone, **770**
Triiodothyronine (T₃), **419**
Trimester(s)
    of gestation, 905
    uterine growth in, 907*f*
Triquetrum, 225*f*
Trisomy 18. *See* Edwards syndrome
Trisomy 21. *See* Down syndrome
Trochanter surface marking, 217*t*
Trochlear nerve (CN IV), 330*f*
Trousseau sign, **431**
True ribs, **226**
Truss, **725**
Tₛ cells. *See* Suppressor T cells
TSEs. *See* Testicular self-examinations (TSEs)
TSH. *See* Thyroid-stimulating hormone (TSH)
TSS. *See* Toxic shock syndrome (TSS)
Tubal ligation, **869**
Tubercle(s)
    of bone, 218*t*
    in tuberculosis, 604
Tuberculin test, **605**
Tuberculosis (TB), **605**, **1179**
Tuberosity, 218*t*
Tuberosity, radial, 218*t*
Tumor(s), 1095, 1096, 1186
    of female reproductive system, 853–855
    of lymphatic/immune system, 661–663
    markers, **1124**
    of skin, 166–169
Tunica (pl. tunicae), 514
Tunica adventitia, 515*f*
Tunica externa, 514
Tunica intima, 514, 515*f*
Tunica media, 514, 515*f*
TUR. *See* Transurethral resection (TUR)

Turbidity, **775**
Turbinates, **222**
Turgor, **153**
Turner syndrome, **928**
Tussis, **585**, **943**
TV. *See* Tidal volume (TV)
Twins
    dizygotic, 915, 915*f*
    monozygotic, 915, 915*f*
Two-dimensional (2D) Doppler ultrasonography, 552
2-hour postprandial glucose test, **923**
2n. *See* Diploid (2n)
Tympanic membrane, **375**
    disorders of, 388–390
Tympanostomy tubes, **389**
Type 1 diabetes, **430**
Type 2 diabetes, **430**
Type I osteoporosis, 1159
Type II osteoporosis, 1159
Typical antipsychotics, 1057

U
UA. *See* Urinalysis (UA)
UCHD. *See* Usual childhood diseases (UCHD)
UGI. *See* Upper gastrointestinal (UGI)
Ulcer(s), 171–172, **172**, 710–712, **712**
    decubitus, 171–172
    duodenal, 711
    gastric, 711
    oral, 708
    peptic, 710–711
Ulcerative colitis, 730–731, **732**, **1117**
Ulna, **226**
Ultrasonographer, 898
Ultrasonography, **117**
Ultrasound, **98**
    diagnostic, 97, 116–118
        medical term parts used in, 95
        procedures, 116
Ultraviolet (UV) radiation, 150
Umbilical arteries, 547, 904
Umbilical cord, **902**
Umbilical hernia, 301, 302*f*
Umbilical region, **61**
Umbilical vein, 547, 904
Undifferentiated-type schizophrenia, **995**
United States Pharmacopeia (USP), 1047
Universal donor, 471
Universal recipient, 471
Upper gastrointestinal (UGI) tract, 695
Upper gastrointestinal series (UGIS), **723**
Upper respiratory infection (URI), **601**
Upper respiratory tract, 576, 577*f*
    disorders of, 600–601
UPPP. *See* Uvulopalatopharyngoplasty (UPPP)
Uptake, **100**
Urea breath test, **123**
Uremia, **779**
Uremic frost, **781**
Ureter(s), **766**, **769**
    intravenous pyelogram of, 113*f*
Ureteritis, **786**
Urethra, **767**, 770, 770*f*
    male, 825, 826*f*
Urethritis, **786**
Urethrocystometry, **114**

Urgency, **777**
URI. *See* Upper respiratory infection (URI)
Urinalysis (UA), 772–775, **775**
Urinary bladder, **766**, 770*f*. *See also* Bladder
    cancer of, **788**
    disorders, 780–790
    intravenous pyelogram of, 113*f*
Urinary incontinence, 1183–1184
Urinary retention, **784**, **1184**
Urinary sediment, microscopic examination of, 772, 774
Urinary system, **53**, 761–813
    across lifespan, 790–791
    aging and, 1183–1184
    anatomy of, 766–772, 766*f*
    cancer of, 787–789, 1118*t*, 1118–1119, 1118*f*
    case study, 792–794
    disorders of, 789–790
    radiography of, 113–114
Urinary tract infections (UTIs), **785**, **1184**
Urination, 766
Urine amylase, 717
Urine formation, 771–772
Urine ketosteroids test, **428**
Urochrome, **775**
Urography, **114**
Urticarial, **175**
USP. See United States Pharmacopeia (USP)
Usual childhood diseases (UCHD), 5
Uterine cancer, **1125**
Uterine cycle, 836–838, **838**
Uterine fibroids, **854**
Uterine sarcoma, **1125**
Uterine tubes, **822**, 830–831, 830*f*
Uterus, **823**, 830, 830*f*
    bimanual examination of, 847
    growth in pregnancy, 906, 907*f*
UTIs. *See* Urinary tract infections (UTIs)
UV. *See* Ultraviolet (UV) radiation
Uveitis, **379**
Uvula, **581**, **693**, 1011
Uvulopalatopharyngoplasty (UPPP), **1012**

V
VA. *See* Visual acuity (VA)
Vaccinations, **946**
Vaccine(s), **652**, **946**
    attenuated, 651
    killed, 651
    sub-unit, 651
    toxoid, 651
Vacuum phenomenon, 262
Vagina, **823**, 830–831, 830*f*
Vaginal barriers, 867–868, **869**
Vaginal birth after cesarean (VBAC), **913**
Vaginal cancer, **853**
Vaginal ring, **869**
Vaginal route, **1051**
Vaginitis, **858**
Vaginoperineotomy, 909
Vagus nerve (CN X), 330*f*
Valsalva maneuver, **725**
Valvular heart disease, 542–543
Valvular insufficiency, **543**
Valvular regurgitation, **543**
Varicella, **180**, **947**
    vaccine, 941*t*, 942*t*
Varicella-zoster virus (VZV), 179, 945

Varicocele, 843, 856
Varicose veins, 547, 1176
Vas deferens, 825
Vascular dementia, 990, 1168
Vascular family, 106
Vascular headache, 333
Vascular murmur, 546
Vascular spasm, 469
Vasculature, disorders of, 543–547
Vasectomy, 869
Vasodilators, 532, 1062
Vasography, 112
Vasopressin, 417. *See also* Antidiuretic hormone (ADH)
VBAC. *See* Vaginal birth after cesarean (VBAC)
VC. *See* Vital capacity (VC)
VDs. *See* Venereal diseases (VDs)
Vein(s), 508, 517t, 518
    coronary, 521f
    disorders of, 543–547
Vein ligation, 547
Vein sclerosing, 547
Vein stripping, 547
Venereal diseases (VDs), 863
Venipuncture, 456, 482
Venography, 111, 547
Venous catheter placement
    nonselective, 104, 106
    selective, 104, 106
Ventral, definition of, 59
Ventricle(s), 332, 513
    of brain, 329, 330f, 332
    cardiac, 511, 512f, 518, 519f
Ventricular septal defect, 529, 933
Venturi mask, 592
Venules, 518
Vermiform appendix, 703, 703f
Vernix caseosa, 183, 913
Verruca vulgaris, 181
Verrucae, 181
Vertebra, 222f
Vertebral body, 63f, 65t, 224
Vertebral column, 222–224
Vertebral foramen, 224
Vertex, 912
Vertigo, 345
Vesicles, 174, 945
Vessel ordering, 106
Vestibule, 375, 832
    of inner ear, 373, 374–375
    vaginal, 831, 832
Vestibulocochlear nerve (CN VIII), 330f, 375

Vibices, 475
Villi, 699
    chorionic, 904, 904f, 905
    intestinal, 698, 699
Viral hepatitis, 863
Viral hepatitis type B (HBV), 859
Viral hepatitis type C (HCV), 859
Virilism, 428
Visceral, definition of, 55
Visceral pericardium, 513, 569
Visceral pleura, 584
Viscous, definition of, 459–460
Vision, 322, 369–373
Vision therapy, 379
Visual acuity (VA), 380
Visual pathway, 371
Vital capacity (VC), 587, 1177
Vital signs, 5, 508, 523–525, 524
Vitamin(s), 705
    imbalances of, 235
Vitamin A, 215
Vitamin B$_{12}$, deficiency of, 473
Vitamin C, 215, 235
Vitamin D, 150, 215, 235, 431
Vitamin P, 909
Vitiligo, 182
Vitrectomy, 382, 385
Vitreous humor, 373
Vocabulary, 9
Vocal cords, 581
    false, 581
    true, 581
Voice box, 580
Vomer, 222
Vomiting, 697, 1068
Vomitus, 721
von Willebrand disease, 486
Vowels, combining, 10
Voyeurism, 1008
Vulva, 823, 831–832
Vulvar cancer, 853
VZV. *See* Varicella-zoster virus (VZV)

W

Wall-eye, 369
Warfarin (Coumadin), 488
Wart(s), 180
    genital, 861f
    plantar, 180, 181
Watchful waiting, 1124
Water intoxication, 1173
WBCs. *See* White blood cells (WBCs)
Wechsler intelligence scales, 983

Wet form of age-related macular degeneration, 1170
Wheal(s), 175, 655
Wheeze, 598
White blood cells (WBCs), 466, 641. *See also* Leukocytes
    population of, 465
White matter, 328
WHO. *See* World Health Organization (WHO)
Whooping cough, 943
Wilms tumor, 788
Wisdom teeth, 707
Witch's milk, 914
Withdrawal method, 869
Within normal limits (WNL), 5
WNL. *See* Within normal limits (WNL)
Wolffian ducts, 870
Womb. *See* Uterus
Word parts, 9–10, 13
Word root, 13
World Health Organization (WHO), 70
Wrist, 225f
    bones of, 225f
    disorders of, 254–255
Wrong-level/wrong-part surgery, 71
Wrong-patient surgery, 71
Wrong-side surgery, 71

X

X chromosome, 870
X-ray imaging, 68
X-rays, 67, 99
Xenograft, 664
Xeroderma, 162, 1155–1156, 1158
Xerostomia, 100
Xiphoid process, 219t, 225f
XO karyotype. *See* Turner syndrome
XXY karyotype. *See* Klinefelter syndrome

Y

Y chromosome, 870
Y-linked inheritance, 918
Yawning, 585
Yolk sac, 903, 904f

Z

Z-tract injection, 1051
Zygomatic bones, 222
Zygote, 898, 902